Viral Outbreaks, Biosecurity, and Preparing for Mass Casualty Infectious Diseases Events

Viral Outbreaks, Biosecurity, and Preparing for Mass Casualty Infectious Diseases Events

TRISH M. PERL

Jay P Sanford Professor of Medicine
Chief of Infectious Diseases
Division of Infectious Diseases
UT Southwestern Medical Center
Dallas, TX, United States

DANIEL MAXWELL

Assistant Professor of Medicine
Infectious Diseases and Critical Care
UT Southwestern, Dallas VA Medical Center
Dallas, TX, United States

ELSEVIER

Elsevier
Radarweg 29, PO Box 211, 1000 AE Amsterdam, Netherlands
125 London Wall, London EC2Y 5AS, United Kingdom
50 Hampshire Street, 5th Floor, Cambridge, MA 02139, United States

ISBN: 978-0-323-54841-0

For information on all Elsevier publications
visit our website at https://www.elsevier.com/books-and-journals

Publisher: Jr Patrick Manley
Acquisitions Editor: Kerry Holland
Editorial Project Manager: Susan Ikeda
Production Project Manager: Erragounta Saibabu Rao
Cover Designer: Miles Hitchen

Typeset by STRAIVE, India

Contents

Contributors

Jean Abbott
Center for Bioethics and Humanities
University of Colorado
Anschutz Medical Campus
Aurora, CO, United States

Bernadette Albanese
Department of Epidemiology
Colorado School of Public Health
Aurora, CO, United States;
University of Colorado Denver
Greenwood Village, CO, United States

Danielle E Anderson
Programme in Emerging Infectious Diseases
Duke-NUS Medical School
Singapore

Brenda Ang
Department of Infectious Diseases
Tan Tock Seng Hospital
Singapore

Anucha Apisarnthanarak
Division of Infectious Diseases
Thammasat University Hospital
Thammasat University
Pathumthani, Thailand;
Division of Infectious Diseases
Department of Medicine
Faculty of Medicine
Thammasat University
Pathumthani, Thailand

Yaseen M. Arabi
College of Medicine
King Saud Bin Abdulaziz University for Health Sciences
King Abdullah International Medical Research Center
Riyadh, Saudi Arabia;
Intensive Care Department
King Abdulaziz Medical City
National Guard Health Affairs
Riyadh, Saudi Arabia

David M. Brett-Major
Department of Epidemiology
College of Public Health
University of Nebraska Medical Center
Omaha, NE, United States;
Global Center for Health Security
University of Nebraska Medical Center
Omaha, NE, United States

Laura Buford
Infection Prevention
Parkland Health
Dallas, TX, United States

Rachel Charney
School of Medicine
Saint Louis University
ST. Louis, MO, United States

Andrew Chou
Department of Surgery and Perioperative Care
UT Austin Dell Medical School/Austin-Travis County EMS
Austin, TX, United States

Theodore J. Cieslak
Departments of Epidemiology and of Environmental Agricultural, and Occupational Health
University of Nebraska Medical Center
College of Public Health
Omaha, NE, United States

James B. Cutrell
Department of Medicine
Division of Infectious Diseases and Geographic Medicine
University of Texas Southwestern Medical Center
Dallas, TX, United States

Jennifer Doren
Communications
Marketing, and Public Affairs
UT Southwestern Medical Center
Dallas, TX, United States

Michel Drancourt
IHU Méditerranée Infection
MEPHI
Aix-Marseille-Université
Marseille, France

Steven J. Drews
Department of Laboratory Medicine & Pathology
Faculty of Medicine and Dentistry
University of Alberta, and Canadian Blood Services
Edmonton, AB, Canada

Karen L. Elkins
LMPCI/DBPAP/OVRR
CBER, FDA
Silver Spring
MD, United States

Laura Evans
Division of Pulmonary
Critical Care and Sleep Medicine
University of Washington
Seattle, WA, United States

Mary M.K. Foote
NYC Department of Health and Mental Hygiene
Long Island City, NY, United States

Esther Y. Golnabi
Department of Pharmacy
University of Texas Southwestern Medical Center
Dallas, TX, United States

Gigi Kwik Gronvall
Johns Hopkins Bloomberg School of Public Health
Department of Environmental Health
and Engineering
Baltimore, MD, United States;
Johns Hopkins Center for Health Security
Baltimore, MD, United States

Charles-Antoine Guay
Department of Medicine
Laval University
Quebec, QC, Canada

Angela L. Hewlett
Global Center for Health Security
University of Nebraska Medical Center
Omaha, NE, United States;
Division of Infectious Diseases
Department of Medicine
College of Medicine
University of Nebraska
Omaha, NE, United States

Crystal K. Hodge
Department of Pharmacy
University of Texas Southwestern Medical Center
Dallas, TX, United States;
University of North Texas Health Science Center
System College of Pharmacy
Fort Worth, TX, United States

Emilio Hornsey
UK Public Health Rapid Support Team
Public Health England
London, England, United Kingdom

Lindsay T. Keegan
Department of Internal Medicine
University of Utah
Salt Lake City, UT, United States

Mark G. Kortepeter
Departments of Epidemiology and of Environmental
Agricultural, and Occupational Health
University of Nebraska Medical Center
College of Public Health
Omaha, NE, United States

James Lawler
National Strategic Research Institute at the University
of Nebraska
Omaha, NE, United States

Nelson Lee
Institute for Pandemics
Dalla Lana School of Public Health
University of Toronto
Toronto, ON, Canada

Justin Lessler
Department of Epidemiology
Johns Hopkins Bloomberg School of Public Health
Baltimore, MD, United States;

Department of Epidemiology
University of North Carolina Gillings School of Public Health
Chapel Hill, NC, United States

Sheri Lewis
Johns Hopkins University Applied Physics Laboratory
Laurel, MD, United States

Charles M. Little
University of Colorado School of Medicine and Colorado School of Public Health
Aurora, CO, United States;
University of Colorado Hospital
Aurora, CO, United States

Rachel E. Lookadoo
Departments of Epidemiology and of Environmental
Agricultural, and Occupational Health
University of Nebraska Medical Center
College of Public Health
Omaha, NE, United States

Al Lulla
Division of Emergency Services
Disaster, and Global Health
Department of Emergency Medicine
UT Southwestern, Dallas, TX, United States

S. Marshal Isaacs
Division of Emergency Services
Disaster, and Global Health
Department of Emergency Medicine
UT Southwestern, Dallas, TX, United States

Grace Ellen Marx
University of Colorado School of Medicine
Denver, CO, United States

C. Mary Healy
Infectious Diseases Section
Baylor College of Medicine
Houston, TX, United States

Daniel N. Maxwell
Infectious Diseases and Critical Care
UT Southwestern, Dallas VA Medical Center
Dallas, TX, United States

Faroukh Mehkri
Division of Emergency Services
Disaster, and Global Health
Department of Emergency Medicine
UT Southwestern, Dallas, TX, United States

Ziad A. Memish
College of Medicine
Alfaisal University
Riyadh, Saudi Arabia;
Research & Innovation Center
King Saud Medical City
Ministry of Health
Riyadh, Saudi Arabia;
Hubert Department of Global Health
Rollins School of Public Health
Emory University
Atlanta, GA, United States

C. Jessica E. Metcalf
Department of Ecology and Evolutionary Biology/ School of Public and International Affairs
Princeton University
Princeton, NJ, United States

Ronna G. Miller
Formerly, Emergency Medicine at UT Southwestern
Dallas, TX, United States

Vikramjit Mukherjee
Division of Pulmonary
Critical Care, and Sleep Medicine
New York University School of Medicine
Bellevue Hospital
New York, NY, United States

Shraddha Patel
Johns Hopkins University Applied Physics Laboratory
Laurel, MD, United States

Trish M. Perl
Department of Medicine, University of Texas Southwestern
Dallas, TX, United States;
Peter O'Donnell Jr School of Public Health
UT Southwestern Medical Center
Dallas, TX, United States;
Division of Infectious Diseases and Geographic Medicine
UT Southwestern Medical Center
Dallas, TX, United States

Jeannine M. Petersen
Division of Vector-Borne Diseases
Centers for Disease Control and Prevention
Fort Collins, CO, United States

Radu Postelnicu
Division of Pulmonary
Critical Care, and Sleep Medicine
New York University School of Medicine
Bellevue Hospital
New York, NY, United States

Connie S. Price
Division of Infectious Diseases
Denver Health Medical Center
Denver, CO, United States;
University of Colorado School of Medicine
Denver, CO, United States

Caroline Quach
Department of Microbiology
Infectiology, and Immunology
University of Montreal
Quebec, QC, Canada

Deepa Raj
Division of Infectious Diseases and
Geographic Medicine
UT Southwestern Medical Center
Dallas, TX, United States

Terri Rebmann
Institute for Biosecurity
College for Public Health and Social Justice
Saint Louis University

James M. Sanders
Department of Pharmacy
University of Texas Southwestern Medical
Center
Dallas, TX, United States;
Department of Medicine
Division of Infectious Diseases and
Geographic Medicine
University of Texas Southwestern Medical
Center
Dallas, TX, United States

Sarah Shalhoub
Department of Medicine
Division of Infectious Diseases
Schulich School of Medicine and Dentistry
University of Western Ontario
London, ON, Canada;
King Fahad Armed Forces Hospital
Jeddah, Saudi Arabia

Emily E. Sickbert-Bennett
Department of Hospital Epidemiology
University of North Carolina Hospitals
Chapel Hill, NC, United States;
Division of Infectious Diseases
UNC School of Medicine
Chapel Hill, NC, United States

Anders Sjöstedt
Department of Clinical Microbiology
Umeå University
Umeå, Sweden

Madhuri M. Sopirala
Infection Prevention
Parkland Health
Dallas, TX, United States;
Division of Infectious Diseases and
Geographic Medicine
Department of Internal Medicine
University of Texas Southwestern Medical Center
Dallas, TX, United States

Mitchell Stripling
NYC Preparedness & Recovery Institute
New York, NY, United States

Kaede V. Sullivan
Department of Pathology and Laboratory Medicine
Lewis Katz School of Medicine at Temple University
Philadelphia, PA, United States

Nuntra Suwantarat
Division of Infectious Diseases
Thammasat University Hospital
Thammasat University
Pathumthani, Thailand;
Chulabhorn International College of Medicine
Thammasat University
Pathumthani, Thailand

Heather Svokos
Employee Communications and Engagement
UT Southwestern Medical Center
Dallas, TX, United States

Geoffrey D. Taylor
Division of Infectious Diseases
Department of Medicine
Faculty of Medicine and Dentistry
University of Alberta
Edmonton, AB, Canada

Lin-fa Wang
Programme in Emerging Infectious Diseases
Duke-NUS Medical School
Singapore

David J. Weber
Department of Hospital Epidemiology
University of North Carolina Hospitals
Chapel Hill, NC, United States;
Division of Infectious Diseases
UNC School of Medicine
Chapel Hill, NC, United States

Matthew Wynia
Center for Bioethics and Humanities
University of Colorado
Anschutz Medical Campus
Aurora, CO, United States;
University of Colorado School of Medicine and Colorado School of Public Health
Aurora, CO, United States

Heather L. Young
Division of Infectious Diseases
Denver Health Medical Center
Denver, CO, United States;
University of Colorado School of Medicine
Denver, CO, United States

Laura B. Zeiser
Department of Epidemiology
Johns Hopkins Bloomberg School of Public Health
Baltimore, MD, United States

Introduction

This book started before the COVID-19 pandemic, and its development was paused while we cared for patients. These experiences molded us all and proved the need for this book. We hope to bridge gaps in knowledge and execution that were revealed and to address the many opportunities for improvement that could and should not be lost. In the context of emerging and reemerging infections and the ethical dilemmas and social strife that they produce, this book addresses two closely related topics: bioterrorism and pandemics. Though not identical, bioterrorism and pandemics are as alike as arson and accidental fires. They strike fear in populations, and they can lead to needless physical and moral injury as well as death. In their wake, they leave mental health struggles, disability, and dramatic economic consequences. Their immediate causes and effects are remarkably similar. It is the intentionality that separates arson and accidental fires, bioterrorism, and outbreaks. Granted, intentional smaller events can spread and change unintentionally. Arson can turn into an accidental conflagration just as bioterror or biowarfare can lead to pandemics. Indeed, the Tatars at Caffa launched plague-infested corpses only as far as their catapults could throw them, but in doing so, they may have inadvertently flung the Black Death from Crimea to Cork, subsequently enveloping Europe in one of the most devastating pandemics in history (See Chapter 1).

Of course, there is a difference that separates large outbreaks from pandemics and bioterrorism that does not separate types of fires—the etiologic agent. Pandemic causes are necessarily contagious and usually quite so, whereas bioterror can be the result of biologic but noninfectious agents, such as ricin or *Clostridium botulinum* toxins. Agents of bioterrorism are often chosen specifically for their ability to produce an effect in a predictable area or population to avoid the unintentional spread already mentioned. This minor difference aside, bioterrorism and pandemics share a great deal of thematic content. As one volume would discuss the prevention and mitigation of fires, similarly this book intends to deal with both the challenges of pandemics and bioterrorism as holistically as possible.

We are the firefighters who are prepared to fight those fires, manage the forests so that the next fire does less damage, and extinguish small fires before the forest is engulfed. Our goals are to address the myriad issues associated with the enormous task of preparedness and help anticipate the needed resources, tools, and skills in case a large outbreak or pandemic arises, or an agent of high consequence is released. In addition, we will outline the theoretical issues and provide practical information so that, in the future, we can avoid some of the medical, societal, and economic disruption and even chaos that can arise in such situations.

How does one prepare for and prevent such events, or at least mitigate the consequences? To answer this question, another overlap merits discussion—that between public health and the healthcare setting. Preparedness within the health sector and the community is the primary strategy to preserve group or societal integrity. In these events, it is difficult to separate public health and healthcare preparation. In fact, in many countries and regions and in certain healthcare settings, healthcare is integrated into the public health sector, requiring a unified strategy to plan for and implement a response to a pathogen of high consequence, an outbreak, or a mass casualty situation. Whether integrated or not, both public health and healthcare facilities are frontline and must be able to: 1. provide appropriate and timely mitigation strategies; 2. negotiate difficult situations and decisions ethically and transparently; 3. communicate effectively and rapidly with large numbers of individuals; and 4. rely on similar supporting services to facilitate decision-making.

In the recent US experience with COVID-19, the response was complicated for both the exposed individuals and those with disease, which required planning and coordination between the care and community settings. The public health authorities had the data and expertise needed to determine how to target treatment and prevention. The CDC and the Advisory Committee on Immunization Practices (ACIP) determined which populations and individuals to target for the initial COVID-19 vaccine doses while it was in short supply. Yet, because the COVID-19 vaccines were initially released under an emergency use authorization (EUA), required special freezers, and distribution was recommended to those most likely to develop severe disease or who were most likely to be exposed, hospitals and healthcare facilities were the ones that could support public health. They had the required freezers to store the vaccine, could provide accessible vaccination sites, had knowledgeable personnel who could navigate and complete the complicated authorizations, and were trained to give vaccines. Hospitals and healthcare facilities cared for and could identify high-risk populations that were the initial populations targeted to receive the vaccine and could easily identify and communicate with both the frontline workers. While we try to separate the aspects that are unique to public health versus the healthcare setting, we recognize the overlap and the redundancy that is needed to facilitate the complicated tasks associated with preparedness. In summary, a holistic approach is again required to respond to these events effectively and to protect the public and healthcare sectors.

This book begins with the extended history of bioterrorism and the role of infectious agents, saving the history of pandemics for their individual agent/disease chapters. We then delve into organism and disease specifics by exploring five selected agents or diseases: anthrax, plague, smallpox, tularemia, and viral hemorrhagic fevers, which comprise a list developed by the Centers for Disease Control and Prevention (CDC) called the category A bioterrorism agents/diseases. We exclude *Clostridium botulinum*, leaving a list of agents with high potential for bioterrorism, outbreaks, and pandemics. These agents have a high associated mortality if undiagnosed or untreated; they are associated with significant mortality, and care of these patients requires sophisticated medical resources. These chapters are followed by a discussion of agents with high pandemic potential but lower likelihood to be used in an intentional attack. We specifically focus on respiratory viruses and the diseases they cause, which have shown time and again their potential to lead to a pandemic. These include influenza and avian influenza strains and the novel coronaviruses, SARS, MERS, and SARS-CoV-2. We end this section with a chapter that addresses the unknown or the designer pathogens that could be created in a laboratory and expresses characteristics that can make them more deadly or more transmissible, whether accidentally or purposefully released. With the groundwork about pathogens laid, we will then cover the systems-based themes of preparedness and response in the public health and healthcare arenas. The long view that needs to be taken is our challenge, the forest we must manage.

In addressing, with a single volume, the challenges of bioterrorism and pandemics, the particular facts and unifying concepts, we can better prepare the reader for the unforeseen challenges that arise in any crisis. Such a work would not be possible without the many contributors to this book. They have persisted over time, responded in crises, and stepped in to fill those gaps. To the authors of these chapters, our experts, we are immensely grateful to you and your fantastic contributions. Each one stepped up to the plate in their own way. They patiently revised and updated their works and contributed tools for us to include. We need to thank Kerry Holland for believing in us and the many project managers, especially Susan Ikeda, whom we have had over the time it has taken to bring this to completion. Finally, our families both at work and home have encouraged and helped us, provided us space and time, made us laugh when needed, and reviewed bits and pieces to make sure we were on track. Of note, we are immensely grateful to the leadership and institutions: UT Southwestern Medical Center, the North Texas Veterans Affairs Medical Center, and Parkland Health and Hospital System, which have reinforced the need for such a book and provided us the academic freedom to realize this project.

In addition to our deepest gratitude, we will end with one wish for humanity and one wish for the reader. For humanity, our wish is to translate pain into learning and complacency into meaningful and sustained preparedness. For the reader, Gorgas observed in 1915 that "In times of stress and danger such as come about as the result of an epidemic [...], many tragic and cruel phases of human nature are brought out, as well as many brave and unselfish ones.[1]" Our wish, should you be found in such times, is that you are brave, unselfish, and, to bolster these virtues, prepared. We hope that this book and its tools play a part in that preparation.

REFERENCES

1. Gorgas WC. Sanitation in Panama. D. Appleton; 1915.

CHAPTER 1

Perspectives on Bioterrorism and Pandemics

DANIEL N. MAXWELL[a] • DEEPA RAJ[b] • TRISH M. PERL[c,d]
[a]Infectious Diseases and Critical Care, UT Southwestern, Dallas VA Medical Center, Dallas, TX, United States • [b]Division of Infectious Diseases and Geographic Medicine, UT Southwestern Medical Center, Dallas, TX, United States • [c]Department of Medicine, University of Texas Southwestern, Dallas, TX, United States • [d]Peter O'Donnell Jr School of Public Health, UT Southwestern Medical Center, Dallas, TX, United States

This book focuses on infectious pathogens of high consequence because of the societal disruption they can cause. While there is considerable overlap between bioterrorist events and pandemics, one means of differentiating them is by differentiating pathogens into two groups depending on their potential to be used as an agent of bioterrorism or their ability to cause large outbreaks or pandemics. The agents of bioterrorism are mostly bacteria or bacterial toxins, and in modern history, the organisms causing pandemics are commonly viruses. Specifically, bacteria or bacterial toxins comprise four of the six top candidates for a bioterror event (Category A agents) and 11 of 12 moderately likely candidate agents (Category B agents) based on the Centers for Disease Control and Prevention (CDC) evaluation.[1] Conversely, pandemics since 1900 have almost exclusively been caused by viruses.[2] Of course, some viruses appear on the list of bioterror agents, but they all have key limiting factors in their pandemic potential (Fig. 1). Smallpox, for example, no longer exists in the wild (see Chapter 7); the filoviruses such as Ebola and Marburg usually require direct contact with contaminated secretions for transmission (see Chapter 6); Hantavirus and *Arenaviridae* such as Lassa and Machupo are primarily transmitted from rodents[3]; and viral encephalitides such as Eastern equine encephalitis are transmitted by mosquitoes or, in rare cases, organ transplantation.[4] Even among the emerging threats such as Nipah virus, reproduction numbers (R_0) are low, roughly 0.33, suggesting an inability to sustain an outbreak. Moreover, the spread is often from clearly infected source patients and via direct contact.[5] With the historical context, increased vigilance is required to ensure the medical community is prepared to act if history repeats itself.

BIOTERRORISM

Bioterrorism refers to the deliberate release of bacteria, viruses, or other biologic agents for the purpose of causing illness or death in humans. An example of one such intentional attack occurred as recently as 2001 when the United States Postal Service was used to distribute envelopes filled with *Bacillus anthracis* (anthrax) spores to several individuals in the US.[6] Hardly a novel concept, bioterrorism attacks and biological warfare, the target of which is military personnel, have been recorded in history as early as 600 BCE when warring factions identified the impact that materials contaminated with infectious agents could have.[7,8] Even earlier records of probable biological warfare date to over 3000 years ago in the Anatolian war.[9] More recent attempts at biological warfare and bioterrorism have led to severe, disfiguring, or otherwise catastrophic illness, thereby significantly increasing public panic around such events (Fig. 1).[7] Hemorrhagic fever viruses were weaponized by the former Union of Soviet Socialist Republics (USSR), or present-day Russia, until 1992. The USSR produced large quantities of Ebola, Lassa, and Marburg viruses[10] and their research found that only a few virions could cause infection in monkeys. Tragically, the epidemic potential of Ebola was later displayed during the

Viral Outbreaks, Biosecurity, and Preparing for Mass Casualty Infectious Diseases Events
https://doi.org/10.1016/B978-0-323-54841-0.00003-2

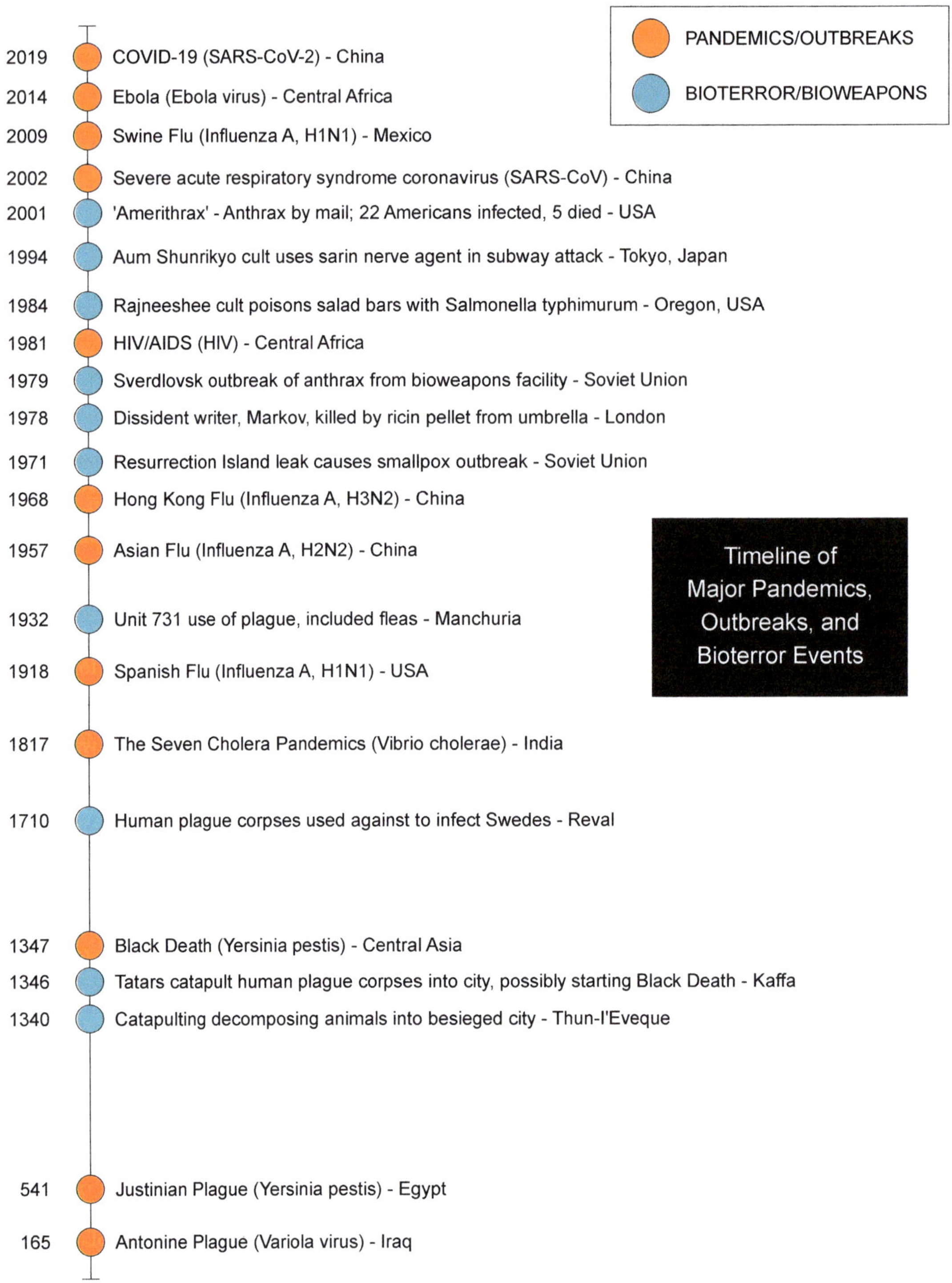

FIG. 1 Timeline of major pandemics, outbreaks, and bioterror events. The *orange circles* represent a pandemic, and the *teal circles* are bioterror events documented over time. Historical notes report events supporting pandemics and bioterror attacks, the latter dating back 2500 to potentially more than 3000 years. This timeline focuses on two millennia of disease with the shift in etiologic agents of pandemics from bacteria in antiquity to viruses in the modern era.

2014 West African Ebola outbreak. In Japan, the Aum Shinrikyo cult attempted to transmit disease to local populations multiple times. Between 1990 and 1995, cult members made three separate efforts to infect specific targets with *B. anthracis.*[11] In 1993, the eight-story building the cult occupied in Tokyo was found to have a liquid suspension of *B. anthracis* that had been aerosolized and spread from the roof.[11] Aum Shinrikyo was also rumored to have sent a team of cult members to the Democratic Republic of the Congo, formerly Zaire, in the midst of the Ebola virus epidemic of the 1990s with a mission of obtaining the virus and then disseminating it to the Japanese population.[7]

Acts of bioterrorism have the potential to be catastrophic in scope, injuring many people in a compressed time period despite limited or indirect exposure. This is due in part to the ease with which some weaponized biological agents can be transmitted from person to person. Small, aerosolized particles, for example, could transmit a large quantity of infectious agents to a wide geographic area, and further spread to second-generation cases would be likely. Aerosolized attacks are particularly treacherous, as infective agents would be dispersed without detection, likely invisible and odorless.[12] Mathematical modeling is an accurate method for estimating the scale of destruction that would result from bioterrorism attacks with different biologic agents and demonstrating the public health response necessary to suppress further transmission. For example, researchers have modeled the effect that an intentional release of variola virus, the causative agent of smallpox, would have on the population. Smallpox is highly contagious and disfiguring, but since 1980 the World Health Organization (WHO) has declared it eradicated following a global vaccination effort. However, vaccination rates wane with the passing years; it is estimated that if 100 people were initially infected, each initial case would infect three subsequent cases. Within 365 days, roughly 4400 individuals would be infected.[13] In another example, the effect of an aerosolized attack with *Francisella tularensis*, the agent responsible for tularemia, if deliberately released in the city of London could expose 2.4 million people, result in roughly 130,000 cases, and have a mortality rate of 18%.[14] A deliberate bioterror attack in large cities with an estimated release of 50 kg of *B. anthracis* spores over an urban population of 5 million could cause 250,000 infections and 100,000 deaths.[12] Regardless of the etiologic agent, a future infectious disease outbreak could result in roughly 865,000 to 9,900,000 hospitalizations, up to 45 million outpatient visits, and $71 to $166 billion in excess costs.[15]

AGENTS OF BIOTERRORISM AND CATEGORIZATION

Multiple strategies are used to rank the risk of agents being used for nefarious purposes. The European Centre for Disease Control summarized the criteria in an analysis and found that most approaches to risk ranking of biologic agents include identifying diseases to be included and assessment criteria, developing weighting criteria, scoring diseases with set criteria, and producing a rank list.[16] The Centers for Disease Control and Prevention (CDC), in the United States, separates bioterrorism agents into three categories (A, B, and C) based on their ease of transmission, severity of illness caused, and ability to be reproduced (Table 1).[17,18] The degree to which the deliberate release of a certain biological agent would prompt reinforced public health preparedness efforts, such as stockpiling vaccinations, enhancing surveillance, or improving diagnostic capacity is also considered.[19] In some cases, a small number of organisms are required to cause infection. Category A agents (Table 1) include the highest priority organisms, which 1. can lead to severe morbidity and mortality, 2. are easily transmissible from person to person, 3. can potentially propagate from person to person leading to secondary and tertiary cases, and 4. could cause social disruption.[20] They are also considered easily aerosolized and weaponized and therefore require special considerations for preparedness and public health responses. Category B agents are moderately transmissible, have lower associated morbidity and mortality, will likely have a less severe impact on public health, and could be used to contaminate food or water.[17] Category C agents are readily available pathogens that could be genetically engineered for dissemination and potentially have devastating effects on morbidity and mortality if weaponized. Because of the extreme human and economic costs incurred by attacks with Category A agents/diseases, we will discuss them further.

PATHOGENS/ORGANISMS

Anthrax

B. anthracis: (see Chapter 3 for in-depth discussion) *B. anthracis* is a naturally occurring, gram-positive, spore-forming, exotoxin-producing bacillus that is ubiquitous in soil around the world.[21] It is the causative agent of anthrax, a zoonotic disease whose spores are environmentally hardy.[22] Disease occurs when humans are exposed to anthrax spores, which can secrete poisonous toxins. Anthrax can cause three forms of disease in humans, the cutaneous and pulmonary are the most likely to be associated with a bioterrorist event.

TABLE 1
CDC Categorization of Bioterrorism Agents[1]

Biological Agent(s)	Disease	Infective Dose
CDC Category A		
Arenaviruses (e.g., *Lassa fever*)	Viral hemorrhagic fevers	1–10 viruses
Bacillus anthracis	Anthrax	8,000–50,000 spores
Clostridium botulinum (toxins)	Botulism	0.001 μg/kg
Filoviruses (e.g., *Ebola virus*)	Viral hemorrhagic fevers	1–10 viruses
Francisella tularensis	Tularemia	10–50 bacteria
Variola major	Smallpox	10–100 viruses
Yersinia pestis	Plague	100–500 bacteria
CDC Category B		
Alphaviruses (e.g., *equine encephalomyelitis*)	Encephalitis	10–100 viruses
Brucella spp.	Brucellosis	10–100 organisms
Burkholderia mallei	Glanders	Very low
Bukholderia pseudomallei	Melioidosis	Very low
Chlamydia psittaci	Psittacosis	Unknown
Coxiella burnetii	Q fever	1–10 organisms
Food safety threats (e.g., *Salmonella* spp.)	Gastroenteritis	Varies
Rickettsia prowazekii	Typhus fever	<10 organisms
Toxins (e.g., from *Ricinus communis*)	Varies	Varies
Water safety threats (e.g., *Vibrio cholerae*)	Varies, commonly gastroenteritis	Varies
CDC Category C		
Emerging infectious threats (e.g., *Nipah virus*)	Varies	Varies

The table lists biologic organisms and toxins with potential for use in a bioterror event as categorized by the CDC based on priority with Category A being the highest priority, Category B of lower priority, and then Category C with lesser priority, which may reflect less CDC = Centers for Disease Control and Prevention.

Cutaneous anthrax: Cutaneous anthrax is the most common form of anthrax and has a low associated morbidity and mortality. This form of disease occurs when spores, most commonly from animal skins or on contaminated surfaces, are touched, penetrate the skin, and germinate. The incubation period is 1–12 days and is followed by the formation of a papule that progresses into a fluid-filled vesicle that then dries, forming a painless eschar with associated regional adenitis, which is the hallmark of this disease.[23]

Gastrointestinal anthrax: Gastrointestinal anthrax, while rare in humans, is transmitted via ingestion of improperly cooked meat from animals infected with *B. anthracis*. The spore germinates within 2–3 days within the gastrointestinal tract leading to both gastrointestinal and systemic symptoms including esophageal or oral ulcers.[24] Symptoms vary, but the diarrhea, which can be bloody, abdominal pain, nausea, and vomiting are typical and can be followed by a syndrome mimicking an acute surgical abdomen, sometimes with cervical lymphadenopathy, dysphagia, and severe gastrointestinal distress.[23,25,26]

Inhalational anthrax: Inhalational anthrax is the most lethal form of infection and results from the inhalation of aerosolized spores that germinate in the lungs. After an incubation period that can last from 1 day to 6 weeks, the presentation of the disease is biphasic. Initially, a nonspecific fever, malaise, and mild respiratory symptoms develop followed by a brief convalescence.[24] Finally, respiratory distress characterized by dyspnea, diaphoresis, and stridor ensues rapidly with a case fatality rate of 90%.[21,24]

Tularemia

F. tularensis: (see Chapter 4 for in-depth discussion) A zoonotic infection distributed worldwide, tularemia is caused by *F. tularensis*, an intracellular, gram-negative coccobacillus.[27] Tularemia exists worldwide and is particularly prevalent in the northern hemisphere. The organism is found in contaminated water and soil, infected insects (ticks, deerflies), and other wild animals and is transmitted via inhalation of contaminated aerosols, contact with infected animals, or ingestion of contaminated water or meat.[12,22] It causes several forms of disease in humans, including pneumonic, ulceroglandular, oculoglandular, oropharyngeal, and typhoidal tularemia.[12] A bioterrorism attack would likely involve inhalation of aerosols, and pneumonic tularemia is the presentation expected.

The incubation period is 3–5 days followed by a presentation similar to community-acquired pneumonia, including cough, dyspnea, and fever,[23] and progresses to pneumonia with bloody sputum, difficulty breathing, and systemic respiratory failure.[12] Sepsis and death can result if appropriate treatment is not initiated.[12]

Plague

Yersinia pestis: (see Chapter 5 for in-depth discussion) Plague is also a zoonotic infection caused by a gram-negative *Enterobacteriaceae*, *Y. pestis*,[21] which occurs in nature worldwide and has been implicated in multiple pandemics throughout the course of history.[12] *Y. pestis* is transmitted to humans through bites from its vector, the flea, and has a natural rodent reservoir.[21] *Y. pestis* infection has three presentations: bubonic, septicemic, and pneumonic.[28]

Bubonic plague: The most common form of *Y. pestis* infection occurs after a bite from an infected flea with an incubation period of 2–8 days. Subsequently, chills, fever, and weakness develop with the formation of the hallmark "buboes," or erythematous, swollen, edematous, and painful lymph nodes primarily in the axilla and groin.[12,22,28] The organism then enters the bloodstream causing endotoxemia, septicemia, disseminated intravascular coagulation, and shock.[21,22] Bubonic plague is not transmitted from person to person unless there is an associated pneumonia, in which case respiratory transmission may occur through droplets, occurring in 5%–15% of cases.[21,24] The case fatality ratio for this form of disease is approximately 14%.[28]

Septicemic plague: Sepsis and septicemia occur in a minority of cases and develop from buboes. Endotoxins lead to disseminated intravascular coagulation, necrosis of small blood vessels, and gangrenous lesions, especially on the tip of the nose, fingers, and toes.[12,22] The case fatality rate is 22%.[28]

Pneumonic plague: Pneumonic plague is rare but the most likely form of disease following a bioterror event associated with an aerosolized release. This form of infection is contagious due to organisms in droplets, and individuals can transmit it until treated with antimicrobials.[21] A brief 2- to 4-day incubation period is followed by chills, dyspnea, headache, myalgias, and fulminant pneumonia.[22] Abdominal pain, diarrhea, nausea, and vomiting often occur.[22] Individuals with the pneumonic infection decline rapidly, with disseminated intravascular coagulation, sepsis, severe respiratory distress, and shock.[21] This form of *Y. pestis* infection has a significant associated mortality of up to 60%.[28]

Viral Hemorrhagic Fever

The agents causing viral hemorrhagic fevers are a large group of taxonomically distinct viruses (see Chapter 6, Table 4). Here we discuss briefly two of the Category A agents/diseases (Filoviruses and Arenaviruses) and then, for completeness, a group of Category B agents/diseases, the alphaviruses.

Filoviruses: (see Chapter 6 for in-depth discussion) Responsible for highly publicized disease outbreaks in Africa in recent years, organisms belonging to the Filoviridae genus are negative-stranded ribonucleic acid (RNA) viruses that can persist in body fluids for extended periods following infection.[29] Both Ebola and Marburg viruses, two viruses that make up the Filoviridae genus, are endemic to Africa and considered zoonotic with animal reservoirs, so naturally occurring infections and outbreaks are reported. The Ebola and Marburg viruses are the etiologic agents for two viral hemorrhagic fevers known as Ebola virus disease and Marburg fever, respectively. There are four known viral subtypes of Ebola and one strain of Marburg, and all but the Reston Ebola species can cause disease in humans.[29,30] Filoviruses are exceedingly contagious and transmitted via contaminated bodily fluids or ingestion of contaminated meat and are associated with significant morbidity and mortality.[24]

Ebola virus disease: The incubation period lasts between 2 and 21 days and is followed by a nonspecific prodrome that can include fever, headache, myalgia, prostration, and vomiting.[22] Petechial hemorrhages precede the maculopapular rash occurring 5 days after infection.[31] In the next week, the infection can lead rapidly to circulatory shock, disseminated intravascular coagulation, and liver and renal dysfunction.[24,27,31] The case fatality ratio for Ebola virus disease ranges from 50% to 90%.[22] Treatments are now available, and a vaccine for the Ebola-Zaire strain is available and effective in preventing infection (see Chapter 25). Postinfection sequelae include lassitude and prolonged shedding of the virus.

Marburg virus disease: The Marburg virus incubates for 2–14 days, during which time an individual is infected but not contagious.[22] The clinical presentation is like Ebola virus disease with headache, sudden-onset fever, myalgia, and prostration followed by the appearance of a non-pruritic maculopapular rash.[22,24] The patient deteriorates rapidly as mucous membrane and conjunctival hemorrhaging begin, followed by disseminated intravascular coagulation and circulatory shock leading to a death rate as high as 70%.[22,27,31] Treatment is supportive and no vaccine is available.

Arenaviruses: (see Chapter 5 for in-depth discussion) Part of the *Arenaviridae* family, these enveloped, single-stranded RNA viruses are responsible for several viral hemorrhagic fevers.[31] The natural host of arenaviruses is a common rat ubiquitous in West Africa that cause many natural arenavirus infections annually.[32,33] Lassa fever caused by Lassa virus is a zoonotic pathogen endemic in West Africa and associated with travel to the region.[34] It is a potential agent of bioterrorism because of its contagiousness and association with morbidity and mortality.[34] It could be aerosolized for widespread release.

Lassa fever is commonly a subclinical infection, although more serious disease can occur.[24] The incubation period lasts between 5 and 16 days and is followed by the gradual appearance of fever, nausea, abdominal pain, cough, chest pain, pharyngitis, and proteinuria.[22] After 7–8 days, craniofacial edema and pleural and pericardial effusions may develop.[22,32] Hemorrhage is less common with this infection, although survivors may become deaf and survivors may shed virus, including via sexual contact, for up to 3 months.[24,34]

Alphaviruses: Belonging to *Togaviridae*, members of the Alphavirus genus cause zoonotic infections primarily in North and South America, such as Eastern equine encephalitis, Venezuelan equine encephalitis, and Western equine encephalitis.[31] While alphaviruses are naturally transmitted to humans by mosquitoes, these pathogens could be weaponized, as strains are readily available and inexpensive.[31] A deliberate release of aerosolized particles of alphaviruses would result in catastrophic disease, as the infective dose for humans is 10–100 virions.[18] Eastern equine encephalitis, Venezuelan equine encephalitis, and Western equine encephalitis have similar clinical presentations except in their neurological sequelae; Eastern equine encephalitis is the most severe infection of the three, causing high morbidity and significant long-term neurological impairment.[27]

Eastern equine encephalitis: An incubation period of 4–10 days is followed by a prodromal phase characterized by sudden fever, malaise, and headache.[35] Leukopenia can occur and progress to leukocytosis.[27] In humans who develop encephalitis, this phase is marked by hematuria and the onset of confusion, somnolence, seizures, and even coma.[35] The mortality is from 50% to 70%, and fatal cases develop facial and brain edema and hemorrhage reported.[31,35]

Venezuelan equine encephalitis: Typically marked by a short incubation period and flu-like illness in naturally occurring cases, this causes neurological sequelae, including ataxia, convulsions, and disorientation.[35] Its case fatality rate is less than 1%, and neurological recovery usually follows nonfatal cases.[35]

Western equine encephalitis: After an incubation period of 2–7 days, infection tends to be mild with nonspecific symptoms including anorexia, fever, headache, malaise, and nausea.[3536] Encephalitis occurs rarely and can result in confusion, tonic-clonic seizures, somnolence, weakness, and coma.[36] The mortality is between 3% and 7%.[36]

Smallpox

Variola virus: (see Chapter 6 for in-depth discussion) The variola virus belongs to the Poxviridae family and causes smallpox, which was declared eradicated globally in 1980.[12] At this time, routine vaccination practices against this infection ceased, leading to a more susceptible population. Stocks of variola virus, however, are known to exist in the United States and Russia and could produce large outbreaks if aerosolized or weaponized given the low infective dose required to cause illness and waning immunity in the general population.

The variola virus enters the body through the nasal and oral mucous membranes and causes three distinct clinical phases of disease: incubation, prodromal illness, and fulminant infection.[22] During the 10- to 14-day incubation period, patients are asymptomatic. The prodromal phase follows for 4 days and is characterized by high fever, malaise, headache, and vomiting. An eruptive rash develops that persists for 7–10 days at which time patients are highly infective.[22] The rash begins in the mouth and spreads to the limbs in a centrifugal pattern, with lesions that progress from macules to papules to vesicles.[23,24] The lesions finally become pustular and scab around the eighth day of the rash, and viral shedding can occur from the onset of the rash until the scabs are separated and healed.[24] In addition to being disfiguring, complications of smallpox include arthritis, blindness, keratitis, corneal ulcers, and osteomyelitis.[27] The case fatality rate is typically 25% if untreated.[23]

PANDEMICS

Pandemics have shaped human populations throughout history.[37] These large-scale outbreaks can span continents and generally involve a new organism or new variant in a particular time frame. They lead to morbidity and mortality among the population, stress healthcare care and healthcare systems, and have economic sequelae. While influenza pandemics have been documented for the past 500 years, the 1918 Spanish flu pandemic is the best documented in modern history leading to 50 million deaths or approximately 2.1% of the world's population at that time.[37] Economically, this pandemic depressed the gross national product by 0.8% and up to 50% in developing countries. The economic impact was felt for two to four decades in some European countries, such as France and Germany. Fear generated from poor health outcomes, personal safety, and uncertainty in the effectiveness of implemented mitigation strategies or available treatments can then lead to economic, social, and political disruption. In fact, models looking at the impact of human behavior during the COVID-19 pandemic showed that fear of infection drove decreased consumption in the population, and this fear had the same economic impact as implementing non-pharmacologic mitigation strategies.[38]

Many of these events have evolved from "spillover" events where an animal pathogen adapts and develops characteristics that allow it to be easily transmitted in the human population.[39] Spillover events are driven by many external factors including humans encroaching on wildlife reservoirs, habitat destruction, changes in climate, animal husbandry practices, consumption of wild animals, and human migration. More recently, climate change and transportation have amplified the ability of organisms to affect the human population. As early as the late 1800s disease, Europeans described large outbreaks of poultry deaths and coined the term "fowl plague." The 1918 Spanish influenza pandemic, likely resulting from a spillover event from waterfowl, affected a fifth of the world's population and may have caused 50 million deaths (Figs. 1 and 4). Interestingly, and unlike Europe, in the United States (US) there were two waves and great variation in mortality geographically depending upon the mitigation strategies used and when they were implemented. Mathematical models used data from 45 cities across the US and correlated 1918 city-specific excess mortality to pre-pandemic mortality to correct for differences in the populations, and socioeconomic characteristics.[40] This analysis found three public health interventions were most effective, yet the effect was dampened if interventions were lifted too early.[41] Those cities (San Francisco, Kansas City, St. Louis, and Milwaukee) that intervened the earliest and retained measures the longest had the lowest mortality rates. These data highlight how public health interventions will impact healthcare systems and their capacity. Ferguson et al. used data from the United Kingdom (UK) and the US to model influenza containment strategies, many of which impact the health care system including the use of antivirals, vaccines, and nonpharmaceutical interventions (NPIs) such as isolation, quarantine, contact tracing, school and workplace closure, and travel restrictions.[42] They also found that case isolation and household quarantine were the two interventions that were most impactful. These models show that if adequate supplies of antivirals are available and given within the first symptomatic day and schools are closed in response, rates could decrease by 40%–50%. To reduce influenza attack rates by 75%, more than 50% of the population would need to receive antivirals, and such estimates could change with poor compliance. Hence, the pressure on the healthcare systems to care for individuals could be immense, and the CDC estimated that in 1999 an influenza pandemic in the US would have led to 89,000–207,000 deaths, 314,000–734,000 hospitalizations, and 18–24 million outpatient visits with an economic cost of $71.3 to $166.5 billion.[43] Overall, the measured impact of past pandemics on human health and the economy has been enormous, and there is no reason to think that they will not be in the future.[12]

PANDEMICS AND RESPIRATORY VIRUSES

Respiratory viruses have led to most modern pandemics due to a number of factors including spillover events, the advent of antibacterial drugs, the global improvement in overall sanitation standards, greater mobility, urbanization, and human populations interfacing with previously uninhabited land. By comparison, many of the viruses that are pathogens of high consequence spread predominantly through routes more amenable to containment, e.g., direct or indirect contact, or are zoonotic in nature. Consequently, when we speak of respiratory viruses within the scope of a potential bioterror event and potential for widespread transmission, we are speaking almost exclusively of pandemics and the potential thereof. This said, the advent of a designer respiratory pathogen that is deliberately released is possible.

The respiratory viruses that have emerged and caused many of the modern outbreaks and pandemics essentially involve only two families: the *Coronaviridae* (Coronaviruses) and the *Orthomyxoviridae* (influenza

TABLE 2
Overview of Influenza Viruses

Influenza Genus	Main Host	Subdivisions/ Lineages	Mild Disease	Severe Disease	Epidemics	Pandemics
Influenza A	Waterfowl, poultry, humans, pigs, horses, seals, whales, domestic animals	Subtyped by HA/NA, primary host (avian, swine, etc.), and, if avian, classified as high/low pathogenicity	X	X	X	X
Influenza B	Humans	Two lineages based on HA: Victoria and Yamagata	X	X	X	
Influenza C	Humans	None	X			
Influenza D	Cattle	None				

Influenza genera, hosts, and categorization are provided along with characteristic severity of human infection and potential for outbreaks and pandemics.
Adapted from Hutchinson EC, Yamauchi Y. *Understanding Influenza*. New York: Springer; 2018:1–21.

viruses). There are three influenza viruses that can infect humans, only two of which cause serious illness: influenza A and influenza B (Table 2). Influenza A is associated with pandemics and has been responsible for at least four pandemics in the 20th and 21st centuries (Fig. 4; see Chapter 8 for more detail). Avian influenza A strains are increasingly recognized (Fig. 4; see Chapter 8 for more detail), especially given the worldwide dissemination of several of the highly pathogenic avian strains, the introduction of some of these strains into multiple mammal species, and the significant increase in reported human cases (Table 3).[44] Several of these strains are considered to have pandemic potential. Regarding coronaviruses, there are only seven known to infect humans, three of which are novel, emerging in the 21st century, and can cause serious human illness (Table 4): SARS-CoV (see Chapter 10), MERS-CoV (see Chapter 11), and SARS-CoV-2 (see Chapter 12).

Influenza pandemics have occurred every 10 to 40 years, and the novel coronaviruses have emerged and led to large outbreaks every 10 years. In 1997, a study published demonstrated the impact of an annual influenza epidemic in 1997–98 in a setting with decreased acute care capacity. An increase in pneumonia and hospitalizations by 10% led to diversions and disruptions in the healthcare system. The measured impact of pandemics on human health and the economy has been enormous.[12] The novel coronavirus strains have zoonotic origins and led to large outbreaks, if not pandemics, the most recent being COVID-19. This latest pandemic brought the challenges of managing large volumes of critically ill patients to the forefront and led some hospitals and health systems to be extremely stretched, which was associated with higher mortality rates.[87,88] Additionally, beyond the immediate care of patients with COVID-19, the decrease in access to care for routine and urgent care was also well described.[89]

RESPIRATORY VIRUSES UNIQUE CHARACTERISTICS

Respiratory viruses have a greater pandemic potential for three reasons: more modes of transmission, a larger surface area to infect, and greater difficulty in controlling spread. The term "respiratory virus" refers to a primary route of transmission via the upper and lower respiratory tracts, but this is not an exclusive route of transmission. Respiratory viruses can be transmitted as aerosols (small particles, certainly <5 μm but still with aerosol behaviors up to 100 μm), droplet sprays (large particles >100 μm), and by direct and indirect contact via fomites.[90] The fine lines between transmission via droplets that can be sprayed one to two meters away or droplets that can be aerosolized have become increasingly evident, especially in the era of modern medicine with devices and treatments that may facilitate aerosolization. This gray zone between clearly airborne small particles at 5 μm and larger droplets at 100 μm is important, and these 5- to 100-μm particles can still hang in the air for 5 s and be inhaled at close distances, so we have categorized them as airborne.[91,92] Regardless, respiratory viruses have a repertoire of transmissibil-

TABLE 3
Overview of Clinical and Epidemiologic Features of Influenza Viruses Including Avian Influenza Subtypes That Have Caused Human Infection

Influenza	Clinical Symptoms	Incubation Period	Mortality and Median Time to Death	Epidemics and Pandemic Potential	Epidemiologic Features	Notes
Influenza A [H1N1, H2N2, and H3N2] [45–48]	Causes moderate to severe symptoms: Fever Myalgia Headache Malaise Chills Nonproductive cough Complications include pneumonia, otitis, sinusitis, and exacerbation of underlying medical conditions	Median 1.4 days Range 1–4 days	Case fatality rate 6% in hospitalized Median time to death = 23 days Mortality increases with age > 65 years; those with underlying medical conditions; pregnancy; children <5 years	Responsible for large flu epidemics, generally seasonal, and has pandemic potential H1N1 and H3N2 Moderate pandemic potential (depends on clade)	Contagious and transmitted via inhalation of infectious droplets Transmission can occur 12 h before symptom onset Birds are the natural reservoir	Seasonal epidemics in temperate climates Severity of illness varies season to season Infection in humans and multiple animal species Classified as avian or swine in origin Vaccine available
Influenza B [45–48]	Milder disease than Influenza A Fever Dry cough Chills Sore throat Myalgias Headache Fatigue Diarrhea and vomiting (More common in children) Complications include pneumonia, otitis, sinusitis, and exacerbation of underlying medical conditions	Median 0.6 days Range 1–4 days	Case fatality rate in hospitalized = 3% 14 days Attributable mortality may be higher for influenza B than influenza A (Odd's ratio = 2.65)	Causes seasonal epidemics No pandemic potential	Contagious and transmitted via inhalation of infectious droplets Accounts for ~1/3 of cases in children Can transmit 12–24 h before symptoms begin Human reservoir	Infects humans (children more than adults) Less antigenic variation than influenza A Vaccine available

(Continued)

TABLE 3
Overview of Clinical and Epidemiologic Features of Influenza Viruses Including Avian Influenza Subtypes That Have Caused Human Infection—cont'd

Influenza	Clinical Symptoms	Incubation Period	Mortality and Median Time to Death	Epidemics and Pandemic Potential	Epidemiologic Features	Notes
Influenza C[49,50]	Cause mild infections Fever Cough Rhinorrhea Wheezing Can cause lower respiratory tract infections	Unknown	Unknown	Not thought to be associated with epidemics	Seropositivity 90% by age 10; primarily affects young children; rarely reported in those over 65 years old Leads to healthcare utilization in adults	Thought to be seasonal Co-infection with other respiratory viruses common Substantial genetic diversity in circulating strains
Influenza D[51]	Unknown	Unknown	Unknown	Not known to cause epidemics	Serologic evidence of infection ranges from 1.3% in those >60; 18% in the general population to 97% in cattle-exposed farmers	Primarily affects cattle with spillover to other species No vaccines currently
H5N1[52–57]	(Symptom frequency varies by clade) ILI[a] Fever, Dry cough, Myalgias Coryza Sore throat Severe dyspnea Headache Nausea, vomiting Diarrhea Rapid progression to bronchiolitis, pneumonia, respiratory distress, and multiorgan dysfunction encephalitis, bleeding also reported	Median 4.3–7 days Range 1–9 days	Mortality: 53% Time to death: Median 9–10 days Range 4–30 days	Highly pathogenic[b] Moderate pandemic potential	Transmission primarily avian to humans with exposure to poultry in farms or live markets, sick poultry, or eating raw poultry products Median age 19–27 years old Human cases worldwide with clusters reported fairly commonly	Infection now reported in multiple mammal species Human-to-human transmission reported with intimate contact Human cases preceded an outbreak in poultry Poultry vaccines used in some countries Inactivated human vaccines developed

H5N6[58–60]	ILI[a] Fever Sore throat Cough Headache Chills Myalgias Dyspnea Blood-tinged sputum Pneumonia Respiratory failure multiorgan failure	2–5 days	Case fatality rate: 55.4%–68.4% Hospital-associated mortality 59% Time to death Median 17 days Range 6–31 days	Highly pathogenic[b] Moderate pandemic potential	Transmission primarily avian to humans with exposure to poultry in farms or live markets, sick poultry, or eating raw poultry products Mean age 37 years old; 50% with comorbid illness Human cases primarily in Asia	94% of reported cases have severe disease. Human-to-human transmission possible
H7N3[61]	Mild ILI[a] Fever Sore throat Cough Headache Chills Myalgias Coryza Diarrhea Conjunctivitis	1–3 days	Mortality 0%	Highly pathogenic[b] Pandemic potential not assessed yet	Transmission primarily avian to humans with exposure to poultry in farms and sick poultry Cases in North and Central America	Infection reported in mammals Tropism for eye Vaccine being tested
H7N7[62–64]	Subclinical disease is common or mild symptoms ILI[a] Fever Headache Cough Rhinorrhea Myalgias Conjunctivitis very common Pneumonia and multiorgan failure (rare)	Median 1–4 days Range 1–10 days	1.1%	Highly pathogenic[b] Moderate pandemic potential	Transmission primarily avian to humans with exposure to poultry in farms and sick poultry Human cases in Europe	Human-to-human transmission reported in family clusters; suggestion of transmission by fomite in one outbreak. Human cases preceded an outbreak in poultry

(*Continued*)

TABLE 3
Overview of Clinical and Epidemiologic Features of Influenza Viruses Including Avian Influenza Subtypes That Have Caused Human Infection—cont'd

Influenza	Clinical Symptoms	Incubation Period	Mortality and Median Time to Death	Epidemics and Pandemic Potential	Epidemiologic Features	Notes
H7N9[44,65,66]	ILI[a] Fever >38 °C, Dry cough Myalgias Conjunctivitis Coryza Sore throat Gastrointestinal symptoms less common Rapid progression to pneumonia, respiratory distress, and multiorgan dysfunction	Median 4 days Range 1–12 days	Mortality ~30% Time to Death: 21 days 12.5–36	Highly pathogenic[b] Moderate to high pandemic potential	More transmissible than A H5N1 as binds to avian and human sialic acid receptors Exposure to poultry, sick poultry, or poultry products Median age 55 years old More likely to have comorbid illness and increased severity Human cases in Asia, North America	Human-to-human transmission in clusters Healthcare-associated transmission (immunocompromised) and non-sustained household transmission China undertook a massive poultry vaccination campaign with combined H5 and H7 strains
H9N2 [44,67,68]	Symptoms generally milder ILI[a] General malaise Headache Nasal discharge Sneezing Sore throat Fever and cough (10%–20% of patients)	2–5 days	Mortality 2.3% (Mortality in a bone marrow transplant recipient)	Low pathogenic[b] Moderate to high pandemic potential	Exposure to poultry, sick poultry, or poultry products Mean age < 4 years old Human cases in Eurasia, Africa, Egypt, Bangladesh	Human-to-human transmission Infection reported in mammals Seroprevalence in Cambodia 1.1%–2.6% Poultry prototype vaccine available

H3N8[69,70]	ILI[a] Fever Chills Sore throat Rhinorrhea Mild symptoms reported thus far in humans	Not known	Mortality 0%	Low pathogenicity[b] (Can cause severe respiratory disease in mammals) Pandemic potential not assessed as of yet	Exposure to poultry, sick poultry, or poultry products Can bind to human sialic acid receptors Resorted from H9N2, avian H3 and N8 viruses Human cases in China	Primary equine influenza but infects other mammals Samples from wet market and environmental samples from cases house positive for H3N8
H10N7[64,71]	Fever Cough Minor upper respiratory tract symptoms conjunctivitis	Not known	Mortality 0%	Low pathogenic[b] Pandemic potential not assessed	Exposure to poultry, sick poultry, or poultry products Eurasia, Australia	Human cases preceded an outbreak in poultry Some pathogenic in mammals
H10N8[c] [64,71]	ILI[a] Fever Running nose Cough Dyspnea Rapid progression to pneumonia	Not known	Mortality 100%	Low pathogenic[b] Moderate pandemic potential	Exposure to poultry, sick poultry, or poultry products Human cases in China, Egypt, and Australia	Infection reported in mammals

[a]ILI = Influenza-like illness: fever >38.5oC and at least one of the following symptoms: cough, myalgia, rhinorrhea, sore throat, or headache.

[b]Highly pathogenic strains have a 90%–100% mortality in poultry within 48 h of infection.

[c]Human cases reported from H7N2 (mild symptoms, related to the outbreak in cat shelter; pandemic potential not assessed), H7N4 (ILI with cough, fever, chills, and pneumonia; poultry exposure; pandemic potential not assessed), and H6N1 (mild pneumonia).

TABLE 4
Overview of Coronaviruses in Humans Clinical and Epidemiological Features of Novel and Epidemic ("Common Cold") Coronaviruses in Humans

Novel Human CoV	Clinical Symptoms	Case Fatality Rate	Incubation Period	Median Time to Death	R_0 Estimate
SARS-CoV-1	Fever Myalgia Headache Malaise Chills Nonproductive cough Dyspnea Respiratory distress Diarrhea (30%–40% of patients)	9.5%	2–11 days	23 days Community attack rate 10%–60%	R_0 = 0.25–6[72]
MERS-CoV	Fever Cough Chills Sore throat Myalgia Arthralgia Dyspnea Pneumonia Diarrhea and vomiting (One-third of patients) Acute renal impairment	36%	2–13 days	14 days	R_0 = 0.95[72]
SARS-CoV-2	**More common:** Fever Cough shortness of breath Myalgia Generalized weakness (fatigue) Chills Chest pain Anosmia Ageusia **Less common:** Diarrhea Nasal congestion Rhinorrhea Sneezing Sore throat Headache Confusion Nausea	~2%[73,74] **Hospitalized cases[a]:** 14%–26% (fatal cases/recovered + fatal cases only)[75–77] 11%–15% (fatal cases/ all hospitalized cases)[76,77] Community attack rate 30%–40%	4–14 days 12.5 days estimated as 95% of distribution[78]	8–20 days[b] **Other info:** Onset to medical visit: 4.6–5.8 days[78] Onset to hospitalization: 7–12.5 days[76,78,79] **Hospitalization to death:** 9–11 days (n = 2)[77]	**Early estimates[c]:** R_0 = 1.4–3.8[80–86] **Later estimates:** R_0 = 2.0–2.5

TABLE 4
Overview of Coronaviruses in Humans Clinical and Epidemiological Features of Novel and Epidemic ("Common Cold") Coronaviruses in Humans—cont'd

Cold or Endemic Human CoV	Clinical Symptoms	Case Fatality Rate	Incubation Period	Median Time to Death	R_0 Estimate
229E	General malaise Headache Nasal discharge Sneezing Sore throat Fever and cough (10%–20% of patients)	N/A	2–5 days	N/A	N/A
OC43	General malaise Headache Nasal discharge Sneezing Sore throat Fever and cough (10%–20% of patients)	N/A	2–5 days	N/A	N/A
NL63	Cough, Rhinorrhea Tachypnea Fever Hypoxia Obstructive laryngitis (croup)	N/A	2–4 days	N/A	N/A
HKU1	Fever Running nose Cough Dyspnea	N/A	2–4 days	N/A	N/A

Clinical and epidemiologic features of coronaviruses. The upper panel displays characteristics of the novel coronaviruses, and the lower panel displays the characteristics of the cold or endemic coronaviruses.
[a]Case fatality rates of hospitalized patients were calculated in two different ways: one as percentage of all hospitalized patients and two as percentage of those with outcomes known at the time of calculation. Some of the known patient outcome rates here were calculated post hoc based on data provided in publications.
[b]Delay from infection to death varies by age and method of calculation.
[c]R0 especially in an initial outbreak can vary widely due to the spectrum of infection, the inclusion of super-spreaders or super-spreading events, delays in obtaining data, and misclassification of cases. Due to the instability of the R0 estimate, its ability to project the trajectory of the outbreak may be more difficult.

ity that other viruses lack, and this repertoire affects recommended mitigation strategies and compliance with those mitigation strategies.

Second, respiratory viruses have a large area to infect. Consider that the human body interacts with its direct environment via three main organ systems: the skin (including mucosa such as the conjunctiva), the respiratory tract (lungs), and the digestive tract (gut). The surface area of each of these organs is roughly 2–25 m^2 for the skin, 30 m^2 for the gut, and 50 m^2 for the lung.[93] Hence, the surface area of the lung is considerably larger than that of the gut and the skin. Moreover, intact skin is specifically structured as to function as a barrier against the entry of pathogens. Furthermore, in the setting of a viral infection, these "surfaces" can be disrupted both micro- and macroscopically.

Third, because of how they are transmitted, controlling the transmission of respiratory viruses is more challenging than other viruses. Humans can influence what enters their gut more easily than what they breathe and enters the lungs. Certainly, fecal-oral contamination is important, and many pathogens, such as norovirus, successfully spread and replicate primarily in the gut as their reservoir or site of infection. Yet, even in children and with certain strains of influenza, fecal-oral contamination is viewed as a secondary mechanism of transmission. With the exception of cholera,[2] the etiology of pandemics has not been gastrointestinal pathogens. This may reflect nonpharmacologic interventions such as isolation, sanitation, etc. that are effective in preventing fecal-oral spread, yet when applied to prevent respiratory pathogen transmission have had variable success. Similarly, limiting global travel and minimizing nosocomial transmission have historically proven factors more difficult for respiratory pathogens. Lastly, there is greater acceptance of hand washing/hand hygiene as a form of mitigation rather than other strategies such as mask-wearing,school closures, and lockdowns. For these and many other reasons, respiratory pathogens have the greatest pandemic potential. The scourges of the 20th century were influenza viruses, and those of the 21st century have thus far been coronaviruses. Furthermore, because of their pandemic potential, respiratory viruses could be targeted for designer pathogen construction and use in a bioterror event, and the evolution of a pathogen may be difficult to trace given how naturally occurring outbreaks or pandemics evolve.

INFLUENZA IN HUMANS (SEE CHAPTERS 8 AND 9 FOR ADDITIONAL DETAILS)

Three influenza strains infect humans: A, B, and C (Fig. 2, Table 3). Influenza C is a rare cause of influenza, and influenza D primarily infects cattle, and though humans have been shown to have antibodies

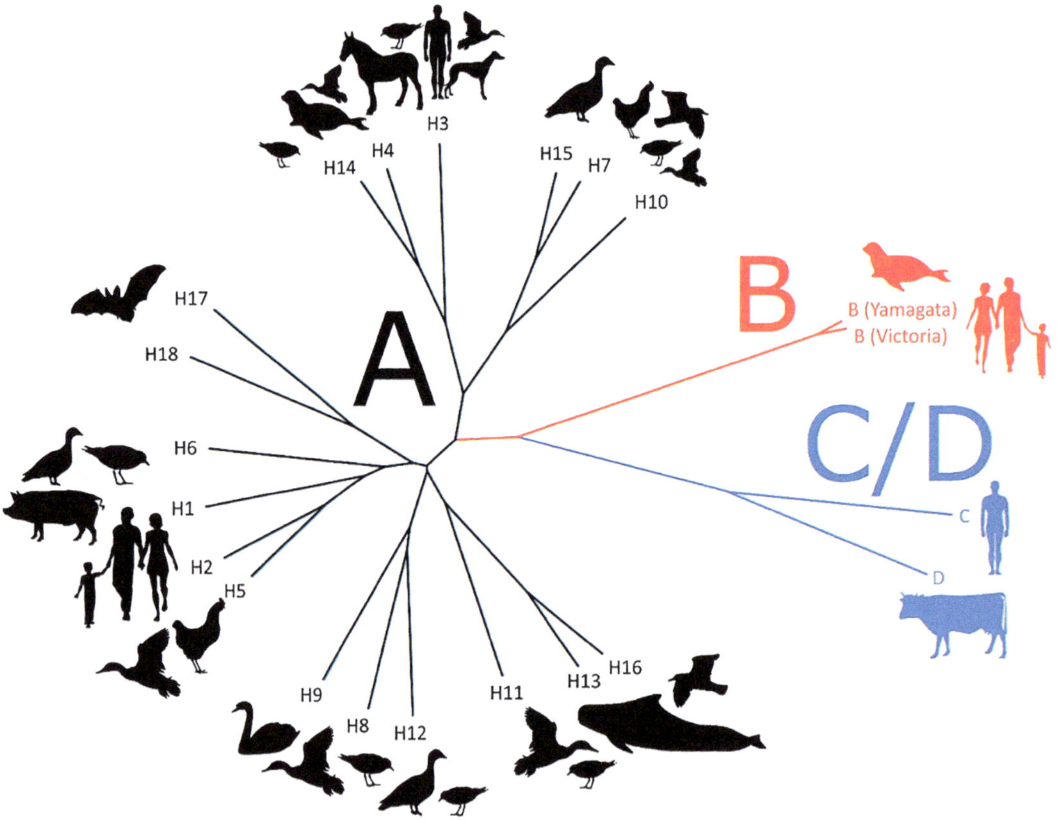

FIG. 2 **Phylogeny of influenza viruses and common species infected.** The phylogenic tree of human and animal influenza viruses demonstrates the four genera (A, B, C, and D) of the orthomyxovirus family. The viruses that may or may not cause infection in waterfowl and avian species may infect certain mammalian hosts. The A genus (*black*) includes viruses with 18 hemagglutinins of which 16 are displayed. The B genus (*red*) contains two lineages Yamagata and Victoria and infects humans and a few mammalian species. Lineage C (*blue*) causes mild disease in humans, and lineage D (*blue*) is primarily a pathogen in cattle and equine species. Used with permission from Hutchinson et al.[94]

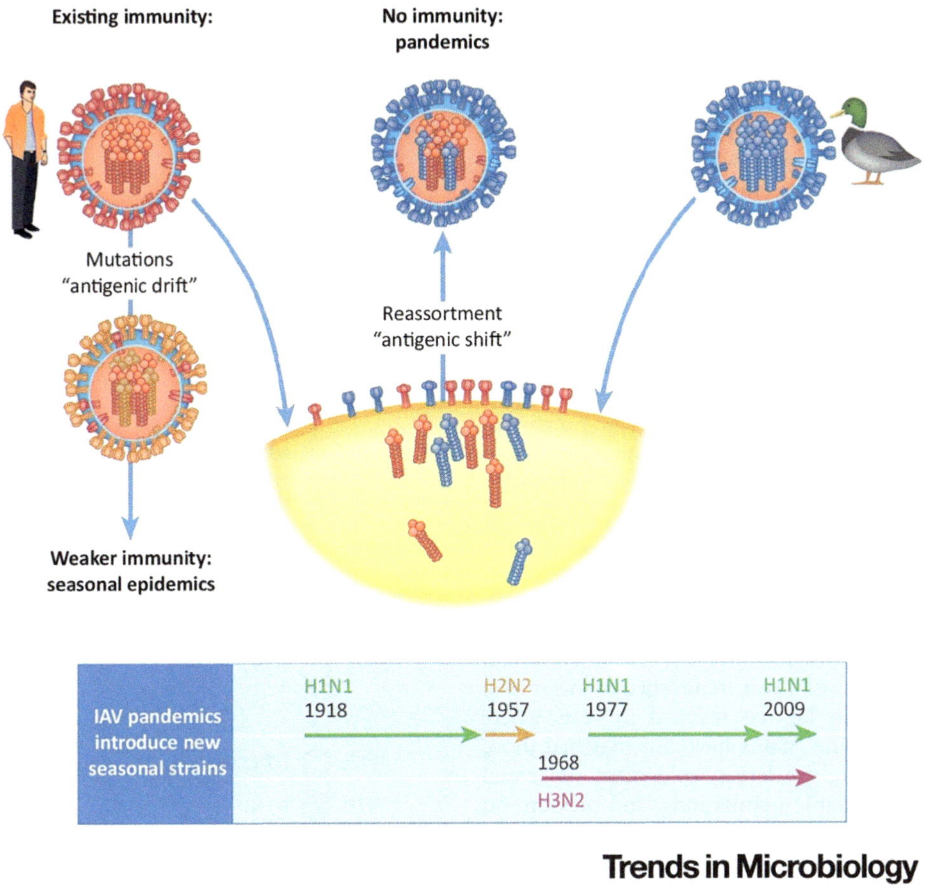

FIG. 3 **Mechanisms by which influenza A viruses mutate: antigenic "Drift" vs "Shift" and associated pandemics.** This figure demonstrates the role of different levels of herd immunity to influenza A strains in a population. Minor viral mutations (upper left) lead to antigenic shift (represented by the *downward arrow*), which leads to seasonal influenza A epidemics. When there is a lack of immunity in the population and changes of either influenza A viral hemagglutinin or neuraminidase with reassortment of the genome with new strains, usually from fowl and pigs, an antigenic shift occurs (*downward arrows* curving toward the center from the human and the duck, then producing the new IAV subtype emerging from this new host with the *upward arrow*), and because there is little immunity in the population, a pandemic occurs. Used with permission from Hutchinson et al.[94]

to this organism, it may simply reflect cross-reaction to prior influenza C infection.[94] Influenza A is subdivided into lineages and/or subtypes. Influenza A and B are subtyped based on two important glycoproteins, hemagglutinin and neuraminidase, abbreviated as HA and NA, respectively, and for influenza A, these are used to identify subtypes and further abbreviated to H and N (Fig. 3). Specifically, an influenza A strain that contains hemagglutinin type 1 and neuraminidase type 1 is labeled as H1N1. This nomenclature is not used for influenza B virus and has only two main divisions, called lineages, Victoria and Yamagata. Influenza C and D lack the HA and NA proteins entirely. The glycoproteins, HA and NA, like the spike protein of SARS-CoV-2, are important in viral pathogenicity and immunity. To date, 18 separate hemagglutinin and 11 separate neuraminidases have been identified. When the hemagglutinin or neuraminidase proteins change slightly, the term "antigenic drift" is used (Fig. 3). This slight variation is responsible for the annual seasonal outbreaks of influenza. However, influenza A can also exhibit "antigenic shift" where the hemagglutinin or the neuraminidase change is from N1 to N2 or H1 to H2, for example. In these cases, the human host does not recognize the "new" virions and does not have immunity.[94] Hence, only influenza A has the potential to cause pandemics, and such shifts led to viruses that had pandemic potential in a population with limited immunity, as occurred in the pandemics in 1918, 1957, 1968, and 2009 (Fig. 3). Unlike influenza B, which is a human pathogen and primarily infects children, the natural host of influenza A strains is waterfowl.Still, infection crosses into avian and mammalian species leading to outbreaks in these animals. Influenza A strains infecting humans are generally reassortments of avian and swine strains; more recently, strains of avian origin are emerging and can cause outbreaks and are of concern based on their potential to cause human pandemics (Fig. 4). These strains have now been associated with human infection cases ranging from asymptomatic infection to severe pneumonia with high fatality rates (Table 3).[94]

Viral drifts and changing immunity have led to recommendations for the annual influenza, which is designed to target the anticipated circulating strains. Because of the lead time required to manufacture vaccines and to vaccinate large populations, experts make predictions about which strains will be predominant and circulating almost a year in advance of the annual flu season.[95,96] This lag has resulted in years where the influenza vaccine strains have not matched those circulating, leading to larger epidemics, increased mortality in vulnerable populations, and pressure on healthcare systems. Hence the benefits of a universal flu vaccine are recognized[97] and such vaccines are under development.[98]

Unlike influenza B, which is a human pathogen and primarily infects children, waterfowl are the natural host of influenza A strains. It is rare to identify infection in waterfowl; however, the virus is transmitted to migratory birds and crosses into other avian and mammalian species leading to outbreaks in these animals.[44] Influenza A strains infecting humans evolve from reassortments of avian and swine strains in general. Although recently strains of pure avian origin have emerged, caused outbreaks, and have potential to cause human pandemics, they have had limited transmissibility. The pace at which influenza subtypes of concern have emerged has increased in recent decades, with a shift toward avian influenza subtypes.[44] New techniques have allowed researchers to determine the origins of these strains, to track their spread through migratory bird flyways, their ability to resort in mammals, and then their predilection to cause large outbreaks in settings with confined birds including farms and wet markets. Hence, surveillance for influenza viruses is complicated and must include avian, mammalian, and

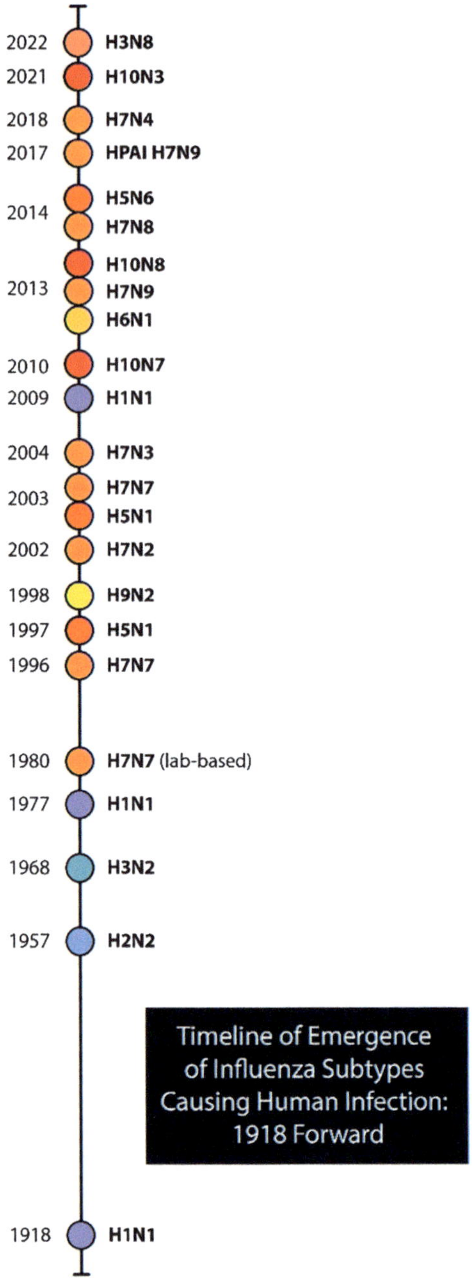

FIG. 4 **Timeline demonstrating the evolution of influenza A subtypes causing human infection: 1918 forward.** Timeline of influenza A subtypes that have evolved and major changes or "antigenic shifts" (*blue/purple* shading in subtypes indicates a resorted influenza virus) that have led to pandemics. The *red/orange/yellow* shading indicates a new avian subtype and the year reported. None of these viruses have led to human pandemics. Avian subtypes were identified more frequently after the mid-1990s.

human strains to best understand their pandemic potential and to develop rational mitigation approaches.

HUMAN CORONAVIRUSES (SEE CHAPTERS 10, 11, AND 12 FOR ADDITIONAL DETAILS)

The coronaviruses are positive-sense, single-stranded RNA-enveloped viruses, which are divided into four genera: Alpha, Beta, Gamma, and Delta (Fig. 5).[99,100] The Alpha coronaviruses circulate in mammals, whereas the delta and gamma coronaviruses mainly infect birds. The two main genera, Alpha-CoV and Beta-CoV, cause human infections, and in the Beta-CoV genera, there are three lineages: A, B, and C. Prior to the emergence of SARS-CoV-2, six human coronaviruses (HCoV) were described: HCoV-NL63, HCoV-229E, HCoV-OC43, and HCoV-HKU1. HCoV-NL63 and HCoV-229E are the oldest of the HCoV and are in the Alpha genera, while HCoV-OC43 and HCoV-HKU1 are Beta-CoV in lineage A. SARS-CoV-1, MERS-CoV, and SARS-CoV-2 are novel coronaviruses in the Beta-CoV genera with SARS-CoV-1 and SARS-CoV-2 in the B lineage and MERS-CoV in the C lineage. Among the HCoV, like SARS-CoV-1, SARS-CoV-2 overlaps with the SAR-CoV-1 genome by 80%. Within the genus beta-coronavirus, the subgenus sarbecovirus denotes those beta-coronaviruses related to the virus SARS-CoV-1.[101]

HCoV-NL63, HCoV-229E, HCoV-OC43, and HCoV-HKU1 are considered endemic and called the cold coronaviruses and usually cause mild upper respiratory tract infections or the common cold (Table 4). Each of the three novel coronaviruses has a wide spectrum of diseases from asymptomatic to severe forms leading to pneumonia, rapidly developing hypoxic respiratory failure, multiorgan involvement, and death. The viruses have high zoonotic potential, and bats are thought to be an important reservoir. For example, until recently the closest

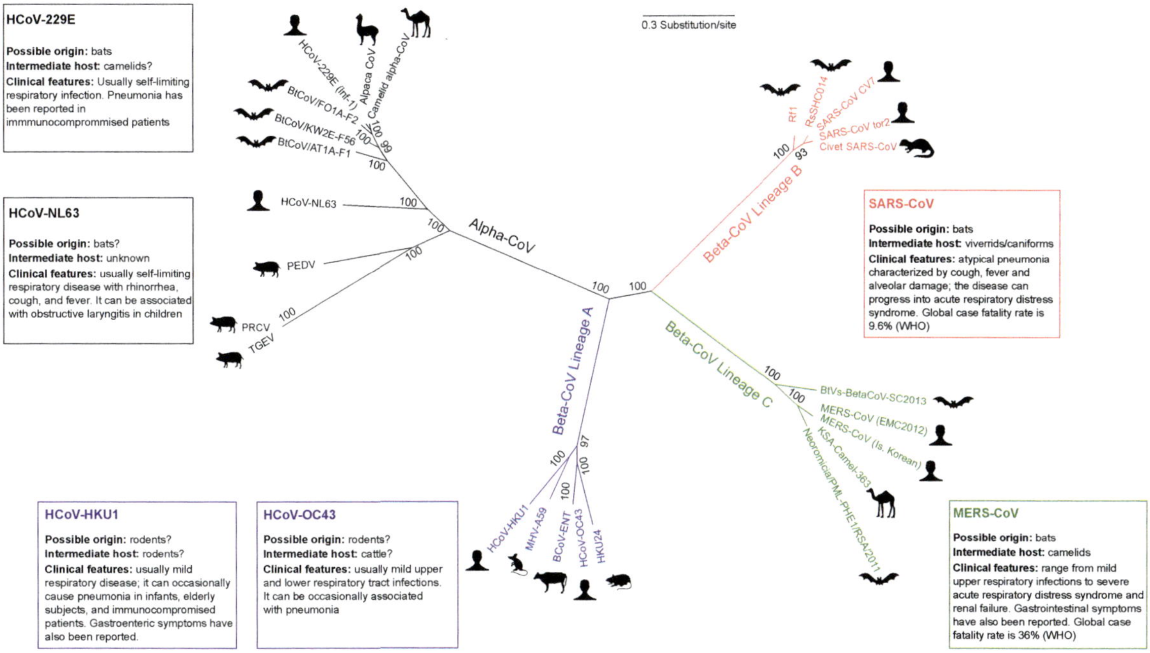

FIG. 5 **Phylogenic tree of known coronaviruses.** The phylogenic tree of human and animal coronaviruses with the four genera (Alpha, Beta, Gamma, and Delta). The delta and gamma lineages are not shown in this figure. The two main genera, Alpha-CoV and Beta-CoV, shown here include three of the four lineages of Beta-CoV: A (in *blue*), B (in *red*), and C (in *green*). The Alpha genus includes two viruses associated with human infection (common cold): HCoV-229E and HCoV-NL63. Otherwise, in the Alpha genus, the viruses are associated with various mammalian hosts. The beta corona genus contains four lineages: A, B, C, and D. All lineages cause infection in a variety of mammalian hosts. In lineage A, the viruses causing human infection (common cold) include OC43 and HKU1 viruses. Lineage B includes the novel coronaviruses associated with the human infections SARS-CoV-1 (SARS) and SARS-CoV-2 (COVID-19). Lineage C includes the virus associated with MERS-CoV (MERS). Used with permission from Forni et al.[100]

known virus to SARS-CoV-2 was the bat coronavirus RaTG13[102] (Fig. 5). Interestingly, in SARS and MERS, an intermediary host played an important role in transmission to humans, the palm civet cat in the case of SARS and the dromedary camel in the case of MERS.

Coronaviruses that have similar nonsegmented genomes are organized similarly yet can evolve rapidly with significant genetic diversity because of the high mutation rates. The first human coronavirus infection was identified in 1965, yet based on phylogenetic analyses, the viruses have existed for thousands of years. Examination of the RNA-dependent RNA polymerase genes suggests these viruses are ancient and emerged over 10,000 years ago, if not longer[100] ,although entered the human population about 1000 years ago.[103] HCoV-NL63, the oldest, emerged approximately 600 years BCE, and HCoV-229E in the 18th century. HCoV-OC43 appeared in the early 1990s and HCoV-HKU1 in the 1950s. None of these are associated with known pandemics, but some experts suggest that the intensity of influenza pandemics increased in the 1700s coinciding with the emergence of HCoV-229E, and the increased frequency of pandemics in the 19th century corresponds to HCoV-OC43 emerging.[103] The novel HCoV, SARS-CoV-1, MERS-CoV, and SARS-CoV-2 emerged in the past 20 years and are the causative agents of systemic acute respiratory syndrome (SARS), Middle Eastern Respiratory Syndrome (MERS), and COVID-19, all of which cause a spectrum of illness but are notable for the severe or even deadly disease they cause in some hosts.[104] They all have been associated with major outbreaks, namely, SARS in 2002, MERS in 2012, and COVID-19 in 2020 (Chapters 10–12, respectively), which infected many healthcare personnel, were transmitted in hospitals and healthcare settings, sometimes dramatically and associated with "super-spreading" events where a single individual or a group of individuals infected multiple other individuals and initiated propagative infection chains.

CONCLUSION

Entire libraries could be dedicated to outbreaks, pandemics, or even to agents of bioterrorism and respiratory viruses. The pathogens, old, new, or yet-to-emerge, can lead to significant harm to populations, disrupt healthcare systems and economies, and cause fear and associated social disruption. It is possible that with time, improved vaccination, or more robust mitigation measures, these agents will not have the impact they have previously had and that we will heed lessons learned, especially from COVID-19. However, after more than a century has passed since the 1918 influenza pandemic and three shots across the bow of human health with SARS-CoV-1, MERS-CoV, and most recently COVID-19, we would do well to not let those lessons fade, but rather to apply and solidify change so that the next great pandemic will be less devastating.

REFERENCES

1. CDC. Bioterrorism Agents/Diseases. CDC; 2018. https://www.cdc.gov/infection-control/hcp/isolation-precautions/appendix-a-table-3.html#cdc_generic_section_1-table-3.
2. Piret J, Boivin G. Pandemics throughout history. *Front Microbiol.* 2020;11, 631736. https://doi.org/10.3389/fmicb.2020.631736.
3. McCormick JB, Fisher-Hoch SP. Lassa Fever. Berlin Heidelberg: Springer; 2002:75–109.
4. Kapadia RK, Chauhan L, Piquet AL, Tyler KL, Pastula DM. An overview of eastern equine encephalitis (EEE). *Neurohospitalist.* 2020;10(3):161–162. https://doi.org/10.1177/1941874420905762.
5. Nikolay B, Salje H, Hossain MJ, et al. Transmission of Nipah virus — 14 years of investigations in Bangladesh. *N Engl J Med.* 2019;380(19):1804–1814. https://doi.org/10.1056/nejmoa1805376.
6. Bush LM, Perez MT. The Anthrax attacks 10 years later. *Ann Intern Med.* 2012;156(1_Part_1):41–44. https://doi.org/10.7326/0003-4819-155-12-201112200-00373.
7. Riedel S. Biological warfare and bioterrorism: a historical review. *Proc (Bayl Univ Med Cent).* 2004;17(4):400–406. https://doi.org/10.1080/08998280.2004.11928002.
8. Barras V, Greub G. History of biological warfare and bioterrorism. *Clin Microbiol Infect.* 2014;20(6):497–502. https://doi.org/10.1111/1469-0691.12706.
9. Trevisanato SI. The 'Hittite plague', an epidemic of tularemia and the first record of biological warfare. *Med Hypotheses.* 2007;69(6):1371–1374. https://doi.org/10.1016/j.mehy.2007.03.012.
10. Borio L, Inglesby T, Peters CJ, et al. Hemorrhagic fever viruses as biological WeaponsMedical and public health management. *JAMA.* 2002;287(18):2391–2405. https://doi.org/10.1001/jama.287.18.2391.
11. Takahashi H, Keim P, Kaufmann AF, et al. Bacillus anthracis incident, Kameido, Tokyo, 1993. *Emerg Infect Dis.* 2004;10(1):117–120. https://doi.org/10.3201/eid1001.030238.
12. Bossi P, Garin D, Guihot A, et al. Biological weapons. *Cell Mol Life Sci.* 2006;63(19):2196–2212. https://doi.org/10.1007/s00018-006-6308-z.
13. Meltzer MI, Damon I, LeDuc JW, Millar JD. Modeling potential responses to smallpox as a bioterrorist weapon. *Emerg Infect Dis.* 2001;7(6):959–969. https://doi.org/10.3201/eid0706.010607.
14. Egan JR, Hall IM, Leach S. Modeling inhalational tularemia: deliberate release and public health response. *Biosecur Bioterror.* 2011;9(4):331–343. https://doi.org/10.1089/bsp.2011.0004.
15. Rebmann T. APIC state-of-the-art report: the role of the infection preventionist in emergency management.

Am J Infect Control. 2009;37(4):271–281. https://doi.org/10.1016/j.ajic.2008.12.002.
16. ECDC. Best Practices in Ranking Emerging Infectious Disease Threats. ECDC; 2015:1–43.
17. Rotz LD, Khan AS, Lillibridge SR, Ostroff SM, Hughes JM. Public health assessment of potential biological terrorism agents. *Emerg Infect Dis.* 2002;8(2):225–230. https://doi.org/10.3201/eid0802.010164.
18. Khardori N. Potential agents of bioterrorism: historical perspective and an overview. In: *Bioterrorism Preparedness;* 2006:1–31.
19. Horton HH, Misrahi JJ, Matthews GW, Kocher PL. Critical biological agents: disease reporting as a tool for determining bioterrorism preparedness. *J Law Med Ethics.* 2002;30(2):262–266. https://doi.org/10.1111/j.1748-720X.2002.tb00392.x.
20. Anderson PD, Bokor G. Bioterrorism: pathogens as weapons. *J Pharm Pract.* 2012;25(5):521–529. https://doi.org/10.1177/0897190012456366.
21. Branda JA, Ruoff K. Bioterrorism. Clinical recognition and primary management. *Am J Clin Pathol.* 2002;117(Suppl):S116–S123. https://doi.org/10.1309/5g7e-f5hq-3g6e-vqmb.
22. Kman NE, Nelson RN. Infectious agents of bioterrorism: a review for emergency physicians. *Emerg Med Clin North Am.* 2008;26(2). https://doi.org/10.1016/j.emc.2008.01.006. 517–47, x-xi.
23. Adalja AA, Toner E, Inglesby TV. Clinical management of potential bioterrorism-related conditions. *N Engl J Med.* 2015;372(10):954–962. https://doi.org/10.1056/NEJMra1409755.
24. Darling RG, Catlett CL, Huebner KD, Jarrett DG. Threats in bioterrorism. I: CDC category a agents. *Emerg Med Clin North Am.* 2002;20(2):273–309. https://doi.org/10.1016/s0733-8627(02)00005-6.
25. Hamutyinei Dhliwayo T, Chonzi P, Madembo C, et al. Anthrax outbreak investigation in Tengwe, Mashonaland West Province, Zimbabwe, 2022. *PloS One.* 2022;17(12), e0278537. https://doi.org/10.1371/journal.pone.0278537.
26. Sirisanthana T, Brown AE. Anthrax of the gastrointestinal tract. *Emerg Infect Dis.* 2002;8(7):649–651. https://doi.org/10.3201/eid0807.020062.
27. Moran GJ, Talan DA, Abrahamian FM. Biological terrorism. *Infect Dis Clin North Am.* Mar 2008;22(1):145–187. vii https://doi.org/10.1016/j.idc.2007.12.003.
28. Rothman RE, Hsieh YH, Yang S. Communicable respiratory threats in the ED: tuberculosis, influenza, SARS, and other aerosolized infections. *Emerg Med Clin North Am.* 2006;24(4):989–1017. https://doi.org/10.1016/j.emc.2006.06.006.
29. Leffel EK, Reed DS. Marburg and Ebola viruses as aerosol threats. *Biosecur Bioterror.* 2004;2(3):186–191. https://doi.org/10.1089/bsp.2004.2.186.
30. Cenciarelli O, Gabbarini V, Pietropaoli S, et al. Viral bioterrorism: learning the lesson of Ebola virus in West Africa 2013-2015. *Virus Res.* Dec 2 2015;210:318–326. https://doi.org/10.1016/j.virusres.2015.09.002.
31. Franz DR, Jahrling PB, Friedlander AM, et al. Clinical recognition and Management of Patients Exposed to biological warfare agents. *JAMA.* 1997;278(5):399–411. https://doi.org/10.1001/jama.1997.03550050061035.
32. Bannister B. Viral haemorrhagic fevers imported into non-endemic countries: risk assessment and management. *Br Med Bull.* 2010;95(1):193–225. https://doi.org/10.1093/bmb/ldq022.
33. Ippolito G, Puro V, Heptonstall J. Hospital preparedness to bioterrorism and other infectious disease emergencies. *Cell Mol Life Sci.* 2006;63(19–20):2213–2222. https://doi.org/10.1007/s00018-006-6309-y.
34. Brosh-Nissimov T. Lassa fever: another threat from West Africa. *Disaster MilMed.* 2016;2:8. https://doi.org/10.1186/s40696-016-0018-3.
35. Zacks MA, Paessler S. Encephalitic alphaviruses. *Vet Microbiol.* 2010;140(3–4):281–286. https://doi.org/10.1016/j.vetmic.2009.08.023.
36. Kumar B, Manuja A, Gulati BR, Virmani N, Tripathi BN. Zoonotic viral diseases of equines and their impact on human and animal health. *Open Virol J.* 2018;12:80–98. https://doi.org/10.2174/1874357901812010080.
37. Kumar S. The global impact of pandemics on world economy and public health response. In: *Computational Approaches for Novel Therapeutic and Diagnostic Designing to Mitigate SARS-CoV-2 Infection;* 2022:43–48. https://doi.org/10.1016/B978-0-323-91172-6.00022-4.
38. Pangallo M, Aleta A, del Rio-Chanona RM, et al. The unequal effects of the health-economy trade-off during the COVID-19 pandemic. *Nat Hum Behav.* 2023;8:264–275. https://doi.org/10.1038/s41562-023-01747-x.
39. Baker RE, Mahmud AS, Miller IF, et al. Infectious disease in an era of global change. *Nat Rev Microbiol.* 2022;20(4):193–205. https://doi.org/10.1038/s41579-021-00639-z.
40. Bootsma MC, Ferguson NM. The effect of public health measures on the 1918 influenza pandemic in U.S. cities. *Proc Natl Acad Sci U S A.* 2007;104(18):7588–7593. https://doi.org/10.1073/pnas.0611071104.
41. Markel H, Lipman HB, Navarro JA, et al. Nonpharmaceutical interventions implemented by US cities during the 1918-1919 influenza pandemic. *JAMA.* 2007;298(6):644–654. https://doi.org/10.1001/jama.298.6.644.
42. Ferguson NM, Cummings DA, Fraser C, Cajka JC, Cooley PC, Burke DS. Strategies for mitigating an influenza pandemic. *Nature.* 2006;442(7101):448–452. https://doi.org/10.1038/nature04795.
43. Meltzer M, Cox N, Fukuda K. The economic impact of pandemic influenza in the United States: priorities for intervention. *Emerg Infect Dis.* 1999;5(5):659–671. https://stacks.cdc.gov/view/cdc/3265.
44. Wille M, Barr IG. Resurgence of avian influenza virus. *Science.* 2022;376(6592):459–460. https://doi.org/10.1126/science.abo1232.
45. CDC. Key Facts About Influenza (Flu); 2022. Updated Oct 24, 2022 https://www.cdc.gov/flu/about/keyfacts.html. Accessed 17 March 2023.

46. Pormohammad A, Ghorbani S, Khatami A, et al. Comparison of influenza type A and B with COVID-19: A global systematic review and meta-analysis on clinical, laboratory and radiographic findings. *Rev Med Virol.* 2021;31(3), e2179.
47. Lessler J, Reich NG, Brookmeyer R, Perl TM, Nelson KE, Cummings DA. Incubation periods of acute respiratory viral infections: a systematic review. *Lancet Infect Dis.* 2009;9(5):291–300.
48. Tran D, Vaudry W, Moore D, et al. Hospitalization for Influenza A Versus B. *Pediatrics.* 2016;138(3).
49. Sederdahl BK, Williams JV. Epidemiology and Clinical Characteristics of Influenza C Virus. *Viruses.* 2020;12(1).
50. Nesmith N, Williams JV, Johnson M, Zhu Y, Griffin M, Talbot HK. Sensitive Diagnostics Confirm That Influenza C is an Uncommon Cause of Medically Attended Respiratory Illness in Adults. *Clin Infect Dis.* 2017;65(6):1037–1039.
51. Liu R, Sheng Z, Huang C, Wang D, Li F. Influenza D virus. *Curr Opin Virol.* 2020;44:154–161.
52. Li YT, Linster M, Mendenhall IH, Su YCF, Smith GJD. Avian influenza viruses in humans: lessons from past outbreaks. *Br Med Bull.* 2019;132(1):81–95.
53. Beigel JH, Farrar J, Han AM, et al. Avian influenza A (H5N1) infection in humans. *N Engl J Med.* 2005;353(13):1374–1385.
54. Abdel-Ghafar AN, Chotpitayasunondh T, Gao Z, et al. Update on avian influenza A (H5N1) virus infection in humans. *N Engl J Med.* 2008;358(3):261–273.
55. WHO. Avian Influenza Weekly Update Number 887; 2023. Updated March 17 https://www.who.int/docs/default-source/wpro- - -documents/emergency/surveillance/avian-influenza/ai_20230203.pdf. Accessed 4 April 2023.
56. Huai Y, Xiang N, Zhou L, et al. Incubation period for human cases of avian influenza A (H5N1) infection, China. *Emerg Infect Dis.* 2008;14(11):1819–1821.
57. Agüero M, Monne I, Sánchez A, et al. Highly pathogenic influenza A(H5N1) viruses in farmed mink outbreak contain a disrupted second sialic acid binding site in neuraminidase, similar to human influenza A viruses. *Euro Surveill.* 2023;28(7):2300109. https://doi.org/10.2807/1560-7917.ES.2023.28.7.2300109. PMID:36795502. PMCID: PMC9936594.
58. Bi Y, Tan S, Yang Y, et al. Clinical and immunological characteristics of human infections with H5N6 avian influenza virus. *Clin Infect Dis.* 2019;68(7):1100–1109.
59. Zhu W, Li X, Dong J, et al. Epidemiologic, clinical, and genetic characteristics of human infections with influenza a(h5n6) viruses, China. *Emerg Infect Dis.* 2022;28(7):1332–1344.
60. Zhang R, Chen T, Ou X, et al. Clinical, epidemiological and virological characteristics of the first detected human case of avian influenza A(H5N6) virus. *Infect Genet Evol.* 2016;40:236–242.
61. Tweed SA, Skowronski DM, David ST, et al. Human illness from avian influenza H7N3, British Columbia. *Emerg Infect Dis.* 2004;10(12):2196–2199.
62. Ry D, van Beest HM, Meijer A, Koopmans M, de Jager CM. Human-to-human transmission of avian influenza A/H7N7, The Netherlands, 2003. *Euro Surveill.* 2005;10(12):3–4.
63. Koopmans M, Wilbrink B, Conyn M, et al. Transmission of H7N7 avian influenza A virus to human beings during a large outbreak in commercial poultry farms in the Netherlands. *Lancet.* 2004;363(9409):587–593.
64. To KK, Tsang AK, Chan JF, Cheng VC, Chen H, Yuen KY. Emergence in China of human disease due to avian influenza A(H10N8)- -cause for concern? *J Infect.* 2014;68(3):205–215.
65. Li Q, Zhou L, Zhou M, et al. Epidemiology of human infections with avian influenza A(H7N9) virus in China. *N Engl J Med.* 2014;370(6):520–532.
66. Zhou L, Li Q, Uyeki TM. Estimated Incubation Period and Serial Interval for Human-to-Human Influenza A(H7N9) Virus Transmission. *Emerg Infect Dis.* 2019;25(10):1982–1983.
67. Um S, Siegers JY, Sar B, et al. Human Infection with avian influenza A(H9N2) Virus, Cambodia, February 2021. *Emerg Infect Dis.* 2021;27(10):2742–2745.
68. Song W, Qin K. Human-infecting influenza A (H9N2) virus: A forgotten potential pandemic strain? *Zoonoses Public Health.* 2020;67(3):203–212.
69. Yang R, Sun H, Gao F, et al. Human infection of avian influenza A H3N8 virus and the viral origins: a descriptive study. *Lancet Microbe.* 2022;3(11):e824–e834.
70. Zhou J, Chen Y, Shao Z, et al. Continuing evolution and transmission of avian influenza A(H3N8) viruses is a potential threat to public health. *J Infect.* 2023;86(2):154–225.
71. CDC. Summary of Influenza Risk Assessment Tool (IRAT) Results; 2023. Updated Feb 23, 2023 https://www.cdc.gov/flu/pandemic-resources/monitoring/irat-virus-summaries.html. Accessed 20 March 2023.
72. Kwok KO, Tang A, Wei VWI, Park WH, Yeoh EK, Riley S. Epidemic models of contact tracing: systematic review of transmission studies of severe acute respiratory syndrome and middle east respiratory syndrome. *Comput Struct Biotechnol J.* 2019;17:186–194.
73. WHO. Coronavirus disease (COVID-19) Weekly Epidemiological Updates and Monthly Operational Updates; 2023. https://www.who.int/emergencies/diseases/novel-coronavirus-2019/situation-reports/. Accessed 23 February 2023.
74. SCMP Graphics. Coronavirus: The Disease. South China Morning Post; 2023. Covid-19 explained. Web site https://multimedia.scmp.com/infographics/news/china/article/3047038/wuhan-virus/index.html?fbclid=IwAR2DnQS17lqbSV2LtRoGbcJvV2EKeGak9L6ZMnnNanvstz6lM4MCT01dsJU. Accessed 23 February 2023.
75. Wu P, Hao X, Lau EHY, et al. Real-time tentative assessment of the epidemiological characteristics of novel coronavirus infections in Wuhan, China, as at 22 January 2020. *Eurosurveillance.* 2020;25(3).
76. Huang C, Wang Y, Li X, et al. Clinical features of patients infected with 2019 novel coronavirus in Wuhan, China. *Lancet.* 2020;395(10223):497–506.

CHAPTER 2

A Brief History of Biological Warfare and Bioterrorism☆

THEODORE J. CIESLAK • RACHEL E. LOOKADOO • MARK G. KORTEPETER
Departments of Epidemiology and of Environmental, Agricultural, and Occupational Health, University of Nebraska Medical Center, College of Public Health, Omaha, NE, United States

The "Amerithrax" incidents in the fall of 2001, occurring on the heels of the attacks of September 11 of that year, brought bioterrorism to the forefront of global consciousness. These incidents, involving the intentional distribution of anthrax-laden mail to US senators and media personalities via the postal system (batches of intentionally contaminated letters were mailed on September 18 and October 9), sickened 22 people, 11 of whom contracted inhalational anthrax, the deadliest form of the disease; five of them died. In response, the US government spent in excess of $41 billion decontaminating Senate office buildings and postal facilities and otherwise mitigating the consequences of the attacks.[1] A massive, sustained increase in biodefense spending remains in place to this day.[2] Media coverage of these events was extensive and dragged on as multiple potential perpetrators were identified and investigated, resulting in widespread ongoing fear among the populace. Seven years would elapse before the alleged perpetrator committed suicide before he could be arrested and charged. "Anthrax" and "bioterror" had become household words.

Despite these newfound fears, the diseases associated with bioterrorism date back to prehistoric times. In fact, some Biblical scholars postulate that the death of Egyptian cattle, described as the fifth plague of the *Book of Exodus*,[3] was caused by anthrax, as were the boils on Egyptians handling these cattle (the sixth plague of Exodus). Numerous examples of the intentional use of biological agents as weapons of war also date to prehistoric and early historic times, predating by many centuries our understanding of toxinology and germ theory. Melanesian tribesmen, from present-day Vanuatu, are believed to have employed arrows dipped into crab burrows, thus contaminating them with *Clostridium tetani*, the causative agent of tetanus.[4] Similarly, Scythian archers, during the Trojan War, dipped their arrows in decomposing cadavers, blood, feces, and snake venom. Hannibal is reported to have ordered his sailors to hurl clay pots filled with venomous snakes onto the decks of enemy ships.[5] Many similarly crude efforts involved attempts by armies to poison battlefield opponents by contaminating food and water sources with cadavers, animal carcasses, and excrement.[6,7]

In 1340, during the Hundred Years' War, the Duke of Normandy ordered that dead horses be catapulted into the besieged city of Thun l'Eveque in an apparent attempt to induce an outbreak of disease. Similarly, in 1346, Mongol forces catapulted the corpses of human plague victims over the walls of Caffa, now Feodosia in present-day Ukraine, leading to the flight of Genoese merchants trading within the besieged city. These merchants may have taken the disease back to Europe with them, thereby assisting in the spread of the plague's second global pandemic, the "Black Death," which killed as much as 60% of Europe's population. The Lithuanian Army also used the corpses of its own dead as weapons, mixing them with garbage and manure and catapulting them into the Bohemian city of Karlstein in 1422.[8] Similar attempts at the use of disease-laden cadavers would continue for another three centuries, through the Russian use, in 1710, of plague-infested corpses against the Swedes at Reval, in modern-day Estonia. Such crude efforts were interspersed with other, almost

☆The views expressed herein are those of the authors and do not necessarily reflect the position of the University of Nebraska or its component entities.

Viral Outbreaks, Biosecurity, and Preparing for Mass Casualty Infectious Diseases Events
https://doi.org/10.1016/B978-0-323-54841-0.00030-5

comical, ones, such as the offering, by the Spaniards to their French adversaries, of wine laced with the blood of leprosy patients[9] and the use, by the Polish Army, of arrows dipped in the saliva of rabid dogs.[10]

The discovery of bacteria by Leeuwenhoek in the 1670s paved the way for the development of "germ theory" by Pasteur and Koch in the 1860s and 1870s. Somewhat ironically, perhaps, the first disease proven, by Koch, to be caused by a microorganism was anthrax. With these discoveries came a burgeoning interest in state-sponsored biological warfare. Throughout the First World War, the Germans used anthrax and glanders to infect sheep, horses, mules, and reindeer destined as food sources or pack animals for Allied armies. They also made attempts to spread plague in Russia and cholera in Italy.[11]

In 1932, Major General Shiro Ishii, a Japanese Army physician working at the Tokyo Army Medical School, established an extensive but crude biological warfare research program in occupied Manchuria and began experimenting on prisoners of war and Manchurian civilians. His operation, known as Unit 731, intentionally infected human subjects with the causative agents of glanders, brucellosis, meningococcal meningitis, dysentery, cholera, anthrax, botulism, smallpox, and, perhaps, dozens of other infectious pathogens. Ishii's favored weapon, however, seems to have been plague, which he disseminated in a number of ways, including the dispersal, among the civilian population of Harbin and other Manchurian cities, of infected fleas. His "experiments" with this disease alone are estimated to have killed as many as 400,000 Manchurian civilians.[12] In fact, prior to the abrupt end of the war following the bombing of Hiroshima and Nagasaki, he had planned to target San Diego in a similar manner.[13]

In 1943, suspicious of Japanese and German efforts, President Franklin Roosevelt authorized the establishment of a secret offensive biological warfare research program at Camp Detrick, Maryland. Following the war and President Harry Truman's withdrawal of the United States from the Geneva Protocol, the modest program continued, experimenting with nonpathogenic surrogate agents such as *Bacillus globigii* and *Serratia marcensces*. The program studied approximately 30 different agents[14] and ultimately resulted in the development of seven antipersonnel and three anticrop weapons[15] (Table 1) before it was terminated by President Richard Nixon in 1969. Coincident with this termination, the US joined British efforts in crafting the Biological Weapons Convention (BWC), a supplement to the Geneva Protocol, which was promulgated in 1972 by the United States, Britain, and the Soviet Union. The BWC entered into force in 1975, with 187 nations ultimately becoming parties to the convention. The BWC prohibits the "development, production, stockpiling, acquisition, and retention" of biological weapons and mandates the destruction of existing arsenals. The history of biological warfare since the ratification of the BWC is, in some ways, a litany of violations of the convention.

TABLE 1
Antipersonnel and Antiagricultural Biological Weapons Declared Under the Auspices of the Biological Weapons Convention

United States	USSR	Iraq
Antipersonnel Agents		
Anthrax	Anthrax	Anthrax
Tularemia	Plague	Botulism
Brucellosis	Tularemia	
Q-Fever	Glanders	
VEE	Brucellosis	
Botulism	Q-Fever	
SEB	Smallpox	
	Marburg	
	VEE	
	Botulism	
	SEB	
Antiagricultural Agents		
Wheat Stem Rust		Camelpox[a]
Rye Stem Rust		
Rice Blast Spore		

VEE, Venezuelan equine encephalitis; *SEB*, staphylococcal enterotoxin B.
[a]It is uncertain whether Iraq intended Camelpox to serve as an antianimal weapon, a surrogate for smallpox, or both.

In 1971, the same year that the Soviet Union joined in efforts to craft the BWC, and 35 years after the nation saw its last case of smallpox, an outbreak involving ten cases of the disease occurred in the Aral Sea port of Aralsk.[16] A scientist working aboard a research vessel proved to be the index case, developing smallpox shortly after returning to Aralsk at the conclusion of her expedition. It is almost certainly no coincidence that the Aral Sea is home to Vozrozhdeniye ("Resurrection") Island, the Soviet Union's secretive biological weapons proving ground. In all likelihood, the release of the variola virus from the island provided the exposure to the scientist. Of particular concern was the form of smallpox seen among the secondary cases: seven immunized individuals survived, but only after developing clinical disease. The three unvaccinated individuals developed fatal hemorrhagic smallpox, historically a very rare form of the disease.[16]

As the Vozrozhdeniye incident did not become known to the West until 2002, it was the 1979 Sverdlovsk outbreak that brought Soviet violations of the BWC into the light of day. It was there that another accidental release occurred, this time from a factory producing anthrax for weaponization. As a result, at least 77 persons living downwind of the factory contracted anthrax, and at least 66 of these died.[17] Some sources suggest that the number of deaths may have been much higher.[18] The outbreak appears to have been the result of a mishap in the facility. A technician there had apparently removed a ventilation filter and neglected to replace it. The lapse resulted in the unfettered release of anthrax spores into the city over the course of several hours.

In 1978, Georgi Markov, a Bulgarian defector and dissident, was killed with a device fashioned from an umbrella used by the Bulgarian Secret Service and allegedly provided by the Soviet KGB to fire a ricin-laced pellet into his thigh.[19] A second Bulgarian dissident, Vladimir Kostov, was similarly attacked in Paris but survived. It was Kostov who, upon hearing of Markov's death, alerted authorities to his own previous umbrella attack, ultimately leading to the exhumation of Markov's remains and the discovery of the nature of his demise. According to disputed CIA accounts, as many as six assassinations may have been carried out in a similar manner, including that of an alleged Polish-American double agent, Boris Korczak, in Tyson's Corner, Virginia.[20]

Although these limited Cold War-era state-sponsored incidents were the result of weapons production and testing mishaps, terrorists and other revenge-minded individuals were also looking to employ biological agents. In 1981, an eco-terrorist group calling itself "Dark Harvest" sent packages of soil to British military and political authorities.[21] The soil, heavily contaminated with anthrax spores, was ostensibly collected from Gruinard Island off the Scottish coast, a British biological weapons testing ground during the Second World War. In 1986, British authorities began an extensive 4-year-long decontamination of the island, removing inches of topsoil and spraying 280 tons of formaldehyde over the remaining topography, finally returning Gruinard to its original owners in 1990.[22]

In 1984, 751 citizens of The Dalles, a small town in Oregon, were infected, nearly simultaneously, with *Salmonella typhimurium*. The outbreak, which could not be attributed to a single contaminated food item or preparer,[23] was eventually determined to have been intentional in nature, spread at local restaurant salad bars by members of the Rajneeshee cult in an apparent attempt to influence local elections by decreasing voter turnout. A prominent member of the cult was trained as a nurse practitioner and possessed a working knowledge of microbiology. A 1996 outbreak of disease due to *Shigella dysenteriae* among laboratory workers at St. Paul Medical Center in Dallas also involved a trained microbiology technician, who injected doughnuts with cultures of *Shigella dysenteriae* and left them in the laboratory's break room. E-mail messages sent by the perpetrator, inviting coworkers to consume the poisoned pastries, as well as surveillance video, led to her ultimate arrest and conviction.[24]

Sadly, medical professionals have played an outsized role in perpetrating biocrimes. From 1964 to 1966, a Japanese physician and bacteriologist intentionally infected over 200 people in multiple attacks employing *Salmonella typhi* and *Shigella dysenteriae*, killing at least four.[25] In 1970, a postgraduate parasitology student in Montreal, in a dispute with his roommates, poisoned them with ova of *Ascaris suum*, a porcine roundworm not normally associated with human pathology, demonstrating the fact that many obscure organisms can prove harmful under certain conditions and in adequate doses.[26] In 1995, a medical oncologist suffering from a severe psychiatric disorder attempted, on multiple occasions, to poison her cardiologist husband by serving him food laced with ricin, a biological toxin derived from castor beans. While he ultimately survived following multiple surgeries and a lengthy intensive care unit stay, the perpetrator reacted by burning down their house, killing two of their three children in the process.[27]

During the early days of the HIV epidemic, several disgruntled individuals attempted to use HIV-tainted blood for purposes of extortion or revenge, intentionally injecting rivals, ex-lovers, and even children (in an apparent attempt to avoid custody payments). A number of incidents involved the threatened or actual contamination of food and retail goods. Still, others involved infected persons acting as "human bombs," purposefully engaging in unprotected sex in the hopes of infecting partners.

In the early 1990s, a Japanese doomsday cult, Aum Shinrikyo, attempted, on multiple occasions, to release anthrax spores and botulinum toxin from the rooftop of a building adjacent to their Tokyo headquarters. They are also believed to have experimented with Q-fever and the spores of poisonous mushrooms, and members of the cult traveled to Zaire in 1993 in an effort to obtain Ebola virus samples.[28] When these attempts proved unsuccessful (they used a vaccine strain of anthrax and a *Clostridium botulinum* strain that produced little toxin), the cult released the nerve agent sarin in crowded residential neighborhoods and in the Tokyo subway system. The latter attack proved successful, resulting in the deaths of 12 and thousands injured. In addition, over 5000 "worried well" overloaded the metropolitan Tokyo healthcare system. Although Aum Shinrikyo is not known to have actually weaponized their Ebola samples, their interest in the virus raised questions regarding its possible use as an aerosolized biological weapon or in a "human bomb" scenario.[29]

A highly infectious virus with extremely high mortality rates, Ebola has the potential for widespread, devastating impact as an agent of bioterrorism. Ebola Virus Disease (EVD) is spread through direct contact with the bodily fluids of someone who is ill or has died from EVD. The average mortality rate for EVD has historically hovered around 50%, but without treatment, it can be as high as 90%.[30] For these reasons, the Centers for Disease Control and Prevention (CDC) has classified Ebola as a Category A agent, the highest level of bioterror threat.

Recent major outbreaks of EVD have occurred in West Africa from 2014 to 2016 and in the Democratic Republic of Congo (DRC) from 2018 to 2020. More recently, sporadic smaller outbreaks have occurred in the DRC, Uganda, and Guinea. With healthcare workers traveling across the globe to assist in these outbreaks, the virus has the potential for global spread. In the wake of these humanitarian response efforts, concerns have been raised that radicalized healthcare workers could potentially inoculate themselves with the Ebola virus and become carriers in order to deliberately infect additional populations.[31] Carriers could then travel to large cities and spread the virus by interacting with people in those locations, or they could potentially commit suicide in a crowded area, thus exposing more individuals to their bodily fluids. This type of "suicide-infector" bears similarities to some of the suicide bombing methods used by the Islamic State (ISIS).[32] There has been no concrete evidence that ISIS has attempted to use Ebola as a biological weapon; however, the potential threat has been enough to raise concerns among policymakers.

In 1998, the CDC responded to the increasing risk of bioterrorism by creating the Bioterrorism Preparedness and Response Program. This program has evolved and is now the CDC Office of Readiness and Response, which administers Public Health Emergency Preparedness (PHEP) cooperative agreements with 50 states, four cities, and eight US territories. These agreements make bioterrorism preparedness a priority for state and local health departments so that the nation as a whole is more prepared for any bioterror events. Additionally, the CDC created the Strategic National Stockpile (SNS), formerly known as the National Pharmaceutical Stockpile, which includes drugs, vaccines, and other medical supplies that may be needed in the event of a large-scale health emergency, such as a pandemic or bioterror attack. In 2018, oversight for the Strategic National Stockpile was transferred to the Administration for Strategic Preparedness and Response (ASPR), an operating agency of the Department of Health and Human Services.

Given the multitude of potential threat agents that might be utilized as biological weapons, health authorities have attempted to categorize them in order to assist in channeling resources to locations where they are most needed. This categorization is based on the understanding that it is impossible to predict the intentions of a terrorist or which organism(s) might be selected for use. Therefore, the focus has been on planning for those agents that might have the greatest effect on public health and medical infrastructure.[33] Criteria used to evaluate the agents included impact on public health (death/disability), potential for large-scale production and delivery over a population, transmission risk, public perception and potential for civil disorder, and public health preparedness needs, including stockpiling of treatments, antidotes, and diagnostic capacity. After bringing together a diverse panel representing the medical, public health, law enforcement, military, and intelligence communities, the CDC designated three levels of threat agents: A, B, and C, where Category A agents are those requiring the most intense preparation (Table 2). This categorization has stood the test of time. In fact, each of the six Category A agents has been used in a nefarious manner; we include, here, a brief summary of each of these agents and provide relevant examples (or allegations) of their intentional use.

Anthrax is a zoonotic infection of herbivores. The causative bacterium, *Bacillus anthracis*, usually infects the animals with its spore form while they graze. Anthrax causes different forms of disease in humans (cutaneous, gastrointestinal, and inhalational) based on the exposure route. Cutaneous disease is the most common manifestation worldwide, but the deadliest form of disease is inhalational. Inhalational anthrax

TABLE 2
CDC Categorization of Bioterror Threats

Category A	Category B	Category C
Anthrax	Brucellosis	*Emerging threats*
Botulism	Glanders	Nipah
Plague	Melioidosis	Hantaviruses
Smallpox	Psittacosis	
Tularemia	Q-Fever	
VHFs	Typhus	
	VEE, EEE, WEE	
	Ricin	
	SEB	
	Epsilon toxin[a]	
	Food & water threats	

VHF, viral hemorrhagic fever; *VEE*, Venezuelan equine encephalitis; *EEE*, Eastern equine encephalitis; *WEE*, Western equine encephalitis; *SEB*, staphylococcal enterotoxin B.
[a]Epsilon toxin of *Clostridium perfringens.*

is not a pneumonia, per se, but rather an infection of the lymphatic system, starting with lymph nodes in the mediastinum, leading to the classic form of the disease, a hemorrhagic mediastinitis, with pleural effusions (also potentially hemorrhagic), subsequent respiratory failure, sepsis, and sometimes hemorrhagic meningitis.

Anthrax is at the top of the potential bioweapon threat lists due to its ability to be produced in large quantities, its stable spore form (allowing the potential for airborne dissemination and long-term storage), and its severe, deadly disease, as was seen in the "Amerithrax" attacks. A large outbreak in Zimbabwe from 1978 to 1984 further demonstrated anthrax's potential for large-scale devastation. The outbreak led to more than 10,000 cases, likely facilitated by multiple factors, such as poor veterinary control, climate changes, and transmission among crowded populations by biting insects. There is also conjecture that deliberate spread was facilitated by allies of the Rhodesian government in a period of unrest with limited control measures, potentially to undermine rebel Zimbabwean ranchers by attempting to kill cattle.

Botulism is caused by any of eight known botulinum toxins, which are produced by species of *Clostridium botulinum*, an anaerobic soil organism. With a dose of 0.7–0.9 μg that can kill approximately 50% of exposed adults (LD_{50}), botulinum toxins are the most potent known neurologic toxins by weight, and exposure to them leads to the inhibition of acetylcholine release at presynaptic vesicles, leading to a descending flaccid paralysis. Their extreme potency makes botulinum toxins attractive bioweapons. Victims may develop cranial nerve deficits, manifested by blurred vision, difficulty swallowing, and difficulty speaking (classically the "4Ds: diplopia, dysarthria, dysphagia, dysphonia"). Other symptoms can also occur, including drooping eyelids, inability to hold the head up, and upper and lower extremity weakness. Patients may die from the inability to manage their oral secretions or suffocation caused by diaphragm paralysis. Studies have demonstrated that botulinum toxins would not likely be effective for wide area dissemination; however, they could be effective with more limited, targeted release on individuals as a weapon of assassination through contaminating food, water, injection, or aerosol release close to the intended victim(s). A potential example of such use is Reinhardt Heydrich, Gestapo chief for Adolf Hitler, who was assassinated under mysterious circumstances. He died shortly after being injured by an explosive device while riding in a vehicle. Botulism has been conjectured as the cause, due to his rapid demise after apparent improvement, from botulinum toxin prepared by the British and delivered during the explosion.[34]

Plague remains one of the longstanding infectious diseases feared by the public, based on known historical devastation. Plague is caused by *Yersinia pestis*, a Gram-negative bacterium, which remains endemic in pockets around the world, including the southern and western parts of the United States. The combination of the fear it engenders, the highly lethal illness it causes, and the ability to aerosolize the agent accounts for its consideration as a potential biological weapon threat. The organism causes severe and highly fatal illness with three primary manifestations: bubonic, septicemic, and pneumonic. Fleas are the vectors that spread bubonic plague, which starts out with severe and painful lymphadenitis (a bubo) but can lead to primary or secondary septicemia. Most feared is pneumonic plague, which can transmit person-to-person, especially in close quarters. Plague is readily treated with antibiotics; however, it can easily be misconstrued for other types of infections, and the treatment window is narrow, such that if the diagnosis is missed, it can be fatal. The Panday plague case provides an example of its purported use as a weapon. Two brothers in India in the early 1930s had an increasingly tense dispute over how to manage their inheritance. The death of the younger Panday by plague after a suspicious injection led to his older brother's conviction for plotting the murder.[35]

Throughout history, smallpox has led to more human illness than any other infectious disease. Caused by the *Variola major* virus, smallpox causes a severe, deep-seated, widely disseminated pustular rash that is more prominent on the face and distal extremities, which has been termed a "centrifugal" rash. The density of the lesions is associated with the severity of illness (more dense = more severe), but average fatality rates were around 30%. The most severe forms, flat type and hemorrhagic, where the lesions never reach their typical forms, had fatality rates near 100%. Survivors were frequently devastated by blindness, disfiguring scars, and bony abnormalities, the latter typically in children. The worldwide successful effort to eradicate smallpox was one of the greatest public health triumphs; however, when vaccinations against this devastating disease were discontinued, it unknowingly rekindled the potential for smallpox to be used as a weapon. Several aspects make smallpox potentially attractive as a bioweapon, including stability in the environment, horrific skin lesions, and potential for transmission from person to person. Having a highly effective vaccine could be viewed positively or negatively depending on the perpetrator. The ability to protect oneself or one's forces could be highly attractive for a perpetrator intent on releasing it on an unsuspecting population. One often-noted example of use in the war occurred during the French and Indian War.[36] British General Sir Jeffrey Amherst proposed to give blankets and handkerchiefs contaminated by smallpox victims under the guise of "gifts" to unsuspecting Native Americans sympathetic to the French. This weapon of opportunity may have led to subsequent outbreaks of smallpox among these susceptible populations.

Tularemia is perhaps the least recognized or appreciated among the Category A threat agents. The causative agent, *Francisella tularensis*, leads to clinical manifestations similar to those of plague, including cutaneous, oropharyngeal, and ocular illnesses, as well as systemic (typhoidal) and pneumonic diseases. Tularemia causes less severe illness than plague (hence it has been called "plague minor") with lower case fatality rates; however, typhoidal and pneumonic tularemia can still have fatality rates of up to 35% if untreated. Features that make tularemia a potential biological weapon include its severity, ability to be grown to large quantities, environmental stability for large area coverage, and a very low infectious dose (<50 organisms). Tularemia often occurs during periods when public health infrastructure has been disrupted, such as in the wake of conflict. Accusations of its use as a weapon have therefore been raised during past wars. A large outbreak associated with reports of thousands of tularemia cases among Soviet and German forces during the WWII battle of Stalingrad led to speculation that the outbreak could have been spread intentionally by the Soviets. Recently, the outbreak was deemed to be more likely due to natural means, and the accusations of intentional use were never substantiated.[37]

Four families of single-stranded RNA viruses cause the syndrome known as viral hemorrhagic fever: Arenaviruses, Bunyaviruses, Filoviruses, and Flaviviruses. Among these, Arenaviruses and Filoviruses are considered potential biological weapon threats. The viruses occur in nature among rodents and bats but differ in the means of human exposure and in their ecologies and epidemiology. The clinical illnesses they cause vary wildly in severity and case fatality but generally involve high fever, prostration, gastrointestinal illness (vomiting, diarrhea, anorexia), and numerous other constitutional symptoms. Although the syndrome name includes the term "hemorrhagic," a minority of patients develop bleeding, and if they do, it is generally oozing from venipuncture sites or from the gums or into the subconjunctiva. If frank hemorrhage occurs, the source is typically in the gastrointestinal tract. Loss of significant amounts of fluid likely contributes significantly to shock and multiorgan failure. These viruses are considered potential bioweapons due to the severity of the disease they cause, their potential for person-to-person spread to close contacts, and the fear they may engender in a population; however, they lack some of the properties of other threats, including stability in aerosol or ease of production. Although there has been some recent progress with Ebola, few have licensed countermeasures for treatment or prevention.

CONCLUSION

Over time, public health authorities have developed methods to reduce casualties and fatalities from viral hemorrhagic fever outbreaks through a combination of early detection, rapid diagnostics, case finding, triage, and the management of patients in controlled care environments (Ebola treatment units) with appropriate infection control measures to reduce spread. Despite the implementation of such methods, when the 2014–16 Ebola outbreak in West Africa began, there were significant new challenges related to a mobile population, cross-border movement, and population resistance to methods instituted to disrupt transmission in an environment where the healthcare system had been severely disrupted by war.

The 2018–20 Ebola outbreak in the eastern DRC brought additional unanticipated challenges,[38] despite the experience gained from the West African epidemic. There was ongoing conflict in the region of the outbreak, with different armed rebel groups in opposition to the government and jockeying for power. Security challenges required parts of the country to be declared off-limits to outbreak responders due to the risk of personal harm, and Ebola treatment units periodically came under attack, leading to temporary disruption of community operations in order to protect healthcare workers. The attacks on the treatment units were unprecedented and significantly hampered the ability to gain control of viral spread.

The activities of targeting Ebola treatment units and aid workers in the DRC that thwarted the response efforts may differ from an intentional attack with a bioweapon, such as the spreading of anthrax in the mail in 2001; however, both actions achieve the same effect, potentially leading to mistrust of the healthcare authorities, sowing disinformation, and ultimately, facilitating the spread of infection. In the end, the objective and result may be to influence policy or further a political agenda. With this view in mind, one might consider the kinds of actions used against Ebola responders in the DRC as acts of bioterrorism. With our eyes on future threats, it is useful to consider the myriad potential ways a perpetrator might select to further disease spread to advance whatever specific goals they are trying to achieve, whether they be political, religious, ideological, or military-related. The methods will change, so we need to be one step ahead and adapt our thinking and ability to recognize the threat in order to be adequately prepared to respond early and effectively, being mindful that the only constant is change.

REFERENCES

1. Miller JD. Postal anthrax aftermath: has biodefense spending made us safer? *Sci Am.* 2008. November 1.
2. Bush LM, Perez MT. The anthrax attacks 10 years later. *Ann Intern Med.* 2012;156:41–44.
3. Exodus 9:6.
4. Carus WS. A Short History of Biological Warfare; From Pre-History to the 21st Century. Government Printing Office; 2017.
5. Rothschild JH. Tomorrow's Weapons: Chemical and Biological. New York: McGraw-Hill; 1964.
6. Christopher GW, Cieslak TJ, Pavlin JL, Eitzen EM. Biological warfare: a historical perspective. *JAMA.* 1997;278:412–417.
7. Mayor A. Greek Fire, Poison Arrows, and Scorpion Bombs: Biological and Chemical Warfare in the Ancient World. Woodstock, NY: Overlook Duckworth; 2003.
8. Geissler E, van Courtland Moon JE. Biological and Toxin Weapons: Research, Development and Use From the Middle Ages to 1945. Oxford University Press; 1999.
9. Marty A. History of the development and use of biological weapons. *Clin Lab Med.* 2001;21:421–434.
10. Frischknecht F. The history of biological warfare: human experimentation, modern nightmares and lone madmen in the 20th century. *EMBO Rep.* 2003;4:S47–S52.
11. Hugh-Jones M. Wickham Steed and German biological warfare research. *Intell Natl Secur.* 1992;7:379–402.
12. Barenblatt D. A Plague Upon Humanity: The Secret Genocide of Axis Japan's Germ Warfare Operation. New York: Harper; 2004.
13. Working R. The trial of Unit 731. *Japan Times.* 2001;(June 5).
14. Roffey R, Tegnell A, Eigh F. Biological warfare in historical perspective. *Clin Microbiol Infect.* 2002;8:450–454.
15. U.S. Army Activity in the U.S. Biological Warfare Program. II; 1977. February 24.
16. Tucker JB, Zilinskas RA. The 1971 Smallpox Epidemic in Aralsk, Kazakhstan, and the Soviet Biological Warfare Program. Monterey, CA: Monterey Institute of International Studies; 2002.
17. Meselson M, Guillemin J, Hugh-Jones M, et al. The Sverdlovsk anthrax outbreak of 1979. *Science.* 1994;266:1202–1208.
18. Wampler R.A., Blanton T.S. Anthrax at Sverdlovsk. National Security Archive Electronic Briefing Book No. 61. 1979 (Accessed 4 December 2024). Available from: https://nsarchive2.gwu.edu/NSAEBB/NSAEBB61.
19. Papaloucas M, Papaloucas C, Stergioulas A. Ricin and the assassination of Georgi Markov. *Pak J Biol Sci.* 2008;11:2370–2371.
20. Douglas JD, Livingston NC. America the Vulnerable: the Threat of Chemical/Biological Warfare. Lanham, MD: Lexington Books; 1987:84–85.
21. Anonymous. Biological warfare: dark harvest. *Time.* 1981. November 9.
22. Johnson MP, Pye S, Allcock L. Dispersal mode and assessments of recovery on the shores of Gruinard, the 'anthrax island'. *Biodivers Conserv.* 2007;17:721–732.
23. Torok TJ, Tauxe RV, Wise RP, et al. A large community outbreak of Salmonellosis caused by intentional contamination of restaurant salad bars. *JAMA.* 1997;278:389–395.
24. Kolavic SA, Kimura A, Simons SL, Slutsker L, Barth S, Haley CE. An outbreak of Shigella dysenteriae type 2 among laboratory workers due to intentional food contamination. *JAMA.* 1996;278:396–398.
25. Anonymous. Deliberate spreading of typhoid in Japan. *Sci J.* 1966;2:11–12.
26. Phills JA, Harrold J, Whiteman GV, Perelmutter L. Pulmonary infiltrates, asthma and eosinophilia due to Ascaris suum infestation in man. *New Engl J Med.* 1972;286:965–970.
27. Carus WS. Bioterrorism and Biocrimes: The Illicit Use of Biological Agents Since 1900. Amsterdam: Fredonia Books; 2002.
28. Olson KB. Aum Shinrikyo: once and future threat? *Emerg Infect Dis.* 1999;5(4):513–516.
29. Maron DF. Weaponized Ebola—is it really a bioterror threat. *Sci Am.* 2014. September 25.

30. World Health Organization. Ebola Virus Disease; 2019. Retrieved from: https://www.who.int/news-room/fact-sheets/detail/ebola-virus-disease.
31. Aquino TL. Radicalized health care workers and the risk of ebola as a bioterror weapon. *J Bioterror Biodefens.* 2016;7(2). https://doi.org/10.4172/2157-2526.1000146.
32. Teckman AM. The bioterrorist threat of ebola in East Africa and implications for global health and security. *Glob Policy.* 2013;4(2).
33. Rotz LD, Khan AS, Lillibridge SR, Ostroff SM, Hughes JM. Public health assessment of potential biological terrorism agents. *Emerg Infect Dis.* 2002;8:225–230.
34. Middlebrook JL, Franz DR. Botulinum toxins. In: Sidell FR, Takafuji ET, Franz DR, eds. *Textbook of Military Medicine: Medical Aspects of Chemical and Biological Warfare.* Washington, DC: Borden Institute; 1997:65.
35. Calcutta High Court: Benoyendra Chandra Pandey and … vs Emperor on 10 January; 1936. Available at https://indiankanoon.org/doc/1586771/. Accessed 30 September 2019.
36. HB Jr G. Colonial Germ Warfare. https://www.history.org/foundation/journal/spring04/warfare.cfm. Accessed 30 September 2019.
37. Croddy E, Krcalova S. Tularemia, biological warfare, and the battle for Stalingrad (1942-1943). *Mil Med.* 2001;100:837–838.
38. Morrison JS. The Ebola Virus Is Winning in Eastern Democratic Republic of the Congo; 2019. September 12 https://www.csis.org/analysis/ebola-virus-winning-eastern-democratic=republic-congo.

CHAPTER 3

Anthrax: Ancient Surge and Current Biothreat

DAVID J. WEBER[a,b] • EMILY E. SICKBERT-BENNETT[a,b]
[a]Department of Hospital Epidemiology, University of North Carolina Hospitals, Chapel Hill, NC, United States • [b]Division of Infectious Diseases, UNC School of Medicine, Chapel Hill, NC, United States

HISTORY

The historical milestones in the recognition of anthrax as a human disease and the discovery of the causative agent, *Bacillus anthracis*, have been well described in review articles.[1–3] The origins of anthrax appear to date back to the establishment of agriculture in the Middle East around 5000 years BC. Since that time, descriptions of what is believed to be anthrax have appeared in ancient Greek, Latin, Hebrew, Chinese, and Hindu texts. Other key historical events have included the description of the disease in animals by Philibert Chabert in 1780, the first observation of anthrax under the microscope by Onesime Delefond in 1838, the cause of anthrax demonstrated by Louis Pasteur and Robert Koch in 1877, the development of the first attenuated anthrax vaccine by Pasteur in 1884, the development of a new vaccine for livestock by Sterne in 1937, the initiation of penicillin therapy in 1944, and the development of alternative antibiotic therapy (e.g., ciprofloxacin) in the 1990s. The history of anthrax as a bioweapon is described later. Given that anthrax may be used as a biothreat, local public health authorities should be notified immediately of any suspected or proven case of anthrax.

The current microbiology, pathogenesis, epidemiology, and clinical features of anthrax have been well described in several review articles.[2,4–12] The clinical presentations of anthrax in children have also been reviewed.[13] The key features of anthrax are described in Table 1.

MICROBIOLOGY

Bacillus anthracis is part of the *B. cereus* group of bacilli.[14] It is a large (1.0 to 1.5 μm by 3.0 to 10.0 μm), spore-forming, Gram-positive rod-shaped bacillus.[14] It is aerobic or facultatively anaerobic. Unlike other *Bacillus* spp. It is nonmotile, nonhemolytic on sheep blood agar, and grows readily at 37 °C. In vitro *B. anthracis* grows as long chains, but in patients, it appears as a single organism or in short chains of two or three bacilli. Colonies are 2 to 5 mm in diameter after 16 to 18 h of incubation, are flat or slightly convex, are irregularly round, are gray to white, and have a "ground glass" appearance. When nutrients are exhausted, *B. anthracis* forms spores. Spores do not form in patient tissues unless the infected body fluids are exposed to ambient air. Spores will germinate when exposed to a nutrient-rich environment, such as blood or tissues of an animal or human.

Bacillus cereus biovar *anthracis* is an emerging bacterium closely related to *B. anthracis* that was first identified as pathogen of chimpanzees and gorillas in 2001 and 2004–05 in Cote d'Ivoire and Cameroon.[15] *B. cereus* biovar *anthracis* exhibits chromosomal characteristics associated with *B. cereus* and contains two virulence plasmids almost identical to those in *B. anthracis.*[15,16] *B. cereus* biovar *anthracis* is widely distributed in Africa and appears to be capable of causing an anthrax-like illness in wildlife and livestock.[15,17] Recently, assays have been developed that allow differentiation of *B. anthracis* and *B. cereus* biovar *anthracis.*[17] *B. cereus* biovar *anthracis* has been included in the list of United States select agents since 2016. While no human infections with *B. cereus* biovar *anthracis* have been reported, antibodies against *B. cereus* biovar *anthracis*-specific antigen pXO2-60 have been detected in selected African populations.[18]

EPIDEMIOLOGY

B. anthracis, the causative agent of anthrax, is primarily a worldwide epizootic or enzootic disease of herbivores (e.g., cattle, goats, and sheep) that acquire the disease

Viral Outbreaks, Biosecurity, and Preparing for Mass Casualty Infectious Diseases Events
https://doi.org/10.1016/B978-0-323-54841-0.00021-4

TABLE 1
At a Glance: Anthrax Caused by *Bacillus anthracis*

Key Features		Clinical Correlation
Microbiology	Aerobic spore-forming Gram-positive bacillus	Spores may survive in the environment for years. Virulent pathogen with a high mortality despite treatment: uncomplicated cutaneous anthrax, <2%; inhalation, ~45%; gastrointestinal, ≥40%; and injection, ~28%. Meningitis is nearly always fatal
Epidemiologyand ecology	Worldwide. Reservoir of *B. anthracis* is the soil. Source of human infection is contaminated soil or water, or infected animals (usually herbivores). Rare cases of human-to-human transmission	Anthrax is an important biothreat. All cases should be reported to local public health and federal authorities
Clinical presentation	Clinical presentation depends on mechanism of infection: inhalation, contact, ingestion, or injection of spores or contaminated products (e.g., food, water, animal products, drugs)	Inhalation leads to hemorrhagic mediastinitis followed by dissemination (bacteremia); contact with nonintact skin (or via invasion of hair follicles) leads to cutaneous anthrax (eschar); ingestion may lead to hemorrhagic adenitis, ascites, and septicemia; direct injection (usually due to intravenous drug abuse) leads to bacteremia
Diagnosis	Culture of skin, blood, ascitic fluid, cerebrospinal fluid. Supportive laboratory evidence consists of positive PCR, IHC staining of tissues, and an antiprotective antigen (PA) immunoglobulin (IgG) detected by enzyme-linked immunosorbent assay (ELISA)	Inhalation anthrax must be distinguished from community-acquired pneumonia and viral respiratory tract illnesses (key suggestive clinical finding is hemorrhagic mediastinitis). Cutaneous anthrax should be considered if the patient has an eschar (painless necrotic ulcer with black depressed crust, often accompanied by regional lymphadenopathy and lymphangitis). Gastrointestinal anthrax can present as oropharyngeal or gastrointestinal anthrax (characterized by abdominal pain, nausea, vomiting, and sometimes diarrhea). Meningeal anthrax presents with classic meningeal symptoms (headache, stiff neck); hemorrhagic meningitis is common
Treatment	Hospitalize patients with systemic anthrax. Prompt administration of antibiotics (see Table 4). In addition to antibacterial therapy, patients should be treated with an antitoxin (raxibacumab or anthrax immunoglobulin)	If anthrax is suspected, initial evaluation should consist of appropriate cultures and other diagnostic tests. Unless contraindicated, all patients with suspected systemic anthrax should have a lumbar puncture to exclude meningitis
Vaccination	Anthrax vaccine adsorbed (AVA) is FDA-approved and CDC-recommended for both pre- and postexposure therapy. It can be obtained from the CDC or local health departments	Preexposure anthrax vaccine is recommended for persons at risk for exposure to *B. anthracis* (e.g., laboratory workers). Postexposure prophylaxis should be offered to persons with documented or suspected exposure to aerosolized *B. anthracis*

from direct contact with contaminated soil.[2,5,7,19–21] However, all mammals, including humans, are susceptible. In the United States, endemic anthrax is a rare disease with only 11 nonoutbreak cases reported between 1989 and 2021 (provisional).[22] In 2003, the United States had 23 cases of anthrax as a result of an intentional release of *B. anthracis* (see later).

The ultimate reservoir of *B. anthracis* is the soil (especially soil with high calcium and pH>6.1), where under proper conditions spores may persist for decades.[20] Dormant spores are highly resistant to adverse environmental conditions, including heat, ultraviolet and ionizing radiation, pressure, and chemical agents, and may persist in the environment for years.[23–25] In a suitable environment, spores reestablish vegetative growth. Vegetative bacteria have poor survival outside of an animal or human host; colony counts decline to an undetectable level within 24 h following inoculation into water.

Classically, human anthrax was described as often a fatal bacterial infection that occurred when *Bacillus anthracis* endospores entered the body through abrasions in the skin (cutaneous anthrax), by inhalation (inhalation anthrax), or by ingestion (gastrointestinal anthrax).[4,5] More recently, a fourth syndrome has emerged that is characterized by severe soft tissue infection in injection drug users (injection anthrax).[9,26] The source of human anthrax is direct contact with infected animal products (e.g., wool, hides, bone) or soil, ingestion of contaminated meat, or inhalation of aerosolized endospores.

Of importance to preparedness and response to the intentional use of *B. anthracis* are rare mechanisms of transmission. First, anthrax ("woolsorter's disease") may be acquired from contaminated fomites. Anthrax has been acquired by playing drums made from contaminated skins including both cutaneous and inhalation anthrax,[27–30] using contaminated animal-hair shaving brushes,[28,31] and using contaminated yarn made from animal fibers.[28] Thus, during an intentional release of anthrax, first responders and emergency medical personnel must be aware that clothes contaminated with *B. anthracis* are capable of causing both cutaneous and inhalation anthrax in unprotected healthcare personnel. Second, laboratory-acquired anthrax has been reported.[32,33] Medical laboratories should follow recommended safety procedures to prevent disease among microbiology personnel (see later). Finally, direct human-to-human transmission of cutaneous anthrax has been reported when people have had direct, unprotected contact with cutaneous lesions of anthrax.[7,34]

CLINICAL FEATURES AND DIAGNOSIS

The clinical manifestations of anthrax depend on the mode of acquisition. Following initial infection, *B. anthracis* may spread via the bloodstream, resulting in sepsis and/or meningitis.[4] Cutaneous anthrax represents greater than 95% of naturally occurring anthrax. Cutaneous anthrax follows deposition of the organisms into the skin via contamination of previous cuts or abrasions.[35–38] The incubation period is generally between 1 and 7 days (range, 1–17 days). An initial pruritic macule or papule enlarges into a round ulcer by the second day. This develops into a painless, black eschar often with extensive local edema. In most cases, the eschar begins to resolve in about 10 days with complete resolution in 6 weeks. However, lymphangitis and painful lymphadenopathy may occur with associated systemic symptoms, and uncommonly cutaneous anthrax may be associated with toxemic shock.[36] Without antibiotic therapy, the mortality rate has been reported to be as high as 20%. With appropriate therapy, the mortality rate is under 1%.

Inhalation anthrax follows deposition of spore-bearing particles into alveolar spaces.[5,30,39–41] Spores are ingested by macrophages that are transported via the lymphatics to mediastinal lymph nodes, where germination occurs after a period of spore dormancy of viable and possibly extended duration. Once germination occurs, clinical symptoms follow rapidly. Replicating *B. anthracis* bacilli releases toxins that lead to hemorrhage, edema, and necrosis. The mortality of inhalation anthrax, even with antibiotic therapy, remains greater than 50%. Symptoms associated with inhalation anthrax commonly include fever and chills, sweats, fatigue, nonproductive cough, dyspnea, chest pain or pleuritic pain, and myalgias. Most patients demonstrate fever and tachycardia. Patients who present with atypical anthrax (nasal or nasopharyngeal, larynx or laryngopharyngeal, primary meningoencephalitis) present with less cough, less chest pain, or are less likely to have an abnormal lung examination than patients with typical inhalation disease.[42] Laboratory findings most commonly include a normal or slightly elevated white blood cell count, often with a left shift, elevated liver transaminases, and hypoxia. The classic radiographic finding of a widened mediastinum is found in approximately 70% of patients. Chest radiographs often demonstrate a pleural effusion and infiltrates or consolidation. The finding of mediastinal widening or pleural effusion on chest radiography is 100% sensitive for inhalation anthrax, 71.8% specific compared with community-acquired pneumonia, and 95.6% specific compared with influenza-like illness. A chest computed tomography (CT) scan is more sensitive for detection of anthrax-associated pulmonary disease than a standard chest radiograph.

Although gastrointestinal anthrax is uncommon, outbreaks continue to be reported from Africa and Asia following ingestion of insufficiently cooked meat.[43,44] The incubation period is 2–5 days. Two clinical forms of disease have been described: oral pharyngeal and abdominal. The oral pharyngeal form of anthrax is characterized by an oral or esophageal ulcer and the development of regional lymphadenopathy, edema, and sepsis. Disease in the lower gastrointestinal tract manifests as primary intestinal lesions, most commonly in the terminal ileum or cecum. Patients present with nausea, vomiting, and malaise that rapidly progresses to bloody diarrhea, development of an acute abdomen, or sepsis.

Since the past two decades, multiple cases of injection anthrax associated with intravenous drug use (principally heroin) have been reported with a case-fatality rate of ~35%.[9,26,45] Many of these cases have presented with severe soft tissue infection with substantial swelling or edema. Erythema and pain were not essential features at presentation, and none of the cases showed the typical eschar (i.e., a black-crusted painless lesion) of cutaneous anthrax.

Anthrax can be diagnosed using a combination of microbiology and pathology testing methods.[5,8,10,46] Specimens should be collected for any patient with symptoms compatible with anthrax, with or without a confirmed epidemiological link to a known or high-risk exposure. The gold standard method for diagnosing is culturing *B. anthracis* from clinical specimens. Ideally, clinical specimens should be collected prior to starting antibiotic therapy. Depending on the clinical syndrome, *B. anthracis* can be cultured from blood, skin lesion exudates, pleural fluid, cerebrospinal fluid, oropharyngeal swab, rectal swab, ascites fluid, and tissues from biopsy or autopsy.[46] In addition to culture, diagnostic techniques include PCR; histopathology, special stains, and immunohistochemistry of tissue biopsy specimens; serology of acute serum (test for anthrax lethal factor) or acute and convalescent serum; plasma (test for anthrax lethal factor).[46] The Centers for Disease Control and Prevention (CDC) provide guidance on which tests should be ordered depending on the clinical syndrome.[46] Testing is available from the CDC via the state health departments. Notify local public health authorities immediately of any suspected or proven case of anthrax.

DIFFERENTIAL DIAGNOSIS

Anthrax often presents a diagnostic dilemma, in part, because it is so rarely seen in developed countries. The differential diagnosis of anthrax has been well described in review articles.[4,6,7,11] The clinical syndromes, causative pathogens (if applicable), and clues for diagnosing anthrax are described in Table 2.

TREATMENT (SEE CHAPTER 19, TABLE 1 FOR ADDITIONAL INFORMATION)

In Vitro Susceptibility

Several caveats should be mentioned in evaluating the reports of the in vitro susceptibility of *B. anthracis* to antibiotics. First, multiple methods for determining the in vitro susceptibility have been used. The Clinical and Laboratory Standards Institute (CLSI) currently recommends that broth microdilution susceptibility testing be performed using cation-adjusted Mueller-Hinton broth (CAMHB) with incubation at 35 + 2 °C ambient air for 16 to 20 h.[47] Second, CLSI provides an

TABLE 2
Differential Diagnosis of Anthrax Clinical Presentations

Clinical Syndrome	Disease (Pathogen {If Applicable})	Diagnostic Clues for Anthrax
• Cutaneous	• Insect bite (e.g., spider) • Staphylococcal skin infection (*S. aureus*) • Erysipelas (*Streptococcus* spp.) • Ecthyma gangrenosum (*Pseudomonas aeruginosa*) • Rat-bite fever (*Streptobacillus moniliformis*, *Spirillum minor*) • Ulceroglandular tularemia (*Francisella tularensis*) • Rickettsialpox (*Rickettsia akari*) • Rickettsial disease with tache noire lesion • Glanders (*P. pseudomalllei*) • Bubonic plague (*Yersinia pestis*) • Cutaneous tuberculosis (*Mycobacterium tuberculosis*) • Leprosy (*M. laprae*) • Buruli ulcer (*M. ulcerans*) • Syphilitic chancre (*Treponema pallidum*) • Necrotizing soft tissue infection • Orf (*parapoxvirus*) • Clostridial infection (*Clostridium* spp.) • Cutaneous fungal infection (Rhizomucor) • Leishmaniasis (*Leshmania* spp.) • *Bacillus cereus*	• Occupational history • History of exposure to *B. anthracis* • Eschar with edema • Painless lesion • Absence of pus (unless secondarily infection) • Gram stain of lesion demonstrates Gram-positive bacillus

TABLE 2
Differential Diagnosis of Anthrax Clinical Presentations—cont'd

Clinical Syndrome	Disease (Pathogen {If Applicable})	Diagnostic Clues for Anthrax
• Injection (subcutaneous)	• Streptococcal cellulitis • Necrotizing fasciitis • Severe soft tissue infection • *Clostridium novyi* A infection • *Vibrio vulnificus* infection	• Injection drug user (especially heroin)
• Gastrointestinal	• Acute abdomen • Acute gastroenteritis • Necrotizing enterocolitis • Flare of inflammatory bowel disease • Typhoid (*Salmonella typhi*) • Paratyphoid (*Salmonella* spp.) • Intestinal tularemia (*F. tularensis*) • Peptic or duodenal ulcer	• History of contaminated meat ingestion • History of occupational or accidental exposure • Positive cultures for *B. anthracis* from blood, vomitus, or stool • Gram stain of ascitic fluid demonstrates Gram-positive bacilli
• Oropharyngeal	• Diphtheria (*Corynebacterium diphtheria*) • Complicated tonsillitis • Vincent angina • Ludwig angina • Parapharyngeal abscess	• Positive cultures for *B. anthracis* from blood, vomitus, or stool • Gram stain of abscess fluid demonstrates Gram-positive bacilli • Positive cultures for *B. anthracis* from blood or abscess
• Inhalation	• Acute viral pneumonia • Acute bacterial pneumonia • Acute mediastinitis • Pneumonic plague (*Y. pestis*) • Pneumonic tularemia (*F. tularemia*) • Histoplasmosis, fibrous mediastinitis (*Histoplasma capsulatum*) • Psittacosis (*Chlamydia psittaci*) • Q fever • Coccidioidomycosis (*Coccidioides immitis*) • *Bacillus cereus* • Ruptured aortic aneurysm • Silicosis • Sarcoidosis	• Widened mediastinum on chest radiograph, chest CT scan, or chest MRI • Gram stain of pleural fluid demonstrates Gram-positive bacilli • Positive culture of sputum, blood, or pleural fluid for *B. anthracis*
• Meningitis	• Viral or aseptic meningitis • Bacterial meningitis (e.g., *S. pneumoniae*) • Subarachnoid hemorrhage • Leaking brain abscess	• Gram stain of cerebral spinal fluid demonstrates Gram-positive bacilli • Positive culture of blood or cerebrospinal fluid for *B. anthracis*

Adapted from Dixon TC, et al. *New Engl J Med.* 1999;341:820; Doganay L, Welsby PD. *Postgrad Med J.* 2006;82:755; World Health Organization. *Anthrax in Humans and Animals*. 4th ed. 2008; Finke E-H, et al. *European J Microbiol and Immunol*. 2020;2:29–63.

interpretative standard (i.e., break points) only for the following agents: penicillin (agents considered susceptible to penicillin are considered susceptible to amoxicillin), tetracycline and doxycycline, and ciprofloxacin and levofloxacin.[47] Third, if MIC susceptibility testing using CLSI methods indicates that *B. anthracis* isolates are susceptible to penicillin, amoxicillin may still be considered for prophylactic use in children and pregnant women.[47]

Testing of clinical isolates of *B. anthracis* has revealed that strains are generally susceptible to first-generation cephalosporins, tetracyclines, quinolones, carbapenems,

TABLE 3
In Vitro Susceptibility of *B. anthracis* to Antimicrobials

Highly Active	Variable Activity	Often Resistant
Tetracyclines	Penicillins	2nd Generation Cephalosporins
• Tetracycline	Macrolides	• Cefuroxime
• Doxycycline[a]	• Erythromycin	• Cefamandole
Macrolides	• Azithromycin	3rd Generation Cephalosporins
• Clarithromycin	Clindamycin	• Cefotaxime
1st Generation Cephalosporins	Aminoglycosides	• Ceftazidime
• Cefazolin	• Gentamicin	• Ceftriaxone
• Cephalothin	• Netilmicin	4th Generation Cephalosporins
Carbapenems	• Amikacin	Cefepime
• Imipenem		Aztreonam
• Meropenem		Trimethoprim-sulfamethoxazole
Glycylcyclines		
• Tigecycline		
Quinolones		
• Ciprofloxacin[a]		
• Levofloxacin[a]		
• Moxifloxacin[a]		
• Ofloxacin		
Rifamycins		
• Rifampin		
Chloramphenicol		
Glycopeptides		
• Vancomycin		
• Dalbavancin		
• Oritavancin		

[a]Although fluoroquinolones are not generally recommended for routine first-line use in pregnant persons and children, multiple studies have found that fluoroquinolones are well tolerated the pediatric population.

clindamycin, chloramphenicol, and vancomycin (Table 3).[48–59] *B. anthracis* also appears to be susceptible to the newer antibiotics tigecycline, linezolid, dalbavancin, and oritavancin.[60–64] Most strains are susceptible to penicillin, but clinical strains may produce a β-lactamase (see later). Most strains are resistant to second- and third-generation cephalosporins, aztreonam, and trimethoprim-sulfamethoxazole. *B. anthracis* may possess genes coding for β-lactamases, and β-lactam resistance may emerge during therapy. For this reason, penicillin or amoxicillin should only be used after appropriate susceptibility testing and only if other agents are unavailable or unsuited for therapy.

ANTIBIOTIC THERAPY

Several caveats should be mentioned when treating anthrax. First, one should consider whether any patient with suspected anthrax may have been exposed via intentional release of *B. anthracis* and hence may have their clothing contaminated with *B. anthracis* spores (see in the following section for management). Second, all patients with suspected systemic anthrax (i.e., systemic symptoms; inhalation, gastrointestinal, injection, or meningeal anthrax) should be admitted to the hospital. Third, patients with suspected anthrax (especially systemic anthrax) should undergo appropriate diagnostic tests as detailed earlier. The key diagnostic methods include pretreatment blood cultures and other appropriate cultures. Fourth, unless contraindicated, all patients with suspected systemic anthrax should undergo a lumbar puncture to exclude meningitis. As noted earlier, local public health authorities should be notified immediately of any suspected or proven anthrax. Rapid diagnosis and early appropriate therapy are key to reducing the substantial mortality associated with anthrax.

A CDC-sponsored expert panel has provided guidance for antibiotic therapy of anthrax in adults.[65] Other publications provide excellent summaries of current treatment recommendations.[12,66] Recommended drugs, doses, and duration are summarized in Table 4. Recommendations are also available for treatment of children[67] and pregnant women.[68] In general, therapy for children is similar to adults, but antibiotics are dosed

TABLE 4
Empiric Treatment for Anthrax: Recommendations of the Centers for Disease Control and Prevention, 2023

Indication (by Syndrome, Pregnancy Status, and Age)	Preferred Therapy[a] (Listed Drugs Joined by "or" Are Considered Equivalent)
Empiric[b] postexposure prophylaxis for nonpregnant adults aged ≥18 years after exposure to *Bacillus anthracis*	Doxycycline OR Ciprofloxacin OR Levofloxacin; PCN-S only (Amoxicillin)[c]
Empiric[b] treatment regimens for nonpregnant adults aged ≥18 years with cutaneous anthrax without signs and symptoms of meningitis	Doxycycline OR Minocycline OR Ciprofloxacin OR Levofloxacin; PCN-S only (Amoxicillin OR Penicillin VK)[c]
Empiric[b] treatment regimens for nonpregnant adults aged ≥18 years with systemic[d] anthrax with or without meningitis[e]	Ciprofloxacin PLUS Meropenem Plus Minocycline
Empiric[b] postexposure prophylaxis for pregnant or lactating persons aged ≥18 years after exposure to *Bacillus anthracis*	Doxycycline OR Ciprofloxacin OR Levofloxacin; PCN-S only (Amoxicillin)[c]
Empiric[b] treatment regimens for pregnant or lactating persons aged ≥18 years with cutaneous anthrax without signs and symptoms of meningitis	Doxycycline OR Ciprofloxacin OR Levofloxacin; PCN-S only (Amoxicillin OR Penicillin VK)[c]
Empiric[b] treatment regimens for pregnant or lactating persons aged ≥18 years with systemic[d] anthrax with or without meningitis	Ciprofloxacin PLUS Meropenem Plus Doxycycline OR Omadacycline[f]
Empiric[b] postexposure prophylaxis for children aged ≥1 month to <18 years after exposure to *Bacillus anthracis*	Ciprofloxacin OR Doxycycline OR Levofloxacin; PCN-S only (Amoxicillin)[c]
Empiric[b] treatment regimens for children aged ≥1 month to <18 years with cutaneous anthrax without signs and symptoms of meningitis[e]	Ciprofloxacin OR Levofloxacin OR Doxycycline OR Minocycline; PCN-S only (Amoxicillin OR Penicillin VK)[c]
Empiric[b] treatment regimens for children aged ≥1 month to <18 years with systemic[d] anthrax with or without meningitis[e]	Ciprofloxacin PLUS Meropenem PLUS Linezolid OR Minocycline

PCN-S, penicillin-susceptible strains.
[a]See Ref.[65] for more details and dose, and for therapy for preterm and full term neonates 32–44 weeks' postmenstrual age (gestational age plus chronologic age).
[b]Definitive therapy should be directed by antibiotic susceptibility test results, when available.
[c]Dosing is via oral route.
[d]"Systemic" was defined as one or more of the following using cutoffs for adults aged ≥18 years: hyperthermia or hypothermia, tachycardia, tachypnea, hypotension, or neutrophilia or neutropenia.
[e]See Ref.[65] for clinical signs and symptoms of anthrax meningitis.
[f]Dosing via intravenous route.

by weight. Similarly, in general, antibiotic therapy for pregnant, postpartum, and lactating women is similar to the therapy recommended for nonpregnant adults. For pregnant, lactating, or postpartum women, ciprofloxacin is the therapy of choice. Other agents that cross the placenta may be used, including levofloxacin, amoxicillin, or penicillin (only for penicillin-susceptible strains).

ANTITOXIN THERAPY

The major virulence factors of *B. anthracis* are a poly-D glutamic acid capsule and a three-component protein exotoxin.[69] The three proteins of the exotoxin are protective antigen, lethal factor, and edema factor. Antitoxins directed against these proteins are important adjunctive therapy to antibiotics for inhalation anthrax.

Prior to the use of antibiotics to treat anthrax, antiserum of animal origin was successfully used to reduce the mortality of anthrax.[70] Currently, two antitoxins are available for use in the United States, raxibacumab and obiltoxaximab. Raxibacumab, which was approved for use by the US Food and Drug Administration (FDA) in 2012, is a human IgG1-gamma antibody directed against protective antigen.[71–73] Raxibacumab is administered as a single intravenous dose after premedication with diphenhydramine. The efficacy of raxibacumab has only been demonstrated in animals since it is not possible to perform such trials in humans given that inhalation anthrax is rare and has a high mortality. Dosing recommendations for raxibacumab have been provided.[74] Obiltoxaximab, which was approved for use by the US FDA in 2016, is also a monoclonal antibody directed against the protective antigen.[72,73,75] As with raxibacumab, all efficacy trials have been completed only in animals. It cannot be used to treat meningitis as it does not cross the blood-brain barrier. Both raxibacumab and obiltoxaximab are stored in the US Strategic National Stockpile for use by federal authorities in the event of an anthrax emergency. Antitoxins should be strongly considered for use along with appropriate antibiotics in patients with inhalation anthrax.[65]

Anthrax immunoglobulin (AIGIV) is derived from the plasma of persons who have been immunized with anthrax vaccine.[71] It is available from the CDC for the treatment of inhalation anthrax in combination with antibiotics. AIGIV has been studied both in animals and in small numbers of human volunteers.[76] Side effects included headache, nausea, and infusion site pain and swelling. AIGIV has been demonstrated to improve the survival of animals when combined with antibiotics. It has also been used to treat small numbers of persons with systemic anthrax (inhalation, gastrointestinal, or injection anthrax).

VACCINES AND PREEXPOSURE PROPHYLAXIS (SEE CHAPTER 20 FOR ADDITIONAL INFORMATION)

The first effective anthrax vaccines were developed in 1880 by William Greenfield and in 1881 by Louis Pasteur.[77] Immunization consisted of a primary inoculation of *B. anthracis* that was incubated at 42–43°C for 15–20 days (type 1 vaccine) and a second inoculation (type 2 vaccine) of a less attenuated *B. anthracis* that had been incubated at 42–43°C for 10–12 days. In 1939, Max Sterne developed a live, attenuated spore vaccine from an avirulent, strain of *B. anthracis*. The currently used veterinary vaccine in the United States is based on the *B. anthracis* Sterne $34F_2$ strain. The currently used vaccine for humans in the United States, anthrax vaccine absorbed (AVA), was licensed by the FDA in 1970 and reapproved by the FDA in 1985. AVA (TioThrax) is licensed for use in persons ages 18 to 65 years who are at high risk for exposure to *B. anthracis*. The dosage approved by the US FDA is 0.5 mL administered intramuscularly (IM) at 0, 1, and 6 months with boosters at 6 and 12 months after completion of the primary series and at 12-month intervals thereafter.[78] It is not approved for use in children or pregnant women. Evidence for the efficacy of the vaccine is derived from studies in animals, immunogenicity data for humans and other mammals, observational data in humans, and a controlled vaccine trial in humans.[77,79–81] The duration of protection after immunization is unknown. The Advisory Committee on Immunization Practices (ACIP) recommends preexposure use of the vaccine in some cases for populations at risk for occupational exposure as follows[77,78]: (1) Routine preexposure vaccination for persons who handle animals or animal products is recommended only for persons for whom previously discussed standards and restrictions are insufficient to prevent exposure to *B. anthracis* spores. (2) Routine vaccination of US veterinarians and animal husbandry technicians is not recommended because of the low incidence of animal anthrax cases in the United States. However, vaccination might be recommended for veterinarians and other persons considered to be at high risk for anthrax exposure if they handle potentially infected animals in research settings or in areas with a high incidence of enzootic anthrax cases. Preexposure vaccination is recommended for laboratorians at risk for repeated exposure to fully virulent *B. anthracis* spores, such as those who (a) work with high concentrations of spores with potential for aerosol production; (b) handle environmental samples that might contain powders and are associated with anthrax investigations; (c) routinely work with pure cultures of *B. anthracis*; (d) frequently work in spore-contaminated areas after a bioterrorism attack; or (e) work in other settings where repeated exposures to *B. anthracis* aerosols may occur. (3) Vaccination is recommended for persons who, as part of their occupation (i.e., researchers and remediation workers), might repeatedly enter areas contaminated with *B. anthracis* spores. (4) Emergency and other responders are not recommended to receive routine preevent anthrax vaccination because of the lack of a calculable risk assessment. However, responder units engaged in response activities that might lead to exposure to aerosolized *B. anthracis* spores may offer their workers voluntary preevent vaccination. For preexposure prophylaxis, five doses of the vaccine are administered (0.5 mL intramuscularly) at 0 weeks, 4 weeks, 6 months, 12 months, and 18 months, with annual boosters to main immunity.

ANTHRAX AS A BIOTHREAT

Response Planning (See Chapter 18, Case Study)

Planning for an intentional release of *B. anthracis* has been reviewed.[82–98] Key aspects of planning for an intentional release of *B. anthracis* are: (1) continued education of clinicians regarding the signs and symptoms of anthrax; (2) inclusion of anthrax in the differential diagnosis of appropriate clinical syndromes; (3) protocols for decontaminating potential victims of an anthrax attack prior to entering the hospital (i.e., "hot" and "cold" zones)[89]; (4) protocols for handling mass casualties (also necessary for responding to emerging disease outbreaks such as avian influenza); (5) protocols for obtaining appropriate clinical specimens to diagnosis anthrax (especially the identification to the species level of all sterile fluids with a positive culture for *Bacillus* spp.); (6) prompt notification of public health authorities for any known or suspected anthrax; (7) protocols for appropriate decontamination of environmental surfaces if contaminated with *B. anthracis* spores; and (8) knowledge of appropriate postexposure prophylaxis treatments (i.e., antibiotics and vaccine).

The clinical management of bioterrorism-related anthrax syndromes has been reviewed.[90] In addition to being able to recognize the clinical syndromes of anthrax, healthcare professionals should be aware of the potential clues of a bioterrorism attack. These were summarized by Khardori as follows: Epidemiological clues include (1) greater caseload than expected of a specific disease, (2) unusual clustering of disease for a specific geographic area, (3) disease occurrence outside of normal transmission season, (4) simultaneous outbreak of different infectious diseases, (5) disease outbreak in humans after recognition of disease in animals, (6) unexplained number of dead birds or animals, and (7) rapid emergence of genetically identical pathogens from different geographic areas. Medical clues include (1) unusual route of infection, (2) unusual age distribution or clinical presentation of a common disease, (3) more severe disease and higher mortality rate than expected, (4) unusual variants of organisms, (5) unusual antimicrobial susceptibility patterns, and (6) a single case of an uncommon disease (a single suspected or proven case of anthrax should lead a clinician to alert public health authorities).[91] For anthrax, infections following exposure to lower-than-expected numbers of spores also may suggest a weaponized strain.

REASONS *BACILLUS ANTHRACIS* REPRESENTS A SUBSTANTIAL THREAT AS A BIOWEAPON

Bacillus anthracis is listed by the Centers for Disease Control and Prevention (CDC) as a category A biothreat agent.[92,93] Category A agents are high-priority agents that pose a risk to national security because of the following: (1) such agents can be easily disseminated or transmitted from person to person; (2) result in high mortality rates and have the potential for major public health impact; (3) might cause public panic and social disruption; and (4) require special action for public health preparedness.[94] Anthrax was designated as the second highest-priority biothreat after smallpox because of the following characteristics (ranked from highest threat {+++} to lowest {0}): public health impact due to disease (++) and death (+++), potential for production and dissemination in quantities that would affect a large population (+++), public perception (+++), and special preparation (+++).[92] There are several important characteristics of *B. anthracis* that make it one of the most likely agents to be used as a bioweapon.[27,94] First, *Bacillus anthracis* spores are easily found in nature, and spores can be inexpensively produced in a laboratory. Second, anthrax spores are highly stable and can persist in the environment for a prolonged period of time. Third, spores can be released by adding powders, sprays, food, or water. Fourth, clinical anthrax is difficult to diagnose in the early phases of disease. Fifth, inhalation anthrax has a high mortality if not immediately recognized and appropriately treated. Finally, *Bacillus anthracis* has been previously used as a weapon. It has been estimated that the release of 50 kg of anthrax along a 2 km line upwind of a population center for 500,000 persons would have a downwind reach of >20 km, incapacitate 125,000 persons, and kill 95,000 persons.[95] Anthrax would have a substantially greater impact than the other biothreats evaluated (i.e., Rift Valley fever, tickborne encephalitis, typhus, brucellosis, Q fever, and tularemia). Further, the number of casualties from a 10 kg release of viable anthrax would kill many people as a Hiroshima-sized nuclear weapon.[96]

Two important features of *B. anthracis* infection that limit the impact of *B. anthracis* when used as a bioweapon are the large dose of natural spores required to cause inhalation anthrax (i.e., 8000 to 50,000 spores) and the fact that, as noted earlier, human-to-human transmission is very rare and limited only to cutaneous infection.[82]

LESSONS LEARNED FROM UNINTENTIONAL AND INTENTIONAL RELEASES

The history of anthrax as a bioweapon has been described in several reviews.[2,78,97,98] Lessons learned from these releases are summarized in Table 5. In January 1917, Baron Otto von Rosen, a Swedish/German/Finnish aristocrat, was apprehended in Karasjok, Finnmark, for suspected involvement in espionage and sabotage.[99] Sugar cubes found in his luggage were ultimately proven to contain *B. arthracis.*[100] The planned intentional use of *B. anthracis* remains unclear, but the likely goal was to disrupt the transport of merchandise by horses and reindeer.

TABLE 5
Lessons Learned From Unintentional and Intentional Releases of *Bacillus anthracis*

Baron Otto von Rosen, Karasjok, Finnmark, Norway (1917)

- *B. anthracis* could be used as a biothreat against animals
- *B. anthracis* could be incorporated into food for use as a bioweapon

Gruinard Island (1942–43)

- *B. anthracis* spores may persist and remain infectious in soil for decades
- Elimination of *B. anthracis* spores from contaminated soil is exceedingly difficult

Japanese Use of B. anthracis in Manchuria (World War II)

- Use of bioweapons, including *B. anthracis*, is capable of killing thousands of people

Release of B. anthracis Spores From a Military Facility in Sverdlovsk, Russia (1979)

- Production of *B. anthracis* spores for military purposes may infect local populations if unintentionally released
- Aerosol dissemination of *B. anthracis* spores may lead to human infection at distances ~4 km (and animals for a much longer distance)
- Aerosol dissemination of *B. anthracis* may cause both inhalation and cutaneous anthrax with a high mortality
- Human infection may occur for up to 6 weeks following aerosol dissemination of *B. anthracis* spores (provides rationale for US recommendations for 60 days of antibiotic postexposure prophylaxis after exposure to *B. anthracis* spores)

Intentional Contamination of Letter With B. anthracis in the United States (2001)

- Contamination of letters may lead to inhalation and cutaneous anthrax
- Contaminated letters may lead to widespread contamination of letter-processing facilities
- Letter-to-letter contamination likely led to indirect transmission of anthrax
- After an intentional release of *B. anthracis*, even one that leads to a small number of infections, thousands of persons might be recommended for postexposure antibiotic prophylaxis
- Many persons provided long-term postexposure antibiotic prophylaxis will develop adverse reactions to the therapy and discontinue therapy
- It is difficult to detect the person responsible for a presumed "lone wolf" attack

During World War II, trials *of B. anthracis* as a potential agent of biological warfare were carried out as part of a British, Canadian, and American research program on Gruinard Island off the west coast of Scotland.[100] Small bombs containing *B. anthracis* spores were suspended from a gantry and detonated, producing widespread contamination of the island's surface. These spores remained viable for decades.[101] Ultimately, the contaminated areas were decontaminated by spraying with a 5% solution of formaldehyde.[102,103] The island was declared safe in 1988 after a local farmer had grazed his flock of sheep on the island for several months with no ill effects.[102,103]

During World War II, Japanese scientists infected prisoners with several different biothreat pathogens, including *B. anthracis*.[98] This research allowed the Japanese army to conduct large-scale trials of biological weapons in Manchuria, which involved the use of bombs to spread pathogens, including *B. anthracis*, which contaminated reservoirs and wells.[2,98] It has been estimated that several thousand people died as a result of these attacks.

The 1979 unintentional release of *B. anthracis* spores from a military bacteriology laboratory in Sverdlovsk, Russia, led to a reported 96 cases of anthrax (79 inhalation anthrax and 17 cases of cutaneous infection), of which 64 resulted in death.[104,105] The onset of infection following release of spores (likely on 2 April) lasted for approximately 6 weeks (4 April to 18 May). Meselson and colleagues reported that the modal incubation period was 9–10 days with a range of 2 to 43 days. Most cases lived or worked in a narrow zone approximately 4 km long, extending from the military facility to the southern city limit. Of note, livestock died of anthrax in villages located along the extended axis of the same zone up to a distance of 50 km.

In 1981, a suspicious package was left on the grounds of a chemical defense establishment in England with an accompanying letter claiming that the package contained anthrax-contaminated soil from Gruinard Island.[2] Analysis of the soil confirmed the presence of *B. anthracis*.

In the mid-1980s, the Aum Shinrikyo cult in Japan began working with *B. anthracis*.[2] On at least three occasions, they released anthrax spores with the intention to cause human illness. However, the *B. anthracis* strain used by Aum Shinrikyo was genetically identical to the Sterne 34F2 strain, which was used in Japan to immunize animals against anthrax and did not cause any human disease.[106]

In 2001, the United States experienced an intentional release of *B. anthracis* via a contaminated letter mailed via the US Postal Service. The investigation by the CDC and other authorities was well described in a series of CDC publications, along with interim recommendations for management.[107–114] Subsequently, the CDC and others published additional reports detailing the mechanisms of anthrax acquisition,[115,116] outcomes of infected persons,[117] side effects of therapies recommended for postexposure prophylaxis (PEP),[118–120] and environmental decontamination methods.[121,122] Overall, 22 cases of anthrax resulted from this intentional release of *B. anthracis*: 11 cases of inhalational anthrax and 11 cases of cutaneous anthrax. The medical costs alone resulting from this release were approximately $177 million.[123] Unexpected features of this attack included the following: (1) the target was the news media; (2) the vehicle for dissemination of *B. anthracis* was mail via the US Postal Service; (3) the source of the *B. anthracis* strain was likely a US weaponized strain; (4) anthrax occurred in US postal workers exposed in main facilities due to widespread environmental contamination and aerosolization of spores; (5) anthrax infections resulted via letter-to-letter contamination; and (6) no person or group claimed responsibility for the attack. Of note, approximately 20% of persons taking PEP developed one or more side effects within 7 to 10 days after initiation of PEP, such as itching, breathing problems; swelling of face, neck, or throat; or seeking medical attention for any adverse event related to taking antibiotic PEP. A subsequent evaluation revealed that among those taking ciprofloxacin, 19% reported severe nausea, vomiting, diarrhea, or abdominal pain; 14 reported fainting, lightheadedness, or dizziness; 7% reported heartburn or acid reflux; and 6% reported rashes, hives, or itchy skin. Overall, 8% discontinued the medication. Persons on doxycycline also reported a high frequency of side effects.

INFECTION PREVENTION AND DECONTAMINATION (SEE CHAPTER 24 FOR ADDITIONAL DETAIL)

As noted earlier, a major concern with an intentional release of anthrax is that exposed patients will arrive at a healthcare facility with skin and/or clothes contaminated with *B. anthracis* spores. This could result in surface contamination of the healthcare facility and/or transmission to healthcare personnel (HCP), patients, or visitors via direct or indirect contact resulting in cutaneous anthrax or aerosolization resulting in inhalation anthrax. The CDC recommends that if there is a possibility of aerosolized powder, HCP should wear protective clothing and a respirator (N95 respirator or powered air purifying respirator).[124] The personnel protective equipment (PPE) recommended could include water-impermeable, chemical-resistant suits, although it was noted that this PPE could prevent evaporative cooling and contribute to dehydration and heat stress; face pieces might aggravate claustrophobia; respirator airflow resistance and the weight of self-contained breathing apparatuses (SCBAs) might aggravate respiratory and heart conditions; and PPE materials might contribute to skin problems.[125] Importantly, it has been shown with surrogate viruses that despite the use of PPE consisting of gloves, a standard isolation gown, and a mask plus a defined protocol for removing the PPE still results in contamination of underlying clothes and skin during removal >70% of the time.[126] Double gloving with the standard isolation gown reduces but does not eliminate contamination of underlying clothes and skin.[127] However, use of PPE is recommended when caring for patients with Ebola (hospital scrubs, Tyvek suit with thumb holes to prevent sliding up the wrist, long-sleeved fluid-resistant gown with thumb holes to prevent sliding up the wrist, 2 pairs of long gloves (covering the wrist completely), Tyvek hood, face shield, N95 respirator, and fluid-resistant boots), plus a defined doffing protocol, trained PPE monitor observing doffing process, and use of hypochlorite washing of gloves provided almost complete protection against contamination of underlying clothes or skin.[128,129] Decontamination of gloves and any potentially contaminated areas of the suit should be undertaken with a sporicidal agent prior to removal.

Only standard precautions are recommended for patients infected with anthrax.[124] However, since transmission through nonintact skin contact with draining lesions is possible, patients with large amounts of uncontained drainage should be managed with contact precautions.[124]

One of the most commonly used antiseptics for hand hygiene by HCP (i.e., alcohol and chlorhexidine gluconate) is not effective in eliminating *Bacillus atrophaeus* spores (a surrogate for *B. anthracis*) from contaminated hands.[130] Physical removal with soap (or chlorhexidine) and water will remove 1.5 to 2.0-$\log_{10}$ organisms. Chlorine-containing towels were also effective in removing 1.3 to 2.2-$\log_{10}$ organisms. Therefore, waterless alcohol antiseptics should not be used for hand hygiene in HCP or laboratory workers if contamination with *B. anthracis* spores is possible.

Spores, including that of *B. anthracis*, are resistant to many commonly used surface disinfectants, such as quaternary ammonium compounds.[131] For surface disinfection, an FDA-approved sporicidal agent such as sodium hypochlorite or aqueous chlorine diozide should be used.[131–134] For an enclosed contaminated area (e.g., emergency room, hospital room), gaseous chlorine dioxide could be used.[135]

The Clinical and Laboratory Standards Institute recommends the following biosafety precautions for clinical laboratories evaluating diagnostic cultures for *B. anthracis*: "Use biosafety level 2 (BSL-2) practices, containment equipment, and facilities for activities using clinical materials and diagnostic quantities of infectious cultures (see Chapter 17 for additional details). Use biosafety level 3 (BSL-3) practices, containment equipment and facilities for work involving production quantities or concentrations of cultures and for activities with a high potential for aerosol production. If BSL-2 or BSL-3 facilities are not available, forward isolates to a referral or public health laboratory with minimum BSL-2 facilities for susceptibility testing."[47] Additional details for BSL-2 and BSL-3 containment in clinical laboratories and research laboratories are available from the US Department of Health and Human Services.[136]

POSTEXPOSURE PROPHYLAXIS IN CASES OF MASS EXPOSURES (SEE CHAPTERS 15 AND 19 FOR ADDITIONAL DETAILS)

Postexposure antibiotic prophylaxis was widely used in the United States after the intentional release of *B. anthracis* via the US Postal Service in 2001. Currently, CDC and the World Health Organization (WHO) recommendations for PEP of exposed but nonsymptomatic persons would consist of an oral antibiotic for up to 60 days.[7,11,12,137] The currently recommended antibiotics are ciprofloxacin or doxycycline. The reason for this prolonged antibiotic course is that while anthrax spores typically take 1 to 6 days to be activated, spores can remain inside the body and can take up to 60 days before they are activated.

Anthrax vaccine absorbed (AVA) was approved by the FDA in 2015 for use after exposure to anthrax for persons ages 18 through 65 years.[138] AVA would be provided as a three-dose series over 4 weeks in addition to a prolonged course of antibiotics (Table 4). Use of the vaccine would be guided by public health authorities. As noted earlier, side effects are common with prolonged use of ciprofloxacin or doxycycline. In a review of 42 persons recommended to take antibiotic PEP after a laboratory incident, 74% of persons who initiated therapy did not complete either the recommended 60 days of antimicrobial therapy or the three-dose vaccine regimen. Among the 29 that discontinued the antimicrobial component of PEP, most (38%) individuals discontinued PEP because of their low perceived risk of infection, 31% discontinued PEP due to adverse events, and 10% cited both low-risk and adverse events as their reason for discontinuation.[139] Most adverse events included gastrointestinal complaints, and none required medical attention.

The most recent recommendations for PEP from the Advisory Committee on Immunization Practices (ACIP) recommend subcutaneous (SC) because SC results in higher antibody concentrations by week 4 than the intramuscular route.[140] For PEP, AVA is provided SC at 0, 2, and 4 weeks along with antibiotics for a prolonged period of time (Table 4a). Dose-sparing regimens could include full-strength doses at only 0 and 2–4 weeks or half-strength doses at 0, 14, and 28 days. All the dose-sparing regimens would stretch the current vaccine supply in case of shortages. Reducing the number of doses might improve patient's compliance. The 2 full-dose strategy will expand the existing vaccine supply by 50%, and the 3 half-dose strategy will expand the supply by 100%. Immediately after a wide-area aerosolized release of *B. anthracis* spores, the preferred dose-sparing PEP regimen might not be apparent until the size of the event is determined. Data suggests that all dose-sparing regimens provide high levels of protection by 2 weeks after the last dose.

ACIP recommends that in immunocompetent adults (e.g., healthy, nonpregnant adults aged 18–65 years), PEP-antibiotics (PEP-Abx) both for the licensed and dose-sparing PEP-vaccine (PEP-Vx) regimens can be discontinued 42 days after initiation of vaccine if AVA is administered on schedule for both the licensed and dose-sparing PEP-vaccine regimens (Table 4a). If the AVA series cannot be completed, then antimicrobial therapy should continue for 60 days. However, the second dose of AVA is critical for producing high antibody concentrations. To account for delays in initial vaccination that might occur because of the emergency situation, antimicrobial administration should be initiated as soon as possible and continued for 42 days after the first dose or 2 weeks after the last dose of the vaccine series, whichever comes last. No data on humans are available to suggest that PEP-antibiotics should be given for >60 days, which is the recommended duration for PEP-antibiotics when given without vaccine. Thus, PEP-antibiotics should not be given for >60 days, regardless of the timing of the last vaccine dose. The shortening of PEP-Abx duration from 60 to 42 days, or 2 weeks after the last dose of vaccine, applies to healthy adults aged 18–65 years. Persons with immunocompromising conditions that might interfere with their ability to develop an adequate immune response or populations for whom data on immune response to AVA are lacking (e.g., children, pregnant women, and adults aged ≥65 years) should continue to receive PEP-Abx for 60 days concurrently with AVA.

AV7909 (AVA plus CpG 7909 adjuvant) is a second-generation anthrax vaccine produced by Emergent BioSolutions that is in a phase 3 trial. The CpG 7909 adjuvant binds to the Toll-like receptor 9 to enhance the immune response to coadministered antigens (primarily *B. anthracis* protective antigen). The PEP schedule, under clinical evaluation for AV7909, is 0.5 mL AVA with 0.25 mg CpG 7909 adjuvant administered IM at 0 and 2 weeks postexposure, combined with antimicrobials. Because of supply concerns and the investigational status of AV7909, AVA should be prioritized over AV7909 for PEP-Vx of potential exposure to aerosolized *B. anthracis* spores. If supplies of AVA are exhausted or unavailable, AV7909 is an option for PEP of persons exposed to aerosolized *B. anthracis* spores under an EUA granted by FDA. As with AVA, antimicrobials should be taken in conjunction with AV7909.

Data indicate that raxibacumab can be coadministered with AVA for PEP without affecting vaccine immunogenicity.[140] No data are available to assess whether obiltoxaximab coadministered with AVA impairs vaccine immunogenicity. Anthrax immunoglobulin (AIGIV) does not have a PEP indication because coadministration of AIGIV and AVA in a rabbit model has been shown to significantly reduce the development of an immune response to AVA.

CONCLUSION

B. anthracis has been repeatedly used as a bioweapon for more than a century. It is one of the most likely pathogens to be used as a biothreat due to its ability to cause infection via aerosolization, the stability of *B. anthracis* spores in the environment, and the lethality of systemic infection. Clinicians should be aware of the differing clinical syndromes of anthrax and include anthrax in their differential diagnosis when appropriate. Healthcare facilities should have policies and procedures in place for managing the intentional release of biothreats. Anthrax vaccine absorbed (AVA) is available for preexposure prophylaxis. Antibiotics plus AVA are available for postexposure prophylaxis.

ACKNOWLEDGMENTS

No conflicts for either author.

REFERENCES

1. Schwartz M, Dr. Jekyll, Mr. Hyde. A short history of anthrax. *Mol Asp Med.* 2009;30(6):347–355.
2. Doganay M, Demiraslan H. Human anthrax as a re-emerging disease. *Recent Pat Antiinfect Drug Discov.* 2015;10(1):10–29.
3. Centers for Disease Control and Prevention. A History of Anthrax. Available at: https://www.cdc.gov/anthrax/resources/history/index.html. Accessed 1 July 2018.
4. Dixon TC, Meselson M, Guillemin J, Hanna PC. Anthrax. *N Engl J Med.* 1999;341(11):815–826.
5. Swartz MH. Recognition and management of anthrax—an update. *N Engl J Med.* 2001;345(22):1621–1626.
6. Doganay L, Welsby PD. Anthrax: a disease in waiting? *Postgrad Med J.* 2006;82(973):754–756.
7. World Health Organization. Anthrax in Humans and Animals. 4th ed. WHO Press; 2008.
8. Sweeney DA, Hicks CW, Cui X, Li Y, Eichacker PQ. Anthrax infection. *Am J Respir Crit Care Med.* 2011;184(12):1333–1341.
9. Hicks CW, Sweeney DA, Cui X, Li Y, Eichacker PQ. An overview of anthrax infection including the recently identified form of disease in injection drug users. *Intensive Care Med.* 2012;38(7):1092–1104.
10. Goel AK. Anthrax: a disease of biowarfare and public health importance. *World J Clin Cases.* 2015;3(1):20–33.
11. Finke EJ, Beyer W, Loderstädt U, Frickmann H. Review: the risk of contracting anthrax from spore-contaminated soil—a military medical perspective. *Eur J Microbiol Immunol (Bp).* 2020;10(2):29–63.
12. Savransky V, Ionin B, Reece J. Current status and trends in prophylaxis and management of anthrax disease. *Pathogens.* 2020;9(5):370.
13. Bravata DM, Holty JE, Wang E, et al. Inhalational, gastrointestinal, and cutaneous anthrax in children: a systematic review of cases: 1900 to 2005. *Arch Pediatr Adolesc Med.* 2007;161(9):896–905.
14. Turenne CY, Snyder JW, Alexander DC. *Bacillus* and other aerobic endospore-forming bacteria. In: Jorgensen JH, Pfaller MA, eds. *Manual of Clinical Microbiology.* Washington, DC: ASM Press; 2015:441–461.
15. Romero-Alvarez D, Peterson AT, Salzer JS, et al. Potential distributions of *Bacillus anthracis* and *Bacillus cereus* biovar anthracis causing anthrax in Africa. *PLoS Negl Trop Dis.* 2020;14(3):e0008131.
16. Klee SR, Brzuszkiewicz EB, Nattermann H, et al. The genome of a Bacillus isolate causing anthrax in chimpanzees combines chromosomal properties of *B. cereus* with *B. anthracis* virulence plasmids. *PLoS One.* 2010;5(7):e10986.
17. Zincke D, Norris MH, Cruz O, et al. TaqMan assays for simultaneous detection of Bacillus anthracis and Bacillus cereus biovar anthracis. *Pathogens.* 2020;9(12):1074.
18. Baldwin VM. You can't *B. cereus*—a review of Bacillus cereus strains that cause anthrax-like disease. *Front Microbiol.* 2020;11:1731.

19. Weber DJ, Rutala WA. Risks and prevention of nosocomial transmission of rare zoonotic diseases. *Clin Infect Dis.* 2001;32(3):446–456.
20. Hugh-Jones M, Blackburn J. The ecology of Bacillus anthracis. *Mol Asp Med.* 2009;30(6):356–367.
21. Beyer W, Turnbull PC. Anthrax in animals. *Mol Asp Med.* 2009;30(6):481–489.
22. Centers for Disease Control and Prevention. Nationally Notifiable Infectious Diseases and Conditions, United States: Weekly Tables; 2021. Available at: https://wonder.cdc.gov/nndss/static/2021/22/2021-22-table1a-H.pdf. Accessed 14 June 2021.
23. Mock M, Fouet A. Anthrax. *Ann Rev Microbiol.* 2001;55:647–671.
24. Nicholson WL, Munakata N, Horneck G, Melosh HJ, Setlow P. Resistance of *Bacillus* endospores to extreme terrestrial and extraterrestrial environments. *Microbiol Mol Biol Rev.* 2000;64(3):548–572.
25. Driks A. The *Bacillus anthracis* spore. *Mol Asp Med.* 2009;30(6):368–373.
26. Zasada AA. Injectional anthrax in human: a new face of the old disease. *Adv Clin Exp Med.* 2018;27(4):553–558.
27. D'Amelio E, Gentile B, Lista F, D'Amelio R. Historical evolution of human anthrax from occupational disease to potentially global threat as bioweapon. *Environ Int.* 2015;85:133–146.
28. Marston CK, Allen CA, Beaudry J, et al. Molecular epidemiology of anthrax cases associated with recreational use of animal hides and yarn in the United States. *PLoS One.* 2011;6(12):e28274.
29. Bennett AM, Pottage T, Parks SR. Is there an infection risk when playing drums contaminated with Bacillus anthracis? *J Appl Microbiol.* 2016;121(3):840–845.
30. Bennett E, Hall IM, Pottage T, Silman NJ, Bennett AM. Drumming-associated anthrax incidents: exposures to low levels of indoor environmental contamination. *Epidemiol Infect.* 2018;(July 4):1–7.
31. Szablewski CM, Hendricks K, Bower WA, Shadomy SV, Hupert N. Anthrax cases associated with animal-hair shaving brushes. *Emerg Infect Dis.* 2017;23(5):806–808.
32. Centers for Disease Control and Prevention. Public health dispatch: update: cutaneous anthrax in a laboratory worker—Texas. *MMWR.* 2002;51(22):482.
33. Singh K. Laboratory-acquired infections. *Clin Infect Dis.* 2009;49(1):142–147.
34. Weber DJ, Rutala WA. Recognition and management of anthrax. *N Engl J Med.* 2002;346(12):943–945.
35. Wenner KA, Kenner JR. Anthrax. *Dermatol Clin.* 2004;22(3):247–256.
36. Doganay M, Metan G, Alp E. A review of cutaneous anthrax and its outcome. *J Infect Public Health.* 2010;3(3):98–105.
37. Aquino LL, Wu JJ. Cutaneous manifestations of category A bioweapon. *J Am Acad Dermatol.* 2011;65(6):1213.e1–1213.e15.
38. Kayabas U, Karahocagil MK, Ozkurt Z, et al. Naturally occurring cutaneous anthrax: antibiotic treatment and outcome. *Chemotherapy.* 2012;58(1):34–43.
39. Shafazand S. When bioterrorism strikes: diagnosis and management of inhalational anthrax. *Semin Respir Infect.* 2003;18(3):134–145.
40. Quintiliani Jr R, Quintiliani R. Inhalational anthrax and bioterrorism. *Curr Opin Pulm Med.* 2003;9(3):221–226.
41. Holty JE, Bravata DM, Liu H, Olshen RA, McDonald KM, Owens DK. Systematic review: a century of inhalational anthrax cases from 1900 to 2005. *Ann Intern Med.* 2006;144(4):270–280.
42. Holty JE, Kim RY, Bravata DM. Anthrax: a systematic review of atypical presentations. *Ann Emerg Med.* 2006;48(2):200–211.
43. Beatty ME, Ashford DA, Griffin PM, Tauxe RV, Sobel J. Gastrointestinal anthrax: review of the literature. *Arch Intern Med.* 2003;163(20):2527–2531.
44. Owen JL, Yang T, Mohamadzadeh M. New insights into gastrointestinal anthrax infection. *Trends Mol Med.* 2015;21(3):154–163.
45. Berger T, Kassirer M, Aran AA. Injection anthrax—new presentation of an old disease. *Euro Surveill.* 2014;19(32):1–11.
46. Centers for Disease Control and Prevention. Recommended specimens for microbiology and pathology for diagnosis of anthrax; 2024. Available at: https://www.cdc.gov/anthrax/specificgroups/lab-professionals/recommended-specimen.html. Accessed 3 November 2024.
47. Clinical and Laboratory Standards Institute. Methods for antimicrobial dilution and disk susceptibility testing of infrequently isolated or fastidious bacteria. M45. 3rd ed; August 2016.
48. Luna VA, King DS, Gulledge J, Cannons AC, Amuso PT, Cattani J. Susceptibility of *Bacillus anthracis, Bacillus cereus, Bacillus mycoides, Bacillus pseudomycoides,* and *Bacillus thuringiensis* to 24 antimicriobials using Sensititre® automated microbroth dilution and Etest® agar gradient diffusion methods. *J Antimicrob Chemother.* 2007;60(3):555–567.
49. Odendaal MW, Pieterson PM, de Vos V, Botha AD. The antibiotic sensitivity patterns of *Bacillus anthracis* isolated from Kruger National Park. *Onderstepoort J Vet Res.* 1991;58(1):17–19.
50. Doganay M, Aydin N. Antimicrobial susceptibility of *Bacillus anthracis. Scand J Infect Dis.* 1991;23(1):333–335.
51. Bryskier A. *Bacillus anthracis* and antibacterial agents. *Clin Microbiol Infect.* 2002;8(8):467–478.
52. Drago L, de Vecchi E, Lombardi A, Nicola L, Valli M, Gismondo MR. Bactericidal activity of levofloxacin, gatifloxacin, penicillin, meropenem and rokitamycin against *Bacillus anthracis* clinical isolates. *J Antimicrob Chemother.* 2002;50(6):1059–1063.
53. Bakici MZ, Eladi N, Bakir M, Bokmetas I, Erandac M, Turan M. Antimicrobial susceptibility of *Bacillus anthracis* in an endemic area. *Scand J Infect Dis.* 2002;34(8):564–566.
54. Cavallo J-D, Ramisse F, Girardet M, Vaissaire J, Mock M, Hernandez E. Antimicrobial susceptibilities of 96 isolates of *Bacillus anthracis* isolated in France between 1994 and 2000. *Antimicrob Agents Chemother.* 2002;46(7):2307–2309.

55. Coker PR, Smith KL, Hugh-Jones ME. Antimicrobial susceptibilities of diverse *Bacillus anthracis* isolates. *Antimicrob Agents Chemother.* 2002;46(12):3843–3845.
56. Frean J, Klugman KP, Arntzen L, Bukofzer S. Susceptibility of *Bacillus anthracis* to eleven antimicrobial agents including novel fluoroquinolones and a ketolide. *J Antimicrob Chemother.* 2003;52(2):297–299.
57. Jones ME, Goguen J, Critchley IA, et al. Antibiotic susceptibility of isolates of *Bacillus anthracis*, a bacterial pathogen with the potential use in biowarfare. *Clin Microbiol Infect.* 2003;9(9):984–986.
58. Turnbull PCB, Sirianni NM, LeBron CI, et al. MICs of selected antibiotics for *Bacillus anthracis*, Bacillus cereus, Bacillus thurigiensis, and Bacillus mycoides from a range of clinical and environmental sources as determined by Etest. *J Antimicrob Chemother.* 2004;42(8):3626–3634.
59. Maho A, Rossano A, Hachler H, et al. Antibiotic susceptibility and molecular diversity of *Bacillus anthracis* strains in Chad: detection of a new phylogenic group. *J Clin Microbiol.* 2006;44(9):3422–3425.
60. Ortatatli M, Karagoz A, Percin D, Kenar L, Kilic S. Antimicrobial susceptibility and molecular subtyping of 55 Turkish *Bacillus anthracis* strains using 25-loci multiple-locus VNTR analysis. *Comp Immunol Microbiol Infect Dis.* 2012;35(4):355–361.
61. Durmaz R, Doganay M, Sahin M, et al. Molecular epidemiology of the *Bacillus anthracis* isolates collected throughout Turkey from 1983 to 2011. *Eur J Clin Microbiol Infect Dis.* 2012;31(10):2783–2790.
62. Heine HS, Purcell BK, Bassett J, Miller L, Goldstein BP. Activity of dalbavancin against *Bacillus anthracis in vitro* and in a mouse inhalation anthrax model. *Antimicrob Agents Chemother.* 2010;54(10):991–996.
63. Heine HS, Bassett J, Miller L, et al. Efficacy of oritavancin in a murine model of *Bacillus anthracis* spore inhalation anthrax. *Antimicrob Agents Chemother.* 2008;52(9):3350–3357.
64. Kreizinger Z, Sulyok KM, Makrai L, et al. Antimicrobial susceptibility of *Bacillus anthracis* strains from Hungary. *Acta Vet Hung.* 2016;64(2):141–147.
65. Bower WA, Yu Y, Person MK, et al. CDC guideline for the prevention and treatment of anthrax, 2023. *MMWR Recomm Rep.* 2023;72:1–47.
66. Sidwa T, Salzer JS, Traxler R, et al. Control and prevention of Anthrax, Texas, USA, 2019. *Emerg Infect Dis.* 2020;26(12):2815–2824.
67. Bradley JS, Peacock G, Krug SE, et al. Pediatric anthrax clinical management. *Pediatrics.* 2014;133(5):e1411–e1436.
68. Meaney-Delman D, Zotti ME, Creanga AA, et al. Special considerations for prophylaxis for and treatment of anthrax in pregnant and postpartum women. *Emerg Infect Dis.* 2014;20(2).
69. Bhatnagar R, Batra S. Anthrax toxin. *Crit Rev Microbiol.* 2001;27(3):167–200.
70. Knudson GB. Treatment of anthrax in man: history and current concepts. *Mil Med.* 1986;151:71–77.
71. Huang E, Pillai SK, Bower WA, et al. Antitoxin treatment of inhalation Anthrax: a systematic review. *Health Secur.* 2015;13(6):365–377.
72. Head BM, Rubinstein E, Meyers AF. Alternative pre-approved and novel therapies for the treatment of anthrax. *BMC Infect Dis.* 2016;16(1):621.
73. Xu W, Ohanjanian L, Sun J, et al. A systematic review and meta-analysis of preclinical trials testing anti-toxin therapies for *B. anthracis* infection: a need for more robust study designs and results. *PLoS One.* 2017;12(8):e0182879.
74. Oosterholt SP, Della Pasqua O. Extrapolation and dosing recommendations for raxibacumab in children from birth to < 18 years of age. *Br J Clin Pharmacol.* 2021;87:4709–4717.
75. Hou AW, Morrill AM. Obiltoxaximab: adding to the treatment arsenal for *Bacillus anthracis* infection. *Ann Pharmacother.* 2017;51(10):908–913.
76. Food and Drug Administration. ANTHRASIL [Anthrax Immune Globulin Intravenous (Human)]. Available at: https://www.fda.gov/vaccines-blood-biologics/approved-blood-products/anthrasil. Accessed 14 June 2021.
77. Centers for Disease Control and Prevention. Use of anthrax vaccine in the United States. Recommendations of the Advisory Committee on Immunization Practices (ACIP), 2019. *MMWR Recomm Rep.* 2010;59:1–30 [No. RR-6].
78. Centers for Disease Control and Prevention. Use of Anthrax Vaccine in the United States. Recommendations of the Advisory Committee on Immunization Practices (ACIP), 2019. *MMWR Recomm Rep.* 2019;68:1–14 [No. RR-4].
79. Kaur M, Singh S, Bhatnagar R. Anthrax vaccines: present status and future prospects. *Expert Rev Vaccines.* 2013;12(8):955–970.
80. Williamson ED, Dyson EH. Anthrax prophylaxis: recent advances and future directions. *Front Microbiol.* 2015;6:1009.
81. Longstreth J, Skiadopoulos MH, Hopkins RJ. Licensure strategy for pre- and post-exposure prophylaxis of biothrax vaccine: the first vaccine licensed using the FDA animal rule. *Expert Rev Vaccines.* 2016;15(12):1467–1479.
82. Franz DR, Jahrling PB, Friedlander AM, et al. Clinical recognition and management of patients exposed to biological warfare agents. *JAMA.* 1997;278(5):399–411.
83. Henderson DA. Bioterrorism as a public health threat. *Emerg Infect Dis.* 1998;4(3):488–492.
84. Henderson DA. The looming threat of bioterrorism. *Science.* 1999;283(5406):1279–1282.
85. Inglesby TV, Henderson DA, Bartlett JG, et al. Anthrax as a biological weapon: medical and public health management. Working Group on Civilian Biodefense. *JAMA.* 1999;281(18):1735–1745.
86. Franz DR. Preparedness for an anthrax attack. *Mol Asp Med.* 2009;30(6):503–510.
87. Christian MD. Biowarfare and bioterrorism. *Crit Care Clin.* 2013;29(3):717–756.
88. Bower WA, Hendricks K, Pillai S, Guarnizo J, Meaney-Delman D. Clinical framework and medical countermeasure use during an anthrax mass-casualty incident. *MMWR Recomm Rep.* 2015;64(4):1–22.

89. Gosden C, Gardener D. Weapons of mass destruction—threats and responses. *BMJ*. 2005;331(7513):397–400.
90. Adalja AA, Toner E, Inglesby TV. Clinical management of potential bioterrorism-related conditions. *N Engl J Med*. 2015;372(10):954–962.
91. Khardori N. Bioterrorism and bioterrorism preparedness: historical perspective and overview. *Infect Dis Clin N Am*. 2006;20(2):179–211.
92. Rotz LD, Khan AS, Lillibridge SR, Ostroff SM, Hughes JM. *Emerg Infect Dis*. 2002;8(2):225–230.
93. Centers for Disease Control and Prevention. Bioterrorism Agents/Diseases. Available at: https://emergency.cdc.gov/agent/agentlist-category.asp. Accessed 14 June 2021.
94. Centers for Disease Control and Prevention. Anthrax: The threat. Available at: https://www.cdc.gov/anthrax/bioterrorism/threat.html. Accessed 14 June 2021.
95. Christopher GW, Cieslak TJ, Pavlin JA, Eitzen Jr EM. Biological warfare. A historical perspective. *JAMA*. 1997;278(5):412–417.
96. Siegrist DW. The threat of biological attack: why concern now? *Emerg Infect Dis*. 1999;5(4):505–508.
97. Szinicz L. History of chemical and biological warfare agents. *Toxicology*. 2005;214:167–181.
98. Barras V, Greub G. History of biological warfare and bioterrorism. *Clin Microbiol Infect*. 2014;20(6):497–502.
99. Redmond C, Pearce MJ, Manchee RJ, Berdal BP. Deadly relic of the great war. *Nature*. 1998;393(6687):747–748.
100. Manchee RJ, Broster MG, Melling J, Henstridge RM, Stagg AJ. *Bacillus anthracis* on Gruinard Island. *Nature*. 1981;294(5838):254–255.
101. Manchee RJ, Broster MG, Anderson IS, Henstridge RM, Melling J. Decontamination of *Bacillus anthracis* on Gruinard Island? *Nature*. 1983;303(5914):239–240.
102. Aldhous P. Biological warfare. Gruinard Island handed back. *Nature*. 1990;344(6269):801.
103. Manchee RJ, Broster MG, Stagg AJ, Hibbs SE. Formaldehyde solution effectively inactivates spores of *Bacillus anthracis* on the Scottish Island of Gruinard. *Appl Environ Microbiol*. 1994;60(11):4167–4171.
104. Meselson M, Guillemin J, Hugh-Jones M, et al. The Sverdlovsk anthrax outbreak of 1979. *Science*. 1994;266(5188):1202–1208.
105. Sepkowitz KA. Anthrax and anthrax anxiety: Sverdlovsk revisited. *Int J Infect Dis*. 2001;5(4):178–179.
106. Tu AT. Aum Shinrikyo's chemical and biological weapons: more than sarin. *Forensic Sci Rev*. 2014;26(2):115–120.
107. Centers for Disease Control and Prevention. Update: investigation of anthrax associated with intentional exposure and interim public health guidelines, October 2001. *MMWR Morb Mortal Wkly Rep*. 2001;50(41):889–893.
108. Centers for Disease Control and Prevention. Recognition of illness associated with the intentional release of a biologic agent. *MMWR Morb Mortal Wkly Rep*. 2001;50(41):893–897.
109. Centers for Disease Control and Prevention. Update: investigation of bioterrorism-related anthrax and interim guidelines for exposure management and antimicrobial therapy, October 2001. *MMWR Morb Mortal Wkly Rep*. 2001;50(42):909–919.
110. Centers for Disease Control and Prevention. Update: investigation of bioterrorism-related anthrax and interim guidelines for clinical evaluation of persons with possible anthrax. *MMWR Morb Mortal Wkly Rep*. 2001;50(43):941–948.
111. Centers for Disease Control and Prevention. Interim guidelines for investigation of and response to *Bacillus anthracis* exposures. *MMWR Morb Mortal Wkly Rep*. 2001;50(44):987–990.
112. Centers for Disease Control and Prevention. Update: investigation of bioterrorism-related anthrax, 2001. *MMWR Morb Mortal Wkly Rep*. 2001;50(45):1008–1010.
113. Centers for Disease Control and Prevention. Update: investigation of bioterrorism-related inhalation anthrax—Connecticut, 2001. *MMWR Morb Mortal Wkly Rep*. 2001;50(47):1049–1050.
114. Centers for Disease Control and Prevention. Update: investigation of bioterrorism-related anthrax--Connecticut, 2001. *MMWR Morb Mortal Wkly Rep*. 2001;50(48):1077–1079.
115. Dull PM, Wilson KE, Kournikakis B, et al. *Bacillus anthracis* aerosolization associated with a contaminated mail sorting machine. *Emerg Infect Dis*. 2002;8(10):1044–1047.
116. Sanderson WT, Stoddard RR, Echt AS, et al. *Bacillus anthracis* contamination and inhalational anthrax in a mail processing and distribution center. *J Appl Microbiol*. 2004;96(5):1048–1056.
117. Centers for Disease Control and Prevention. Follow-up of deaths among U.S. postal service workers potentially exposed to *Bacillus anthracis*—District of Columbia, 2001-2002. *MMWR Morb Mortal Wkly Rep*. 2003;52(39):937–938.
118. Centers for Disease Control and Prevention. Surveillance for adverse events associated with anthrax vaccination-US Department of defense, 1998-2000. *MMWR Morb Mortal Wkly Rep*. 2000;49(16):341–345.
119. Centers for Disease Control and Prevention. Update: investigation of bioterrorism-related anthrax and adverse events from antimicrobial prophylaxis. *MMWR Morb Mortal Wkly Rep*. 2001;50(44):973–976.
120. Centers for Disease Control and Prevention. Update: adverse events associated with anthrax prophylaxis among postal employees—New Jersey, New York City, and the District of Columbia metropolitan area, 2001. *MMWR Morb Mortal Wkly Rep*. 2001;50(47):1051–1054.
121. Teshale EH, Painter J, Burr GA, et al. Environmental sampling for spores of *Bacillus anthracis*. *Emerg Infect Dis*. 2002;8(10):1083–1087.
122. Sanderson WT, Hein MJ, Taylor L, et al. Surface sampling methods for *Bacillus anthracis* spore contamination. *Emerg Infect Dis*. 2002;8(10):1145–1151.
123. Chugh T. Bioterrorism: clinical and public health aspects of anthrax. *Curr Med Res Pract*. 2019;9(3):110–111.
124. Siegel JD, Rhinehart E, Jackson M, Chiarello L. Guidelines for Precautions: Preventing Transmission of Infectious

Agents in Healthcare Settings; 2007. Available at: https://www.cdc.gov/anthrax/specificgroups/health-care-providers/index.html. Accessed 10 July 2018.
125. Centers for Disease Control and Prevention. Notice to Readers: Occupational Health Guidelines for Remediation Workers at Bacillus anthracis-Contaminated Sites—United States, 2001–2002. *MMWR Morb Mortal Wkly Rep.* 2002;51(35):786–789.
126. Casanova L, Alfano-Sobsey E, Rutala WA, Weber DJ, Sobsey M. Virus transfer from personal protective equipment to healthcare employees' skin and clothing. *Emerg Infect Dis.* 2008;14(8):1291.
127. Casanova LM, Rutala WA, Weber DJ, Sobsey MD. Effect of single- versus double-gloving on virus transfer to health care workers' skin and clothing during removal of personal protective equipment. *Am J Infect Control.* 2012;40(4):369–374.
128. Casanova LM, Teal LJ, Sickbert-Bennett EE, et al. Assessment of self-contamination during removal of personal protective equipment for Ebola patient care. *Infect Control Hosp Epidemiol.* 2016;37(10):1156–1161.
129. Casanova LM, Erukunuakpor K, Kraft CS, et al. Assessing viral transfer during doffing of Ebola-level personal protective equipment in a biocontainment unit. *Clin Infect Dis.* 2018;66(6):945–949.
130. Weber DJ, Sickbert-Bennett E, Gergen MF, Rutala WA. Efficacy of selected hand hygiene agents used to remove *Bacillus atrophaeus* (a surrogate of *Bacillus anthracis*) from contaminated hands. *JAMA.* 2003;289(10):1274–1277.
131. Yim JH, Song KY, Kim H, Bae D, Chon JW, Seo KH. Effectiveness of calcium hypochlorite, quaternary ammonium compounds, and sodium hypochlorite in eliminating vegetative cells and spores of *Bacillus anthracis* surrogate. *J Vet Sci.* 2021;22(1):e11. 017/dmp.2018.113.
132. Spotts Whitney EA, Beatty ME, Taylor Jr TH, et al. Inactivation of *Bacillus anthracis* spores. *Emerg Infect Dis.* 2003;9(6):623–627.
133. Chatuev BM, Peterson JW. Analysis of the sporicidal activity of chlorine dioxide disinfectant against *Bacillus anthracis* (Sterne strain). *J Hosp Infect.* 2010;74(2):178–183.
134. Stratilo CW, Crichton MK, Sawyer TW. Decontamination efficacy and skin toxicity of two decontaminants against *Bacillus anthracis. PLoS One.* 2015;10(9):e0138491.
135. Lowe JJ, Gibbs SG, Iwen PC, Smith PW, Hewlett AL. Decontamination of a hospital room using gaseous chlorine dioxide: *Bacillus anthracis, Francisella tularensis*, and *Yersinia pestis. J Occup Environ Hyg.* 2013;10(10):533–539.
136. Centers for Disease Control and Prevention. Biosafety in microbiology and biomedical laboratories (BMBL). 6th ed; 2020. Available at: https://www.cdc.gov/labs/pdf/SF__19_308133-A_BMBL6_00-BOOK-WEB-final-3.pdf. Accessed 14 June 2021.
137. Centers for Disease Control and Prevention. How to prevent anthrax. Available at: https://www.cdc.gov/anthrax/medical-care/prevention.html. Accessed 14 June 2021.
138. Centers for Disease Control and Prevention. Anthrax vaccine recommendations. Available at: https://www.cdc.gov/vaccines/vpd/anthrax/hcp/recommendations.html. Accessed 14 June 2021.
139. Nolen LD, Traxler RM, Kharod GA, et al. Postexposure prophylaxis after possible anthrax exposure: adherence and adverse events. *Health Secur.* 2016;14(6):419–423.
140. Skoura N, Wang-Jairaj J, Della Pasqua O, et al. Effect of raxibacumab on immunogenicity of Anthrax vaccine adsorbed: a phase 4, open-label, parallel-group, randomised non-inferiority study. *Lancet Infect Dis.* 2020;20(8):983–991.

CHAPTER 4

Tularemia: A Bioterrorist Threat and Public Health Concern

KAREN L. ELKINS[a] • JEANNINE M. PETERSEN[b] • ANDERS SJÖSTEDT[c]
[a]LMPCI/DBPAP/OVRR, CBER, FDA, Silver Spring, MD, United States • [b]Division of Vector-Borne Diseases, Centers for Disease Control and Prevention, Fort Collins, CO, United States • [c]Department of Clinical Microbiology, Umeå University, Umeå, Sweden

OVERVIEW AND HISTORY

In 1912, two US Public Health Service (PHS) officers, George McCoy and Charles Chapin, isolated a microbe that sickened squirrels in Tulare County, California, and named it *Bacterium tularense*.[1,2] The small, Gram-negative organism was difficult to culture but could be grown on the right consistency of coagulated egg yolk, on which it exhibited a range of coccoid, irregular, or globular forms. Soon thereafter, the same microbe was associated with human illness in the form of abscesses around the eye of a meat cutter in an Ohio restaurant.[3] Well before the microbiological discoveries, the disease that came to be known as tularemia was described in other regions of the world. "Yato-Byo" or "wild hare disease" was defined by 1818 in Japan; local terminology later evolved to "Ohara's disease," following classic studies in the early 1900s by Dr. Hachiro Ohara that identified a number of human cases, especially following handling of wild rabbits for food.[4] In Norway, a human disease dubbed lemming fever was described in the 1890s, a couple of centuries after recognition of a similar disease in the lemmings themselves.

Serological studies using serum from Dr. Chapin, who appears to have been an asymptomatic victim of infection, linked together bacteria isolated from cases in different parts of the United States as the same.[5] Serological cross-reactions also resulted in renaming the bacterium *Pasteurella tularensis* in the 1920s, a designation that remained until DNA hybridization studies in the 1960s indicated the organism had little in common with *Pasteurella*. The organism gained its current name, *Francisella tularensis*, in recognition of Dr. Edward Francis. Francis, also a PHS officer, conducted extensive studies of the organism and human infections in the United States throughout the first quarter of the 20th century—so much so that he contracted tularemia himself at least 4 times.[5–7]

These historical features serve to illustrate a key characteristic of *F. tularensis*: the bacterium is among the most highly infectious zoonotic agents known, moving from animals or contaminated materials to humans efficiently and quickly. By the mid-20th century, tularemia was endemic in some areas of the world and thus a significant regional public health problem; Russia experienced large-scale epidemics, especially during World War II.[8] For reasons that are not well studied but may include improvements in housing and hygiene as well as decreased reliance on hunting for food, the incidence of tularemia worldwide declined over the second half of the last century. Tularemia's most recent claim to fame arose because of its notorious, and exploitable, infectivity: *F. tularensis* was weaponized by at least three countries (the United States, the USSR, and Japan[9]). In the United States, *F. tularensis* remains a Tier 1 select agent (http://www.selectagents.gov/SelectAgentsandToxinsList.html) due to concerns regarding its potential nefarious use. Fortunately, the explosion of biodefense research in the United States after the 9/11 and anthrax letter attacks has provided new understanding of the pathogenesis of disease caused by this fascinating pathogen. This chapter will therefore summarize current scientific knowledge about the microbiology, immunology, epidemiology, and ecology of *Francisella* spp., as well as clinical features and management of human infections caused by *F. tularensis* (Table 1).

Viral Outbreaks, Biosecurity, and Preparing for Mass Casualty Infectious Diseases Events
https://doi.org/10.1016/B978-0-323-54841-0.00008-1

TABLE 1
At a Glance: Tularemia, Caused by *Francisella tularensis*

	Key Features	Clinical Correlations
Microbiology	Gram-negative fastidious bacterium Intracellular; replicates primarily in macrophages Major subspecies = *F. tularensis* subsp. *tularensis* (North America only) *F. tularensis* subsp. *holarctica* (Northern Hemisphere)	Replication and resulting tissue destruction are important in pathogenesis *F. tularensis* subsp. *tularensis* infections are more severe
Immunology	Innate responses such as cytokine production likely contribute to symptoms Th1 T cells dominate successful responses to infection; serum antibodies are useful for diagnosis	Experimental evidence suggests bacterial immune evasion strategies contribute to pathogenesis
Epidemiology and ecology	Zoonotic; infects a wide variety of mammals, invertebrates, and arthropods Humans infected by many routes following contact with infected animals or by arthropod bite, or ingestion or inhalation of contaminated materials Primary mode of transmission can vary geographically	No documented cases of human-to-human transmission
Clinical presentation	Incubation time varies but averages 3 to 5 days Specific symptoms follow route of infection, e.g., ulcers and regional lymph node swelling after introduction via skin Ulceroglandular form is the most common; respiratory form is the most serious	Fever, malaise, myalgia, cough, and headache are usually common to all forms
Diagnosis	Serology, PCR of infected tissue, and/or direct culture	Challenging; rare disease; initial symptoms often nonspecific
Treatment	Gentamicin for most serious disease, or streptomycin Doxycycline for less severe disease Ciprofloxacin for mass casualty settings (see Table 2 for dosing, duration, and special considerations)	Streptomycin problematic Tetracyclines associated with relapse
Vaccination	In Western countries, no approved vaccines; LVS is investigational In Russia and FSU countries, live attenuated strains are used for outbreaks	Main prevention strategy is avoiding contact with infected animals and materials

MICROBIOLOGY AND HOST RESPONSE

F. tularensis is a Gram-negative, pleomorphic, facultative intracellular bacterium.[10] Its aerobic growth is fastidious and requires rich media that include cysteine. DNA hybridization studies,[11] 16S RNA analyses, single nucleotide polymorphism (SNP) analyses,[12] and whole genome sequencing studies[13] all indicate that *F. tularensis* isolates are highly similar. *F. novicida* and *F. philomiragia* strains, which are very rare human pathogens, are genetically quite closely related to *F. tularensis*.[12]

F. tularensis isolates have an atypical lipopolysaccharide that is poorly endotoxic[14] and a carbohydrate-rich capsule,[15] both of which are associated with unusual long-chain fatty acids.[14,16] The virulence of *F. tularensis* remains incompletely understood, but like many intracellular pathogens, it causes tissue damage and disease by replicating within macrophages and other cells of the reticuloendothelial system, not by overt toxin production or endotoxemia.[17–19] *Francisella* genes organized in a pathogenicity island[20,21] produce products that allow the bacterium to escape from phagosomes after cell invasion, avoid phagolysosomal fusion, and replicate within the cytoplasm of mammalian cells. Some pathogenicity island gene products comprise an unusual Type VI secretion system whose structure and specific functions are the subjects of ongoing study.[22,23]

In experimental animals, host innate and adaptive immune responses to virulent *F. tularensis* strains appear to be substantially delayed as compared to responses to attenuated strains such as the "Live Vaccine Strain," or LVS (derived from *F. tularensis* subsp. *holarctica*[24]), supporting the concept that part of the bacterium's pathogenesis includes active immune evasion.[25,26] Both *F. tularensis* infection and vaccination with LVS eventually result in innate immune responses that are characterized by pro-inflammatory responses of macrophages, dendritic cells, and neutrophils that include production of TNF-α, IL-12, and AIM-2-dependent inflammasome activation for IL-1β production.[27,28] These drive development of Th1 T lymphocyte responses with production of IFN-γ and related Th1 cytokines; in rodent cells, these mediators trigger the production of nitric oxide, which is toxic to bacteria.[27] Specific antibody responses accompany vaccination and infection[27] and rise in serum antibody levels have been used as the basis for diagnosis[29] (see later). In animal studies, T-cell-mediated immune responses appear to predominate and be critical for successful control of *F. tularensis* infections, with antibodies potentially contributing a relatively minor role.[27]

EPIDEMIOLOGY AND ECOLOGY

Tularemia is endemic throughout much, but not all, of the Northern Hemisphere; until its recent description from Australia, *F. tularensis* had not been reported from the Southern Hemisphere.[7,30,31] Human cases, which are rare, are widely but not evenly distributed throughout Eurasia and the United States[7] The number of cases fluctuates annually and is frequently linked to population densities of animal hosts.[32,33] From 2010 through 2014, an average annual incidence of $\leq$0.20 cases per 100,000 persons was reported for the European Union/European Economic Area and the United States.[34,35]

Human tularemia cases result from infection by either *F. tularensis* subsp. *holarctica* (Type B) or subsp. *tularensis* (Type A), and subpopulations of both that differ in virulence, erythromycin sensitivity, and/or geographic distribution have been further identified.[36] A third subspecies, *F. tularensis* subsp. *mediasiatica*, has been described in animals and ticks in Central Asia and Russia but is not associated with human infections. *F. tularensis* subsp. *holarctica* predominates worldwide, occurring throughout the Northern Hemisphere and also Australia, whereas *F. tularensis* subsp. *tularensis* is more narrowly distributed in North America.[7,30,31] Characterization of isolates from 316 human cases in the United States from 1964 to 2004 identified 66% as *F. tularensis* subsp. *tularensis*.[37]

An unusually large number of animal species, both invertebrates and vertebrates, are susceptible to *F. tularensis* infection.[38,39] Human cases may follow tularemia epizootics in lagomorphs and rodents, which are considered to play key roles in bacterial amplification.[40,41] Tularemia is not typically an urban disease; human infections are more commonly associated with settings where contact with infected wildlife or arthropod vectors is more likely.[34,35] As with other zoonotic diseases, the risk of exposure is greater in persons who spend a great deal of time outdoors. Hunters, wildlife specialists, hikers, campers, veterinarians, and others with animal or arthropod exposure are all at increased risk of infection. Seasonal patterns may vary by region. In Europe and the United States, most cases occur in the warmer months of May through September and are often linked to bites from infected arthropods,[35,42,43] unlike infections due to direct or indirect contact with infected animals that are not seasonal.[42,44] Healthy persons of all ages are susceptible to *F. tularensis* infection; however, in many countries, the frequency of cases is typically higher in males,[35,42,43] which is thought to be related to both occupational and leisure activities. Exceptions are observed in Kosovo and Turkey, where the occurrence of tularemia cases is higher in females and linked to more frequent contact with contaminated water or food.[44,45]

Humans are dead-end hosts for *F. tularensis* and are incidentally infected via a number of exposure routes.[7,46] The organism can enter the body by many routes, including the skin, mucous membranes, or lungs, after direct or indirect contact with infected animals or arthropod vectors. Transmission of *F. tularensis* via direct contact with infected animals results from activities such as hunting or skinning wildlife, ingesting undercooked game meat, and close contact with domestic animals (e.g., cats or dogs). Infected ticks, deer flies, horseflies, and mosquitoes can directly transmit the organism by bite. Contamination of the environment by infected animals can lead to transmission of the organism via indirect contact. Examples include drinking water contaminated by infected animal carcasses, ingesting food contaminated by infected animals, or inhaling infectious dust or aerosols during farming or landscaping activities. Curiously, there is no evidence that tularemia can be transmitted from person to person. For this reason, standard precautions are recommended in hospitals, and isolation is not required.

All modes of transmission can occur worldwide; however, the dominant mode of infection may often be unique to a given geographic region.[43,46] Tick bites are a common mode of transmission,[46,47] but in Scandinavia the primary mode appears to be mosquito bites, especially during outbreaks.[48,49] Mosquito transmission is not common in other regions of Europe and is not known to occur in North America. Waterborne cases of tularemia most often occur in areas without chlorinated municipal water systems, via ingestion of contaminated well water or streams/springs compromised by infected animals. Infections with *F. tularensis*, *F. novicida*, and *F. philomiragia* have all been reported in individuals following near-drowning episodes.[11,50–52] The latter examples may result from persistent bacteria in the water, which is a postulated habitat of *Francisella* species.[7,53] In general, waterborne transmission is uncommon in most parts of the world, although Turkey and Kosovo are two striking exceptions. In Turkey from 2005 to 2009 and Kosovo from 2001 to 2010, almost all cases presented as the oropharyngeal form.[44,45] In Norway, the oropharyngeal form is also relatively common and was the most common form recorded in 2011, when a record number of cases occurred.[32] Despite the proximity to lakes and rivers as a strong risk factor for tularemia in Sweden,[54] there have been very few cases of oropharyngeal tularemia reported in Sweden or Finland. Similarly, very few cases of oropharyngeal tularemia have been reported in North America. Direct inhalation of the organism has been reported throughout Europe and the United States. Risk factors associated with direct inhalation in Scandinavia include farm work.[48] In the United States, mowing and brush cutting were linked with a pneumonic outbreak of tularemia in Martha's Vineyard.[55]

Human cases are often sporadic, although outbreaks of tularemia involving tens to thousands of cases have occurred. For example, over 900 suspected infections occurred throughout Kosovo in 1999–2000 due to war-torn conditions.[56] A disrupted agricultural environment and unprotected food and water sources likely resulted in a rapid increase in rodent populations favorable for epizootic spread of tularemia in rodents and consequent widespread environmental contamination with *F. tularensis*. Large outbreaks of tularemia due to inhalation of the organism have been reported in the Nordic countries. The largest occurred in Sweden in 1966–67 with more than 2700 cases, most likely due to aerosol generation from handling hay contaminated with dead voles.[57]

F. tularensis strains demonstrate limited genetic diversity worldwide, with *F. tularensis* considered a monomorphic pathogen. Nonetheless, both phenotypic and genotypic characteristics have been used to characterize the worldwide geographic distribution of *F. tularensis* populations.[36,46] *F. tularensis* subsp. *tularensis* strains possess citrulline ureidase activity, but *F. tularensis* subsp. *holarctica* strains do not. Erythromycin-sensitive *F tularensis* subsp. *holarctica* strains are reported in Western Europe and North America, whereas erythromycin-resistant *F tularensis* subsp. *holarctica* strains are distributed across eastern Europe and Russia, and erythromycin-sensitive *F. tularensis* subsp. *holarctica* biovar japonica strains occur in Japan, China, and Turkey. High-resolution genotypic typing of strains, based on canonical SNPs identified from whole genome sequencing, has been widely used to determine the worldwide phylogeography of *F. tularensis* strains.[46,58] Characterization of *F. tularensis* strains from naturally occurring focal outbreaks due to arthropod bite and inhalation has demonstrated the presence of more than one strain and even subspecies as a cause of human illness.[59–61] These findings are suggestive that the polyclonal origin of strains may be common for naturally occurring outbreaks of tularemia.

CLINICAL PRESENTATION, NATURAL HISTORY, AND DIAGNOSIS

The clinical manifestations of tularemia reflect the route of infection but exhibit common features. Regardless of the route of infection, an incubation period of 3 to 5 days usually follows, although the incubation time may vary widely; in a large Swedish study, incubation ranged from 7 h to 11 days.[62] Onset of symptoms occurs thereafter, often rather abruptly with flu-like symptoms including fever, malaise, myalgia, cough, and headache.[49,62,63] More uncommon presentations include dyspnea, nausea, diarrhea, vomiting, and sore throat.[49,62]

Other clinical manifestations are highly dependent on the route of bacterial entrance. Infection acquired through skin or mucous membranes results in the ulceroglandular form, as evidenced by a cutaneous ulcer at the site of the arthropod bite that is surrounded by inflammation and eventually prominent enlargement of adjacent draining lymph nodes. The ulcer may be inconspicuous and is often mistaken for a normal tick bite or mosquito bite, but otherwise develops at the same time as general symptoms and becomes pustular and ulcerates within a few days. It soon heals, leaving a more or less visible scar. The primary ulceration may be noticed only by physical examination, whereas the lymph node enlargement more frequently is a cause for medical attention. If appropriate treatment is not given within a 2-week period, the risk of abscess development may reach 20%.[64]

The term glandular tularemia refers to a similar clinical presentation, although without a primary skin lesion. In most parts of the world, more than 80% of cases are represented by the ulceroglandular and glandular forms.[49,62] The uncommon oculoglandular form is likely transmitted via physical inoculation, e.g., via the patient's fingers, and presents with conjunctivitis and preauricular lymph node enlargement. The oropharyngeal form of tularemia results from the intake of contaminated food or water and presents with exudative stomatitis and pharyngitis, often with tonsillar involvement and a very marked regional, often unilateral, neck lymphadenitis.[65] Intake of contaminated food or water may also result in the intestinal form, characterized by intestinal pain, vomiting, and diarrhea.[66]

The respiratory form of tularemia is the most serious form of the disease. In Europe, mortality from infection with *F. tularensis* subsp. *holarctica* strains is very low, but in the United States, where infections result from either *F. tularensis* subspecies, a case-fatality rate of up to 35% was noted before effective antibiotics were available.[67] Today, antibiotic regimens have reduced the fatality rate in the United States to less than 2%.[9,37] Symptoms of respiratory tularemia may vary, and patients may present with systemic illness and fever, but not necessarily with prominent signs of pneumonic disease.[63] Respiratory infection caused by *F. tularensis* subsp. *tularensis* is by far the most serious form of tularemia and has been extensively described in the literature.[63,67–71] Onset may be abrupt with a chill, fever, dyspnea, cough, chest pain, bradycardia, and profuse sweating. However, the development of pulmonary signs can be greatly delayed; some individuals may even experience relatively mild disease, and one review concluded that physicians may easily misdiagnose the disease.[69] Nonetheless, in a majority of cases, pulmonary symptoms predominate.[69] In a review of respiratory tularemia patients from Arkansas, pneumonia was diagnosed in 31% of patients with ulceroglandular tularemia and in 83% of patients with the typhoidal variant; in all but one patient, parenchymal infiltrates were demonstrated, and in a third of the cases, also pleural effusion.[63]

During the large Swedish outbreak of respiratory tularemia in 1966–67, detailed medical information was obtained from 140 of over 2700 patients, and only 7% showed pneumonia.[57] During an outbreak of 53 cases in Finland in 1982, 11% were classified as mild (fever <1 week) and 34% as severe (fever >3 weeks).[72] All presented with fever, and most had headache, myalgia, and arthralgia; approximately half reported dry cough, pleural pain, and dyspnea. Notably, only 10% of the patients had typical pneumonic symptoms.[72] In a recent follow-up of 58 cases of respiratory tularemia in northern Finland from 2000 to 2012, respiratory symptoms were absent in 47% of patients, and 7% had normal chest X-rays.[71] X-ray findings usually reveal lung infiltrates, pleuritis, and often hilar lymph node enlargement.[62,72] Collectively, the studies demonstrate that during respiratory tularemia caused by *F. tularensis* subsp. *holarctica*, prototypical symptoms of pneumonia are not that common, and even X-ray findings may be normal. Even during *F. tularensis* subsp. *tularensis* respiratory infections, signs and symptoms may be atypical and pneumonia delayed or not even present.

The term typhoidal tularemia has been used to describe a clinical presentation with rather severe systemic manifestations, such as high fever, hepatomegaly, splenomegaly, and possibly septicemia, but lacking characteristic regional symptoms such as cutaneous or mucosal lesions, or regional lymphadenitis.[9] The route of infection is unclear, but this form is likely an unusual manifestation of respiratory tularemia.

A substantial number of unusual manifestations have also been described, which reflect the versatility of *F. tularensis* as a human pathogen. The manifestations include pleuritis,[9,73,74] aortitis,[75] uveitis,[76] fascial cellulitis,[77] middle ear infection,[78] otomastoiditis,[79] facial paresis,[79] dacryocystitis,[80] pseudoptosis,[81] inflammatory neck mass,[82] dental abscess,[83] rhombencephalitis,[84] Parinaud's syndrome,[85] endocarditis,[86] and Guillain-Barre syndrome.[73,87] Tularemia pleuritis shows striking biochemical and cellular characteristics of the pleural fluid with tuberculous pleurisy.[88] Also, pulmonary tularemia may show much resemblance to lung cancer.[89] Curiously, 3 cases of mastoiditis were observed in the same region in France during a 6-year period and likely contracted while canyoneering in a river.[79]

F. tularensis subsp. *tularensis* may cause other severe clinical manifestations, such as rhabdomyolysis and septic shock,[90] and gastrointestinal symptoms, such as vomiting, diarrhea, and abdominal pain.[9] A number of atypical presentations have also been reported after infection with *F. tularensis* subsp. *holarctica*. In a Swedish study of 250 patients, 16.2% encountered complications. Prolonged fatigue of greater than 1 month after termination of antibiotic treatment was present among 5.1%; lymph node suppuration occurred in 3.8%, while lymph node incision was performed in 2.1%.[62] Venous thrombosis occurred in 0.9% of the patients.

A variety of dermatological manifestations have been reported in conjunction with tularemia. In a Turkish study of 151 patients, erythema multiforme was the most common, followed by ulcers (6.0%), urticaria (3.3%), erythema nodosum (2.6%), and cellulitis (0.7%).[91] A similar variety of skin manifestations was also described in a study from former Czechoslovakia and in another one from Sweden.[62,92] A study from the United States noted that skin lesions of tularemia patients may be mistakenly diagnosed as herpes simplex or varicella zoster infection.[93]

Tularemia during pregnancy is rare.[94] Most cases have occurred without any adverse pregnancy outcomes; however, a case that occurred in the first trimester resulted in intrauterine fetal death.[95] Thus, tularemia during pregnancy requires special consideration, since the therapeutic options are limited (discussed further).[96]

Due to the diversity of disease manifestations, clinical diagnosis of tularemia may be challenging (see Chapter 17 for additional details). This is especially the case for a physician with little experience treating the disease or for clinical presentations other than ulceroglandular tularemia (Fig. 1). Even in the latter case, diagnosis may be difficult and not immediately obvious until lymph node enlargement becomes prominent. Diagnosis is often confirmed by serology.[46] Polymerase chain reaction (PCR) assays have been utilized most frequently with ulcer exudates for the diagnosis of ulceroglandular tularemia. More limited applications have also shown the utility of PCR for detection of *F. tularensis* DNA in pharyngeal swabs, lymph node aspirates, and respiratory specimens.[46]

Culture provides a conclusive diagnosis of infection. Its frequency of use as a confirmatory method varies; ~50% and ~ 10% of tularemia cases in the United States and Europe, respectively, are diagnosed by culture.[42,46] Because of the rarity as well as the sporadic nature of most tularemia cases, the organism is not easily identified upon culture recovery. Due to the low infectious dose for *F. tularensis,* laboratory workers have an increased risk of exposure, particularly when manipulating cultures.

TREATMENT, PREVENTION, AND VACCINATION

Historically, treatment of tularemia has relied on the use of aminoglycosides, tetracyclines, and chloramphenicol (see Chapter 19 for additional details). Since their introduction, aminoglycosides have been the first line of treatment for severe cases, since they are bactericidal and demonstrate low relapse rates. The drugs of choice are gentamicin or streptomycin, since their efficacy against tularemia and high cure rate have been proven for many decades (Table 2).[97,98] Due to streptomycin's marked ototoxicity, it is very rarely used today and, in fact, is not available in many countries. It is still an option for the rare cases of tularemia meningitis in combination with antibiotics with good cerebrospinal fluid penetration. For other forms of tularemia, gentamicin is the recommended form of treatment.[97] There are practical disadvantages of using aminoglycosides, since they require parenteral administration and continuous monitoring of serum levels; therefore, they are preferentially used for serious forms of tularemia and in cases where there are few alternatives, such as treatment of children and pregnant women.[94,99] In contrast to aminoglycosides, the widely used tetracyclines have the drawback of being bacteriostatic, and relapses are relatively common, at least when given in standard doses. Still, due to its excellent pharmacokinetics, the preferred tetracycline, doxycycline, has for many decades been the most commonly used treatment for less severe cases of tularemia, such as uncomplicated ulceroglandular tularemia (see Table 2 for details).

Besides aminoglycosides and tetracyclines, quinolones demonstrate excellent in vitro efficacy against *F. tularensis,* and minimal inhibitory concentrations are extremely low for strains of subsp. *tularensis* and *holarctica.*[98,100] In addition, several studies have demonstrated excellent clinical efficacy of ciprofloxacin,[47,101,102] moxifloxacin,[103] and levofloxacin.[104] Thus, clinical evidence and microbiological data strongly support that ciprofloxacin, and possibly moxifloxacin and levofloxacin, are drugs of choice for treatment of uncomplicated tularemia and as a second line of treatment for severe infections.[9,99] However, quinolones are not approved in the United States by the Food and Drug Administration (FDA). Nonetheless, newer treatment guidance in the United States recommends oral levofloxacin or ciprofloxacin for skin and soft tissue infection due to *F. tularensis.*[105] Accumulating evidence also indicates that ciprofloxacin may be an alternative for the treatment of children and pregnant women.[94,101] Oral administration of ciprofloxacin, or alternatively doxycycline, is the drug of choice for treatment in a mass casualty setting.[9] Penicillins, cephalosporins, macrolides, lincosamides, and trimoxazole all lack proven efficacy for treatment of tularemia, even though *F. tularensis* exhibits susceptibility in vitro to parental cephalosporins. As noted earlier, there is widespread natural resistance against erythromycin among strains of *F. tularensis* subsp. *holarctica.*[100,106]

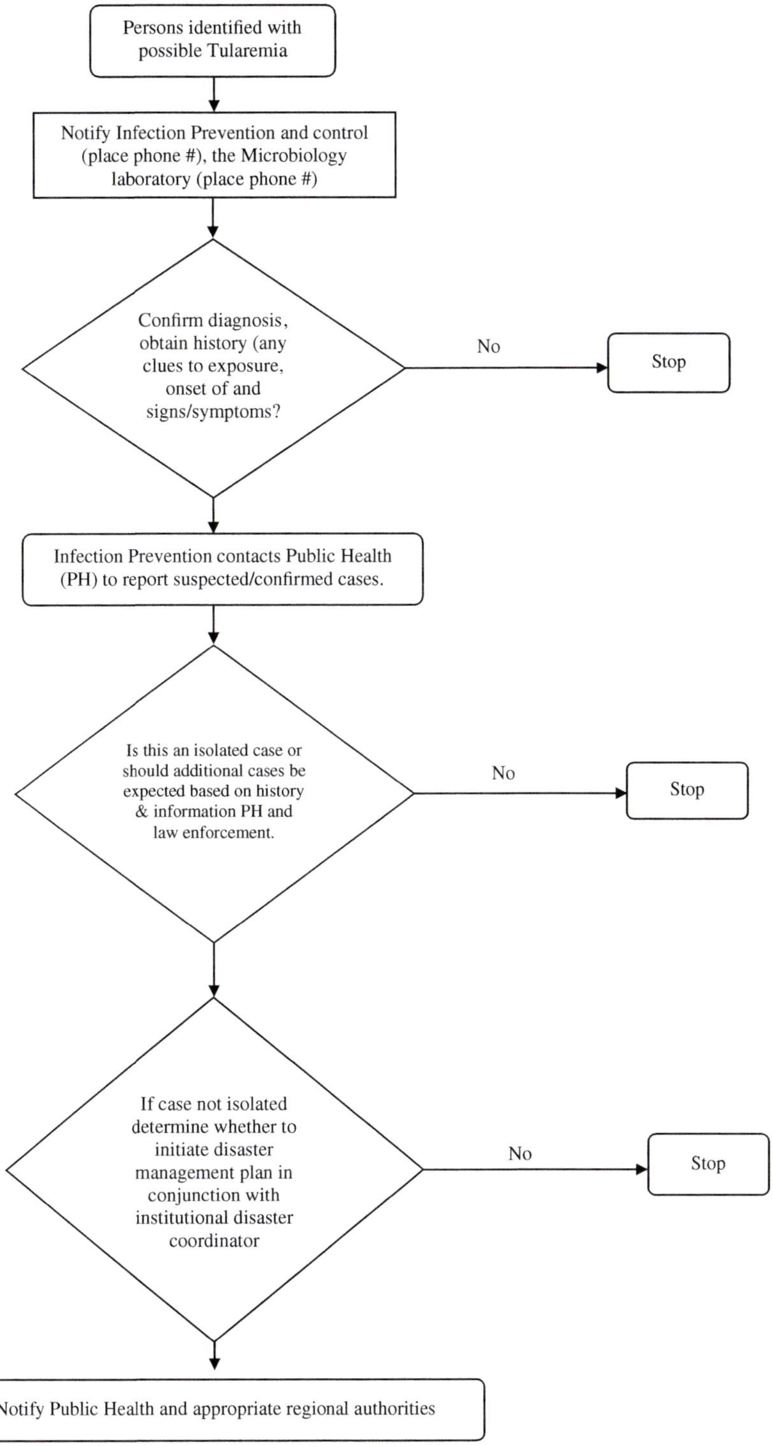

FIG. 1 Steps in assessing a patient with suspected *F. tularensis* infection including notifications of key personnel to facilitate safe care and activate infection prevention and control and public health processes. If bioterrorism is suspected, both public health authorities and law enforcement may provide additional information about potential exposure or history to obtain. Standard precautions are utilized but no transmission-based precautions are required.

TABLE 2
Preferred and Alternative Treatment and Prophylaxis for Tularemia (*F. tularensis*)

Indication/ Population	Recommended Antibiotics and Dosages	Alternative	Notes
SERIOUS DISEASE			
Adults (includes pregnant women)	• Streptomycin 10 mg/kg IM q 12h (1 g IM q12h)[a] × 7–10 days OR • Gentamicin 5 mg/kg/day IM/qd or IV divided q8h[a] × 7–10 days	Ciprofloxacin 500 mg PO or 400 mg IV q 12 h × 7–10 days	If fluoroquinolone is used, consider it with an aminoglycoside. In addition to ciprofloxacin, levofloxacin and moxifloxacin have been used in clinical settings Once-daily dosing of gentamicin is acceptable (with desired levels of at least 5 µg/mL)
Children	• Streptomycin 15–20 mg/kg IM q 12 (1 g IM q12h)[a] × 7–10 days OR • Gentamicin 5 mg/kg/day IM or IV divided q 8–12 h (not to exceed 2 g/d) and with desired levels of at least 5 µg/mL[a] × 7–10 days	Ciprofloxacin 15 mg/kg/dose IV q 12 h × 7–10 days	Once-daily dosing could be considered in consultation with a pediatric infectious disease specialist and a pharmacist
MENINGITIS			
Adults (includes pregnant women)	• Streptomycin 10 mg/kg IM q 12 h (1 g IM q12h)[a] OR Gentamicin 5 mg/kg/day IM/qd or IV divided q8h[a] • PLUS either ciprofloxacin 500 mg po OR 400 mg IV q 12 h[a] OR doxycycline 100 mg IV or po q 12 h OR chloramphenicol 15–25 mg/kg IV q 6 h (not to exceed 4 g/d) × 14–21 d		Once-daily dosing of gentamicin is acceptable (with desired levels of at least 5 µg/mL)
Children	• Gentamicin 5 mg/kg/day IM/qd or IV divided q8h (with desired levels of at least 5 µg/mL)[a] PLUS either ciprofloxacin 20–30 mg/kg/d IV divided q 8–12 h (not to exceed 1.2 g/d) OR doxycycline 2.2–4.4 mg/kg/d IV divided q 12 h (not to exceed 200 mg/d) × 14–21 d		Once-daily dosing could be considered in consultation with a pediatric infectious disease specialist and a pharmacist
MILD TO MODERATE DISEASE			
Adults (includes pregnant women)	• Ciprofloxacin 500 mg po BID × 10–14 days OR • Doxycycline 100 mg po BID × 14–21 d	Streptomycin 10 mg/kg IM q 12 h (1 g IM q12h) OR Gentamicin 5 mg/kg/day IM/qd[a] could be considered in pregnant females × 14 days	Relapses have been reported with doxycycline
Children	• Gentamicin 5 mg/kg/day IM/qd or IV divided q8h[a] OR • Ciprofloxacin 20–40 mg/kg/d PO divided q 12 h (not to exceed 1.5 g/d) × 10–14 d		Once-daily dosing could be considered in consultation with a pediatric infectious disease specialist and a pharmacist

TABLE 2
Preferred and Alternative Treatment and Prophylaxis for Tularemia (*F. tularensis*)—cont'd

Indication/ Population	Recommended Antibiotics and Dosages	Alternative	Notes
MASS CASUALTY/POSTEXPOSURE PROPHYLAXIS			
Adults (includes pregnant women)	• Ciprofloxacin 500 mg po BID × 14 d OR doxycycline 100 mg po BID × 10–14 d	Streptomycin 10 mg/kg IM q 12 h (1 g IM q12h) OR Gentamicin 5 mg/kg/day IM/qd[a] could be considered in pregnant females × 14 days	Because relapses have been reported with doxycycline some experts prefer ciprofloxacin
Children	• Doxycycline (for children ≥8 years) × 14 days o Weight < 45 kg: 2.2 mg/kg PO q12h (maximum daily dose, 200 mg) o Weight ≥ 45 kg: use adult dosing	• Ciprofloxacin 15 mg/kg PO q12h (maximum daily dose, 1 g) × 14 days	

PO, oral; *IV*, intravenous; *IM*, intramuscular; *q*, every; *BID*, twice daily; *qd*, daily; *h*, hours; *g*, grams; *mg*, milligrams; *kg*, kilograms.
[a]Dosing assumes normal renal function; adjust as appropriate for renal impairment.

No tularemia vaccines are approved in Western countries, despite some history of tularemia vaccine development. In the United States, vaccines comprised of *F. tularensis* bacteria killed by various methods were used in at-risk populations such as field workers between the 1930s and 1950s, but with little obvious or lasting success.[6,107] On the other hand, the USSR developed a number of live attenuated strains from *F. tularensis* subsp. *holarctica* isolates by in vitro passage and antisera exposure.[8,108,109] Mass vaccination campaigns in Russia in the late 1940s using these strains appear to have reduced the incidence of disease.[8,109] Live attenuated strains, including one designated Strain 15, are still produced by the Gamaleia Institute in Moscow and remain in use today in Russia and other former Soviet Union (FSU) republics, mostly for outbreak control.[109] Beginning in the 1950s, the US Department of Defense (DoD) developed and explored the use of LVS, which was derived from a mixture of attenuated Russian vaccine strains, as a vaccine primarily for military use. Lots of LVS were produced under contracts for DoD and more recently for the US National Institutes of Health, with a view toward potential civilian use.[110,111] Safety and immunogenicity studies of LVS performed under US FDA Investigational New Drug (IND) status have been reported.[111–113] Not surprisingly, given the low incidence of tularemia in the United States and elsewhere, LVS has not been evaluated for efficacy in field trials. Remarkably, naïve and LVS-vaccinated volunteers were subjected to parenteral and aerosol challenge with virulent *F. tularensis* in the late 1950s. Outcomes depended on vaccination doses and the stringency of the challenge doses, but in general, vaccination improved challenge outcomes. At present, licensing of a tularemia vaccine awaits evaluation either in field trials, which are difficult to envision, or by further safety studies coupled with establishing efficacy in appropriate animal models, as is now an option in the United States under the FDA's "Animal Rule."[114,115] Until such efforts come to fruition, control of tularemia outside of Russia and FSU countries will continue to rely on efficient diagnosis and drug treatment.

SUMMARY

Due to the threat of intentional misuse of *F. tularensis*, vigilance for unusual presentations or unexpected cases of tularemia is important (Fig. 1). For example, a cluster of pneumonic cases in an urban setting might raise suspicion. Given the severity of illness associated with primary respiratory tularemia, particularly those due to *F. tularensis* subsp. *tularensis* strains, an increase in respiratory tularemia cases, in particular, should prompt an investigation to identify the source of exposure and verify consistency with natural occurrence. As discussed, the primary clinical manifestation of aerosolized *F. tularensis* is expected to be respiratory disease and systemic infection, if not treated. Aerosols might also contaminate the eye, resulting in oculoglandular tularemia.

Awareness of the local epidemiology is critical for identifying unusual or unexpected routes of *F. tularensis* transmission that may present. Recovery of isolates from naturally occurring cases of tularemia provides an understanding of strain types and antimicrobial susceptibility profiles in endemic areas, which is important for differentiating between naturally occurring cases and those that may arise from an intentional release. Clearly, unusual presentations or cases of tularemia should prompt an increased effort to recover isolates for strain typing, antimicrobial susceptibility monitoring, and appropriate response interventions.

ACKNOWLEDGMENTS

Grant support was obtained from the Swedish Medical Research Council (K2012-3469 and K2013-8621), Västerbottens läns landsting (Spjutspetsmedel, VLL-582571, Centrala ALF medel, VLL-463691), and the Medical Faculty, Umeå University, Umeå, Sweden.

REFERENCES

1. McCoy GW, Chapin CW. Further observations on a plague like disease of rodents with a preliminary note on the causative agent *Bacterium tularense*. *J Infect Dis.* 1912;10:61–72.
2. McCoy G, Chapin CV. *Bacterium tularense*—the cause of a plague-like disease of rodents. *Public Health Bull.* 1912;53:17–23.
3. Wherry WB, Lamb BH. Infection of man with *Bacterium tularense*. *J Infect Dis.* 1914;15:331–340.
4. Ohara S. Studies on Yato-Byo (Ohara's disease, tularemia in Japan), report I. *Jpn J Exp Med.* 1954;24:69–85.
5. Francis E. A summary of the present knowledge of tularemia. *Medicine.* 1928;7:411–426.
6. Foshay L. Tularemia. *Ann Rev Micro.* 1950;4:313–330.
7. Sjöstedt A. Tularemia: history, epidemiology, pathogen physiology, and clinical manifestations. *Ann N Y Acad Sci.* 2007;1105:1–29.
8. Sändstrom G. The tularaemia vaccine. *J Chem Tech Biotechnol.* 1994;59:315–320.
9. Dennis DT, Inglesby TV, Henderson DA, et al. Tularemia as a biological weapon: medical and public health management. *JAMA.* 2001;285(21):2763–2773.
10. Nano FE, Elkins KL. Francisella. In: Borriello S, Murray P, Funke G, eds. *Topley and Wilson's Microbiology and Microbial Infections.* vol. 2. London: Hodder Arnold; 2005:1752–1760.
11. Hollis DG, Weaver RE, Steigerwalt AG, Wenger JD, Moss CW, Brenner DJ. *Francisella philomiragia* comb. nov. (formerly *Yersinia philomiragia*) and *Francisella tularensis* biogroup novicida (formerly *Francisella novicida*) associated with human disease. *J Clin Microbiol.* 1989;27(7):1601–1608.
12. Forsman M, Sandström G, Sjöstedt A. Analysis of 16S ribosomal DNA sequences of *Francisella* strains and utilization for determination of the phylogeny of the genus and for identification of strains by PCR. *Int J Syst Bacteriol.* 1994;44:38–46.
13. Dwibedi C, Birdsell D, Larkeryd A, et al. Long-range dispersal moved *Francisella tularensis* into Western Europe from the east. *Microb Genom.* 2016;2(12):e000100.
14. Gunn JS, Ernst RK. The structure and function of *Francisella* lipopolysaccharide. *Ann N Y Acad Sci.* 2007;1105:202–218.
15. Bandara AB, Champion AE, Wang X, et al. Isolation and mutagenesis of a capsule-like complex (CLC) from *Francisella tularensis*, and contribution of the CLC to *F. tularensis* virulence in mice. *PLoS One.* 2011;6(4):e19003.
16. Kanistanon D, Powell DA, Hajjar AM, et al. Role of *Francisella* lipid a phosphate modification in virulence and long-term protective immune responses. *Infect Immun.* 2012;80(3):943–951.
17. Bröms JE, Sjöstedt A, Lavander M. The role of the *Francisella tularensis* pathogenicity island in type VI secretion, intracellular survival, and modulation of host cell signaling. *Front Microbiol.* 2010;1:136.
18. Jones BD, Faron M, Rasmussen JA, Fletcher JR. Uncovering the components of the *Francisella tularensis* virulence stealth strategy. *Front Cell Infect Microbiol.* 2014;4:32.
19. Celli J, Zahrt TC. Mechanisms of *Francisella tularensis* intracellular pathogenesis. *Cold Spring Harb Perspect Med.* 2013;3(4):a010314.
20. Nano FE, Schmerk C. The *Francisella* pathogenicity island. *Ann N Y Acad Sci.* 2007;1105:122–137.
21. Nano FE, Zhang N, Cowley SC, et al. A *Francisella tularensis* pathogenicity island required for intramacrophage growth. *J Bacteriol.* 2004;186(19):6430–6436.
22. Bröms JE, Meyer L, Sun K, Lavander M, Sjöstedt A. Unique substrates secreted by the type VI secretion system of *Francisella tularensis* during intramacrophage infection. *PLoS One.* 2012;7(11):e50473.
23. Bröms JE, Meyer L, Lavander M, Larsson P, Sjöstedt A. DotU and VgrG, core components of type VI secretion systems, are essential for *Francisella* LVS pathogenicity. *PLoS One.* 2012;7(4):e34639.
24. Eigelsbach HT, Downs CM. Prophylactic effectiveness of live and killed tularemia vaccines. *J Immunol.* 1961;87:415–425.
25. Bosio CM, Bielefeldt-Ohmann H, Belisle JT. Active suppression of the pulmonary immune response by *Francisella tularensis* Schu4. *J Immunol.* 2007;178(7):4538–4547.
26. Gillette DD, Curry HM, Cremer T, et al. Virulent type A *Francisella tularensis* actively suppresses cytokine responses in human monocytes. *Front Cell Infect Microbiol.* 2014;4:45.
27. Cowley SC, Elkins KL. Immunity to *Francisella*. *Front Microbiol.* 2011;2:26.
28. Dotson RJ, Rabadi SM, Westcott EL, et al. Repression of inflammasome by *Francisella tularensis* during early stages of infection. *J Biol Chem.* 2013;288(33):23844–23857.

29. Tärnvik A, Chu MC. New approaches to diagnosis and therapy of tularemia. *Ann N Y Acad Sci.* 2007;1105:378–404.
30. Eden JS, Rose K, Ng J, et al. *Francisella tularensis* ssp. *holarctica* in ringtail possums, Australia. *Emerg Infect Dis.* 2017;23(7):1198–1201.
31. Jackson J, McGregor A, Cooley L, et al. *Francisella tularensis* subspecies *holarctica*, Tasmania, Australia, 2011. *Emerg Infect Dis.* 2012;18(9):1484–1486.
32. Larssen KW, Bergh K, Heier BT, Vold L, Afset JE. All-time high tularaemia incidence in Norway in 2011: report from the national surveillance. *Eur J Clin Microbiol Infect Dis.* 2014;33(11):1919–1926.
33. Rodriguez-Pastor R, Escudero R, Vidal D, et al. Density-dependent prevalence of *Francisella tularensis* in fluctuating vole populations, northwestern Spain. *Emerg Infect Dis.* 2017;23(8):1377–1379.
34. Centers for Disease Control. Tularemia; 2017. [Internet]. November 29, 2016 https://www.cdc.gov/tularemia/statistics/index.html. Accessed 15 November 2017.
35. European Centre for Disease Prevention and Control. Tularaemia—Annual Epidemiological Report 2016 [2014 Data]; 2017 [Internet] https://ecdc.europa.eu/en/publications-data/tularaemia-annual-epidemiological-report-2016-2014-data. Accessed 15 November 2017.
36. Petersen JM, Molins CR. Subpopulations of *Francisella tularensis* ssp. tularensis and holarctica: identification and associated epidemiology. *Future Microbiol.* 2010;5(4):649–661.
37. Staples JE, Kubota KA, Chalcraft LG, Mead PS, Petersen JM. Epidemiologic and molecular analysis of human tularemia, United States, 1964-2004. *Emerg Infect Dis.* 2006;12(7):1113–1118.
38. Hopla CE. The ecology of tularemia. *Adv Vet Sci Comp Med.* 1974;18:25–53.
39. Keim P, Johansson A, Wagner DM. Molecular epidemiology, evolution, and ecology of *Francisella*. *Ann N Y Acad Sci.* 2007;1105:30–66.
40. Larssen KW, Afset JE, Heier BT, et al. Outbreak of tularaemia in Central Norway, January to March 2011. *Euro Surveill.* 2011;16(13):1–3.
41. Gurycova D, Vyrostekova V, Khanakah G, Kocianova E, Stanek G. Importance of surveillance of tularemia natural foci in the known endemic area of Central Europe, 1991-1997. *Wien Klin Wochenschr.* 2001;113(11–12):433–438.
42. Centers for Disease Control and Prevention. Tularemia—United States, 2001-2010. *MMWR Morb Mortal Wkly Rep.* 2013;62(47):963–966.
43. Hestvik G, Warns-Petit E, Smith LA, et al. The status of tularemia in Europe in a one-health context: a review. *Epidemiol Infect.* 2015;143(10):2137–2160.
44. Gurcan S. Epidemiology of tularemia. *Balkan Med J.* 2014;31(1):3–10.
45. Grunow R, Kalaveshi A, Kuhn A, Mulliqi-Osmani G, Ramadani N. Surveillance of tularaemia in Kosovo, 2001 to 2010. *Euro Surveill.* 2012;17(28):1–7.
46. Maurin M, Gyuranecz M. Tularaemia: clinical aspects in Europe. *Lancet Infect Dis.* 2016;16(1):113–124.
47. Centers for Disease Control and Prevention. Tularemia—Missouri, 2000-2007. *MMWR Morb Mortal Wkly Rep.* 2009;58(27):744–748.
48. Eliasson H, Lindback J, Nuorti JP, Arneborn M, Giesecke J, Tegnell A. The 2000 tularemia outbreak: a case-control study of risk factors in disease-endemic and emergent areas, Sweden. *Emerg Infect Dis.* 2002;8(9):956–960.
49. Rossow H, Sissonen S, Koskela KA, et al. Detection of *Francisella tularensis* in voles in Finland. *Vector Borne Zoonotic Dis.* 2014;14(3):193–198.
50. Brett ME, Respicio-Kingry LB, Yendell S, et al. Outbreak of *Francisella novicida* bacteremia among inmates at a Louisiana correctional facility. *Clin Infect Dis.* 2014;59(6):826–833.
51. Wenger JD, Hollis DG, Weaver RE, et al. Infection caused by *Francisella philomiragia* (formerly *Yersinia philomiragia*). A newly recognized human pathogen. *Ann Intern Med.* 1989;110:888–892.
52. Ughetto E, Hery-Arnaud G, Cariou ME, et al. An original case of *Francisella tularensis* subsp. *holarctica* bacteremia after a near-drowning accident. *Infect Dis (Lond).* 2015;47(8):588–590.
53. Desvars-Larrive A, Liu X, Hjertqvist M, Sjostedt A, Johansson A, Ryden P. High-risk regions and outbreak modelling of tularemia in humans. *Epidemiol Infect.* 2017;145(3):482–490.
54. Desvars A, Furberg M, Hjertqvist M, et al. Epidemiology and ecology of tularemia in Sweden, 1984-2012. *Emerg Infect Dis.* 2015;21(1):32–39.
55. Feldman KA, Enscore RE, Lathrop SL, et al. An outbreak of primary pneumonic tularemia on Martha's Vineyard. *N Engl J Med.* 2001;345(22):1601–1606.
56. Reintjes R, Dedushaj I, Gjini A, et al. Tularemia outbreak investigation in Kosovo: case control and environmental studies. *Emerg Infect Dis.* 2002;8(1):69–73.
57. Dahlstrand S, Ringertz O, Zetterberg B. Airborne tularemia in Sweden. *Scand J Infect Dis.* 1971;3:7–16.
58. Vogler AJ, Birdsell D, Price LB, et al. Phylogeography of *Francisella tularensis*: global expansion of a highly fit clone. *J Bacteriol.* 2009;191(8):2474–2484.
59. Petersen JM, Carlson JK, Dietrich G, et al. Multiple *Francisella tularensis* subspecies and clades, tularemia outbreak, Utah. *Emerg Infect Dis.* 2008;14(12):1928–1930.
60. Johansson A, Larkeryd A, Widerstrom M, et al. An outbreak of respiratory tularemia caused by diverse clones of *Francisella tularensis*. *Clin Infect Dis.* 2014;59(11):1546–1553.
61. Svensson K, Back E, Eliasson H, et al. Landscape epidemiology of tularemia outbreaks in Sweden. *Emerg Infect Dis.* 2009;15(12):1937–1947.
62. Eliasson H, Back E. Tularaemia in an emergent area in Sweden: an analysis of 234 cases in five years. *Scand J Infect Dis.* 2007;39(10):880–889.
63. Evans ME, Gregory DW, Schaffner W, McGee ZA. Tularemia: a 30-year experience with 88 cases. *Medicine.* 1985;64:251–269.
64. Stuart B, Pullen R, Tularemia pneumonia. Review of American literature and twenty-three cases,

with observations at autopsy in one. *Am J Med Sci.* 1935;55:223–236.

65. Steinrucken J, Graber P. Oropharyngeal tularemia. *CMAJ.* 2014;186(1):E62.
66. Cerny Z. Tularemia—history, epidemiology, clinical aspects, diagnosis and therapy. *Cas Lek Cesk.* 2002;141(9):270–275.
67. Dienst Jr FT. Tularemia: a perusal of three hundred thirty-nine cases. *J La State Med Soc.* 1963;115:114–127.
68. Tärnvik A, Berglund L. Tularaemia. *Eur Respir J.* 2003;21(2):361–373.
69. Matyas BT, Nieder HS, Telford 3rd SR. Pneumonic tularemia on Martha's Vineyard: clinical, epidemiologic, and ecological characteristics. *Ann N Y Acad Sci.* 2007;1105:351–377.
70. Thomas LD, Schaffner W. Tularemia pneumonia. *Infect Dis Clin N Am.* 2010;24(1):43–55.
71. Vayrynen SA, Saarela E, Henry J, Lahti S, Harju T, Kauma H. Pneumonic tularaemia: experience of 58 cases from 2000 to 2012 in Northern Finland. *Infect Dis (Lond).* 2017;49(10):758–764.
72. Syrjala H, Kujala P, Myllyla V, Salminen A. Airborne transmission of tularemia in farmers. *Scand J Infect Dis.* 1985;17(4):371–375.
73. Syrjala H, Koskela P, Kujala P, Myllyla V. Guillain-Barre syndrome and tularemia pleuritis with high adenosine deaminase activity in pleural fluid. *Infection.* 1989;17(3):152–153.
74. Kohlmann R, Wolf PJ, Gatermann SG. Pleuropulmonary tularemia in a 63-year-old hunter in Germany. *Dtsch Med Wochenschr.* 2014;139(11):534–537.
75. Briere M, Kaladji A, Douane F, et al. *Francisella tularensis* aortitis. *Infection.* 2016;44(2):263–265.
76. Terrada C, Azza S, Bodaghi B, Le Hoang P, Drancourt M. Rabbit hunter uveitis: case report of tularemia uveitis. *BMC Ophthalmol.* 2016;16(1):157.
77. Arslan F, Karagoz E, Zemheri E, Vahaboglu H, Mert A. Tick-related facial cellulitis caused by *Francisella tularensis*. *Infez Med.* 2016;24(2):140–143.
78. Gurkov R, Kisser U, Splettstosser W, Hogardt M, Krause E. Tularaemia of middle ear with suppurative lymphadenopathy and retropharyngeal abscess. *J Laryngol Otol.* 2009;123(11):1252–1257.
79. Guerpillon B, Boibieux A, Guenne C, et al. Keep an ear out for *Francisella tularensis*: otomastoiditis cases after canyoneering. *Front Med (Lausanne).* 2016;3:9.
80. Celik T, Yuksel D, Kosker M, Turkoglu EB. Unilateral acute dacryocystitis associated with oculoglandular tularemia: a case report. *Semin Ophthalmol.* 2013;28(2):91–93.
81. Celik T, Kosker M, Kirboga K. An atypical case of tularemia presented with pseudoptosis. *Infection.* 2014;42(4):785–788.
82. Uzun MO, Yanik K, Erdem M, Kostakoglu U, Yilmaz G, Tanriverdi CY. Epidemiological and clinical characteristics and management of oropharyngeal tularemia outbreak. *Turk J Med Sci.* 2015;45(4):902–906.
83. Tunga U, Bodrumlu E, Acikgoz A, Acikgoz G. A case of tularemia presenting as a dental abscess: case report. *Oral Surg Oral Med Oral Pathol Oral Radiol Endod.* 2007;103(1):e33–e35.
84. Barbaz M, Piau C, Tadie JM, et al. Rhombencephalitis caused by *Francisella tularensis*. *J Clin Microbiol.* 2013;51(10):3454–3455.
85. Altuntas EE, Polat K, Durmus K, Uysal IO, Muderris S. Tularemia and the oculoglandular syndrome of Parinaud. *Braz J Infect Dis.* 2012;16(1):90–91.
86. Yeom JS, Rhie K, Park JS, et al. The first pediatric case of tularemia in Korea: manifested with pneumonia and possible infective endocarditis. *Korean J Pediatr.* 2015;58(10):398–401.
87. Ylipalosaari P, Ala-Kokko TI, Tuominen H, Syrjala H. Guillain-Barre syndrome and ulceroglandular tularemia. *Infection.* 2013;41(4):881–883.
88. Pettersson T, Nyberg P, Nordstrom D, Riska H. Similar pleural fluid findings in pleuropulmonary tularemia and tuberculous pleurisy. *Chest.* 1996;109(2):572–575.
89. Fachinger P, Tini GM, Grobholz R, Gambazzi F, Fankhauser H, Irani S. Pulmonary tularaemia: all that looks like cancer is not necessarily cancer—case report of four consecutive cases. *BMC Pulm Med.* 2015;15:27.
90. Klotz SA, Penn RL, Provenza JM. The unusual presentations of tularemia. Bacteremia, pneumonia, and rhabdomyolysis. *Arch Int Med.* 1987;147(2):214.
91. Senel E, Satilmis O, Acar B. Dermatologic manifestations of tularemia: a study of 151 cases in the mid-Anatolian region of Turkey. *Int J Dermatol.* 2015;54(1):e33–e37.
92. Cerny Z. Skin manifestations of tularemia. *Int J Dermatol.* 1994;33(7):468–470.
93. Byington CL, Bender JM, Ampofo K, et al. Tularemia with vesicular skin lesions may be mistaken for infection with herpes viruses. *Clin Infect Dis.* 2008;47(1):e4–e6.
94. Yesilyurt M, Kilic S, Celebsmall i UB, Gul S. Tularemia during pregnancy: report of four cases. *Scand J Infect Dis.* 2013;45(4):324–328.
95. Ata N, Kilic S, Ovet G, Alatas N, Celebi B. Tularemia during pregnancy. *Infection.* 2013;41(4):753–756.
96. Kosker M, Celik T, Yuksel D. Treatment of tularemia during pregnancy. *J Infect Dev Ctries.* 2015;9(1):118–119.
97. World Health Organization. WHO Guidelines on Tularaemia. Geneva, Switzerland: WHO; 2007.
98. Johansson A, Urich SK, Chu MC, Sjostedt A, Tarnvik A. In vitro susceptibility to quinolones of *Francisella tularensis* subspecies tularensis. *Scand J Infect Dis.* 2002;34(5):327–330.
99. Boisset S, Caspar Y, Sutera V, Maurin M. New therapeutic approaches for treatment of tularaemia: a review. *Front Cell Infect Microbiol.* 2014;4:40.
100. Ikaheimo I, Syrjala H, Karhukorpi J, Schildt R, Koskela M. In vitro antibiotic susceptibility of *Francisella tularensis* isolated from humans and animals. *J Antimicrob Chemother.* 2000;46(2):287–290.
101. Johansson A, Berglund L, Gothefors L, Sjöstedt A, Tärnvik A. Ciprofloxacin for treatment of tularemia in children. *Pediatr Infect Dis J.* 2000;19(5):449–453.

102. Perez-Castrillon JL, Bachiller-Luque P, Martin-Luquero M, Mena-Martin FJ, Herreros V. Tularemia epidemic in northwestern Spain: clinical description and therapeutic response. *Clin Infect Dis.* 2001;33(4):573–576.
103. Meric M, Willke A, Finke EJ, et al. Evaluation of clinical, laboratory, and therapeutic features of 145 tularemia cases: the role of quinolones in oropharyngeal tularemia. *APMIS.* 2008;116(1):66–73.
104. Aranda EA. Treatment of tularemia with levofloxacin. *Clin Microbiol Infect.* 2001;7(3):167–168.
105. Stevens DL, Bisno AL, Chambers HF, et al. Practice guidelines for the diagnosis and management of skin and soft tissue infections: 2014 update by the Infectious Diseases Society of America. *Clin Infect Dis.* 2014;59(2):e10–e52.
106. Karlsson E, Golovliov I, Larkeryd A, et al. Clonality of erythromycin resistance in *Francisella tularensis. J Antimicrob Chemother.* 2016;71(10):2815–2823.
107. Tärnvik A. Nature of protective immunity to *Francisella tularensis. Rev Infect Dis.* 1989;11:440–451.
108. Tigertt WD. Soviet viable *Pasteurella tularensis* vaccines. A review of selected articles. *Bacteriol Rev.* 1962;26:354–373.
109. Feodorova VA, Sayapina LV, Corbel MJ, Motin VL. Russian vaccines against especially dangerous bacterial pathogens. *Emerg Microbes Infect.* 2014;3(12):e86.
110. Pasetti MF, Cuberos L, Horn TL, et al. An improved *Francisella tularensis* live vaccine strain (LVS) is well tolerated and highly immunogenic when administered to rabbits in escalating doses using various immunization routes. *Vaccine.* 2008;26(14):1773–1785.
111. El Sahly HM, Atmar RL, Patel SM, et al. Safety, reactogenicity and immunogenicity of *Francisella tularensis* live vaccine strain in humans. *Vaccine.* 2009;27(36):4905–4911.
112. Waag DM, McKee Jr KT, Sandstrom G, et al. Cell-mediated and humoral immune responses after vaccination of human volunteers with the live vaccine strain of *Francisella tularensis. Clin Diagn Lab Immunol.* 1995;2(2):143–148.
113. Waag DM, Sändstrom G, England MJ, Williams JC. Immunogenicity of a new lot of *Francisella tularensis* live vaccine strain in human volunteers. *FEMS Immunol Med Microbiol.* 1996;13(3):205–209.
114. Snoy PJ. Establishing efficacy of human products using animals: the US Food and Drug Administration's "animal rule". *Vet Pathol.* 2010;47(5):774–778.
115. Elkins KL, Kurtz SL, De Pascalis R. Progress, challenges, and opportunities in *Francisella* vaccine development. *Expert Rev Vaccines.* 2016;15(9):1183–1196.

CHAPTER 5

Plague: The *Yersinia pestis* Infection

MICHEL DRANCOURT
IHU Méditerranée Infection, MEPHI, Aix-Marseille-Université, Marseille, France

HISTORY

Plague is a deadly zoonosis caused by *Yersinia pestis*.[1] It is a reportable and quarantinable disease covered by national and international health regulations. Plague pandemics have had huge impacts on past demography and social organizations, as recorded by historical European documents. *Y. pestis* has been a long companion of populations detected in Bronze Age individuals[2] and was then responsible for the 6th-century Justinian plague[3] and the medieval Black Death plague, which claimed one-third of the European population.[4,5] The current pandemic began in Asia at the end of the 19th and opened the microbiological area of plague after Alexandre Yersin first isolated the culprit bacterium in 1894 in Hong Kong.[6] This third pandemic now involves the Old and New Worlds. *Yersinia pestis* genotyping indicates that ancient *Y. pestis* organisms belonged to the Orientalis biotype, suggesting that this biotype was responsible for all three historical pandemics and that it may have the unique capability to rapidly spread in human populations over large geographic areas.[5,7] Central Asia plateau seems to give birth to all pandemics, which can be understood as the spreading of clones of the *Y. pestis*, which itself derives from a common ancestor with *Yersinia pseudotuberculosis*, its closest pathogenic parent expressing a different pattern of epidemiology and clinical pictures.[8,9]

MICROBIOLOGY

Y. pestis is classified among the enteric bacteria belonging to the gamma-proteobacteria. It is a nonsporulated, aerobic, Gram-negative, oxidase-negative, urease-negative, catalase-positive bacillus growing at 28°C, pH 7.4. Biochemical profiling distinguishes nine subspecies, including *Y. pestis* subsp. *pestis* and additional subspecies *angola*, *altaica*, *caucasica*, *hissarica*, *quinghaiensis*, *talassica*, *ulegeica*, and *xilingolensis*, whose pathogenicity remains unknown after their isolation from various rodent species in Angola (subspecies *angola*) and Central Asia.[10] *Yersinia pestis* subsp. *pestis* organisms' biotypes Antiqua are glycerol and nitrate reduction-positive, Medievalis are glycerol-positive and nitrate reduction-negative, and Orientalis are glycerol-negative and nitrate reduction-positive. Microtus biotype organisms have been proposed to include rhamnose-positive rodent strains, while rhamnose-positive, Antiqua-like isolates occasionally isolated from patients in China could form a fifth biotype: Intermedium.[11] *Y. pestis* 4.6–4.65 Mb genome may have emerged by reductive evolution from the 4.72 Mb-*Y. pseudotuberculosis* genome.[8] It comprises one circular chromosome along with a 70–75-kb plasmid (termed pCD1, pCad, pVW, pYV, or pLcr plasmid) encoding a type III secretion system (Yops for "*Yersinia* Outer Proteins") and V antigen. Also, a 100–110-kb plasmid (termed pFra/Tox, pFra, pTox, pMT1, or pYT plasmid) encodes the capsular F1 glycoprotein antigen and the toxin Ymt. A 9.5-kb plasmid (termed pPst, pPla, pPCP1, or pYP plasmid) encodes the plasminogen activator Pla, promoting the systemic spread of *Y. pestis* and pesticin, a bacteriocine involved in iron capture in mammalian hosts.[1] The chromosome-encoded lipopolysaccharide endotoxin is also a major factor in pathogenicity. *Y. pestis* subsp. *pestis* Orientalis isolates are unique in their capacity to stabilize a bacteriophage into the chromosome.[12] The organisms' characteristics, which encompass virulence factors, membrane proteins, protease, and the iron capture system, allow it to evade the immune system and replicate in the lymph nodes and lungs.[13]

EPIDEMIOLOGY AND NATURAL HISTORY

Y. pestis can be regarded as a telluric organism sporadically reemerging first in rodent populations and then in individuals and populations in contact with such infected animals. Plague is, therefore, regularly reemerging in so-called plague foci in all continents except Antarctica and Oceania (Table 1). In particular,

Viral Outbreaks, Biosecurity, and Preparing for Mass Casualty Infectious Diseases Events
https://doi.org/10.1016/B978-0-323-54841-0.00007-X

TABLE 1
At a Glance: Key Features of *Yersinia pestis* and Plague

	Key Features	Clinical Correlations
Microbiology	Vector-borne, Gram-negative, fastidious bacterium evolved from *Yersinia pseudotuberculosis* by genome reduction and plasmid acquisition, comprising several biotypes	Vector-borne transmission and intense replication resulting in tissue destruction are important in pathogenesis
Epidemiology and ecology	• Zoonotic infection: *Y. pestis* infects a wide variety of mammals, and dogs are resistant • Humans infected by – Contact with infected animals – Arthropod bite – Inhalation of contaminated materials – Ingestion of contaminated materials • Three major clinical forms – Bubonic – Septicemic – Pneumonia • Primary mode of transmission can vary geographically	Contact and respiratory isolation of suspected/confirmed pulmonary plague cases
Clinical presentation	• Incubation time varies but averages 3–5 days • Specific symptoms follow route of infection – Mainly painful regional lymph nodes (buboes) after vector-borne inoculation – Respiratory form is the most serious	Fever, malaise, myalgia, cough, and headache are usually common to all forms
Diagnosis	Lateral flow assay, PCR on infected tissue, and/or direct culture	– Collect buboes' pus – Collect sputum
Treatment	Fluoroquinolones and gentamicin for septicemic and pneumonic plague or fluoroquinolones or tetracycline with gentamicin for bubonic plague Fluoroquinolones and cephalosporins effective in animal models Use droplet isolation for 48 h after appropriate antimicrobials are initiated	– Fluoroquinolones or tetracycline combined with gentamicin – Supportive therapy – Postexposure fluoroquinolones or tetracycline
Vaccination	• Live-attenuated EV76 strain as vaccine • No evaluation in controlling epidemics	– Avoiding contact with infected animals and materials – Avoiding contact with vectors: protective clothes, repellents – Adequate meat cooking

salt soils may preserve *Y. pestis* in some geographic areas, as observed in Algeria.[14] Contaminated soil may be a primary source of infection for burrowing rodents.[15] More than 200 species of rodents can be infected by *Y. pestis*, with plague-resistant species being regarded as reservoirs for *Y. pestis*.[1,10] Several ectoparasites, including ticks, have been found to be naturally infected with *Y. pestis*, but fleas are thought to be the vector of primary importance.[1] Also, the human lice *Pediculus humanus* has been found to be infected, including both the head lice and the body lice, and is a potential vector of *Y. pestis* for interhuman transmission of plague.[16,17] Carnivores can be infected after ingestion of contaminated rodents. Dogs and canids are resistant to plague.[18]

The complex life cycle of *Y. pestis* involving soil, ectoparasites, and mammals results in a variable prevalence of animal plague (enzoonosis) with sudden outbreaks of dying-off in plague-susceptible animals (epizoonoses). It remains endemic in many countries and has been reported in 21 countries in the Americas, Africa, and Asia over the past few decades.[4] During the last 15 years, eight geographic areas have experienced outbreaks of human plague after silent periods of

30–50 years: India in 1994, Zambia in 1996, Indonesia in 1997, Algeria in 2003 and 2009, Congo in 2005, Uganda in 2006, and Libya and China in 2009. Africa reports approximately 97% of the world's cases and plague is still active in Madagascar, as illustrated by the 2017–18 outbreak.[4,19] In the United States, activities with close extended contact with pet dogs (such as sleeping in bed with a pet dog) were significantly associated with plague.[20] In Europe, human cases have not been recently reported, but animal plague presently exists along the western banks of the Caspian Sea.

CLINICAL PRESENTATION AND DIAGNOSIS (SEE CHAPTER 17 FOR ADDITIONAL DETAILS)

Y. pestis is either inoculated through direct contact with a *Y. pestis*-infected animal carcass or more frequently by an animal ectoparasite. The incubation period is usually 3–7 days, and plague primarily presents a discrete inflammatory skin lesion at the site of inoculation along with an enlarged, painful regional lymph node called a "buboe," hence the bubonic form of plague. In addition to the bubo, which is a manifestation of inflammation, bubonic plague is characterized by chills, fever, myalgias, arthralgias, and weakness. The femoral and inguinal lymph nodes are the most frequently involved (bubo is Greek for "groin"), followed in frequency by axillary and cervical nodes. The bubo of plague is clinically distinguishable from enlarged lymph nodes owing to other causes by its association with systemic signs of toxemia and its rapid onset. Moreover, an outbreak of buboes is pathognomonic of plague. Bubonic plague usually rapidly responds to appropriate antibiotic therapy with the lymph node remaining enlarged and tender for 1 week. If untreated with an effective antibiotic, the patient will become increasingly toxic and will develop a septicemic form of plague, with a mortality risk of 50%–90%. Human ectoparasite transmission may have been underappreciated in the human-to-human transmission that may have played a key role during historical epidemics.[21,22] Transmission by the anthropophilic flea *Pulex irritans* and by the human body-louse *Pediculus humanus* has been suggested during familial cases of plague,[23,24] the latter being supported by experimental evidence.[25,26] In the case of the inoculation through skin lacerations after handling (typically skinning) dead animals or animal bites, bubonic or septicemic plague may be declared.[18,27] Overwhelming bacterial growth in the lymph node precedes the *Y. pestis* dissemination via the lymphatic and blood vessels to the spleen and liver, causing rapidly fatal septicemia, with dissemination in the lung resulting in secondary pneumonic plague, and in the meninges and cerebrospinal fluid (CSF), causing meningitis. *Y. pestis* rapidly multiplies in human tissues because it protects itself from the human immune system by serum resistance and evasion from innate immune functions.

Y. pestis may also infect after inhalation of *Y. pestis*-contaminated droplets when in close contact with an infected animal such as a cat[28] or a coughing patient (<1.5 m), leading to primary pneumonia (pneumonic plague) with an incubation period of 1–3 days after exposure to the patient. The patient will suddenly present with fever, chest pain, and bloody sputum in this deadly form with fatality rates >40% within 3 days of infection. Septicemic plague with invasion of the bloodstream can occur after the ingestion of *Y. pestis*-contaminated raw or poorly cooked food including goat and camel meat and liver.[18] However, septicemic plague most often follows the bubonic presentation and features a rapidly progressive, overwhelming toxemia. The patient may present with gastrointestinal symptoms including nausea, vomiting, diarrhea, and abdominal pain. Lack of immediate supportive therapy combined with ineffective antibiotic treatment renders septicemic plague fatal (Table 2). Rare clinical forms include meningeal plague, pharyngitis in patients who consumed raw or poorly cooked contaminated meat, such as camel meat, and features anterior cervical lymphadenitis. Pleuritis, endophthalmitis, and myocarditis are exceptional forms of plague.

Once plague is suspected, a few clinical specimens should be collected for rapid diagnosis while at the same time effective treatment is undertaken. If possible, obtain blood (3 sets of cultures in succession), sputum, urine, and lymph node fluid (aspirated using saline)[18] for culture (gold standard) and molecular tests including conventional PCR. The latter can be performed in qualified laboratories. Any ectoparasite found on the patient's body and clothes, as well as specimens from any animal suspected to be a potential source of infection, should also be collected. Clinical and environmental specimens should be handled in a Biosafety Level (BSL)-2 laboratory, but handling and culture of *Y. pestis* requires a BSL-3 laboratory. Plague is usually a reportable infection and quarantinable disease covered by national and international health regulations requiring reporting to public health authorities.

Point of care diagnostics use PCR-based assays[29] along with a commercially available dipstick immunochromatographic assay detecting the F1 capsular antigen.[30] This dipstick assay, which takes a few minutes,

TABLE 2
Preferred and Alternative Treatment and Prophylaxis for Plague (*Y. pestis*)

Indication/ population	Recommended antibiotic and dosages	Alternative	Notes
SEPTICEMIC/PNEUMONIC			
Adults	• Gentamicin 5 mg/kg IM or IV q24h OR 2 mg/kg loading dose followed by 1.7 mg/kg q8h OR • Streptomycin 1 g IM q12h	• Levofloxacin 500 mg IV or PO q24h OR • Ciprofloxacin 400 mg IV q8-12h OR 500–750 mg PO q12h OR • Doxycycline 100 mg IV or PO q12h OR 200 mg IV or PO q24h OR • Moxifloxacin 400 mg IV or PO q24h OR • Chloramphenicol 25 mg/kg IV q6h	Streptomycin availability limited so gentamicin is preferred. If meningitis suspected, use an agent that penetrates the central nervous system such as chloramphenicol.
Pregnant women	• Gentamicin 5 mg/kg IM or IV q24h OR 2 mg/kg loading dose followed by 1.7 mg/kg q8h	• Ciprofloxacin 400 mg IV q8-12h OR 500–750 mg PO q12h OR • Doxycycline 100 mg IV or PO q12h OR 200 mg IV or PO q24h	

Children	• Gentamicin 2.5 mg/kg/ dose IM or IV q8h OR
	• Streptomycin 15 mg/kg IM q12h (maximum 2 g/ day)
		• Levofloxacin 8 mg/kg/dose IV or PO q12h (max 250 mg per dose) OR
		• Ciprofloxacin 15 mg/kg/dose IV q12h (maximum 400 mg/dose) OR 20 mg/kg/dose PO q12h (maximum 500 mg/dose) OR
		• Doxycycline
		  ○ Weight <45 kg: 2.2 mg/kg IV or PO q12h (maximum daily dose, 200 mg)
		  ○ Weight ≥45 kg: Same as adult dose OR
		• Chloramphenicol (for children >2 years) 25 mg/kg IV q6h (maximum daily dose, 4 g)
			All recommended antimicrobials have relative contraindications for use in children; however, use is justified in life-threatening situations.

BUBONIC			
Adults (includes pregnant women)	• Doxycycline 100 mg IV or PO q12h OR 200 mg IV or PO q24h OR • Levofloxacin 500 mg IV or PO q24h OR • Ciprofloxacin 400 mg IV q8-12h OR 500–750 mg PO q12h OR • Moxifloxacin 400 mg IV or PO q24h OR • Chloramphenicol 25 mg/ kg IV q6h	Combination therapy of multiple classes recommended for severe bubonic plague.	Gentamicin penetrates poorly into abscesses so not preferred.

TABLE 2
Preferred and Alternative Treatment and Prophylaxis for Plague (*Y. pestis*)—cont'd

Indication/ population	Recommended antibiotic and dosages	Alternative	Notes

Children	• Doxycycline
	  ◦ Weight <45 kg: 2.2 mg/kg IV or PO q12h (maximum daily dose, 200 mg)
	  ◦ Weight ≥45 kg: Same as adult dose OR
	• Chloramphenicol (for children >2 years) 25 mg/kg IV q6h (maximum daily dose, 4 g) OR
	• Levofloxacin 8 mg/kg/dose IV or PO q12h (max 250 mg per dose) OR
	• Ciprofloxacin 15 mg/kg/dose IV q12h (maximum 400 mg/dose) OR 20 mg/kg/dose PO q12h (maximum 500 mg/dose)
		Combination therapy of multiple classes recommended for severe bubonic plague.	All recommended antimicrobials have relative contraindications for use in children; however, use is justified in life-threatening situations.

MASS CASUALTY/POSTEXPOSURE PROPHYLAXIS			
Adults (includes pregnant women)	• Doxycycline 100 mg PO q12h or 200 mg PO q24h	• Moxifloxacin 400 mg PO q24h OR • Ciprofloxacin 500–750 mg PO q12h OR • Levofloxacin 500 mg PO q24h	Daily dosing options for ease of mass distribution

Children	• Doxycycline
	  ◦ Weight <45 kg: 2.2 mg/kg PO q12h (maximum daily dose, 200 mg)
	  ◦ Weight ≥45 kg: Same as adult dose OR
	• Ciprofloxacin 20 mg/kg/dose PO q12h (maximum 500 mg/dose)
		• Levofloxacin 8 mg/kg/dose PO q12h (max 250 mg per dose)	Doxycycline preferred for children >8 yrs

PO, oral; *IV*, intravenous; *IM*, intramuscular; *q*, every; *BID*, twice daily; *qd*, daily; *h*, hours; *g*, grams; *mg*, milligrams; *kg*, kilograms; *H*, hours; *yrs*, years.

has been applied to urine, whole blood, bubo pus, and sputum. A 98.4% specificity and 90.1% sensitivity are reported for serum samples, and 100% sensitivity and specificity are reported for lymph node fluid. Direct microscopic examination of clinical specimens after Gram staining is another technique to rapidly diagnose plague when Gram-negative bacilli exhibiting a characteristic bipolar staining with a "hairpin appearance" are detected. Isolation and culture of *Y. pestis* are performed by incubating cultures at 32°C under 5% CO_2 atmosphere for 1–4 days. Because slow growth is observed on MacConkey agar, other selective media, including the cefsulodin-Irgasan-novobiocin (CIN) and beef heart-Irgasan-novobiocin (BIN) agar, have been developed.[31] The identification of *Y. pestis* can be achieved rapidly using immunochromatographic detection of the F1antigen on colonies.[32] Rapid identification using peptidic profiling by mass spectrometry is also effective[33] and has to be confirmed by appropriate molecular identification. Phage typing is also used to confirm the identification of *Y. pestis*.[34] Antibiotic susceptibility testing should be performed as a few antibiotic-resistant strains have emerged in Madagascar.[35] One strain was reported as resistant to eight antimicrobial agents, including those recommended for therapy (streptomycin, chloramphenicol, and tetracycline) and prophylaxis (sulfonamide and tetracycline), as well as ampicillin, kanamycin, and spectinomycin. A second strain was only resistant to streptomycin. In these resistant strains, all of the resistance genes were carried by conjugative plasmids of approximately 150 and 40 kb, respectively.[35] Ampicillin and tetracycline-resistant isolates have been identified in fleas and rats in Madagascar,[35] whereas the 150-kd plasmid backbone was shown to be broadly disseminated among multidrug-resistant zoonotic pathogens associated with agriculture.[36] Experimental data indicate that *Y. pestis* strains resistant to fluoroquinolones could be easily selected in the laboratory, but such strains were identified clinically.

TREATMENT AND PREVENTION CONSIDERATIONS (SEE CHAPTER 19 FOR ADDITIONAL DETAILS)

There are few examples of the use of *Y. pestis* as a bioterrorism agent. The classical historical example is (dating back to 1346) of Tartars hurdling plague-laden cadavers over the walls in order to introduce plague into the then Italian-run city of Caffa (situated on the banks of the Black Sea) and is the rare example for centuries.[37] More recently, Japanese used *Y. pestis* as a weapon during World War II,[38] while former the Soviet Union laboratories stocked it potentially as a biologic weapon.[39] Indeed, *Y. pestis* has been classified among the category A bioterrorism agents because of its proven droplet/airborne transmission and the fear that aerosolization could lead to massive contamination across a population. However, reevaluation of this risk using modeling strategies indicates that the number of secondary cases per primary inhalational case is likely 1.3,[40,41] suggesting that it would be impossible to sustain ongoing transmission and a plague outbreak.[42] Rapid administration of an effective antibiotic to patients with suspected plague is mandatory (Table 2). Gentamicin alone, or in combination with a tetracycline, is of current use.[43] Fluoroquinolones and cephalosporins are effective in animal models. However, recent guidance suggests their clinical efficacy, going beyond a single reported case of plague successfully treated with ciprofloxacin.[18,44] The Centers for Disease Control and Prevention recently published updated guidance recommending fluoroquinolones and aminoglycosides as first-line therapy for pneumonic and septicemic plague and fluoroquinolones, doxycycline, and aminoglycosides for bubonic and pharyngeal plague in both adults and children.[44] This new guidance also provides therapeutic recommendations for pregnant and breastfeeding women and neonates. Antibiotics should be initiated as early as possible, and treatment should be continued for 10–14 days. Patients generally improve within 2–3 days but may remain febrile for up to a week. Supportive therapy, including fluid resuscitation and use of pressors, should be undertaken in cases of septic shock and septicemic plague. Patients suspected and diagnosed with pneumonic plague should be placed in transmission-based isolation (droplet/respiratory) for 48 h after appropriate antibiotic treatment has been initiated.[44]

Plague prevention obviously relies on avoiding unprotected contact with any apparently sick and dead animals in endemic areas; reporting such animals to the health authorities and avoiding exposure to rats and fleas from diseased rats or other rodents, including use of protective clothes and repellents to avoid exposure to ectoparasites when outdoors; applying insect repellent containing *N,N*-diethyl-meta-toluamide (DEET) to legs and ankles; applying repellents and insecticides to clothes and outer bedding; and adequately cooking meat coming from wild and domestic animals such as goats and camels.[45]

While a few vaccines are available (live-attenuated *Y. pestis* EV76 strain; formalin-inactivated whole-cell plague; heat-killed whole-cell plague; F1 fraction) to be administrated by aerosol (EV76), subcutaneously (EV76; heat-killed CSL vaccine; CSL Ltd., Victoria, Australia) or intramuscularly (formalin-inactivated Greer vaccine; Greer Laboratories Inc., NC, United States),[46] there is no real evaluation of their role in controlling plague outbreaks.[46] Nevertheless, new-generation vaccines are under development and being tested in nonhuman primates.[47] Postexposure prevention is based on the administration of tetracycline or trimethoprim-sulfamethoxazole,[43] with doxycycline or ciprofloxacin being reasonable first-line choices in the management of bioterrorism agents, including *Y. pestis*.[7,48]

The control of a human plague outbreak mainly relies on surveillance strategies, the rapid confirmation of the diagnosis and treatment of confirmed and suspected cases, the killing of any human ectoparasite as well as killing animal fleas using appropriate and licensed insecticides, and the contact and respiratory isolation of patients suspected or diagnosed with pulmonary plague by implementing standard isolation procedures until at least 48 h after the initiation of antibiotic treatment (Table 1).[44]

REFERENCES

1. Perry RD, Fetherston JD. *Yersinia pestis*—etiologic agent of plague. *Clin Microbiol Rev.* 1997;10:35–66.
2. Andrades Valtueña A, Mittnik A, Key FM, et al. The stone age plague and its persistence in Eurasia. *Curr Biol.* 2017;27:3683–3691.
3. Drancourt M, Raoult D. Molecular history of plague. *Clin Microbiol Infect.* 2016;22:911–915.
4. Barbieri R, Signoli M, Chevé D, et al. *Yersinia pestis*: the natural history of plague. *Clin Microbiol Rev.* 2020;34(1): e00044-19. https://doi.org/10.1128/CMR.00044-19. PMID:33298527. PMCID: PMC7920731.
5. Drancourt M, Roux V, Dang LV, et al. Genotyping, Orientalis-like *Yersinia pestis*, and plague pandemics. *Emerg Infect Dis.* 2004;10:1585–1592.
6. Yersin A. La peste bubonique à Hong Kong. *Ann Inst Pasteur.* 1894;8:662–667.
7. Inglesby TV, Dennis DT, Henderson DA, et al. Plague as a biological weapon: medical and public health management. Working Group on Civilian Biodefense. *JAMA.* 2000;283:2281–2290.
8. Achtman M, Zurth K, Morelli G, et al. *Yersinia pestis*, the cause of plague, is a recently emerged clone of *Yersinia pseudotuberculosis*. *Proc Natl Acad Sci USA.* 1999;96:14043–14048.
9. Achtman M, Morelli G, Zhu P, et al. Microevolution and history of the plague bacillus, *Yersinia pestis*. *Proc Natl Acad Sci USA.* 2004;101:17837–17842.
10. Anisimov AP, Lindler LE, Pier GB. Intraspecific diversity of *Yersinia pestis*. *Clin Microbiol Rev.* 2004;17:434–464.
11. Li Y, Cui Y, Hauck Y, et al. Genotyping and phylogenetic analysis of *Yersinia pestis* by MLVA: insights into the worldwide expansion of Central Asia plague foci. *PLoS One.* 2009;4:e6000.
12. Derbise A, Chenal-Francisque V, Pouillot F, et al. A horizontally acquired filamentous phage contributes to the pathogenicity of the plague bacillus. *Mol Microbiol.* 2007;63:1145–1157.
13. Demeure CE, Dussurget O, Mas Fiol G, Le Guern AS, Savin C, Pizarro-Cerdá J. *Yersinia pestis* and plague: an updated view on evolution, virulence determinants, immune subversion, vaccination, and diagnostics. *Genes Immun.* 2019;20(5):357–370. https://doi.org/10.1038/s41435-019-0065-0. Epub 2019 Apr 3 PMID: 30940874. PMCID:PMC6760536.
14. Malek MA, Bitam I, Levasseur A, et al. *Yersinia pestis* halotolerance illuminates plague reservoirs. *Sci Rep.* 2017;7:40022.
15. Mollaret HH, Karimi Y, Eftekhari M, Baltazard M. Burrowing plague. *Bull Soc Pathol Exot Filiales.* 1963;56:1186–1193.
16. Drali R, Shako JC, Davoust B, Diatta G, Raoult D. A new clade of African body and head lice infected by *Bartonella quintana* and *Yersinia pestis*-Democratic Republic of the Congo. *Am J Trop Med Hyg.* 2015;93:990–993.
17. Piarroux R, Abedi AA, Shako JC, et al. Plague epidemics and lice, Democratic Republic of the Congo. *Emerg Infect Dis.* 2013;19:505–506.
18. Butler T. Plague into the 21st century. *Clin Infect Dis.* 2009;49:736–742.
19. Mead PS. Plague in Madagascar—a tragic opportunity for improving public health. *N Engl J Med.* 2018;378:106–108.
20. Gould LH, Pape J, Ettestad P, et al. Dog-associated risk factors for human plague. *Zoonoses Public Health.* 2008;55:448–454.
21. Dean KR, Krauer F, Walløe L, et al. Human ectoparasites and the spread of plague in Europe during the second pandemic. *Proc Natl Acad Sci USA.* 2018. Jan. 16. pii: 201715640. https://doi.org/10.1073/pnas.1715640115.
22. Drancourt M, Houhamdi L, Raoult D. *Yersinia pestis* as a telluric, human ectoparasite-borne organism. *Lancet Infect Dis.* 2006;6:234–241.
23. Blanc G, Baltazard M. Recherches expérimentales sur la peste. L'infection du pou de l'homme, Pediculus corporis de Geer. *CR Acad Sci.* 1941;213:849–851.
24. Blanc G, Baltazard M. Rôle des ectoparasites humains dans la transmission de la peste. *Bull Acad Med.* 1942;125: 446–448 [in French].
25. Ayyadurai S, Sebbane F, Raoult D, Drancourt M. Body lice, *Yersinia pestis* orientalis, and black death. *Emerg Infect Dis.* 2010;16:892–893.
26. Houhamdi L, Lepidi H, Drancourt M, Raoult D. Experimental model to evaluate the human body louse as a vector of plague. *J Infect Dis.* 2006;194:1589–1596.
27. Melman SD, Ettestad PE, VinHatton ES, et al. Human case of bubonic plague resulting from the bite of a wild Gunnison's prairie dog during translocation from a plague-endemic area. *Zoonoses Public Health.* 2018;65:e254–e258.
28. Gage KL, Dennis DT, Orloski KA, et al. Cases of cat-associated human plague in the Western US, 1977-1998. *Clin Infect Dis.* 2000;30:893–900.
29. Stewart A, Satterfield B, Cohen M, et al. A quadruplex real-time PCR assay for the detection of *Yersinia pestis* and its plasmids. *J Med Microbiol.* 2008;57:324–331.
30. Chanteau S, Rahalison L, Ralafiarisoa L, et al. Development and testing of a rapid diagnostic test for bubonic and pneumonic plague. *Lancet.* 2003;361:211–216.
31. Ber R, Mamroud E, Aftalion M, et al. Development of an improved selective agar medium for isolation of *Yersinia pestis*. *Appl Environ Microbiol.* 2003;69:5787–5792.
32. Tomaso H, Thullier P, Seibold E, et al. Comparison of hand-held test kits, immunofluorescence microscopy, enzyme-linked immunosorbent assay, and flow cytometric analysis for rapid presumptive identification of *Yersinia pestis*. *J Clin Microbiol.* 2007;45:3404–3407.
33. Couderc C, Nappez C, Drancourt M. Comparing inactivation protocols of Yersinia organisms for identification with matrix-assisted laser desorption/ionization time-of-flight mass spectrometry. *Rapid Commun Mass Spectrom.* 2012;26:710–714.

34. Sergueev KV, Nikolich MP, Filippov AA. Field and clinical applications of advanced bacteriophage-based detection of *Yersinia pestis*. *Adv Exp Med Biol.* 2012;954:135–141.
35. Galimand M, Carniel E, Courvalin P. Resistance of *Yersinia pestis* to antimicrobial agents. *Antimicrob Agents Chemother.* 2006;50:3233–3236.
36. Welch TJ, Fricke WF, McDermott PF, et al. Multiple antimicrobial resistance in plague: an emerging public health risk. *PLoS One.* 2007;2:e309.
37. Wheelis M. Biological warfare at the 1346 siege of Caffa. *Emerg Infect Dis.* 2002;8:971–975.
38. Harris SH. Factories of Death: Japanese Biological Warfare 1932–45 and the American Cover-Up. New York: Routledge; 1994.
39. Alibek K, Handelman S. Biohazard: The Chilling True Story of the Largest Covert Biological Weapons Program in the World—Told From the Inside by the Man Who Ran It. New York: Random House; 1999.
40. Gani R, Leach S. Epidemiologic determinants for modeling pneumonic plague outbreaks. *Emerg Infect Dis.* 2004;10:608–614.
41. Kool JL. Risk of person-to-person transmission of pneumonic plague. *Clin Infect Dis.* 2005;40:1166–1172.
42. Drancourt M, Raoult D. Investigation of pneumonic plague. *Madagascar Emerg Infect Dis.* 2018;24:183.
43. Boulanger LL, Ettestad P, Fogarty JD, et al. Gentamicin and tetracyclines for the treatment of human plague: review of 75 cases in New Mexico, 1985–1999. *Clin Infect Dis.* 2004;38:663–669.
44. Nelson CA, Meaney-Delman D, Fleck-Derderian S, Cooley KM, Yu PA, Mead PS. Antimicrobial treatment and prophylaxis of plague: recommendations for naturally acquired infections and bioterrorism response. *MMWR Recomm Rep.* 2021;70(No. RR-3):1–27. https://doi.org/10.15585/mmwr.rr7003a1external icon.
45. Porto-Fett AC, Juneja VK, Tamplin ML, Luchansky JB. Validation of cooking times and temperatures for thermal inactivation of *Yersinia pestis* strains KIM5 and CDC-A1122 in irradiated ground beef. *J Food Prot.* 2009;72:564–571.
46. Jefferson T, Demicheli V, Pratt M. Vaccines for preventing plague. *Cochrane Database Syst Rev.* 1998;CD000976.
47. Liu L, Wei D, Qu Z, et al. A safety and immunogenicity study of a novel subunit plague vaccine in cynomolgus macaques. *J Appl Toxicol.* 2018;38:408–417.
48. Brouillard JE, Terriff CM, Tofan A, Garrison MW. Antibiotic selection and resistance issues with fluoroquinolones and doxycycline against bioterrorism agents. *Pharmacotherapy.* 2006;26:3–14.

## CHAPTER 6

Viral Hemorrhagic Fevers (VHFs): An Archetype for Risk Management and High-Consequence Pathogens

DAVID M. BRETT-MAJOR[a,b] • ANGELA L. HEWLETT[b,c]
[a]Department of Epidemiology, College of Public Health, University of Nebraska Medical Center, Omaha, NE, United States • [b]Global Center for Health Security, University of Nebraska Medical Center, Omaha, NE, United States • [c]Division of Infectious Diseases, Department of Medicine, College of Medicine, University of Nebraska, Omaha, NE, United States

INTRODUCTION AND A PERSPECTIVE ON CONVERGENT PATHOGEN EVOLUTION

Viral Hemorrhagic Fevers (VHFs) are caused by a diverse array of viruses, referred to by striking elements of the patient and caregiver experience—in particular, bleeding. While bleeding is observed in sentinel severe cases presenting late for care, in pregnancy, and to varying degrees in other patients, in some ways, it is as much a misnomer to consider the pathogens virologically linked as to ascribe bleeding as the only, or even main, consequence for most patients. Nonetheless, viral hemorrhagic fever outbreak experiences are similar enough to merit grouping, and each of the viruses has relevant vascular tropism. The term VHF emerged from the yellow fever experience in the early days of virology research.[1] And much like the assignation of filterable agents for viruses, it became a broad category name in an era when pathogen-specific features were less easily characterized.

The commonly associated VHF threats are primarily caused by four viral families, including filoviruses, arenaviruses, bunyaviruses, and flaviviruses (Tables 1 and 2). While all of these represent enveloped RNA viruses, they possess positive, negative, and ambisense genomes and are both segmented and nonsegmented.[43] In fact, there are at least five different species of Ebola virus alone. Each of the organisms and the clinical syndromes care unit tends to emerge in different parts of the world with their unique geographical distribution, epidemiologic characteristics, clinical features, and management challenges.

The reservoirs and habits of crossing into people—when known—are surprisingly different among the VHF viruses from insects to rodents and bats. In general, the viruses replicate in the cytoplasm, are pantropic, and infect dendritic cells, monocytes, and macrophages early in the infection. And yet, in any given person becoming infected with any of them, there is an influenza-like prodrome characterized by fever and sometimes other symptoms such as headache, fatigue, muscle or joint pain, and rash. After a few days when the virus has replicated and escaped the reticuloendothelial system, there is wide dissemination throughout the body, sepsis, and organ injury. The virus permeates secretions, and person-to-person transmission may occur, usually with direct contact with secretions, respiratory droplets, or uncommonly aerosolization.

What Makes All These Pathogens That Seem So Different Get Transmitted in Similar Fashions and Cause Similar Symptoms?

Part of the answer lies in how sepsis manifests, the common pathway for how a severe infection impacts a patient.[44,45] In engineering terms, inflammation occurs in a poorly damped system where inflammation occurs quickly yet resolves slowly. Even injured tissue can induce local inflammatory cascades resulting in systemic inflammation with consequences in all organs. In sepsis, these inflammatory cascades and related tissue injury can lead to the consumption of coagulation factors and endovascular injury resulting in disseminated intravascular coagulation (DIC).

Another part of the answer is that VHF pathogens all have mechanisms that directly assault endovascular

Viral Outbreaks, Biosecurity, and Preparing for Mass Casualty Infectious Diseases Events
https://doi.org/10.1016/B978-0-323-54841-0.00017-2

TABLE 1
At a Glance: Viral Hemorrhagic Fevers (VHFs)

	Key Features	Clinical Correlations
Microbiology	Other viruses may be identified that result in the clinical phenotype. Those listed here are enveloped with RNA genomes of various constructs[2–5] *Arenaviruses* (e.g., Lassa fever, Machupo, Junin) *Bunyaviruses* (e.g., Crimean-Congo hemorrhagic fever, Rift Valley fever) *Filoviruses* (e.g., Ebola, Marburg) *Flaviviruses* (e.g., yellow fever, Omsk hemorrhagic fever, dengue) *Hantaviruses* (e.g., hemorrhagic fever with renal syndrome)	While differential cellular tropism exists, VHF pathogens widely disseminate in tissues
Immunology	Entry via a vector into the skin or by mucous membranes results in dissemination via the reticuloendothelial system and viremia. Consequently, pathogens are available to the innate, humoral, and cell-mediated systems. In some instances, such as Ebola or Marburg disease, viral reproduction results in secretory glycoprotein, which has immunosuppressive and antibody-capture effects.[6–8] *Arenaviruses* display nuclear protein immune disruption.[9] Ebola virus, in particular, has been observed to persist in immune-privileged sanctuary sites.[10] This may occur in other instances, such as occasionally with dengue virus[11]	Any part of the body may experience insult from a VHF. Contributions to disease from the pathogen and the immune response may occur. The role of immune privileged site persistence in recrudescence as well as onward transmission may be underappreciated in some VHF
Epidemiology and ecology	There is an association between bats and bushmeat with Marburg disease. Less is known about Ebola disease crossover zoonotic events. Ticks transmit Crimean-Congo hemorrhagic fever as well as Omsk hemorrhagic fever virus and could be a vector for New World arenaviruses. Mosquitoes transmit Rift Valley fever, yellow fever, and dengue viruses. *Arenaviruses* and *hantaviruses* typically have a peri-domestic rodent involved in zoonotic crossover, generally via food source contamination or aerosolization from animals in farming. The range of mammals involved in amplification and environmental persistence of many VHF is underestimated. Humans are amplifying hosts but usually not direct vectors in transmission of yellow fever and dengue viruses	VHF events range from sporadic sentinel cases with clusters to sustained human-to-human transmission events. Some VHF events typically have substantial epizootic features, in particular, Rift Valley fever in sheep (Table 3)
Clinical presentation	Incubation time varies from days to weeks. However, onset of symptoms beyond 2–3 weeks is very unusual for any of the known VHF pathogens	Most patients present with or first experience an influenza-like illness
Diagnosis	Serologic and nucleic acid systems are the mainstay of diagnosis, requiring blood sampling for early detection of disease. Culture requires highly specialized laboratory facilities with requisite biosecurity capability	As the pathogen typically enters the reticuloendothelial system before viremia, symptoms may be present for more than 2 days before a blood test might be positive

TABLE 1
At a Glance: Viral Hemorrhagic Fevers (VHFs)—cont'd

	Key Features	Clinical Correlations
Treatment	Usual aggressive strategies for sepsis are undertaken in these patients, mindful of organ damage and titrating volume and electrolyte needs, as well as pain management, nutrition, patient safety, and other requirements. Ribavirin commonly is employed against *arenaviruses* and increasingly *hantaviruses*.[35–37] Dosing should be done in accordance with the latest guidelines, as there remain questions regarding toxicity and optimum use. A range of experimental biologic therapies exist for Zaire Ebola virus, and there are small molecules under study against *filoviruses* and other related threats[38,39]	Clinicians should pursue the latest guidelines and contact established VHF facility networks as the role of targeted therapeutics is evolving. Safe and effective care requires a system of care approach for survival, comfort, and safety. See Table 3, Chapter 19
Vaccination	A variety of experimental vaccines are at several stages of product development. However, few of them are broadly licensed at the time of this writing for any VHF disease other than yellow fever and Ebola Zaire. rVSV-ZEBOV has been employed in ring vaccination and primary prevention for healthcare personnel in West and Central Africa, with thousands of doses administered.[40,41] In late 2019, it was approved by the European Commission (EC) and the US Food and Drug Administration (FDA). A vaccine is employed in South America against Junin virus, a New World arenavirus[42]	While in some instances, such as yellow fever, Ebola Zaire, and hopefully soon others, early vaccination is an important strategy. The dominant need for prevention and mitigation is awareness and application of interruption of transmission. That could entail vector control, IPC, food safety, or other measures depending upon the threat

targets. Attacking the circulatory system directly affects all tissues with more severe disease, potentially with vascular leak, distributive shock, and bleeding. Though surprisingly little is known about explicit pathogenesis, several suggestive mechanisms have been identified, some shared and some varied among the VHF pathogens. Yellow fever virus, a flavivirus, is effective at entering human endothelial cells and eliciting an aggressive Th1 cytokine response, in particular with IL-6 thought to activate fibrinogen.[46] Not surprisingly, the infection is associated with significant hepatic dysfunction.[47] Another flavivirus, dengue, has a nonstructural protein (NS1) that interrupts the endothelial glycocalyx and adds to a milieu of diverse endothelial and inflammatory cells and platelet factors that disrupt hemostasis.[48] Infections caused by both of these viruses are associated with low platelet counts and platelet dysfunction.[49] In some instances, the pathogen-vector relationship further contributes in surprising ways. For example, Langat virus, a third flavivirus, enters into endothelial cells in vitro facilitated by tick exosomes.[50] Filoviruses have long been understood to replicate in endothelial cells and to attract inflammatory cells to them, though the relative contributions of DIC and endothelial injury in making a patient bleed remains a matter of debate.[51,52] Patients with Crimean-Congo hemorrhagic fever virus, a bunyavirus, have robust markers for both endothelial dysfunction and inflammation.[53]

These VHF pathogens, with both shared and distinct mechanisms despite very different origins, have converged into a common phenotype from the perspective of a patient and those near them: an ILI, transmitted by blood, body fluids, or vectors, leading in some patients to sepsis and, potentially, bleeding (Tables 1, 3, and 4). This provides opportunities for syndromic-triggered patient and community management approaches but also portends consequences for how those at risk and those affected react to the possibility of a VHF in their midst.

TABLE 2

Selected Viral Hemorrhagic Fevers, Viral Characteristics, Vector, and Geographic Distribution

Family	Genus	Virus	Infection/Disease	Vector	Additional Sources	Geographic Distribution	Epidemiologic Considerations
Filoviridae (negative-sense ssRNA)	Filovirus	Ebola virus (6 species)	Ebola hemorrhagic fever	Bat	Contact with nonhuman primate; direct contact with bodily secretions	Africa	Burial workers, healthcare workers
		Marburg (1 species)	Marburg hemorrhagic fever	Bat	Contact with nonhuman primate; direct contact with bodily secretions; caves, mines	Africa	Burial workers, healthcare workers
Arenaviridae (negative-sense ssRNA)	Arenavirus	Lassa (Old World)	Lassa fever	Rodent (*Mastomys* species of rat)		West Africa	
		Junin (New World)	Argentine hemorrhagic fever	Rodent (vesper mouse)		South America, primarily Argentina	Harvest season
		Machupo (New World)	Bolivian hemorrhagic fever	Rodent (*Calomys*)	Contact with infected individuals	South America	Dry season; occurs with high rodent densities
		Sabia (New World)	Brazilian hemorrhagic fever	Rodent		South America	
		Guanarito (New World)	Venezuelan hemorrhagic fever	Rodent		South America	November to January, when increased agricultural activity

Bunyaviridae (negative-sense ssRNA)	Nairovirus	Crimean-Congo virus	Crimean-Congo hemorrhagic fever	Tick	Slaughtering of domestic animals; direct contact with bodily secretions	Africa, Balkans, Europe, Eurasia	Herders, slaughterhouses, and livestock workers
	Phlebovirus	Rift Valley fever virus	Rift Valley fever	Mosquito (*Aedes aegypti*)	Slaughtering of domestic animals	Africa, Arabian Peninsula	Herders, slaughterhouses, and livestock workers
	Hantavirus	Hantaan, Puumal, Seoul, and Dobrava viruses	Hemorrhagic fever with renal syndrome	Rodents		Eurasia	Aerosols of rodent urine
	Hantavirus	Sin Nombre, Andes, Cholo viruses	Hantavirus cardiopulmonary syndrome	Rodents		North, Central, and South America	Aerosols of rodent urine
Flaviviridae (positive-sense ssRNA)	Flavivirus	Dengue	Dengue fever	Mosquito (*Aedes aegypti*)		Africa, tropical and subtropical Americas, Asia, Caribbean, and Pacific	
		Yellow fever	Yellow fever	Mosquito (*Aedes aegypti*)		Africa, tropical Americas	
		Omsk hemorrhagic fever	Omsk hemorrhagic fever	Tick	Contact with muskrat-infected water	Central Asia, western Siberia	
		Kyasanur	Kyasanur Forest disease	Tick		India (Karnataka state)	

TABLE 3
Overview of Clinical and Epidemiologic Features of Selected[a] Viral Hemorrhagic Fevers (VHFs)

Disease (Virus)	Endemic Region/ Mortality	Natural Reservoir-Vector/Exposed Population/ Incubation Period	Mode of Transmission	Signs and Symptoms
Argentine hemorrhagic fever; (Junin virus)[12–15]	Central Argentina Mortality: 15%–30%	Rodents (corn mouse) Farmworkers 6–14 days	Direct contact (e.g., bite) Contact with excreta-contaminated substances (e.g., food, grain) or inhalation of aerosols of rodent excreta (e.g., dust)	20% asymptomatic *Prodromal phase* (1 week): chills, malaise, anore headache, myalgia (lower back), moderate fever, retro-orbital pain, nausea, vomiting, epigastric pain, photophobia, dizziness, constipation, mild diarrheal, hemorrhagic, or neurological symptom Relative bradycardia and orthostatic hypotensio are frequent *Neurologic-hemorrhagic phase* (20%–30%): sev hemorrhagic or neurologic manifestations, shock and superimposed bacterial infections *Convalescence phase* (1–3 months): asthenia, irritability, memory changes, hair loss
Crimean-Congo Hemorrhagic Fever (CCHF) (Nairovirus)[12,16,17]	Central and Eastern Europe, Central Asia, the Middle East, East, West, and South Africa Mortality: 30%–50%	Ixodid tick; domestic and wild animals, including cattle, goats, sheep, and rabbits Animal herders, livestock owners and workers, abattoir workers, veterinarians 2–7 days	Bite of an infected tick Contact with blood, body fluids, and tissue from infected patients or livestock	Abrupt onset of fever, myalgia, conjunctivitis, dizziness, neck pain, nuchal rigidity, headache, retro-orbital pain, photophobia, irritability, mood swings, nausea, vomiting, diarrhea, abdominal pain (right upper quadrant); agitation leading to sleepiness, depression, and lassitude *Clinical signs*: tachycardia, lymphadenopathy, hepatosplenomegaly, petechial rash, uncontrolle bleeding, and organ failure including kidney, live, respiratory failure
Dengue Fever (Dengue virus, 5 serotypes)[18–20]	Africa, tropical and subtropical North, South and Central America, Caribbean islands, Asia, and Australia (rare) Mortality: 1%–5%	Aedes mosquito (*Aedes. aegypti* or *Aedes albopictus*) 4–10 days	Bite from an infected mosquito Peripartum vertical transmission, blood transfusion, organ transplantation, needle stick injuries	75% asymptomatic *Febrile phase* (2–7 days): Sudden high-grade fev facial flushing, retro-orbital pain, skin erythema, myalgia, arthralgia, headache, nausea, vomiting, minor hemorrhagic manifestations (petechia, hematuria, epistaxis...), maculopapular rash *Critical phase* (24–48 h, 5% of patients): defervescence, leukopenia, thrombocytopenia, followed by plasma leakage, hemorrhage, organ impairment, shock *Recovery phase*: gradual reabsorption of extravascular compartment fluid (48–72 h)
Ebola Virus Disease (formerly called Ebola Hemorrhagic Feber) (Ebolavirus)[21,22]	Sub-Saharan Africa; primarily central Africa but also Western Africa Mortality: 25%–90%	Thought to be primates, fruit bats 2–21 days	Transmission to the index case is probably via contact with infected animals Human-to-human transmission from contact with infected blood, body fluids, or corpses	While asymptomatic cases occur, classically, sudden onset of high fever, fatigue, and body ac ("dry" symptoms) Followed by nausea, vomiting, diarrhea, fluid los up to 5–10 L/day ("wet" symptoms), maculopapu rash, hiccups Some patients will progress to shock, hypovolen and hemorrhagic events (conjunctival bleeding, petechiae, gastrointestinal bleeding, mucosal hemorrhage) Rare neurologic events (confusion, convulsions) and occasional bacterial coinfections

Diagnosis	Treatment	Prevention and Precautions	Comments
RT-PCR in blood or tissue Serology	Convalescent plasma given in the first week of illness decreases mortality Ribavirin and Favipiravir have in vitro activity against Junin virus	Live attenuated vaccine (Candid #1) licensed in Argentina is 95% effective In healthcare: Standard Precautions (human-to-human transmission not documented)	Other New World arenaviruses include Chapare, Machupo (Bolivian HF), and Sabia (Brazilian HF) with similar presentations Bolivian and Venezuelan HF have been associated with nosocomial outbreaks Reservoir is thought to be rodents for infections caused by Chapare and Sabia viruses
Viral antigen, RNA (RT-PCR) in blood or tissue Serology Virus isolation by cell culture[b]	Supportive care Ribavarin has in vitro and animal antiviral effects, but efficacy in humans is controversial	Tick bite avoidance; use of appropriate personal protective equipment (PPE) during animal slaughter and butchery of livestock; avoidance of contact with blood and body fluids In healthcare: contact and droplet to prevent blood-borne exposures	Human-to-human transmission including to healthcare personnel documented (contact with blood/body fluids of the infected patient)
RNA (RT-PCR) in blood NS1 antigen detection (days 0–7) Serology Virus isolation by cell culture[b]	Supportive care	Mosquito bite prevention Standard precautions Dengavaxia vaccine for seropositive persons over the age of 9 years; additional vaccines in clinical trials	Risk of severe disease associated with reinfection, 3rd trimester of pregnancy, and infants whose mothers were previously exposed Severe dengue is defined by the presence of one or more of the following symptoms – Severe plasma leakage leading to shock or fluid accumulation with respiratory distress – Severe bleeding (defined by physician) – Severe organ impairment: elevated transaminases $\geq$1000 IU/L, impaired consciousness, or heart impairment
RT-PCR in blood or body fluid may repeat after 72 h Serology virus isolation by cell culture[b] Postmortem antigen detection on skin biopsy	Supportive care Monoclonal antibodies and other experimental treatments under trial	Avoidance of contact with blood and body fluids; safe burial practice; avoidance of bushmeat and contact with nonhuman primates and bats In healthcare: contact and droplet to prevent blood-borne exposures Vaccinations for the Zaire strain of Ebola are available in the United States, Europe, and several African countries	Both isolated and large, sustained outbreaks with human-to-human transmission have occurred with sexual transmission reported including contact with blood and body fluids and sexual contact

(Continued)

TABLE 3
Overview of Clinical and Epidemiologic Features of Selected[a] Viral Hemorrhagic Fevers (VHFs)—cont'd

Disease (Virus)	Endemic Region/ Mortality	Natural Reservoir-Vector/Exposed Population/ Incubation Period	Mode of Transmission	Signs and Symptoms
Lassa Fever (Lassa virus)[23,24]	West and Central Africa Mortality: 1% (15% if hospitalized with severe clinical presentation)	Rodents 2–21 days	Contact with excreta or materials contaminated with excreta of an infected multimammate rat (*Mastomys* spp.) Inhalation of aerosols of excreta of multimammate rat Contact with blood or body fluids from infected patients, or sexual contact	80% asymptomatic Gradual onset of fever, general weakness, and malaise After a few days, headache, sore throat, muscle pain, chest pain, nausea, vomiting, diarrhea, cou and abdominal pain Severe cases: facial swelling, pulmonary edema, bleeding from the mouth, nose, vagina, or gastrointestinal tract and low blood pressure, shock, seizures, tremors, disorientation, and con Deafness in 1/3 of patients can persist after recovery
Marburg Hemorrhagic Fever (Marburg virus)[25,26]	Africa Mortality: 24% in Europe and the United States, 82% in low-income countries	Fruit bats Human-to-human transmission (contact with blood and bodily fluids) Burial ceremonies 3–21 days (typically 5–10 days)	Contact with infected animals Human-to-human transmission: direct contact with droplets or body fluids, or contact with equipment and other objects contaminated with infectious blood or tissues	Abrupt flu-like symptoms followed by lethargy, nausea, vomiting, abdominal pain, severe watery diarrhea, coughing, headache, hypotension, maculopapular rash, ± hemorrhagic manifestatic of various severity. Patients described as "ghost-like" Fatal cases progress to more severe symptoms days 7–14
Omsk Hemorrhagic Fever (Omsk hemorrhagic fever virus)[25,27,28]	Western Siberia Mortality: 0.5%–3%	Rodents (muskrat), ticks 3–8 days	Tick bite Contact with an infected muskrat	High continuous fever (39°C to 40°C) in all cases myalgia, cough, hyperemia (especially of the pharynx) ± petechial rash (5–12 days) Followed by recovery, or a more severe second febrile phase with meningeal signs and nonseve hemorrhagic manifestations (5–14 days). Lungs a kidneys are also commonly affected
Rift Valley Fever (Rift Valley Fever Virus)[25,29]	Africa and Arabian Peninsula[30]	Livestock, mosquitoes 2–6 days	Contact with blood and body fluids of infected animals Bite of an infected mosquito Aerosol transmission in laboratories	90% of patients suffer mild symptoms only (flu-li symptoms, sometimes biphasic fever) Severe cases (8%–10%): ocular complications (uveitis, retinitis, vasculitis, retinal hemorrhages), severe hepatic disease, neurologic disease with delayed onset (headache, excessive salivation, partial paralysis), hemorrhagic fever (<1%)

Diagnosis	Treatment	Prevention and Precautions	Comments
RT-PCR Serology Antigen detection Viral isolation by cell culture[b]	Ribavirin early in the course Supportive care	Rodent control, hygiene interventions Health care setting: contact and droplets precautions, face shield	Human-to-human transmission documented, including sexually transmitted
RT-PCR (blood and tissues) Serology Isothermal assay for RNA amplification	Supportive treatment	Protect pigs from fruit bats in endemic areas Use gloves, appropriate clothing, and masks with exposure to mines or caves inhabited by fruit bat colonies Healthcare setting: contact + droplets precautions Prompt and safe burial using protective equipment	No licensed vaccines are available but several vaccines have shown potential to protect nonhuman primates from Marburg virus infection
RT-PCR Serology	Supportive care Strict bed rest	Tick bite prevention Safe laboratory practices	Tick-born encephalitis vaccine could confer cross-protection but was not formally demonstrated No human-to-human transmission has been documented but infections due to lab contamination have been described
RT-PCR Serology Antigen detection Viral isolation by cell culture[b]	Supportive treatment Ribavirin has in vitro efficacy	Mosquito bite prevention Appropriate personal protective equipment when working with animals in endemic areas Livestock vaccination	No human-to-human transmission documented High rates of miscarriage and vertical transmission were reported with acute infection during pregnancy Three licensed veterinary vaccines are being used; human vaccines are under development

(Continued)

TABLE 3
Overview of Clinical and Epidemiologic Features of Selected[a] Viral Hemorrhagic Fevers (VHFs)—cont'd

Disease (Virus)	Endemic Region/ Mortality	Natural Reservoir-Vector/Exposed Population/ Incubation Period	Mode of Transmission	Signs and Symptoms
Venezuelan Hemorrhagic Fever (Guanarito virus)[12,15,31,32]	Northwestern Venezuela Mortality: 26%–33%	Rodents 14–21 days	Direct contact (e.g., bite) with infected rat or mouse, or their excreta Contact with materials (e.g. food) contaminated with excreta from infected rats or mice Inhalation of aerosols of excreta (often in dust) of rat or mouse	Fever, malaise, headache, arthralgia, sore throat vomiting, abdominal pain, diarrhea, convulsions, and a variety of hemorrhagic manifestations
Yellow Fever (Yellow fever virus in Flavivirus family)[25,33,34]	Africa, South America Mortality: 20%–60%	Mosquitoes (*Aedes aegypti*) 3–6 days	Bite from an infected mosquito	*Viremic period* (3–5 days): fever, malaise, photophobia, irritability, nausea, vomiting *Remission period* (1–2 days) *Period of intoxication* (20%–60% of patients): liver, renal failure, hemorrhages, jaundice, thrombocytopenia, multiorgan dysfunction

HF, hemorrhagic fever; *RT-PCR*, reverse transcriptase polymerase chain reaction; *IU*, international units; *L*, liter.
[a]Other less common VHF, or those mentioned elsewhere in the chapter, that were not included in this table are: Alkhurma hemorrhagic fever, Bolivian hemorrhagic fever, Chapare hemorrhagic fever, Hantavirus pulmonary syndrome, Hemorrhagic fever with renal syndrome, Kyasanur Forest disease, Lujo hemorrhagic fever, Lymphocytic choriomeningitis, Sabia-associated hemorrhagic fever, Tick-borne encephalitis.
[b]Viral culture of these pathogens can be conducted in a small number of referral laboratories with appropriate biosafety and biosecurity capabilities.
Author: Elisa Pichlinski, MD.

SAFE AND EFFECTIVE CARE

A key element of the epidemiologic control of VHF is its early recognition. VHFs are zoonotic in nature, and in endemic areas, the presence of disease-specific reservoirs and/or vectors in the natural environment signals the plausibility of human infections (Tables 1–3).[64] Initial human cases of VHF typically occur after contact with infected animals or insects, which occur via bites or contact with infected tissues or fluids on mucous membranes or nonintact skin.[65] If the sentinel case of VHF is recognized, then further cases, whether zoonotic, secondary human-to-human, or human-mosquito-human, as occurs in yellow fever and dengue, can be caught early or prevented. This recognition and subsequent provision of safe and effective care, however, is fraught with potential barriers: lack of access to medical care, patient refusal to present to a healthcare facility, lack of screening based on case definition, inadequate staffing, incomplete training of staff in infection prevention and control practices (IPC), and lack of equipment and supplies, including personal protective equipment (PPE) and diagnostics. Unlike the respiratory patho-

Diagnosis	Treatment	Prevention and Precautions	Comments
RT-PCR Virus isolation by cell culture[b]	Ribavirin Supportive care	No vaccine available Healthcare setting: standard precautions	Controversial human-to-human transmission yet standard precautions are currently recommended Seasonal (peak November to January)
RT-PCR (blood, serum, urine) Serology Virus isolation by cell culture[b]	Supportive care	Avoidance of mosquitoes Vaccine available In the healthcare setting: standard precautions	NS1 antigen detection is promising for early diagnosis; however, data is limited

gens discussed in this book, even with the most modern diagnostics, VHF pathogens are not reliably detected until after a patient has been symptomatic, usually for a couple of days. This lag in diagnosis is exacerbated in resource-limited settings where a sample must be moved by logistics chains with variable reliability and then assessed at a site distant from the potential VHF event (see Chapter 18, case study). Healthcare centers must be able to isolate the patient presumptively when VHF is suspected and to provide clinical care until the diagnosis is confirmed.

Although the sentinel case of VHF generally occurs in an area endemic or at risk for the disease, other settings often face a similar need to identify infected patients with presumptive VHF as the result of travel to affected areas.[66] These individuals often are termed Persons Under Investigation (PUIs), assuming an appropriate epidemiologic history and a compatible clinical illness. Identification tools prepared in advance by health facilities, including travel screening and process maps, can be helpful in the management of PUIs (see Fig. 8, Chapter 13, for example).[67] Depending on the

TABLE 4
Signs and Symptoms of Selected[a] Viral Hemorrhagic Fevers (VHFs)

Disease (Virus)	Onset and Phases of Illness	General Symptoms	Cardiopulmonary Symptoms	Gastrointestinal, Genitouri Symptoms
Argentine Hemorrhagic Fever (Junin virus)[13,15]	Prodromal phase: insidious onset, lasts 1 week after onset of symptoms	Chills, malaise, anorexia, moderate hyperthermia (38°C to 39°C)	Relative bradycardia, orthostatic hypotension No pulmonary abnormalities	Nausea, vomiting, epigastric mild diarrhea or constipation Very rare: hepatomegaly, splenomegaly Frequently found at the end the phase: superimposed ora candidiasis
	Neurologic-hemorrhagic phase (20%–30% of cases): 8–12 days after onset of symptoms	Shock: septic from superimposed bacterial infections (pneumonia, bacteremia), hypovolemic from capillary leak syndrome		
	Convalescence phase: 1–3 months Survivors usually recover completely			
Crimean-Congo Hemorrhagic Fever (CCHF) (Nairovirus)[16,54]	Abrupt onset	Fever		Nausea, vomiting, diarrhea, abdominal pain
	Beginning around the 4th day of illness and lasting for 2 weeks	Multiorgan failure		
	Long-term effects	Unknown, slow recovery		

Skin and Mucous Membrane Findings	Hematologic Symptoms	Neurologic, Ophthalmologic, Ears/ Nose/Throat Symptoms	Musculoskeletal Symptoms *Pregnancy Considerations*
Flushing of the face, neck, and upper chest; petechiae in the axillary regions; upper chest; and arms Congested gums may bleed spontaneously, or under slight pressure Enanthem with petechiae and small vesicles almost over the soft palate (almost always found on physical examination) Very rare: jaundice	Enlarged cervical lymph nodes (laterocervical regions) Metrorrhagia	Headache, photophobia, dizziness Retro-orbital pain, conjunctival congestion, periorbital edema At the end of prodromal phase: irritability, lethargy, fine tremor of the hand and tongue, moderate ataxia, cutaneous hyperesthesia, decrease in deep tendon reflexes, and muscular tonicity	Myalgia (particularly lower back)
	Bleeding: hematemesis, hemoptysis, epistaxis, hematomas, metrorrhagia, hematuria	Confusion, marked ataxia, irritability, tremors Followed by delirium, generalized convulsions, and coma	
Hair loss (temporary)		Asthenia, irritability, memory changes Late neurological syndrome (10% of cases treated with immune plasma): begins after a symptom-free period; febrile symptoms may recur; cerebellar signs; cranial nerve palsies	
Flushed face, petechiae on the palate, jaundice		Dizziness, headache, sore eyes, photophobia, confusion Severe cases: changes in mood and sensory perception Conjunctival injection Sore/red throat	Muscle aches, back pain and stiffness, backache, joint pain
Petechial rash	Bruising, generalized bleeding of the gums and orifices, uncontrolled bleeding at injection sites		

(Continued)

TABLE 4
Signs and Symptoms of Selected[a] Viral Hemorrhagic Fevers (VHFs)—cont'd

Disease (Virus)	Onset and Phases of Illness	General Symptoms	Cardiopulmonary Symptoms	Gastrointestinal, Genitouri Symptoms
Dengue Fever (Dengue virus, 5 serotypes)[19,55,56]	Febrile phase: abrupt onset, lasts 2–7 days	High-grade fever, anorexia		Nausea, vomiting After a few days: enlarged ar tender liver Uncommon: gastrointestinal bleeding
	Critical phase (24–48 h): starts with defervescence[c], usually on days 3–7 of illness	Temperature drops to 37.5°C to 38°C, increase in capillary permeability with plasma leakage, hypovolemic shock, narrow pulse pressure, multiorgan failure	Pleural effusions, myocarditis	Ascites, severe hepatitis, pancreatitis (uncommon)
	Recovery phase: in the following 48–72 h	Gradual resorption of extravascular compartment fluid, improvement in general well-being, hemodynamic stabilization followed by diuresis	Bradycardia, electrocardiographic changes Respiratory distress from massive pleural effusion and ascites Associated with excessive intravenous fluids: pulmonary edema, congestive heart failure	Gastrointestinal symptoms re
Ebola Virus Disease (formerly Ebola Hemorrhagic Fever) (Ebolavirus)[22,57,58]	Early febrile or mild stage (0–3 days): abrupt onset	High fever, malaise, fatigue		
	Gastrointestinal involvement (3–10 days)		Rare: cough, dyspnea, chest pain	Nausea, vomiting, diarrhea: r severe with fluid loss up to 5 day Rare: abdominal pain, hiccup (10%–30%)
	Complicated stage (7–12 days): varied symptoms across different outbreaks	Hypovolemic and distributive shock, multiorgan failure		Gastrointestinal bleeding, dysphagia
Lassa Fever (Lassa Fever virus)[23,59]	Gradual onset	Fever, malaise		
	After a few days		Chest pain, cough	Nausea, vomiting, diarrhea, abdominal pain
	Severe cases	Shock, multiorgan failure	Pleural effusion, respiratory distress	Gastrointestinal bleeding, rep vomiting
	Recovery			

Skin and Mucous Membrane Findings	Hematologic Symptoms	Neurologic, Ophthalmologic, Ears/Nose/Throat Symptoms	Musculoskeletal Symptoms *Pregnancy Considerations*
Facial flushing, skin erythema, petechiae, macular or maculopapular rash Positive tourniquet test[b]	Mild mucosal membrane bleeding, hematuria Uncommon: massive vaginal bleeding	Severe headache, retro-orbital eye pain Conjunctival injection Sore throat, injected pharynx	Generalized body aches, myalgia, arthralgia
	Disseminated intravascular coagulation, severe hemorrhagic manifestations	Encephalitis	*Risk of preeclampsia is 12% and vertical transmission has been documented, but its significance is still uncertain*
Rash of "isles of white in the sea of red," generalized pruritus			
		Weakness, lethargy	Body aches
		Rare: conjunctival injection	Rare: localized muscle or joint pain
Petechiae, maculopapular rash may arise on days 5–7 and include palms/soles. Subsequent desquamation portends better prognosis.	Hemorrhagic events, mucosal bleeding, oozing after venipuncture	Rare: confusion, delirium, convulsions Conjunctival bleeding Throat pain, oral ulcers	*Maternal death estimated at 68% (relative risk of death 1.18 compared with nonpregnant women), fetal loss at 77%, and neonatal death at 98%*
		General weakness	*Spontaneous abortion in 95% of infected pregnant patients*
		Headache Sore throat	Muscle pain
Facial swelling	Hemorrhagic manifestations	Seizures, tremors, encephalitis, coma	Back pain *High mortality rates in the third trimester of pregnancy*
Transient hair loss		Transient gait disturbance, deafness in 25% of cases (half recover partially within 1–3 months)	

(Continued)

TABLE 4
Signs and Symptoms of Selected[a] Viral Hemorrhagic Fevers (VHFs)—cont'd

Disease (Virus)	Onset and Phases of Illness	General Symptoms	Cardiopulmonary Symptoms	Gastrointestinal, Genitouri Symptoms
Marburg Hemorrhagic Fever (Marburg virus)[25,26]	Abrupt onset	Chills, high fever, malaise, hypotension, "ghost-like" drawn features, deep-set eyes, expressionless face	Cough	Nausea, vomiting, abdomina severe watery diarrhea
	After 5–7 days	Sustained high fever, hemorrhagic shock		Hematemesis, gastrointestin bleeding Orchitis reported in late phas (15 days)
Omsk Hemorrhagic Fever (Omsk hemorrhagic fever virus)[25,27]	Early symptoms, worsening over the first 3–4 days of disease 50%–70% of patients recover after 1–2 weeks	Malaise, high continuous fever (39°C to 40°C) in all cases, dehydration	Cough, arterial hypotension, bradycardia, hemoptysis	Gastrointestinal symptoms, enlarged liver Gastrointestinal bleeding Intermittent hematuria (days and 15–25)
	Second phase, starting at the beginning of 3rd week (30%–50%)—recurrence of primary symptoms—lasts 5–14 days	Continued high fever, chills		Nausea
	Recovery	Generally favorable, with rare complications	Prolonged asthenia	
Rift Valley Fever (Rift Valley Fever Virus)[25,60]	Uncomplicated with onset 2–7 days	Flu-like symptoms, biphasic fever		
	8%–10% develop more severe symptoms			Severe hepatic disease
	Convalescence	May take several weeks		
Venezuelan Hemorrhagic Fever (Guanarito virus)[15]	Acute, often mild, resolves within 1–2 weeks	Fever, chills, generalized malaise	Coughing	Nausea, vomiting, diarrhea

Skin and Mucous Membrane Findings	Hematologic Symptoms	Neurologic, Ophthalmologic, Ears/ Nose/Throat Symptoms	Musculoskeletal Symptoms *Pregnancy Considerations*
Maculopapular rash		Lethargy, severe headache	Myalgia
	Mucosal bleeding, metrorrhagia, bleeding from venipuncture sites	Confusion, irritability, aggression	
Skin hemorrhages, hyperemia of the face, neck, and chest, petechial rash on the abdomen and extremities	Mucosal bleeding Increased intensity of bleeding after a few days	Skin hyperesthesia Acute scleral injection Bright colorization and light edema of mouth and throat, dryness of mucous membranes (especially tongue), putrid odor from the mouth, labial fissures and crusts, Continuous gingivitis, hyperemia of soft palate and tonsils, uvular edema, necrosis of the pharynx surface (rare)	Muscle pain, pain in lower-leg joints, and calf muscles
Reddening of the face, petechial rash, bruises at site of pressure or injection	Mucosal bleeding	New symptoms of meningitis (headache and meningism) Scleral injection	
Hair loss		Weakness, hearing loss, behavioral and psychological difficulties (poor memory, impaired ability to concentrate)	
		Dizziness, weakness	Back pain
Jaundice	Hemorrhagic disease (2–4 days after onset of illness)	Neurologic disease (typically delayed 1–4 weeks): severe headache, hallucinations, disorientation, vertigo, excessive salivation, weakness or partial paralysis, encephalitis, seizures, coma Ocular complications (<10%) after 1–3 weeks: uveitis, retinitis, vasculitis, retinal hemorrhages	
		Most ocular lesions disappear after 10–12 weeks, except lesions on the macula (half will have permanent vision loss) Neurologic deficits may be severe and long-lasting	
Macular rash		Severe headache, photophobia. Mild to severe neurological signs (children, adults >50 years) Sore throat	Myalgia (legs and lumbosacral region), arthralgia (wrists and ankles) *Fetal encephalitis, placental damage, abortion/stillbirth, severe congenital neurological anomalies*

(Continued)

TABLE 4
Signs and Symptoms of Selected[a] Viral Hemorrhagic Fevers (VHFs)—cont'd

Disease (Virus)	Onset and Phases of Illness	General Symptoms	Cardiopulmonary Symptoms	Gastrointestinal, Genitouri Symptoms
Yellow Fever (Yellow fever virus in Flavivirus family)[25,61,62]	Viremic period (3–5 days), sudden onset Followed by a remission period (~1 day)	Estimates that 55% are asymptomatic, 33% mild, 12% severe Of the affected, fever, malaise, and fatigue. Fatigue may last several months		Nausea, vomiting
	Period of intoxication (20%–60% of patients)	Shock, multiorgan failure, high fever		Liver failure Renal failure

[a]Other less common VHF, or those mentioned elsewhere in the chapter, that were not included in this table are: Alkhurma hemorrhagic fever, Bolivian hemorrhagic fever, Chapare hemorrhagic fever, Hantavirus pulmonary syndrome, Hemorrhagic fever with renal syndrome, Kyasanur Forest disease, Lujo hemorrhagic fever, Lymphocytic choriomeningitis, Sabia-associated hemorrhagic fever, Tick-borne encephalitis.
[b]Tourniquet test: inflate a blood pressure cough on the upper arm of the patient to a point midway between the systolic and the diastolic blood pressure and maintain it for 5 minutes. Deflate the cuff and wait 2 more minutes. 10 or more petechiae per square inch represents a positive test.[63]
[c]Some patients progress without defervescing.
Author: Elisa Pichlinski, MD.

transmissibility of the VHF in question, PUIs should be isolated, and an aggressive IPC posture adopted by healthcare personnel (HCP), which includes PPE appropriate to the intended tasks. It is important to note that while a patient is under investigation for VHF, alternative diagnoses and coinfections should be evaluated, and the clinical care should continue. This is a particular concern in resource-limited settings, where healthcare facility closures and patient diversion into VHF suspect case management are common during VHF emergencies.[30,68] Patients with complications of pregnancy and conditions associated with bleeding, such as severe liver disease, are especially vulnerable when this occurs.

CLINICAL MANIFESTATIONS

A wide spectrum of clinical illnesses, ranging from asymptomatic or mild disease to severe disease with shock, circulatory failure, and death, has been observed in patients with VHF (Tables 3 and 4). Although some specific clinical manifestations of VHF infection may vary depending on the infecting virus and the host, the general clinical syndrome is similar.[69] After an incubation period of days to weeks depending upon the pathogen, patients initially present with an influenza-like syndrome with nonspecific symptoms including fever, malaise, fatigue, and anorexia.[70,71] Other symptoms, including headache, neck pain, conjunctivitis, pharyngitis, jaundice, cough, photophobia, and rash, occur in select VHF. Crimean-Congo Hemorrhagic Fever (CCHF), for instance, has a particular association with facial rash, in contrast to the commonly described diffuse, fine, papular rash described with Ebola disease.[72] These initial symptoms may then progress to include gastrointestinal symptoms, with nausea, vomiting, diarrhea, and abdominal pain.[73] Profound fluid losses may lead to volume depletion and significant electrolyte disturbances. Rhabdomyolysis has also been observed.[74] More severe cases may develop vascular leakage, hemodynamic instability, multiorgan failure, superimposed bacterial sepsis, encephalitis, shock, and death.[75] Despite the use of the term VHF, overt hemorrhage is the exception and not the norm in many VHFs, and while it may be present, early bleeding is usually a late clinical manifestation. The likelihood of hemorrhage varies in each VHF, though predicting it is tainted by observation bias. When present, hemorrhage usually manifests as mucosal bleeding, particularly from the gastrointestinal tract, including melena, hematochezia, and hematemesis.[76] Oozing from intravenous lines or puncture sites, gum

Skin and Mucous Membrane Findings	Hematologic Symptoms	Neurologic, Ophthalmologic, Ears/Nose/Throat Symptoms	Musculoskeletal Symptoms *Pregnancy Considerations*
	Headache, photophobia, irritability		Myalgia
Jaundice	Hemorrhages, vasculopathy, disseminated intravascular coagulation		

bleeding, and epistaxis can also occur. More severe disease is seen in those who are pregnant, the extremes of age, and with conditions associated with a compromised immune system.

DIAGNOSIS (SEE CHAPTER 17 FOR ADDITIONAL DETAILS)

Both the initial nonspecific presentation and the wide spectrum of clinical illness among VHF patients often result in an extensive list of differential diagnoses. Thus, a high index of clinical suspicion for VHF must be based on both clinical and epidemiologic data. A comprehensive history and a thorough physical examination should be obtained in all patients. The epidemiologic history should consist of country or region of residence, travel history, exposures to ill or deceased persons, healthcare exposure, occupational exposures, history of animal contact and insect bites, and sexual history. VHF should be considered in patients with a concerning epidemiologic history who present with a clinical syndrome compatible with VHF and within the appropriate incubation period. Other potential diagnoses should also be investigated based on the epidemiology and clinical presentation. Coinfections such as malaria are common in areas endemic for VHF.[77]

If VHF is suspected, specimens should be obtained for laboratory analysis to confirm the diagnosis as well as to best manage the patient's sepsis. Diagnostic options for VHF include serological demonstration of viral antibodies and reverse transcriptase polymerase chain reaction (RT-PCR) for nucleic acid detection (see Chapter 17). If support from a high containment referral laboratory is available, electron microscopy or culture also may be undertaken.[78,79] However, more distributable technologies are employed in routine diagnostics in most settings. Increasingly, these have included rapid diagnostic tests (RDTs), such as automated and other field deployable PCR and dipstick immunoassays, especially when screening patients for select VHFs in resource-limited settings.[80,81]

In general, laboratory findings in VHF reflect a patient's sepsis with disseminated inflammation and organ dysfunction, though some nuances have been observed. Leukopenia and thrombocytopenia have been observed in many VHF patients, while leukocytosis is common in Hantavirus hemorrhagic fever with renal syndrome. Manifestations of disseminated intravascular coagulopathy (DIC) can be seen in coagulation studies.[82,83] Electrolyte abnormalities are commonly observed in patients with VHF, particularly hypokalemia, hypomagnesemia, hypocalcemia, and hyponatremia, though when renal injury is present, hyperkalemia may occur. These disturbances have been hypothesized to result in fatal arrhythmias in otherwise responding patients, emphasizing the importance of clinical laboratory monitoring whenever feasible.[76] Transaminase elevations, elevated creatine kinase, and lactate levels have been reported, along with elevated creatinine and hypoalbuminemia.[84] Yellow fever patients may have a striking hepatic injury.[85] Metabolic acidosis is observable in all stages of illness, either through compensatory tachypnea or frank perturbations on chemistry and blood gas analysis. Blood cultures may reveal secondary infection with bacterial or fungal pathogens, most likely due to gut translocation. Malaria coinfection has been present frequently, in some instances in almost half of cases.[86,87] Additionally, patients with severe disease may develop or acquire secondary infections while under care, including from usual nosocomial pathogens, invasive enteric gram-negative rods, commensals, and in endemic areas, malaria and arboviral diseases.

TREATMENT

Supportive Care

An aggressive system of care approach as is done for any critically ill patient with sepsis is the cornerstone of therapy for VHF. Careful risk-benefit analysis should guide all interventions in patients with VHF, weighing the potential benefit of the intervention against the risk to HCPs. Volume and electrolyte repletion by oral and intravenous means with careful monitoring of fluid balance and electrolyte status are critical. Third-spacing, including pulmonary edema, has been observed with aggressive hydration and must be managed. Medications like acetaminophen or paracetamol can be given to reduce fever and pain. Nonsteroidal antiinflammatory medications are avoided due to their antiplatelet effect, though admittedly without clear evidence of the scale of potential impact. Some patients experience profound visceral pain indicating the use of more potent analgesia such as opioids. Volume loss can be reduced by the use of antiemetic and antidiarrheal medications to control secretions, though the risk of concomitant enteric bacterial infection should be considered.[88,89] Blood products, including packed red blood cells, platelets, and fresh frozen plasma, may be used to treat bleeding complications.[84] Laboratory analysis is an important aspect of supportive care and can guide correction of electrolyte disturbances, evaluation of complications, and clinical monitoring of patients with VHF. Serum viral load monitoring is often employed both for clinical decision-making as well as for meeting local requirements for discharge from isolation care. Vasopressors, inotropes, and antiarrhythmic agents can be utilized for hypotension and cardiac complications, including via peripheral access, when required to do so.[90] Nutritional support, including the use of total parenteral nutrition (TPN), may be used if available. In resource-limited settings where families are often responsible for providing food and other necessities for patients, special arrangements for even basic nutrition must be made. When concomitant bacterial infection is suspected, early use of appropriate broad-spectrum antibiotics is advised. Field isolation units with limited clinical laboratory capabilities sometimes employ routine broad-spectrum antibacterial therapy for all new VHF patients, also citing risks of bacterial translocation in the course of illness. Similar systematic treatment or rapid assay test-and-treat approaches are taken against malaria. Supplemental oxygen may be necessary for patients exhibiting hypoxia, though this usually is secondary to volume repletion, secondary infection, or other complications such as from VHF in pregnancy. Nonpharmacologic aggressive supportive interventions for critically ill patients, including mechanical ventilation, dialysis, and placement of central venous or arterial catheters, have been utilized in the management of patients with VHF in resourced settings and are being advocated increasingly in less constrained settings when focused support is available.[91–94]

Patients hospitalized with VHF should be monitored closely for the development of healthcare-associated infections, like central-line or IV catheter-associated infections, ventilator-associated pneumonia, and urinary tract infections, as well as for patient safety issues such as falls when HCP access to the patient may be limited in some settings.

Therapeutic Agents (See Chapter 19 for Additional Details)

There are only a few Food and Drug Administration (FDA)-approved therapeutic agents for the management of most VHFs. Many experimental therapeutics were utilized in the 2014–16 epidemic of Ebola virus disease (EVD) in West Africa, as well as the larger of two outbreaks that began in the Democratic Republic of the Congo in 2018. Initially, these investigational agents were administered to individual or small numbers of patients through emergency use authorization or uncontrolled trials, making it difficult to draw any conclusions regarding efficacy. Then, larger, controlled trials and an observational study signaled benefit from two biologic (monoclonal antibody) agents for the treatment of EVD, leading to the first EVD therapeutic approval by the FDA, the three-antibody cocktail of atoltivimab, maftivimab, and odesivimab-ebgn, followed by another monoclonal antibody, ansuvimab-zykl.[95,96] These products are specifically approved for *Zaire ebolavirus*. Convalescent serum has been utilized for EVD but has not been shown to decrease mortality.[97] However, it is used in the management of the Junin virus.[42] Small molecules are under study for filoviruses and continue to be of interest because of the presence of such viruses in compartments less available to circulating antibodies.[38] Ribavirin is used to treat select VHFs, most notably Lassa fever, New World arenaviruses, and Crimean-Congo hemorrhagic fever, backed by varying degrees of evidence.[98]

INFECTION PREVENTION AND CONTROL AND WASTE MANAGEMENT (SEE CHAPTERS 24 AND 25 FOR ADDITIONAL DETAILS)

Successful infection prevention and control practices enabling effective public health action and clinical care require a layered approach recognizing the roles of policies, procedures, HCPs, environmental staff, and the public. Whether for a suspected or confirmed VHF event, in either high or low-resourced settings, for community or healthcare facility interactions, the overall strategy is to separate low and high-risk situations in both structure and function. This allows staffing, equipping, and employing areas in predictable ways that can be sustained, reproduced, monitored, assessed, and adapted or corrected. In general, an individual HCP starts at low risk, gradually increasing the IPC posture as transmission of the VHF pathogen is more likely, and then only de-escalates when appropriate risk mitigation has occurred, in the case of a VHF suspected or confirmed patient contact, usually in the form of decontamination and doffing. Within this, the selection and utilization of appropriate personal protective equipment (PPE) is an important step in minimizing VHF transmission during direct patient care, waste management, and any other activity performed in the healthcare environment. Choices should be based upon a risk assessment that includes available PPE guidance for the specific pathogen, the care environment, training of HCP, and the acuity and clinical status of the patient.[99,100] When in close contact with a patient or within a designated high-risk area, PPE should protect the skin and mucous membranes from exposure to bodily fluids or potentially contaminated items and surfaces. Examples of PPE for VHF include everything from that employed in standard precautions to powered-air purifying respirators and coveralls. Choice of PPE depends on the potential for pathogen transmission and may also vary depending on the clinical status of the patient, including the amount of bodily fluids (vomitus, diarrhea) or potential for aerosol generation as might occur during an invasive procedure. Donning and doffing of PPE requires significant attention to detail, as these are potential modes for breaks in infection control technique that could result in transmission. Incorporating standard practices, initial and maintenance training that addresses rehearsed tasks and procedures, as well as donning and doffing partners or trained observers, helps mitigate risk by ensuring that all steps are performed appropriately.[30,101]

In patient care areas, control of bodily fluids using emesis bags, fecal management systems, or bedside commodes is an important environmental infection control modality, especially within-hospital isolation care wards with limited space and environmental management accommodations. Patient care facilities should have detailed protocols for spill cleanup and plans for the safe disposal of contaminated medical waste. These should be tested in advance of an event, as the handling of contaminated medical waste can result in the transmission of VHF pathogens. All persons handling waste should be trained in waste management protocols and wear appropriate PPE for the designated tasks. Protocols should include the packaging, storage, and ultimate management of both solid and liquid waste, including contaminated linens, PPE, and general medical waste. Solid waste disposal strategies may include incineration or autoclaving. Liquid waste can be disposed of in the sewer system or properly sited and laid pits or leach fields; however, some facilities utilize pretreatment strategies with disinfectant prior to disposal.[102] Solidifiers can be used to facilitate liquid waste disposal. When septic systems are used, and in smaller sewer systems, the potential impact of chlorine and other disinfectants should be considered. VHF-experienced water and sanitation and environmental hygiene experts should participate in planning and operations of VHF event management regardless of setting. Protocols for the terminal cleaning of the patient care facility generally include environmental surface cleaning and decontamination utilizing a hospital-grade disinfectant. Medical equipment for which single-patient use is not feasible should be thoroughly cleaned according to manufacturer guidelines, ensuring that appropriate decontamination procedures are followed. Some facilities in resourced settings use ultraviolet germicidal irradiation or vaporized hydrogen peroxide as an additional step in environmental decontamination.[103] Processes for the cleaning and decontamination of transport vehicles have been described.[104,105] Supervision by individuals trained in infection control, training and education of staff, documentation of each procedure, and tracking of waste are all important concepts to maintain the highest standards of environmental infection control.

For patients, families, communities, and response teams, facilitation of transparency, communication, visitation, psychosocial support, reintegration planning, and clinical medicine-public health coordination are important aspects of planning and executing a VHF event response. In a clinical context, simple measures such as designated visitation areas, availability of telephones or other electronic communication tools, and counselor support can make a strikingly positive difference in overall effectiveness and response team: community relationship.

HIGH-LEVEL CONTAINMENT CARE (SEE CHAPTER 26 FOR ADDITIONAL DETAILS)

In resourced settings, High-Level Containment Care (HLCC), also called biocontainment care units, may be available for patients with person-to-person transmissible VHF (see Chapter 26). The original HLCC, or "biocontainment" unit, located at the US Army Medical Research Institute of Infectious Diseases (USAMRIID), opened in 1971 but was decommissioned in 2012. The unit had specialized protocols and engineering controls. It was designed to manage patients who were exposed to or infected with highly hazardous communicable diseases (HHCD).[106] Currently, there are multiple HLCC facilities across the globe, many of which have cared for patients with VHF. HLCC units feature trained teams of HCPs; defined and practiced infection prevention and control protocols; specialized equipment; engineering controls designed to limit exposure to pathogens; laboratory capabilities with the purpose of providing ICU-level care to patients with HHCD; and, established methods of coordination with their communities.[107,108a] In these settings, the use of occupational health programmed vaccination is gaining interest, particularly with respect to Ebola virus disease and the rVSV-EBOV vaccine.[108b]

HEALTH SYSTEM IMPACT IN RESOURCED AND RESOURCE-LIMITED SETTINGS (SEE CHAPTERS 15 AND 24 FOR ADDITIONAL DETAILS)

Significant and often broad issues affecting the healthcare system may arise during an outbreak of VHF observed in both resource-limited and well-resourced settings. During an outbreak, the community may view the healthcare center as a place of danger, whether this is perceived or real. Due to these concerns, ill patients with symptoms concerning VHF may avoid the healthcare center, which contributes to the perpetuation of the outbreak through unidentified and uninterrupted chains of transmission in the community. Community-based work and isolation care centers have drawn violence, in some instances freezing the ability to perform necessary response functions. The optics of public health and clinical actions in response may become blurred in an emergency, with an unpopular public health action triggering anger or avoidance at healthcare facilities and vice versa.[109] HCPs may refuse to come to work due to concern for their personal or their families' well-being, an increased risk of exposure, recognizing insufficient or untrusted preparations at their facility, stigma, or possibly due to becoming ill themselves.[68] This may have long-term consequences for staffing.[110] In resourced settings with a single or small number of VHF cases, it has been observed that other patients may avoid the healthcare facility caring for VHF patients, resulting in a tarnished reputation and loss of revenue for the facility.[111] Public health programs, including contract tracing for VHF, may be interrupted, resulting in ill patients that are not detected. Disruptions in non-VHF programmatic elements, including vaccination, maternal health, and malaria-control programs, may be seen in resource-limited settings. Disruption of routine healthcare services may also occur, especially during a large outbreak where local healthcare facilities may limit their services, become VHF treatment centers, or close altogether. The entirety of these impacts on the health system may result in additional morbidity and mortality outside of that which occurs directly from VHF, though the extent of attributable mortality is a subject of debate.[112,113] Regardless, focused planning and operational activity are required for maintenance of usual healthcare services and public health programming during a VHF event.

SOCIETAL IMPACT AND INTERVENTIONS (SEE CHAPTERS 13, 15, AND 18 FOR ADDITIONAL DETAILS)

When the World Health Organization undertook to construct a research and development priority list against pathogens not otherwise covered under existing large-scale programming, it incorporated the idea of societal impact in two ways.[114] First, the internal scoring mechanism used to facilitate expert discussion rounds included a category of questions on societal impact.

Second, and perhaps more importantly, when a broad array of stakeholders was asked to contribute potential pathogens for consideration, the idea of pathogens that matter was captured. This process started in late 2014, as the scale and disruptive power of health emergencies were being felt from the Ebola virus disease epidemic in West Africa. In retrospect, research groups from a variety of disciplines have tried to understand what impact resulted to an already fragile subregion. By the end of the epidemic in June 2016, there were nearly 29,000 EVD cases with over 11,000 deaths reported across Liberia, Sierra Leone, Guinea, and Nigeria.[115]

Most experts believe these observations underestimate the totals. Mixed economic and social costs to West Africa were high. One group estimated more than a 53 billion USD cost, including almost 19 billion USD in related non-Ebola deaths.[116] These happen from a range of factors including healthcare site abandonment and disruption of long-term public health programs such as antimalaria efforts. World Bank estimates of pure economic costs are lower but still range in the billions of dollars and, importantly, show interrupted and down turned development in the subregion.[117] These broad-stroke numbers do not convey the striking impact in individual communities. In eastern Sierra Leone, movement was restricted with hours-long waits at road checkpoints placed to conduct screening. This stalled market activity and impacted available goods, increasing local anger toward responders, even when from their own communities. A study in Liberia showed that household income fell in communities regardless of whether they directly experienced Ebola virus disease or not.[118] Villages and communes across the subregion had varying experiences with the disease, some without recognized cases at all and others with devastating mortality. This sporadic, severe impact contributed to fear, stigma, and resistance to being identified as having a case.

A year-plus-long Ebola virus disease emergency afflicted the eastern Democratic Republic of Congo (DRC) in 2018–20. Nearly 3500 cases with 2300 deaths occurred, with the full scope of economic impact yet undetermined.[119] Smaller resurgences continue. Ebola there emerged in the context of a complex emergency with insurgencies and other varied political and economic interests. It has not helped peace and development.[120] Of course, VHF other than Ebola has a significant societal impact as well. Recurrent Lassa fever outbreaks across West Africa seem to be growing in frequency and scope, with increases in host and geographic range.[121,122] Capturing costs for distributed, recurring, focused outbreaks such as these is challenging. In contrast, Rift Valley fever has livestock value chain impacts that are more amenable to tracing. A 2007 outbreak in Kenya resulted in 32 million USD lost.[123] Still, human epizootic cases, livestock decapitalization, and the threat of hunger add to the complexity of how the community and the economy react to such an outbreak.

SURVIVORSHIP AND COMMUNITY RECOVERY (SEE CHAPTER 21 FOR ADDITIONAL DETAILS)

Long-term sequelae may occur from any severe infection, and VHF diseases are no different. The increasing pace of recognized VHF-related health emergencies has resulted in a greater understanding of these problems and their consequences. For many years, events were recognized so sporadically and in the context of such persistent stigma that little was understood about what happens to patients and their communities in the out-years of an event. Systematic assessments of Ebola survivors, for instance, did not arrive in the indexed literature until more than 20 years following its identification.[124,125] Larger events observed over longer periods of time meant a greater subclinical, mild, and moderate case load, affording a larger fraction of survivorship. The 2014–16 West Africa Ebola virus disease emergency led to several long-term studies of survivors. A retrospective cohort of over a thousand Guinean EVD survivors assessed against population-level data had a fivefold increased risk of death out to 1 year post discharge from isolation care, after which it seemed to normalize.[126] A similarly sized case cohort with contact controls followed prospectively in Liberia and assessed sequelae a year from discharge.[127] Complaints of urinary frequency, headache, muscle and joint pain, uveitis, memory loss, and other neurological findings on exam were more common among survivors. While the impact of longer-term sequelae remains to be observed, an assessment of survivors 2 years after an Ebola outbreak in Bundibugyo yielded similar results, including functional impact.[128] Differential features for survivors among the various filoviruses are not known.

The most studied of the sequelae from Lassa fever is sensorineural hearing loss. Estimates of prevalence among survivors vary widely, though it may occur in up to a third of patients.[129] This has been noted in Ebola as well.[130] Work in a guinea pig model for Lassa fever virus suggests a vasculitis in survivors to explain the constellation of muscle, joint, and hearing symptoms in survivors.[131] Omsk hemorrhagic fever virus, a tick-borne flavivirus, is associated with a long recovery period but then, less commonly, a constellation of hearing loss, hair loss, and behavioral and neurological sequelae.[132]

Like patients, communities take time to heal and may suffer long-term consequences from a VHF emergency. In disasters like the West Africa EVD epidemic, paths to recovery are complex whether focused on health system reassembly and performance or on broader views of community wellness such as wealth and social resilience.[133,134] Research on disaster recovery from any cause is scant; research focused on small communities even more so. Communities impacted by EVD and Lassa fever may acquire the appearance of normalcy quickly, but manpower deficits, orphans, negative attitudes toward affected communities, and other more subtle challenges persist in ways difficult to quantify. Less is known about the impact and durability of harm in remote communities or slums affected by, for example, Junin virus.

Unfortunately, for VHF, past performance seems to predict future performance. Excepting dengue's cosmopolitan behavior and strain iteration-linked population burden of hemorrhagic fever, geographic zones become well associated with the comparatively small number of VHF outbreaks that occur.[135,136] Arenaviruses in the Old and New Worlds and Omsk hemorrhagic fever virus are being understood to either have a range of mammalian hosts more broad or more species fitting a range of hosts than previously thought, allowing an expanding geographic range.[132,137–140] Crimean-Congo hemorrhagic fever has also spread and diversified strikingly throughout Asia, the Middle East, and now Africa.[141] For the tick- and mosquito-borne threats, mammalian hosts might not even be required given evidence of transovarian transmission across generations of vectors.[142,143] And, like dengue, both Ebola and Marburg viruses display antibody-dependent enhancement in laboratory conditions. Prior exposure to a VHF could mean either some protection from a future event, a more severe reemergence, or both, depending on the population subset.[144–146]

In the nearer term, welcoming infected persons back into communities for healing, reconciliation, and community wellness is the challenge of recrudescence of disease from sanctuary and immune-privileged sites such as the central nervous system and testes. HCPs returning to well-resourced settings have manifested recrudescent disease.[147,148] Though, in general, survivors have undergone cataract surgery and other related procedures without signs of infection.[149] While viral persistence in semen had been known, viral nucleic acid persistence in semen for nearly 2 years in a Liberian cohort surprised many, and a sexual transmission-associated recrudescent outbreak may have occurred in Liberia.[127,150–152] The Zika experience suggests that this probably is not a unique phenomenon among the filoviruses but rather something to consider for any disseminated virus causing a VHF.[151]

Patients and communities require focused management in recovery from a VHF emergency that is personal, social, and economic. Both health and non-health strategies are important for reintegration and recovery and are mindful of each level of need and risk.

HEALTH SECURITY APERTURE ON VHF—PUBLIC HEALTH INTERDICTION

VHF has entered the general consciousness regarding what it means to be unsafe. *The Hot Zone* by Richard Preston, the movie *Outbreak*, and a Nigerian film on its 2014 Ebola virus disease emergency called *93 Days* reflect the enlarging popular association between VHF and safety and security. The most striking popular notice, however, is the opening scene of Marvel's feature film *Captain America: Civil War*, where the Avengers seek to interrupt capture of a single Ebola virus-infected blood sample from a fanciful, sophisticated, specially designed, single-tube vault in a public health laboratory in Lagos, Nigeria. As the details of this chapter relate, a VHF emergency strikingly impacts affected patients and communities and can achieve consequences in at risk, unaffected communities and global marketplaces. VHF pathogens do this even though their sustained person-to-person transmission capabilities are much lower than those of the respiratory transmitted viruses such as Severe Acute Respiratory Syndrome coronavirus (SARS-CoV), SARS-CoV-2, or smallpox.[153] In part, this is due to a fallacy—universal acquisition of the disease by those exposed and complete mortality—driven by a decades-long history of sporadic events observed late in their course among isolated populations by few experts.[154] Even when not equipped with antipathogen-directed therapeutics, larger events are starting to force a slow evolution toward more moderate thinking that events while impactful are not catastrophic, and aggressive action matters.[155]

That a single VHF event is so disruptive raises concerns that a relevant pathogen could be used as a tool for harm. According to one senior defector, the Soviets actively worked on the development of Ebola, Marburg, Machupo, and Junin virus variants as weapons for use in assassination and larger conflict, with a Marburg virus submitted for approval.[156] In VHF, distinguishing a natural from a deliberate event early in an emergency would be very difficult, as in both instances these outbreaks may not be detected from the initial cases but rather secondary clusters of severe disease. A variety of national and international efforts exist to counter the proliferation of natural events into deliberate event opportunities. In the United States, these include biosafety and biosecurity regulations under the Select Agents program, global engagement activities for improved disease detection and characterization, biosecurity, reduction of dual-use research of concern, and raising multidisciplinary awareness.[157–159] For state actors, the Biological Weapons Convention governs roles and responsibilities of the international community regarding counter-proliferation.[160] This treaty has been in force since 1975. In 2004, the UN Security Council Committee 1540 was established to address these issues in the context of nonstate actors.[161] National programming on dual-use research of concern requires a more nuanced conversation among researchers, funding entities, journals, and industry as innovation remains needed in the characterization of high-consequence pathogen risks and development of appropriate countermeasures.[162,163]

Unfortunately, this combination of historical community impact and security threat optics has sometimes resulted in transference, exacerbating the idea of the infected patient as a threat, contributing to aggressive biosecurity postures and narratives around isolation care that degrade community and patient trust regarding intent. This may have contributed to the stunting of clinical management tools and best practices for better patient outcomes seen in VHF regardless of pathogen. On the other hand, thinking roundly about the threat in terms of risk management offers advantages to planning and executing prevention and mitigation to preserve health and societal outcomes against VHF (Fig. 1) or any other high-consequence threat.

Like other special pathogens, medical countermeasure development against VHF has been plagued by sporadic opportunities to develop sufficient understanding to develop effective products, conduct advanced clinical trials, and avoid the pitfalls of technologies narrowly focused against individual pathogens.[164,165] A major challenge in advancing therapeutic products against VHF has been difficulty executing appropriately rigorous clinical trials against a background of aggressive, safe, and effective care. Some of this is caused by a necessarily high infection prevention and control posture that increases the activation

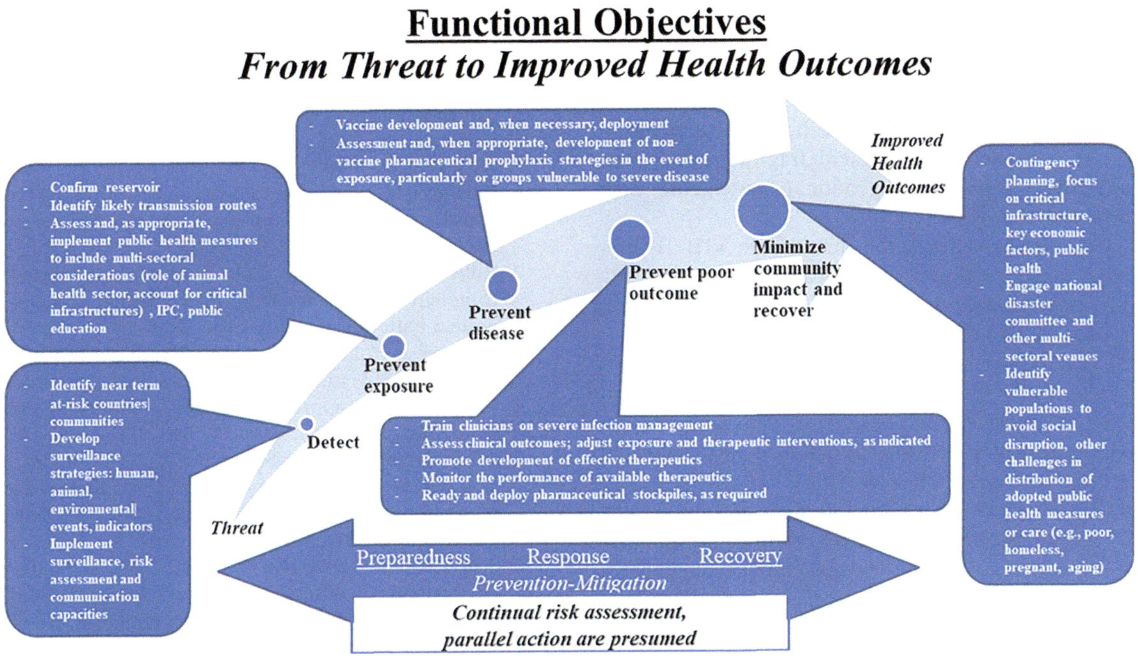

FIG. 1 This figure denotes health emergency and disaster risk management objectives related to each step in the process of preventing and mitigating an emerging infectious disease threat. The objectives to the left of the diagram focus on risk identification and characterization and then move to prevention. As the threat is increasingly realized in communities (right side of figure), the objectives focus on community actions with the goal of improving outcomes. The arc represents the various steps considered in a response with examples in the bubbles.

energy required to execute the trial at bedside and the laboratory, a problem being attacked by some movements to be ready earlier than the start of an outbreak. Another problem has been the niche researcher base driven by IPC and security requirements, which leaves datasets less robust and a broad reticence to do important repetitive work to verify results. This is best demonstrated in the context of ribavirin, where there is some literature supporting its use against Hantaan virus and Lassa fever virus, but push and pull on safety, efficacy, best use, and extrapolations to closely related viruses.[35,36,98,166] A strong therapeutic misconception is applied in this context, such as aggressive use of ribavirin against Lassa fever virus without sufficient attention to advanced critical care approaches.[167] Nonetheless, the Ebola virus disease experience has been large enough in scale in recent years to result in substantial movement in products near licensure, at least with effect against particular strains.

All these challenges create conundrums for those attempting to construct stockpiles for use in broad prevention and mitigation efforts. Vaccine and therapeutic agent selection is currently narrowed by pathogens, despite the larger threat coming from a wide array of pathogens. Diagnostic advances with multipathogen film arrays, distributable lateral flow assays, and portable sequencing technologies have promise but have their own early and mid-developmental challenges with fully exploiting the potential use cases, such as validity false positives due to persistent nucleic acid fragments and confounding by pathogen genetic or antigenic drift, shift, or heterogeneity.[168–170]

On a granular level, the threat from VHF is interdicted by conventional public health action:

(1) Characterization of modes of zoonotic crossover or accidental or deliberate release.
(2) Layered steps to limit the occurrence of such events, especially the enculturation of universal precautions, biosafety, and biosecurity principles.
(3) Contingency readiness to enhance performance in response and resilience.
(4) Early case identification and management.
(5) Rapid risk assessment and scaling upwards of the response to enable robust contact tracing and monitoring.
(6) Culturally lucid social mobilization and risk communication with mutually reinforcing clinical care and public health activities.
(7) Interruption of usual VHF event propagation modalities such as with enhanced screening on presentation and within healthcare facilities, applying a low threshold for case investigations, and broadly engaging traditional healer avenues as well as employing safe and dignified burial practices.
(8) Targeting opportunities for decreasing exposures such as food storage and peri-domestic animals and vector exposures, relevant to the particular VHF threat.
(9) Recovery.[171]

This is analogous to the challenge of managing all high-consequence threats and fitting a patient- and community-centered outcome approach such as that depicted in Fig. 1. In total, cogency in health security regarding VHF requires whole-of-society approaches that recognize the broad spate of risks and yet pursue a wide array of opportunities for each actor to enhance general health emergency risk management.

REFERENCES

1. Maegraith B. Yellow fever in West Africa, 1942. *Trans R Soc Trop Med Hyg.* 1946;39(4):347.
2. Knipe DM, Howley PM, eds. *Fields Virology.* 6th ed. Philadelphia, PA: Wolters Kluwer/Lippincott Williams & Wilkins Health; 2013. 2 p.
3. Avšič-Županc T, Saksida A, Korva M. Hantavirus infections. *Clin Microbiol Infect Off Publ Eur Soc Clin Microbiol Infect Dis.* 2019;21S:e6–16.
4. Brisse ME, Ly H. Hemorrhagic fever-causing arenaviruses: lethal pathogens and potent immune suppressors. *Front Immunol.* 2019;10:372.
5. Hartman A. Rift valley fever. *Clin Lab Med.* 2017;37(2):285–301.
6. Pallesen J, Murin CD, de Val N, et al. Structures of Ebola virus GP and sGP in complex with therapeutic antibodies. *Nat Microbiol.* 2016;1(9):16128.
7. Sullivan NJ, Peterson M, Yang Z, et al. Ebola virus glycoprotein toxicity is mediated by a dynamin-dependent protein-trafficking pathway. *J Virol.* 2005;79(1):547–553.
8. Bukreyev A, Volchkov VE, Blinov VM, Netesov SV. The GP-protein of Marburg virus contains the region similar to the "immunosuppressive domain" of oncogenic retrovirus P15E proteins. *FEBS Lett.* 1993;323(1–2):183–187.
9. Loureiro ME, Zorzetto-Fernandes AL, Radoshitzky S, et al. DDX3 suppresses type I interferons and favors viral replication during Arenavirus infection. *PLoS Pathog.* 2018;14(7), e1007125.
10. Schindell BG, Webb AL, Kindrachuk J. Persistence and sexual transmission of filoviruses. *Viruses.* 2018;10(12):683. https://doi.org/10.3390/v10120683. PMID: 30513823; PMCID: PMC6316729.
11. Lalle E, Colavita F, Iannetta M, et al. Prolonged detection of dengue virus RNA in the semen of a man returning from Thailand to Italy, January 2018. *Euro Surveill Bull Eur Sur Mal Transm Eur Commun Dis Bull.* 2018;23(18), 18-00197. https://doi.org/10.2807/1560-7917.ES.2018.23.18.18-00197. PMID: 29741153; PMCID: PMC6053624.

12. Advisory Committee on Dangerous Pathogens. Management of Hazard Group 4 Viral Haemorrhagic Fevers and Similar Human Infectious Diseases of High Consequence; 2015. gov.uk.
13. Enria DA, Briggiler AM, Sanchez Z. Treatment of Argentine hemorrhagic fever. *Antivir Res.* 2008;78(1):132–139.
14. Ambrosio A, et al. Argentine hemorrhagic fever vaccines. *Hum Vaccin.* 2011;7(6):694–700.
15. Spickler AR. Viral Hemorrhagic Fevers Caused by Arenaviruses; 2010. http://www.cfsph.iastate.edu/DiseaseInfo/factsheets.php.
16. Crimean-Congo Haemorrhagic Fever: Origins, Reservoirs, Transmission and Guidelines; 2014. Available from: https://www.gov.uk/guidance/crimean-congo-haemorrhagic-fever-origins-reservoirs-transmission-and-guidelines.
17. Centers for Disease Control and Prevention (CDC). Crimean-Congo Hemorrhagic Fever; 2024. Available from: https://www.cdc.gov/vhf/crimean-congo/index.html.
18. Dengue vaccine: WHO position paper—July 2016. *Wkly Epidemiol Rec.* 2016;91(30):349–364.
19. World Health Organization (WHO). Dengue Guidelines for Diagnosis, Treatment, Prevention and Control; 2009. Available from: http://apps.who.int/iris/bitstream/handle/10665/44188/9789241547871_eng.pdf?sequence=1.
20. Centers for Disease Control and Prevention (CDC). Dengue. Available from: https://www.cdc.gov/dengue/index.html.
21. Centers for Disease Control and Prevention (CDC). Ebola (Ebola Virus Disease). Available from: https://www.cdc.gov/vhf/ebola/index.html.
22. Malvy D, et al. Ebola virus disease. *Lancet.* 2019;393(10174):936–948.
23. World Health Organization (WHO). Lassa Fever. Available from: https://www.who.int/health-topics/lassa-fever#tab=tab_1.
24. Centers for Disease Control and Prevention (CDC). Lassa Fever. CDC; 2024. https://www.cdc.gov/lassa-fever/about/.
25. Iannetta M, et al. Viral hemorrhagic fevers other than Ebola and Lassa. *Infect Dis Clin N Am.* 2019;33(4):977–1002.
26. World Health Organization (WHO). Marburg Haemorrhagic Fever. Available from: https://www.afro.who.int/health-topics/marburg-haemorrhagic-fever.
27. Růžek D, et al. Omsk haemorrhagic fever. *Lancet.* 2010;376(9758):2104–2113.
28. Centers for Disease Control and Prevention (CDC). Omsk Hemorrhagic Fever (OHF). CDC; 2013. https://www.cdc.gov/omsk-fever/about/.
29. Centers for Disease Control and Prevention (CDC). Rift Valley Fever (RVF). CDC; 2024. website https://www.cdc.gov/rift-valley-fever/about/.
30. Brett-Major DM, Jacob ST, Jacquerioz FA, et al. Being ready to treat Ebola virus disease patients. *Am J Trop Med Hyg.* 2015;92(2):233–237.
31. McLay L, et al. Targeting virulence mechanisms for the prevention and therapy of arenaviral hemorrhagic fever. *Antivir Res.* 2013;97(2):81–92.
32. Velasquez R, del Valle M, Rodriguez S, et al. Detection of Guanarito virus by one step RT-PCR. Revista de la Sociedad Venezolana de. *Microbiologia.* 2017;37(2):82–86.
33. Centers for Disease Control and Prevention (CDC). Yellow Fever. CDC; 2024. https://www.cdc.gov/yellow-fever/about/.
34. Domingo C, et al. Yellow fever in the diagnostics laboratory. *Emerg Microbes Infect.* 2018;7(1):129.
35. Rusnak JM, Byrne WR, Chung KN, et al. Experience with intravenous ribavirin in the treatment of hemorrhagic fever with renal syndrome in Korea. *Antivir Res.* 2009;81(1):68–76.
36. Eberhardt KA, Mischlinger J, Jordan S, Groger M, Günther S, Ramharter M. Ribavirin for the treatment of Lassa fever: a systematic review and meta-analysis. *Int J Infect Dis IJID Off Publ Int Soc Infect Dis.* 2019;87:15–20.
37. Moreli ML, Marques-Silva AC, Pimentel VA, da Costa VG. Effectiveness of the ribavirin in treatment of hantavirus infections in the Americas and Eurasia: a meta-analysis. *Virusdisease.* 2014;25(3):385–389.
38. Tchesnokov EP, Feng JY, Porter DP, Götte M. Mechanism of inhibition of ebola virus RNA-dependent RNA polymerase by remdesivir. *Viruses.* 2019;11(4):326. https://doi.org/10.3390/v11040326. PMID: 30987343; PMCID: PMC6520719.
39. Patel JS, Quates CJ, Johnson EL, Ytreberg FM. Expanding the watch list for potential Ebola virus antibody escape mutations. *PLoS One.* 2019;14(3), e0211093.
40. Henao-Restrepo AM, Camacho A, Longini IM, et al. Efficacy and effectiveness of an rVSV-vectored vaccine in preventing Ebola virus disease: final results from the Guinea ring vaccination, open-label, cluster-randomised trial (Ebola Ça Suffit!). *Lancet Lond Engl.* 2017;389(10068):505–518.
41. Wells CR, Pandey A, Parpia AS, et al. Ebola vaccination in the Democratic Republic of the Congo. *Proc Natl Acad Sci USA.* 2019;116(20):10178–10183.
42. Leske A, Waßmann I, Schnepel K, et al. Assessing cross-reactivity of Junín virus-directed neutralizing antibodies. *Antivir Res.* 2019;163:106–116.
43. International Committee on Taxonomy of Viruses. Taxonomic Information International Committee on Taxonomy of Viruses; 2019. [Internet]. [cited 2019 Sep. 23]. Available from: https://talk.ictvonline.org/taxonomy/.
44. Cohen J. The immunopathogenesis of sepsis. *Nature.* 2002;420(6917):885–891.
45. van der Poll T, van de Veerdonk FL, Scicluna BP, Netea MG. The immunopathology of sepsis and potential therapeutic targets. *Nat Rev Immunol.* 2017;17(7):407–420.
46. Khaiboullina SF, Rizvanov AA, Holbrook MR, St Jeor S. Yellow fever virus strains Asibi and 17D-204 infect human umbilical cord endothelial cells and induce novel changes in gene expression. *Virology.* 2005;342(2):167–176.

47. Ho Y-L, Joelsons D, Leite GFC, et al. Severe yellow fever in Brazil: clinical characteristics and management. *J Travel Med.* 2019;26(5), taz040. https://doi.org/10.1093/jtm/taz040. PMID: 31150098.
48. Malavige GN, Ogg GS. Pathogenesis of vascular leak in dengue virus infection. *Immunology.* 2017;151(3):261–269.
49. Michels M, Alisjahbana B, De Groot PG, et al. Platelet function alterations in dengue are associated with plasma leakage. *Thromb Haemost.* 2014;112(2):352–362.
50. Zhou W, Woodson M, Neupane B, et al. Exosomes serve as novel modes of tick-borne flavivirus transmission from arthropod to human cells and facilitates dissemination of viral RNA and proteins to the vertebrate neuronal cells. *PLoS Pathog.* 2018;14(1), e1006764.
51. Schnittler HJ, Mahner F, Drenckhahn D, Klenk HD, Feldmann H. Replication of Marburg virus in human endothelial cells. A possible mechanism for the development of viral hemorrhagic disease. *J Clin Invest.* 1993;91(4):1301–1309.
52. Geisbert TW, Young HA, Jahrling PB, et al. Pathogenesis of Ebola hemorrhagic fever in primate models: evidence that hemorrhage is not a direct effect of virus-induced cytolysis of endothelial cells. *Am J Pathol.* 2003;163(6):2371–2382.
53. Doğan HO, Büyüktuna SA, Kapancik S, Bakir S. Evaluation of the associations between endothelial dysfunction, inflammation and coagulation in Crimean-Congo hemorrhagic fever patients. *Arch Virol.* 2018;163(3):609–616.
54. Centers for Disease Control and Prevention (CDC). Crimean-Congo Hemorrhagic Fever (CCHF): Signs and Symptoms; 2013. Available from: https://www.cdc.gov/vhf/crimean-congo/symptoms/index.html.
55. Centers for Disease Control and Prevention (CDC). Dengue: Clinical Presentation; 2023. Available from: https://www.cdc.gov/dengue/healthcare-providers/clinical-presentation.html.
56. Pouliot SH, et al. Maternal dengue and pregnancy outcomes: a systematic review. *Obstet Gynecol Surv.* 2010;65(2):107–118.
57. Rojas M, et al. Ebola virus disease: an emerging and re-emerging viral threat. *J Autoimmun.* 2020;106, 102375.
58. Kayem ND, et al. Ebola virus disease in pregnancy: a systematic review and meta-analysis. *Trans R Soc Trop Med Hyg.* 2022;116(6):509–522.
59. Centers for Disease Control and Prevention (CDC). Lassa Fever: Signs and Symptoms; 2014. Available from: https://www.cdc.gov/vhf/lassa/symptoms/index.html.
60. Centers for Disease Control and Prevention (CDC). Rift Valley Fever: Signs and Symptoms; 2020. Available from: https://www.cdc.gov/vhf/rvf/symptoms/index.html.
61. Centers for Disease Control and Prevention (CDC). Yellow Fever Virus: Symptoms, Diagnosis, & Treatment; 2022. Available from: https://www.cdc.gov/yellowfever/symptoms/index.html.
62. Johansson MA, Vasconcelos PF, Staples JE. The whole iceberg: estimating the incidence of yellow fever virus infection from the number of severe cases. *Trans R Soc Trop Med Hyg.* 2014;108(8):482–487.
63. Centers for Disease Control and Prevention (CDC). Tourniquet Test. CDC; 2018. Available from: ourniquet test: inflate a blood pressure cough on the upper arm of the patient to a point midway between the systolic and the diastolic blood pressure and maintain it for 5 minutes. Deflate the cuff and wait 2 more minutes. 10 or more petechiae per square inch represents a positive test https://www.cdc.gov/dengue/training/cme/ccm/page73112.html. Available from: ourniquet test: inflate a blood pressure cough on the upper arm of the patient to a point midway between the systolic and the diastolic blood pressure and maintain it for 5 minutes. Deflate the cuff and wait 2 more minutes. 10 or more petechiae per square inch represents a positive test.
64. Swanepoel R, Smit SB, Rollin PE, et al. Studies of reservoir hosts for Marburg virus. *Emerg Infect Dis.* 2007;13(12):1847–1851.
65. Blumberg L, Enria D, Bausch DG. Viral haemorrhagic fevers. In: *Manson's Tropical Infectious Diseases.* Elsevier; 2014:171–194.e2. [Internet]. [cited 2019 Sep. 23]. Available from: https://linkinghub.elsevier.com/retrieve/pii/B9780702051012000170.
66. Wood SM, Brett-Major DM. Risk mitigation for travelers: managing endemic and emerging threats. *Pol Arch Intern Med.* 2019;129(9):612–619. https://doi.org/10.20452/pamw.14946. Epub 2019 Aug 28. PMID: 31456592.
67. Wadman MC, Schwedhelm SS, Watson S, et al. Emergency department processes for the evaluation and management of persons under investigation for ebola virus disease. *Ann Emerg Med.* 2015;66(3):306–314.
68. Brett-Major D. A Year of Ebola: Durable Lessons; and, Essays on Our Ancient Relationship With Infectious Diseases. Navigating Health Risks, LLC; 2017 [278 pp, ISBN-10: 099836516 5I; SBN-13: 978-0998365169].
69. Hidalgo J, Richards GA, Jiménez JIS, Baker T, Amin P. Viral hemorrhagic fever in the tropics: report from the task force on tropical diseases by the World Federation of Societies of Intensive and Critical Care Medicine. *J Crit Care.* 2017;42:366–372.
70. Bah EI, Lamah M-C, Fletcher T, et al. Clinical presentation of patients with Ebola virus disease in Conakry, Guinea. *N Engl J Med.* 2015;372(1):40–47.
71. McCormick JB, King IJ, Webb PA, et al. A case-control study of the clinical diagnosis and course of Lassa fever. *J Infect Dis.* 1987;155(3):445–455.
72. Duygu F, Sari T, Gunal O, Barut S, Atay A, Aytekin F. Cutaneous findings of crimean-congo hemorrhagic fever: a study of 269 cases. *Jpn J Infect Dis.* 2018;71(6):408–412.
73. Leligdowicz A, Fischer WA, Uyeki TM, et al. Ebola virus disease and critical illness. *Crit Care Lond Engl.* 2016;20(1):217.
74. Cournac JM, Karkowski L, Bordes J, et al. Rhabdomyolysis in ebola virus disease. Results of an observational study in a treatment center in guinea. *Clin Infect Dis Off Publ Infect Dis Soc Am.* 2016;62(1):19–23.
75. Wolf T, Kann G, Becker S, et al. Severe Ebola virus disease with vascular leakage and multiorgan failure: treat-

ment of a patient in intensive care. *Lancet Lond Engl.* 2015;385(9976):1428–1435.
76. Fowler RA, Fletcher T, Fischer WA, et al. Caring for critically ill patients with ebola virus disease. Perspectives from West Africa. *Am J Respir Crit Care Med.* 2014;190(7):733–737.
77. Waxman M, Aluisio AR, Rege S, Levine AC. Characteristics and survival of patients with Ebola virus infection, malaria, or both in Sierra Leone: a retrospective cohort study. *Lancet Infect Dis.* 2017;17(6):654–660.
78. Raabe V, Koehler J. Laboratory diagnosis of Lassa fever. *J Clin Microbiol.* 2017;55(6):1629–1637.
79. Isaäcson M. Viral hemorrhagic fever hazards for travelers in Africa. *Clin Infect Dis Off Publ Infect Dis Soc Am.* 2001;33(10):1707–1712.
80. Pemba CM, Kurosaki Y, Yoshikawa R, et al. Development of an RT-LAMP assay for the detection of Lassa viruses in southeast and south-central Nigeria. *J Virol Methods.* 2019;269:30–37.
81. Dhillon RS, Srikrishna D, Kelly JD. Deploying RDTs in the DRC Ebola outbreak. *Lancet Lond Engl.* 2018;391(10139):2499–2500.
82. Mourya DT, Viswanathan R, Jadhav SK, Yadav PD, Basu A, Chadha MS. Retrospective analysis of clinical information in Crimean-Congo haemorrhagic fever patients: 2014-2015, India. *Indian J Med Res.* 2017;145(5):673–678.
83. Koskela SM, Joutsi-Korhonen L, Mäkelä SM, et al. Diminished coagulation capacity assessed by calibrated automated thrombography during acute Puumala hantavirus infection. *Blood Coagul Fibrinolysis Int J Haemost Thromb.* 2018;29(1):55–60.
84. Uyeki TM, Mehta AK, Davey RT, et al. Clinical management of ebola virus disease in the United States and Europe. *N Engl J Med.* 2016;374(7):636–646.
85. Monath TP, Vasconcelos PFC. Yellow fever. *J Clin Virol Off Publ Pan Am Soc Clin Virol.* 2015;64:160–173.
86. Li T, Mbala-Kingebeni P, Naccache SN, et al. Metagenomic next-generation sequencing of the 2014 ebola virus disease outbreak in the Democratic Republic of the Congo. *J Clin Microbiol.* 2019;57(9), e00827-19. https://doi.org/10.1128/JCM.00827-19. PMID: 31315955; PMCID: PMC6711896.
87. Sow A, Loucoubar C, Diallo D, et al. Concurrent malaria and arbovirus infections in Kedougou, southeastern Senegal. *Malar J.* 2016;15:47.
88. Chertow DS, Uyeki TM, DuPont HL. Loperamide therapy for voluminous diarrhea in Ebola virus disease. *J Infect Dis.* 2015;211(7):1036–1037.
89. Chertow DS, Kleine C, Edwards JK, Scaini R, Giuliani R, Sprecher A. Ebola virus disease in West Africa—clinical manifestations and management. *N Engl J Med.* 2014;371(22):2054–2057.
90. World Health Organization. Optimized Supportive Care for Ebola Virus Disease: Clinical Management Standard Operating Procedure. WHO; 2019. [Internet]. [cited 2019 Sep. 23]. Available from: https://apps.who.int/iris/bitstream/handle/10665/325000/9789241515894-eng.pdf?sequence=1.
91. Sueblinvong V, Johnson DW, Weinstein GL, et al. Critical care for multiple organ failure secondary to ebola virus disease in the United States. *Crit Care Med.* 2015;43(10):2066–2075.
92. Johnson DW, Sullivan JN, Piquette CA, et al. Lessons learned: critical care management of patients with Ebola in the United States. *Crit Care Med.* 2015;43(6):1157–1164.
93. Connor MJ, Kraft C, Mehta AK, et al. Successful delivery of RRT in Ebola virus disease. *J Am Soc Nephrol.* 2015;26(1):31–37.
94. Fischer WA, Crozier I, Bausch DG, et al. Shifting the paradigm—applying universal standards of care to Ebola virus disease. *N Engl J Med.* 2019;380(15):1389–1391.
95. Woods A. Two experimental Ebola drugs are saving lives in the Congo. *New York Post.* 2019. August. [Internet]. 13 [cited 2019 Sep. 23]. Available from: https://nypost.com/2019/08/13/two-experimental-ebola-drugs-are-saving-lives-in-the-congo/.
96. World Health Organization. Notes for the Record: Consultation on Monitored Emergency Use of Unregistered and Investigational Interventions for Ebola Virus Disease (EVD). WHO; 2018. [Internet]. [cited 2019 Sep 23]. Available from: https://www.who.int/emergencies/ebola/MEURI-Ebola.pdf?ua=1.
97. van Griensven J, Edwards T, de Lamballerie X, et al. Evaluation of convalescent plasma for Ebola virus disease in guinea. *N Engl J Med.* 2016;374(1):33–42.
98. McCormick JB, King IJ, Webb PA, et al. Lassa fever. Effective therapy with ribavirin. *N Engl J Med.* 1986;314(1):20–26.
99. Centers for Disease Control and Prevention. Guidance on Personal Protective Equipment (PPE) To Be Used by Healthcare Workers during Management of Patients with Confirmed Ebola or Persons under Investigation (PUIs) for Ebola who are Clinically Unstable or Have Bleeding, Vomiting, or Diarrhea in U.S. Hospitals, Including Procedures for Donning and Doffing PPE [Internet]. Ebola Virus Disease: For Public Health Planners: Personal Protective Equipment; 2019. [cited 2019 Sep. 23]. Available from: https://www.cdc.gov/vhf/ebola/healthcare-us/ppe/guidance.html.
100. World Health Organization. EBOLA STRATEGY: Ebola and Marburg Virus Disease Epidemics: Preparedness, Alert, Control and Evaluation; 2014. [Internet]; Aug [cited 2019 Sep. 23]. Report No.: WHO/HSE/PED/CED/2014.05. Available from: https://www.who.int/csr/resources/publications/ebola/manual_EVD/en/.
101. Fischer WA, Hynes NA, Perl TM. Protecting health care workers from Ebola: personal protective equipment is critical but is not enough. *Ann Intern Med.* 2014;161(10):753–754.
102. Lowe JJ, Olinger PL, Gibbs SG, et al. Environmental infection control considerations for Ebola. *Am J Infect Control.* 2015;43(7):747–749.

103. Jelden KC, Gibbs SG, Smith PW, et al. Nebraska Biocontainment Unit patient discharge and environmental decontamination after Ebola care. *Am J Infect Control.* 2015;43(3):203–205.
104. Isakov A, Miles W, Gibbs S, Lowe J, Jamison A, Swansiger R. Transport and management of patients with confirmed or suspected ebola virus disease. *Ann Emerg Med.* 2015;66(3):297–305.
105. Schilling S, Follin P, Jarhall B, et al. European concepts for the domestic transport of highly infectious patients. *Clin Microbiol Infect Off Publ Eur Soc Clin Microbiol Infect Dis.* 2009;15(8):727–733.
106. Kortepeter MG, Kwon EH, Hewlett AL, Smith PW, Cieslak TJ. Containment care units for managing patients with highly hazardous infectious diseases: a concept whose time has come. *J Infect Dis.* 2016;214(Suppl. 3):S137–S141.
107. Garibaldi BT, Chertow DS. High-containment pathogen preparation in the intensive care unit. *Infect Dis Clin N Am.* 2017;31(3):561–576.
108. (a)Hewlett AL, Varkey JB, Smith PW, Ribner BS. Ebola virus disease: preparedness and infection control lessons learned from two biocontainment units. *Curr Opin Infect Dis.* 2015;28(4):343–348. (b)https://www.cdc.gov/vhf/ebola/clinicians/vaccine/index.html.
109. Marcis FL, Enria L, Abramowitz S, Saez A-M, Faye SLB. Three acts of resistance during the 2014–16 West Africa Ebola Epidemic. *J Humanit Aff.* 2019;1(2):23–31.
110. Wolf L, Ulrich CM, Grady C. Emergency nursing, ebola, and public policy: the contributions of nursing to the public policy conversation. *Hast Cent Rep.* 2016;46(Suppl. 1):S35–S38.
111. Mangan D. Ebola Hits Texas Hospital in the Pocketbook. CNBC; 2014. [Internet] [cited 2019 Sep 23]. Available from: https://www.cnbc.com/2014/10/22/ebola-hits-texas-hospital-in-the-pocketbook.html.
112. Kuehne A, Lynch E, Marshall E, et al. Mortality, morbidity and health-seeking behaviour during the ebola epidemic 2014-2015 in monrovia results from a mobile phone survey. *PLoS Negl Trop Dis.* 2016;10(8), e0004899.
113. Vygen S, Tiffany A, Rull M, et al. Changes in health-seeking behavior did not result in increased all-cause mortality during the Ebola outbreak in Western Area, Sierra Leone. *Am J Trop Med Hyg.* 2016;95(4):897–901.
114. Blueprint for R&D Preparedness and Response to Public Health Emergencies Due to Highly Infectious Pathogens: Workshop on Prioritization of Pathogens. World Health Organization; 2015. [Internet]. Dec. [cited 2019 Sep. 23]. Available from: https://www.who.int/blueprint/what/research-development/meeting-report-prioritization.pdf?ua=1.
115. Ebola Virus Disease. World Health Organization; 2016. [Internet]. Jun. [cited 2019 Sep. 23]. Available from: https://apps.who.int/iris/bitstream/handle/10665/208883/ebolasitrep_10Jun2016_eng.pdf;jsessionid=D4909DCD1F28771714924 0027FD4F415?sequence=1.
116. Huber C, Finelli L, Stevens W. The economic and social burden of the 2014 Ebola outbreak in West Africa. *J Infect Dis.* 2018;218(suppl_5):S698–S704.
117. 2014-2015 West Africa Ebola Crisis: Impact Update. World Bank Group; 2016. [Internet]. 2016 May [cited 2019 Sep. 23]. Available from: http://pubdocs.worldbank.org/en/297531463677588074/Ebola-Economic-Impact-and-Lessons-Paper-short-version.pdf.
118. Gatiso TT, Ordaz-Németh I, Grimes T, et al. The impact of the Ebola virus disease (EVD) epidemic on agricultural production and livelihoods in Liberia. *PLoS Negl Trop Dis.* 2018;12(8), e0006580.
119. World Health Organization. Ebola health update—DRC; 2019. [Internet]. Emergencies—Diseases—Ebola.[cited 2021 Mar. 09]. Available from: https://www.who.int/emergencies/diseases/ebola/drc-2019.
120. Brett-Major DM. Peace is a better focus than Ebola in the DRC. *Health Secur.* 2019;17(3):251–252.
121. WHO Regional Office for Africa. WHO supports five countries to fight Lassa fever outbreaks. *WHO Africa [News].* 2019. [Internet]. [cited 2019 Sep. 23]. Available from: https://www.afro.who.int/news/who-supports-five-countries-fight-lassa-fever-outbreaks.
122. Olayemi A, Cadar D, Magassouba N, et al. New hosts of the lassa virus. *Sci Rep.* 2016;03(6):25280.
123. Rich KM, Wanyoike F. An assessment of the regional and national socio-economic impacts of the 2007 Rift Valley fever outbreak in Kenya. *Am J Trop Med Hyg.* 2010;83(2 Suppl):52–57.
124. De Roo A, Ado B, Rose B, Guimard Y, Fonck K, Colebunders R. Survey among survivors of the 1995 Ebola epidemic in Kikwit, Democratic Republic of Congo: their feelings and experiences. *Trop Med Int Health.* 1998;3(11):883–885.
125. Kibadi K, Mupapa K, Kuvula K, et al. Late ophthalmologic manifestations in survivors of the 1995 Ebola virus epidemic in Kikwit, Democratic Republic of the Congo. *J Infect Dis.* 1999;179(Suppl. 1):S13–S14.
126. Keita M, Diallo B, Mesfin S, et al. Subsequent mortality in survivors of Ebola virus disease in Guinea: a nationwide retrospective cohort study. *Lancet Infect Dis.* 2019;19(11):1202–1208. https://doi.org/10.1016/S1473-3099(19)30313-5. Epub 2019 Sep 4. PMID: 31494017.
127. PREVAIL III Study Group, Sneller MC, Reilly C, et al. A longitudinal study of Ebola sequelae in Liberia. *N Engl J Med.* 2019;380(10):924–934.
128. Clark DV, Kibuuka H, Millard M, et al. Long-term sequelae after Ebola virus disease in Bundibugyo, Uganda: a retrospective cohort study. *Lancet Infect Dis.* 2015;15(8):905–912.
129. Mateer EJ, Huang C, Shehu NY, Paessler S. Lassa fever-induced sensorineural hearing loss: a neglected public health and social burden. *PLoS Negl Trop Dis.* 2018;12(2), e0006187.
130. Ficenec SC, Schieffelin JS, Emmett SD. A review of hearing loss associated with Zika, Ebola, and Lassa fever. *Am J Trop Med Hyg.* 2019;101(3):484–490.

131. Liu DX, Perry DL, DeWald LE, et al. Persistence of Lassa virus associated with severe systemic arteritis in convalescing guinea pigs (Cavia porcellus). *J Infect Dis.* 2019;219(11):1818–1822.
132. Růžek D, Yakimenko VV, Karan LS, Tkachev SE. Omsk haemorrhagic fever. *Lancet Lond Engl.* 2010;376(9758):2104–2113.
133. Edelstein M, Angelides P, Heymann DL. Ebola: the challenging road to recovery. *Lancet Lond Engl.* 2015;385(9984):2234–2235.
134. Tambo E, Chengho CF, Ugwu CE, Wurie I, Jonhson JK, Ngogang JY. Rebuilding transformation strategies in post-Ebola epidemics in Africa. *Infect Dis Poverty.* 2017;6(1):71.
135. Huang X, Yue Y, Li D, et al. Antibody-dependent enhancement of dengue virus infection inhibits RLR-mediated Type-I IFN-independent signalling through upregulation of cellular autophagy. *Sci Rep.* 2016;6:22303.
136. Mizumoto K, Ejima K, Yamamoto T, Nishiura H. On the risk of severe dengue during secondary infection: a systematic review coupled with mathematical modeling. *J Vector Borne Dis.* 2014;51(3):153–164.
137. Lalis A, Evin A, Janier M, Koivogui L, Denys C. Host evolution in Mastomys natalensis (Rodentia: Muridae): an integrative approach using geometric morphometrics and genetics. *Integr Zool.* 2015;10(6):505–514.
138. Mylne AQN, Pigott DM, Longbottom J, et al. Mapping the zoonotic niche of Lassa fever in Africa. *Trans R Soc Trop Med Hyg.* 2015;109(8):483–492.
139. Briggiler A, Sinchi A, Coronel F, et al. New transmission scenarios of the Argentine hemorrhagic fever since the introduction of the live attenuated junin virus vaccine (Candid #1): an experience in migrant workers. *Rev Peru Med Exp Salud Publica.* 2015;32(1):165–171.
140. Sayler KA, Barbet AF, Chamberlain C, et al. Isolation of Tacaribe virus, a Caribbean arenavirus, from host-seeking Amblyomma americanum ticks in Florida. *PLoS One.* 2014;9(12), e115769.
141. Spengler JR, Bergeron É, Spiropoulou CF. Crimean-Congo hemorrhagic fever and expansion from endemic regions. *Curr Opin Virol.* 2019;34:70–78.
142. Lwande OW, Paul GO, Chiyo PI, et al. Spatio-temporal variation in prevalence of Rift Valley fever: a post-epidemic serum survey in cattle and wildlife in Kenya. *Infect Ecol Epidemiol.* 2015;5:30106.
143. Gargili A, Estrada-Peña A, Spengler JR, Lukashev A, Nuttall PA, Bente DA. The role of ticks in the maintenance and transmission of Crimean-Congo hemorrhagic fever virus: a review of published field and laboratory studies. *Antivir Res.* 2017;144:93–119.
144. Kuzmina NA, Younan P, Gilchuk P, et al. Antibody-dependent enhancement of ebola virus infection by human antibodies isolated from survivors. *Cell Rep.* 2018;24(7):1802–1815.e5.
145. Furuyama W, Marzi A, Carmody AB, et al. Fcγ-receptor IIa-mediated Src signaling pathway is essential for the antibody-dependent enhancement of ebola virus infection. *PLoS Pathog.* 2016;12(12), e1006139.
146. Nakayama E, Tomabechi D, Matsuno K, et al. Antibody-dependent enhancement of Marburg virus infection. *J Infect Dis.* 2011;204(Suppl. 3):S978–S985.
147. Jacobs M, Rodger A, Bell DJ, et al. Late Ebola virus relapse causing meningoencephalitis: a case report. *Lancet Lond Engl.* 2016;388(10043):498–503.
148. Shantha JG, Crozier I, Varkey JB, et al. Long-term management of panuveitis and Iris heterochromia in an Ebola survivor. *Ophthalmology.* 2016;123(12):2626–2628.e2.
149. Shantha JG, Mattia JG, Goba A, et al. Ebola Virus Persistence in Ocular Tissues and Fluids (EVICT) Study: reverse transcription-polymerase chain reaction and cataract surgery outcomes of ebola survivors in Sierra Leone. *EBioMedicine.* 2018;30:217–224.
150. Christie A, Davies-Wayne GJ, Cordier-Lassalle T, et al. Possible sexual transmission of Ebola virus—Liberia, 2015. *MMWR Morb Mortal Wkly Rep.* 2015;64(17):479–481.
151. D'Ortenzio E, Matheron S, Yazdanpanah Y, et al. Evidence of sexual transmission of Zika virus. *N Engl J Med.* 2016;374(22):2195–2198.
152. Mate SE, Kugelman JR, Nyenswah TG, et al. Molecular evidence of sexual transmission of Ebola virus. *N Engl J Med.* 2015;373(25):2448–2454.
153. Cieslak TJ, Herstein JJ, Kortepeter MG, Hewlett AL. A methodology for determining which diseases warrant care in a high-level containment care unit. *Viruses.* 2019;11(9):773. https://doi.org/10.3390/v11090773. PMID: 31443440; PMCID: PMC6784089.
154. Centers for Disease Control and Prevention. Years of Ebola virus disease outbreaks. In: *History of Ebola Virus Disease*; 2019. [Internet]. [cited 2019 Sep. 23]. Available from: https://www.cdc.gov/vhf/ebola/history/chronology.html.
155. Brett-Major DM. Thinking about Ebola. *J R Coll Physicians Edinb.* 2015;45(1):15–17.
156. Alibek K, Handelman S. Biohazard: The Chilling True Story of the Largest Covert Biological Weapons Program in the World, Told From the Inside by the Man Who RAN It. New York: Dell Publishing Company; 2000.
157. Centers for Disease Control and Prevention. Division of Select Agents and Toxins. Center for Preparedness and Response; 2018. [Internet]. [cited 2019 Sep. 23]. Available from: https://www.cdc.gov/cpr/dsat.htm.
158. Cooperative Threat Reduction Directorate. Defense Threat Reduction Agency. [Internet]. [cited 2019 Sep. 23]. Available from: https://www.dtra.mil/Mission/Mission-Directorates/Cooperative-Threat-Reduction/.
159. Building Bridges for a More Biosecure World. Biosecurity Engagement Program; 2019. [Internet]. [cited 2019 Sep. 23]. Available from: https://www.bepstate.net/.
160. The Biological Weapons Convention. The United Nations Office at Geneva; 2024. [Internet]. [cited 2019 Sep. 23]. Available from: https://www.unog.ch/80256EE600585943/(httpPages)/04FBBDD6315AC720C1257180004B1B2F?OpenDocument. [Internet]. [cited 2019 Sep. 23]. Available from:.

161. 1540 Committee. United Nations; 2024. [Internet] [cited 2019 Sep. 23]. Available from: https://www.un.org/en/sc/1540/.
162. National Institutes of Health Office of Intramural Research. Dual-Use Research; 2019. [Internet]. [cited 2019 Sep. 23]. Available from: https://oir.nih.gov/sourcebook/ethical-conduct/special-research-considerations/dual-use-research.
163. Report of the WHO Informal Consultation on Dual Use Research of Concern. World Health Organization; 2013. [Internet]. Feb [cited 2019 Sep. 23]. Available from: https://www.who.int/csr/durc/durc_feb2013_full_mtg_report.pdf?ua=1.
164. Brett-Major D, Lawler J. Catching chances: the movement to be on the ground and research ready before an outbreak. *Viruses.* 2018;10(8):439.
165. Brett-Major DM, Racine T, Kobinger GP. Consequences of pathogen lists: why some diseases may continue to plague us. *Am J Trop Med Hyg.* 2019;100(5):1052–1055.
166. Malinin OV, Platonov AE. Insufficient efficacy and safety of intravenous ribavirin in treatment of haemorrhagic fever with renal syndrome caused by Puumala virus. *Infect Dis Lond Engl.* 2017;49(7):514–520.
167. Ilori EA, Furuse Y, Ipadeola OB, et al. Epidemiologic and clinical features of Lassa fever outbreak in Nigeria, January 1-May 6, 2018. *Emerg Infect Dis.* 2019;25(6):1066–1074.
168. Gay-Andrieu F, Magassouba N, Picot V, et al. Clinical evaluation of the BioFire FilmArray® BioThreat-E test for the diagnosis of Ebola Virus Disease in Guinea. *J Clin Virol Off Publ Pan Am Soc Clin Virol.* 2017;92:20–24.
169. Wonderly B, Jones S, Gatton ML, et al. Comparative performance of four rapid Ebola antigen-detection lateral flow immunoassays during the 2014-2016 Ebola epidemic in West Africa. *PLoS One.* 2019;14(3), e0212113.
170. Kafetzopoulou LE, Pullan ST, Lemey P, et al. Metagenomic sequencing at the epicenter of the Nigeria 2018 Lassa fever outbreak. *Science.* 2019;363(6422):74–77.
171. A Global Strategy to Eliminate Yellow Fever Epidemics (EYE) 2017–2026. World Health Organization; 2018. [Internet]. [cited 2019 Sep. 23]. Available from: https://apps.who.int/iris/bitstream/handle/10665/272408/9789241513661-eng.pdf?ua=1.

## CHAPTER 7

Smallpox and Mpox

JAMES LAWLER
National Strategic Research Institute at the University of Nebraska, Omaha, NE, United States

HISTORY

The origins of smallpox are unknown. The first case may have emerged in early agricultural communities of northeast Africa around 10,000 BC, coinciding with the first human populations dense enough to propagate transmission.[1] Multiple references to smallpox exist in ancient Chinese and Indian writings.[2] Egyptian mummies dating back to 1570–1085 BC bear the earliest preserved evidence of pock-like lesions, including the Egyptian pharaoh Ramses V, who died in 1156 BC.[1,3,4] By the late 1500s, smallpox had spread across India, China, and Europe. As cities grew in both size and population density, recurrent smallpox outbreaks swept through them, leaving up to 30% of the infected dead.[5] European conquistadors introduced smallpox to immunologically naïve indigenous populations of the Americas in the early 1500s, largely contributing to the demise of the Incan, Aztec, and other native civilizations.[4]

Smallpox was the first infectious disease to be intentionally eradicated from the natural world, an extraordinary public health achievement made possible through efforts of the World Health Organization (WHO).[a] The 1958 World Health Assembly approved a resolution to globally eliminate smallpox, and by 1966, the WHO allocated $2.4 million per year to the Intensified Smallpox Eradication Program with goals of its elimination in 10 years.[5,6] At the time, smallpox was still endemic in Brazil, most countries in sub-Saharan Africa, Pakistan, Afghanistan, India, Bangladesh, Nepal, and Indonesia, with 10 million cases and 2 million deaths reported in 1967.[5,6] Three principles guided the eradication effort: (1) smallpox vaccination for at least 80% of the population in endemic countries; (2) weekly surveillance-containment reports on smallpox incidence with response teams dispatched to locate additional cases and vaccinate any contacts (ring vaccination); and (3) distribution of surveillance case reports including effective tactics for surveillance-containment to program participants.[6] Communities worldwide were largely welcoming of smallpox immunization programs, enabling health officials to vaccinate over 500 participants daily when supported by local leadership.[6] Freeze-dried vaccines, a novel development that avoided the need for a cold chain, were logistically critical for programmatic success.[5,6] The last case of naturally occurring smallpox was diagnosed in Somalia in 1977, with one subsequent infection related to a laboratory exposure in England in 1978.[2,5,6] Endemic countries completed two additional years of search and surveillance before eradication certification was granted, and in 1980, the World Health Assembly triumphantly declared "Smallpox is dead."[5,6]

The history of smallpox also includes its use as an agent of biological warfare. During the French Indian War in 1763, evidence suggests that English troops donated smallpox-contaminated blankets to Native Americans who were allied with the French army, instigating a smallpox outbreak among the indigenous people.[7] The Geneva Protocol of 1925 was the first major international agreement to ban biological weapons; nevertheless, the USSR, Japan, the United States, the United Kingdom, and other countries maintained programs for weaponization of various pathogens.[5] Most Western countries appear to have finally abandoned their biological weapons programs prior to, or as a result of, the more comprehensive Biological Weapons Convention of 1972. However, several nation-states continued pursuing biological weapons, most notably the Soviet Union. Previous deputy director of the Soviet Union's civilian bioweapons program, Ken Alibek, has claimed the Soviet government produced and stockpiled mass quantities of smallpox for use in missiles and bombs.[8] Perhaps ironically, it was a Soviet scientist, V.M. Zhadanov, who first proposed global smallpox eradication to the World Health Assembly in 1958.[9] The biological warfare program was reportedly dissembled in 1992 following the collapse of the USSR, but concerns persist as to whether smallpox was smug-

[a]Rinderpest, a viral infection of cattle and other ungulates, is the only other disease declared globally eradicated (in 2010).

Viral Outbreaks, Biosecurity, and Preparing for Mass Casualty Infectious Diseases Events
https://doi.org/10.1016/B978-0-323-54841-0.00022-6

gled outside of Russia or remains a biological weapons threat from other sources or programs.[5,7] Despite a World Health Assembly recommendation to destroy all remaining smallpox virus reservoirs, laboratories at the State Research Center of Virology and Biotechnology (VECTOR) in Russia and the Centers for Disease Control and Prevention (CDC) in the United States officially retain smallpox virus stocks.[5] Other secret or unknown collections likely exist, as evidenced by the 2014 discovery of vials of variola virus in a Food and Drug Administration (FDA) storage closet on the campus of the National Institutes of Health in Bethesda, MD. Finally, modern technology allows for de-novo construction of orthopoxviruses, as was recently done with the horsepox virus, highlighting the realistic risk that synthetic biology presents to biosecurity.

MICROBIOLOGY, PATHOPHYSIOLOGY, AND IMMUNOLOGY

Smallpox is caused by the variola virus, a large, double-stranded DNA virus with brick-shaped morphology when viewed under an electron microscope. Variola falls within the *Orthopoxvirus* genus, which also includes vaccinia (utilized for smallpox vaccine development) and other enzootic and zoonotic poxviruses such as Mpox (formerly known as monkeypox), camelpox, and cowpox.[10] Two separate strains of variola virus, variola major and variola minor, are responsible for the two epidemiologically distinct forms of smallpox disease that were recognized by the early 20th century (Table 1).

Variola virions primarily entered the body through the upper and lower respiratory tract, less commonly following skin inoculation (or variolation), conjunctival contact, or transplacental transmission.[2,11] The virus initially replicated within the respiratory epithelium and local macrophages and lymphatic tissue, leading to a transient primary viremia without symptoms or lesions.[2] After spreading to other lymph nodes and the reticuloendothelial system, the virus continued to replicate, eventually prompting a secondary viremia that led to the onset of epithelial lesions, initially within the pharynx, larynx, tongue, trachea, and esophagus (in descending frequency; Table 2).[2,12] Maturation and rupture of lesions within the oropharynx released high levels of variola virus into saliva and airway secretions.[2] Simultaneously, characteristic pock lesions developed on the skin due to invasion of the epidermis by variola-infected macrophages, leading to adjacent epidermal cell infection.[2] Cytopathic findings caused by variola have been described in organs such as the liver, spleen, kidney, lymph nodes, bone marrow, testes, and the central nervous system.[12] In the hemorrhagic form of the disease, hemorrhages have been noted within the skin, gastric mucus membrane, kidney pelvis, myocardium, endocardium, and submucosa of the pharynx and larynx.[2]

Variola virus elicits both a humoral and cellular immunological response. Two to three weeks after infection, hemagglutinin-inhibiting antibodies, neutralizing antibodies, and complement-fixation antibodies are detectable, but their clinical significance is unknown.[13] In other poxvirus species, cytotoxic T cells play a role in limiting early viral cellular transmission,[14] and patients with T-cell deficiencies are more likely to develop disseminated vaccinia infection following vaccination.[15] Inflammatory responses from polymorphic nuclear cells (PMNs), monocytes, and macrophages cannot alone contain a poxvirus infection, but in combination with T cells, they slow infection progression and promote viral clearance.[14] Level and duration of immunity are very similar between smallpox survivors and those vaccinated for smallpox, with T cells slowly diminishing over time and antibody levels decreasing over several decades.[16] Yet, given the limitations in immunology during the time of natural smallpox, no specific markers or antibody levels have been documented to confer smallpox immunity.[13]

Prior to eradication, laboratory tests for smallpox and Mpox included viral culture, electron microscopy, and serology.[10] Today, PCR is the standard approach for diagnosis and can be used to rapidly detect and differentiate between *Orthopoxvirus* genus members.[17]

EPIDEMIOLOGY

Eradication of smallpox was possible because humans were the only natural host. Although human-to-monkey transmission was documented, no viral reservoirs for variola exist in animals.[11] Variola is highly infectious, requiring as few as one virus particle to produce infection.[18] Smallpox was primarily transmitted through airway secretions and droplets after oropharyngeal lesions opened to release variola virions.[2,19,20] In some well-documented cases, smallpox outbreaks demonstrated clear airborne transmission with index patients who were suffering from respiratory symptoms.[2,21] Additionally, airborne variola was cultured within a smallpox isolation hospital.[22] However, cough was an infrequent smallpox symptom.[2] Skin lesion fluid and scabs contained infectious particles that contaminated the environment with rupture or shedding.[23] Smallpox has been transmitted following contact with contaminated bedding and

TABLE 1
Comparison of Rash Syndromes With Prodromes

	Variola (Smallpox)	Varicella (Chickenpox)	Mpox (Formerly Monkeypox)
Incubation	10–14 days (range 7–19; average 12 days)	10–21 days	7–14 days (range 5–21; average 12 days)
Prodrome	**2–4 days before rash** (abrupt-onset fever, chills, malaise, severe headache, backache, delirium, vomiting, diarrhea, abdominal pain, and, rarely, convulsions in children)	**None or minimal rash and symptoms occur simultaneously (within 12 h)**	**Variable**. Often **1–3 days** (fever, malaise, headache, lymphadenopathy, back pain, myalgia, then rash)
Distribution	**Centrifugal** (starts and concentrates on face, hands, and arms); commonly involves palms and soles	**Centripetal** (concentrated centrally on head and trunk); rarely involves palms and soles	Variable; at inoculation site, then generally **centrifugal**; commonly involves palms and soles
Evolution	**Synchronous** (in each body region)	**Asynchronous**, rapid evolution, various stages of lesions occur together	**Asynchronous;** lesions appear simultaneously, recent experience with Clade II has been more variable
Rash	Begins with enanthem—red papular lesions (palate, tongue, and pharynx). Within 24 h, exanthem appears—macular lesions on the skin progressing from clear, fluid-filled vesicles to opaque, fluid-filled pustules with central umbilication and scabs	Small erythematous macules begin on face, trunk, and proximal limbs with rapid sequential progression (within 14 h) to papules, vesicles, and pustules with central umbilication	Rash begins as macular (days 1–3); progressing to papular (days 3–4); then vesicular (days 4–5); to pustular (days 5–7) before scabbing (~days 12) and desquamating
Time to scabs	10–14 days; detaching in 3–4 weeks	4–7 days; detaching in less than 2 weeks	5–10 days; detaching in 2–4 weeks
Infectivity	From rash onset until all scabs detach; scabs and fomites can be infectious	1–2 days prior to rash until lesions are scabbed	? Onset of symptoms and 1–2 days prior to rash until lesions scabbed
Other epidemiologic clues	Consider bioterrorism exposure or laboratory exposure	Nonimmune host, exposure to children or infected individual	Travel to region with active or endemic disease and contact with forest rodents Pet rodents (e.g., prairie dogs from endemic region), Contact (including sexual) with infected individuals Preparation of "bush" meat very rare

clothing as well as handling the remains of individuals who died from smallpox.[24]

Cases of smallpox were routinely underreported prior to eradication, leading to an overall underestimation of incidence.[2] In the 1950s, an estimated 50 million people worldwide were infected with smallpox yearly, likely declining to 10–15 million cases per year by 1967 during eradication efforts.[2] Cases were generally dispersed throughout small villages, often transmitted slowly through a family unit.[2] Recurrent attacks were rare in persons previously infected with smallpox who had cleared the virus.[11]

Smallpox had two epidemiological subtypes, variola major and variola minor. Variola major was more common with a case fatality rate of 20% or more in those unvaccinated.[2] Case fatality rates for variola major from

TABLE 2
At a Glance: Smallpox, Caused by Variola Virus

	Key Features	Clinical Correlations
Microbiology	Variola virus, large double-stranded DNA in the Orthopoxvirus genus Replicates initially within the respiratory epithelium, local macrophages, and lymphatic tissue Major clades = *V. major* = *V. minor*	Replication and resulting viremia Cytopathic effects in all organs *V. major* associated with more severe disease and higher mortality
Immunology	Elicits both a humoral and cellular response; T cells play role in limiting early viral cellular response	2–3 weeks after infection hemagglutinin-inhibiting, neutralizing, and complement-fixation antibodies form; individuals with T-cell deficiencies have increased risk of disseminated disease
Epidemiology and ecology	Humans are infected by many routes following contact with infected humans or contact with a contaminated fomite or inhalation of contaminated air particles Primary mode of transmission can vary depending on host	Documented cases of human-to-human transmission; transmission via airborne route can occur
Clinical presentation	Incubation time varies but averages 10–14 days; range of 7–19 days Symptoms often cannot distinguish between the *V. major* and *V. minor* clades.[a] Symptoms, signs, and clinical findings are further classified as ordinary-type, flat-type, modified-type, and hemorrhagic-type. Rash appears after a 2–3-day prodrome. Rash has centrifugal distribution and synchronized progression	Abrupt-onset fever, chills, malaise, severe headache, backache, delirium, vomiting, diarrhea, abdominal pain, and rarely, convulsions in children
Diagnosis	Clinical, PCR of infected tissue	Challenging; rare disease, initial symptoms often nonspecific
Treatment	Supportive care AND Tecovirimat is FDA-approved for treatment. Cidofovir has in vitro activity but is associated with significant side effects, so an alternative Vaccinia immune globulin (VIG) for patients with severe immunodeficiency in T-cell function, pregnant individuals, and those less than 8 years old Postexposure prophylaxis: vaccinia live vaccine (ACAM2000) or live nonreplicating viral vaccine (Imvamune or Imvanex)	If a vaccine is considered, it is most effective within 72 h of exposure
Vaccination	Vaccinia live vaccine (ACAM2000) for those over 18 years old Live nonreplicating vaccinia vaccine (Imvamune or Imvanex)	ACAM2000 is not recommended for immunocompromised. If there is high-risk exposure and no alternative, consult experts Contraindications to vaccines exist; however, the benefits outweigh the risks in the exposure and during "outbreaks"

[a]Clinical signs, symptoms, and course do not commonly differentiate between whether a patient has *V. minor* and *V. major*—other than, *V. minor* is like a less severe form of *V. major*. However, there is a lot of overlap. In the past, epidemiologic features of large outbreaks, including the case fatality rate, were used to distinguish between the two clades.

a study involving 23,546 cases in India from 1974 to 1975 were highest in children less than 1 year old (43% overall), followed by adults over 50 years old (37% overall).[25] The secondary attack rate, or proportion of susceptible persons infected with variola major after exposure to an index case within a household, was observed as 58% in unvaccinated contacts and nearly 4% in vaccinated contacts.[b,2] Pregnant women were more susceptible to severe illness and death regardless of immunization status, with a case fatality rate of 27% in the vaccinated and 61% in the unvaccinated.[11] Variola minor was clinically indistinguishable from variola major and was most easily recognized across a population, having a case fatality rate of less than 1%. Variola minor at times was severe in children less than 1 year old, with case fatality rates ranging from 5% to nearly 13%.[2]

Variola major had several stereotypical clinical manifestations described as ordinary-type (including confluent, semiconfluent, and discrete subtypes based on rash distribution), modified-type, flat-type, and hemorrhagic-type.

The most common variant of variola major was ordinary-type smallpox, totaling 88% of cases with a 30% overall case fatality rate among the unvaccinated.[11] Ordinary-type smallpox occurred across a spectrum of severity, often classified into three subtypes. Nearly a quarter of total cases (23%) were considered confluent with a case fatality rate of 62% in the unvaccinated.[2,11] Semiconfluent ordinary-type smallpox occurred as frequently (24% of total cases) but had lower case fatality rates (37% in unvaccinated patients).[2,11] The most common and least severe subtype was discrete ordinary-type smallpox (42% of total cases), with a case fatality rate of 9% in those without vaccination.[2,11]

Modified-type smallpox was a mild form of disease more often affecting vaccinated individuals, with no recorded deaths.[2,11] Those with the modified subtype shed less virus and usually remained ambulatory within their communities, at times being blamed for importations into other countries.[2]

Flat-type smallpox occurred relatively infrequently (7% of cases) but had a devastating case fatality rate (97%) in those without immunization.[2,11] Cases were rarely, if ever, recorded in individuals with primary and secondary vaccinations.[11]

Hemorrhagic-type smallpox was relatively uncommon, yet almost invariably fatal. Early hemorrhagic-type smallpox, defined as having hemorrhages that preceded the appearance of a vesicular rash, was the most infrequent manifestation of smallpox at 0.7% of unvaccinated cases.[2] Case fatality rates were essentially 100% regardless of immunization status.[2,11] Pregnant women were disproportionately affected by early hemorrhagic-type smallpox, comprising 16% of total cases.[11] Late hemorrhagic-type smallpox occurred in less than 2% of cases with a case fatality rate of 90%–95% among those with or without vaccination.[2,11]

CLINICAL PRESENTATION

Smallpox disease was characterized by a stereotypical presentation of disfiguring skin lesions or "pocks." Rao[11] described the most widely accepted picture of variola major as presenting with several variations, classified as ordinary-type (with confluent, semiconfluent, and discrete subtypes), modified-type, flat-type, and hemorrhagic-type.

Ordinary-type smallpox was the most common variant of variola major. This type had an incubation period of 7–19 days (averaging 12 days) until symptom onset.[2] A prodromal phase consists of abrupt-onset fever, chills, malaise, splitting headache, backache, delirium, vomiting, diarrhea, abdominal pain, and rarely, convulsions in children.[2,11] This prodrome was an important differentiating feature, distinguishing the clinical presentation of early smallpox from the mimicry of other diseases such as varicella. In the subsequent 1 to 4 days, constitutional symptoms generally subsided, and the earliest red papular lesions presented on the palate, tongue, and pharynx, called enanthem.[2,11] Within 24 h, macular lesions emerged on the skin (exanthem), eventually progressing to clear, fluid-filled vesicles that later developed into opaque, fluid-filled pustules.[2,11] Skin lesions first appeared on the face, rapidly spreading in a "centrifugal" pattern to the distal extremities, including palms and soles, and trunk.[2,11,24] Lesions remained most concentrated in a centrifugal pattern (i.e., peripherally) rather than the centripetal concentration of lesions in the trunk, as is varicella. Within a body area, lesions evolve slowly together through the rash stages.[11] Smallpox pustules were round, well-circumscribed, firm, and "shotty" to touch, numbering from a few to hundreds or thousands per patient.[2,11] Lesions progressed to umbilication and scabbing, and fever often reemerged until scabs formed

[b]Note that true vaccination status was not always easily determined in many lesser-developed regions. Investigating teams generally used presence of a classical vaccination scar as documentation of prior vaccination. However, in preeradication campaign times, vaccine quality control was poor with frequent bacterial contamination. Some scars may have resulted from bacterial rather than vaccinia infection.

over all pustules.[2,11] Three to four weeks into the rash, scabs generally shed, except for lesions on the palms and soles that retained "seeds" for several additional weeks.[2] Once all scabs were detached, patients were no longer capable of transmitting the infection.[2]

Based on the density of the rash, ordinary-type smallpox was further classified as confluent, semi-confluent, or discrete. Confluent ordinary-type smallpox was described as continuous lesions, typically on extensor surfaces and the face.[11] Semiconfluent ordinary-type smallpox presented with discrete lesions on the body and confluent lesions on the face alone.[11] Discrete ordinary-type smallpox was the most common type, presenting with unaffected skin between lesions.[11]

Modified-type smallpox presented with constitutional symptoms but with few or no lesions.[11] If lesions did appear, they had an accelerated clinical course that erratically followed the typical distribution patterns, were relatively superficial, did not umbilicate, and formed scabs earlier.[11]

Flat-type smallpox was defined by lesions that remained level to the skin rather than forming vesicles. This type brought more severe constitutional symptoms that persisted during the rash stages.[11] Lesions typically did not form in the centrifugal pattern, and many showed hemorrhages at their base.[11] Pustules generally formed only on palms and soles.[11]

Hemorrhagic-type smallpox was defined by hemorrhages on the skin and/or mucus membranes and was divided into early and late types based on the timing of hemorrhage presentation before or after the vesicular skin rash, respectively.[11] The prodromal phase was extended to 4 to 6 days for the early variant and 3 to 4 days for the late variant (compared to 1 to 4 days in ordinary-type smallpox) and accompanied by more severe constitutional symptoms that persisted as the skin rash appeared.[11] Hemorrhage was commonly located in the subconjunctiva, and other bleeding sites included skin lesions (less common in early variant), gums, nasal cavity, gastrointestinal tract, urinary tract, and vagina.[11]

Variola minor was initially not recognized as a different disease (and virus), as it presented similarly to discrete ordinary-type smallpox or modified-type smallpox but with a case fatality rate of less than 1%. Distinguishing variola minor from major required epidemiological data from the outbreak for definitive diagnosis until restriction fragment typing allowed differentiation of virus.[2] Genomic sequencing later confirmed that variola minor was caused by a distinct clade of virus. Illness in variola minor similarly started with sudden onset constitutional symptoms (e.g., fever, headache, backache) but was generally less acute, and patients often remained ambulatory.[2] Skin lesion distribution and appearance were like variola major but with an accelerated progression, as vesicles appeared by day three and transformed into pustules within the next day.[2] Secondary fever during the pustular stage was uncommon except in those who were severely ill.[2] Scabbing began within a week of rash appearance.[2] Variola minor cases with hemorrhagic complications were exceptionally rare.[2]

NATURAL HISTORY OF DISEASE

Smallpox imparted various sequelae and complications following infection. Respiratory complications were common and included pulmonary edema (particularly in hemorrhagic- and flat-types), interstitial pneumonitis, and viral or bacterial pneumonia.[2,11,12] Less frequently, complications such as stomach dilation and sloughing of intestinal mucosa as a tubular cast occurred; these were poor prognostic signs with high mortality.[2,11] Encephalitis affected one in five hundred of Rao's[11] cases of variola major. Corneal ulceration and keratitis at times lead to vision loss.[11,24] Less than 2% of Rao's[11] cases experienced arthritis and osteomyelitis, rarely resulting in loss of function. Pockmark scars commonly persisted as a hallmark of prior infection, and shedding of scabs prompted secondary bacterial skin infections, abscesses, and septicemia.[2,11,12]

The mechanisms of death from smallpox remain unclear, though late and severe disease was classically described as a "general toxemia."[24] Death generally occurred between days 10 and 16 after the onset of the rash.[2] Pathologic evidence suggests that death may have resulted from the consequence of cytopathic effects from the variola virus rather than from secondary bacterial complications or immune complex deposition.[12] However, the role of dysregulated immune response, as characterizes other forms of sepsis, should not be discounted. Direct and insensible fluid loss from skin disruption and capillary leak led to intravascular volume depletion, secondary shock, and renal failure.[12,26] Tubulointerstitial nephritis also contributed to renal failure.[12,26] Airway pseudomembranes from mucosal lesions created barriers for ventilation and nutrition, and viral pneumonia decreased oxygenation.[12] In flat- and hemorrhagic-type smallpox, death was similar to "septic shock," compounded by bleeding diathesis, resembling disseminated intravascular coagulation (DIC) for those with the hemorrhagic-type.[26] Secondary complications that did rarely contribute to mortality include encephalitis and osteomyelitis.[12]

MPOX

Mpox (formerly known as monkeypox) is a human febrile exanthem similar to smallpox (Table 1), albeit generally milder, caused by infection with another virus of the genus *Orthopoxvirus*. In 2022, the WHO renamed monkeypox, Mpox, and this new name is currently included in the online version of the International Classification of Diseases (ICD) with plans to officially add it to the 2023 release of the ICD-11 update. Mpox virus was first isolated in 1958 from captive monkeys imported from Malaysia suffering from a vesicular-pustular rash.[27] Several Mpox outbreaks were subsequently recognized in captive monkey populations imported from Asia, but the first human case of Mpox was recorded in Zaire in 1970, initially misidentified as smallpox.[28]

Mpox traditionally has been characterized as a zoonotic disease of West and Central Africa, although our understanding of the disease is changing due to the global epidemic that began in 2022. Despite its name, the Mpox virus is most commonly identified in small mammal reservoirs, which are thought to be its most important reservoir and source of species jumping to humans. Various animals have been found to be infected with the virus, including monkeys, great apes, squirrels, and anteaters.[2] Around 400 human cases of Mpox were recorded in tropical rainforest regions of Africa between 1980 and 1986, mostly in small villages, which was thought to be the principal endemic region for the disease.[2] In historical studies, the disease was primarily obtained from environmental exposure, and human-to-human transmission was less common. An estimated 70% of Mpox cases in the former Zaire (current Democratic Republic of the Congo) could be traced to an animal source, with the remaining 30% presumably transmitted from person to person.[2] In a study of 282 patients with Mpox in the former Zaire, case fatality rates were 11% among those unvaccinated for smallpox, and no deaths were recorded in those with previous immunizations.[29] Children under 15 years old constituted more than 90% of cases, with no deaths in those who were 10 years or older.[29]

Characterization of Mpox has likely been misshaped by experts' historical bias. Description of disease from the Congo River Basin dominated reports prior to 2022, although milder clinical disease was reported from Nigeria and other parts of West Africa. Eventually, two separate clades of the virus were recognized; one from the Congo Basin (Clade I) that presented with disease resembling smallpox and had a case fatality ratio (CFR) of roughly 10%, and a second from West Africa (Clade II) that had a much milder clinical course and CFR of 1%–2% (Table 3). In 2003, a West African Mpox virus caused the first outbreak in the United States with 47 confirmed human cases.[30] All case patients shared exposure to prairie dogs from a pet shop that had been initially infected by rodents imported from Ghana; no human-to-human transmission was documented.[31]

The reemergence (or at least enhanced recognition) of Mpox in Nigeria in 2017, with a suggested increase in human-to-human transmission, served as the harbinger for the global epidemic that ensued in 2022. In addition to being the largest epidemic of Mpox to date, the 2022 outbreak has been characterized by almost exclusively human-to-human transmission, particularly among men who have sex with men (MSM), and a milder and more protean clinical course.

The classical understanding of clinical Mpox (primarily Congo Basin or Clade 1) was as a disease that presented like discreet, ordinary-type smallpox. Illness begins with 1 to 3 days of prodromal signs and symptoms that include fever, headache, backache, and malaise.[29] Distinctive from smallpox, generalized lymphadenopathy is more prominent in Mpox during the prodromal phase, particularly in the neck and inguinal regions.[2,29] Usually a few days following fever onset, lesions start to appear in the oral cavity and on the face, progressing peripherally to involve the palms and soles.[2,29] Few to thousands of lesions develop rapidly and evolve together from macules to vesicles to pustules before umbilication and desquamation, usually after a course of 3 to 4 weeks.[2,29] The severity of illness is generally proportional to the density of lesions.[29] No cases of Mpox resembling flat- or hemorrhagic-type smallpox have been recorded.[29]

Mpox virus infection in the 2022 global outbreak has been characterized by milder disease, more predominant genital lesions, and unpredictable timing of systemic symptoms relative to exanthem. In a large US study, fever remained a feature in almost two-thirds of cases. Lesions themselves tend to be stereotypical of orthopoxvirus infection although the distribution was more limited in some cases. Such a widespread outbreak with more than 75,000 cases worldwide has confirmed the milder nature of infection with the West African (now termed Clade II) strain in non-African populations. The predominant mode of transmission in this outbreak, through sexual contact, may also play a role in the modified clinical manifestations and severity. Rather than the previously reported 1%–2% case fatality ratio for West African Mpox, as of November 2022, the lethality of the 2022 outbreak has been more than 20-fold lower.

Complications and sequelae following human Mpox infection have been notably more common among those unvaccinated for smallpox, including secondary bacterial skin infections, fluid depletion from vomiting and diarrhea, keratitis, corneal scarring, pneumonia, septicemia, and encephalitis.[29] A recent report of severe cases of

TABLE 3
At a Glance: Mpox[a] Caused by *Monkeypox Virus*

	Key Features	Clinical Correlations
Microbiology	Large double-stranded DNA in the Orthopoxvirus genus Clade I (formerly called Congo Basin, Central Africa) Clade II (formerly called West African). Clade II has 2 subclades, IIa and IIb (variant associated with 2022 outbreak)	Clade I is associated with a higher mortality (approximately 10%–11%) Clade II mortality of ≤1%
Immunology	Extrapolated from mousepox, rabbit pox, and other orthopox infections in mammals. Elicits a humoral and cellular response. T-cell immunity limits viral cellular response	2–3 weeks after infection, hemagglutinin-inhibiting, neutralizing, and complement-fixation antibodies form; individuals with T-cell deficiencies have increased risk of disseminated disease
Epidemiology and ecology	Classically described as zoonotic disease of West and Central Africa. Recently, Mpox has become primarily a disease associated with human sexual transmission. Humans are infected by many routes following contact with infected humans (including sexual) or contact with infected small mammal reservoirs (scratch, bite, contact with bodily fluids) Primary modes of transmission include sexual, close contact, or large droplet; indirect contact through fomites	Associated with contact with small mammalian (forest rodents) reservoirs in endemic countries Documented cases of human-to-human, transmission including sexual transmission Traditionally affects males more than females
Clinical presentation	Incubation time varies but averages 7–14 days, range of 5–21 days Prodrome generally proceeds as rash; prodrome can be mild to more severe	Fever, malaise, headache, lymphadenopathy, back pain, myalgia, then rash
Diagnosis	Clinical, PCR of infected tissue	Challenging; rare disease, initial symptoms often nonspecific
Treatment	Supportive care Tecovirimat is effective in primate models and is currently undergoing human clinical trials Vaccinia immune globulin (VIG) for patients with severe immunodeficiency in T-cell function, pregnant individuals, and those less than 8 years old Postexposure prophylaxis: nonreplicating viral vaccine (MVA) is preferred, but live (ACAM) is reasonable for clade 1 for postexposure prophylaxis	Contraindications to vaccination exist, but the risk is often outweighed by the benefits in the significantly exposed and during "outbreaks"; vaccinia vaccine (ACAM2000) is not recommended because risks may outweigh benefits
Vaccination	Attenuated, nonreplicating vaccinia vaccine (MVA) for those over 18 years old; live vaccine (ACAM) may be used for pre and postexposure prophylaxis	ACAM2000 is not recommended for immunocompromised

[a]Formerly called Monkeypox and renamed by the WHO in 2022.

Mpox in the United States noted the severe dermatologic manifestations and diffuse organ involvement including the lungs, eyes, brain, or spinal cord primarily occurring in those with significant immune suppression (HIV/AIDS, organ transplantation) or pregnancy.[c]

[c]https://www.cdc.gov/mmwr/volumes/71/wr/pdfs/mm7144e1-H.pdf.

VACCINATION FOR ORTHOPOXVIRUSES

The smallpox vaccine was the world's first true immunization, although variolation (inoculation of material from smallpox lesions into the skin of smallpox-naïve persons) had been practiced for centuries in China and India (see Chapter 20 for more details). English physician Edward Jenner was the first to publish on immunization; in 1796, he inoculated a farm boy with material from a human cowpox lesion and later exposed the boy to smallpox, demonstrating immunity when the boy did not fall ill.[32]

Live vaccinia virus was utilized in vaccines during the smallpox eradication campaign but carried risks of severe adverse events, including death.[2,33] The predominant strain of vaccine used in the United States was the New York City Board of Health strain called Dryvax (Wyeth Laboratories). Within the United States in 1968, there were 74 complications and one death per 1 million vaccinations administered.[34] Complications were more common after primary immunization, particularly for infants under 1 year, and included postvaccinia encephalitis, progressive vaccinia, eczema vaccinatum, generalized vaccinia, accidental infection, and erythema multiforme, including Stevens-Johnson syndrome.[34,35] Smallpox vaccination within the United States was terminated for civilians by 1972 and the military by 1989, and global vaccine production discontinued with the decline of natural smallpox.[33] In recent times, the risk of smallpox release by accident or in an act of bioterrorism, especially following the synthetic production of an *Orthopoxvirus* in 2018, as well as declining levels of population immunity, have driven the revitalization of vaccine development and stockpiling as well as evaluation of potential treatments.[36,37]

Dryvax, praised for its success during eradication, was reintroduced in 2002 via the US Smallpox Vaccination Program for military personnel and at-risk public health and healthcare workers.[38] Adverse events were anticipated, but cardiac complications such as pericarditis and myocarditis, i.e., myopericarditis, that had been previously underrecognized have since been causally associated with Dryvax.[38–41]

Second-generation smallpox vaccines employ clones of live vaccinia strains that are grown on cell cultures to improve quality and safety in manufacturing.[33,42] In 2007, the US FDA approved a second-generation vaccination, ACAM2000 (Acambis), to replace Dryvax.[36,43] Complications associated with ACAM2000 are similar to those in previous vaccines and include myopericarditis, progressive vaccinia, and generalized vaccinia.[44–46] ACAM2000 should not be given to those with atopic dermatitis or other skin conditions such as eczema and psoriasis, autoimmune diseases, who are pregnant, or who have immunosuppressive states.[47] This is a considerable limitation if widespread civilian immunization were warranted.[33]

The search for improved safety profiles, particularly for immunodeficient populations, has prompted the development of third- and fourth-generation smallpox vaccinations. Third-generation vaccines are highly attenuated live vaccine strains.[33] In 2019, a third-generation vaccine using Modified Vaccinia Ankara (MVA), named JYNNEOS (Bavarian Nordic A/S), received FDA licensure for prevention of smallpox and Mpox.[48] Although newly approved, MVA vaccine origins are in the 1960s, when it was developed as a safer alternative smallpox vaccine through a repeated passage through chick embryo fibroblasts. MVA is a replication-deficient virus and was intended to be delivered by subcutaneous injection, leaving no residual scar. In clinical trials, the MVA vaccine has not demonstrated an increased risk of myopericarditis and appears safe for those with immunodeficiencies and atopic dermatitis.[49–56] Practical shortcomings of MVA vaccines include the current need for two immunizations at least 4 weeks apart to achieve target neutralizing antibody levels and a refrigeration requirement for storage.[33] Another highly attenuated third-generation vaccine, called LC16m8, has shown promise in safety, efficacy, and potential outbreak response. LC16m8 does not require refrigeration, produces a skin reaction at the vaccination site, and replicates within the body, which may deter the need for multiple vaccinations.[33,57–59] Thus far, fourth-generation vaccines that contain noninfectious viral subunits or nonreplicating molecules have demonstrated protective immunity in animal models with *Orthopoxviruses*.[60–62]

The international community gained considerable practical experience with MVA vaccine in response to the 2022 global epidemic of Mpox. Because of the milder nature of disease and low CFR in this outbreak, public health experts determined that adverse events associated with traditional first- and second-generation smallpox vaccines generally outweighed benefit, and the focus of pre and postprophylactic vaccination shifted to the MVA vaccine. In the United States, more than 1 million first and second doses of the MVA vaccine were given between May and the end of October 2022. The vaccine was approved for subcutaneous administration, but a rapid emergency use authorization (EUA) allowed for intradermal delivery of 1/5th of the subcutaneous volume, stretching supply fivefold. Not without controversy, this decision was based upon a single study of 146 persons that indicated comparable neutralizing antibody titers and safety profiles. Nevertheless, intradermal administration provided a much-needed boost in available vaccines that appeared to be critical in reining in the outbreak, with CDC data providing the first real-world evidence of MVA effectiveness in preventing orthopoxvirus disease. In an analysis of case incidence among vaccinated and unvaccinated persons over a 35-day span around August

2022, the CDC found a 14-fold decrease in Mpox infection among persons who had received at least one dose of MVA vaccine at least 2 weeks prior. Smallpox vaccine can be given up to 1 week after exposure (prior to rash appearance) as a prophylactic measure to prevent illness or reduce symptoms.[63] As of 2017, the WHO stockpiles 2.4 million smallpox vaccines with an additional 31 million doses pledged for international aid from various national stockpiles.[64] The Strategic National Stockpile (SNS) can provide smallpox vaccines for every person within the United States.[33]

In addition to active vaccination, passive vaccination with vaccinia immune globulin remains an important tool in preventing severe orthopoxvirus infection. Vaccinia immune globulin (VIG) was originally collected in the 1950s to treat vaccination complications. As the name implies, it is simply the pheresed plasma of recently vaccinated individuals containing high levels of antiorthopoxvirus antibodies.[65] VIG was previously administered intramuscularly and showed significant benefit in treating the more common complications of smallpox vaccination and infection with vaccinia virus.[2] More recently, an intravenous infusion is available that achieves higher serum antibody titers. VIG can be used for prophylaxis prior to vaccination (ACAM or Dryvax) for those with contraindications (e.g., eczema), for postexposure prophylaxis of orthopoxvirus in exposed contacts, and for treatment of vaccine complications including progressive vaccinia but notably excluding postvaccinia encephalitis and, with exceptions, keratitis.[65] Henry Kempe demonstrated convincingly in two studies that VIG was an effective adjunct to postexposure vaccination in reducing incidence of smallpox. VIG should be considered as an addition to postexposure vaccination in persons who have high-risk exposure with late identification, in immunocompromised hosts who may have blunted response to vaccination, and in pregnant women.

TREATMENT OF ORTHOPOXVIRUS INFECTION (SEE CHAPTER 20 FOR ADDITIONAL DETAIL)

No effective antiviral drugs were available for treatment of naturally occurring smallpox prior to eradication. Promising antivirals have since emerged, in large part due to concerns about the use of orthopoxviruses as biological weapons.

Tecovirimat has quickly become the gold standard antiviral drug for orthopoxvirus infection. Tecovirimat is a novel antiviral drug that specifically inhibits proteins involved in envelope formation necessary to create mature infectious orthopoxviruses. Studies proved the drug effective for postexposure prophylaxis and treatment of nonhuman primates with Mpox viruses at doses that were well tolerated in human Phase 1, and in 2018, tecovirimat became the first drug approved by the FDA for treatment of smallpox.[66–69]

Tecovirimat (under its previous name of ST-246) had been made available for compassionate use on multiple occasions prior to approval in 2018, but its true test in humans came during the 2022 global Mpox outbreak. The United States had already purchased 2 million courses of tecovirimat for the SNS and, therefore, was the country with the most available drug for treatment of Mpox.[68] As of November 2022, healthcare providers have treated more than 4800 Mpox patients under the CDC's expanded access protocol, with anecdotal reports confirming the drug is well tolerated. Clinical trial data for efficacy in accelerating lesion healing and resolution of symptoms are expected in 2023.

Scientists have explored other antiviral drugs for treatment of orthopoxvirus infections, but results are less promising. Cidofovir is an FDA-approved drug for the treatment of cytomegalovirus (CMV) and can prevent mortality in animal models of orthopoxvirus infection when given early. Due to significant nephrotoxicity of cidofovir, scientists have explored brincidofovir, a lipid conjugate of cidofovir, as an option, as it has more favorable safety and tolerability in humans. Brincidofovir did demonstrate efficacy in animal studies of *Orthopoxvirusess*, but its therapeutic window remains narrow. It remains a second-line choice for most experts and has not received FDA approval as a treatment for orthopoxviruses.[66,68,70–73] Additional antivirals continue to undergo evaluation as potential medications against smallpox to anticipate and combat the potential emergence of drug-resistant variola strains.[66]

INFECTION PREVENTION AND CONTROL FOR ORTHOPOXVIRUSES (SEE CHAPTER 24 FOR ADDITIONAL DETAIL)

Precise understanding of transmissibility of variola and other orthopoxviruses remains difficult. Estimates gauging infectious doses of variola range down to a single virus particle.[18,d] However, it is also true that smallpox transmission generally occurs in situations of more sustained and intensive contact, such as with household cohabitants and caregivers.[2]

[d]https://doi.org/10.1177/153567600400900302.

Nosocomial transmission of smallpox and Mpox constitutes a particular concern. Smallpox and Mpox patients with more severe disease have higher lesion-associated virus shedding and shed virus from the naso- and oropharynx, in saliva, and in stool[2]. Although potentially a less common mechanism, aerosol transmission of smallpox clearly occurred with shocking efficiency in instances such as the Meschede outbreak.[21,e] Mpox DNA is also detected in air samples in patient care areas as well as relatively heavy surface environmental contamination. Although confirmed healthcare personnel infections in the 2022 Mpox epidemic are rare, well-documented infections from likely environmental fomites are well documented in patrons of a tattoo parlor and two healthcare workers involved in a home visit. A recent systematic review of the literature between 2000 and May 2022 found only a single transmission in a well-resourced setting.[f]

As with all effective infection prevention and control (IPC) regimes, prevention of smallpox and Mpox infection in healthcare personnel and bystanders should begin with the hierarchy of controls (see Fig. 1; Chapters 15 and 24 for more detail). Patients should be isolated in individual rooms with closed doors away from other patients and busy traffic areas. Negative pressure isolation rooms are preferred, but if unavailable, windows and other sources of fresh air can be used to enhance ventilation. Access to Mpox patient rooms should be limited to essential personnel, and staff should be appropriately trained in IPC for orthopoxvirus infection. While waste for West African/Clade II Mpox virus patients can be managed by standard medical waste streams, waste for Congo Basin/Clade I Mpox virus and variola virus patients should be separated and handled as highly hazardous. Linens should be handled separately for all orthopoxviruses. We disposed of all linens and provider gowns contacting Mpox patients during the 2022 outbreak, as hospital laundry workers were at particular risk of infection from smallpox.[2]

Preexposure vaccination for healthcare providers at high risk to care for Mpox or smallpox cases should be considered—as was done in some clinics providing care to men who have sex with men communities in 2022—especially as lower-risk vaccine (i.e., MVA) is now available. To care for smallpox patients, staff with prior history of vaccination should be preferentially chosen to staff clinical care, if possible. For unvaccinated staff providing patient care, or those who come in contact with a patient or the patient care environment, immediate vaccination is advisable and requires an assessment of the type of exposure and the potential risk to the provider (Fig. 1) and also may require a fever watch (Fig. 2).

Personal protective equipment and infection prevention and control (IPC) practices remain debatable, but a combination of airborne and contact barrier precautions is common for more ill patients and is what our group recommends for all patient contact. For patients with prominent features of respiratory disease or undergoing potential aerosol-generating procedures, such as endotracheal intubation, teams should consider maximal respiratory protection with N95 or P3 respirators (with face shields), powered air-purifying respirators (PAPRs), or equivalent.

Environmental cleaning and disinfection are an important component of IPC for Mpox and smallpox, and staff should perform spot cleaning of high-risk surfaces frequently. Terminal cleaning and disinfection are essential as part of outpatient and inpatient room turnover to minimize risk to subsequent patients and staff. Standard hospital protocols for cleaning and disinfection should suffice, but particular attention should be paid to high-risk surfaces and insuring waste and linen disposal is properly undertaken.

Mpox is contagious, and the recent experience demonstrates that effective vaccination of high-risk individuals and the use of personal protective equipment limited transmission of the virus. On the other hand, smallpox is one of the most infectious agents that could be used as an agent of bioterrorism and could elicit large epidemics, if not pandemics, because the population lacks immunity. Should a case of smallpox be discovered, the public health response would include a myriad of interventions to protect the general population and those who are immunocompromised. Case finding, diagnosis, contract tracing, quarantine, and isolation of the exposed and infected and widescale vaccination would be implemented. Mathematical models can and would be used to facilitate decision-making and prioritization of interventions (see case study Chapter 18) in the hope of limiting transmission and minimizing the size of an outbreak.

[e]https://www.ncbi.nlm.nih.gov/pmc/articles/PMC2427800/.
[f]https://www.cambridge.org/core/journals/infection-control-and-hospital-epidemiology/article/monkeypox-transmission-following-exposure-in-healthcare-facilities-in-nonendemic-settings-low-risk-but-limited-literature/98E48E5050C7D97CB2C37CD114F49515.

Name:
DOB:
Contact telephone and email:
Date of exposure:

Summary of Exposure: ______________________________

____

____

____

Exposure Algorithm: (Circle Type of Exposure, and Endpoint of Algorithm)

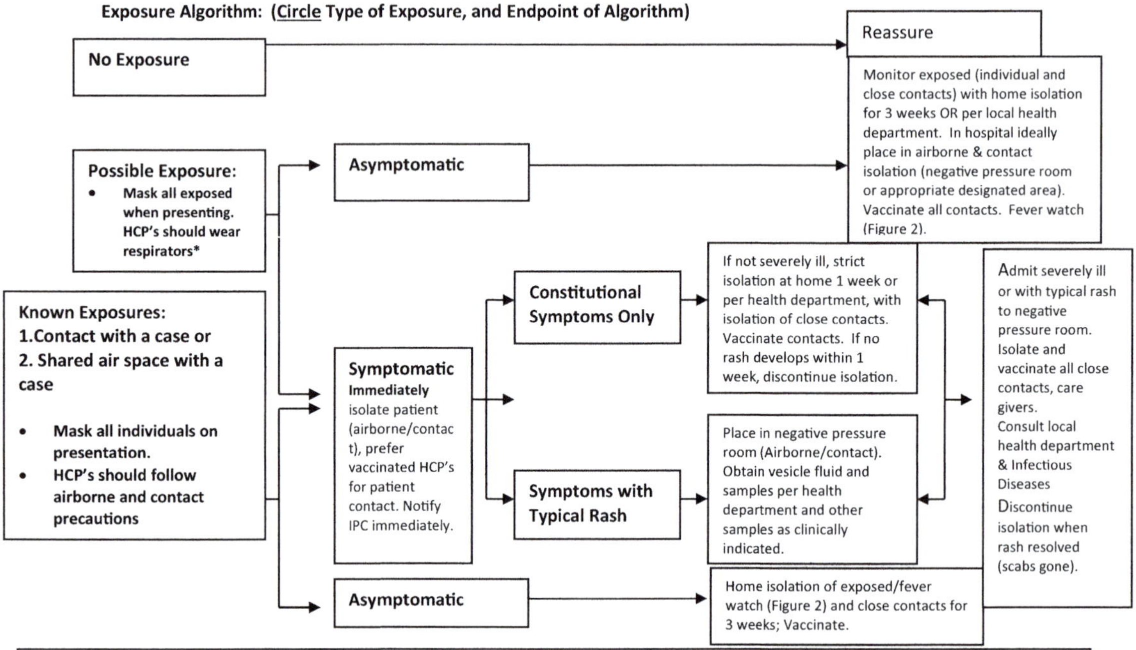
No Exposure
Reassure
Possible Exposure:
• Mask all exposed when presenting. HCP's should wear respirators*
Known Exposures:
1.Contact with a case or
2. Shared air space with a case
• Mask all individuals on presentation.
• HCP's should follow airborne and contact precautions
Asymptomatic
Monitor exposed (individual and close contacts) with home isolation for 3 weeks OR per local health department. In hospital ideally place in airborne & contact isolation (negative pressure room or appropriate designated area). Vaccinate all contacts. Fever watch (Figure 2).
Symptomatic
Immediately
isolate patient (airborne/contact), prefer vaccinated HCP's for patient contact. Notify IPC immediately.
Constitutional Symptoms Only
If not severely ill, strict isolation at home 1 week or per health department, with isolation of close contacts. Vaccinate contacts. If no rash develops within 1 week, discontinue isolation.
Symptoms with Typical Rash
Place in negative pressure room (Airborne/contact). Obtain vesicle fluid and samples per health department and other samples as clinically indicated.
Admit severely ill or with typical rash to negative pressure room. Isolate and vaccinate all close contacts, care givers. Consult local health department & Infectious Diseases
Discontinue isolation when rash resolved (scabs gone).
Asymptomatic
Home isolation of exposed/fever watch (Figure 2) and close contacts for 3 weeks; Vaccinate.

Typical Features of Chickenpox (Varicella) vs. Smallpox (Variola)

Chickenpox	Smallpox
Respiratory and skin contact	Respiratory and Skin Contact
Usual mild prodrome	Usual severe prodrome
Incubation 12-21 days	Incubation 5-21 days
Fever typically rises with rash	Fever typically falls with rash
Multistage rash, truncal	Uniform rash, extremities, face, palms, soles

Location of Follow-up:________________ Date/Time of Follow-up:________________ (Follow-up for 60+days)

PLEASE COMPLETE REPORTS FOR ALL PATIENTS AND SEND TO IPAC AND HEALTH DEPARTMENT

*Respirators include N95 or equivalent (fit tested) or powered air purified respirator (PAPR) or equivalent

Glossary: DOB=date of birth; HCP= health care personnel; IPC=infection prevention and control

FIG. 1 Potential management of suspected smallpox/Mpox exposure in a healthcare setting.

Example of Post-Exposure Monitoring for Orthopox Infections

Name/MRN:														
Date(s) of Exposure:														
Post-Exposure Day	1	2	3	4	5	6	7	8	9	10	11	12	13	14
Date:														
Temp 8AM (°F)														
Temp 8PM(°F)														
Symptoms Present– Please check if symptom is present on each day														
Malaise														
Headache														
Sore throat														
Cough														
Lymphadenopathy (swollen nodes)														
Back pain														
Myalgia														
Intense fatigue														
Sores in mouth														
Sores on tongue														
Rash														
Rash on face														
Vesicular rash														
Scabs														

➢ If you have any questions or concerns regarding symptoms, please contact (XXX-XXX-XXXX)

FIG. 2 Form to use for postexposure monitoring for Orthopox Infections.

REFERENCES

1. Hopkins DR, Lythcott GI. Princes and Peasants: Smallpox in History. Chicago: University of Chicago Press; 1983.
2. Fenner F, Henderson DA, Arita I, Jezek Z, Ladnyi ID. Smallpox and Its Eradication. Geneva, Switzerland: World Health Organization; 1988.
3. Lyons AS, Petrucelli RJ. Medicine: An Illustrated History. New York: Harry N. Abrams; 1978.
4. Riedel S. Edward Jenner and the history of smallpox and vaccination. *Proc (Bayl Univ Med Cent)*. 2005;18(1):21–25. https://doi.org/10.1080/08998280.2005.11928028.
5. Geddes AM. The history of smallpox. *Clin Dermatol*. 2006;24(3):152–157.
6. Henderson DA. The eradication of smallpox—an overview of the past, present, and future. *Vaccine*. 2011;29:D7–D9.
7. Henderson DA, Inglesby TV, Bartlett JG, et al. Smallpox as a biological weapon: medical and public health management. *JAMA*. 1999;281(22):2127–2137.
8. Alibek K, Handelman S. Biohazard: The Chilling True Story of the Largest Covert Biological Weapons Program in the World, Told From the Inside by the Man Who Ran It. New York: Random House; 1999.
9. Shchelkunov GA, Shchelkunov SN. 40 years without smallpox. *Acta Nat*. 2017;9(4):4–12.
10. Fenner F, Wittek R, Dumbell KR. The Orthopoxviruses. San Diego, CA: Academic Press; 1989.
11. Rao AR. Smallpox. Bombay: Kothari Book Deposit; 1972.
12. Martin DB. The cause of death in smallpox: an examination of the pathology record. *Mil Med*. 2002;167(7):546–551.
13. Moore ZS, Seward JF, Lane JM. Smallpox. *Lancet*. 2006;367(9508):425–435.
14. Buller RM, Palumbo GJ. Poxvirus pathogenesis. *Microbiol Rev*. 1991;55(1):80–122.
15. Fulginiti VA, Papier A, Lane JM, et al. Smallpox vaccination: a review, part II. Adverse events. *Clin Infect Dis*. 2003;37(2):251–271.
16. Hammarlund E, Lewis MW, Hansen SG, et al. Duration of antiviral immunity after smallpox vaccination. *Nat Med*. 2003;9(9):1131–1137.
17. Espy MJ, Cockerill III FR, Meyer RF, et al. Detection of smallpox virus DNA by LightCycler PCR. *J Clin Microbiol*. 2002;40(6):1985–1988. https://doi.org/10.1128/jcm.40.6.1985-1988.2002.
18. Nicas M, Hubbard AE, Jones RM, Reingold AL. The infectious dose of variola (smallpox) virus. *Appl Biosaf*. 2004;9(3):118–127.
19. Downie AW, Vincent LS, Meiklejohn G, et al. Studies on the virus content of mouth washings in the acute phase of smallpox. *Bull World Health Organ*. 1961;25(1):49–53.
20. Sarkar JK, Mitra AC, Mukherjee MK, De SK, Mazumdar DG. Virus excretion in smallpox: 1. Excretion in the throat, urine, and conjunctiva of patients. *Bull World Health Organ*. 1973;48(5):517.

21. Wehrle PF, Posch J, Richter KH, Henderson DA. An airborne outbreak of smallpox in a German hospital and its significance with respect to other recent outbreaks in Europe. *Bull World Health Organ.* 1970;43(5):669–679.
22. Thomas G. Air sampling of smallpox virus. *Epidemiol Infect.* 1974;73(1):1–8.
23. Mitra AC, Sarkar JK, Mukherjee MK. Virus content of smallpox scabs. *Bull World Health Organ.* 1974;51(1):106–107.
24. Dixon CW. Smallpox. London: Churchill; 1962.
25. Basu RN, Jezek Z, Ward NA. The Eradication of Smallpox From India. New Delhi, India: World Health Organization, South East Asia Regional Office; 1979.
26. Koplan JP, Foster SO. Smallpox: clinical types, causes of death, and treatment. *J Infect Dis.* 1979;140(3):440–441. https://doi.org/10.1093/infdis/140.3.440.
27. Magnus PV, Andersen EK, Petersen KB, Birch-Andersen A. A pox-like disease in cynomolgus monkeys. *Acta Pathol Microbiol Scand.* 1959;46(2):156–176.
28. Ladnyj ID, Ziegler P, Kima E. A human infection caused by monkeypox virus in Basankusu territory, Democratic Republic of the Congo. *Bull World Health Organ.* 1972;46(5):593–597.
29. Ježek Z, Szczeniowski M, Paluku K, Mutombo M. Human monkeypox: clinical features of 282 patients. *J Infect Dis.* 1987;156(2):293–298.
30. Reynolds MG, Yorita KL, Kuehnert MJ, et al. Clinical manifestations of human monkeypox influenced by route of infection. *J Infect Dis.* 2006;194(6):773–780.
31. Centers for Disease Control and Prevention (CDC). Update: Multistate Outbreak of Monkeypox—Illinois, Indiana, Kansas, Missouri, Ohio, and Wisconsin, 2003; 2003. Retrieved from https://www.cdc.gov/mmwr/preview/mmwrhtml/mm5227a5.htm.
32. Jenner E. An Inquiry Into the Causes and Effects of the Variolae Vaccinae, a Disease Discovered in Some of the Western Counties of England, Particularly Gloucestershire, and Known by the Name of the Cow Pox. 2nd ed. London: Sampson Low; 1800.
33. Lane JM. The current and future landscape of smallpox vaccines. *Glob Biosecurity.* 2019;1(1).
34. Lane JM, Ruben FL, Neff JM, Millar JD. Complications of smallpox vaccination, 1968: national surveillance in the United States. *N Engl J Med.* 1969;281(22):1201–1208.
35. Neff JM, Lane JM, Pert JH, Moore R, Millar JD, Henderson DA. Complications of smallpox vaccination: national survey in the United States, 1963. *N Engl J Med.* 1967;276(3):125–132.
36. Nalca A, Zumbrun EE. ACAM2000: the new smallpox vaccine for United States strategic national stockpile. *Drug Des Devel Ther.* 2010;4:71–79. https://doi.org/10.2147/dddt.s3687.
37. Osterholm M. An unfortunate need to revisit smallpox preparedness. *Glob Biosecurity.* 2019;1(1).
38. Poland GA, Grabenstein JD, Neff JM. The US smallpox vaccination program: a review of a large modern era smallpox vaccination implementation program. *Vaccine.* 2005;23(17–18):2078–2081.
39. Casey CG, Iskander JK, Roper MH, et al. Adverse events associated with smallpox vaccination in the United States, January-October 2003. *JAMA.* 2005;294(21):2734–2743.
40. Halsell JS, Riddle JR, Atwood JE, et al. Myopericarditis following smallpox vaccination among vaccinia-naive US military personnel. *JAMA.* 2003;289(24):3283–3289.
41. Morgan J, Roper MH, Sperling L, et al. Myocarditis, pericarditis, and dilated cardiomyopathy after smallpox vaccination among civilians in the United States, January–October 2003. *Clin Infect Dis.* 2008;46(Supplement_3):S242–S250.
42. Monath TP, Caldwell JR, Mundt W, et al. ACAM2000 clonal vero cell culture vaccinia virus (New York City Board of Health strain)—a second-generation smallpox vaccine for biological defense. *Int J Infect Dis.* 2004;8:31–44.
43. Food and Drug Administration (FDA). ACAM2000; 2019. Retrieved from https://www.fda.gov/vaccines-blood-biologics/vaccines/acam2000.
44. Beachkofsky TM, Carrizales SC, Bidinger JJ, Hrncir DE, Whittemore DE, Hivnor CM. Adverse events following smallpox vaccination with ACAM2000 in a military population. *Arch Dermatol.* 2010;146(6):656–661.
45. McNeil MM, Cano M, Miller ER, Petersen BW, Engler RJ, Bryant-Genevier MG. Ischemic cardiac events and other adverse events following ACAM2000® smallpox vaccine in the vaccine adverse event reporting system. *Vaccine.* 2014;32(37):4758–4765.
46. Neff J, Modlin J, Birkhead GS, et al. Monitoring the safety of a smallpox vaccination program in the United States: report of the joint smallpox vaccine safety working group of the advisory committee on immunization practices and the armed forces epidemiological board. *Clin Infect Dis.* 2008;46(Supplement_3):S258–S270.
47. Centers for Disease Control and Prevention (CDC). Contraindications to Vaccination; 2016. Retrieved from https://www.cdc.gov/smallpox/clinicians/vaccination-contraindications1.html.
48. Food and Drug Administration (FDA). JYNNEOS; 2019. Retrieved from https://www.fda.gov/vaccines-blood-biologics/jynneos.
49. Greenberg RN, Overton ET, Haas DW, et al. Safety, immunogenicity, and surrogate markers of clinical efficacy for modified vaccinia Ankara as a smallpox vaccine in HIV-infected subjects. *J Infect Dis.* 2013;207(5):749–758.
50. Greenberg RN, Hurley MY, Dinh DV, et al. A multicenter, open-label, controlled phase II study to evaluate safety and immunogenicity of MVA smallpox vaccine (IMVAMUNE) in 18-40 year old subjects with diagnosed atopic dermatitis. *PLoS One.* 2015;10(10):e0138348. https://doi.org/10.1371/journal.pone.0138348.
51. Greenberg RN, Hay CM, Stapleton JT, et al. A randomized, double-blind, placebo-controlled phase II trial investigating the safety and immunogenicity of modified vaccinia Ankara smallpox vaccine (MVA-BN(R)) in 56-80-year-old subjects. *PLoS One.* 2016;11(6):e0157335. https://doi.org/10.1371/journal.pone.0157335.
52. Overton ET, Stapleton J, Frank I, et al. Safety and immunogenicity of modified vaccinia Ankara-Bavarian Nordic smallpox vaccine in vaccinia-naive and experienced human immunodeficiency virus-infected individuals: an open-label, controlled clinical phase II trial.

In: *Paper presented at the Open Forum Infectious Diseases.* 2; 2015 [2].
53. Overton ET, Lawrence SJ, Wagner E, et al. Immunogenicity and safety of three consecutive production lots of the non-replicating smallpox vaccine MVA: a randomised, double blind, placebo-controlled phase III trial. *PLoS One.* 2018;13(4).
54. Pittman PR, Hahn M, Lee HS, et al. Phase 3 efficacy trial of modified vaccinia Ankara as a vaccine against smallpox. *N Engl J Med.* 2019;381(20):1897–1908. https://doi.org/10.1056/NEJMoa1817307.
55. von Sonnenburg F, Perona P, Darsow U, et al. Safety and immunogenicity of modified vaccinia Ankara as a smallpox vaccine in people with atopic dermatitis. *Vaccine.* 2014;32(43):5696–5702. https://doi.org/10.1016/j.vaccine.2014.08.022.
56. Zitzmann-Roth E, von Sonnenburg F, de la Motte S, et al. Cardiac safety of modified vaccinia Ankara for vaccination against smallpox in a young, healthy study population. *PLoS One.* 2015;10(4):e0122653. https://doi.org/10.1371/journal.pone.0122653.
57. Kennedy JS, Gurwith M, Dekker CL, et al. Safety and immunogenicity of LC16m8, an attenuated smallpox vaccine in vaccinia-naive adults. *J Infect Dis.* 2011;204(9):1395–1402. https://doi.org/10.1093/infdis/jir527.
58. Kenner J, Cameron F, Empig C, Jobes DV, Gurwith M. LC16m8: an attenuated smallpox vaccine. *Vaccine.* 2006;24(47–48):7009–7022. https://doi.org/10.1016/j.vaccine.2006.03.087.
59. Kidokoro M, Tashiro M, Shida H. Genetically stable and fully effective smallpox vaccine strain constructed from highly attenuated vaccinia LC16m8. *Proc Natl Acad Sci USA.* 2005;102(11):4152–4157. https://doi.org/10.1073/pnas.0406671102.
60. Buchman GW, Cohen ME, Xiao Y, et al. A protein-based smallpox vaccine protects non-human primates from a lethal monkeypox virus challenge. *Vaccine.* 2010;28(40):6627–6636. https://doi.org/10.1016/j.vaccine.2010.07.030.
61. Golden JW, Josleyn M, Mucker EM, et al. Side-by-side comparison of gene-based smallpox vaccine with MVA in nonhuman primates. *PLoS One.* 2012;7(7):e42353. https://doi.org/10.1371/journal.pone.0042353.
62. Hooper JW, Thompson E, Wilhelmsen C, et al. Smallpox DNA vaccine protects nonhuman primates against lethal monkeypox. *J Virol.* 2004;78(9):4433–4443. https://doi.org/10.1128/JVI.78.9.4433-4443.2004.
63. Centers for Disease Control and Prevention (CDC). Treatment; 2019. Retrieved from https://www.cdc.gov/smallpox/clinicians/treatment.html.
64. World Health Organization (WHO). Operational Framework for the Deployment of the WHO Smallpox Vaccine Emergency Stockpile in Response to a Smallpox Event. Geneva: World Health Organization; 2017.
65. Wittek R. Vaccinia immune globulin: current policies, preparedness, and product safety and efficacy. *Int J Infect Dis.* 2006;10(3):193–201.
66. Delaune D, Iseni F. Drug development against smallpox: present and future. *Antimicrob Agents Chemother.* 2020;64(4):e01683-19. https://doi.org/10.1128/AAC.01683-19.
67. Grosenbach DW, Honeychurch K, Rose EA, et al. Oral tecovirimat for the treatment of smallpox. *N Engl J Med.* 2018;379(1):44–53. https://doi.org/10.1056/NEJMoa1705688.
68. Meyer H, Ehmann R, Smith GL. Smallpox in the post-eradication era. *Viruses.* 2020;12(2):138. https://doi.org/10.3390/v12020138.
69. Russo AT, Grosenbach DW, Brasel TL, et al. Effects of treatment delay on efficacy of tecovirimat following lethal aerosol monkeypox virus challenge in cynomolgus macaques. *J Infect Dis.* 2018;218(9):1490–1499. https://doi.org/10.1093/infdis/jiy326.
70. Chittick G, Morrison M, Brundage T, Nichols WG. Short-term clinical safety profile of brincidofovir: a favorable benefit–risk proposition in the treatment of smallpox. *Antivir Res.* 2017;143:269–277. https://doi.org/10.1016/j.antiviral.2017.01.009.
71. Parker S, Touchette E, Oberle C, et al. Efficacy of therapeutic intervention with an oral ether–lipid analogue of cidofovir (CMX001) in a lethal mousepox model. *Antivir Res.* 2008;77(1):39–49. https://doi.org/10.1016/j.antiviral.2007.08.003.
72. Rice AD, Adams MM, Lampert B, et al. Efficacy of CMX001 as a prophylactic and presymptomatic antiviral agent in New Zealand white rabbits infected with rabbitpox virus, a model for Orthopoxvirus infections of humans. *Viruses.* 2011;3(2):63–82. https://doi.org/10.3390/v3020063.
73. Rice AD, Adams MM, Wallace G, et al. Efficacy of CMX001 as a post exposure antiviral in New Zealand white rabbits infected with rabbitpox virus, a model for Orthopoxvirus infections of humans. *Viruses.* 2011;3(1):47–62. https://doi.org/10.3390/v3010047.

## CHAPTER 8

Preparing for Influenza Epidemics and Pandemics

NELSON LEE[a] • STEVEN J. DREWS[b] • GEOFFREY D. TAYLOR[c,*]
[a]Institute for Pandemics, Dalla Lana School of Public Health, University of Toronto, Toronto, ON, Canada • [b]Department of Laboratory Medicine & Pathology Faculty of Medicine and Dentistry, University of Alberta, and Canadian Blood Services, Edmonton, AB, Canada • [c]Division of Infectious Diseases, Department of Medicine, Faculty of Medicine and Dentistry, University of Alberta, Edmonton, AB, Canada

INFLUENZA VIROLOGY

Influenza are negative-sense single-stranded ribonucleic acid (RNA) viruses and fall under the Baltimore Classification V. These viruses belong to the family *Orthomyxoviridae*, the genus *Influenzavirus A*, and make up three species of importance to humans: the influenza A, B, and C viruses.[1] Influenza A viruses can be further divided into 18 Hemagglutinin (HA) subtypes and 11 Neuraminidase (NA) subtypes and widely exist in animals.[2,3] Their quick pace of evolution (compared with influenza B and C) and propensity for genetic reassortment have resulted in annual epidemics and posed constant pandemic threats to humans.[3] Influenza B viruses also cause annual epidemics, but infections are largely restricted to humans (with some minor exceptions), with low pandemic potential; influenza C viruses generally cause sporadic, mild respiratory infections (Table 1). Their virology has been reviewed elsewhere.[1]

The Influenza Virion

Influenza A virions are enveloped and usually round in structure, 80–120 nm in diameter, and occasionally filamentous. The lipid bilayer envelope contains multiple proteins, including hemagglutinin (HA), neuraminidase (NA), and matrix (M2). M1 forms the matrix, which sits below the lipid bilayer and associates with viral ribonuclear proteins (vRNP).[8] Within the virion are a nuclear export protein (NEP) and proteins associated with the genome [proteins nucleoprotein (NP), a polymerase complex (PA, PB1, and PB2)] (https://viralzone.expasy.org/). The core of the virus, the vRNP, consists of negative-stranded viral RNA wrapped around both the NP and low concentrations of NEP. The RNA polymerase complex (PB1, PB2, and PA) is located at one end of the vRNP.[9,10]

The genome of influenza viruses is linear and segmented[1] and is divided into eight distinct segments (PB2, PB1, PA, HA, NP, NA, M, and NS). These RNA genomes are under pressure of genetic drift (single nucleotide polymorphisms [SNPs]) and genetic shift (large segment reassortment).[11,12] SNPs can lead to changes in virulence, susceptibility to antiviral agents, and as well as antigenic mismatches that may contribute to decreased vaccine effectiveness.[13–15] Genetic reassortment may result in large epidemics and pandemics (e.g., $H1N1_{pdm09}$), as populations are immunologically naïve and susceptible to infection.[16] Influenza A viruses infect and circulate in humans, pigs, birds (e.g., ducks and chickens), and other mammals (e.g., cats, horses, seals, and whales), and cross-species transmission is known to occur.[2,3] Animal-to-human transmission has been reported for a large number of virus subtypes (especially the avian and swine origin viruses, e.g., H7N9, H3N2v, H5N1, H5N6, H7N7, and H10N8); for some, adaptations for more efficient human infection have been shown.[3,17] Although the risk of transmission appears low for other viruses (e.g., H5N8), it cannot be completely excluded. Human-to-human transmission of the avian viruses is generally limited and nonsustained, but human clusters have been well reported

* Dr. Geoff Taylor sadly passed away after the completion of this work. He was the founder of the infection prevention and control surveillance program at the University of Alberta Hospital. His contributions are deeply missed by the infectious diseases community.

Viral Outbreaks, Biosecurity, and Preparing for Mass Casualty Infectious Diseases Events
https://doi.org/10.1016/B978-0-323-54841-0.00019-6

TABLE 1
At a Glance: Influenza

	Key Features	Clinical Correlations
Microbiology/ Virology	Negative-sense, single-stranded RNA virus in the family *Orthomyxoviridae*, genus *Influenza virus A* Three species of human importance: Influenza A, B, and C viruses The virus has two surface proteins: hemagglutinin (HA), classified (H1–H18), and neuraminidase (NA), classified (N1–N11), which are essential for viral entry and release. The matrix (M) is another protein in the lipid bilayer.	Influenza A virus antigenic "drifts" yearly when there are minor changes in the HA or NA proteins leading to yearly epidemics; antigenic "shifts" in the HA or NA proteins through reassortment lead to viruses associated with pandemics. Influenza B has only been associated with epidemics. The NA and polymerase acidic protein (PA) are the targets for the most commonly used class of antivirals used to treat influenza.
Immunology	Influenza viruses kill epithelial cells and damage the tight junctions at the epithelial-endothelial barrier. Innate responses with high levels of proinflammatory cytokine production likely contribute to symptoms.	Fluid leakage into the alveolar space results in respiratory insufficiency. Uncontrolled inflammation leads to rapidly progressive illness with multiorgan failure.
Epidemiology and Ecology	Zoonotic—wild aquatic birds and waterfowl are major natural hosts for influenza A viruses, and different subtypes can infect poultry and mammals. Human—humans become infected following close contact with infected humans.	Human-to-human transmission is efficient for seasonal viruses. Outbreaks are common in daycare, schools, communal settings, and healthcare, especially long-term care facilities.
Clinical Presentation	Incubation period is 1.5–2 days; generation time varies by variant and between 2.3 and 3.6 days. Spectrum of illness from asymptomatic to severe infection with complications (Table 2). In severe cases, rapid progression to pneumonia, respiratory failure, and multiorgan failure. Severe disease is more common in the very young and elderly. Specific symptoms include fever, dry cough, breathing difficulties, body aches, and gastrointestinal symptoms.	Gastrointestinal symptoms are more common in children. In the elderly, fever may be absent.
Diagnosis	PCR of upper or lower respiratory secretions is the primary diagnostic mode (highest sensitivity and specificity; antigen tests have lower sensitivity; culture in rare instances (slow) M1 gene is a common target for NAAT tests.	Testing is most sensitive early in illness.
Treatment	Supportive therapy and neuraminidase inhibitor treatment (oseltamivir, peramivir, and zanamivir) or polymerase inhibitor (baloxavir) (Chapter 19, table 1 for dosing) for individuals at risk of complications and those hospitalized. Treat bacterial or fungal co or superinfections if they arise.	Early use of antiviral treatments may reduce complications and improve clinical outcomes.
Vaccination	Vaccination is the primary mode of prevention. The vaccine contains four strains (two A and two B) and is modified yearly to target the circulating influenza A and B strains.	Recommended for all individuals 6 months and older.

NAAT: nucleic acid amplification tests; generation time: the time interval between the infections of the infector and infectee in a transmission chain.

with H5N1 and H7N9 infections.[17,18] Continuous surveillance at the human-animal interface and close monitoring for virus adaptation to efficient human transmissions are essential for pandemic preparedness.

Virus Life Cycle and Potential Targets for Diagnostics and Therapeutics

Life cycle of influenza A virus infection includes binding and entry into the host cell, vRNP entry into the host nucleus, viral genome transcription and replication, vRNP export from the nucleus, virion assembly, and budding from the host cell membrane.[8] The HA assembles as a homotrimer that forms spikes on the bilayer. The two subunits, the receptor binding domain (HA1, "head") and the fusion peptide (HA2, "stalk"), are linked by disulfide bonds. The HA binds to host cells by $\alpha^{2,3}$ and $\alpha^{2,10}$ sialic acid via a receptor binding site (preferential binding of avian and human viruses to these linkages, respectively, and their distribution along the respiratory epithelium affect host affinity); it is also a key site for antibody neutralization, with important implications on "universal" vaccine and sero-therapeutics development (e.g., through antibodies that target the more conserved stalk region).[19,20] Fusion of the virus and endosome membranes opens the M2 ion channel, acidifying the viral core, releasing the vRNP from M1, and allowing the vRNP into the cytoplasm of the host.[21] Gating of this channel depends on protonation of a His37 residue, low pH, and as per quantum mechanics/molecular mechanics (QM/MM) molecular dynamic (MD) simulations.[22] The M2 ion channel is the target of adamantanes, a class of antivirals affected by widespread resistance caused by the S31N mutation (e.g., H3N2, $H1N1_{pdm09}$), with few exceptions.[13,23,24] The M1 gene (more conserved than HA) is a commonly used diagnostic target in nucleic acid amplification tests.[25,26]

The viral RNA-dependent RNA polymerase (RdRp), including PB1, PB2, and PA subunits, is responsible for genome replication.[27] Its efficiency is impacted by mutations that change the conformational flexibility of the M1 in a manner that remains unclear.[28] The RdRp primes viral transcription using a four-step process of "cap snatching."[20] The virus can also highjack the host RNA splicing machinery, allowing for splicing of targets in genome segments 7 (M1 and M2) and 8 (NS1 and NEP).[29] Production of M2-ion channel mRNA uses a 3′ splice site on segment 7.[30] A novel class of antivirals designed to inhibit the polymerase, thus viral replication in influenza A and B, is already in clinical development (Section Clinical aspects and treatment).[23,31] Viral vRNPs are exported from the host cell nucleus,[32,33] and viral proteins (e.g., HA and NA) are packaged at the budozone of the host cell membrane.[34] Budding virions will be bound to sialic acids on glycoproteins and glycolipids, and utilize NA for release from the host cell surface. The NA is the target site of the main class of antivirals to date, the neuraminidase inhibitors (NAIs).[23] Mutations of NA, such as H275Y in H1N1 and H5N1 and R292K in H3N2 and H7N9 viruses, are shown to confer high-level resistance to NAIs such as oseltamivir.[23,24,35]

Pathogenesis

Influenza infection may lead to a variety of disease presentations from mild upper respiratory symptoms to severe respiratory illness.[16,36] In influenza pneumonia, damage to the lung microvascular endothelium can occur due to a combination of direct viral actions and indirectly through the host inflammatory responses.[37] Influenza viruses kill epithelial cells, damage the tight junctions at the epithelial-endothelial barrier, and reduce sodium pump activity, allowing for the influx of neutrophils and macrophages into the interstitium.[38,39] These processes involve the inflammasome (a component of the innate immune response in myeloid cells consisting of caspase 1, NALP, and PYCARD), epithelial cell-produced cytokines (e.g., TNF, IL-6, and IL-8), neutrophil extracellular traps (NETs), and reactive oxygen and nitrogen-producing endothelial cells and leukocytes, which could be potential targets for therapeutic intervention.[37,38,40,41] Fluid linkage into the alveolar lumen results in respiratory insufficiency.[37,38,42]

Laboratory Detection (See Chapter 17 for Additional Details)

Upper respiratory tract samples (e.g., nasal swab, throat swab, nasopharyngeal swab/aspirate/wash) are commonly used for detection of influenza and other respiratory viruses.[5,43] Sampling should be performed as soon as possible, ideally within 2–3 days after illness onset, as virus level declines with time. Notably in influenza pneumonia, viral load is substantially higher and viral replication much more prolonged in the lower respiratory tract; thus, testing of lower respiratory samples (e.g., tracheal aspirates, BAL, or even sputum) should be considered to avoid false-negative results.[5,43,44] For emerging virus strains, standard, contact, and airborne precautions should be implemented during specimen collection and transported according to current recommendations.[44] Further, nonrespiratory specimen types, including stool, cerebrospinal fluid, urine, and blood, have been shown to contain detectable (and potentially viable) viruses in such infections.[45]

Rapid antigen detection assays are shown to have significantly lower sensitivity (15%–56%) compared with reverse-transcription polymerase chain reaction (PCR) for the diagnosis of influenza A, though they are reasonably specific (99%–100%).[5,43,46–52] Newer generation assays have shown improved sensitivity (67%–81%) and specificity (98%–100%).[50,53–56] Similar performance characteristics have been reported for direct fluorescence antigen (DFA) detection assays for seasonal viruses, but it is technically more demanding.[5] Due to their low accuracy, antigen assays are not recommended for detection of emerging virus strains.[5,43,44]

PCR is considered the test of choice for influenza due to its high sensitivity and specificity, greater time window for detection, and rapid results. It can detect all influenza A subtypes with the universal primers (targeting the M-gene, as for influenza B) or individual subtypes using specific primers (e.g., H1, H3, H5, H7).[43] Such information may allow rapid identification of emerging strains (e.g., $H1N1_{pdm09}$ and H7N9 are initially "untypable" using existing primers), which could be followed by genome sequencing for characterization.[5,25,43] Multiplex PCR assays allow simultaneous panel detection of influenza and noninfluenza respiratory viruses for etiological investigation of respiratory infections.[43] Newer molecular "point-of-care" assays (that potentially can include HA and NA subtyping) may provide more rapid results to assist clinical management.[43,57,58] Isothermal assays allow for faster turnaround times but may have lower sensitivity (73%–94%) and specificity (63%–100%) compared with PCR.[58–61] Notably, these assays can vary in their ability to detect or subtype emerging influenza virus strains, and further study is required.[58,62]

Virus culture, due to its low sensitivity and slow results (even with shell vial culture technique), is now rarely used for diagnosis,[5,46] but for virus propagation for strain characterization and antiviral susceptibility testing.[63] Cell culture of emerging strains should only be performed in reference laboratories equipped with appropriate biosafety-level facilities.[44] Influenza resistance testing includes genotypic and phenotypic methods, as reviewed elsewhere.[23,24,64] Testing of baseline and samples subsequent to treatment may allow differentiation between primary and secondary resistance.[23,24] Known resistance-associated mutations, such as H275Y of neuraminidase that confers high-level oseltamivir resistance in H1N1 viruses, can be directly detected by molecular assays in clinical samples to guide management.[5,23,43,65] Newer techniques such as pyrosequencing can show relative proportions of wild-type and multiple resistant mutations, and be directly applied to clinical samples. The latest next-generation sequencing (NGS, also known as massively parallel sequencing) has the advantage of unprecedented sequencing depth, which will allow simultaneous detection of influenza virus quasi-species harboring resistance mutations at low frequencies ($<1\%$); its clinical applications are promising.[23,24] Phenotypic methods include chemiluminescent and fluorescent-based NAI assays, providing results on the degree of susceptibility (e.g., IC_{50} and IC_{90} values) to an individual antiviral agent, but definitions for "resistance," i.e., values predictive of clinical failure, are evolving.[23,64]

EPIDEMIOLOGY

Pandemics and Epidemics

Despite decades of intense observation and research, many questions remain unanswered regarding the global epidemiology of influenza; consequently, the onset, virology, and severity of influenza outbreaks are, to a large extent, unpredictable.[66] Since 1918, four well-characterized pandemics (1918–19, 1957–58, 1968–70, 2009–10) caused by genetically reassorted influenza A viruses have occurred at intervals of 10–40 years.[67,68] Historically, several other pandemics might have been attributed to influenza, but influenza B is never known to cause a pandemic.[66,67] It is unclear that influenza pandemics occur more frequently or spread more rapidly in the modern era, due to increased human travel, though in some instances, initial cases in a country have been linked to travelers arriving from destinations where widespread transmission has occurred.[69] Nevertheless, it seems unlikely that border controls would indefinitely protect a country from the introduction of pandemic influenza. Asia has usually been identified as the originating source of pandemic viruses; however, the 2009–10 pandemic, resulting from a novel H1N1 strain, was first recognized in Mexico,[16,67,68,70] indicating the importance of global surveillance. Typically, pandemics occur in multiple waves, with second or third waves, for unknown reasons, producing greater morbidity and mortality than the initial wave.[68] Further, the population groups most severely affected during pandemics often differ from those in "typical" influenza seasons (affecting the elderly and those with underlying conditions). For example, during the 2009–10 pandemic, children and young and middle-aged adults (up to 25% without any preexisting condition) experienced the greatest disease burden, which could be attributable to preexisting cross-immunity in older individuals who had been exposed to previous antigenically-related viruses.[16] Importantly, during pandemics, a very large proportion of the global population is infected, leading to possible socioeconomic and healthcare crises. The 2009–10 pandemic, compared with historical ones, was relatively mild; and despite partial blunting by the eventual availability of an effective vaccine, an estimated 20.2% of the US population became infected in the first 9 months, including 53% of school-age children.[16,70] Also, it is estimated that 100,000–400,000 excess deaths had occurred globally in the first year.[68]

During each fall-winter season in temperate climates, an upsurge of influenza cases occurs (seasonal influenza).[66] The reasons behind this seasonality are unclear; besides antigenic "drift" (or "shift" in some instances), social (e.g., increased indoor person-person interaction) and climatic factors (e.g., humidity, temperature) have also been implicated.[66,71,72] Unlike in a pandemic, when there is a single infecting strain of influenza A virus, seasonal influenza is commonly caused by cocirculation or sequential circulation of multiple influenza A and/or B virus strains. Despite improvements in global surveillance and its methods, prediction of the onset, severity, and predominating virus strain in these epidemics or pandemics remains challenging. New risk assessment tools that include multiple virological, clinical, and public health elements have been proposed.[68,73] Use of an antigenically mismatched strain for vaccine production, which must begin before their occurrence, has contributed to major year-to-year variations in vaccine efficacy.[15,63] Notably, even a modestly severe influenza season can place major stress on public health and acute-care resources; thus, surge capacity built into existing healthcare systems should be considered as part of epidemic and pandemic preparedness.

Influenza Transmission and Outbreaks in Institutional and Community Settings (See Chapter 18, Case Study for H1N1)

Outbreaks of influenza are common and occur in a variety of closed settings, especially hospitals and long-term care facilities for the elderly, but also in social settings. Crowdedness, poor ventilation, inadequate hygiene measures, and low vaccination coverage (or responsiveness) are likely important contributing factors.[74,75] Influenza viruses are predominantly transmitted from person to person by the contact-droplet route. However, in controlled experimental settings, typically using ferret models, airborne transmission of influenza can be demonstrated.[76] Human-to-human particle transmission by expelled respiratory particles does occur, but the role of biologic factors such as infective dose will require further clarification.[77] Long-distance transmission of influenza by respiratory aerosols in naturally occurring human influenza likely occurs, but observational studies are often confounded by alternate explanations.[78,79] A special circumstance of airborne transmission in healthcare settings concerns the performance of procedures such as tracheal intubation, noninvasive ventilation, endotracheal suction, and bronchoscopy, among others, which produce aerosols with aerodynamic diameter below 5 μm (aerosol-generating medical procedures—AGMP).[79–83] The transmission risk of these procedures has been mostly assessed through simulation models; nevertheless, clinical evidence supports several AGMPs as increasing transmission risk.[81,82,84]

Influenza transmission in acute-care or long-term care settings often leads to a major burden of disease and disruption of clinical services, at times when healthcare systems are stressed by surging numbers of patients during seasonal peaks. In a 7-year multihospital Canadian survey, using a conservative definition of healthcare acquisition, 17.3% of hospital patients with virologically confirmed influenza had acquired the infection in a healthcare setting (39.5% in acute care, 60.5% in long-term care facilities).[74] The season with the lowest proportion of hospital-acquired infections was 2009–10 (6.6%). Likely related to older age and comorbid conditions of patients, such infections are associated with substantial mortality (8.1%).[74,75] Efforts on real-time hospital surveillance for influenza and other respiratory viral infections may lead to earlier recognition of these outbreaks, ensuring timely implementation of control measures.[85] In the community, influenza outbreaks are most frequently reported in schools, workplaces, as well as in correctional facilities, sports teams, cruise ships, and aircraft, where there is a grouping of a large number of susceptible individuals and multiple opportunities for interactions, facilitating virus transmission.[78,85–89]

Preparedness, Personal Protection, and Response to Influenza Outbreaks (See Chapters 13, 24, 25)

Given the abrupt onset and rapid disease transmission in influenza epidemics and pandemics, it is imperative to have advanced planning at the global, national, and local hospital levels, in order to deploy swift responses to mitigate impacts and deal with potential clinical consequences (see Chapter 18 for additional details).[68,90] Building surge capacity into existing healthcare systems is emphasized. These pandemic preparedness plans should be updated regularly based on the latest epidemiological information and public health research. In the community, medical consultants to workplaces, corporations, and schools should devise their response strategies in consultation with local public health officials. School closure and social distancing are most likely to be considered in the early stages of an epidemic or pandemic when attack rates are high and an effective vaccine is not yet available; however, how they would impact the magnitude or duration of community outbreaks will require further research.[91–93]

During hospital outbreaks, the evidence base concerning the most effective approach remains insufficient. Unit closure, isolation precautions, nonimmunized staff furlough, and antiviral postexposure prophylaxis are often implemented with variable reported success.[94] Healthcare personnel (HCP) caring for influenza patients are at risk of acquiring the infection themselves; risk factors including performance of AGMP and low adherence to infection control recommendations.[95] Immunization may provide important protection, but vaccine efficacy is variable from year to year, and voluntary vaccine uptake is often poor.[96] Further, in the initial wave of a pandemic, a vaccine may not be available, and the willingness to receive a new vaccine could be low.[97] Several studies support the concept of vaccinating HCPs in hospitals and long-term care facilities as a strategy to prevent transmission to patients or residents. This has led many hospitals to require annual vaccination of their clinical staff, a strategy that has been endorsed by several professional organizations.[98,99] In institutions that have mandatory immunization policies, there is a markedly increased uptake of vaccination by HCP compared to voluntary vaccination.[100] However, this strategy remains controversial.[101] Personal protective equipment (PPE) may provide additional protection to HCPs providing care for influenza patients. Despite some evidence of airborne transmission of influenza, it has not been possible to demonstrate that enhanced respiratory protection (such as the use of NIOSH-certified N-95 respirators or equivalent) provides additional protection beyond a surgical/procedure mask.[102–104] A reasonable compromise is to restrict N-95 respirators or equivalent use to HCPs performing AGMP on patients.[68,85,90]

At present, vaccination remains the main strategy for influenza control, as reviewed elsewhere (see Chapter 20).[105] Its limited efficacy (ranging from 10% to 60%), due to multiple factors such as antigen mismatch (including novel virus strains), poor immunogenicity in certain subgroups (e.g., elderly, immunocompromised), prior virus/vaccine exposure history, slow production, etc., emphasizes the importance of research on the development of an "universal" vaccine and new production techniques (e.g., cell-based vaccines, recombinant vaccines) to meet the challenges of future influenza epidemics and pandemics.[4,106,107]

CLINICAL ASPECTS AND TREATMENT

Clinical Manifestations and Severity

Clinical presentations of influenza are diverse and nonspecific, including pulmonary and extrapulmonary manifestations and exacerbations of underlying chronic cardiorespiratory and metabolic conditions (Table 2).[5,108,109] Fever may be absent in the elderly, the immunosuppressed, and with antipyretic use, and upper respiratory infection (URI) symptoms such as sore throat and rhinorrhea are uncommon (<1/3) in patients hospitalized for severe infections.[5,108] Late presentation is frequent in such cases (overall: median 2, IQR 1–5 days; pneumonia: median 4, IQR 2–6 days).[5,16,108,110] For surveillance purposes, the WHO case definition for influenza-like illness (ILI) is an acute respiratory infection with fever of ≥38°C and cough, onset within 10 days; and for severe acute respiratory infections (SARI), ILI cases requiring hospitalization.[7] However, their sensitivities and specificities for diagnosing influenza are low; therefore, laboratory confirmation should be considered in suspected cases (see Section Laboratory detection).

Pneumonia is the main complication of influenza, which accounts for >35%–45% of hospital admissions of seasonal or pandemic H1N1 virus infections, and 10%–25% may develop acute respiratory failure requiring ventilatory support.[5,7,108,109] Respiratory failure can also result from acute worsening of underlying cardiorespiratory conditions (e.g., acute pulmonary edema), posing diagnostic and management challenges. In some patients, acute respiratory distress syndrome (ARDS) ensues, leading to refractory hypoxemia; concurrent systemic and extrapulmonary complications (e.g., multiorgan failure, hemophagocytosis) further contribute to high morbidity and mortality (15%–50%).[5,6,16,111] Advanced ventilation strategies and extracorporeal membrane oxygenation (ECMO) therapy may be necessary for life support, meaning that surge capacity in critical care services should be considered an integral part of epidemic and pandemic preparedness.[16,112–114]

TABLE 2
Clinical Manifestations and Complications of Influenza

Pulmonary	Extrapulmonary	Exacerbation of Underlying Conditions
Pneumonia (viral, bacterial, mixed viral-bacterial) e.g., *S. pneumoniae, S. aureus, H. influenzae, S. pyogenes*; gram-negative bacilli including *Ps. aeruginosa*[a] **Acute airway diseases** (bronchitis/bronchiolitis) **Diffuse alveolar damage** (acute respiratory distress syndrome, ARDS) **Others** (e.g., hemoptysis, empyema, pleural effusion; pneumothorax, pneumomediastinum)	**Systemic** (sepsis/shock, acute renal failure, multiorgan failure) **Cardiac** (myocarditis) **Neurologic** (encephalopathy, encephalitis; myelitis, Guillain-Barré syndrome)[b] **Hematological** (leucopenia, thrombocytopenia; hemophagocytosis, thromboembolism) **Musculoskeletal** (myositis, rhabdomyolysis) **Gastrointestinal** (diarrhea, liver derangement)	**Cardiorespiratory** (e.g., COPD, asthma, bronchiectasis, lung fibrosis; heart failure, ischemic heart disease, arrhythmia) **Neurological** (e.g., seizures, cerebrovascular disease, delirium) **Metabolic** (e.g., renal failure, diabetic keto-acidosis or hyperosmolarity)

[a]Antibacterial treatment for suspected superinfections should provide appropriate coverage against *S. pneumoniae* and *S. aureus* (methicillin-sensitive/resistant, guided by local epidemiological data); Gram-negative pathogens should also be considered in patients with chronic lung diseases, immunosuppression, and hospital/ventilator-associated pneumonias.[4] Fungal infections (e.g., aspergillosis) have been reported to complicate influenza pneumonia.[5]

[b]A whole range of neurological conditions have been associated with influenza. Possible mechanisms include direct viral invasion, metabolic derangement, and immune-mediated injury.[6] Acute necrotizing encephalitis is a rapidly progressive disease with high morbidity and mortality, typically involving children of East Asian ethnicity.[7] Neuropsychiatric events (confusion, abnormal behavior) may occur in pediatric and adolescent patients with or without receiving oseltamivir treatment and require monitoring as listed in the drug warning label.

Current evidence suggests that complication and fatality risks are highest with avian influenza, followed by pandemic, and lowest with seasonal virus infections, as determined by complex interactions of virus (e.g., virulence, receptor binding, cytokine induction) and host (e.g., preexisting or cross-immunity, age, comorbidity, immunosuppression) factors.[5,16,115] Pregnancy, obesity, and genetic variants of immune-related genes (e.g., SNPs of interferon-induced transmembrane protein 3 (IFITM3), toll-like receptors (TLRs), and complement-decay accelerating factor (CD55)) are newly identified risk factors for severe influenza disease.[16,116–118] Over-representation of pregnant women in critically ill and fatal pandemic influenza cases (6%–10%; mostly in the third trimester) emphasizes the need for enhanced preventive and intervention efforts in this vulnerable group.[16,119]

Secondary bacterial infection is an important contributing factor to influenza severity. It is evident in about 5%–15% of patients requiring hospitalization (up to 35% in ICU patients) and is significantly associated with increased mortality risk by at least two-fold.[120,121] Differentiation from viral pneumonia can be difficult, and empirical antibiotics that provide adequate coverage may be required (Table 2). Recent advances in rapid molecular detection of bacterial pathogens and the use of biomarkers (e.g., procalcitonin) may assist in ruling in/out coinfections, which deserve further study.[43,122]

Management of Severe Influenza Infections (see Chapter 19 for Additional Details)

At present, neuraminidase inhibitors (NAIs; oseltamivir, zanamivir, and peramivir) are the only class of antiviral approved by the US FDA and most other health authorities for the treatment of uncomplicated influenza in adults and children (Table 3 and Chapter 19, table 1).[123] Amid concerns over lack of randomized, placebo-controlled trial data in treating severe infections, available evidence does provide support for its effectiveness in reducing adverse outcomes. A meta-analysis of nine placebo-controlled trials (N=4328, influenza-infected outpatients) showed reduced risk of lower respiratory tract complications (RR 0.56, 95% CI 0.42–0.75) and hospital admissions with oseltamivir treatment; mild gastrointestinal side effects

TABLE 3
Current and Potential Treatments for Influenza Virus Infections

	Status/Stage of Development	Indications/Efficacy and Safety Remarks	Reference
Neuraminidase Inhibitors			
Oseltamivir (PO)	Approved[a]	Treatment of uncomplicated influenza A and B infections. Chemoprophylaxis. Data from controlled trials on complicated and severe infections are lacking. Gastrointestinal side effects (nausea, vomiting) are most common.	16,119,122,123
Zanamivir (Inh.)	Approved[a]	Treatment of uncomplicated influenza A and B infections. Chemoprophylaxis. Active against oseltamivir-resistant (H275Y) virus. Lack of systemic availability for severe infections. Risk of bronchospasm[b]	5,23,122
Peramivir (IV)	Approved[a]	Treatment of uncomplicated influenza A and B infections (single-dose). RCTs showed comparable clinical and virologic efficacy and safety profile to oseltamivir in hospitalized patients (multidosing regimens). Cross-resistance with oseltamivir.	122,124,125
Zanamivir (IV)	Phase III	RCTs (multidosing) showed comparable clinical and virologic efficacy and safety profile to oseltamivir in hospitalized patients. Active against oseltamivir-resistant (H275Y) virus.	23,126
Laninamivir (Inh.)	Phase II/III	Approved in Japan for treatment of uncomplicated influenza infections and chemoprophylaxis. RCTs (single-dose) showed comparable clinical and virologic efficacy and safety profile to oseltamivir in ambulatory patients. Active against oseltamivir-resistant (H275Y) virus.	23,127
M2 Inhibitors			
Amantadine, rimantadine (PO)	–	Not recommended due to widespread resistance in all circulating viruses: A(H3N2), $A(H1N1)_{pdm09}$, B. RCT of oseltamivir-ribavirin-amantadine combination failed to show clinical benefit.	23,24,128
Polymerase Inhibitors			
Favipiravir (PO)	Phase III	Limited approval in Japan for "novel or reemerging," and drug-resistant influenza viruses. Preliminary results from RCTs (multidosing *vs* placebo) on uncomplicated influenza showed virologic efficacy. Teratogenicity concern based on animal data.	129,130
Baloxavir/S-033188 (PO)	Phase III	Preliminary results from RCT (single-dose *vs* placebo) on uncomplicated influenza showed clinical and virologic efficacy and a comparable safety profile to oseltamivir.	131
Pimodivir/ JNJ63623872 (PO)	Phase IIb	Preliminary results from RCT (multidosing *vs* placebo) on uncomplicated influenza showed virologic efficacy and comparable safety profile to oseltamivir.	130,132
Host-targeted Agents			
Nitazoxanide (PO)	Phase III	Phase IIb RCT (multidosing *vs* placebo) on uncomplicated influenza showed clinical and virologic efficacy. Phase III RCT (multidosing *vs* oseltamivir) results are pending.	130,133

TABLE 3
Current and Potential Treatments for Influenza Virus Infections—cont'd

	Status/Stage of Development	Indications/Efficacy and Safety Remarks	Reference
DAS181 (Inh.)	Phase I/II	RCT (multidosing *vs* placebo) showed virologic efficacy. Caution in asthmatic patients and longer treatment course due to respiratory adverse effects. Clinical development on parainfluenza virus infection treatment is ongoing.	130,134
Serotherapy			
Immune plasma (IV)	Phase II	RCT showed improved clinical status at day 7 in hospitalized patients treated with immune plasma and oseltamivir compared with oseltamivir alone. No major safety signal was recorded. Phase III clinical trial is ongoing.	135
Monoclonal antibodies (IV)	Phase I/II	At least five antibodies are undergoing clinical development, all targeting the haemagglutinin stalk. Efficacy and safety data are limited at present.	129,136

Route of administration: oral (PO), intravenous (IV), inhalational (Inh.); RCT: randomized-controlled trial.

[a]Oseltamivir and zanamivir are approved by the US FDA for treatment of uncomplicated influenza within 2 days of illness onset in persons aged >14 days and > 7 years, respectively, and for chemoprophylaxis >1 year and > 5 years, respectively. CDC recommends no age restriction for oseltamivir treatment and chemoprophylaxis in persons aged >3 months [CDC]. There is resistance concern with half-dose chemoprophylaxis regimens (see text). Single-dose peramivir is approved for uncomplicated influenza treatment within 2 days of onset in persons aged >2 years; clinical trials using multiple-dosing regimens among hospitalized patients showed noninferiority to oseltamivir.[124,125]

[b]There is delivery challenge to pulmonary sites with inhalational zanamivir (Diskhaler), and the powder may cause ventilator blockade (Lee, 2012); nebulized aqueous zanamivir is an investigational agent with limited access.[137] Inhalational zanamivir is contraindicated in patients with underlying respiratory diseases (e.g., COPD, asthma) because of the risk of bronchospasm and in those with milk protein allergy. Intravenous zanamivir is of limited access through a pharmaceutical compassionate use program.[126]

were experienced by about 8%–10%.[138] Another meta-analysis of 74 observational studies reported net benefits of NAI over no treatment in reducing risks of hospitalization (OR 0.75, 95% CI 0.66–0.89) and mortality (OR 0.23, 95% CI 0.13–0.43).[139] A global effort to meta-analyze Individual Patient Data of 29,234 pandemic H1N1 influenza cases showed lower death risks in hospitalized adults (OR 0.75, 95% CI 0.64–0.87), pregnant women (OR 0.46, 95% CI 0.23–0.89), and the critically ill (OR 0.72, 95% CI 0.56–0.94) with NAI compared with no treatment.[110] It is also associated with reduced hospitalizations in high-risk outpatients (OR 0.24, 95% CI 0.20–0.30).[140] However, maximal benefit of NAI can only be expected if initiated within 2 days from illness onset (in <50% of patients, largely because of late presentation); and with each day of delay, there is approximately 20% increase in risk for adverse outcomes in hospitalized patients.[108,110,120,141] Available data suggest that there may be a lower but significant benefit with treatment started within 5 days for severe seasonal and pandemic influenza and within 1 week for avian influenza, due to longer durations of viral shedding.[108,110,120,141–144] Although NAI efficacy is likely limited in patients presented with advanced disease and ARDS,[144] treatment is still recommended as a small benefit cannot be ruled out.[120,123,142]

While a standard dose (75 mg bid) 5-day course of oseltamivir is recommended for uncomplicated influenza, the dosage and duration are less certain when treating severe diseases. Controlled trials have failed to show clinical or virological benefit with higher-dose (150 mg bid) treatment, attributable to high oseltamivir carboxylate plasma levels achieved with standard dosing (>1000-folds above the 50% inhibitory concentration (IC_{50}) of most influenza A viruses), especially in the older individuals and the renally impaired, including those who are critically ill.[124,145] Higher-dose treatment, however, may deserve further study for influenza B and novel viruses with higher IC_{50}, and in neuroinvasive infections because of limited penetration into the CNS.[111,145] Intravenous peramivir provides immediate, high-concentration drug delivery and is well tolerated. Clinical trials using multiple-dosing regimens for severe lower respiratory tract diseases have shown noninferiority to oseltamivir in influenza A and virologic advantage in influenza B infections.[125,146] It can be an option in treating the seriously ill and in situations where oral therapy is considered infeasible. Inhalational zanamivir is not recommended for pneumonia treatment due to delivery challenges to pulmonary sites and risk of ventilator blockade.[5] Notably, in patients with influenza pneumonia, only about 40% achieve RNA clearance in the upper respiratory tract after 5 days of NAI and far fewer in the lower tract, and viral rebound has been reported with premature termination.[123,125,147,148] Therefore, a longer duration of therapy of at least 10 days has been suggested for influenza pneumonia, novel viruses, and in the immunocompromised, guided by careful clinical and virological monitoring.[16,148]

Surveillance data have indicated that primary resistance to oseltamivir is generally rare (<3%) among the currently circulating A(H3N2), $A(H1N1)_{pdm09}$, and B virus strains.[23,24,35,149] Secondary resistance, largely due to the H275Y mutation in $A(H1N1)_{pdm09}$ viruses that increases IC_{50} by 200- to 1200-fold, has been described among immunocompromised patients (e.g., transplant, hematological oncology; comprising one-third of reported resistant cases), young children <5 years old, and in individuals who received half-dose oseltamivir prophylaxis. Close monitoring of virologic response is advisable when treating the immunosuppressed.[16,23,24] The H275Y mutant shows cross-resistance to peramivir but remains susceptible to zanamivir (and non-NAI treatments except adamantanes, described later). Notably, its replicative and transmission "fitness," as well as virulence are preserved; and major nosocomial and community outbreaks have been reported.[23,24] The global outbreak of H275Y oseltamivir-resistant A(H1N1) although lasted briefly during 2007–08, was a great cause of concern and highlighted the need to include drug resistance and expanded therapeutic options in pandemic preparedness.[24,126]

Therapies Recently Approved or in Clinical Development

Potential therapies in clinical development are summarized in Table 3. Intravenous zanamivir may provide a systemic form of treatment, and neuraminidase inhibition is unaffected by the H275Y mutation. This investigational formulation has limited access, although, through a previous compassionate access program, it had been used for viral suppression and "rescue therapy" in patients suspected/confirmed with oseltamivir resistance.[5,23] A randomized, double-blind phase III trial among hospitalized patients ($N=635$) showed comparable clinical and virological responses and safety profiles to oral oseltamivir; treatment-emergent H275Y mutations ($N=4$) was identified exclusively in the oseltamivir group.[127] Laninamivir, an inhalational NAI given as a single-dose therapy, has been shown in randomized trials to be noninferior to a 5-day course of oral oseltamivir in ambulatory patients and has received approval in Japan.[23,150] Similar to zanamivir, its resistance barrier is generally high and is unaffected by the H275Y mutation, making it a potential candidate for postexposure prophylaxis.[151]

Viral polymerase inhibitors are a novel class of anti-influenza agents. Favipiravir (T-705) is a competitive substrate inhibitor of the RNA-dependent RNA polymerase that is broadly active against a range of RNA viruses, including influenza A, B, C, and the NAI-resistant strains, as demonstrated in *in vitro* and animal studies.[129,130] To date, there is limited data on clinical efficacy and safety, and results from two completed phase III trials have not been published.[132] Recent data suggest that the desired plasma concentration could be difficult to achieve in the clinical setting.[152] It received limited approval in Japan in 2014 for infections caused by "novel or reemerging" influenza viruses and those resistant to available antivirals. Pimodivir (JNJ63623872, formerly VX-787) inhibits the PB2 subunit (by binding to the cellular capped RNAs as part of the "cap snatching" process) of influenza A viruses including NAI-resistant strains (it is not active against influenza B viruses); synergism with NAI has been shown *in vitro*.[130,131] Preliminary data from a phase IIb trial in uncomplicated influenza indicate significant viral load reduction compared with placebo, which is more pronounced when combined with oseltamivir,[132,133] and similar results in hospitalized adults.[153] However, the development of pimodivir was halted due to a phase 3 interim analysis that showed pimodivir plus standard of care NAI did not have added clinical benefit compared to standard of care alone in hospitalized patients.[154] Baloxavir marboxil (S-033188, a prodrug) is a small-molecule inhibitor of the cap-dependent endonuclease of influenza A and B viruses. In mouse models, it has been shown to reduce influenza viral load and improve survival.[130] Data from a phase III, randomized, placebo-controlled trial ($N=1064$) show that single-dose oral baloxavir is associated with shorter symptom and viral shedding durations when compared with placebo and greater initial viral titer reduction when compared with oseltamivir.[134] Another randomized-controlled trial in adolescent and adult outpatients at high risk for influenza complications showed that baloxavir led to faster time to symptom improvement and reduced risk of complications compared with placebo.[155] There was no statistically significant difference between baloxavir and oseltamivir regarding time to symptom improvement, except among influenza B patients where baloxavir resulted in faster improvement. Single-dose baloxavir showed significant postexposure prophylactic efficacy in preventing influenza in household contacts of patients with influenza.[156] Treatment-emergent mutations potentially associated with reduced susceptibility to these polymerase inhibitors have been reported, and further studies are required to determine their significance.[133,134,157] Baloxavir was approved by FDA in 2018 for treating uncomplicated flu in patients 12 years of age and older who have been symptomatic for no more than 48 h and extended to include post-exposure prevention of influenza for patients 12 years of age and older after contact with an infected individual in 2020.

Nitazoxanide (active metabolite tizoxanide), an approved antiparasitic agent with a known safety profile, is found to possess a broad range of antiviral activities, including blockade of influenza viral haemagglutinin assembly, maturation, and trafficking in host cells, and induction of interferons.[23] Synergism with NAI has been shown *in vitro* against avian influenza and oseltamivir-resistant virus strains.[129,130] A Phase IIb/III, randomized, placebo-controlled trial on uncomplicated influenza showed significant viral suppression and reduction in illness duration by 1.0–1.5 days.[128] Further results from phase III trials comparing with oseltamivir are pending.[132] A recent randomized-controlled trial ($n=257$) showed that nitazoxanide in addition to standard of care did not reduce the duration of hospital stay in severe influenza-like illness.[158] Other host-targeted treatments, such as DAS181 (recombinant sialidase fusion protein), are also undergoing clinical development.[129,132,159] Although a triple combination of oseltamivir-amantadine-ribavirin has failed to show clinical benefit over oseltamivir monotherapy (despite reduced viral shedding on day 3),[136] based on encouraging results from experimental studies, various combination therapies, including NAI, polymerase inhibitors, and host-targeted agents, have been proposed.[129,133]

Serotherapy, such as convalescent plasma and hyperimmune intravenous immunoglobulin [IVIG], has been used in cases of SARS-coronavirus and avian and pandemic influenza virus infections (H5N1, H7N9, $H1N1_{pdm09}$) reporting probable benefits.[135,160] A randomized phase II trial comparing donor immune plasma (with hemagglutination inhibition antibody titers ≥80) plus NAI vs NAI alone among hospitalized influenza patients ($N=98$) has shown trends toward improved clinical outcomes if given within 5 days of illness.[161] However, subsequent trials on immune plasma or hyperimmune IVIG failed to demonstrate significant clinical benefits in hospitalized patients.[162,163] The mechanisms of action (e.g., virus neutralization, immune modulation), the effective antibody titer, and the risk-benefit ratio should deserve further study.[135] Development of humanized monoclonal antibodies that are broadly neutralizing (both group 1 and group 2 influenza viruses) and target the more conservative regions of the virus (e.g., anti-hemagglutinin stalk) might circumvent some of the practical challenges of serotherapy, such as emerging virus strains and donor availability, without evoking adverse host immune responses (e.g., complement activation in antibody-dependent enhancement).[130,132,135,160]

Immunomodulatory adjunctive therapy (e.g., macrolides, mTOR inhibitors, nonsteroidal anti-inflammatory agents, statins) is an area of active research that has been reviewed elsewhere.[160,164] Notably, systemic corticosteroids administered in high doses have been associated with secondary infections, prolonged viral shedding, and increased mortality in patients with seasonal, pandemic, and avian influenza infections and should be avoided.[160,165]

Pharmacological Preventive Strategies

NAI (oseltamivir, inhalational zanamivir) has been shown in clinical studies to decrease the risk of symptomatic secondary transmission (OR/RR range 0.1–0.5)[166] and is used for postexposure prophylaxis and outbreak control to reduce its magnitude and duration.[137,167] However, evidence suggests that the use of the half-dose oseltamivir prophylactic regimen in $A(H1N1)_{pdm09}$ infections might lead to the emergence of the H275Y-resistant strain (possibly related to subtherapeutic dosing in already established infections), which is readily transmissible.[23,24] Therefore, widespread or routine use of NAI for chemoprophylaxis is generally not recommended.[7,123] Alternative approaches include preemptive treatment (i.e., close monitoring and early initiation of treatment dose at the first occurrence of symptoms), chemoprophylaxis for individuals at high risk of complications if it can be started within 48 h of exposure, and considering an antiviral based on the target virus's resistance potential (e.g., zanamivir for $A(H1N1)_{pdm09}$, oseltamivir for A(H3N2)), which have been suggested and require careful scenario-based evaluation.[7,123,168] Importantly, chemoprophylaxis should be considered in the context of multiple interventions that are necessary to curtail an institutional outbreak (see Section Preparedness, Personal Protection and Response to Influenza Outbreaks).

REFERENCES

1. Drews SJ. The taxonomy, classification, and characterization of medically important viruses. In: Loeffelholz MJHRLYSAPBA, ed. *Clinical Virology Manual.* 5th ed. Washngton, D.C.: American Society for Microbiology; 2016.
2. Centers for Disease Control and Prevention (CDC). Transmission of Influenza Viruses From Animals to People; 2018. https://www.cdc.gov/flu/about/viruses/transmission.htm. [Last acess: 25th January 2018].
3. Uyeki TM, Katz JM, Jernigan DB. Novel influenza A viruses and pandemic threats. *Lancet.* 2017;389(10085):2172–2174.
4. Lambert LC, Fauci AS. Influenza vaccines for the future. *N Engl J Med.* 2010;363(21):2036–2044.
5. Lee N, Ison MG. Diagnosis, management and outcomes of adults hospitalized with influenza. *Antivir Ther.* 2012;17(1 Pt B):143–157.
6. Sellers SA, Hagan RS, Hayden FG, Fischer 2nd WA. The hidden burden of influenza: a review of the extra-pulmonary complications of influenza infection. *Influenza Other Respi Viruses.* 2017;11(5):372–393.
7. World Health Organization (WHO). Influenza; 2018. http://www.who.int/influenza/en/ (last access: 25th January, 2018).
8. Samji T. Influenza A: understanding the viral life cycle. *Yale J Biol Med.* 2009;82(4):153–159.
9. Nayak DP, Balogun RA, Yamada H, Zhou ZH, Barman S. Influenza virus morphogenesis and budding. *Virus Res.* 2009;143(2):147–161.
10. Nayak DP, Hui EK, Barman S. Assembly and budding of influenza virus. *Virus Res.* 2004;106(2):147–165.
11. Ormond L, Liu P, Matuszewski S, et al. The combined effect of oseltamivir and favipiravir on influenza A virus evolution. *Genome Biol Evol.* 2017;9(7):1913–1924.
12. Lowen AC. Constraints, drivers, and implications of influenza A virus reassortment. *Annu Rev Virol.* 2017;4(1):105–121.
13. Higgins RR, Eshaghi A, Burton L, Mazzulli T, Drews SJ. Differential patterns of amantadine-resistance in influenza A (H3N2) and (H1N1) isolates in Toronto, Canada. *J Clin Virol.* 2009;44(1):91–93.
14. Lee HK, Tang JW, Loh TP, Oon LL, Koay ES. Predicting clinical severity based on substitutions near epitope A of influenza A/H3N2. *Infect Genet Evol.* 2015;34:292–297.
15. Skowronski DM, Chambers C, Sabaiduc S, et al. A perfect storm: impact of genomic variation and serial vaccination on low influenza vaccine effectiveness during the 2014-2015 season. *Clin Infect Dis.* 2016;63(1):21–32.
16. Writing Committee of the WHO Consultation on Clinical Aspects of Pandemic (H1N1) 2009 Influenza, Bautista E, Chotpitayasunondh T, et al. Clinical aspects of pandemic 2009 influenza A (H1N1) virus infection. *N Engl J Med.* 2010;362(18):1708–1719.
17. Blanton L, Wentworth DE, Alabi N, et al. Update: influenza activity—United States and Worldwide, May 21-September 23, 2017. *MMWR Morb Mortal Wkly Rep.* 2017;66(39):1043–1051.
18. Artois J, Jiang H, Wang X, et al. Changing Geographic Patterns and Risk Factors for Avian Influenza A(H7N9) Infections in Humans, China. *Emerg Infect Dis.* 2018;24(1):87–94.
19. Raymond DD, Bajic G, Ferdman J, et al. Conserved epitope on influenza-virus hemagglutinin head defined by a vaccine-induced antibody. *Proc Natl Acad Sci U S A.* 2018;115(1):168–173.
20. Pflug A, Gaudon S, Resa-Infante P, et al. Capped RNA primer binding to influenza polymerase and implications for the mechanism of cap-binding inhibitors. *Nucleic Acids Res.* 2017. https://doi.org/10.1093/nar/gkx1210. [Epub ahead of print].
21. Lee J, Kim J, Son K, d'Alexandry d'Orengiani AP, Min JY. Acid phosphatase 2 (ACP2) is required for membrane fusion during influenza virus entry. *Sci Rep.* 2017;7:43893.
22. Dong H, Fiorin G, DeGrado WF, Klein ML. Proton release from the histidine-tetrad in the M2 channel of the influenza A virus. *J Phys Chem B.* 2014;118(44):12644–12651.
23. Lee N, Hurt AC. Neuraminidase inhibitor resistance in influenza—a clinical perspective. *Curr Opin Infect Dis.* 2018; [in press].
24. Hurt AC, Chotpitayasunondh T, Cox NJ, et al. Antiviral resistance during the 2009 influenza A H1N1 pandemic: Public health, laboratory, and clinical perspectives. *Lancet Infect Dis.* 2012;12:240–248.
25. Pabbaraju K, Tellier R, Wong S, et al. Full-genome analysis of avian influenza A(H5N1) virus from a human, North America, 2013. *Emerg Infect Dis.* 2014;20(5):887–891.
26. Pabbaraju K, Wong S, Wong AA, et al. Design and validation of real-time reverse transcription-PCR assays for detection of pandemic (H1N1) 2009 virus. *J Clin Microbiol.* 2009;47(11):3454–3460.
27. Reich S, Guilligay D, Cusack S. An in vitro fluorescence based study of initiation of RNA synthesis by influenza B polymerase. *Nucleic Acids Res.* 2017;45(6):3353–3368.
28. Hutchinson EC, Fodor E. Nuclear import of the influenza A virus transcriptional machinery. *Vaccine.* 2012;30(51):7353–7358.
29. Dubois J, Terrier O, Rosa-Calatrava M. Influenza viruses and mRNA splicing: doing more with less. *MBio.* 2014;5(3):e00070-14.
30. Moss WN, Dela-Moss LI, Priore SF, Turner DH. The influenza A segment 7 mRNA 3′ splice site pseudoknot/hairpin family. *RNA Biol.* 2012;9(11):1305–1310.
31. Zhou Z, Liu T, Zhang J, Zhan P, Liu X. Influenza A virus polymerase: an attractive target for next-generation anti-influenza therapeutics. *Drug Discov Today.* 2018. https://doi.org/10.1016/j.drudis.2018.01.028. [Epub ahead of print].
32. Li J, Yu M, Zheng W, Liu W. Nucleocytoplasmic shuttling of influenza A virus proteins. *Viruses.* 2015;7(5):2668–2682.
33. Paterson D, Fodor E. Emerging roles for the influenza A virus nuclear export protein (NEP). *PLoS Pathog.* 2012;8(12):e1003019.

34. Leser GP, Lamb RA. Lateral organization of influenza virus proteins in the budozone region of the plasma membrane. *J Virol.* 2017;91(9).
35. Chaudhry A, Bastien N, Li Y, et al. Oseltamivir resistance in an influenza A (H3N2) virus isolated from an immunocompromised patient during the 2014-2015 influenza season in Alberta, Canada. *Influenza Other Respi Viruses.* 2016;10(6):532–535.
36. Leung NH, Xu C, Ip DK, Cowling BJ. Review article: the fraction of influenza virus infections that are asymptomatic: a systematic review and meta-analysis. *Epidemiology.* 2015;26(6):862–872.
37. Armstrong SM, Mubareka S, Lee WL. The lung microvascular endothelium as a therapeutic target in severe influenza. *Antiviral Res.* 2013;99(2):113–118.
38. Short KR, Kroeze EJBV, Fouchier RAM, Kuiken T. Pathogenesis of influenza-induced acute respiratory distress syndrome. *Lancet Infect Dis.* 2014;14(1):57–69.
39. Wonderlich ER, Swan ZD, Bissel SJ, et al. Widespread virus replication in alveoli drives acute respiratory distress syndrome in aerosolized H5N1 influenza infection of macaques. *J Immunol.* 2017;198(4):1616–1626.
40. Pinar A, Dowling JK, Bitto NJ, et al. PB1-F2 peptide derived from avian influenza A virus H7N9 induces inflammation via activation of the NLRP3 inflammasome. *J Biol Chem.* 2017;292(3):826–836.
41. Zhu L, Liu L, Zhang Y, et al. High level of neutrophil extracellular traps correlates with poor prognosis of severe influenza A infection. *J Infect Dis.* 2018;217(3):428–437.
42. Armstrong SM, Darwish I, Lee WL. Endothelial activation and dysfunction in the pathogenesis of influenza A virus infection. *Virulence.* 2013;4(6):537–542.
43. Torres A, Lee N, Cilloniz C, Vila J, Van der Eerden M. Laboratory diagnosis of pneumonia in the molecular age. *Eur Respir J.* 2016;48(6):1764–1778.
44. Centers for Disease Control and Prevention (CDC). Interim Guidance on Testing, Specimen Collection, and Processing for Patients with Suspected Infection With Novel Influenza A Viruses With the Potential to Cause Severe Disease in Humans; 2018. https://www.cdc.gov/flu/avianflu/severe-potential.htm. (Last acess: 25th January 2018).
45. Zhu Z, Liu Y, Xu L, et al. Extra-Pulmonary Viral Shedding in H7N9 Avian Influenza Patients. *J Clin Virol.* 2015;69:30–32.
46. Gharabaghi F, Hawan A, Drews SJ, Richardson SE. Evaluation of multiple commercial molecular and conventional diagnostic assays for the detection of respiratory viruses in children. *Clin Microbiol Infect.* 2011;17(12):1900–1906.
47. Koul PA, Mir H, Bhat MA, et al. Performance of rapid influenza diagnostic tests (QuickVue) for influenza A and B Infection in India. *Indian J Med Microbiol.* 2015;33(Suppl):26–31.
48. Lucas PM, Morgan OW, Gibbons TF, et al. Diagnosis of 2009 pandemic influenza A (pH1N1) and seasonal influenza using rapid influenza antigen tests, San Antonio, Texas, April-June 2009. *Clin Infect Dis.* 2011;52(Suppl 1):S116–S122.
49. Moesker FM, van Kampen JJ, Aron G, et al. Diagnostic performance of influenza viruses and RSV rapid antigen detection tests in children in tertiary care. *J Clin Virol.* 2016;79:12–17.
50. Nam MH, Jang JW, Lee JH, Cho CH, Lim CS, Kim WJ. Clinical performance evaluation of the BD veritor system flu A+B assay. *J Virol Methods.* 2014;204:86–90.
51. Stebbins S, Stark JH, Prasad R, et al. Sensitivity and specificity of rapid influenza testing of children in a community setting. *Influenza Other Respi Viruses.* 2011;5(2):104–109.
52. Hatchette TF, Bastien N, Berry J, et al. The limitations of point of care testing for pandemic influenza: what clinicians and public health professionals need to know. *Can J Public Health.* 2009;100(3):204–207.
53. Bruning AH, van DK, van Eijk HW, et al. Evaluation of a rapid antigen detection point-of-care test for respiratory syncytial virus and influenza in a pediatric hospitalized population in the Netherlands. *Diagn Microbiol Infect Dis.* 2014;80(4):292–293.
54. Hazelton B, Nedeljkovic G, Ratnamohan VM, Dwyer DE, Kok J. Evaluation of the sofia influenza A + B fluorescent immunoassay for the rapid diagnosis of influenza A and B. *J Med Virol.* 2015;87(1):35–38.
55. Leonardi GP, Wilson AM, Mitrache I, Zuretti AR. Comparison of the sofia and veritor direct antigen detection assay systems for identification of influenza viruses from patient nasopharyngeal specimens. *J Clin Microbiol.* 2015;53(4):1345–1347.
56. Tuttle R, Weick A, Schwarz WS, et al. Evaluation of novel second-generation RSV and influenza rapid tests at the point of care. *Diagn Microbiol Infect Dis.* 2015;81(3):171–176.
57. Brendish NJ, Malachira AK, Armstrong L, et al. Routine molecular point-of-care testing for respiratory viruses in adults presenting to hospital with acute respiratory illness (ResPOC): a pragmatic, open-label, randomised controlled trial. *Lancet Respir Med.* 2017;5(5):401–411.
58. Merckx J, Wali R, Schiller CC, et al. Diagnostic accuracy of novel and traditional rapid tests for influenza infection compared with reverse transcriptase polymerase chain reaction: a systematic review and meta-analysis. *Ann Intern Med.* 2017;167(6):394–409.
59. Chapin KC, Flores-Cortez EJ. Performance of the molecular Alere I influenza A&B test compared to that of the xpert flu A/B assay. *J Clin Microbiol.* 2015;53(2):706–709.
60. Hazelton B, Gray T, Ho J, Ratnamohan VM, Dwyer DE, Kok J. Detection of influenza A and B with the Alere i Influenza A & B: a novel isothermal nucleic acid amplification assay. *Influenza Other Respi Viruses.* 2015;9(3):151–154.
61. Nie S, Roth RB, Stiles J, et al. Evaluation of Alere i Influenza A&B for rapid detection of influenza viruses A and B. *J Clin Microbiol.* 2014;52(9):3339–3344.

62. Hatchette TF, Drews SJ, Bastien N, et al. Detection of influenza H7N9 virus: all molecular tests are not equal. *J Clin Microbiol.* 2013;51(11):3835–3838.
63. Skowronski DM, Chambers C, Sabaiduc S, et al. Beyond antigenic match: possible agent-host and immuno-epidemiological influences on influenza vaccine effectiveness during the 2015-2016 season in Canada. *J Infect Dis.* 2017;216(12):1487–1500.
64. World Health Organization (WHO). Laboratory methodologies for testing the antiviral susceptibility of influenza viruses: Neuraminidase inhibitor (NAI); 2018. http://www.who.int/influenza/gisrs_laboratory/antiviral_susceptibility/nai_overview/en/. (Last access: 25th January, 2018).
65. Wong S, Pabbaraju K, Wong A, Fonseca K, Drews SJ. Development of a real-time RT-PCR assay for detection of resistance to oseltamivir in influenza A pandemic (H1N1) 2009 virus using single nucleotide polymorphism probes. *J Virol Methods.* 2011;173(2):259–265.
66. Nguyen-van-Tam J. Epidemiology of influenza. In: Nicholson KG, Webster RG, Hay AJ, eds. *Textbook of Influenza.* Blackwell Science Ltd; 1998:181–206.
67. Potter C. Chronicle of influenza pandemics. In: Nicholson KG, Webster RG, Hay AJ, eds. *Textbook of influenza.* Blackwell Science Ltd; 1998:3–18.
68. World Health Organization. Pandemic influenza risk management. In: *Global Influenza Program, A WHO guide to inform & harmonize national & international pandemic preparedness and response*; 2024 [WHO/WHE/IHM/GIP/2017.1].
69. Cummings MJ, Bakamutumaho B, Yang W, et al. Emergence, epidemiology, and transmission dynamics of 2009 pandemic A/H1N1 influenza in Kampala, Uganda, 2009-2015. *Am J Trop Med Hyg.* 2018;98(1):203–206.
70. Reed C, Katz J, Hancock K, Balish A, Fry A. Prevalence of seropositivity to pandemic influenza A/H1N1 virus in the United States following the 2009 pandemic. *PloS One.* 2012;7(10):e48187.
71. Shaman J, Kandula S, Yang W, Karspeck A. The use of ambient humidity conditions to improve influenza forecast. *PLoS Comput Biol.* 2017;13(11):e1005844.
72. Gomez-Barroso D, Leon-Gomez I, Delgado-Sanz C, Larrauri A. Climatic factors and influenza transmission, Spain, 2010-2015. *Int J Environ Res Public Health.* 2017;14(12):E1469.
73. Burke SA, Trock SC. Use of influenza risk assessment tool for prepandemic preparedness. *Emerg Infect Dis.* 2018;24(3):471–477.
74. Taylor G, Mitchell R, McGeer A, et al. Healthcare-associated influenza in Canadian hospitals from 2006 to 2012. *Infect Control Hosp Epidemiol.* 2014;35(2):169–175.
75. Taylor G, Abdesselam K, Pelude L, et al. Epidemiological features of influenza in Canadian adult intensive care unit patients. *Epidemiol Infect.* 2016;144(4):741–750.
76. Belser J, Eckert A, Tumpey T, Maines T. Complexities in ferret influenza virus pathogenesis and transmission models. *Microbiol Mol Biol Rev.* 2016;80(3):733–744.
77. Yan J, Grantham M, Pantelic J, et al. Infectious virus in exhaled breath of symptomatic seasonal influenza cases from a college community. *Proc Natl Acad Sci U S A.* 2018. pii: 201716561. https://doi.org/10.1073/pnas.1716561115. [Epub ahead of print].
78. Moser MR, Bender TR, Margolis HS, Noble GR, Kendal AP, Ritter DG. An outbreak of influenza aboard a commercial airliner. *Am J Epidemiol.* 1979;110(1):1–6.
79. Lei H, Li Y, Xiao S, et al. Routes of transmission of influenza A H1N1, SARS CoV and norovirus in air cabin: comparative analyses. *Indoor Air.* 2017. https://doi.org/10.1111/ina.12445. [Epub ahead of print].
80. Tang JW, Li Y, Eames I, Chan PK, Ridgway GL. Factors involved in the aerosol transmission of infection and control of ventilation in healthcare premises. *J Hosp Infect.* 2006;64(2):100–114.
81. Chan MTV, Chow BK, Le T, et al. Exhaled air dispersion during bag-mask ventilation and sputum suctioning—implications for infection control. *Sci Rep.* 2018;8(1):198.
82. Hui DS, Chow BK, Chu LCY, et al. Exhaled air and aerosolized droplet dispersion during application of a jet nebulizer. *Chest.* 2009;135(3):648–654.
83. Wong BCK, Lee N, Yuguo L, et al. Possible role of aerosol transmission in a hospital outbreak of influenza. *Clin Infect Dis.* 2010;51(10):1176–1183.
84. Tran K, Cimon K, Severn M, Pessoa-Silva CL, Conly J. Aerosol-generating procedures and risk of transmission of acute respiratory infections: a systematic review. *PloS One.* 2012;7(4):e35797.
85. Coleman BL, Ng W, Mahesh V, et al. Active surveillance for influenza reduces but does not eliminate hospital exposure to patients with influenza. *Infect Control Hosp Epidemiol.* 2017;38(4):387–392.
86. Besney J, Moreau D, Jacobs A, et al. Influenza outbreak in a Canadian correctional facility. *J Infect Prev.* 2017;18(4):193–198.
87. Fernandes EG, de Souza PB, de Oliveira ME, et al. Influenza B outbreak on a cruise ship off the Sao Paulo Coast, Brazil. *J Travel Med.* 2014;21(5):298–303.
88. Wang L, Chu C, Yang G, et al. Transmission characteristics of different students during a school outbreak of (H1N1) pdm09 influenza in China, 2009. *Sci Rep.* 2014;4:5982.
89. Kousoulis AA, Sergentanis TN, Tsiodras S. 2009 H1N1 flu pandemic among professional basketball players: data from 18 countries. *Infez Med.* 2014;22(4):302–308.
90. Public Health Agency of Canada. Canadian Pandemic Influenza Preparedness: Planning Guidance for the Health Sector. https://www.canada.ca/en/public-health/services/flu-influenza/canadian-pandemic-influenza-preparedness-planning-guidance-health-sector.html.
91. Cauchemez S, Ferguson NM, Wachtel C, et al. Closure of schools during an influenza pandemic. *Lancet Infect Dis.* 2009;9(8):473–481.
92. Jackson C, Mangtani P, Hawker J, Olowokure B, Vynnycky E. The effects of school closures on influenza outbreaks and pandemics: systematic review of simulation studies. *PloS One.* 2014;9(5):e97297.

93. Kelso J, Milne G, Kelly H. Simulation suggests that rapid activation of social distancing can arrest epidemic development due to a novel strain of influenza. *BMC Public Health.* 2009;9:117.
94. Ocampo W, Geransar R, Clayden N, et al. Environmental scan of infection prevention and control practiced for containment of hospital acquired infectious diseases outbreaks in acute care hospital settings across Canada. *Am J Infect Control.* 2017;45(10):1116–1126.
95. Kuster SP, Coleman BL, Raboud J, et al. Risk factors for Influenza Among Health Care Workers During 2009 Pandemic, Toronto, Ontario, Canada. *Emerg Infect Dis.* 2013;19(4):606–615.
96. Chor JS, Pada SK, Stephenson I, et al. Seasonal influenza vaccination predicts pandemic H1N1 vaccination uptake among healthcare workers in three countries. *Vaccine.* 2011;29(43):7364–7369.
97. Chor JS, Ngai KL, Goggins WB, et al. Willingness of Hong Kong healthcare workers to accept pre-pandemic influenza vaccination at different WHO alert levels: two questionnaire surveys. *BMJ.* 2009;339:b3391.
98. Talbot T, Babcock H, Caplan A, et al. Revised SHEA position pater: influenza vaccination of healthcare personnel. *Infect Control Hosp Epidemiol.* 2010;31(10):987–995.
99. Bryce E, Embree J, Evans G, et al. AMMI Canada position paper: 2012 mandatory influenza immunization of healthcare workers. *Can J Infect Dis Med Microbiol.* 2012;23(4):e93–e95.
100. Black CL, Yue MPS, Ball SW, et al. Influenza vaccination coverage among health care personnel—United States, 2016-17 influenza season. *MMWR Morb Mortal Wkly Rep.* 2017;66(38):1009–1015.
101. De Serres G, Skowronski DM, Ward BJ, et al. Influenza vaccination of healthcare workers: critical analysis of the evidence for patient benefit underpinning policies of enforcement. *PloS One.* 2017;12(1):e0163586.
102. Loeb M, Dafoe N, Mahony J, et al. Surgical mask vs N95 respirator for preventing influenza among healthcare workers: a randomized trial. *JAMA.* 2009;302(17):1865–1871.
103. MacIntyre CR, Chughtai AA, Rahman B, et al. The efficacy of medical masks and respirators against respiratory infection in healthcare workers. *Influenza Other Respi Viruses.* 2017;11(6):511–517.
104. Smith JD, MacDougall CC, Johnstone J, Copes RA, Schwartz B, Garber GE. Effectiveness of N95 respirators versus surgical masks in protecting health care workers from acute respiratory infection: a systematic review and meta-analysis. *CMAJ.* 2016;188(8):567–574.
105. Treanor JJ. Clinical Practice. Influenza Vaccination. *N Engl J Med.* 2016;375(13):1261–1268.
106. Osterholm M, Kelley N, Sommer A, Belongia E. Efficacy and effectiveness of influenza vaccines: a systematic review and meta-analysis. *Lancet.* 2012;12(1):36–44.
107. Skowronski DM, Chambers C, Sabaiduc S, et al. Beyond antigenic match: possible agent-host and immuno-epidemiological influences on influenza vaccine effectiveness during the 2015-2016 season in Canada. *J Infect Dis.* 2017;216(12):1487–1500.
108. Lee N, Chan PK, Lui GC, et al. Complications and outcomes of pandemic 2009 influenza A (H1N1) virus infection in hospitalized adults—How do they differ from those in seasonal influenza? *J Infect Dis.* 2011;203(12):1739–1747.
109. Reed C, Chaves SS, Perez A, et al. Complications among adults hospitalized with influenza: a comparison of seasonal influenza and the 2009 H1N1 pandemic. *Clin Infect Dis.* 2014;59(2):166–174.
110. Muthuri SG, Venkatesan S, Myles PR, et al. Effectiveness of neuraminidase inhibitors in reducing mortality in patients admitted to hospital with influenza A H1N1pdm09 virus infection: a meta-analysis of individual participant data. *Lancet Respir Med.* 2014;2(5):395–404.
111. Lee N, Wong CK, Chan PK, et al. Acute encephalopathy associated with influenza A infection in adults. *Emerg Infect Dis.* 2010;16(1):139–142.
112. Kumar A, Zarychanski R, Pinto R, et al. Critically ill patients with 2009 influenza A(H1N1) infection in Canada. *JAMA.* 2009;302(17):1872–1879.
113. Dominguez-Cherit G, De la Torre A, Rishu A, et al. Influenza A (H1N1pdm09)-related critical illness and mortality in Mexico and Canada, 2014. *Crit Care Med.* 2016;44(10):1861–1870.
114. Australia and New Zealand Extracorporeal Membrane Oxygenation (ANZ ECMO) Influenza Investigators, Davies A, Jones D, et al. Extracorporeal membrane oxygenation for 2009 influenza A(H1N1) acute respiratory distress syndrome. *JAMA.* 2009;302(17):1888–1895.
115. Wang C, Yu H, Horby PW, et al. Comparison of patients hospitalized with influenza A subtypes H7N9, H5N1, and 2009 pandemic H1N1. *Clin Infect Dis.* 2014;58(8):1095–1103.
116. Mertz D, Kim TH, Johnstone J, et al. Populations at risk for severe or complicated influenza illness: systematic review and meta-analysis. *BMJ.* 2013;347:f5061.
117. Lee N, Cao B, Ke C, et al. IFITM3, TLR3, and CD55 genes SNPs and cumulative genetic risks for severe outcomes in chinese patients with H7N9/H1N1pdm09 influenza. *J Infect Dis.* 2017;216(1):97–104.
118. Allen EK, Randolph AG, Bhangale T, et al. SNP-mediated disruption of CTCF binding at the IFITM3 promoter is associated with risk of severe influenza in humans. *Nat Med.* 2017;23(8):975–983.
119. Siston AM, Rasmussen SA, Honein MA, et al. Pandemic 2009 influenza A(H1N1) virus illness among pregnant women in the United States. *JAMA.* 2010;303(15):1517–1525.
120. Lee N, Leo YS, Cao B, et al. Neuraminidase inhibitors, superinfection and corticosteroids affect survival of influenza patients. *Eur Respir J.* 2015;45(6):1642–1652.
121. Chertow DS, Memoli MJ. Bacterial coinfection in influenza: a grand rounds review. *JAMA.* 2013;309(3):275–282.
122. Branche AR, Walsh EE, Vargas R, et al. Serum procalcitonin measurement and viral testing to guide

antibiotic use for respiratory infections in hospitalized adults: a randomized controlled trial. *J Infect Dis.* 2015;212(11):1692–1700.
123. Centers for Disease Control and Prevention (CDC). Influenza Antiviral Medications; 2018. https://www.cdc.gov/flu/professionals/antivirals/summary-clinicians.htm (last access: 25th January, 2018).
124. South East Asia Infectious Disease Clinical Research Network. Effect of double dose oseltamivir on clinical and virological outcomes in children and adults admitted to hospital with severe influenza: double blind randomised controlled trial. *BMJ.* 2013;346:f3039.
125. Lee N, Chan PKS, Tam WWS, et al. Virologic response to peramivir treatment in adults hospitalized for influenza-associated lower respiratory tract infections. *Int J Antimicrob Ag.* 2016;48(2):215–219.
126. Dharan NJ, Gubareva LV, Meyer JJ, et al. Infections with oseltamivir-resistant influenza A(H1N1) virus in the United States. *JAMA.* 2009;301:1034–1041.
127. Marty FM, Vidal-Puigserver J, Clark C, et al. Intravenous zanamivir or oral oseltamivir for hospitalised patients with influenza: an international, randomised, double-blind, double-dummy, phase 3 trial. *Lancet Respir Med.* 2017;5(2):135–146.
128. Haffizulla J, Hartman A, Hoppers M, et al. Effect of nitazoxanide in adults and adolescents with acute uncomplicated influenza: a double-blind, randomised, placebo-controlled, phase 2b/3 trial. *Lancet Infect Dis.* 2014;14:609–618.
129. Dunning J, Baillie JK, Cao B, Hayden FG. Antiviral combinations for severe influenza. *Lancet Infect Dis.* 2014;14:1259–1270.
130. Naesens L, Stevaert A, Vanderlinden E. Antiviral therapies on the horizon for influenza. *Curr Opin Pharmacol.* 2016;30:106–115.
131. Byrn RA, Jones SM, Bennett HB, et al. Preclinical activity of VX-787, a first-in-class, orally bioavailable inhibitor of the influenza virus polymerase PB2 subunit. *Antimicrob Agents Chemother.* 2015;59(3):1569–1582.
132. McKimm-Breschkin JL, Jiang S, Hui DS, Beigel JH, Govorkova EA, Lee N. Prevention and treatment of respiratory viral infections: presentations on antivirals, traditional therapies and host-directed interventions at the 5th ISIRV Antiviral Group conference. *Antiviral Res.* 2018;149:118–142.
133. Finberg RW, Lanno R, Anderson D, Fleischhackl R, et al. Phase 2b study of pimodivir 1 (JNJ-63623872) as monotherapy or in combination with oseltamivir in treatment of acute uncomplicated seasonal influenza A: TOPAZ trial. *J Infect Dis.* 2019;219(7):1026–1034.
134. Hayden FG, Sugaya N, Hirotsu N, et al. Baloxavir marboxil for uncomplicated influenza in adults and adolescents. *N Engl J Med.* 2018;379(10):913–923.
135. Lee N, Hui DSC. Potential and challenges of serotherapy for severe influenza. *Lancet Respir Med.* 2017;5(8):e27.
136. Beigel JH, Bao Y, Beeler J, et al. Oseltamivir, amantadine, and ribavirin combination antiviral therapy versus oseltamivir monotherapy for the treatment of influenza: a multicentre, double-blind, randomised phase 2 trial. *Lancet Infect Dis.* 2017;17(12):1255–1265.
137. Lee VJ, Yap J, Cook AR, et al. Oseltamivir ring prophylaxis for containment of 2009 H1N1 influenza outbreaks. *N Engl J Med.* 2010;362(23):2166–2174.
138. Dobson J, Whitley RJ, Pocock S, Monto AS. Oseltamivir treatment for influenza in adults: a meta-analysis of randomised controlled trials. *Lancet.* 2015;385(9979):1729–1737.
139. Hsu J, Santesso N, Mustafa R, et al. Antivirals for treatment of influenza: a systematic review and meta-analysis of observational studies. *Ann Intern Med.* 2012;156(7):512–524.
140. Venkatesan S, Myles PR, Leonardi-Bee J, et al. Impact of outpatient neuraminidase inhibitor treatment in patients infected with influenza A(H1N1)pdm09 at high risk of hospitalization: an individual participant data metaanalysis. *Clin Infect Dis.* 2017;64(10):1328–1334.
141. Lee N, Choi KW, Chan PK, et al. Outcomes of adults hospitalised with severe influenza. *Thorax.* 2010;65(6):510–515.
142. Louie JK, Yang S, Acosta M, et al. Treatment with neuraminidase inhibitors for critically ill patients with influenza A (H1N1)pdm09. *Clin Infect Dis.* 2012;55(9):1198–1204.
143. Fry AM, Goswami D, Nahar K, et al. Efficacy of oseltamivir treatment started within 5 days of symptom onset to reduce influenza illness duration and virus shedding in an urban setting in Bangladesh: a randomised placebo-controlled trial. *Lancet Infect Dis.* 2014;14(2):109–118.
144. Chan PKS, Lee N, Zaman M, et al. Determinants of antiviral effectiveness in H5N1 avian influenza. *J Infect Dis.* 2012;206(9):1359–1366.
145. Lee N, Hui DSC, Zuo Z, et al. A prospective intervention study on higher-dose oseltamivir treatment in adults hospitalized with influenza A and B infections. *Clin Infect Dis.* 2013;57(11):1511–1519.
146. De Jong MD, Ison MG, Monto AS, et al. Evaluation of intravenous peramivir for treatment of influenza in hospitalized patients. *Clin Infect Dis.* 2014;59:e172–e285.
147. Lee N, Chan PK, Hui DS, et al. Viral loads and duration of viral shedding in adult patients hospitalized with influenza. *J Infect Dis.* 2009;200(4):492–500.
148. Lee N, Chan PK, Wong CK, et al. Viral clearance and inflammatory response patterns in adults hospitalized for pandemic 2009 influenza A(H1N1) virus pneumonia. *Antivir Ther.* 2011;16(2):237–247.
149. Whitley RJ, Boucher CA, Lina B, et al. Global assessment of resistance to neuraminidase inhibitors, 2008–2011: the Influenza Resistance Information Study (IRIS). *Clin Infect Dis.* 2013;56:1197–1205.
150. Watanabe A, Chang SC, Kim MJ, Chu DW, Ohashi Y, MARVEL Study Group. Long-acting neuraminidase inhibitor laninamivir octanoate versus oseltamivir for treatment of influenza: a double-blind, randomized, non-inferiority clinical trial. *Clin Infect Dis.* 2010;51:1167–1175.

151. Kashiwagi S, Watanabe A, Ikematsu H, Uemori M, Awamura S, Laninamivir Prophylaxis Study Group. Long-acting neuraminidase inhibitor laninamivir octanoate as post-exposure prophylaxis for influenza. *Clin Infect Dis.* 2016;63(3):330–337.
152. Wang Y, Zhong W, Salam A, et al. Phase 2a, open-label, dose-escalating, multi-center pharmacokinetic study of favipiravir (T-705) in combination with oseltamivir in patients with severe influenza. *EBioMedicine.* 2020;62:103125.
153. O'Neil B, Ison MG, Hallouin-Bernard MC, et al. A phase 2 study of pimodivir (JNJ-63623872) in combination with oseltamivir in elderly and nonelderly adults hospitalized with influenza A infection: OPAL study. *J Infect Dis.* 2020.
154. PRNewswire. Janssen to Discontinue Pimodivir Influenza Development Program; 2020. https://www.prnewswire.com/news-releases/janssen-to-discontinue-pimodivir-influenza-development-program-301122958.html.
155. Ison MG, Portsmouth S, Yoshida Y, et al. Early treatment with baloxavir marboxil in high-risk adolescent and adult outpatients with uncomplicated influenza (CAPSTONE-2): a randomised, placebo-controlled, phase 3 trial. *Lancet Infect Dis.* 2020;20(10):1204–1214.
156. Ikematsu H, Hayden FG, Kawaguchi K, et al. Baloxavir marboxil for prophylaxis against influenza in household contacts. *N Engl J Med.* 2020;383(4):309–320.
157. Uehara T, Hayden FG, Kawaguchi K, et al. Treatment-emergent influenza variant viruses with reduced baloxavir susceptibility: impact on clinical and virologic outcomes in uncomplicated influenza. *J Infect Dis.* 2020;221(3):346–355.
158. Gamiño-Arroyo AE, Guerrero ML, McCarthy S, et al. Efficacy and safety of nitazoxanide in addition to standard of care for the treatment of severe acute respiratory illness. *Clin Infect Dis.* 2019;69(11):1903–1911.
159. Moss RB, Hansen C, Sanders RL, Hawley S, Li T, Steigbigel RT. A phase II study of DAS181, a novel host directed antiviral for the treatment of influenza infection. *J Infect Dis.* 2012;206:1844–1851.
160. Hui DS, Lee N, Chan PK, Beigel JH. The role of adjuvant immunomodulatory agents for treatment of severe influenza. *Antiviral Res.* 2018;150:202–216.
161. Beigel JH, Tebas P, Elie-Turenne MC, et al. Immune plasma for the treatment of severe influenza: an open-label, multicentre, phase 2 randomised study. *Lancet Respir Med.* 2017;5(6):500–511.
162. Beigel JH, Aga E, Elie-Turenne MC, et al. Anti-influenza immune plasma for the treatment of patients with severe influenza A: a randomised, double-blind, phase 3 trial. Lancet. *Respir Med.* 2019;7(11):941–950.
163. Davey Jr RT, Fernández-Cruz E, Markowitz N, et al. Anti-influenza hyperimmune intravenous immunoglobulin for adults with influenza A or B infection (FLU-IVIG): a double-blind, randomised, placebo-controlled trial. Lancet. *Respir Med.* 2019;7(11):951–963.
164. Lee N, Wong CK, Chan MCW, et al. Anti-inflammatory effects of adjunctive macrolide treatment in adults hospitalized with influenza: a randomized controlled trial. *Antiviral Res.* 2017;144:48–56.
165. Lee N, Hui DSC. Dexamethasone in community-acquired pneumonia. *Lancet.* 2011;378(9795):979–980.
166. Doll MK, Winters N, Boikos C, Kraicer-Melamed H, Gore G, Quach C. Safety and effectiveness of neuraminidase inhibitors for influenza treatment, prophylaxis, and outbreak control: a systematic review of systematic reviews and/or meta-analyses. *J Antimicrob Chemother.* 2017;72(11):2990–3007.
167. Ye M, Jacobs A, Khan MN, et al. Evaluation of the use of oseltamivir prophylaxis in the control of influenza outbreaks in long-term care facilities in Alberta, Canada: a retrospective provincial database analysis. *BMJ Open.* 2016;6(7):e011686.
168. Public Health England (PHE). PHE Guidance on Use of Antiviral Agents for the Treatment and Prophylaxis of Seasonal Influenza; 2023. Version 11.0, November 2021. https://www.gov.uk/government/publications/influenza-treatment-and-prophylaxis-using-anti-viral-agents (last access: May 23, 2023).

CHAPTER 9

Avian Influenza

NUNTRA SUWANTARAT[a,b] • ANUCHA APISARNTHANARAK[a,c]
[a]Division of Infectious Diseases, Thammasat University Hospital, Thammasat University, Pathumthani, Thailand • [b]Chulabhorn International College of Medicine, Thammasat University, Pathumthani, Thailand • [c]Division of Infectious Diseases, Department of Medicine, Faculty of Medicine, Thammasat University, Pathumthani, Thailand

INTRODUCTION

Avian influenza A viruses rarely infect humans; however, over the past 20 years, avian influenza A has emerged, causing illness with minimal to no symptoms to severe pneumonias and death and frequently associated with poultry outbreaks. This has led to heightened awareness and international surveillance, and impacted public health practices and care in healthcare systems.[1–7] These strains cause mild to fatal infection in poultry, occasionally transmitting to humans who were in contact with infected birds, poultry, their products, or their environments.[1–3,7–10]

In 1997, Hong Kong reported a cluster of 18 cases of influenza A H5N1 human infections.[11] Six (35%) of the cases died. The investigation matched the human viruses to those isolated from poultry found at the local wet markets. These findings led public health officials to cull millions of birds. Since this time, sporadic human cases of avian influenza continue to be reported. Between January 2003 and 2023, 868 cases of human H5N1 have been reported with 457 deaths and a case fatality rate of 53%.[12] In a recent twist and cause for consternation, an outbreak of highly pathogenic A (H5N1) was reported at a mink farm, demonstrating the virus is capable of infecting mammals.[13] Minks are in the same family as ferrets, and ferrets are a host that develops influenza infection and is used to study influenza, leading to a concern that this virus could evolve into one more adapted to human infection. One of the mutations noted in this outbreak strain enhances the polymerase activity in mammalian host cells, which could facilitate more robust transmission and has implications for public health. Of the 12 humans exposed to these animals in this cluster, one developed symptoms and tested negative for influenza.

The clinical experience of these infections is relatively limited and based on case reports and some outbreak investigations. Importantly, human infections with highly pathogenic strains have a very high reported mortality rate, yet the likelihood of sustained human-to-human transmission of these viruses remains low.[1–3,7–15] While the mortality rate may be inflated due to reporting biases, the pandemic potential remains especially given recent transmission in large poultry containment facilities and the emergence of strains that can bind to both avian and human sialic acid receptors. Hence, public health authorities continue to investigate the possible modes of transmission and improve surveillance to better estimate the mortality in humans and animals and implement prevention mechanisms.

Because of the pandemic potential of these viruses, guidelines, detailed information about ongoing outbreaks and circulating viruses, and recommendations from international public health organizations such as the World Health Organization (WHO), the Centers for Disease Control and Prevention (CDC), and the European Centre for Disease Prevention and Control (ECDC) provide up-to-date recommendations for diagnosis, investigation, and treatment when cases are found.[1,7,8,16,17] However, care of these patients remains a challenge and in order to prevent patient-to-patient and patient-to-healthcare personnel (HCPs) transmission. We summarize the current concepts in microbiology, epidemiology, diagnosis, and risk factors for transmission of avian influenza A infection. Furthermore, we discuss effective treatment and infection prevention strategies in healthcare settings for this emerging and evolving infection.

Viral Outbreaks, Biosecurity, and Preparing for Mass Casualty Infectious Diseases Events
https://doi.org/10.1016/B978-0-323-54841-0.00028-7

MICROBIOLOGY AND IMMUNOLOGY

Avian influenza is caused by a negative sense, single-stranded RNA virus in the family *Orthomyxoviridae* and an influenza A virus that routinely circulates in waterfowl and poultry (see Chapter 7 for further details). The genome encodes for eight nonstructural proteins. Influenza A virus has two enveloped proteins, hemagglutinin (HA), classified as H1 through H18, and neuraminidase (NA), classified as N1 through N11, that are used to characterize the subtypes. These surface proteins are essential for viral entry into the cell and release. However, errors are common in the viral RNA-dependent polymerase, leading to mutations. Mutations in these proteins, which are important for neutralizing antibody responses, can lead to alterations in the host's immune response. The subtypes that are circulating at a given time and geographic area and infect humans and animals are evolving and vary. These viruses infect a variety of animals, including humans, mammals, and birds; however, the natural reservoir for the influenza A virus is wild waterfowl yet have now become entrenched in domestic poultry. To date, 16 combinations of HA and 9 NA have been described in wild bird populations.[11] Currently, two influenza subtypes are circulating among humans (H1N1 and H3N2). Yet, among animals, many other subtypes have been identified including, influenza A virus subtypes H17N10 and H18N11, which have been isolated from bats; H7N7 and H3N8 have been reported in horses; and H3N8 has caused infection in horses and dogs.[14,15,17]

The pathogenesis of avian influenza is not completely understood and may vary from strain to strain. These viruses replicate efficiently in animal models, and some subtypes such as A (H7N3), which can cause human infections, have a tropism for specific tissues such as the eye. The hemagglutinin determines the specificity for binding to α2,36 sialic acid in avian cell receptors and then to human α2,6-sialic acid receptors.[11] Avian influenza viruses bind to receptors in bronchoalveolar cells, the respiratory tract tissues, and renal and intestinal tissues that express sialic acid.[18] In addition, the hemagglutinin subunits also cleave proteases within the cells, which influences viral dissemination. However, the receptors that bind avian strains are primarily found in the lower lung, which is one reason human infections are thought to be rare.[11] Importantly, several viral polymerases mediate virulence in animals, including ferrets, and it is alteration in the PB2 genes and adaption of these proteins that enhance mammalian adaption. Furthermore, avian viruses are adapted to higher temperatures, i.e., 37°C vs the lower temperature of 33°C found in the human lung.[11] This said, a single mutation and substitution in the Glu627Lys of the PB2 protein can change the temperature adaptabilities of these viruses.[11]

AVIAN INFLUENZA A VIRUS LINEAGES AND PATHOGENICITY

Avian influenza viruses cause mild infection in waterfowl; however, they can develop mutations and evolve in domestic poultry, so they are classified as highly pathogenic (HPAI) and low pathogenic (LPAI) types based on the severity of illness and mortality rates in poultry.[11] Both HPAI and LPAI viruses can spread rapidly through poultry flocks.[19,20] Poultry infected with LPAI viruses do not develop symptoms or have mild illness.[11] Infection of poultry with HPAI viruses can cause severe disease in these animals with a 90% to 100% mortality within 48h of infection. The highly pathogenic avian influenza A lineages that are currently circulating are A (H5N1), A (H7N9), and A (H5N6). Of these, the A (H5N1) subtypes have become the dominant strain in 2023 and have replaced other A (H5Nx) strains that have been circulating with introductions in most continents.[21] The trajectory of this change demonstrates the impact of the recent introductions into the bird populations, and outbreaks were linked to migration along the flyways (Fig. 1). Avian influenza A viruses have crossed the species barrier and infected humans (known as avian-original influenza), especially subtypes H5 (H5N1, H5N6), H7 (H7N3, H7N7, H7N9), H9 (H9N2), and H10 (H10N8) viruses (Table 1).[1–3,7,12,19,20,22–24] A more recent report from China of a mild human H3N10 infection with fever, chills, sore throat, and rhinorrhea in humans was notable as the virus is composed of resorted genes from H9N2, avian H3, and N8 viruses.[25,26]

EPIDEMIOLOGY, CLINICAL FINDINGS, AND SIGNIFICANCE AND TRANSMISSION

Two major avian influenza A subtypes cause most human infections and are associated with outbreaks; avian influenza A (H5N1) and A (H7N9).[1,6–8] However, the list of avian strains infecting humans is expanding. Isolated human cases of LPAI including A (H9N2), A (H10N7), and A (H10N8) have been reported.[11,12,24,27] Other viral subtypes, to a lesser extent, such as A (H10N7, H10N8), A (H10N7), A (H6N8), and H7 subtypes have caused human infection and outbreaks.[19,20,24,27] In humans, the spectrum of infection for both LPAI and HPAI viruses is from mild to severe. The 1997 outbreak of avian influenza A (H5N1) that occurred in Hong Kong was the first to identify human infection with an as-

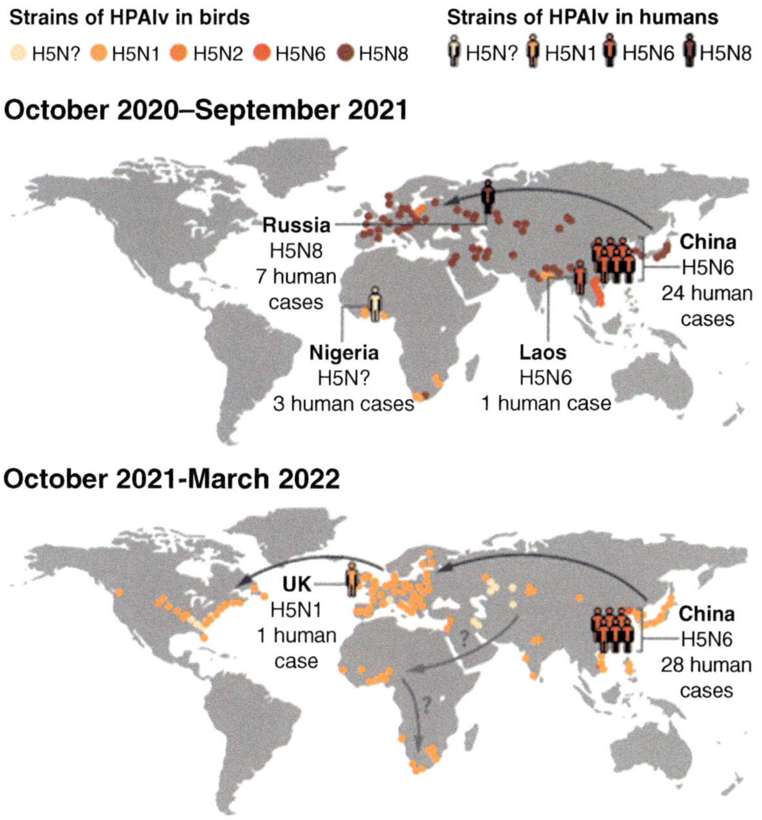

FIG. 1 Spread of H5Nx highly pathogenic avian influenza since 2014. Since 2014, H5Nx highly pathogenic avian influenza has spread worldwide with increased outbreaks of A H5N1 in both poultry and wild avian species in 2021 and 22. Human cases were reported. The migratory bird flyways antedate outbreaks. Outbreaks are indicated by *arrows*. Map lines delineate study areas and do not necessarily depict accepted national boundaries.

sociated large poultry outbreak, which was controlled with the culling of over one million poultry, fowl, and other avian species.[28] Subsequently, prevention policies and early detection surveillance strategies were implemented, and no new human cases of H5N1 were detected in Hong Kong until February 2003. Sporadic infections continue to be described in other Asian countries, Europe, and North America.[29] The reemergence of the viral subtype and its rapid evolution have raised awareness about pandemic potential of an avian influenza strain.[14,15,20,21] In 2013, a novel, avian influenza A (H7N9) virus emerged in poultry markets in China. Over 100 infected persons were identified.[4,5] Since then, 1568 human cases have been reported with a case fatality rate of 39%. As a result of over 759 human cases in 2017, healthcare-associated and non-sustained household transmission, China undertook a massive poultry vaccination campaign with combined H5 and H7 strains. Wet markets were closed, and only two human A (H7N9) infections were reported in 2018. Another subtype emerges in Sichuan China in May of 2014, with the first human case of A (H5N6).[21] As of February 2023, 32 of 84 (39%) cases died.[29] The high mortality rates are notable with these human cases of avian influenza, especially in A (H5N1).[19,20,23–32] Sporadic human cases and outbreaks of avian strains, new subtypes, and subclades, especially of A (H5N1), have been reported in Europe (Netherlands), the Middle East, Africa (Egypt and others), and North and South America, with these strains affecting both migratory bird and poultry populations globally.[20,21]

The incubation period for avian influenza is longer than seasonal influenza and is usually 2–5 days but can extend to 17 days.[33] For human A (H7N9), the incubation period on average is 5 days with a range of one to 10 days. Symptoms are varied from a mild upper respiratory tract infection with fever and cough and can progress to severe pneumonia. The fever is typically

TABLE 1
Summary of Avian Influenza A Virus Lineages

Avian Influenza A virus Lineages	First Reported (Year, Country)	Common Subtype Caused Disease in Human	Demographics of Poultry Infection	Clinical Presentation in Human	Mortality (Approximately)
Subtype H3 (H3N8)	- 2022 China	- H3N8	- H3N8 viruses have been associated with disease in dogs, horses, pigs, donkeys, and seals	- a 4-year-old boy who consumed chickens from the backyard. - Severe pneumonia, acute respiratory failure	Two human infections reported with no death
Subtype H5 (H5N1, H5N2, H5N3, H5N4, H5N5, H5N6, H5N7, H5N8, and H5N9)	- 1997 Hong Kong (H5N1) and again in 2003 - 2014–2022 China	- H5N1 (multiple clades) - H5N6	- LPAI reported worldwide - Asian lineage HPAI H5N1 reported in Asia and the Middle East (16 countries)	Severe pneumonia, acute respiratory distress syndrome (H5N1)	50%–60%
Subtype H7 (H7N1, H7N2, H7N3, H7N4, H7N5, H7N6, H7N7, H7N8, and H7N9)	2004 Netherlands (H7N7) - 2013 China (H7N9) - 2018 China (H7N4)	- H7N9 (most common) H7N2, H7N3, H7N4, H7N7	- LPAI reported in China (H7N9). the Netherlands, Middle East, and Africa (H7N7)	- Severe respiratory illness (H7N9) - Mild to moderate respiratory tract infection, including conjunctivitis and upper respiratory (H7N2, H7N3, H7N7)	30%–40% with H7N9; extremely low with H7N3, H7N7
Subtype H9 (H9N1, H9N2, H9, N3, H9, N4, H9N5, H9N6, H9, N7, H9N8, and H9, N9)	- 1991 Hong Kong (H9N2)	- H9N2 (mild respiratory tract infection)	- LPAI reported in Asia, Europe, the Middle East, and Africa	Mild respiratory tract infection (rare sporadic human infections)	2%–3%
Subtype H10 (H10N7, H10N8)	- 2013 China (H10N8)	H10N8 Fatal pneumonia	LPAI in China, Egypt, Eurasia, Australia	Mild respiratory disease (H10N7) to severe pneumonia (H10N8) depending on clade	0% (H10N7) and 100% (H10N8) few cases reported

Note: *HPAI*, highly pathogenic avian influenza; *LPAI*, low-pathogenic avian influenza.

greater than 38 °C. Coryza and sore throat are less common. Gastrointestinal symptoms include diarrhea, nausea, and vomiting and are more frequent in A (H5N1) subtypes. With H7 subtypes conjunctivitis is common. In severe cases with pneumonia, cases typically present with severe dyspnea and rapidly develop respiratory failure and multiorgan failure. Other complications include encephalitis, bleeding, secondary bacterial infections, and shock. With some subtypes (i.e., A (H5N1), A (H7N9)), mild to moderate illness appears rare, yet in others, such as A (H7N7) and A (H9N2), disease is typically subclinical or mild. Chest radiography usually reveals bilateral, diffuse interstitial infiltrates, patchy infiltrates, or ground glass opacities. Other laboratory findings are nonspecific with leukopenia being a feature. Mortality is generally attributed to severe lower hypoxic respiratory failure in the setting of acute severe pneumonia. While pneumonia caused by influenza A (H7N9) virus is severe, the mortality of 30% is less than that of A (H5N1) infection.[4–6] Like epidemic influenza, surviving patients develop serum antibody responses 10–14 days after symptoms onset.[2,4–6,20,28]

In general, influenza viruses are transmitted from person to person primarily via droplets or via direct or indirect (fomite) contact with contaminated secretions or surfaces. Occasionally, airborne transmission of the influenza virus is reported, especially when particles are aerosolized, such as with aerosol-generating medical procedures. However, human infections with avian influenza strains commonly result from direct or indirect contact with infected live or dead poultry, a contaminated environment, or inoculation into the pharynx or gastrointestinal tract.[1–3,14,15] In fact, most cases of the human A (H5N1) and A (H7N9) virus infection are linked to exposure to slaughtering or handling poultry or poultry markets.[1–3] A few cases have been linked to the consumption of raw, contaminated poultry blood. Serologic surveys support that while these infections are rare, those exposed to poultry and others with illness are at higher risk than the general population. A recent meta-analysis of seroprevalence data for A (H5N1) found 0%–0.5% of those exposed to poultry and 0.4%–1.8% of those exposed to human A (H5N1) or infected birds had antibodies compared to none or extremely low frequencies in the general population.[24] Whereas, a seroprevalence survey in Cambodia found that 1.1% of the general population had neutralizing antibodies to H9N2 and that more than doubled among those with extensive poultry exposure to 2.6%.[21,34,35] Risk from another large longitudinal cohort study in China demonstrated that the risk of seropositivity increased with age and duration of exposure.[36]

Although rare, human-to-human transmission of avian influenza (H5N1) has occurred via intimate contact, such as among household contacts where protections such as masks and other barrier precautions were not used. Transmission has not been described from casual social contact.[9,10,30] Recently, transmission in healthcare settings has been reported with two clusters where patients were on the same ward. One reported an immunocompromised patient with A (H7N9) and A (H1N1)pdm09 infected another immunocompromised patient after exposure for 6 days.[37] Genetic sequences were identical for both isolates. All 103 contacts were negative for A (H7N9). A second patient-to-patient transmission of A (H7N9) was supported by genetically similar isolates.[38] One patient had visited a poultry market, and the A (H7N9) isolates from the patient and market were genetically similar. PCR of environmental site samples detected A (H7N9). No specific antibodies were detected in 38 contacts. In both nosocomial clusters, the patients were hospitalized in the same ward with the index case.[37,38] Furthermore, Apisarnthanarak et al.[30] reported no evidence of seroconversion among 25 HCPs who were exposed to a patient with H5N1 virus infection at a tertiary care hospital in Thailand. These data suggest that the risk to HCPs for occupational acquisition of H5N1 virus infection remains low, but patient-to-patient transmission can occur in rare instances.

OUTBREAK SUMMARY AND CURRENT SITUATION

As a result of the avian outbreaks and human cases in Hong Kong and other areas in Asia and the concern about the pandemic potential of these viruses if not recognized in a timely fashion, the International Health Regulations required reporting of all human infections caused by a new or novel influenza subtype to the WHO beginning in 2005.[1,2] This requirement includes the reporting of any animal and noncirculating seasonal influenza A viruses, in essence targeting strains considered epidemiologically important. Information from these notifications, including genetic analysis of strains and identification of important mutations that will alter viral fitness, is critical to understanding the epidemiology, to inform risk assessments, and to characterize transmission dynamics of influenza at the human-animal interface. These data help public health authorities monitor for genetic changes and evidence for transmission, determine the best infection prevention and control strategies, identify effective treatment strategies, and inform and update national and international guidelines. The overall public health risk from currently known avian influenza viruses and those emerging at the human-animal interface has not changed, and the likelihood of sustained human-to-human transmission of these viruses remains low. Further human infections with viruses of animal origin are expected, and ongoing research and communication can enhance our understanding.[1,2,14–16] Currently, two major lineages A (H5N1) and A (H7N9) viruses are circulating in migratory birds, causing outbreaks in domesticated poultry and occasional human infection. Recently, China reported three cases of human infection with avian influenza A (H3N8) virus.[12,22]

Avian influenza A (H5N1)

Though all influenza A (H5) subtype viruses have the potential to cause disease in humans, thus far human cases have been limited to influenza A (H5N1) and A (H5N6) viruses reported to WHO. According to reports received by the World Organization for Animal Health (OIE), various influenza A (H5) subtypes continue to be detected in birds in Africa, Europe, and Asia.[1,2,20] The first known human avian influenza A (H5N1) outbreak occurred in Hong Kong in 1997. The outbreak was notable for the described epidemiology. At that time, six of 18 (33%) people with confirmed H5N1 infection died.[28] Over one million chickens were culled with significant economic implications. After this outbreak, prevention policies and early detection strategies were put into place, but no new cases of H5N1 were detected in Hong Kong until February 2003, when two cases were reported, of which one died.[2,3,29] In 2015, the number of influenza A (H5N1) virus outbreaks in poultry and human infections increased in Egypt and other African countries.[2] The virus has further spread and at an accelerated pace into Europe and now North America causing over 400 million chickens to be culled.[21] Rapid spread in 2021–2022 is likely multifactorial with recent mutations and new subtypes being more fit, increased outbreaks including in high-density production facilities, an ability to infect a broader range of avian species, and the introduction into migratory bird populations (Fig. 1). Since its introduction into the United States and Canada, less than 2 years ago, over 60 million birds have been affected and significant economic losses have occurred.[39,40] New clades have emerged, and the viruses have diverged geographically. Each clade has individual antigenic profiles that do not appear to provide cross-reacting neutralizing antibodies.[11] The outbreak of highly pathogenic A (H5N1) at a Spanish mink farm and now new outbreaks reported in sea lions in Argentina and Uruguay demonstrate transfer into several mammalian species.[13] Furthermore, human avian influenza cases have been reported in both the United States of America (USA) and Ecuador, prompting many countries to consider mass poultry vaccination.[39,40] As of 5 January 2023, 868 laboratory-confirmed human cases of avian influenza A (H5N1) virus infection, including 457 deaths, have been reported from 16 countries (number of cases, death); including Azerbaijan (8, 5), Bangladesh (8, 1), Cambodia (56, 37), Canada (1,1), China (54, 32), Djibouti (1,0), Egypt (359, 120), Indonesia (200, 168), Iraq (3,2), Laos (3, 2), Myanmar (1, 0), Nigeria (1, 1), Pakistan (3,1), Spain (2, 0), Thailand (25, 17), Turkey (12, 4), United Kingdom (1, 0), USA (1, 0), and Vietnam (127, 64).[2]

Avian Influenza A (H5N6) and Other A (H5 Viruses)

Since 2014, 83 laboratory-confirmed human cases of avian influenza A (H5N6) virus infection, including 33 deaths, were reported in the Western Pacific Region.[12] The virus emerged in 2008, and it was in 2014 that the first human case was reported. According to the animal health authorities in China, by 2017, influenza A (H5N6) viruses had become the prominent viruses in poultry in many provinces in the country, including those that have reported human cases. All patients had exposure to live poultry before illness onset, and no further human cases were reported among three close contacts of this case.[1,2,20] More recently, A (H5N8) has circulated in poultry and has resulted in a few human cases, including in poultry workers in Russia.[11]

Avian Influenza A (H7N9)

In March 2013, a novel avian influenza A (H7N9) was described in China.[4,5] Between 2013 and March 2, 2023, a total of 1568 laboratory-confirmed human infections with avian influenza A (H7N9) virus, including 616 deaths (CFR: 39%), were reported to the WHO. The majority of the H7N9 avian influenza cases were reported from China. Deaths were also reported from Taiwan, Hong Kong, Malaysia, and Canada. The last human avian influenza A (H7N9) cases in the Western Pacific Region were in 2019.[12]

The initial epidemiologic investigators demonstrated that patients came from multiple regions in China and that the mean age of cases was older (61 years old). Most patients had poultry exposure and were hospitalized.[5] There were four small family clusters with generally two to four people, which may have been caused by human-to-human transmission. Death generally occurs within 3 weeks of illness onset. Over 2500 contacts were traced, and of those, 28 (1%) developed respiratory symptoms, yet testing did not identify influenza. Yang et al.[31] reported on epidemiological and clinical characteristics of humans with avian influenza A (H7N9) infection in Guangdong, China, 2013–2017. Of the 256 cases, 39.0% of patients died, and 65.6% of patients were admitted to an intensive care unit. High-risk populations identified were the elderly and the groups with high-frequency exposure to live poultry. To mitigate the impact of this and other subtypes, agricultural authorities in China have employed vaccination of domestic poultry against infection with avian influenza A (H7) and A (H5) viruses. Though this virus has pandemic potential, the risk assessment has not changed, and to date, A (H7N9) viruses have not exhibited sustained human-to-human transmission, significant changes in viral properties, or the epidemiology of human infections. Still, rapid information sharing and dissemination remain essential to detect key changes and facilitate rapid risk assessments with increased confidence.[1,2,7,20,31] These events, along with the experience from the SARS outbreak in 2003, have led to vast improvements in the Chinese government's awareness of and capacity to respond to health emergencies, which include rapid communication and disclosure of information, abilities to detect and confirm an emerging virus within 1 month of identification, and enhanced capacity to collect clinical information.[6]

Avian Influenza A (H9N2)

Avian influenza A (H9N2) viruses are enzootic in poultry in China. Generally, this is associated with mild illness in poultry. Between 1999 and 2003 in Hong Kong and possibly because of heightened surveillance, an avian influenza A (H9N2) virus was isolated from several children with mild, self-limiting illnesses.[32,41] As of March 2, 2023, 84 laboratory-confirmed human cases of A (H9N2) virus infection and two deaths have been reported to WHO from China. Cases have now been reported in Bangladesh, Africa, Eurasia, and Egypt.[5] Cases are younger and most commonly children. Most cases have mild respiratory symptoms, and because of the mild symptom profile, the cases may not be diagnosed. This is supported by a meta-analysis that found that the seroprevalence by hemagglutinin inhibition among avian-exposed individuals ranged from 1% to 43% (median 9%) consistent with the WHO estimates.[42] Most cases provide histories of exposure to live poultry or contaminated environments, and the deaths have occurred in patients with severe underlying diseases.[1,2,12,20,32,41] Human-to-human transmission is reported. The importance of these viruses is that they have been a source of genes that are resorted in avian viruses and contain genes that facilitate viral replication in human cells and may have the ability to bind to human cells.[11] This strain is considered one of the parent strains in the recently reported H3N8 cases reported from China.[25,26]

Other Avian Influenza A

As of February, human infections have been reported from other avian strains and include two cases of A (H10N3) and a single case of A (H7N4) (in 2018) both from China.[12] Three human cases of A (H3N8) with one death case have been reported from China since March 2022.[22,25,26] All patients had a history of live poultry exposures. Two patients presented with severe acute respiratory distress syndrome. The fatal case was a 56-year-old woman who had multiple comorbidities.[22]

PANDEMIC INFLUENZA CONCERNS

Avian influenza, influenza A, has three of four properties necessary to cause a serious pandemic: it can infect humans and nearly all are immunologically naive, and many strains are highly lethal. However, this virus lacks the ability to be transmitted in a sustained fashion between humans.[14,15] Since the avian influenza A (H5N1) outbreaks in 2003 and 2021–2022, and avian influenza A (H7N9) in 2013, influenza experts have warned that influenza pandemics historically occur every 11 to 42 years with the worst pandemic in recorded medical history between 1918 and 19 (the Spanish flu (H1N1)). The last pandemic was in 2009, when H1N1 reemerged and contained fragments of swine, avian, and human influenza. H5N1 influenza viruses have demonstrated that they can acquire new properties by mutational adaption of the avian strain, as with the Spanish influenza, or by genetic reassortment through dual infection with human and avian strains, as occurred in 1957 (Asian influenza), 1968 (Hong Kong influenza), and 2009 H1N1pdm2009.

H5N1, on the other hand, is of avian origin, and nearly all cases have resulted from direct contact with poultry with rare human-to-human transmission.[9,10] Those who are skeptical about an H5N1 pandemic point out that genetic changes to facilitate efficient human-to-human transmission are unlikely to occur as the virus has not acquired this property while circulating. If correct, H5N1 will remain primarily an avian pathogen that sporadically causes human infection requiring close contact with sick poultry.[14,15,30] In an effort to predict the potential pandemic risk posed by influenza A viruses, including avian subtypes that are not currently circulating in people, the CDC and international animal and human health experts developed the Influenza Risk Assessment Tool (IRAT). Currently, avian influenza H7N9 [A/Hong Kong/125/2017] stain has the highest pandemic risk (Table 2).[27]

TABLE 2
Example of Influenza Risk Assessment Tool (IRAT) for Various Strains of Avian Influenza A

Virus	Most Recent Date Evaluation	Potential Emergence Risk	Potential Impact Risk	Overall Summary
H7N9 [A/Hong Kong/125/2017]	May 2017	6.5	7.5	Moderate-High
H7N9 [A/Shanghai/02/2013]	April 2016	6.4	7.2	Moderate-High
H9N2 Y280 lineage [A/Anhui-Lujiang/13/2018]	July 2019	6.2	5.9	Moderate
H9N2 G1 lineage [A/Bangladesh/0994/2011]	February 2014	5.6	5.4	Moderate
H5N6 Clade 2.3 4 4b [A/Sichuan/06681/2021]	October 2021	5.3	6.3	Moderate
H5N1 Clade 1 [A/Vietnam/1203/2004]	November 2011	5.2	6.6	Moderate
H5N6 [A/Yunnan/14564/2015] - like	April 2016	5.0	6.6	Moderate
H10N8 [A/Jiangxi-Donghu/346/2013]	February 2014	4.3	6.0	Moderate
H7N9 [A/chicken/Tennessee/17–007431-3/2017]	October 2017	3.1	3.5	Low
H7N9 [A/chicken/Tennessee/17–007147-2/2017]	October 2017	2.8	3.5	Low

Note: The summary average risk score for the virus to achieve sustained human-to-human transmission was low-moderate (less than 5), moderate risk range (less than 7), high-risk range (more than 8). **H7N9: Asian avian [A/Hong Kong/125/2017]** Low-pathogenic avian influenza (LPAI) H7N9 viruses were first reported from China in March 2013. These viruses were first scored using the IRAT in April 2013 and then annually in 2014, 2015, and 2016 with no change in overall risk scores. A risk assessment of H7N9 [A/Hong Kong/125/2017] was conducted in May 2017. The overall IRAT risk assessment score for this virus falls into the moderate-high risk category and is similar to the scores for the previous H7N9 viruses. **H7N9: Avain [A/Shanghai/02/2013].** On March 31, 2013, the China Health and Family Planning Commission notified the World Health Organization (WHO) of three cases of human infection with influenza H7N9. These LPAIs were rescored most recently in April 2016 with no substantive change in risk scores since May 2013. **H9N2: Avian Influenza A (H9N2) Y280 lineage [A/Anhui-Lujiang/39/2018].** Low-pathogenic avian influenza A (H9N2) viruses are enzootic in poultry in many countries in Africa, Asia, the Middle East, and Europe. Since the late 1990s, when the first human infections with avian influenza A (H9N2) virus were identified, detection of this virus has been reported infrequently in humans and in swine and other mammals. In 2018, there were seven reported human infections, most with known exposure to poultry and with the majority involving viruses of the Y280 lineage. **H9N2: Avain G1 lineage [A/Bangladesh/0994/2011].** Human infections with influenza AH9N2 virus have been reported sporadically; cases reportedly exhibited mild influenza-like illness. Historically, these LPAIs have been isolated from wild and domestic birds. In response to these reports, a risk assessment of this H9N2 influenza virus was conducted in 2014. **H5N6: Highly Pathogenic Avian Influenza A (H5N6) clade 2.3.4.4b [A/Sichuan/06681/2021].** Since 2014, 52 human infections with highly pathogenic avian influenza (HPAI) A (H5N6) clade 2.3.4.4b virus (H5N6 2.3.4.4b) have been reported to the World Health Organization, with 26 human infections reported in 2021 as of 19 November, all but one reported from China. Most infected persons reported exposure to poultry or poultry environments prior to infection. The majority of infections have resulted in severe illness requiring hospitalization, with 9 deaths in 2021. In addition, surveillance reports indicate the detection of A (H5N6) 2.3.4.4b in poultry, waterfowl, and environmental samples. In 2013, a HPAI A (H5N6) virus was first detected in poultry in China. From 2016 to 2019, A (H5N6) clade 2.3.4.4b virus was reported in wild birds and in domestic poultry from multiple countries throughout Asia, Europe, and Africa. However, during 2020–2021, A (H5N6) clade 2.3.4.4b virus was only reported in birds in four countries in Asia. H**5N1: Clade 1 [A/Vietnam/1203/2004].** The first human cases of HPAI H5N1 virus were reported in Hong Kong in 1997. Since 2003, highly pathogenic H5N1 avian influenza viruses have caused over 850 laboratory-confirmed human cases; mortality among these cases was high. A risk assessment of this H5N1 clade 1 virus was conducted in 2011. **H5N6: [A/Yunnan/14564/2015 (H5N6-like)].** Between January 2014 and May 2019, there were 23 human cases of H5N6 highly pathogenic avian influenza reported, and 14 of the cases were fatal. Avian outbreaks of this virus were first reported in China in 2013. Subsequently, avian outbreaks have been reported in several countries through 2019. **H10N8: Avian H10N8 [A/Jiangxi-Donghu/346/2013].** Three human infections with influenza A (H10N8) virus were reported by the China Health and Family Planning Commission in 2013 and 2014. All cases were hospitalized and two died. Historically, low-pathogenicity avian influenza H10 and N8 viruses have been recovered from birds. A risk assessment of the H10N8 influenza was conducted in 2014. **H7N9: Low-Pathogenicity North American avian [A/chicken/Tennessee/17–007431-3/2017].** Surveillance conducted in March 2017 during the investigation of a highly pathogenic avian influenza (HPAI) A (H7N9) virus in commercial poultry in Tennessee revealed the contemporaneous presence of North American lineage low-pathogenicity avian influenza (LPAI) A (H7N9) virus in commercial and backyard poultry flocks in Tennessee and three other states. The outbreak in poultry appeared limited with no further detections in subsequent surveillance. There were no reports of human cases associated with this virus. **H7N9: Highly Pathogenic North American avian [A/chicken/Tennessee/17–007147-2/2017].** In March 2017, the US Department of Agriculture (USDA) reported the detection of a highly pathogenic avian influenza (HPAI) A (H7N9) virus in 2 commercial poultry flocks in Tennessee. Full genome sequence analysis indicated that all eight gene segments of the virus were of North American wild bird lineage and genetically distinct from the lineage of influenza A (H7N9) viruses infecting poultry and humans in China since 2013. The outbreak investigation revealed that a related North American low-pathogenicity avian influenza A (H7N9) was circulating in poultry prior to the detection of the HPAI A (H7N9). There were no reports of human cases associated with this virus.

Centers for Disease Control Prevention. *Summary of Influenza Risk Assessment Tool (IRAT) Results*. https://www.cdc.gov/flu/pandemic-resources/monitoring/irat-virus-summaries.htm [Accessed 20

DIAGNOSIS AND LABORATORY INVESTIGATION (SEE CHAPTER 17 FOR ADDITIONAL DETAILS)

Case definitions for avian influenza A virus infection is important to standardize patient characteristics and help classify potential individuals as confirmed, probable, and cases under investigation.[43] Clinical presentation of avian influenza A virus infections in humans (especially avian influenza A H5N1 and H7N9) range from mild to severe, with signs and symptoms described earlier.[16,43]

Laboratory confirmation is a critical investigation for early diagnosis of avian influenza A virus infection. Several methods have been established for avian influenza A virus direct detection from patients' clinical specimens, including swabs from the upper respiratory tract (nose or throat) and lower respiratory tract specimens. Testing is more accurate when the swab is collected during the first few days of illness. Special precautions for collecting and transferring specimens to testing laboratories vary for different counties, and local guidance should be reviewed and followed. Nucleic acid testing, antigen testing, and viral cultures and isolations must be performed in specialized reference laboratories with the appropriate biosafety facilities.[20,43,44]

The microneutralization assay is a serological test that is highly sensitive and specific for detecting viral-specific neutralizing antibodies to influenza A viruses in human and animal sera, potentially including the detection of human antibodies to avian subtypes.[19,44]

A rise in antibody titers greater than or equal to four-fold between acute-phase and convalescent-phase sera may establish the diagnosis of a recent influenza infection. These tests can also be used in epidemiological studies to assess vaccine immunity and to detect asymptomatic infection. The detection of influenza antibodies as a testing strategy has several advantages. First, it primarily detects antibodies to the influenza viral HA protein and thus can identify functional strain-specific antibodies in human and animal sera. Second, since infectious viruses are used to develop the assay, new assays can be developed quickly for specific viruses once the emergence of a novel subtype is recognized. The technique, however, can be time-consuming. For example, viral cell culture is needed to determine the inhibition of cytopathogenic effect formation in MDCK cell culture, and the turnaround time for this study may exceed 3–4 weeks.[19,44,45] A newer technique, microneutralization assay using microtiter plates in combination with an ELISA to detect virus-infected cells, can yield results within 2 days.[45]

Interpretation of low-level titers in such assays is an area of active research. For example, current understanding suggests that the detection of anti-H5 micro-NT titers of <1: 80 is a false-positive result.[46] The question remains whether demonstrating microneutralization assays of low-titer antibodies against avian influenza virus A (H5N1) in an endemic area in patients with plausible poultry, environmental, or human exposure to H5N1 is indicative of infection. Apisarnthanarak et al.[47] detected low anti-H5 micro-NT titers in six intensive care unit patients with severe community-acquired pneumonia (a total of 242 patients). Prior exposure to poultry was the sole independent risk factor for these low-titer antibodies (adjusted OR 42.41; 95% CI 22.45–64.51; $P<0.001$). As the result may indicate prior H5N1 exposure and not acute viral infection, additional studies are needed to enhance our understanding of anti-H5 seroprevalence and the significance of low anti-H5 micro-NT titers in healthy and ill populations.

Risk Factors and Evidence of Infection in HCPs

To date, there are two reports of avian influenza transmission to patients,[1,2,37,38] and no data showing efficient transmission to high-risk groups such as HCPs (Table 3). Apisarnthanarak et al.[30] reported no evidence of seroconversion among 25 HCPs who were exposed to a patient with H5N1 virus infection at a Thai tertiary care hospital. None of the 141 contacts of the patients in the two hospital clusters described earlier developed A (H7N9) infection.[37,38] These data suggest low risks for occupational acquisition of A (H5N1) virus infection among HCPs. However, given the high case fatality rate in humans (more than 50%), the types of aerosol-generating procedures done in hospitals, the high burden of viruses secreted by ill patients, and the multiple potential infected body fluids, the risks for transmission to HCPs merit further investigation.[1,2,14,15]

INFECTION PREVENTION AND CONTROL STRATEGIES (SEE CHAPTER 25 FOR ADDITIONAL DETAILS)

The WHO encourages all countries to continue ongoing national health preparedness activities, of which avian influenza surveillance is essential. This includes surveillance for severe acute respiratory

TABLE 3
Number of Total Cases and HCP/Patient Affected Cases of Avian Influenza; Risk Factors and Infection Prevention and Control Recommendations

Emerging Diseases	Year and Country of the First Outbreak	Number of Total Cases	Number of Deaths (% of Total cases)	Number of HCPs/Patient Transmissions (% of Total Cases)	Risks of Infection to HCPs	Infection Prevention and Control Recommendations
AVIAN INFLUENZA A						
- H5N1	1997 and 2003, Hong Kong	868[a]	457[a] (53%)	None	- HCPs are at low occupational risk for acquisition of H5N1 infection[c]	- Use standard/ contact/droplet precautions with eye protection (some countries may recommend the use of respirators)
- H7N9	2013, China	1568[b]	616[b] (39%)	None/2 (50%)	- Potential for pandemic influenza outbreak - Human-to-human transmission of avian influenza A occurred to 2 patients in separate exposures. The patients shared space on the same ward. Other risk factors were not identified. In one cluster, both the infector and infectee were immunocompromised. Otherwise, transmission has occurred only via intimate contact without the use of barrier, and in household clusters.	- Use airborne precautions and isolation room, especially with aerosol-generating procedures. - Follow pandemic avian influenza preparedness plans, especially in developing countries - Employ strategies to rapidly create temporary isolation facilities, restrict access in HCPs, and screen and identify cases early using ID specialists - Monitor infection prevention & control practices - Monitor HCPs and exclude them from work 7 days (H5N1), and 10 days (H7N9) after exposure - Perform active disease surveillance for other cases with active screening and serology or PCR testing. - Follow laboratory standards when handling patient specimens - Use adjuvanted vaccine to prevent avian influenza A (H5N1) in people with high-risk exposures and in pandemic if indicated. - H7N9 vaccination has been developed, and its use is supported by WHO and CDC.

Note: *HCPs*, healthcare personnel; *N/A*, not available; *ID*, infectious disease; *WHO*, World Health Organization; *CDC*, Center of Diseases and Control.
[a]Laboratory-confirmed cases of human infection with avian influenza A (H5N1) as of January 26, 2023.
[b]Laboratory-confirmed cases of human infection with avian influenza A (H7N9) in China as of March 2, 2023.

illnesses with reporting of human infections.[41,43,44] Surveillance should include close monitoring for evidence of human-to-human transmission, nosocomial transmission, or improved "fitness" in humans that could signal pandemic potential.[7,14,15,48] Key strategies for control of avian influenza outbreaks include the ability to rapidly respond and be flexible in the response as data emerge. National and regional health authorities and veterinary experts can facilitate case finding, identify potential sources, implement mitigation strategies, educate communities, and deploy resources, including HCPs if needed.[14,15,48–50] In developing countries, pandemic avian influenza preparedness plans should align with their resources and the various potential settings. Planning for healthcare facilities includes infectious diseases and infection prevention and control specialists along with healthcare administrative support, specialists to rapidly create temporary isolation facilities, policies, and systems to follow and restrict exposed HCPs, and protocols for triage, screening, testing, isolation, and treatment. Infection prevention and control specialists can screen and identify cases early, provide for continuous monitoring to ensure adherence to optimal infection-control practices, and support regular feedback of protocol compliance data to HCPs.[7,49,50] To prevent nosocomial transmission of avian influenza to HCPs and patients, planning for a case and the potential for a pandemic from an avian influenza A strain should be considered and include heightened protective measures (Fig. 2).[1,2,41,43,44]

Finally, vaccine research and development are a key component to facilitate mitigation and prevention. Avian influenza A vaccines have been developed to prevent transmission of influenza in poultry and humans, especially during a pandemic.[43] Currently, there are several avian influenza A vaccines (Northern and Southern hemispheres: H5N1, H5 non-A [H5N1], H7, H7N9, H9N2, H3N2, H1) circulating in the endemic areas and beyond. A vaccine for avian influenza A, H3N8 (Southern hemisphere), is being developed with the CDC.[51]

Treatment

As with seasonal influenza viruses, most influenza A (H7N9) and A (H5N1) viruses are susceptible to the neuraminidase inhibitors (oseltamivir, peramivir, and zanamivir) but resistant to the adamantanes (amantadine and rimantadine).[52] Therefore, amantadine and rimantadine are not recommended for the treatment of novel avian influenza A virus infections. Among patients hospitalized with avian influenza A (H5N1) virus infections, observational studies suggest that early treatment reduces disease severity and mortality.[52,53] Clinical benefits are greatest when antiviral treatment is administered early, especially within 48 h of influenza illness onset. Although earlier antiviral treatment results in greater clinical benefit, observational studies support the use of antiviral agents in hospitalized patients even if started more than 48 h after symptom onset, including in critically ill patients.[53–56] Neuraminidase inhibitor treatment with oseltamivir, peramivir, and zanamivir has been used for severely ill persons infected with A (H7N9) viruses, but the effectiveness remains undetermined in severe disease.[57,58] Because antiviral resistance has developed in Asian H5N1 and H7N9 influenza viruses isolated from some human cases, monitoring for antiviral resistance among these viruses is crucial and ongoing.[52]

Some previous studies have reported the benefit of using higher oseltamivir doses (150 mg twice daily) in patients with uncomplicated influenza. Others, however, have found no significant improvement in clinical or virological outcomes compared with a standard dose (75 mg twice daily). Despite a lack of definite evidence, several authorities have suggested the use of double-dose oseltamivir for severe influenza.[52,56] In the largest randomized treatment trial of severe avian influenza A in 326 patients at 13 Indonesian, Singaporean, Thai, and Vietnamese hospitals, there was no clinical or virological benefit to doubling the dose of oseltamivir compared to standard dosing.[59] The study enrolled a heterogeneous population that included children, and 5.2% of the patients were infected with avian H5N1 virus. A subgroup analysis that controlled for patient age, virus type and subtype, and time to treatment did not demonstrate additional virological efficacy with high-dose oseltamivir in any subgroup.[59]

Future Research

Influenza transmission dynamics is another active area of active research, and previous studies show limited aerosol transmission of avian influenza A strains.[60,61] Yan J et al.[61] tested for infectious virus in various respiratory samples from 142 volunteers with confirmed influenza infection during the 2012–2013 flu season. They found influenza virus was present in 89% of the nasopharyngeal (NP) samples and 39% of fine aerosol samples. Geometric mean RNA copy numbers for fine and coarse aerosol samples

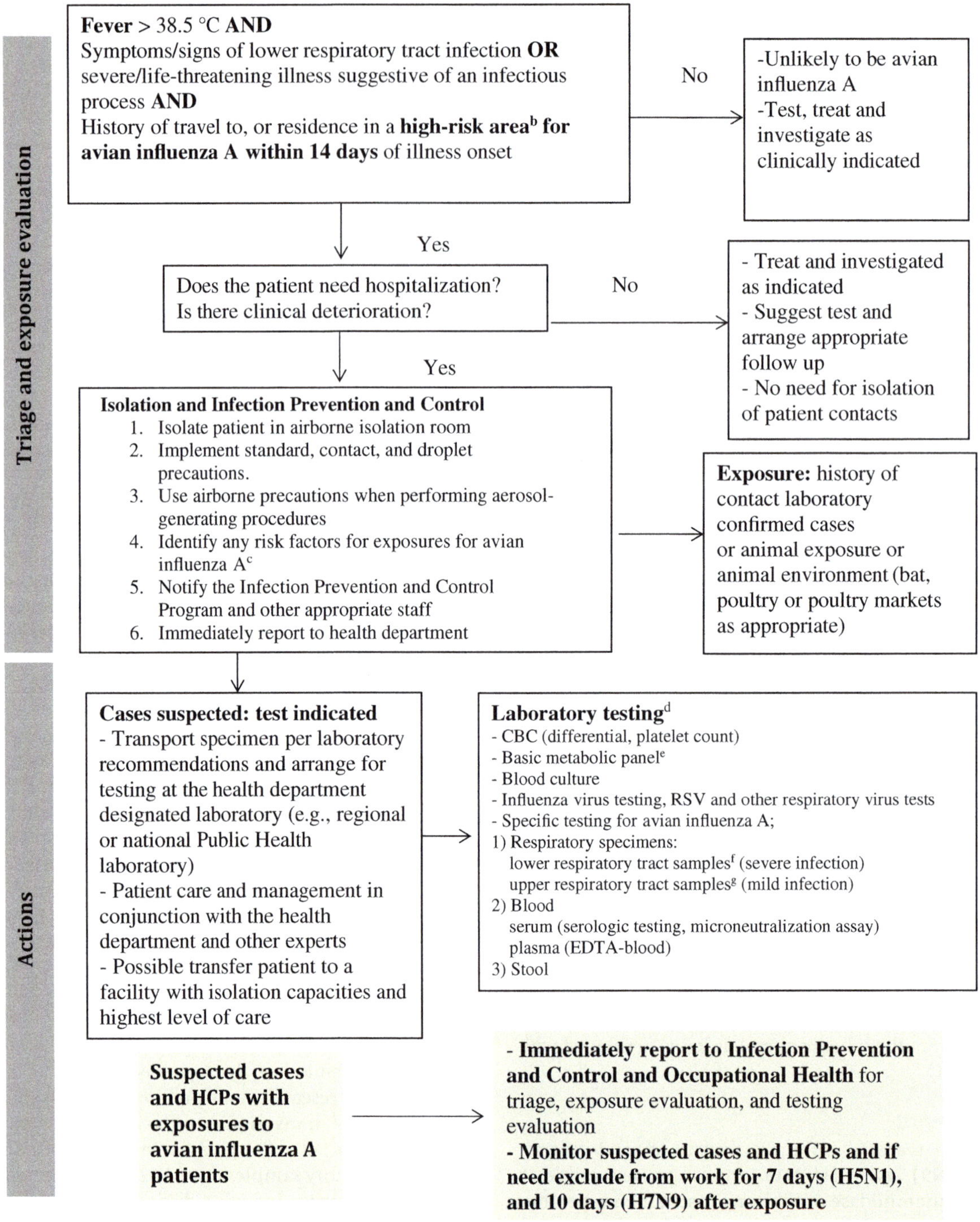

FIG. 2 See Figure legend on opposite page.

(Continued)

were 3.8×104 and 1.2×104 per 30 min, respectively, compared with 8.2×10^8 per NP swab. The amount of viral shedding in fine aerosol samples declined with the number of days after symptom onset and was increased in males and with coughing, although shedding did occur without coughing or sneezing. Further study on aerosol transmission of avian influenza A virus transmission will be critical to refining current infection prevention and control practices and policies.

Lastly, given the emergence of drug-resistant influenza A strains, further research on novel antiviral treatment is ongoing. One potential antiviral target is the type II transmembrane serine proteases (TTSPs). TTSPs are activated via proteolytic cleavage of influenza hemagglutinin in a wide range of influenza virus subtypes, including avian influenza viruses, both in vitro and in vivo. Consequently, TTSP inhibition is a potential novel broad-spectrum antiviral against various influenza virus subtypes.[62] Moreover, an anti-neuraminidase monoclonal antibody (NA mAb) has potential uses in drug-resistant A (H7N9) virus. When delivered intraperitoneally and intranasal administration to mice within 24 h of infection, it was 100% protective against mortality.[63]

SUMMARY

In the few decades since its emergence, avian influenza A has had an enormous impact on the poultry industry and human and animal medical and public health practices globally. Though primarily a disease of poultry and other avian species, these viruses have now spread to mammals and can be transmitted to humans in contact with these poultry and the environment. With the recent increases in poultry outbreaks and the spread of these viruses into new geographic areas, the potential risk of these viruses becoming more fit exists. While the overall public health risk from the currently recognized avian influenza viruses has not changed, given the lack of sustained human-to-human transmission of these viruses, avian influenza infection when it occurs in humans has a high mortality rate. That said, the recent rapid spread of H5N1 and the human cases that have emerged in Russia, the United Kingdom, and Nigeria signal a potential threat to humans. Thus, international collaboration to monitor changing genetics and epidemiology in wild and domestic avian species, mammals and humans is critical. In addition to rapidly transmitting information about emerging avian viruses, investigating for evidence of transmission, implementing infection prevention and control measures in healthcare, and implementing prevention strategies in poultry populations remain critical to have appropriate situational awareness and to proactively respond to an imminent threat. If an outbreak were to occur, it is critical to understand viral characteristics and the mechanisms of transmission, the options for prophylaxis, treatment, vaccination, and other countermeasures to prevent the ongoing spread and impact public safety.

CONFLICT OF INTEREST

None.

FIG. 2, CONT'D Algorithm for evaluation of and infection prevention and control recommendations for suspected avian influenza cases, and HCPs exposure to avian influenza A infected patients. Note: HCPs, healthcare personnel; RSV, respiratory syncytial virus; rRT-PCR, real-time reverse transcription polymerase chain reaction. [b]High-risk area for avian influenza A.[16,43,44] [c]Risk of exposures for avian influenza A.[16,43,44] [d]Laboratory testing for suspected patients with avian influenza A.[43,44] [e]Sodium, potassium, chloride, bicarbonate, calcium, blood urea nitrogen, creatinine, and glucose concentrations. [f] Broncheoalveolar lavage, tracheal aspirate, pleural fluid. [g]Nasopharyngeal and oropharyngeal swabs.(Adapted from World Health Organization. *Influenza at the Human-Animal Interface*, summary and assessment, 6 January 2023 to 26 January 2023. https://www.who.int/publications/m/item/influenza-at-the-human-animal-interface-summary-and-assessment-26-jan-2023 [Accessed 19 February 2023]; World Health Organization. *Cumulative Number of Confirmed Human Cases for Avian Influenza A (H5N1) Reported to WHO, 2003-2023*. https://www.who.int/publications/m/item/cumulative-number-of-confirmed-human-cases-for-avian-influenza-a(h5n1)-reported-to-who-2003-2022-5-jan-2023 [Accessed 19 February 2023]; Centers for Disease Control and Prevention. *Case Definitions for Investigations of Human Infection with Avian Influenza Viruses in the United States.* https://www.cdc.gov/flu/avianflu/case-definitions.html?CDC_AA_refVal=https%3A%2F%2Fwww.cdc.gov%2Fflu%2Favianflu%2Fhpai%2Fcase-definitions.htm [Accessed 19 February 2023]; Centers for Disease Control and Prevention. *Interim Guidance on Testing and Specimen Collection for Patients with Suspected Infection with Novel Influenza A Viruses Associated with the Potential to Cause Severe Disease in Humans*. https://www.cdc.gov/flu/avianflu/severe-potential.htm [Accessed 19 February 2023].)

REFERENCES

1. World Health Organization. Influenza at the Human-Animal Interface, Summary and Assessment, 6 January 2023 to 26 January 2023. https://www.who.int/publications/m/item/influenza-at-the-human-animal-interface-summary-and-assessment-26-jan-2023. Accessed 19 February 2023.
2. World Health Organization. Cumulative Number of Confirmed Human Cases for Avian Influenza A (H5N1) Reported to WHO, 2003–2023; 2023. https://www.who.int/publications/m/item/cumulative-number-of-confirmed-human-cases-for-avian-influenza-a(h5n1)-reported-to-who-2003-2022-5-jan-2023. Accessed 19 February 2023.
3. World Health Organization. H5N1 Highly Pathogenic Avian Influenza: Timeline of Major Events; 2014. 4 December http://www.who.int/influenza/human_animal_interface/H5N1_avian_influenza_update20141204.pdf?ua=1. Accessed 19 February 2023.
4. Gao HN, Lu HZ, Cao B, et al. Clinical findings in 111 cases of influenza a (H7N9) virus infection. *N Engl J Med.* 2013;368:2277–2285.
5. Li Q, Zhou L, Zhou M, et al. Epidemiology of human infections with avian influenza a(H7N9) virus in China. *N Engl J Med.* 2014;370:520–532.
6. Wang Y. The H7N9 influenza virus in China- -changes since SARS. *N Engl J Med.* 2013;368:2348–2349.
7. Suwantarat N, Apisarnthanarak A. Risks to healthcare workers with emerging diseases: lessons from MERS-CoV, Ebola, SARS, and avian flu. *Curr Opin Infect Dis.* 2015;28(4):349–361.
8. Sarikaya O1, Erbaydar T. Avian influenza outbreak in Turkey through health personnel's views: a qualitative study. *BMC Public Health.* 2007;7:330.
9. Kandun IN, Wibisono H, Sedyaningsih ER, et al. Three Indonesian clusters of H5N1 virus infection in 2005. *N Engl J Med.* 2006;355:2186–2194.
10. Ungchusak K, Auewarakul P, Dowell SF, et al. Probable person-to-person transmission of avian influenza a (H5N1). *N Engl J Med.* 2005;352:333–340.
11. Li YT, Linster M, Mendenhall IH, Su YCF, Smith GJD. Avian influenza viruses in humans: lessons from past outbreaks. *Br Med Bull.* 2019;132(1):81–95. https://doi.org/10.1093/bmb/ldz036.
12. World Health Organization. Avian Influenza Weekly Update Number 885; 2023. 3 March https://www.who.int/docs/default-source/wpro- - -documents/emergency/surveillance/avian-influenza/ai_20230224.pdf?sfvrsn=5f006f99_111. Accessed 19 March 2023.
13. Agüero M, Monne I, Sánchez A, et al. Highly pathogenic avian influenza a(H5N1) virus infection in farmed minks, Spain, October 2022. *Euro Surveill.* 2023;28(3):2300001.
14. Bartlett JG. Planning for avian influenza. *Ann Intern Med.* 2006;145:141–144.
15. Martinello RA. Preparing for avian influenza. *Curr Opin Pediatr.* 2007;19:64–70.
16. World Health Organization. Interim Guidance for Infection Control Within Healthcare Settings When Caring for Confirmed Cases, Probable Cases, and Cases Under Investigation for Infection with Novel Influenza A Viruses Associated with Severe Disease. http://www.cdc.gov/flu/avianflu/h7n9-infection-control.htm. Accessed 19 March 2023.
17. European Centre for Disease Prevention and Control. Country Preparedness Plans on Zoonotic Influenza. https://www.ecdc.europa.eu/en/avian-influenza-humans/country-preparedness-plans-avian-influenza-humans. Accessed 20 March 2023.
18. Uyeki TM. Human infection with highly pathogenic avian influenza A (H5N1) virus: review of clinical issues. *Clin Infect Dis.* 2009;49(2):279–290.
19. Atmar RT, Linstrom SE. Influenza viruses. In: Jorgensen JH, Pfaller MA, eds. *Manual of Clinical Microbiology.* vol. 2. 11th ed. Washington, DC: ASM Press; 2015:1470–1486.
20. Centers for Disease Control and Prevention. *Influenza A Viruses.* https://www.cdc.gov/flu/avianflu/influenza-a-virus-subtypes.htm [Accessed 19 February 2023].
21. Wille M, Barr IG. Resurgence of avian influenza virus. *Science.* 2022;376:459–460.
22. World Health Organization. Avian Influenza A(H3N8) - China https://www.who.int/emergencies/disease-outbreak-news/item/2023-DON456 [Accessed 14 April 2023].
23. Tweed SA, Skowronski DM, David ST, et al. Human illness from avian influenza H7N3, British Columbia. *Emerg Infect Dis.* 2004;10(12):2196–2199.
24. To KK, Tsang AK, Chan JF, Cheng VC, Chen H, Yuen KY. Emergence in China of human disease due to avian influenza A(H10N8)- -cause for concern? *J Infect.* 2014;68(3):205–215.
25. Yang R, Sun H, Gao F, et al. Human infection of avian influenza a H3N8 virus and the viral origins: a descriptive study. *Lancet Microbe.* 2022;3(11):e824–e834.
26. Zhou J, Chen Y, Shao Z, et al. Continuing evolution and transmission of avian influenza a(H3N8) viruses is a potential threat to public health. *J Infect.* 2023;86(2):154–225.
27. Centers for Disease Control Prevention. *Summary of Influenza Risk Assessment Tool (IRAT) Results.* https://www.cdc.gov/flu/pandemic-resources/monitoring/irat-virus-summaries.htm [Accessed 20 March 2023].
28. Chan PK. Outbreak of avian influenza a (H5N1) virus infection in Hong Kong in 1997. *Clin Infect Dis.* 2002;34(Suppl 2):S58–S64.
29. Hien TT, de Jong M, Farrar J. Avian influenza — a challenge to global health care structures. *N Engl J Med.* 2004;351:2363–2365.
30. Apisarnthanarak A, Erb S, Stephenson I, et al. Seroprevalence of anti-H5 antibody among Thai health care workers after exposure to avian influenza (H5N1) in a tertiary care center. *Clin Infect Dis.* 2005;40:e16–e18.
31. Yang Y, Zhong H, Song T, et al. Epidemiological and clinical characteristics of humans with avian influenza a (H7N9) infection in Guangdong, China, 2013–2017. *Int J Infect Dis.* 2017;65:148–155.

32. Guan Y, Shortridge KF, Krauss S, Webster RG. Molecular characterization of H9N2 influenza viruses: were they the donors of the "internal" genes of H5N1 viruses in Hong Kong? *Proc Natl Acad Sci.* 1999;96:9363–9367.
33. World Health Organization. Influenza (Avian and Other Zoonotic) https://www.who.int/news-room/fact-sheets/detail/influenza-(avian-and-other-zoonotic) [Accessed 19 March 2023].
34. Um S, Siegers JY, Sar B, et al. Human infection with avian influenza a(H9N2) virus, Cambodia, February 2021. *Emerg Infect Dis.* 2021;27(10):2742–2745.
35. Song W, Qin K. Human-infecting influenza a (H9N2) virus: a forgotten potential pandemic strain? *Zoonoses Public Health.* 2020;67(3):203–212.
36. Quan C, Wang Q, Zhang J, et al. Avian influenza a viruses among occupationally exposed populations, China, 2014-2016. *Emerg Infect Dis.* 2019;25(12):2215–2225.
37. Chen H, Liu S, Liu J, et al. Nosocomial co-transmission of avian influenza A(H7N9) and A(H1N1)pdm2009 viruses between 2 patients with hematologic disorders. *Emerg Infect Dis.* 2016;22(4):598–607.
38. Fang CF, Ma MJ, Zhan BD, et al. Nosocomial transmission of avian influenza a (H7N9) virus in China: epidemiological investigation. *BMJ.* 2015;351, h5765.
39. Reuters. Bird Flu Alarm Drives World Towards Once-Shunned Vaccines https://www.reuters.com/business/healthcare-pharmaceuticals/bird-flu-alarm-drives-world-towards-once-shunned-vaccines-2023-02-17/ [Accessed 19 March 2023].
40. Wired. The Bird Flu Outbreak Has Taken an Ominous Turn; 2023:32–33. https://www.wired.com/story/the-bird-flu-outbreak-has-taken-an-ominous-turn/. Accessed 19 March 2023.
41. Butt KM, Smith GJ, Chen H, et al. Human infection with an avian H9N2 influenza a virus in Hong Kong in 2003. *J Clin Microbiol.* 2005;43(11):5760–5767.
42. Khan SU, Anderson BD, Heil GL, Liang S, Gray GC. A systematic review and Meta-analysis of the Seroprevalence of influenza a(H9N2) infection among humans. *J Infect Dis.* 2015;212(4):562–569.
43. Centers for Disease Control and Prevention. *Case Definitions for Investigations of Human Infection with Avian Influenza Viruses in the United States* https://www.cdc.gov/flu/avianflu/case-definitions.html?CDC_AA_refVal=https%3A%2F%2Fwww.cdc.gov%2Fflu%2Favianflu%2Fhpai%2Fcase-definitions.htm [Accessed 19 February 2023].
44. Centers for Disease Control and Prevention. *Interim Guidance on Testing and Specimen Collection for Patients with Suspected Infection with Novel Influenza A Viruses Associated with the Potential to Cause Severe Disease in Humans.* https://www.cdc.gov/flu/avianflu/severe-potential.htm [Accessed 19 February 2023].
45. World Health Organization. *Serological Diagnosis of Influenza by Microneutralization Assay.* https://www.who.int/publications/i/item/serological-diagnosis-of-influenza-by-microneutralization-assay [Accessed 19 February 2023].
46. Rowe T, Abernathy RA, Hu-Primmer J, et al. Detection of antibody to avian influenza a (H5N1) virus in human serum by using a combination of serologic assays. *J Clin Microbiol.* 1999;37:937–943.
47. Apisarnthanarak A, Puthavathana P, Mundy LM. Detection by microneutralization of antibodies against avian influenza virus in an endemic avian influenza region. *Clin Microbiol Infect.* 2010;16(9):1354–1357.
48. Manabe T, Pham TP, Kudo K, et al. Impact of education and network for avian influenza H5N1 in human: knowledge, clinical practice, and motivation on medical providers in Vietnam. *PloS One.* 2012;7, e30384.
49. Apisarnthanarak A, Warren DK, Fraser VJ. Issues relevant to the adoption and modification of hospital infection-control recommendations for avian influenza (H5N1 infection) in developing countries. *Clin Infect Dis.* 2007;45:1338–1342.
50. Apisarnthanarak A, Mundy LM. Infection control for emerging infectious diseases in developing countries and resource-limited settings. *Infect Control Hosp Epidemiol.* 2006;27:885–887.
51. World Health Organization. Zoonotic Influenza: Candidate Vaccine Viruses and Potency Testing Reagents. https://www.who.int/teams/global-influenza-programme/vaccines/who-recommendations/zoonotic-influenza-viruses-and-candidate-vaccine-viruses [Accessed 19 February 2023].
52. Centers for Disease Control and Prevention. *Interim Guidance on the Use of Antiviral Medications for Treatment of Human Infections with Novel Influenza A Viruses Associated with Severe Human Diseases* https://www.cdc.gov/flu/avianflu/novel-av-treatment-guidance.htm [Accessed 19 March 2023].
53. Adisasmito W, Chan PK, Lee N, et al. Effectiveness of antiviral treatment in human influenza A(H5N1) infections: analysis of a Global Patient Registry. *J Infect Dis.* 2010;202(8):1154–1160.
54. McGeer A, Green KA, Plevneshi A, et al. Antiviral therapy and outcomes of influenza requiring hospitalization in Ontario, Canada. *Clin Infect Dis.* 2007;45(12):1568–1575.
55. Lee N, Choi KW, Chan PK, et al. Outcomes of adults hospitalized with severe influenza. *Thorax.* 2010;65(6):510–515.
56. Lee N, Cockram CS, Chan PK, Hui DS, Choi KW, Sung JJ. Antiviral treatment for patients hospitalized with severe influenza infection may affect clinical outcomes. *Clin Infect Dis.* 2008;46(8):1323–1324.
57. Hu Y, Lu S, Song Z, et al. Association between adverse clinical outcome in human disease caused by novel influenza a H7N9 virus and sustained viral shedding and emergence of antiviral resistance. *Lancet.* 2013;381(9885):2273–2279.
58. Ho PL, Sin WC, Chan JF, Cheng VC, Chan KH. Severe influenza A H7N9 pneumonia with rapid virological response to intravenous zanamivir. *European Resp J.* 2014;44(2):535–537.

59. Southeast Asia Infectious Disease Clinical Research Network. Effect of double dose oseltamivir on clinical and virological outcomes in children and adults admitted to hospital with severe influenza: double blind randomized controlled trial. *BMJ*. 2013;346:3039.
60. Xu L, Bao L, Deng W, et al. Novel avian-origin human influenza a(H7N9) can be transmitted between ferrets via respiratory droplets. *J Infect Dis*. 2014;209(4):551–556. Available from: doi.org/10.1093/infdis/jit474.
61. Yan J, Grantham M, Pantelic J, et al. Infectious virus in exhaled breath of symptomatic seasonal influenza cases from a college community. *Proc Natl Acad Sci*. 2018;115(5):1081–1086.
62. Shin WJ, Seong BL. Type II transmembrane serine proteases as potential target for anti-influenza drug discovery. *Expert Opin Drug Discovery*. 2017;12(11):1139–1152.
63. Wilson JR, Belser JA, DaSilva J, et al. An influenza a virus (H7N9) anti-neuraminidase monoclonal antibody protects mice from morbidity without interfering with the development of protective immunity to subsequent homologous challenge. *Virology*. 2017;511:214–221.

CHAPTER 10

Severe Acute Respiratory Syndrome (SARS)

BRENDA ANG[a] • LIN-FA WANG[b] • DANIELLE E ANDERSON[b]
[a]Department of Infectious Diseases, Tan Tock Seng Hospital, Singapore • [b]Programme in Emerging Infectious Diseases, Duke-NUS Medical School, Singapore

HISTORY AND BACKGROUND

Before 2003, coronaviruses were thought to cause mild respiratory infections in adults and children. Four human coronaviruses (HCoV-229E, HCoV-NL63, HCoV-HKU1, and HCoV-OC43) are endemic and, in addition to causing the common cold in adults, are now known to cause more severe disease in the very young, the elderly, and the immunosuppressed. In late 2002, a mysterious and new infection emerged that ultimately was found to be due to a novel coronavirus. As reports and data were gathered, its severity was evident, and on March 12, 2003, the World Health Organization (WHO) issued a global alert describing the severe cases of atypical pneumonia. They noted the dramatic transmission rates in healthcare settings. In a remarkable scientific feat by the end of March 2003, a novel 2b beta coronavirus was confirmed as the causative agent responsive for the SARS infections. Its genome sequence was not related to previously identified human coronaviruses.

China

In November 2002, cases of highly contagious and severe atypical pneumonia were described in the Guangdong province of southern China, some of which were reported in ProMED mail alerts. The illness was more prevalent among healthcare personnel (HCP) and their family members, and those who developed severe disease, pneumonia, and respiratory failure commonly had a rapidly fatal course. The health authorities in the province initially ascribed these infections, which looked like atypical pneumonias, to chlamydia, yet concern increased among the public around the mysterious illness, which resulted in rapid deterioration and death.[1] By February 14, 2003, 305 cases of which 105 (34.4%) occurred in HCPs, and five deaths due to an unknown respiratory illness had been reported to the WHO.[2]

Only much later did retrospective analysis unravel the outbreak's origins.[3] The first wave began with the index case from Foshan, a city 24 km from Guangzhou, reported on November 16, 2002. He infected his wife, two sisters, and seven hospital staff who had participated in his care. The second case was a chef who worked in a restaurant in Shenzhen and had regular contact with wild game used for meals he prepared. Lookback and case finding identified cases of "severe disease-causing atypical pneumonia" in five cities surrounding Guangzhou between November and December 2002. The second wave began in January 2003 when ill patients with severe pneumonias were transferred to major cities of Guangdong province for access to facilities with more sophisticated medical care.

The ability for a contagious respiratory disease to spread through a single individual, the impact of air travel in facilitating transmission, and the dramatic ability for transmission to amplify in healthcare settings became the stark lessons learned as SARS spread internationally throughout Asia, North and South America, and Europe. This outbreak reportedly cost the Asian economies between $11 and $18 billion with a loss of up to 2% of their gross national product.[4,5] International travel fell between 50% and 70%.[6]

Hong Kong

On February 21, 2003, a week after the report to the WHO, a 65-year-old physician from Guangdong who cared for patients with atypical pneumonia checked into the 9th floor of Hotel M in Hong Kong. Upon arrival at the hotel, he was symptomatic. The doctor was admitted to Kwong Wah Hospital with pneumonia and transferred to an ICU, where he subsequently died on

Viral Outbreaks, Biosecurity, and Preparing for Mass Casualty Infectious Diseases Events
https://doi.org/10.1016/B978-0-323-54841-0.00011-1

March 5. He is considered the index case and unwittingly exposed and infected at least 12 other guests and visitors, many of whom had rooms on the hotel's 9th floor. This led to additional transmission within Hong Kong and rapid worldwide dissemination as these visitors, incubating a highly contagious infection caused by a virus that had not yet been identified, returned to their home countries (Fig. 1).[7]

On March 5, a patient from Hanoi was transferred to the Prince of Wales Hospital, and 5 days later, 18 healthcare personnel (HCP) working on a medical ward reported respiratory symptoms; all had been exposed to the case and admitted on March 5. An investigation revealed that over 50 HCPs had febrile illnesses in the preceding few days, and by March 11th, 23 (46%) of them were admitted and 8 (35%) had developed pneumonia.[8] Overall, the attack rate was 41% with 30/74 (40.5%) individuals developing SARS on one ward alone.[9] Because of poor ventilation, overcrowding, and potentially a "super-spreader," ultimately, 156 individuals with SARS were linked to the index case.[10]

Ultimately in Hong Kong, there were 1755 SARS cases, of which 25% were HCP, and 299 (17%) died. The outbreak in Hong Kong can be divided into three phases. The initial phase involved the index case and transmission within hospitals, especially at and as illustrated by the Prince of Wales Hospital. The second phase began in April, where infections were transmitted

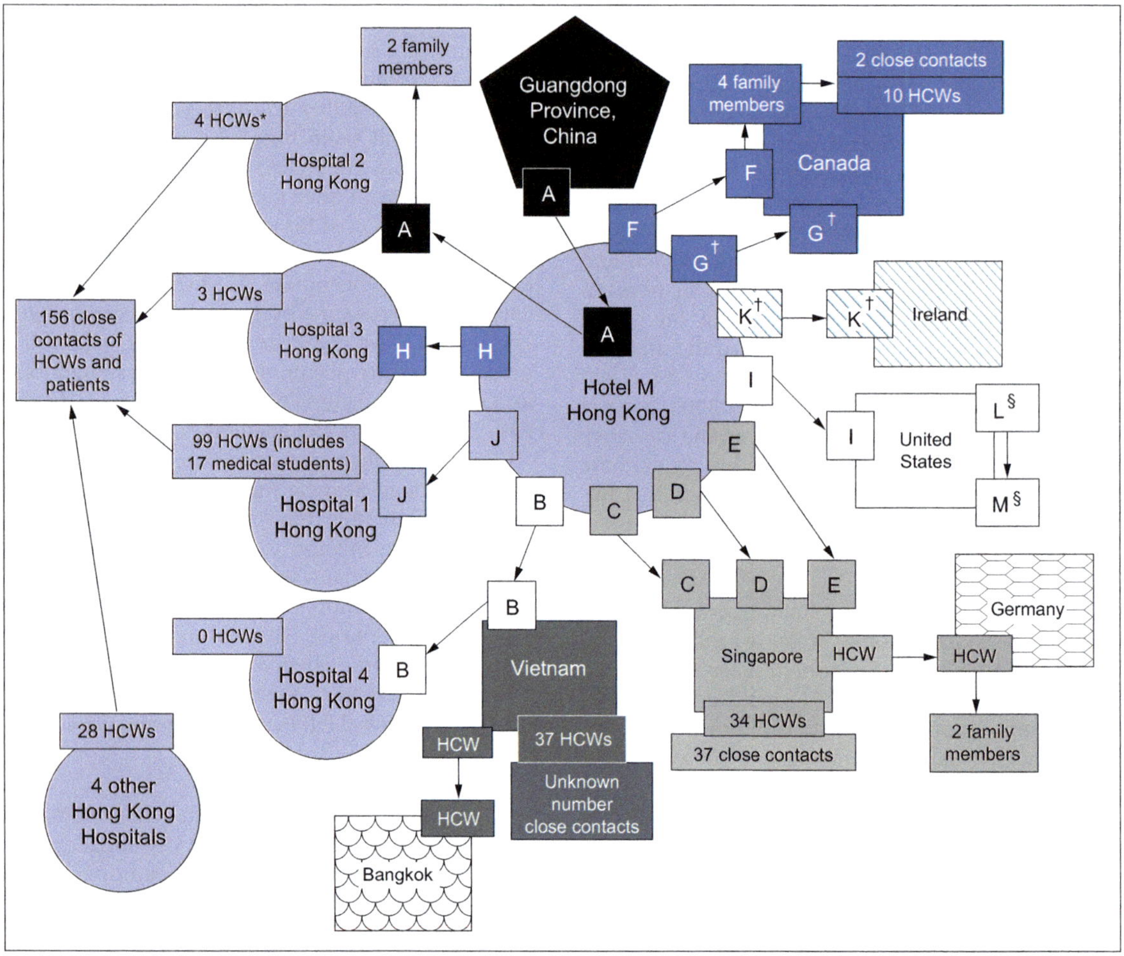

* Health-care workers.
† All guests except G and K stayed on the 9th floor of the hotel. Guest G stayed on the 14th floor, and Guest K stayed on the 11th floor.
§ Guests L and M (spouses) were not at Hotel M during the same time as index Guest A but were at the hotel during the same times as Guests G, H, and I, who were ill during this period.

FIG. 1 Worldwide spread of SARS from Hotel M, Hong Kong, 2003.

into the community by those who were hospitalized or working in healthcare settings. The third phase during May and June was characterized by decreasing cases as public health and hospital-based prevention strategies were implemented.

Two characteristics of these outbreaks are revealed by the early epidemiology in Hong Kong. First is the importance of super-spreading events, and second is the role of intrahospital transmission because patients sought care from multiple facilities or because of transfers among healthcare institutions. The event on the 9th floor of Hotel M characterizes what is now called "super-spreading events," where one individual who is extremely infectious transmits to multiple other individuals, and the number of individuals is higher than what is expected. In other words, not all individuals are equally infectious. Mathematical models have now shown that in Hong Kong, 2.7 cases resulted from every index case when super-spreading events were not included.[10] The second characteristic occurred because patients sought care from multiple facilities or because of transfers among healthcare institutions. For example, the second wave in Guangdong province and the first wave in Hong Kong (Prince of Wales Hospital) occurred after infectious patients were transferred for a higher level of care but were not suspected of being infectious.

Vietnam

The Vietnam French Hospital of Hanoi, a private 60-bed hospital, contacted the Hanoi WHO office on February 28. A patient who had stayed at Hotel M in Hong Kong returned to Hanoi on February 26 and presented with high fever, dry cough, myalgia, and a sore throat, and the clinicians suspected avian influenza A. On March 5, he was medically evacuated to Hong Kong. Within 2 days, approximately 20 of the Vietnam French Hospital staff presented with pneumonia, and some were critically ill, progressing to acute respiratory distress syndrome.[11] Early on 60 cases were recognized of which half were HCPs. Dr. Carlo Urbani, a WHO official, investigated the illness, implemented prevention and control measures, and notified the WHO of the significance of the outbreak under investigation. Working with the Ministry of Health in Vietnam, the French Hospital was temporarily closed, and two wards of the Bach Mai Hospital were set up as isolation units. Dr. Urbani and five other HCPs succumbed to the illness; however, their legacy was Vietnam's open, swift, and decisive response, which led to rapid containment of the outbreak, minimizing economic and reputational damage.

Singapore

On March 1, 2003, a Singaporean woman who also had stayed at Hotel M and was returning from a holiday was admitted to Tan Tock Seng Hospital (TTSH) with atypical pneumonia. Two other Singaporeans who had also stayed at Hotel M were hospitalized on March 2 and 3 at TTSH and the Singapore General Hospital, respectively. On March 6, because the WHO had reported an outbreak in Hanoi, the Singapore Ministry of Health (MOH) instructed hospital staff to isolate any patients returning from Hong Kong with pneumonia or respiratory symptoms. This index Singaporean case transmitted the infection to HCPs, family, and friends. To limit transmission, the MOH declared TTSH the "SARS" hospital on March 22, and all patients with suspected SARS were cohorted there. As part of the process, TTSH had robust lab testing, screening of HCPs and patients, set up isolation wards, cohorted patients, provided HCPs with personal protective equipment (PPE), and monitored HCPs. Patients who did not fulfill a diagnosis of SARS were admitted to other local hospitals. None the less, patients with unrecognized infection or those not suspected to have SARS had already transmitted to other individuals and propagated transmission within hospitals and nursing homes.[12]

A recurring theme emerged in Singapore. Mathematical modeling of the SARS-CoV-1 transmission dynamics demonstrated that 75% of infections in Singapore were attributable to super-spreading events.[10] Among the first 201 cases in Singapore, 81% did not transmit to others, and five individuals infected 10 or more people. Subsequent work demonstrated that delaying hospital admission and isolation by 4 days may have fueled these super-spreading events.[10]

Taiwan

A Taiwanese businessman who had visited Guangdong on February 5 returned to Taipei via Hong Kong. He developed symptoms on February 25, was hospitalized on March 8, and was diagnosed with SARS-CoV-1 on March 14. Between March 14 and 21, Taiwan reported 28 probable SARS cases, which were primarily sporadic among business travelers who were mostly cared for in academic medical centers. Importantly, four cases resulted from secondary transmission (one HCP and three family contacts). The number of probable SARS cases in Taiwan more than tripled to 89 between April 22 and May 1, as an unrecognized SARS case in another hospital exposed multiple staff, other patients, visitors, and HCPs who were not adequately protected.[13] By May 22, 3 weeks later, Taiwan reported multiple SARS clusters within hospitals resulting from the initial case. The importance of nosocomial transmission and intrahospital transmission became increasingly evident with this experience. Taiwan, like other countries, implemented multiple mitigation strategies, including infection prevention and control training, thorough contact tracing and quarantine, and airport and border screening, which were successful in limiting further transmission.

Canada

A Canadian returned to Toronto after visiting Hong Kong and staying at Hotel M. She became ill on February 23 and died on March 5. Her son and four other family members caring for her at home became ill and were admitted to several hospitals in the Toronto area. On March 13, 2003, 1 day after the WHO issued its first global alert about "atypical pneumonia," Toronto Public Health reported Toronto's first case of SARS.[14] Prior to its recognition, transmissions to HCPs, hospital visitors, and patients had occurred and fueled the first phase of the outbreak, which chiefly affected these groups at four hospitals. Among the initial 225 SARS cases identified in this first phase, all but three were epidemiologically linked to the index case. Again, intrahospital transmission characterized the transmission, and SARS spread to 11 (58%) of the acute care facilities in the region.[15] Canada also responded with robust infection prevention and control measures, aggressive case finding, quarantine and isolation, screening in healthcare settings, and testing. As a result, cases decreased, and the WHO removed Toronto from the list of areas with recent local transmission on May 14, 2003, and the Ontario provincial government lifted the public health emergency order on May 17. However, an unsuspected hospitalised SARS case transmitted to patients, visitors, and HCPs and led to a second wave of SARS. Again, this wave was associated with transfers to other hospitals, which was finally controlled with hospital-based active patient surveillance, screening of HCPs and visitors, ongoing isolation and quarantine, and limiting the movement of HCPs. Toronto Public Health implemented mitigation measures dropping the number of cases of SARS in hospitals and households from 20 (13%) in phase one to zero.[15] The second phase of the outbreak was driven by hospital-based exposures with 68 (88%) cases having an exposure to a hospital unit compared to 25 (17%) in the initial phase. Importantly, the impact of education and training was evident by the second wave, as exposures in the ICUs dropped from 13 (9%) during phase one to zero in the second phase. The outbreak in Canada was the largest outside Asia, and its toll was notable. Ultimately, Toronto Public Health investigated 2132 potential SARS cases and 23,103 contacts. Finally, there was a tremendous impact on the healthcare workforce, which manifested in a variety of mental health disorders and post-traumatic stress disorder and resulted in many of the HCPs leaving healthcare.

EPIDEMIOLOGY

Early in its emergence, SARS was unnamed, had no diagnostic criteria, and no diagnostic laboratory tests, leaving HCPs and healthcare facilities using epidemiologic risk factors, exposure information, and symptoms to identify potential cases. Initially, the foremost risk factor in patients with pneumonia was travel to an affected geographic area such as China and Hong Kong. As family members and HCPs became infected, criteria were amended to include contacts of known cases. As is common in outbreaks, the definition for this new syndrome evolved as new information and new epidemiological risk factors were identified.[16]

Retrospective serologic data suggests that the origins of the SARS-CoV-1 virus were an animal source with transmission to humans in wet market settings. Early in the outbreak, one key epidemiologic link was exposure to these animal markets. Additional serologic data linked to SARS-CoV-1 provided support for occupational exposure with animal handlers and masked palm civets. Later, the ultimate reservoir was found to be Chinese horseshoe bats, which carry a SARS-like virus with a high degree of homology to both the isolated human and civet cat SARS viruses. The exact transmission link has not been clarified.

After the initial species jump, SARS-CoV-1 spread primarily through human-to-human transmission. Infected secretions were transmitted through droplets in general but were also opportunistically aerosolized with certain types of medical procedures, including the use of high-flow oxygen, nebulization of medications, and intubation. Hence, transmissions were reported in healthcare facilities, then homes, workplaces, and on public transportation could be explained by these transmission mechanisms. At the beginning of the outbreak, regardless of the region, and prior to implementation of appropriate infection prevention and control procedures, most infections occurred among HCPs, especially nurses, respiratory therapists, and intensive care unit physicians who had extensive patient and patient secretion exposure. In addition, transmission between patients and from patients to visitors occurred. Nosocomial transmission accelerated outbreaks, and in Hong Kong, almost half the reported SARS-CoV-1 cases were acquired in a healthcare setting. In Taiwan and Toronto, 55% and 72% of cases were acquired in healthcare settings.[17] Ultimately, HCPs accounted for 23.1% of all cases, and the ratio of infections in females to males was five to four. Of Singapore's 238 cases, 67.6% were among females, and about half were among those between 25 and 44 years old, with infections in HCPs constituting 40.8% of the total cases.[12]

Initial clusters were primarily in larger acute care hospitals offering higher levels of care, then affecting community hospitals, nursing homes, and eldercare facilities. The later occurred because symptoms were atypical and illness was unrecognized. Spread between household contacts led to secondary household attack rates that ranged from 4.6% in Beijing,[18] 6.2% in Singapore,[19] to 25% in Toronto.[15] The higher attack rate in healthcare settings compared to households may be attributed to patients visiting hospitals in the later phase of illness when they had a higher viral burden, increased coughing, and required more manipulation of the respiratory tract and procedures. Once transmission was understood and PPE was widely used, healthcare case transmission decreased significantly. Likewise, transmission in communities and infection rates decreased as public health implemented enhanced screening, contact tracing, isolation and quarantine, and other mitigation strategies.

In Singapore, for example, community transmission occurred in a large vegetable wholesale market and among a group of friends who gathered for a mahjong game.[12] One of the largest community outbreaks occurred in Hong Kong at the Amoy Gardens, a residential 19-building complex, eventually accounting for 18.8% of total SARS cases.[20] The distribution of affected cases was peculiar. Cases were concentrated in one apartment block with smaller proportions of cases in two neighboring blocks. The source of infection was subsequently ascribed to the sewage system, faulty plumbing, and ventilation. Investigations after the outbreak revealed that reflux of air from the soil pipe into the bathroom through the floor drain could have contained aerosolized droplets of SARS-CoV-1 from contaminated sewage. Contamination from the soil pipe, into the bathroom and bathroom exhaust fan, then vented into the light well between adjacent apartment units, which could be aerosolized into other units and spread infection.[20] Furthermore, wind patterns facilitated transmission to the second and third apartment blocks. More than 10 years after the outbreak, Yu showed that this airborne spread could have accounted for infections in nearby residential complexes that were a distance of 200 m away.[21]

Not surprisingly, transmission was also reported on aircraft, although the risk differed, depending on proximity to an infected person, the duration of exposure, and whether the infected person was symptomatic. Transmission was highest among those within two rows of an infected traveler and on longer flights (over 3.5 h). Olsen reported on a flight carrying 119 passengers, one of whom was symptomatic, which led to laboratory-confirmed SARS-CoV in 16 (13.4%) of these passengers. In addition, six (5%) others likely developed SARS based on symptoms but were not tested.[22] In contrast, no transmission was shown among passengers seated in close proximity to an index patient who had traveled extensively on seven flights.[23] Of note, in this case, the case was only symptomatic while on five flights, and only one of those flights was over 3 h. Furthermore, only a small portion of potential contacts were included.

CLINICAL FEATURES AND PRESENTATION

The time from exposure to symptom onset (incubation period) varied considerably, ranging from 2 to 16 days with a mean incubation period of 4.6 days (95% CI 3.8–5.8).[24,25] This variability reflects differences in the routes of transmission, the extent of and type of exposure, the infectiousness of the infectee and the viral inoculum, and perhaps biases in symptom reporting.[26] In many cases, estimates of the incubation period relied on statistical assumptions because most patients were unaware of when their exposure occurred or what type of exposure they had had. The WHO estimated the maximum incubation period was 10 days.[27]

The mean time from onset of clinical symptoms to hospital admission was between three and 5 days, with longer times earlier in the epidemic.[25] As hospitals moved toward early identification and expended criteria for isolation, the interval between the onset of symptoms and isolation in the hospital was reduced from 6.8 days in the week of March 3, to 2.9 days for the week of March 31, to 1.3 days for the week of April 21.[28]

Initial Symptomology

SARS affected all age groups with a spectrum of illness. Children tended to have mild symptoms, while adolescents and adults presented with mild to severe illness.[29] The most common sign of SARS-CoV-1 infection was fever, defined as a body temperature of >38.0°C (100.4°F), leading the WHO to include fever as a key criterion for suspected or probable SARS-CoV-1 cases.[30] The prodrome is a constellation of influenza-like symptoms, including chills or rigors, myalgias, malaise, headache, and nonproductive cough were other major presenting symptoms, whereas rhinorrhea and sore throat were seen less frequently.[8,25,31] Watery diarrhea was a significant symptom reported among some cases. This symptom was well characterized in the Amoy Gardens outbreak in Hong Kong and tended to occur 2–7 days after symptoms began. Anorexia was reported in the elderly, who may not mount a febrile response. Generally, 7–10 days into symptoms, dyspnea and symptoms of pneumonia develop. Cases presenting with atypical pneumonia rarely had crackles or wheezing heard on auscultation.

Peiris described a triphasic clinical course: Week 1 was characterized by fever and myalgias; Week 2 was associated with recurrence of fever, diarrhea, and oxygen desaturation with worsening radiological findings; and then approximately 20% progressed to the third phase when acute respiratory distress syndrome requiring ventilatory support developed.[32] The peak viral load occurred around the 10th day of illness, which also correlates with the most prominent radiographic changes. The proportion (between 20% and 30%) requiring ICU management was similar in two early case series from Hong Kong and Canada, with about two-thirds of ICU patients requiring mechanical ventilation.[8,25] A high incidence of spontaneous miscarriage, preterm delivery, and intrauterine growth retardation were reported.[33] Perinatal infections were not described.

Laboratory Findings

Diagnosis is primarily based on quantitative RT-PCR tests. The sensitivity depends on the technology used. In general, nasopharyngeal and blood samples are preferred for diagnostic testing although PCR has been on both stool and urine.[32] In addition, antibodies to the SARS-CoV-1 virus (IgG) can be measured. Not surprisingly, SARS-CoV-1-infected patients (most cases) demonstrated absolute lymphopenia and thrombocytopenia.[8,24,34] Progressive lymphopenia was found in the peripheral blood of 153/157 (98%) patients infected with SARS-CoV-1, reaching the lowest point in the second week postinfection. The lymphocyte counts generally returned to normal in the third week, although one-third of the patient's lymphopenia persisted up to 5 weeks postinfection.[35] Interestingly, resolution of lymphopenia and thrombocytosis correlated with recovery. Liver function tests, primarily the transaminases, were abnormal in approximately one-third of patients.

Radiographic Findings

Despite the paucity of lung findings on physical examination, chest radiographs were nonspecific and consistent with findings of viral pneumonia. Chest radiographs could have minimal to diffuse ground-glass opacities and focal consolidations. In severe illness, these would rapidly and progressively involve all lobes and both lung fields, eventually ending with an ARDS picture.[36–38] Computer tomography demonstrated intralobular thickening and ground-glass findings in the peripheral lung fields and the lower lobes.

Atypical Clinical Presentations

Atypical clinical presentations of SARS were reported, and some patients presented with minimal or no fever, or with diarrhea but no pneumonia. Other patients, especially those with comorbid conditions and other infections, already had developed fever and chest infiltrates. Delayed recognition and diagnosis in these patients fostered further transmission with some cases becoming "super-spreaders."[39] As a result of this information, the WHO further revised the case definition in May 2003.[2] While most SARS cases were adults, children were also infected, but their clinical course was much milder with less florid radiological changes and faster disease resolution.[29,40]

Asymptomatic Infection

As noted earlier, there was a spectrum of illnesses reported with a subset of patients who rapidly deteriorated. Concerns lingered about whether infected people could be asymptomatic or mildly symptomatic, and whether they could transmit the virus. In a retrospective study, Leung et al. followed over 1000 close contacts of SARS patients, and only 0.19% demonstrated antibodies to SARS-CoV (immunoglobulin G), supporting that this virus rarely manifested as a subclinical infection.[41]

Mortality

The overall case fatality rate of SARS-CoV at the end of the outbreak was 9.5% but ranged from 0% to 40%. Mortality rates varied by age, with a lower mortality rate observed in people younger than 24 years old and a higher mortality in those above 65 years and those with comorbidities. Mortality rates also differed geographically, where different treatment regimens and availability of ICU facilities impacted outcomes.[27] Mortality was highest in those who were pregnant (25%).[33] No known deaths occurred in children. Factors associated with poor prognosis included advanced age, higher SARS-CoV-1 plasma and nasopharyngeal viral loads, comorbid illnesses including diabetes mellitus and concomitant hepatitis B infection, and certain laboratory findings, including a high LDH, a high neutrophil count, or low CD4 and CD8 on admission.[42]

INFECTION PREVENTION AND CONTROL (SEE CHAPTER 25 FOR MORE DETAIL)

When SARS-CoV emerged, it was known to be causing serious illness, and nothing was known about transmission. It was hypothesized to be transmitted via the respiratory route by direct or indirect contact of the mucosae from infectious respiratory droplets.[43,44] Initial precautions in healthcare facilities focused on the use of PPE, frequent use of hand hygiene, and limiting exposure to potential cases. Simultaneously, there were efforts on case identification, isolation, cohorting of patients, contact tracing, and quarantine of exposed persons. Rapid communication with and training of staff were vital. Prevention strategies evolved as more information was known later.

SARS-CoV-1 was detected in multiple body fluids, which may contribute to its more dramatic transmission in certain settings, such as healthcare. Virus was detected in respiratory secretions, urine, stool, and tears.[4] SARS-CoV-1 could survive in respiratory specimens for more than 7 days at room temperature and up to 3 weeks at 4°C. SARS-CoV survived for 4 days in diarrheal stool samples with an alkaline pH helping explain the outbreak in Amoy Gardens.[45] In addition, using PCR testing, SARS-CoV-1 virus or viral particles were identified in the air of rooms housing patients with SARS and from surfaces including bedside tables, television remote control, and a nursing station refrigerator.[46] Another study demonstrated that approximately a quarter of samples collected in areas housing patients were contaminated with SARS-CoV, and areas with patients who were most infectious had the highest environmental contamination and positivity rates. SARS-CoV survived better on disposable gowns than cotton gowns.[47] Such data supported the infection prevention guidance, which included respiratory protection (mask or respirator), gowns, and gloves with maximized ventilation. WHO generally recommended droplet and contact precautions, while the CDC recommended airborne and contact precautions. Both organizations encouraged respirators and airborne precautions for aerosol-generating procedures. In addition, frequent cleaning of surfaces and hand hygiene were strongly promoted.

Using computation transmission dynamic techniques and multiagent mathematical modeling of the hospital-based outbreak at the Prince of Wales Hospital in Hong Kong, investigators demonstrated that transmission of viruses was predominantly driven by the respiratory route (including airborne route) with the risk of transmission based on location in the room.[9,48] The risk of transmission was greatest (65%) for a patient or HCP working in the same bay as a patient.[9] It decreased to 52% for patients or HCPs in an adjacent bay and was only 18% if a patient or HCP was in a distant bay but on the same hospital ward. In addition, risk was associated with time of exposure, where the risk of transmission was greatest when the patient was considered most infectious.

Within several months of the SARS being recognized by the public health community, additional data from outbreaks and other information emerged that helped refine infection prevention precautions needed to protect patients and HCPs. In Vietnam, hospital A (Vietnam French Hospital, see earlier) with extensive nosocomial SARS-CoV-1 transmission including 28 patients and HCPs was closed to new admissions other than sick hospital workers.[49] Two units of a second hospital B were prepared to receive patients. Staff received infection prevention training, PPE was provided, hand hygiene stations were built, patients were screened, cohorted, and isolated, and access to the units was limited. HCPs wore PPE while caring for the 33 patients who were admitted. Compliance with PPE was monitored. Among the 117 HCPs, no SARS cases were reported.

Subsequent data elucidated the risks of HCPs acquiring SARS. In Hong Kong, 143 HCP control subjects who did not develop SARS were compared to 72 who acquired SARS while working. Those with more than 2h of infection prevention and control training were 97% less likely to acquire SARS (OR=0.03 95% CI 0.001–0.20).[50] Risk factors for nosocomial transmission of SARS-CoV-2 include resuscitation (OR=3.81, 95% CI 1.04–13.87), HCP working with symptoms (OR=10.55, 95% CI 2.28–48.87), patients requiring more than 6L/min O_2 therapy (OR=4.30, 95% CI 1.00–18.43), patients with noninvasive positive pressure ventilation (OR=11.82, 95% CI 1.97–70.80), and less than 1m between patient beds (OR=6.98, 95% CI 1.68–28.75).[17] Data from a cohort of nurses revealed that the risk of acquiring SARS infection increased by 6% per shift worked and being in a patient room for more than 4h. Other activities that increased the risk of HCP acquiring infection included intubation and suctioning before intubation, the use of a nebulizer, and manipulation of an oxygen mask.[51] Facilities with staff changing, washing, and showering decreased the risk of nosocomial transmission by 88% (OR=0.12, 95% CI 0.02–0.97).[52]

HCP protection while working with SARS patients became critical to maintaining patient care and reassuring staff. While PPE use was popularized during the Middle Ages and hand hygiene was introduced in the 19th century, the effectiveness of these strategies in protecting HCP from this novel infection was not known. During SARS, several cohort and case–control studies examined several interventions. Seto et al. found the risk of SARS-CoV-1 acquisition among HCPs was increased if an HCP did NOT use hand hygiene (OR = 5, 95% CI 1–19), use gloves (OR = 2, 95% CI 0.6–7), wear gowns (OR = undefined $P = 0.006$), or use medical/surgical masks or respirators (OR = 13, 95% CI 3–60).[43] While medical/surgical masks reduced the risk of acquiring SARS infection, there was no difference found between masks and N95 respirators in this small study. Importantly, the use of **all** measures significantly reduced the risk of acquiring SARS, and the authors concluded that in the absence of aerosol-generating procedures, surgical masks and contact precautions were adequate to prevent SARS-CoV infection among HCP. Loeb et al. compared PPE use in a cohort of 43 nurses, 8 of whom developed SARS.[53] Among this group, the risk of acquiring nosocomial SARS was reduced if one consistently used gloves (OR = 0.45, 95% CI 0.14, 1.46), gowns (OR = 0.36, 95% CI 0.10, 1.24), and an N95 or surgical mask (OR = 0.23, 95% CI 0.07, 0.78). A slight increase in protection was observed in nurses who used N95 masks compared to surgical masks, but the increase was not statistically significant. Those who had sustained close contact or participated in high-risk procedures (e.g., endotracheal intubation) had a higher risk of contracting SARS-CoV.[46,54] These findings heightened the concern about airborne spread of particles, which was later demonstrated as a likely mode of transmission by Booth and colleagues.[55] In addition, using fluid dynamics to study a hospital-based outbreak, investigators provided support to epidemiologic investigation further demonstrating that airborne transmission was the primary mode of transmission associated with a super-spreading event and that fomites contribute minimally.[48]

Case Study TTSH

Singapore's index patient was initially housed in an open general ward and only isolated 5 days after admission, following an alert from the MOH. Based on information from their counterparts in Hong Kong, the MOH recommended that patients be placed in respiratory isolation and that HCPs use medical/surgical masks for all patient contact. Following the global alert issued by the WHO on March 12, 2003, about a severe form of pneumonia of unknown origin, PPE was changed to high-filtration respirators (e.g., N95 or FFP3), gowns, and gloves. Initially, TTSH applied these precautions only to staff in certain high-risk areas, such as the Communicable Disease Centre, the ICU, and the Emergency Department.[56] However, this evolved when TTSH was designated as Singapore's SARS hospital. A SARS-CoV diagnostic test had yet to be developed, and because of expanded clinical diagnostic criteria, many patients were classified as potential SARS cases. HCPs wore gowns, gloves, and respiratory protection that were changed in between every patient. Eye protection was not routinely used. After April 1 and once the use of gowns, gloves, and medical/surgical masks for all patient contact, no new HCP infections were reported.[57] This again changed because of SARS transmission to frontline HCPs described in Canada, and respirators (e.g., N-95, FFP3) became mandatory for all HCP contacts with patients.[58] The issue of the best respiratory protection (surgical masks vs respirators) was controversial at the time and remains unresolved to this day.

In preoutbreak times, each hospital would have a limited supply of respirators (e.g., N-95, FFP3), usually reserved for protection when caring for cases of tuberculosis, measles, and chickenpox, all infections known to be spread by small particles. As the demand for masks was unprecedented, unorthodox, and innovative ways to conserve masks were developed. By mid-March at TTSH when only 200 N95 masks were available in the hospital, the decision was made to use masks for prolonged periods of time and to allow HCPs to reuse their own personal masks. Strict criteria were written to protect HCPs and care for masks but also to stipulate how often each HCP would be provided a new mask (Table 1).[59]

Mask shortages were experienced in other countries, and the CDC formulated guidelines on their safe reuse, suggesting the use of a surgical mask over an N95 respirator. Studies have shown inconsistent use of PPE and inadequate training to be associated with increased risk of infection.[50] In TTSH, mass mask fit training sessions were held, education was enhanced with posters placed outside isolation wards and ICUs, and guidance was communicated with videos.

Other measures included increasing the separation between patients. As there is an increased risk of contracting SARS after being a patient, attempts were made to increase the distance between chairs and seating in waiting areas and between patient beds in the Emergency Department bays and inpatient wards.[48,54] While generally accepted that SARS-CoV-1 was spread by contact with droplets from infected patients/visitors or staff, there was uncertainty about transmission via fomites and potential contamination of environmental surfaces. For this reason, various products, including sodium hypochlorite (bleach), household detergent,

TABLE 1
Recommendations on the Use of Masks, Gowns and Gloves During SARS, Based on Ward or Job, TTSH, Singapore, March 2003

	Key Features	Clinical Correlations
Microbiology	SARS Coronavirus 1 family *Coronaviridae*, which are enveloped, positive-sense single-stranded RNA viruses divided into four genera: *alpha, beta, gamma, and delta.* This virus was in a novel group in the beta genera (2b β CoV).	Novel virus, so humans had no immunity
Immunology	The virus was found to bind to the ACE2 receptor on ciliated airway cells.	Respiratory tract is major site of SARS infection and cause of disease morbidity
Epidemiology and Ecology	Zoonotic: Origin and reservoir are bats, most abundantly from the genus *Rhinolophus* (horseshoe bats). Intermediary hosts were civet cats and raccoon dogs found in wild animal markets in southern China. Humans infected by direct contact with or exposure to secretions of these animals, and human-to-human transmission.	Initial infections were a jump from animals to humans. Subsequent propagation was via human-to-human transmission
Clinical Presentation	Incubation period ranged from 2 to 16 days with a mean of 4.6 days. All age groups were affected, but the disease was milder in younger age groups.	Symptoms were fever, cough, chills, myalgias, and malaise. Diarrhea was significant in the Amoy Gardens outbreak
Diagnosis	Serology, PCR of infected tissue, and/or direct culture. PCR of blood, nasopharyngeal aspirates, stool, urine.	Challenging; rare disease, initial symptoms often nonspecific Challenging as a new disease, initial symptoms like any respiratory infection
Treatment	Initial treatments were all experimental and done before in vitro or in vivo tests on SARS-CoV were performed—ribavirin, steroids, lopinavir/ritonavir. Convalescent plasma was also used.	Initial therapies showed promise from observation, though no prospective randomized studies were carried out. Passive immunity from convalescent plasma showed good results.
Vaccination	No vaccine was created as the outbreak was controlled within a few months.	Main prevention strategy is avoidance of contact with animal hosts and IPC measures when dealing with infected persons.

and some approved disinfectants, were evaluated for efficacy and found that SARS-CoV-1 could be inactivated quite easily with many commonly used disinfectants.[60]

MICROBIOLOGY

The initial cases of severe atypical pneumonia described in China in November 2022 were thought to be caused by an avian influenza A strain due to the similarity of patient symptoms, signs, laboratory, and radiologic findings involved in the 1997 outbreak in Hong Kong.[61] Paramyxoviruses were initially implicated when paramyxovirus-like particles were observed by electron microscopy, and subsequently, human metapneumovirus was detected in some patients and considered a potential pathogen. The WHO called upon 11 laboratories in nine countries to join a collaborative multicenter research project, and in a remarkable scientific feat by late March, laboratories in Hong Kong, the United States, and Germany identified and characterized a novel coronavirus (SARS-CoV-1) as the etiologic agent for SARS.[44,62,63]

The virus identified as the causative agent of SARS was in the family *Coronaviridae*, which are enveloped, positive-sense single-stranded RNA viruses that are divided into four genera: *alpha, beta, gamma,* and *delta.*[42] This virus was in a novel branch in the beta genera (2b β CoV). The genome was distinct from other previously described coronaviruses which cause infection and/or disease in both humans and animals. Importantly, part of the genome of this virus encodes for structural proteins including spike (S), envelope (E), membrane

(M), and nucleocapsid (N), which are important for the virus receptor attachment. The virus was found to bind to the ACE2 receptor on ciliated airway cells.[64]

Animal Reservoir

Epidemiologic and subsequent serologic data suggested demonstrated higher antibody levels in those with occupational exposures to wet markets, which was then considered a potential source of transmission of the SARS-CoV-1 virus from an animal to a human host. These seroprevalence epidemiologic studies initially pointed to the palm civet cat, a threatened species, as a source, and after the SARS-CoV-1 virus was isolated, SARS-CoV-like viruses were also isolated from palm civets and raccoon dogs from wild animal markets in the Guangdong Province of China. These findings suggested that these animals could be the intermediary host and source of human infections. As a result, massive numbers of palm civets were culled in January 2004 in an attempt to prevent the reemergence of SARS-CoV-1 in Guangdong. Subsequent studies revealed no evidence of widespread infection in wild or farmed palm civet cats.[65] Experimental infection of palm civets with two different human isolates of SARS-CoV resulted in overt clinical signs of infection, rendering the animals unlikely to be the natural reservoir host.[66] Multiple international teams spent the next decade hunting for the origin of SARS-CoV and serendipitously found many SARS-CoV-related viruses in bats, most abundantly from the genus *Rhinolophus* (Chinese horseshoe bats).[67,68] The most conclusive evidence resulted from the isolation of a coronavirus from bats in China that was more than 98% identical to the SARS-CoV-1 genome sequence and capable of using the ACE2 receptor, which allows the virus to bind to human cells.[69]

TREATMENT (SEE CHAPTER 19 FOR MORE DETAIL)

Treatment was primarily supportive. Strategies included the management of atypical pneumonias and respiratory distress syndromes using antibiotics for atypical pneumonia and/or antivirals such as oseltamivir for the potential of influenza. Critically ill patients received supportive care, and noninvasive or invasive assisted ventilation was instituted for those with respiratory failure. Immune-modulatory agents were used ad hoc and within clinical trials when it became apparent that organ damage might be attributable to excessive inflammatory reaction.

Antiviral Drugs

Multiple antiviral agents were used to treat patients with SARS, including ribavirin, protease inhibitors, and interferons. When influenza was excluded as the etiologic agent causing SARS, ribavirin was one of the first antiviral drugs tried in these patients. Ribavirin has broad-spectrum activity, preventing replication of many RNA and DNA viruses in vitro, including myxo-, paramyxo-, arena-, bunya-, herpes-, adeno-, pox-, and retroviruses. Ribavirin may be used in combination with other antiviral therapy, such as interferon. In addition, ribavirin analogs previously developed for the treatment of hepatitis C and other viral diseases (e.g., Viramidine) were potential treatments for SARS-CoV-1.[70] Due to the rapidly unfolding situation, ribavirin treatment differed across teams and countries; it was used in various doses and for various durations, and in combination with steroids or other immunotherapies.

Patients were treated with these regimens before in vitro or in vivo tests on SARS-CoV-1 activity were performed. One study reported that ribavirin reduced the viral load in five of eight patients; however, this was not supported by subsequent data.[71] Aside from the risk of teratogenicity to HCPs, ribavirin given at low doses (400–600 mg/day) was ineffective, and at higher doses it was associated with significant side effects, including anemia in 27%–59% of patients, elevated transaminases, bradycardia, hypocalcemia, and hypomagnesemia.[25,72,73] The situation was further complicated once in vitro data from ribavirin studies became available, and conflicting results were again observed. Ribavirin did not inhibit SARS-CoV replication in Vero-E6 (African green monkey kidney) cells at therapeutically achievable concentrations but did inhibit replication in fetal rhesus kidney cells in concentrations above the mean plasma levels in treated individuals.[74] These findings suggested that multiple cell types should be used to evaluate the activity of antiviral agents against emerging viruses such as SARS-CoV-1.

To find an effective treatment for SARS-CoV infection, researchers screened >10,000 compounds for activity against SARS-CoV-1. Compounds screened included calpain inhibitors, SARS-CoV protease inhibitors, entry inhibitors, and HIV-1 protease inhibitors. Traditional therapies, including Chinese medicine and herbal remedies, were investigated, and a compound from the licorice root (glycyrrhizin) was found to be active against SARS-CoV in vitro although the mechanism of action is unclear.[74]

Chen et al. noted that none of the HIV (0/19) patients hospitalized close to other SARS patients contracted the infection, yet 6/28 (21%) of HCPs were infected.[75] In a multicenter, retrospective matched cohort study from Hong Kong, 75 SARS patients were treated with lopinavir and low-dose ritonavir in addition to a standard treatment protocol including antibiotics, ribavirin, and corticosteroids. The use of lopinavir/ritonavir as initial treatment was associated with a lower overall mortality rate (2.3%) and intubation rate (0%), compared with a matched cohort of subjects who did not receive lopinavir/ritonavir. However, there was no difference in the subgroup who received lopinavir/ritonavir as rescue therapy, suggesting that only early use of lopinavir/ritonavir was effective against SARS-CoV-1.[76]

Steroids

Corticosteroids were the mainstay of immunomodulatory therapy for SARS-CoV-1, and timely use often led to early improvement in terms of subsidence of fever, improved oxygenation, and resolution of radiographic infiltrates. Steroid use was rationalized to interfere in acute viral respiratory infections and negate damage from early response cytokines such as interferon-gamma (IFN-c), tumor necrosis factor, interleukin-1 (IL-1), and interleukin-6 (IL-6) that contribute to tissue injury.[77] The hypothesis was that poor clinical outcomes observed during the second phase of illness resulted from immunopathological damage from an overexuberant host response.[78]

There were many inconsistencies among steroid treatment timing, dosing, and duration of corticosteroid use that could account for differences in outcomes. It was suggested that initiation of corticosteroid treatment should coincide with the onset of an excessive immune response, gauged by radiological changes and increased oxygen requirements, generally occurring at the end of the second week of illness. The fear was that early use of steroids may increase the viral load or prolong the viral replicative phase, while delayed steroids may not avert the cytokine storm and prevent immunopathological lung damage. The use of steroid treatment in the first five SARS patients in Singapore did not demonstrate a benefit,[79] so this treatment was not continued. Others reported the effects of prolonged courses of high-dose steroids, which included secondary infections, psychosis, and avascular necrosis.[71,80–82]

Convalescent Plasma

Convalescent plasma became one of the most promising medical therapies used during the SARS outbreak. Plasma containing high titers of neutralizing antibodies was donated by recovered SARS patients and used for passive immunization of patients who continued to deteriorate. When administered to SARS patients, human convalescent plasma, especially early in the illness, had a beneficial effect.[83–85] Convalescent plasma in one study increased discharge rates and decreased mortality (OR = 0.25, 95% CI 0.14, 0.45).[84]

PUBLIC HEALTH MITIGATION STRATEGIES AND MEASURES (SEE CHAPTER 13 FOR MORE DETAILS)

Identifying Patients and Quarantining Contacts

Measures to contain SARS-CoV-1 took two major forms: isolation of symptomatic cases to prevent further transmission and quarantine and close observation of asymptomatic contacts of SARS cases to assure rapid isolation should signs or symptoms develop. The earlier the index cases could be isolated, the fewer contacts risked getting infected.[86] Multiple approaches were employed to identify and assess both cases and contacts depending on the local epidemiology and resources. The approaches varied, and in some countries they focused on healthcare-based transmission, while in other countries the focus was on community transmission. Strategies to identify cases included large-scale screening efforts. In Singapore, monitoring of temperature to detect an early indication of infection was implemented in workplaces and schools.[57] Temperature screening was set up at border crossings and airports to identify persons who might have SARS-CoV-1, though this was not thought to be very effective.[87,88] However, all the efforts ascertaining and isolating case patients, combined with rapid identification and management of contacts, were highly effective in interrupting SARS transmission in several countries.[15,89,90]

To manage those requiring isolation required rethinking patient care models. In the initial stages of the outbreak, attempts were made to admit all suspect/confirmed cases to negative-pressure isolation rooms with anterooms. However, these attempts were stymied as most hospitals did not have isolation capacity that matched the need. This led to innovative strategies to manage ventilation in patient rooms as well as in wards caring for these patients, including the rapid installation of exhaust fans to create negative pressure,[91–93] the use of tents as screening facilities (Fig. 2), or repurposing of existing facilities. In Hong Kong, the government constructed 558 new state-of-the-art SARS isolation rooms supporting more than 1300 beds in 14 hospitals. The construction of these state-of-the-art facilities

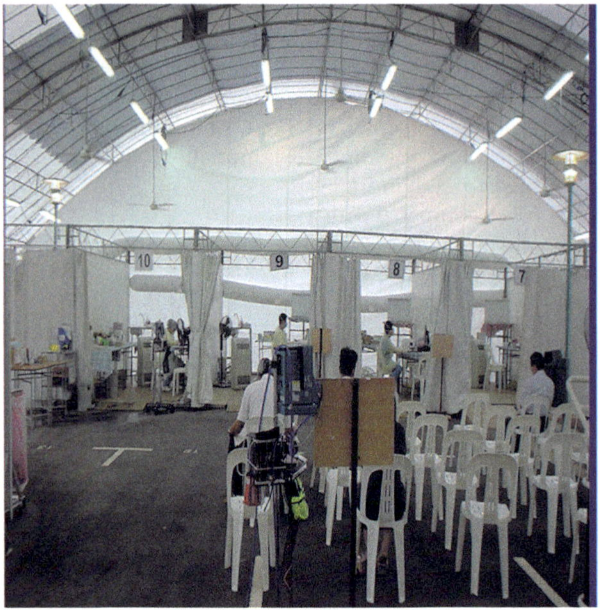

FIG. 2 Tents used as screening facilities, TTSH, Singapore, 2003.

was completed by the end of 2003.[94] In another example, China built an infectious diseases hospital, the world's largest in a record-breaking time.[95]

Some countries set up screening clinics to facilitate the patient influx. Importantly, however, quarantine was used in a targeted fashion, which decreased the frustration among the general population and healthcare workers. Communication also became key, and it was rational, factual, and frequent. Such efforts were coupled with educational campaigns to inform the public about prevention strategies and the signs and symptoms of infection. This included promoting hand hygiene, use of physical distancing, personal hygiene practices, and avoidance of crowds and healthcare facilities when possible. Multiple modalities were used to target different populations and included newspapers, television, and the Internet. There was extensive involvement of public health officials in contact tracing, enforcing quarantine, community outreach, and public education. In healthcare facilities, education targeted symptom recognition, testing strategies, and the proper use of PPE. Some health authorities stopped visitation to healthcare facilities to reduce transmission risks. In addition to heightened awareness of the importance of infection control precautions and their compliance, response to the SARS epidemic extended beyond healthcare facilities. These communication and educational efforts were also meant to quell fear and reassure the general public and HCPs.

The magnitude of interruption of daily life varied. In some regions, schools were closed, masking was required in public, and public transportation was limited. Other localities were more draconian in their approach, placing many individuals in quarantine.[12,18]

PUBLIC HEALTH AND INTERNATIONAL IMPACT

SARS-CoV caused widespread disruptions not only to healthcare facilities but to whole communities. In the initial wave, HCPs were shunned on public transport and at restaurants, and some were even evicted from their homes by landlords. Some hospitals reduced elective surgeries and routine activities, impacting timely access to care.[96] Attendance at emergency departments and clinics was sharply reduced as the public stayed away out of fear of infection (Fig. 3).[97,98]

When it became apparent by mid-March 2003 that this new infectious disease was spreading, health ministries of affected countries set up SARS task forces at central and regional levels to coordinate surveillance, response, and communication activities. In Vietnam, Singapore, Hong Kong, Taiwan, and Canada, SARS became a notifiable disease by the end of March with cases reported to the WHO as they were identified.[99] WHO actively sent out advisories and updated travel alerts to various countries when there were reports of cases.[100,101] Beyond the public health sector, the

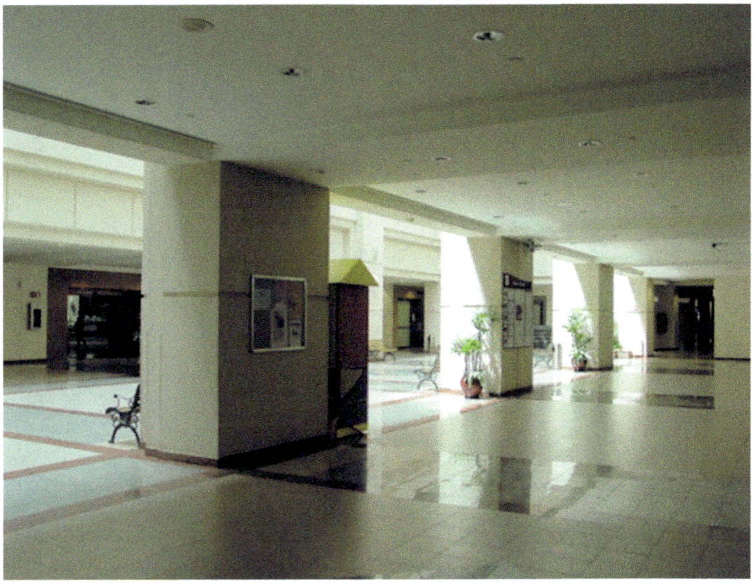

FIG. 3 Completely empty hospital lobby during SARS, March–April 2003, TTSH.

remarkable international scientific collaboration led to the identification of a previously unknown and novel virus in 3 weeks. The 11 scientific laboratories in nine countries that collaborated and identified the virus, sequenced it, and subsequently went on to screen potential candidate therapeutics and develop vaccines provided an incredible service to humanity.

Despite these herculean efforts, international travel to affected countries fell sharply by 50%–70%, with dramatic impacts on tourism, hotel occupancy, and related service businesses.[6] The impact on economies was significant with the Asian Development Bank estimating reductions in the gross domestic product ranging from 2.6% in Hong Kong, 1% in China, 0.49% in Taiwan, and 0.47% in Singapore.[102] With all these monumental efforts, the outbreak was controlled, and WHO declared its end in July 2003. The final toll was 8096 cases in 29 countries, with 774 (9.6%) deaths (Table 2).[103]

RESURGENCE

The question that remained on all minds was "Will SARS-CoV reemerge and when?" Such fears were reignited with incidents of laboratory-acquired SARS-CoV-1 infection. In September 2003, a graduate student working on West Nile Virus acquired SARS-CoV-1 in a Biosafety Level 3 (BSL3) laboratory in Singapore.[104] Subsequent lab-acquired SARS-CoV-1 infections were reported in Taiwan on December 17, 2003, and on March 25 and April 17, 2004, in Beijing, China.[105–107] All incidents were thoroughly investigated to assure that there was not a resurgence of the infection. The incident at the National Institute of Virology in Beijing was particularly concerning as experiments using live and inactivated SARS-CoV-1 were performed in the facility. However, the two researchers infected did not work with SARS-CoV-1. This raised questions about the Institute's biosafety procedures, especially given the propensity for this infection to be transmitted among humans and that these lab-acquired infections could have easily spread into the community (Table 3).

Following the four incidents of laboratory-acquired SARS-CoV infection, the WHO issued post-outbreak biosafety guidelines and strongly recommended BSL3 as the minimum containment level to do laboratory work with live SARS-CoV-1. Member States were urged to maintain a thorough inventory of laboratories working with and/or storing live SARS-CoV-1 and to ensure that necessary biosafety standards were in place and followed.[108]

LESSONS LEARNED, DEVELOPMENTS, AND PREPARATION FOR THE NEXT OUTBREAK

Countries that had experienced SARS-CoV-1 outbreaks learned valuable lessons in improving both outbreak detection and response, facilitating communication,

TABLE 2

Summary of Probable SARS Cases With Onset of Illness From 1 November 2002 to 31 July 2003. 2003, World Health Organization: Geneva

	CUMULATIVE NUMBER OF CASES									
	Female[a]	Male[a]	Total	Median Age (Range)	Number of Deaths[b,c]	Case Fatality Ratio (%)	Number of Imported Cases (%)	Number of HCP[d] Affected (%)	Date Onset First Probable Case	Date Onset Last Probable Case
Australia	4	2	6	15 (1–45)	0	0	6 (100)	0 (0)	26-Feb-03	01-Apr-03
Canada	151	100	251	49 (1–98)	43	17	5 (2)	109 (43)	23-Feb-03	12-Jun-03
China	2674	2607	5327	Not available	349	7	Not applicable	1002 (19)	16-Nov-02	03-Jun-03
China, Hong Kong	977	778	1755	40 (0–100)	299	17	Not applicable	386 (22)	15-Feb-03	31-May-03
China, Macao	0	1	1	28	0	0	1 (100)	0 (0)	05-May-03	05-May-03
China, Taiwan	218	128	346	42 (0–93)	37	11	21 (6)	68 (20)	25-Feb-03	15-Jun-03
France	1	6	7	49 (26–61)	1	14	7 (100)	2 (29)[e]	21-Mar-03	03-May-03
Germany	4	5	9	44 (4–73)	0	0	9 (100)	1 (11)	09-Mar-03	06-May-03
India	0	3	3	25 (25–30)	0	0	3 (100)	0 (0)	25-Apr-03	06-May-03
Indonesia	0	2	2	56 (47–65)	0	0	2 (100)	0 (0)	06-Apr-03	17-Apr-03
Italy	1	3	4	30.5(25–54)	0	0	4 (100)	0 (0)	12-Mar-03	20-Apr-03
Kuwait	1	0	1	50	0	0	1 (100)	0 (0)	09-Apr-03	09-Apr-03
Malaysia	1	4	5	30 (26–84)	2	40	5 (100)	0 (0)	14-Mar-03	22-Apr-03
Mongolia	8	1	9	32 (17–63)	0	0	8 (89)	0 (0)	31-Mar-03	06-May-03
New Zealand	1	0	1	67	0	0	1 (100)	0 (0)	20-Apr-03	20-Apr-03
Philippines	8	6	14	41 (29–73)	2	14	7 (50)	4 (29)	25-Feb-03	05-May-03
Republic of Ireland	0	1	1	56	0	0	1 (100)	0 (0)	27-Feb-03	27-Feb-03
Republic of Korea	0	3	3	40 (20–80)	0	0	3 (100)	0 (0)	25-Apr-03	10-May-03
Romania	0	1	1	52	0	0	1 (100)	0 (0)	19-Mar-03	19-Mar-03
Russian Federation	0	1	1	25	0	0	Not available	0 (0)	05-May-03	05-May-03

Singapore	161	77	238	35 (1–90)	33	14	8 (3)	97 (41)	25-Feb-03	05-May-03
South Africa	0	1	1	62	1	100	1 (100)	0 (0)	03-Apr-03	03-Apr-03
Spain	0	1	1	33	0	0	1 (100)	0 (0)	26-Mar-03	26-Mar-03
Sweden	3	2	5	43 (33–55)	0	0	5 (100)	0 (0)	28-Mar-03	23-Apr-03
Switzerland	0	1	1	35	0	0	1 (100)	0 (0)	09-Mar-03	09-Mar-03
Thailand	5	4	9	42 (2–79)	2	22	9 (100)	1 (11)	11-Mar-03	27-May-03
United Kingdom	2	2	4	59 (28–74)	0	0	4 (100)	0 (0)	01-Mar-03	01-Apr-03
United States[e]	13	14	27	36 (0–83)	0	0	27 (100)	0 (0)	24-Feb-03	13-Jul-03
Viet Nam	39	24	63	43 (20–76)	5	8	1 (2)	36 (57)	23-Feb-03	14-Apr-03
Total			**8096**		**774**	**9.6**	**142**	**1706**		

[a]Case classification by sex is unknown for 46 cases.
[b]Includes only cases whose death is attributed to SARS.
[c]Since 11 July 2003, 325 cases have been discarded in Taiwan, China. Laboratory information was insufficient or incomplete for 135 discarded cases, of which 101 died.
[d]Includes HCPs who acquired illness outside of healthcare settings.
[e]Due to differences in case definitions, the United States has reported probable cases of SARS with onsets of illness after 5 July 2003.
Source: https://www.who.int/publications/m/item/summary-of-probable-sars-cases-with-onset-of-illness-from-1-november-2002-to-31-july-2003

TABLE 3
Example of a Protocol to Determine PPE Use by Healthcare Ward or Setting During SARS: Recommendations for the Use of Masks, Gowns, and Gloves

Categories of Healthcare Personnel (HCPs)	N95 Masks (FFP3, Respirator)	Gowns	Gloves
Group 1: HCPs with Direct Patient Contact (Inpatient Areas)			
Group 1A: SARS ICU	Change mask every 24 h or when contaminated by blood/body fluid/secretions or when damaged.	Change gown after every direct patient contact.	Change gloves in between patients.
Group 1B: SARS General ward	Change mask every 24 h or when contaminated by blood/body fluid/secretions or when damaged.	Change gown after every direct patient contact.	Change gloves in between patients.
Group 1C: SARS Pediatrics	Change mask every 24 h or when contaminated by blood/body fluid/secretions or when damaged.	Change gown after every direct patient contact.	Change gloves in between patients.
Group 1D: Quarantine and other hospital wards	Change mask every 24 h or when contaminated by blood/body fluid/secretions or when damaged.	Change gown after every direct patient contact.	Change gloves in between patients.
Group 1E: Unknown SARS wards (not known to have a patient)	Change mask every 24 h or when contaminated by blood/body fluid/secretions or when damaged.	Gowns should be worn when there is direct bodily contact with patient/patient's environment (e.g., bed sponging of patient). Change gowns between cubicles. Aprons can be worn when no bodily contact is expected (e.g., handing patient newspaper, and serving medication)	Change gloves in between patients.
Group 1F: Cleaners/Housekeepers	Change mask every 24 h or when contaminated by blood/body fluid/secretions or when damaged.	Change gown after cleaning every patient room/cubicle/toilet/sluice room, etc. For the mid-day emptying of rubbish, the operative may wear the same set of PPE for the entire ward and remove the PPE when the rubbish is cleared.	Change gloves in between every room/cubicle.
Group 2: HCPs in the Ambulatory Care			
Group 2A: ED/Radiology, etc.	Change mask every 24 h or when contaminated by blood/body fluid/secretions or when damaged.	Change gowns when contaminated by blood/body fluid/secretions.	Change gloves in between patients.
Group 2B: Medical Center/Clinics/Outpatient areas	Change mask every 24 h or when contaminated by blood/body fluid/secretions or when damaged.	Change gowns when contaminated by blood/body fluid/secretions.	Change gloves in between patients.
Group 2C: Laboratory	Change mask every 24 h or when contaminated by blood/body fluid/secretions or when damaged.	Change gowns when contaminated by blood/body fluid/secretions/upon leaving workstation.	Change gloves when contaminated by blood/body fluid/secretion.

TABLE 3
Example of a Protocol to Determine PPE Use by Healthcare Ward or Setting During SARS: Recommendations for the Use of Masks, Gowns, and Gloves—cont'd

Categories of Healthcare Personnel (HCPs)	N95 Masks (FFP3, Respirator)	Gowns	Gloves
Group 2D: Transport staff	Change mask every 24 h or when contaminated by blood/body fluid/secretions or when damaged.	Change gowns in between patients.	Change gloves in between patients.
Group 3: HCPs Providing Support Services			
Group 3A: Delivery man from store, pharmacy staff delivering supplies to ward, etc.	Change mask only when damaged.	NA	NA
Group 3B: Engineers covering SARS areas	Change mask every 24 h or when contaminated by blood/body fluid/secretions or when damaged.	Change gowns for every patient room.	Change gloves in between patients.
Group 4: HCPs in Administration			
Group 4: Administrative staff	Change mask only when damaged.	NA	NA

PPE = Personal Protective Equipment; HCP=Healthcare Personnel; ED = Emergency Department; ICU=Intensive Care Unit; NA = Not Applicable.

and planning for resources, their distribution, and utilization. With the recognition that changes were required in disease surveillance and reporting and with communication among healthcare sectors, governments, and the public, processes, policies, and infrastructure were developed in various countries.

China launched new reforms aiming to establish a sound public health system with infrastructure and expertise to support disease prevention and control activities, supervision for those activities, and a public health emergency response system covering both urban and rural areas. As such, it established the world's largest reporting system for infectious disease epidemics and public health emergencies. All types of health institutions at all levels could directly report cases of infections, clusters, outbreaks, and public health emergencies at the national level. The result was dramatic in that after a healthcare institution detected and diagnosed an infection, the reporting time decreased on average from 5 days to 4 h.[109]

The Hong Kong government adopted a clearly defined, tiered command structure to prepare for and respond to future outbreaks and consolidated all health protection functions under a new centralized agency. In parallel, they made a massive investment into research preparedness, enhancing public health testing and reporting infrastructure with real-time dialogue between the scientific and policy-making communities. In 2004, the Legislative Council approved funding for the establishment of the first Infectious Diseases Centre (IDC) in Hong Kong at Princess Margaret Hospital, which officially opened on June 22, 2007. This state-of-the-art healthcare facility is a standalone building with 108 negative-pressure single rooms equipped with high-efficiency particulate air filters; isolation beds; a BSL-3 laboratory, radio-diagnostics, and imaging services; a control and command center; and an operating theater, delivery suite, and ICU all built to manage and care for patients infected with patients of high consequence. In addition to providing clinical management, the IDC also serves as a training and research center for infectious diseases and infection prevention and control professionals.[110]

As SARS started in hospitals with a severe impact on HCP, much more attention was paid to occupational safety and protection from infectious diseases. In Singapore, to enhance surveillance and also have an additional early warning strategy, a web-based sickness surveillance system was developed and allowed HCPs who were too unwell to come to work to voluntarily submit data. Monitoring for unusual numbers or trends of employee illness and facilitated investigations were undertaken by infection prevention and control teams if required.[111] Another sentinel surveillance system was developed to monitor cases of sudden Severe Illness and Death from Possible Infectious Causes (*SIDPIC*) and implemented in government and MOH-run hospitals. Also created was the Disease Outbreak Response Condition (DORSCON) framework with different color coding for different levels of size and severity of outbreaks (Fig. 4).[112] Plans for the construction of a new Communicable Disease Centre were revived and eventually resulted in the National Centre of Infectious Diseases, a 330-bed purpose-built and state-of-the-art isolation facility that opened in 2019.

The Taiwanese government reapproached its response and undertook a fundamental reorganization of the Center for Disease Control, recruiting experts in infection prevention and control and public health, and established a new unit, the Central Epidemic Command Center, to help monitor outbreaks and manage the response. In addition, they instituted a four-tiered pandemic risk notification system with divided alert phases to facilitate the response.[113]

In Canada, public health and epidemic control systems were largely overhauled after a sweeping set of recommendations to Canada's federal, provincial, and territorial leaders in a report entitled "Learning from SARS, Renewal of Public Health in Canada."[114] This led to the construction of a fully digital institution, the Humber River Hospital, which opened in 2015 with greater number of isolation rooms.[115] In addition, in an effort to enhance the reach and effectiveness of infection prevention and control, Canada implemented standards to assure there were adequate numbers of infection preventionists in healthcare facilities. Perhaps one of the greatest contributions was developing a national (and international) collaborative multispecialty research network that could facilitate the rapid initiation of clinical trials through preparing study protocols with appropriate methodology in advance, working with research ethics infrastructure, and developing communication systems to connect with frontline clinicians.

Vaccines

The development of a vaccine against SARS-CoV-1 became a priority after the pandemic for both human and animal hosts. Various vaccine formulations targeting SARS-CoV-1 were developed, but in animal

Colour	Nature of Disease	Impact on Daily Life	Advice to Public
Green	Disease is mild OR Disease is severe but does not spread easily from person to person (e.g. MERS, H7N9)	Minimal disruption e.g. border screening, travel advice	• Be socially responsible: if you are sick, stay home • Maintain good personal hygiene • Look out for health advisories
Yellow	Disease is severe and spreads easily from person to person but is occurring outside Singapore. OR Disease is spreading in Singapore but is **(a)** typically mild i.e. only slightly more severe than seasonal influenza. Could be severe in vulnerable groups. (e.g. H1N1 pandemic) ***OR*** **(b)** being contained	Minimal disruption e.g. additional measures at border and/or healthcare settings expected, higher work and school absenteeism likely	• Be socially responsible: if you are sick, stay home • Maintain good personal hygiene • Look out for health advisories
Orange	Disease is severe AND spreads easily from person to person, but disease has not spread widely in Singapore and is being contained (e.g. SARS experience in Singapore).	Moderate disruption e.g. quarantine, temperature screening, visitor restrictions at hospitals.	• Be socially responsible: if you are sick, stay home • Maintain good personal hygiene • Look out for health advisories • Comply with control measures
Red	Disease is severe AND is spreading widely.	Major disruption e.g. school closures, work from home orders, significant number of deaths.	• Be socially responsible: if you are sick, stay home • Maintain good personal hygiene • Look out for health advisories • Comply with control measures • Practise social distancing: avoid crowded areas

FIG. 4 Disease Outbreak Response Condition (DORSCON) Framework, Ministry of Health, Singapore.

trials, results were inconclusive, and in some cases, vaccinated animals displayed significant disease upon challenge.[116] Some candidate vaccines were tested in preclinical models; however, research funding for ongoing development slowly disappeared, and none were FDA-approved. The development approaches, however, were helpful in advancing certain formulations, including protein subunit vaccines, virus-like particle vaccines, DNA vaccines, viral vector vaccines, whole-inactivated vaccines, and live-attenuated vaccines.[117]

Animal Models

An imperative to understand pathogen and viral pathogenesis, evaluate candidate vaccines and antiviral drugs, and assess their effectiveness includes developing appropriate animal models. There were many challenges in developing good animal models for SARS-CoV-1. First, an ideal animal model mimics human disease by sharing the route of infection and disease severity with comparable morbidities and mortality rates. Second, to achieve these characteristics, the physiologic and anatomic mechanisms of viral attachment such as viral cell receptors should mimic those of humans and be similarly distributed.[118] Finally, some congruity between findings facilitates their incorporation into the scientific knowledge needed to further critical research. In the case of SARS, there was not one definitive model. Young, inbred mice supported viral replication but did not display clinical signs of infection, while older inbred mice, knockout mice, and transgenic mice developed generalized illness, had robust viral growth, and pronounced lung pathology consistent with pneumonia and acute lung injury.[118] Viral replication was supported in golden Syrian hamsters and ferrets, and histologic changes in the lungs were observed in both species. Nonhuman primates (Rhesus macaques, Cynomolgus macaques, African green monkeys, and common marmosets) are susceptible to SARS-CoV-1 infection, but clinical signs, viral replication, and pathology varied between these species challenging interpretation of the various findings.

Infection Prevention and Control

For many years, infection prevention and control have been given scant attention in medical centers, considered a low priority for education and training, and issues with compliance or best practice were addressed in a limited and fragmented manner if at all. Infection prevention and control professionals and the programs they oversee are responsible for surveillance for healthcare-associated infections, including pathogens of consequence, information provision, education and training, guideline and policy development, and planning for infectious disease emergencies and surge capacity. In some institutions, these activities also include employee and occupational health as it pertains to infectious pathogens and their prevention. The SARS outbreak raised many questions with regard to issues that affect both patients and employees. For example, debates about the routes of transmission of emerging infectious diseases, and in this case SARS-CoV-1, and whether transmission was via a droplet or an airborne route developed and have continued for years and are still not decisively resolved. This debate was fueled by the morbidity and mortality suffered by HCPs who acquired SARS-CoV-1 and focused attention on infection prevention and control practices, the use of PPE, and the role of education and training in prevention of SARS-CoV-1 acquisition and transmission. SARS-CoV-1 clearly demonstrated that infection control was not only about implementing but being trained on the components of the guidelines and complying with those guidelines. For example, it was not good enough to put on PPE, but knowing how to don and doff PPE was critical. Furthermore, the authority of the infection prevention and control groups, the support for adequate numbers of trained professionals, and the platform to implement best practices and effective programs needed to be strengthened globally.[119]

PREPARATION FOR THE NEXT OUTBREAK

Responses from the medical and scientific communities as well as public health authorities to understand and control SARS-CoV within a short time were remarkable. Yet, the challenge was to maintain the readiness and prepare for the next novel pathogen that could disrupt society. Why was/is this necessary? Ultimately, because the sources of many viruses, including coronavirus, are bats, and they are ubiquitous and are the reservoirs.[120] Many genetically diverse SARS-related coronaviruses (SARS-rCoV) have been isolated from multiple species of bats worldwide.[121,122] This includes a large reservoir of SARS-rCoV and similar viruses in horseshoe bats (genus *Rhinolophus*), and the Chinese horseshoe bat is strongly suspected to be the source of SARS-CoV-1 with the masked civet cat, the intermediary host.[123] This said, should an intermediary host become infected with a novel virus and brought to market, there is a great potential for humans and animals to mix in settings like "wet markets" in many parts of Asia.[124] Hence, if we consider coronaviruses as an example, they are known to undergo genetic recombination, which may lead to new variants, a potential time bomb ripe for new outbreaks of infectious diseases.[125]

Super-spreading events and the role of intrahospital transfers were identified by careful case tracing. Hospitals and healthcare facilities were consistently the fulcrums of transmission, which was then complicated by expansion, and international transmission was facilitated by airplane travel. While this highlights the opportunities for planning, it also provides insight into how successful the response was using basic scientific public health knowledge and resources. Early in the SARS outbreak, without diagnostic tests and with relatively nonspecific clinical presentations, clinicians who carefully obtained epidemiologic history were able to ascertain cases correctly and provide appropriate clinical management. Adherence to basic infection prevention and control (use of PPE) and public health measures including careful contract tracing, aggressive isolation, and quarantine strategies led to global control of an epidemic within 4 months. This occurred using the clinical acumen of clinicians, the best guesses of the transmission by infection prevention experts, and without a rapid diagnostic test, a vaccine, or effective therapy.[126]

Even though the outbreak was declared over in 6 months, continued research was needed to fill the gaps. There remain activities and actions that may not have merited the "squeeze." Did all the palm civets need to be culled, and did broad public health actions, such as stopping, travel decrease transmission? Was there an adequate understanding of the infectivity and pathogenesis of the virus from molecular and immunological standpoints? Is there a need for a vaccine? There is still an urgent and ongoing need for better detection of early disease, more robust research on optimal infection prevention and control practices, and better antivirals and therapeutics, immune-modulating agents, and effective vaccines. Emerging infectious diseases will continue for the foreseeable future, and there are many painful lessons and bright spots from this first novel coronavirus.

REFERENCES

1. Rosling L, Rosling M. Pneumonia causes panic in Guangdong province. *BMJ*. 2003;326(7386):416.
2. World Health Organization. Severe Acute Respiratory Syndrome (SARS):Status of the Outbreak and Lessons for the Immediate Future. Geneva: World Health Organization; 2003.
3. Zhong NS, et al. Epidemiology and cause of severe acute respiratory syndrome (SARS) in Guangdong, People's Republic of China, in February, 2003. *The Lancet*. 2003;362(9393):1353–1358.
4. Peiris M. Severe Acute Respiratory Syndrome. Wiley & Sons; 2008.
5. General Accounting Office. EMERGING INFECTIOUS DISEASES: Asian SARS-CoV-1 Outbreak Challenged International and National Responses; 2004. *Report to the Chairman*, Subcommittee on Asia and the Pacific, Committee on International Relations, House of Representatives, April 2004. Available from: https://www.gao.gov/products/gao-04-564.
6. International Air Transport Association. Economics' Chart of the Week—What Can We Learn From Past Pandemic Episodes? IATA; 2020. Available from: https://www.iata.org/en/iata-repository/publications/economic-reports/what-can-we-learn-from-past-pandemic-episodes/.
7. Centers for Disease Control and Prevention. *Update: Outbreak of Severe Acute Respiratory Syndrome—Worldwide*, 2003, in *MMWR*. Centers for Disease Control and Prevention; 2003:241–248.
8. Lee N, et al. A major outbreak of severe acute respiratory syndrome in Hong Kong. *N Engl J Med*. 2003;348(20):1986–1994.
9. Yu IT, et al. Temporal-spatial analysis of severe acute respiratory syndrome among hospital inpatients. *Clin Infect Dis*. 2005;40(9):1237–1243.
10. Stein RA. Super-spreaders in infectious diseases. *Int J Infect Dis*. 2011;15(8):e510–e513.
11. Reilley B, et al. SARS and Carlo Urbani. *N Engl J Med*. 2003;348(20):1951–1952.
12. Goh KT, et al. Epidemiology and control of SARS in Singapore. *Ann Acad Med Singapore*. 2006;35(5):301–316.
13. Centers for Disease Control and Prevention. Severe acute respiratory syndrome—Taiwan, 2003. *MMWR Morb Mortal Wkly Rep*. 2003;52(20):461–466. Available from: https://www.cdc.gov/mmwr/preview/mmwrhtml/mm5220a1.htm.
14. National Advisory Committee on SARS and Public Health. *Learning From SARS—Renewal of Public Health in Canada*, in *SARS in Canada: Anatomy of an Outbreak*; 2003. Available from: https://www.canada.ca/content/dam/phac-aspc/migration/phac-aspc/publicat/sars-sras/pdf/chapter2-e.pdf.
15. Svoboda T, et al. Public health measures to control the spread of the severe acute respiratory syndrome during the outbreak in Toronto. *N Engl J Med*. 2004;350(23):2352–2361.
16. Foo CL, Tham KY, Seow E. Evolution of an emergency department screening questionnaire for severe acute respiratory syndrome. *Acad Emerg Med*. 2004;11(2):156–161.
17. McDonald LC, et al. SARS in healthcare facilities, Toronto and Taiwan. *Emerg Infect Dis*. 2004;10(5):777–781.
18. Centers for Disease Control and Prevention. *Efficiency of quarantine during an epidemic of severe acute respiratory syndrome—Beijing, China*, 2003. *MMWR Morb Mortal Wkly Rep*. 2003;52(43):1037–1040. Available from: https://www.cdc.gov/mmwr/preview/mmwrhtml/mm5243a2.htm.
19. Goh DL, et al. Secondary household transmission of SARS, Singapore. *Emerg Infect Dis*. 2004;10(2):232–234.

20. McKinney KR, Gong YY, Lewis TG. Environmental transmission of SARS at Amoy gardens. *J Environ Health.* 2006;68(9):26–30. quiz 51-2.
21. Yu IT, et al. Severe acute respiratory syndrome beyond Amoy gardens: completing the incomplete legacy. *Clin Infect Dis.* 2014;58(5):683–686.
22. Olsen SJ, et al. Transmission of the severe acute respiratory syndrome on aircraft. *N Engl J Med.* 2003;349(25):2416–2422.
23. Breugelmans JG, et al. SARS transmission and commercial aircraft. *Emerg Infect Dis.* 2004;10(8):1502–1503.
24. Tsang KW, et al. A cluster of cases of severe acute respiratory syndrome in Hong Kong. *N Engl J Med.* 2003;348(20):1977–1985.
25. Booth CM, et al. Clinical features and short-term outcomes of 144 patients with SARS in the greater Toronto area. *JAMA.* 2003;289(21):2801–2809.
26. Donnelly CA, et al. Epidemiological determinants of spread of causal agent of severe acute respiratory syndrome in Hong Kong. *Lancet.* 2003;361(9371):1761–1766.
27. World Health Organization. Update 49—SARS Case Fatality Ratio, Incubation Period. Geneva: World Health Organization; 2003. Available from: https://www.who.int/emergencies/disease-outbreak-news/item/2003_05_07a-en.
28. Tan CC. SARS in Singapore—key lessons from an epidemic. *Ann Acad Med Singapore.* 2006;35(5):345–349.
29. Hon KL, et al. Clinical presentations and outcome of severe acute respiratory syndrome in children. *Lancet.* 2003;361(9370):1701–1703.
30. World Health Organization. Case Definitions for Surveillance of Severe Acute Respiratory Syndrome (SARS)—Case Definitions (Revised 1 May 2003). Geneva: World Health Organization; 2003. Available from: https://www.who.int/publications/m/item/case-definitions-for-surveillance-of-severe-acute-respiratory-syndrome-(sars).
31. Chan PK, et al. Severe Acute Respiratory Syndrome-associated Coronavirus infection. *Emerg Infect Dis.* 2003;9(11):1453–1454.
32. Peiris JS, et al. Clinical progression and viral load in a community outbreak of coronavirus-associated SARS pneumonia: a prospective study. *Lancet.* 2003;361(9371):1767–1772.
33. Wong SF, et al. Pregnancy and perinatal outcomes of women with severe acute respiratory syndrome. *Am J Obstet Gynecol.* 2004;191(1):292–297.
34. Poutanen SM, et al. Identification of severe acute respiratory syndrome in Canada. *N Engl J Med.* 2003;348(20):1995–2005.
35. Wong RS, et al. Haematological manifestations in patients with severe acute respiratory syndrome: retrospective analysis. *BMJ.* 2003;326(7403):1358–1362.
36. Lai EK, et al. Severe acute respiratory syndrome: quantitative assessment from chest radiographs with clinical and prognostic correlation. *AJR Am J Roentgenol.* 2005;184(1):255–263.
37. Grinblat L, et al. Severe acute respiratory syndrome: radiographic review of 40 probable cases in Toronto, Canada. *Radiology.* 2003;228(3):802–809.
38. Hsieh SC, et al. Radiographic appearance and clinical outcome correlates in 26 patients with severe acute respiratory syndrome. *AJR Am J Roentgenol.* 2004;182(5):1119–1122.
39. Fisher DA, et al. Atypical presentations of SARS. *Lancet.* 2003;361(9370):1740.
40. Chiu WK, et al. Severe acute respiratory syndrome in children: experience in a regional hospital in Hong Kong. *Pediatr Crit Care Med.* 2003;4(3):279–283.
41. Leung GM, et al. SARS-CoV antibody prevalence in all Hong Kong patient contacts. *Emerg Infect Dis.* 2004;10(9):1653–1656.
42. Hui DSC, Zumla A. Severe acute respiratory syndrome: historical, epidemiologic, and clinical features. *Infect Dis Clin North Am.* 2019;33(4):869–889.
43. Seto WH, et al. Effectiveness of precautions against droplets and contact in prevention of nosocomial transmission of severe acute respiratory syndrome (SARS). *Lancet.* 2003;361(9368):1519–1520.
44. Drosten C, et al. Identification of a novel coronavirus in patients with severe acute respiratory syndrome. *N Engl J Med.* 2003;348(20):1967–1976.
45. World Health Organization. Update 47—Studies of SARS Virus Survival, Situation in China. Geneva: World Health Organization; 2003. Available from: https://www.who.int/emergencies/disease-outbreak-news/item/2003_05_05-en.
46. Scales DC, et al. Illness in intensive care staff after brief exposure to severe acute respiratory syndrome. *Emerg Infect Dis.* 2003;9(10):1205–1210.
47. Dowell SF, et al. Severe acute respiratory syndrome coronavirus on hospital surfaces. *Clin Infect Dis.* 2004;39(5):652–657.
48. Xiao S, et al. Role of fomites in SARS transmission during the largest hospital outbreak in Hong Kong. *PLoS One.* 2017;12(7), e0181558.
49. Le DH, et al. Lack of SARS transmission among public hospital workers, Vietnam. *Emerg Infect Dis.* 2004;10(2):265–268.
50. Lau JT, et al. SARS transmission among hospital workers in Hong Kong. *Emerg Infect Dis.* 2004;10(2):280–286.
51. Hui DS. Severe acute respiratory syndrome (SARS): lessons learnt in Hong Kong. *J Thorac Dis.* 2013;5(Suppl 2):S122–S126.
52. Yu IT, et al. Why did outbreaks of severe acute respiratory syndrome occur in some hospital wards but not in others? *Clin Infect Dis.* 2007;44(8):1017–1025.
53. Loeb M, et al. SARS among critical care nurses, *Toronto. Emerg Infect Dis.* 2004;10(2):251–255.
54. Varia M, et al. Investigation of a nosocomial outbreak of severe acute respiratory syndrome (SARS) in Toronto, *Canada. CMAJ.* 2003;169(4):285–292.
55. Booth TF, et al. Detection of airborne severe acute respiratory syndrome (SARS) coronavirus and environmental contamination in SARS outbreak units. *J Infect Dis.* 2005;191(9):1472–1477.

56. Seow E. SARS: experience from the emergency department, Tan Tock Seng Hospital, Singapore. *Emerg Med J.* 2003;20(6):501–504.
57. Ministry of Health. Special feature: severe acute respiratory syndrome (SARS). In: *Communicable Diseases Surveillance in Singapore 2003*; 2003. Available from: https://www.moh.gov.sg/docs/librariesprovider5/resources-statistics/reports/special_feature_sars.pdf.
58. Kamming D, Gardam M, Chung F. Anaesthesia and SARS. *Br J Anaesth.* 2003;90(6):715–718.
59. Ang B. Tan Tock Seng Hospital SARS Task Force:Infection Control and Use of Personal Protective Equipment; 2003.
60. Rabenau HF, et al. Efficacy of various disinfectants against SARS coronavirus. *J Hosp Infect.* 2005;61(2):107–111.
61. World Health Organization. WHO Issues a Global Alert About Cases of Atypical Pneumonia. Geneva: World Health Organization; 2003. Available from: https://www.who.int/news/item/12-03-2003-who-issues-a-global-alert-about-cases-of-atypical-pneumonia.
62. Peiris JS, et al. Coronavirus as a possible cause of severe acute respiratory syndrome. *Lancet.* 2003;361(9366):1319–1325.
63. Ksiazek TG, et al. A novel coronavirus associated with severe acute respiratory syndrome. *N Engl J Med.* 2003;348(20):1953–1966.
64. Li W, et al. Angiotensin-converting enzyme 2 is a functional receptor for the SARS coronavirus. *Nature.* 2003;426(6965):450–454.
65. Tu C, et al. Antibodies to SARS coronavirus in civets. *Emerg Infect Dis.* 2004;10(12):2244–2248.
66. Wu D, et al. Civets are equally susceptible to experimental infection by two different severe acute respiratory syndrome coronavirus isolates. *J Virol.* 2005;79(4):2620–2625.
67. Lau SK, et al. Severe acute respiratory syndrome coronavirus-like virus in Chinese horseshoe bats. *Proc Natl Acad Sci U S A.* 2005;102(39):14040–14045.
68. Hu D, et al. Genomic characterization and infectivity of a novel SARS-like coronavirus in Chinese bats. *Emerg Microbes Infect.* 2018;7(1):154.
69. Ge XY, et al. Isolation and characterization of a bat SARS-like coronavirus that uses the ACE2 receptor. *Nature.* 2013;503(7477):535–538.
70. De Clercq E. Potential antivirals and antiviral strategies against SARS coronavirus infections. *Expert Rev Anti Infect Ther.* 2006;4(2):291–302.
71. Wang WK, et al. Temporal relationship of viral load, ribavirin, interleukin (IL)-6, IL-8, and clinical progression in patients with severe acute respiratory syndrome. *Clin Infect Dis.* 2004;39(7):1071–1075.
72. Sung JJ, et al. Severe acute respiratory syndrome: report of treatment and outcome after a major outbreak. *Thorax.* 2004;59(5):414–420.
73. Knowles SR, et al. Common adverse events associated with the use of ribavirin for severe acute respiratory syndrome in Canada. *Clin Infect Dis.* 2003;37(8):1139–1142.
74. Cinatl J, et al. Development of antiviral therapy for severe acute respiratory syndrome. *Antiviral Res.* 2005;66(2–3):81–97.
75. Chen XP, Cao Y. Consideration of highly active antiretroviral therapy in the prevention and treatment of severe acute respiratory syndrome. *Clin Infect Dis.* 2004;38(7):1030–1032.
76. Chan KS, et al. Treatment of severe acute respiratory syndrome with lopinavir/ritonavir: a multicentre retrospective matched cohort study. *Hong Kong Med J.* 2003;9(6):399–406.
77. Yu WC, Hui DS, Chan-Yeung M. Antiviral agents and corticosteroids in the treatment of severe acute respiratory syndrome (SARS). *Thorax.* 2004;59(8):643–645.
78. Peiris JS, et al. Clinical progression and viral load in a community outbreak of coronavirus-associated SARS pneumonia: a prospective study. *Lancet.* 2003;361(9371):1767–1772.
79. Hsu LY, et al. Severe acute respiratory syndrome (SARS) in Singapore: clinical features of index patient and initial contacts. *Emerg Infect Dis.* 2003;9(6):713.
80. Franks TJ, et al. Lung pathology of severe acute respiratory syndrome (SARS): a study of 8 autopsy cases from Singapore. *Hum Pathol.* 2003;34(8):743–748.
81. Zhao FC, Guo KJ, Li ZR. Osteonecrosis of the femoral head in SARS patients: seven years later. *Eur J Orthop Surg Traumatol.* 2013;23(6):671–677.
82. Zhao R, et al. Steroid therapy and the risk of osteonecrosis in SARS patients: a dose-response meta-analysis. *Osteoporos Int.* 2017;28(3):1027–1034.
83. Zhang Z, et al. Purification of severe acute respiratory syndrome hyperimmune globulins for intravenous injection from convalescent plasma. *Transfusion.* 2005;45(7):1160–1164.
84. Mair-Jenkins J, et al. The effectiveness of convalescent plasma and hyperimmune immunoglobulin for the treatment of severe acute respiratory infections of viral etiology: a systematic review and exploratory meta-analysis. *J Infect Dis.* 2015;211(1):80–90.
85. Yeh KM, et al. Experience of using convalescent plasma for severe acute respiratory syndrome among healthcare workers in a Taiwan hospital. *J Antimicrob Chemother.* 2005;56(5):919–922.
86. Lipsitch M, et al. Transmission dynamics and control of severe acute respiratory syndrome. *Science.* 2003;300(5627):1966–1970.
87. St John RK, et al. Border screening for SARS. *Emerg Infect Dis.* 2005;11(1):6–10.
88. Glass K, Becker NG. Evaluation of measures to reduce international spread of SARS. *Epidemiol Infect.* 2006;134(5):1092–1101.
89. Chau PH, Yip PS. Monitoring the severe acute respiratory syndrome epidemic and assessing effectiveness of interventions in Hong Kong special administrative region. *J Epidemiol Community Health.* 2003;57(10):766–769.
90. Hsieh YH, et al. Quarantine for SARS, Taiwan. *Emerg Infect Dis.* 2005;11(2):278–282.

91. Tai DY. SARS: how to manage future outbreaks? *Ann Acad Med Singapore.* 2006;35(5):368–373.
92. Fung CP, et al. Rapid creation of a temporary isolation ward for patients with severe acute respiratory syndrome in Taiwan. *Infect Control Hosp Epidemiol.* 2004;25(12):1026–1032.
93. Loutfy MR, et al. Hospital preparedness and SARS. *Emerg Infect Dis.* 2004;10(5):771–776.
94. Li Y, et al. An evaluation of the ventilation performance of new SARS isolation wards in nine hospitals in Hong Kong. *Indoor Built Environ.* 2007;16(5):400–410.
95. Sars hospital opens in China. In: *The Guardian*; 2003. Available from: https://www.theguardian.com/world/2003/may/02/china.sars.
96. Schull MJ, et al. Effect of widespread restrictions on the use of hospital services during an outbreak of severe acute respiratory syndrome. *CMAJ.* 2007;176(13):1827–1832.
97. Chen TA, Lai KH, Chang HT. Impact of a severe acute respiratory syndrome outbreak in the emergency department: an experience in Taiwan. *Emerg Med J.* 2004;21(6):660–662.
98. Man CY, et al. Impact of SARS on an emergency department in Hong Kong. *Emerg Med.* 2003;15(5–6):418–422.
99. Ahmad A, Krumkamp R, Reintjes R. Controlling SARS: a review on China's response compared with other SARS-affected countries. *Trop Med Int Health.* 2009;14(Suppl 1): 36–45.
100. World Health Organization. WHO extends its SARS-related travel advice to Beijing and Shanxi Province (China) and to Toronto (Canada), 23 April 2003. *Wkly Epidemiol Rec.* 2003;78(17):137–138. Available from: https://apps.who.int/iris/bitstream/handle/10665/232151/WER7817_137-138.PDF?sequence=1.
101. World Health Organization. WHO recommended measures for persons undertaking international travel from areas affected by severe acute respiratory syndrome (SARS). *Wkly Epidemiol Rec.* 2003;78(14):97–99. Available from: https://www.who.int/publications/i/item/weekly-epidemiological-record-78-97-120.
102. Lee JW, McKibbin WJ. Estimating the global economic costs of SARS. In: Knobler S, Mahmoud A, Lemon S, et al., eds. *Institute of Medicine (US) Forum on Microbial Threats.* Washington (DC): National Academies Press (US); 2004. Learning from SARS: Preparing for the Next Disease Outbreak: Workshop Summary.
103. World Health Organization. Summary of Probable SARS Cases With Onset of Illness From 1 November 2002 to 31 July 2003. Geneva: World Health Organization; 2003. Available from: https://www.who.int/publications/m/item/summary-of-probable-sars-cases-with-onset-of-illness-from-1-november-2002-to-31-july-2003.
104. Lim PL, et al. Laboratory-acquired severe acute respiratory syndrome. *N Engl J Med.* 2004;350(17):1740–1745.
105. Normile D. SARS experts want labs to improve safety practices. *Science.* 2003;302(5642):31.
106. Normile D. Mounting lab accidents raise SARS fears. *Science.* 2004;304(5671):659–661.
107. Normile D. Second lab accident fuels fears about SARS. *Science.* 2004;303(5654):26.
108. World Health Organization. China's Latest SARS Outbreak Has Been Contained, But Biosafety Concerns Remain—Update 7. Geneva: World Health Organization; 2004. Available from: https://www.who.int/emergencies/disease-outbreak-news/item/2004_05_18a-en.
109. Wang L, et al. The development and reform of public health in China from 1949 to 2019. *Global Health.* 2019;15(1):45.
110. Wong ATY, et al. From SARS to avian influenza preparedness in Hong Kong. *Clin Infect Dis.* 2017;64(Suppl_2):S98–S104.
111. Sadarangani S, et al. Use of healthcare worker sickness absenteeism surveillance as a potential early warning system for influenza epidemics in acute care hospitals. *Ann Acad Med Singapore.* 2010;39(4):341–342.
112. Ministry of Health. Pandemic Preparedness; 2014. Available from: https://https://www.moh.gov.sg/diseases-updates/being-prepared-for-a-pandemic.
113. Yen MY, et al. From SARS in 2003 to H1N1 in 2009: lessons learned from Taiwan in preparation for the next pandemic. *J Hosp Infect.* 2014;87(4):185–193.
114. National Advisory Committee on SARS and Public Health. *Learning from SARS: Renewal of Public Health in Canada—Report of the National Advisory Committee on SARS and Public Health*; 2003. Available from: https://www.canada.ca/en/public-health/services/reports-publications/learning-sars-renewal-public-health-canada.html.
115. How Humber River Hospital was Designed With Pandemics In Mind; 2020. Available from: https://www.hrhfoundation.ca/blog/how-humber-river-hospital-was-designed-with-pandemics-in-mind/.
116. Cheng VC, et al. Severe acute respiratory syndrome coronavirus as an agent of emerging and reemerging infection. *Clin Microbiol Rev.* 2007;20(4):660–694.
117. Li YD, et al. Coronavirus vaccine development: from SARS and MERS to COVID-19. *J Biomed Sci.* 2020;27(1):1–23.
118. Gretebeck LM, Subbarao K. Animal models for SARS and MERS coronaviruses. *Curr Opin Virol.* 2015;13:123–129.
119. Shaw K. The 2003 SARS outbreak and its impact on infection control practices. *Public Health.* 2006;120(1):8–14.
120. Li W, et al. Bats are natural reservoirs of SARS-like coronaviruses. *Science.* 2005;310(5748):676–679.
121. Drexler JF, et al. Genomic characterization of severe acute respiratory syndrome-related coronavirus in European bats and classification of coronaviruses based on partial RNA-dependent RNA polymerase gene sequences. *J Virol.* 2010;84(21):11336–11349.
122. Tong S, et al. Detection of novel SARS-like and other coronaviruses in bats from Kenya. *Emerg Infect Dis.* 2009;15(3):482–485.
123. Hu B, et al. Discovery of a rich gene pool of bat SARS-related coronaviruses provides new insights into the origin of SARS coronavirus. *PLoS Pathog.* 2017;13(11), e1006698.

124. Woo PC, Lau SK, Yuen KY. Infectious diseases emerging from Chinese wet-markets: zoonotic origins of severe respiratory viral infections. *Curr Opin Infect Dis.* 2006;19(5):401–407.
125. Woo PC, et al. Comparative analysis of 22 coronavirus HKU1 genomes reveals a novel genotype and evidence of natural recombination in coronavirus HKU1. *J Virol.* 2006;80(14):7136–7145.
126. Weinstein RA. Planning for epidemics—the lessons of SARS. *N Engl J Med.* 2004;350(23):2332–2334.

CHAPTER 11

Middle East Respiratory Syndrome

SARAH SHALHOUB[a,b] • ZIAD A. MEMISH[c,d,e] • YASEEN M. ARABI[f,g]
[a]Department of Medicine, Division of Infectious Diseases, Schulich School of Medicine and Dentistry, University of Western Ontario, London, ON, Canada • [b]King Fahad Armed Forces Hospital, Jeddah, Saudi Arabia • [c]College of Medicine, Alfaisal University, Riyadh, Saudi Arabia • [d]Research & Innovation Center, King Saud Medical City, Ministry of Health, Riyadh, Saudi Arabia • [e]Hubert Department of Global Health, Rollins School of Public Health, Emory University, Atlanta, GA, United States • [f]College of Medicine, King Saud Bin Abdulaziz University for Health Sciences, King Abdullah International Medical Research Center, Riyadh, Saudi Arabia • [g]Intensive Care Department, King Abdulaziz Medical City, National Guard Health Affairs, Riyadh, Saudi Arabia

INTRODUCTION

Middle East Respiratory Syndrome Coronavirus (MERS-CoV) is a novel betacoronavirus that was first reported in 2012.[1] It was isolated from respiratory samples of a middle-aged man from the city of Bisha who was admitted to a hospital in Jeddah, Kingdom of Saudi Arabia (KSA), with severe and fatal pneumonia. Failure to identify a causative organism using bacterial cultures and respiratory viral multiplex PCR prompted the treating physician to perform viral cultures on respiratory samples, which revealed cytopathic effects. The samples were sent to the Erasmus Medical Center in the Netherlands, and genetic sequencing revealed a novel coronavirus. It was initially named human betacoronavirus 2c EMC, after Erasmus Medical Center. The announcement of the discovery of the novel coronavirus prompted researchers from Zarqa, Jordan, to test for MERS-CoV from two saved samples obtained from patients who had succumbed to an acute respiratory disease. These two patients were among 13 individuals who had developed severe pneumonia with an unidentified etiology in April 2012. The stored samples tested positive for MERS-CoV real-time reverse transcription polymerase chain reaction (rRT-PCR).[2] Subsequently, several names were given to the same virus (human betacoronavirus 2c England-Qatar, human betacoronavirus 2C Jordan-N3, betacoronavirus England 1). To avoid the lack of uniformity in naming the virus, the Coronavirus Study Group (CSG) of the International Committee on Taxonomy of Viruses eventually named the virus MERS-CoV after global consensus, as all the initial cases were geographically linked to the Middle East.[3]

Coronaviruses are known to cause human disease, and the endemic viruses (HCoV-229E, HCoV-NL63, HCoV-HKU1, and HCoV-OC43) are associated with mild respiratory symptoms and are a cause of the common cold. MERS-CoV was the second novel coronavirus to be recognized in the 21st century, emerging after SARS-CoV, which caused an international outbreak in 2002–03, followed more recently by SARS-CoV-2, which caused the coronavirus disease 19 (COVID-19) pandemic.

EPIDEMIOLOGY

Following the first report of the confirmed MERS-CoV case in Jeddah in September of 2012 and the retrospective report that followed from the Jordan cluster from March-April 2012, the number of reported cases increased, and the majority were acquired in the Arabian Peninsula (Saudi Arabia, the United Arab Emirates, and Qatar). There were also cases who traveled to several continents, including Europe, the United States of America, North Africa, and the Far East.

As of May 2024, the WHO has been notified of 2613 laboratory-confirmed cases of MERS-CoV infection in 27 countries. To date, the case fatality rate is 36% (943/2613) and notably lower than that reported in published case series (Fig. 1).[4,5] This may represent reporting bias in which the cases reported in cohort studies include those that usually require hospitalization

Viral Outbreaks, Biosecurity, and Preparing for Mass Casualty Infectious Diseases Events
https://doi.org/10.1016/B978-0-323-54841-0.00004-4

and are more likely to be tested. In general, surveillance systems that identify symptomatic individuals may not capture pauci- or asymptomatic individuals, which may contribute to an overestimation of the overall reported mortality rate for MERS.

Much of the reported MERS cases are sporadic and endemic to certain geographic regions in the Middle East. Except for a large outbreak in the Republic of South Korea in 2015,[6–8] the number of cases transmitted to other countries by travel has been limited. In the United States, two cases were reported in travelers from KSA[9,10]; other countries that reported travel-associated cases include the United Kingdom, France, Germany, Italy, Greece, Austria, Turkey, Lebanon, Yemen, Tunisia, Algeria, the Netherlands, China, Malaysia, Thailand, the Philippines, Egypt, and Bahrain.[11–16] Notably, cases of MERS have declined substantially in 2020 and 2021, with only 66 cases reported. This decline is probably at least partially related to the community-wide precautions taken with the COVID-19 pandemic.[17]

Ninety-eight percent of cases are reported in adults, defined as 14 years or older. Infection in children is rare; the reason for this is unknown.[18,19] Over 65% of confirmed reported cases occur in males.[20] Community clusters have been reported mostly in individuals where index cases were exposed either directly or indirectly to camels or camel products.[21–23] Some clusters were also likely related to transmission from asymptomatic cases.[23] However, the majority increase in the number of reported cases is related to hospital or healthcare-related outbreaks resulting from nosocomial transmission in places with shared ventilation such as open emergency departments, hemodialysis units, and medical wards.[24–27] The geographic areas of risk are likely linked to a number of factors; most importantly, overcrowding, lack of screening and early case identification, concentration of high-risk patients with multiple comorbidities, and failure to isolate confirmed cases, particularly in emergency departments.[24,27,28] Additionally, in experimental studies, the virus survives the longest on surfaces in low temperature and humidity environments for up to 5 days, similar to conditions in hospitals. This finding was confirmed in clinical settings where MERS-CoV was recovered from

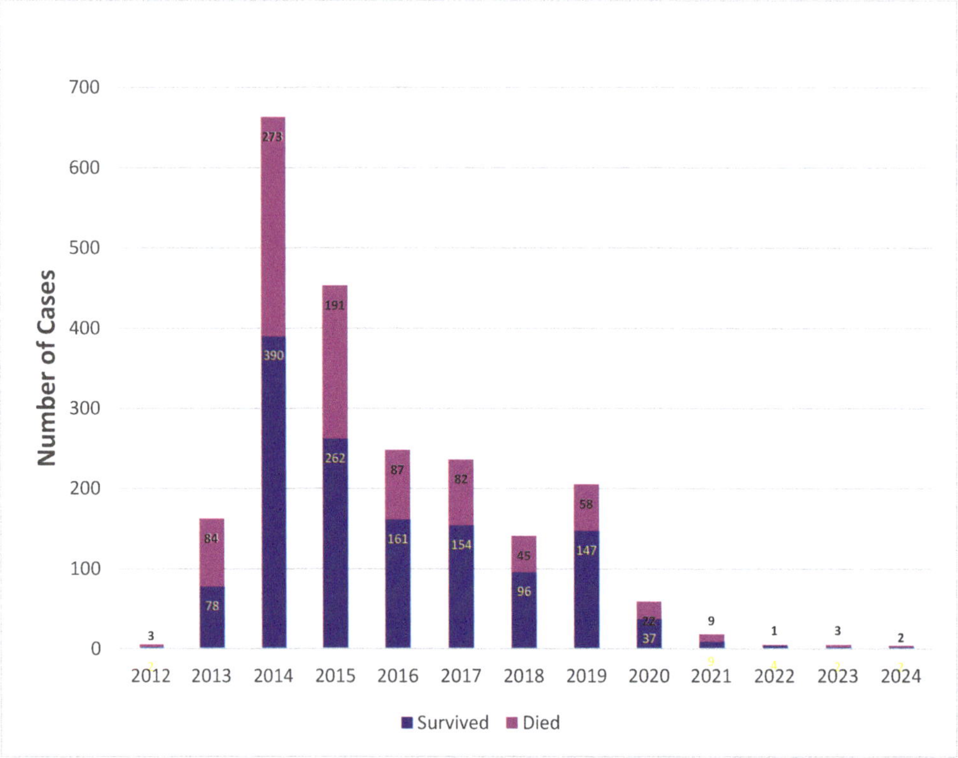

FIG. 1 Epidemic curve of MERS-CoV cases in KSA, total 2204 cases and 860 deaths reported (2012-April 2024). The figure was generated using data published by the WHO.[4]

environmental samples around MERS cases for extended periods of time.[29–32] However, with an effective reproduction number (R0) of <1, the epidemic potential of MERS-CoV is considered low, and amplification into an outbreak is unlikely unless viral mutations that render it more fit emerge.[32,33]

The seroprevalence of MERS-CoV antibodies, when measured, is less than 2.3% of the population in western KSA.[34] Community transmission is rare, and the secondary transmission rate between humans has been estimated to be 4% in community cluster cases.[20] Most transmissions have been reported in family clusters when individuals are exposed to an infectious case. Yet, in mass gatherings, such as during Hajj, where there was a major concern for transmission due to the theoretical epidemic potential, no MERS cases were identified. This finding is in the setting of intensive surveillance and the implementation of other pre- and post-Hajj prevention strategies.[35] Surveillance after returning from Hajj uncovered MERS-CoV from two patients returning to Germany. However, history of contact with camels presented a probable source for MERS-CoV.[16]

ANIMAL HOSTS OF MERS-COV

MERS-CoV is a zoonotic disease and may have several natural hosts. How it is transmitted among these hosts and to humans is not fully understood.

BATS

Bats are the known natural hosts for several coronaviruses and are considered one of the main reservoirs for the betacoronaviruses that resemble MERS-CoV and have been considered as a potential candidate for interspecies transmission. Fecal bat samples were collected from the surrounding geographic area where an index human case was identified in the Bisha area of KSA. Importantly, 190 nucleotide fragments of MERS-CoV RNA from an Egyptian tomb bat coronavirus were genetically identical to those of the first patient MERS-CoV genome isolate.[36] Closely related coronaviruses were isolated from South African vesper, leading some to consider them as the origin of the virus.[37,38] Still, MERS-CoV has not been detected in bats, and contact of human MERS cases with bats has not been reported.

CAMELS

While camels are thought to be one of the sources, and perhaps an intermediary source, of MERS-CoV infections, their role in human infections is not fully understood.[38,39] A number of confirmed MERS cases in humans were identified in individuals with a clear exposure history to camels.[39]

Evidence of Past Infection

MERS-CoV neutralizing antibodies were found in sera collected from dromedary camels from the Arabian Peninsula, North and East Africa, and Pakistan, as well as Jordan.[40–49] The seroprevalence of MERS-CoV in camels from the Gulf region is higher than in camels in Europe.[43] Additionally, MERS-CoV antibodies were detected in stored camel sera from as early as the 1990s.[45,46,48,49]

Evidence of Active Infection

Active infection is defined as a documented rise in MERS-CoV neutralizing antibody titers in addition to positive RT-PCR in symptomatic camels.[50,51] To confirm whether MERS-CoV can induce clinical infection in camels, Adney and colleagues experimentally inoculated camels with MERS-CoV. As a result, clinical manifestations of a mild upper respiratory tract infection, namely fever and rhinorrhea, occurred. Viable MERS-CoV was isolated in cultures of nasal swab samples from those camels, and seroconversion was documented 14 days postinoculation.[50] Samples collected from multiple anatomical sites from camels were found positive for MERS-CoV RT-PCR. Samples obtained from nasal swabs carried the highest frequency of positivity as well as the highest viral loads, as reflected by the lower cycle threshold values compared to oral and rectal swabs.[50–52]

This suggests that clinical presentations in camels vary from asymptomatic to symptomatic, generally with mild respiratory symptoms. Severe respiratory tract manifestations have not been reported in dromedary camels. It is noteworthy that prior infection may not offer a long-lasting immunity as MERS-CoV RT-PCR was documented in nasal secretions of camels that have prior evidence of MERS-CoV infection, evidenced by seropositivity.[51]

Evidence of Camel-to-Human Transmission

In 2013, human MERS-CoV infection was confirmed after exposure to an infected camel in Jeddah, KSA. Analysis of the whole human-derived virus and 15% of the camel-derived virus sequence yielded identical nucleotide polymorphism signatures suggestive of cross-species transmission.[53,54] Moreover, two other and unrelated confirmed human cases had a significant epidemiological history of visiting a camel slaughterhouse in Qatar.[55] A subsequent investigation took place where nasal, oral, and rectal swabs were collected from pre and postmortem camels. Up to 29% of samples tested for MERS-CoV RT-PCR were positive.[52] Rooting the phylogenetic tree of MERS-CoV in relation to coronaviruses isolated from bats and dromedary camels suggests that MERS-CoV developed in camels where they acted as a mixing vessel for the virus before transmitting it to humans.[56]

MERS-CoV full genomes were isolated from camels and were successfully replicated in human cells in vitro suggesting camels as a potential source of human MERS-CoV infection.[57] Camel milk, which is a popular drink among some people who live in the Arabian Peninsula, tested positive for MERS-CoV RT-PCR yet the role of contaminated milk in transmission to humans remains unclear.[42]

While there are pieces that need to be clarified, this elegant body of evidence to date strongly supports camels as a likely source of MERS-CoV infection for humans.

Occupational Studies

A national serological survey in Saudi Arabia demonstrated a very low seroprevalence of MERS-CoV in the general population, which may explain why community transmission is a minimal feature of this infection.[47] Importantly, the seroprevalence was 15 times higher among camel shepherds and 23 times higher among slaughterhouse workers compared to the general population. Seropositive individuals failed to recall symptoms of an MERS-CoV-like infection.[53] Hence, individuals who have close contact with dromedary camels were more likely to have MERS-CoV neutralizing antibodies than those who do not. These data further support that a spectrum of illness exists and includes those who are asymptomatic or minimally symptomatic.[55] The overall low national seroprevalence of MERS-CoV in an endemic country like KSA could be explained by the fact that IgG antibodies against MERS-CoV are not persistent. For example, another study failed, however, to identify MERS-CoV neutralizing antibodies in sera of slaughterhouse workers or shepherds who were in direct contact with infected camels in Western and Southern provinces of Saudi Arabia.[47,58,59]

MERS-COV AND OTHER ANIMALS

To test the ability of MERS-CoV to infect other animals, artificial nasal inoculation of sheep, goats, and horses did not result in clinical symptoms or viral shedding.[60] Apart from neutralizing MERS-CoV antibody detection in young goats, none of the other tested species had evidence of MERS-CoV infection 4 weeks following inoculation.[60] In a seroprevalence study in Jordan that included a variety of animals, camels, goats, and cattle. Only camels were found to harbor MERS-CoV antibodies, whereas goats and cattle were notably negative for neutralizing antibodies.[41]

Virology

Coronaviruses are enveloped RNA viruses that cause community-acquired respiratory tract infections in humans. MERS-CoV is a novel positive-sense, single-stranded RNA virus with a genomic size of 30,000 nucleotides.[61] It is a member of the Coronaviridae family (order: Nidovirales; family: Coronaviridae; subfamily: Coronavirinae; genus: *Betacoronavirus*; lineage: C). It is the first betacoronavirus of the lineage C group known to infect humans.[1,62,63] It is phylogenetically distinct from previously known betacoronavirus species such as the bat coronaviruses HKU4, HKU5 from the C lineage, human coronavirus HKU1 and OC43, from the lineage A group, the SARS from the lineage B group, and HKU9 from the D lineage as well SARS-CoV-2.[63,64]

MERS-CoV is further classified into two clades: clade A (the earliest cluster of infection: EMC/2012 and Jordan N3/2012) and clade B (new clusters that are genetically distinct from clade A).[32] Replication takes place in the host-cell cytoplasm. The virus gains entry by binding its spike glycoprotein to the functional receptor dipeptidyl (DPP4), also known as CD26, on the host-cell surface. Binding is mediated by a receptor-binding domain on the S1 subunit of the spike (S) proteins on the virus' surface.[65,66] The membrane fusion and entry are facilitated by the S2 subunit by the actions of 2 heptad repeat domains (HR1 and HR2) and a fusion protein.[67]

DPP4 is expressed on epithelial and endothelial cells of several human organs including respiratory (type l and type ll alveolar cells, ciliated and nonciliated bronchial epithelium, endothelium), renal, intestinal, and liver cells. This wide expression may explain the multisystem involvement of severe MERS manifested by severe pneumonia and respiratory distress, gastrointestinal symptoms, elevated liver enzymes, and renal failure. The virus was also found to bind to DPP4 receptors in other species, such as camels, sheep, goats, and nonhuman primates.[63]

CONFIRMING MERS-COV INFECTION

MERS-CoV infection is confirmed by the gold standard MERS-CoV reverse transcription polymerase chain reaction (RT-PCR) from a respiratory tract sample.

Additionally, rising antibody titer can be used to confirm infection; however, its' value in establishing a diagnosis during the acute phase may be limited.

MOLECULAR TESTING

The recommended RT-PCR assay includes a screening assay targeting the upstream region of E protein gene[68] and a confirmatory assay targeting the open reading frame 1a (ORF 1a) or open reading frame 1b (ORF 1b). ORF assays are generally less sensitive than the screening assay but are more specific.[68,69] World Health Organization[5] recommends performing the screening assay first; if positive, the confirmatory (ORF 1a or ORF 1b) assay should then be performed.[69] If the confirmatory assay is positive, then MERS-CoV infection is confirmed. If the (ORF 1a) assay is negative and the case and epidemiologic context are both highly suggestive then repeating the confirmatory test is suggested, or performing sequencing assays (RdRpSeq or NSeq) should be done.[69]

SEROLOGY

Serologic testing to confirm MERS-CoV infection includes enzyme-linked immunosorbent assay,[70] indirect fluorescent antibody (IFA), and a serum neutralization assay.[69] WHO and CDC require evidence for seroconversion in at least one screening assay (i.e., IFA, ELISA) and confirmation by a neutralization assay in a minimum of two samples taken 14 to 21 days apart to confirm the diagnosis. The first sample should be collected within 14 days after the onset of symptoms.[69,71,72] A single sample with a positive screening assay (IFA or ELISA) and confirmation by a neutralization assay in a single specimen would constitute a probable case.[73,74]

False-positive tests may occur as a result of cross-reactivity with other betacoronaviruses such as OC43 or HKU1 if IFA testing is done alone.[69]

VIRAL CULTURE

Although MERS-CoV has been isolated in cell cultures from respiratory tract specimens, performing routine viral cultures for diagnostic purposes is not recommended, as viral cultures for MERS-CoV require high bio-safety level facilities.[75]

VIRAL KINETICS

Lower respiratory tract samples have a higher viral load compared to nasopharyngeal swabs and thus have a better yield in confirming the diagnosis.[76,77] Shedding in respiratory tract samples, for longer than 30 days, was documented in asymptomatic patients, patients with a compromised immune system, and critically ill patients, particularly in those who received corticosteroids[20,77,78] (Arabi, 2017 #22).[79] Positive RT-PCR from blood samples obtained at the time of diagnosis was indicative of a severe outcome, evidenced by a greater need for mechanical ventilation and extracorporeal membrane oxygenation and a possibly higher mortality.[77,80]

CLINICAL PRESENTATION

As confirmed cases began to emerge and the number of reported cases to the WHO started increasing, the need for case definitions to provide needed guidance to public health officials and practitioners became obvious. Definitions for possible, probable, and definite cases have been established to help clinicians as well as standardize reporting.[5] The initial reports of patients with confirmed MERS described severe and potentially fatal pneumonia in hospitalized patients in the Middle East, which led the WHO and CDC to include a travel history to the Middle East, hospitalization, and severe pneumonia to define cases.[73] Those definitions were crucial to facilitate rapid detection of possible cases and facilitate isolation to avoid hospital outbreaks.[81] As more reports emerged, hospitalization was removed from the revised WHO interim case definitions.[5]

Subsequently, and upon performing epidemiological and cluster investigations, confirmed MERS was documented in asymptomatic or minimally symptomatic patients who have no animal contact.[19–21] This further emphasized the possibility of human-to-human transmission, particularly after demonstrating viral shedding in recovering individuals, which may extend to 3 and in some cases 5 weeks.[78,79,82,83]

In 2013, a number of descriptive cohort studies provided much-needed information that helped elucidate MERS clinical presentation.[84] Assiri and colleagues reported clinical characteristics of 47 confirmed MERS cases. National and international authorities such as the WHO, CDC, and the Ministry of Health of Saudi Arabia incorporated these data into their updated case definitions.

Ninety-eight percent of confirmed MERS cases presented with fever (Table 1). Consequently, the presence of fever was strongly emphasized and included as a prerequisite in those case definitions. Subsequent cohort studies, however, described variable clinical presentations of cases where absence of fever or respiratory symptoms was documented.[77,85,87] Case definitions

TABLE 1
Clinical and Laboratory Characteristics of Confirmed MERS Cases in Different Cohort Studies

Clinical or Laboratory Feature	Assiri[84] ($n=47$)	Al-Tawfiq[85] ($n=17$)	AlGhamdi[86] ($n=51$)	Shalhoub[77] ($n=32$)	Saad[87] ($n=70$)	Arabi[88] ($n=330$)
Fever	98%	40%	49%	84%	61.5%	75%
Cough	83%	86%	80%	84%	54%	69%
SOB	72%	67%	NA	70%	60%	75%
Sputum	36%	NA	NA	70%	24%	39%
Myalgia	32%	7%	NA	NA	20%	19.4%
Vomiting	21%	7%	23%	13%	30%	18%
Diarrhea	26%	7%	25%	19%	30%	12%
Death	59%	76%	37%	75%	60%	66%
Leukopenia ($<4\times10^9$/L)	14%	0%	54%	54%	NA	20%
Lymphopenia ($<1.5\times10^9$/L)	34%	35%	35%	NA	NA	NA
Thrombocytopenia ($<150\times10^9$/L)	36%	NA	NA	29%	NA	39%
Increased LDH (>280 U/L)	49%	47%	47%	63%	NA	NA
Increased Alt (>40 U/L)	11%	18%	18%	45%	31%	39%
Abnormal chest X-ray	100%	100%	100%	81%	90%	100%

SOB, shortness of breath; *LDH*, lactate dehydrogenase; *Alt*, alanine aminotransferase.

were updated to accommodate those variable clinical presentations.

Therefore, MERS has a wide range of clinical presentations that range from absence of symptoms or mild upper respiratory tract symptoms to severe pneumonia with multiple organ failure.[89,90] That realization was crucial to avoid diagnostic delays which particularly occurred in older individuals who often had atypical presentations that either stemmed from their lack of fever at presentation or overlapped with other medical conditions or bacterial infections.

Most patients present after a median incubation period of 5.2 days (95% CI 1.9–14.7 days) with fever and respiratory tract symptoms that include the following: cough, which is most commonly dry, productive of sputum, or in a minority of cases accompanied by hemoptysis as well as shortness of breath.[24] Twelve to 30% of cases in MERS cohorts presented with gastrointestinal symptoms that included vomiting or diarrhea or both. Some also presented with abdominal pain in the presence or absence of respiratory symptoms.[78,87,91,92] Patients may also present with fatigue and myalgia sometimes in the absence of significant respiratory manifestations (Table 1).[78,85] The latter two presentations caused cases to be missed initially since they were not originally recognized as possible clinical manifestations of MERS.

Diagnostic delays have been reported, particularly in elderly patients with atypical presentations (i.e., lack of fever at presentation or overlap with other medical conditions or bacterial infections).[93]

NATURAL COURSE OF MERS

As the clinical presentation is highly variable and ranges from no symptoms to rapidly progressive pneumonia, the natural course of MERS is variable as well. Where complete recovery is expected in asymptomatic cases, a longer, more difficult course is expected in symptomatic, particularly high-risk, cases.

The median time from symptom onset to death ranges from 16.5 to 20.5 days in cohort studies.[85,87] The median time to viral clearance, documented by negative RT-PCR on respiratory specimens, is 11 days (range 6 to 38 days). However, it could be longer, particularly in immunocompromised cases and in patients on steroids.[77,83].

In patients who survived, the median time from symptom onset to discharge from hospital in a cohort study was 27 days (range 20 to 31.5 days).[87]

LABORATORY FINDINGS

Laboratory findings typically include a normal or low white blood cell count (WBC) and lymphopenia. However, elevated WBC has been reported in some cohorts, particularly in the presence of coexisting bacterial infections.[77,84,85,87] Elevated aminotransferases, and more commonly, lactate dehydrogenase and acute kidney injury were reported as well (Table 1). Despite all the knowledge gained during the last 10 years when MERS-CoV emerged, it remains almost impossible to differentiate the clinical presentations of patients with MERS-CoV from patients presenting with other severe viral respiratory infections.[85]

RISK FACTORS FOR MERS, SEVERITY, AND MORTALITY

Risk factors for acquiring MERS depend on whether the exposure was in the community or the healthcare setting. However, factors predicting disease progression are similar. A hospital-based case-control study was done to compare those with MERS to control patients without infection who were admitted with pneumonia. Cases of confirmed MERS were significantly more likely to have diabetes mellitus (DM), obesity, and end-stage renal disease.[85] In a serologic investigation of extended family contacts of a confirmed MERS case, close contact, including contact with respiratory secretions, male gender, older age, and the presence of comorbid medical conditions were identified at a higher frequency in those that acquired MERS compared to those who did not.[88] Another case-control study aimed to elucidate the risk factors of acquiring MERS in the community and revealed that contact with dromedary camels or simply being in close proximity to camels posed a significant risk factor in acquiring MERS.[94]

Hospital outbreaks have been linked to delayed diagnosis of MERS cases, underrecognition of hospital-acquired cases, and lack of proper isolation and compliance with infection prevention practices leading to exposures among health care workers (HCWs), visitors, and other patients (Table 3). In a serologic surveillance study to screen HCWs for evidence of MERS-CoV infection, only HCWs who had close contact with confirmed MERS cases and did not appropriately use personal protective equipment (PPE) had serologic evidence of MERS-CoV infection.[91,95]

Furthermore, multiple studies identified older age, diabetes mellitus (DM), end-stage renal disease, heart disease, and smoking as risk factors for severity and increased mortality.[78,87,92,96–98] An important laboratory marker among confirmed MERS-CoV cases for increased severity and possibly mortality was a positive plasma MERS-CoV RT-PCR.[77] Lower cycle threshold values of MERS-CoV RT-PCR in nasopharyngeal swabs, which are inversely related to virus load, as well as lack of seroconversion, were significantly associated with death in a cohort of confirmed MERS cases.[77,87,88,99,100]

Management, Current Knowledge and Future Directions

Supportive management consists of oxygen therapy, fluids, and noninvasive or invasive mechanical ventilation as required.[88,96,101] Treatment strategies to date have focused on treating the virus and modulating the immune response. A cohort study demonstrated that corticosteroid therapy was not associated with a difference in mortality after adjusting for time-varying confounders. Moreover, it was associated with delayed MERS-CoV clearance.[83]

MERS-CoV was found to reduce the production of IFN-a and IFN-b.[97] On the other hand, interferon-a was found to inhibit the MERS-CoV-induced cytopathic response and viral replication,[102] particularly when combined with ribavirin.[103] Subsequent encouraging data from rhesus macaques that were treated with interferon-α2b and ribavirin 8 h after inoculation with MERS-CoV showed a lack of progression to pneumonia compared to no treatment.[104] Additionally, IC50 values were determined for different interferon compounds against MERS-CoV. The respective IC50 for IFN-β over IFN-α2b and IFN-α2a were 1.37, 21.4, and 160.8 U/mL, highlighting a probable favorable efficacy of IFN-β over IFN-α2b followed by IFN-α2a.[105] This evidence was supplemented by several retrospective small cohort studies that used different types of interferons for MERS treatment (Table 2). None of those studies revealed a sustained significant difference in survival, but interpretation is limited by the study design and small samples. In a large cohort study that included 349 critically ill patients with MERS-CoV pneumonia, none of the studied interferon types (rIFN-α2a, rIFN-α2b, or rIFN-β1a; none received rIFN-β1b) with or without ribavirin was associated with a reduction in 90-day mortality or faster viral clearance, after adjusting for time-varying confounders.[108] Recently, the MIRACLE randomized controlled trial demonstrated that a combination of recombinant interferon beta-1b and lopinavir-ritonavir resulted in lower 90-day mortality compared to placebo among patients who had been hospitalized with MERS, especially when treatment was started within 7 days after symptom onset.[109,110]

Other agents with potential antiviral activities, such as cyclosporine and mycophenolic acid, have been

TABLE 2
Use of Different Interferon Types in Human Studies

	AlTawfiq[106]	Omrani[107]	Shalhoub[77]	AlGhamdi[86]	Arabi[108]	Arabi[109]
Design	Single arm cohort	Retrospective comparative	Retrospective comparative	Retrospective cohort	Retrospective cohort	Randomized controlled trial
Intervention[a]	IFN-α2b	None vs IFN-α2a (180 μg × 2 w) + ribavirin[b] (8–10 d)	IFN-α2a + ribavirin vs IFN-β1a + ribavirin[c]	IFN-β in 23 IFN-α in 8 Mycophenolate in 8 Ribavirin in 7	RBV and/or rIFN-α2a, rIFN-α2b, or rIFN-β1a; none received rIFN-β1b	Interferon Beta-1b and Lopinavir-Ritonavir
Number	5	24 vs 20	13 vs 11	51	Of 349 patients, 144 (41.3%) patients received RBV/rIFN	95 patients
Primary endpoint	Survival	Survival at 14 days Survival at 28 days	In-hospital mortality	Overall mortality	90-day mortality	90-day mortality
Results (%) of primary end point	0%	70 vs 29%, $P=0.004$ 30 vs 17%, $P=0.054$	85 vs 64%, $P=0.24$	37%		
Comment	Median time from diagnosis to treatment was 19 days	Renal failure cases were excluded	Mortality observed in all renal failure cases	Confounded by using different combinations of antivirals-conclusions could not be made	After adjusting for baseline and time-varying confounders, RBV/rIFN was not associated with changes in 90-day mortality (adjusted odds ratio, 1.03 [95% confidence interval {CI}, 0.73–1.44]; $P=0.87$)	Risk difference of −19 percentage points (upper boundary of the 97.5% confidence interval [CI], −3; one-sided $P=0.024$)

[a]All patients received supportive therapy as required at baseline.
[b]Ribavirin 2 g loading, then 1200 Q8H for 4 days, then 600 Q8H for 4–6 days.
[c]Loading dose of 2 g orally followed by 600 mg orally every 12 h.

tested but have produced conflicting results so far and therefore have not demonstrated proven benefits in humans.[102,105] In a univariate analysis in a cohort of 51 patients, interferon beta as well as mycophenolate mofetil were predictors of survival. However, multivariate analysis rendered those results insignificant.[86]

Blocking DPP4 by antibodies was found to inhibit MERS-CoV binding and thus entry into the human bronchial epithelial cells.[65] A synthetic peptide (HR2P) that was developed to block the HR1 domain on the S2 subunit of the MERS-CoV virus has demonstrated potent antiviral effects in vitro.[63,111] An intranasal formulation of this drug (HR2P-M2) has been developed and was shown to be effective in protecting mice. Using HR2P in combination with interferon beta enhanced the protective effect.[112] Those peptides are yet to be tested on humans. A broad-spectrum antiviral (remdesivir), which is currently approved to treat SARS-CoV-2 infection, has been studied to treat MERS-CoV.[113] Human polyclonal immunoglobulin G from transchromosomic bovines has been shown to inhibit MERS-CoV in vivo and has undergone a phase 1 randomized double-blind, placebo-controlled trial for safety in human volunteers.[114,115]

VACCINE DEVELOPMENT

Different vaccine candidates have been explored. Achieving a balance between efficacy and safety is pivotal before a vaccine can be utilized. Spike protein has been an important target for vaccine development. Recent evidence that explored using the HR1 region and S1-subunit as potential vaccine targets revealed promising results, where immunization against S1-subunit elicited a balanced T-helper-1/T-helper-2 response and a high level of IgG isotypes in mice without compromising safety.[116,117] Recombinant adenovirus 5-based vaccine platform expressing a MERS-CoV S1-CD40L fusion protein yielded promising immunogenicity and potential efficacy in a transgenic human dipeptidyl peptidase mouse model.[118] There is no data on the utility of vaccines in humans yet. A recently published open-label, nonrandomized, dose-escalation, phase Ib trial demonstrated the safety and tolerability of a ChADOx1, a chimpanzee adenovirus vaccine vector targeted against MERS-CoV.[119] Cell and antibody-mediated immune responses were found to be stable at 6 months of follow-up.[119]

This study followed an earlier study conducted in the United Kingdom that similarly demonstrated the safety and tolerability of the ChADOx1 vectored vaccine.[120]

GLS-5300 is a DNA vaccine that expresses a full-length MERS-CoV S-glycoprotein antigen and has shown promising immunogenicity in mice and camels. A phase-1 human trial that included 75 participants assigned to 3 different doses has shown tolerability and immunogenicity against MERS-CoV.[121]

Promising data on camel vaccines were recently published. A modified vaccinia virus Ankara (MVA) vaccine that expresses the MERS-CoV spike protein has been shown to reduce MERS-CoV shedding in vaccinated compared to nonvaccinated camels.[122] This vaccine platform was also tested in a phase I study in humans that included a total of 26 study participants who were assigned to receive a high or a low dose of the vaccine followed by an identical booster dose 28 days later.[123] These cases were compared to healthy controls that did not receive the vaccine. Immunogenicity was assessed using neutralizing antibodies to assess humoral immune response as well as an IFN-γ-linked ELISpot testing to assess cell-mediated immune response. Both dose series were safe and immunogenic in this study.[123]

None of these vaccines have been licensed yet for human use; phase 2 studies to further examine these encouraging results on those different vaccines are awaited.

PREVENTION AND CHALLENGES

Since almost 45% of cases are acquired in healthcare settings (Table 3), early recognition and rapid isolation of suspected MERS cases, particularly in crowded areas of high-risk patients such as emergency departments

TABLE 3
MERS-CoV-Related Nosocomial Outbreak Reports

Setting and Population	HA Transmissions	Risk Factors for Infection	Contributing Factors
Al-Hasa, KSA; 3 hospitals; hemodialysis, ICU, in-patient units; HCWs[24]	23 confirmed cases, 11 probable cases; 2 HCWs	Male, age ≥ 50, DM, ESRD; HCW	Insufficient infection prevention measures; intra-facility transfers
Jordan; 1 Hospital April, 2012[2]	9 cases; 6 HCWs	HCW	Poor compliance with PPE; delayed case identification
3 ICUs, Riyadh & Al-Hasa, KSA, 12/2012–8/2013[124]	12 probable or confirmed cases; 1 HCW	Comorbid illness, HCW	Poor compliance with PPE; delayed case identification
Jeddah, KSA, 3–5/2014[27]	123 cases: 78 HCWs	Comorbid illness, renal dialysis, HCW	Insufficient infection control measures; delayed case identification
Korea: 44 hospitals, 5–7/2015[7]	186 cases; 13% HCWs; 44% caregivers	HCW, ED crowding, delayed isolation, extensive family visitation, sharing room or ward of the index patient	Insufficient infection control measures; delayed case identification; intra-hospital transfers
Riyadh, 1 Hospital, 6–9/2015[25]	130 confirmed or probable cases; 43 HCWs	ED crowding, uncontrolled patient movement, extensive family visitation, delayed isolation	Poor compliance with infection control recommendations, delayed case identification

HA, healthcare associated; *KSA*, Kingdom of Saudi Arabia; *HCW*, healthcare workers; *ED*, emergency department; *DM*, diabetes mellitus; *ESRD*, end-stage renal diseases.

and hemodialysis units is crucial. Several healthcare-associated outbreaks were fueled by unrecognized cases not being isolated and causing ongoing transmission. Furthermore, these unrecognized cases have been transferred between facilities augmenting transmission. For this reason, screening patients for symptoms, providing masks to those with respiratory symptoms waiting in triage areas, and following infection prevention and control precautions, including wearing personal protective equipment, are key to preventing the devastating consequences of healthcare outbreaks.[2,23,26,123] Moreover, in addition to case identification, tracing contacts, and identifying suspected cases as early as possible can prevent further MERS-CoV spread and potential outbreaks.[93] Once identified, the Saudi Ministry of Health recommends that suspected and confirmed cases be placed in droplet isolation, ideally in a single room airborne isolation is mandated for critically ill patients or those requiring aerosol-generating procedures. If a single room is not available, suspected cases may be cohorted and should be placed at least 1.2 m apart. HEPA filters may be used in the absence of negative pressure or single isolation rooms and should be turned on maximum power near the head of the patient although efficacy was not proven.[125]

These isolation guidelines vary, and in some countries, airborne and droplet or airborne and contact precautions are recommended. Maintaining cases in isolation for the appropriate duration of time is also an important practice. This further supported the potential of human-to-human transmission, particularly after demonstrating viral shedding in recovering individuals, which could extend up to 5 weeks.[79,81,84]

On the other hand, screening for possible cases has imposed major challenges on healthcare institutions' resources as the clinical and laboratory presentation of MERS overlaps with several other infections. Isolation rooms are limited in number, which necessitates around-the-clock molecular laboratory support to confirm or rule out MERS-CoV infection in suspected cases. Such molecular tests require equipment, laboratory space, and trained personnel and are considerably expensive. This is particularly relevant since most hospitals require two consecutive negative molecular tests, in confirmed cases, before isolation can be discontinued.[126,127] This exerts tremendous pressure on emergency departments in healthcare institutions dealing with patients presenting with respiratory symptoms in countries endemic to MERS-CoV. In KSA, for example, in 1 year, 57,363 persons with suspected MERS-CoV infection were identified and tested, but only 384 (0.7%) tested positive.[128] There is an urgent need to develop a highly sensitive and specific rapid point-of-care testing that can be applied in emergency rooms and outpatient clinics to rapidly identify and properly isolate MERS-CoV cases.

At the community level, healthcare authorities such as the Centers for Disease Prevention and Control (CDC), WHO, and the Saudi Ministry of Health have issued educational materials and started awareness campaigns to the public to educate them on recognizing signs and symptoms suggestive of MERS-CoV and simple measures of protection and isolation until seeking medical advice to avoid the spread of MERS-CoV within the community.[74,129] During 2017, the majority of reported cases have been sporadic community-acquired cases with either direct or indirect contact with camels or camel products.[10] Enforcing precautions in the community that include hand washing, wearing a mask, and protective clothing before and after camel or camel product contact in farms and slaughterhouses, which are recommended by the Saudi Ministry of Health, has been challenging as well, possibly due to cultural factors.[128,130–132] Certain measures have been taken to limit potential community outbreaks, such as the relocation of camel markets as well as the banning of camels from holy areas and intensive surveillance during Hajj.[131] However, the significant reduction in the rate of reported cases is encouraging, as healthcare institutions in the Middle East and other affected areas are now better equipped with knowledge to avoid future outbreaks. The significant drop in the number of reported MERS-CoV cases during the years of the SARS-CoV-2 pandemic further emphasizes the importance of infection prevention and control measures in decreasing community-acquired respiratory viral infections, including MERS-CoV.

REFERENCES

1. Zaki AM, van Boheemen S, Bestebroer TM, Osterhaus AD, Fouchier RA. Isolation of a novel coronavirus from a man with pneumonia in Saudi Arabia. *N Engl J Med.* 2012;367(19):1814–1820 [in eng] https://doi.org/10.1056/NEJMoa1211721.
2. Al-Abdallat MM, Payne DC, Alqasrawi S. Hospital-associated outbreak of Middle East respiratory syndrome coronavirus: a serologic, epidemiologic, and clinical description. *Clin Infect Dis.* 2014;59(9):1225–1233 [in eng] https://doi.org/10.1093/cid/ciu359.
3. de Groot RJ, Baker SC, Baric RS. Middle East respiratory syndrome coronavirus (MERS-CoV): announcement of the Coronavirus Study Group. *J Virol.* 2013;87(14):7790–7792 [in eng] https://doi.org/10.1128/jvi.01244-13.
4. WHO. Middle East respiratory syndrome coronavirus-Kingdom of Saudi Arabia. *Disease Outbreak News.* 2024. https://www.who.int/emergencies/disease-outbreak-news/item/2024-DON516.

5. WHO. Middle East Respiratory Syndrome Outbreak Toolbox; 2024. https://www.who.int/emergencies/outbreak-toolkit/disease-outbreak-toolboxes/mers-outbreak-toolbox.
6. Hui DS, Perlman S, Zumla A. Spread of MERS to South Korea and China. *Lancet Respir Med.* 2015;3(7):509–510 [in eng] https://doi.org/10.1016/s2213-2600(15)00238-6.
7. Ha KM. A lesson learned from the MERS outbreak in South Korea in 2015. *J Hosp Infect.* 2016;92(3):232–234 [in eng] https://doi.org/10.1016/j.jhin.2015.10.004.
8. Lee SI. Costly lessons from the 2015 Middle East respiratory syndrome coronavirus outbreak in Korea. *J Prev Med Public Health.* 2015;48(6):274–276 [in eng] https://doi.org/10.3961/jpmph.15.064.
9. CDC. CDC Announces First Case of Middle East Respiratory Syndrome Coronavirus Infection in the United States; 2014. https://www.cdc.gov/media/releases/2014/p0502-US-MERS.html.
10. WHO. Middle East Respiratory Syndrome Coronavirus-Kingdom of Saudi Arabia. *Disease Outbreak News.* 2025. https://www.who.int/emergencies/disease-outbreak-news/item/2025-DON560.
11. Seddiq N, Al-Qahtani M, Al-Tawfiq JA, Bukamal N. First confirmed case of Middle East respiratory syndrome coronavirus infection in the Kingdom of Bahrain: in a Saudi gentleman after cardiac bypass surgery. *Case Rep Infect Dis.* 2017;2017:1262838 [in eng] https://doi.org/10.1155/2017/1262838.
12. Puzelli S, Azzi A, Santini MG. Investigation of an imported case of Middle East Respiratory Syndrome Coronavirus (MERS-CoV) infection in Florence, Italy, May to June 2013. *Euro Surveill.* 2013;18(34). http://www.ncbi.nlm.nih.gov/pubmed/23987829.
13. Kraaij-Dirkzwager M, Timen A, Dirksen K. Middle East respiratory syndrome coronavirus (MERS-CoV) infections in two returning travellers in the Netherlands, May 2014. *Euro Surveill.* 2014;19(21) [in eng].
14. Abroug F, Slim A, Ouanes-Besbes L. Family cluster of Middle East respiratory syndrome coronavirus infections, Tunisia, 2013. *Emerg Infect Dis.* 2014;20(9):1527–1530 [in eng] https://doi.org/10.3201/eid2009.140378.
15. Guery B, Poissy J, el Mansouf L. Clinical features and viral diagnosis of two cases of infection with Middle East respiratory syndrome coronavirus: a report of nosocomial transmission. *Lancet.* 2013;381(9885):2265–2272 [in eng] https://doi.org/10.1016/s0140-6736(13)60982-4.
16. Reuss A, Litterst A, Drosten C, et al. Contact investigation for imported case of Middle East respiratory syndrome, Germany. *Emerg Infect Dis.* 2014;20(4):620–625. https://doi.org/10.3201/eid2004.131375. PMID: 24655721; PMCID: PMC3966395.
17. WHO. Middle East Respiratory Syndrome. MERS Situation Update; 2024. www.emro.who.int/health-topics/mers-cov/mers-outbreaks.html#:~:text=MERS%20situation%20update%2C%20January%202023,(CFR)%20of%2036%25.
18. Khuri-Bulos N, Payne DC, Lu X. Middle East respiratory syndrome coronavirus not detected in children hospitalized with acute respiratory illness in Amman, Jordan, march 2010 to September 2012. *Clin Microbiol Infect.* 2014;20(7):678–682 [in eng] https://doi.org/10.1111/1469-0691.12438.
19. Memish ZA, Al-Tawfiq JA, Assiri A. Middle East respiratory syndrome coronavirus disease in children. *Pediatr Infect Dis J.* 2014;33(9):904–906 [in eng] https://doi.org/10.1097/inf.0000000000000325.
20. Memish ZA, Al-Tawfiq JA, Makhdoom HQ. Screening for Middle East respiratory syndrome coronavirus infection in hospital patients and their healthcare worker and family contacts: a prospective descriptive study. *Clin Microbiol Infect.* 2014;20(5):469–474 [in eng] https://doi.org/10.1111/1469-0691.12562.
21. Memish ZA, Cotten M, Watson SJ. Community case clusters of Middle East respiratory syndrome coronavirus in Hafr Al-Batin, Kingdom of Saudi Arabia: a descriptive genomic study. *Int J Infect Dis.* 2014;23:63–68 [in eng] https://doi.org/10.1016/j.ijid.2014.03.1372.
22. Drosten C, Meyer B, Müller MA. Transmission of MERS-coronavirus in household contacts. *N Engl J Med.* 2014;371(9):828–835 [in eng] https://doi.org/10.1056/NEJMoa1405858.
23. Omrani AS, Matin MA, Haddad Q, Al-Nakhli D, Memish ZA, Albarrak AM. A family cluster of Middle East respiratory syndrome coronavirus infections related to a likely unrecognized asymptomatic or mild case. *Int J Infect Dis.* 2013;17(9):e668–e672 [in eng] https://doi.org/10.1016/j.ijid.2013.07.001.
24. Assiri A, McGeer A, Perl TM. Hospital outbreak of Middle East respiratory syndrome coronavirus. *N Engl J Med.* 2013;369(5):407–416 [in eng] https://doi.org/10.1056/NEJMoa1306742.
25. Balkhy HH, Alenazi TH, Alshamrani MM. Description of a hospital outbreak of Middle East respiratory syndrome in a large tertiary care hospital in Saudi Arabia. *Infect Control Hosp Epidemiol.* 2016;37(10):1147–1155 [in eng] https://doi.org/10.1017/ice.2016.132.
26. Memish ZA, Al-Tawfiq JA, Assiri A. Hospital-associated Middle East respiratory syndrome coronavirus infections. *N Engl J Med.* 2013;369(18):1761–1762 [in eng] https://doi.org/10.1056/NEJMc1311004.
27. Oboho IK, Tomczyk SM, Al-Asmari AM. 2014 MERS-CoV outbreak in Jeddah—a link to health care facilities. *N Engl J Med.* 2015;372(9):846–854 [in eng] https://doi.org/10.1056/NEJMoa1408636.
28. Shalhoub S, Abdraboh S, Palma R, AlSharif H, Assiri N. MERS-CoV in a healthcare worker in Jeddah, Saudi Arabia: an index case investigation. *J Hosp Infect.* 2016;93(3):309–312 [in eng] https://doi.org/10.1016/j.jhin.2016.04.002.
29. Khan RM, Al-Dorzi HM, Al Johani S. Middle East respiratory syndrome coronavirus on inanimate surfaces: a risk for health care transmission. *Am J Infect Control.* 2016;44(11):1387–1389 [in eng] https://doi.org/10.1016/j.ajic.2016.05.006.

30. van Doremalen N, Bushmaker T, Munster VJ. Stability of Middle East respiratory syndrome coronavirus (MERS-CoV) under different environmental conditions. *Euro Surveill.* 2013;18(38). https://doi.org/10.2807/1560-7917.es2013.18.38.20590 [in eng].
31. Bin SY, Heo JY, Song MS. Environmental contamination and viral shedding in MERS patients during MERS-CoV outbreak in South Korea. *Clin Infect Dis.* 2016;62(6):755–760 [in eng] https://doi.org/10.1093/cid/civ1020.
32. Cotten M, Watson SJ, Zumla AI. Spread, circulation, and evolution of the Middle East respiratory syndrome coronavirus. *mBio.* 2014;5(1). https://doi.org/10.1128/mBio.01062-13 [in eng].
33. Breban R, Riou J, Fontanet A. Interhuman transmissibility of Middle East respiratory syndrome coronavirus: estimation of pandemic risk. *Lancet.* 2013;382(9893):694–699 [in eng] https://doi.org/10.1016/s0140-6736(13)61492-0.
34. Degnah AA, Al-Amri SS, Hassan AM. Seroprevalence of MERS-CoV in healthy adults in western Saudi Arabia, 2011-2016. *J Infect Public Health.* 2020;13(5):697–703 [in eng] https://doi.org/10.1016/j.jiph.2020.01.001.
35. Gautret P, Charrel R, Benkouiten S. Lack of MERS coronavirus but prevalence of influenza virus in French pilgrims after 2013 Hajj. *Emerg Infect Dis.* 2014;20(4):728–730 [in eng] https://doi.org/10.3201/eid2004.131708.
36. Memish ZA, Mishra N, Olival KJ. Middle East respiratory syndrome coronavirus in bats, Saudi Arabia. *Emerg Infect Dis.* 2013;19(11):1819–1823 [in eng] https://doi.org/10.3201/eid1911.131172.
37. Ithete NL, Stoffberg S, Corman VM. Close relative of human Middle East respiratory syndrome coronavirus in bat, South Africa. *Emerg Infect Dis.* 2013;19(10):1697–1699 [in eng] https://doi.org/10.3201/eid1910.130946.
38. Annan A, Baldwin HJ, Corman VM. Human betacoronavirus 2c EMC/2012-related viruses in bats, Ghana and Europe. *Emerg Infect Dis.* 2013;19(3):456–459 [in eng] https://doi.org/10.3201/eid1903.121503.
39. Haagmans BL, Al Dhahiry SH, Reusken CB. Middle East respiratory syndrome coronavirus in dromedary camels: an outbreak investigation. *Lancet Infect Dis.* 2014;14(2):140–145 [in eng] https://doi.org/10.1016/s1473-3099(13)70690-x.
40. Saqib M, Sieberg A, Hussain MH. Serologic evidence for MERS-CoV infection in dromedary camels, Punjab, Pakistan, 2012-2015. *Emerg Infect Dis.* 2017;23(3):550–551 [in eng] https://doi.org/10.3201/eid2303.161285.
41. Reusken CB, Ababneh M, Raj VS. Middle East respiratory syndrome coronavirus (MERS-CoV) serology in major livestock species in an affected region in Jordan, June to September 2013. *Euro Surveill.* 2013;18(50):20662 [in eng] https://doi.org/10.2807/1560-7917.es2013.18.50.20662.
42. Reusken CB, Farag EA, Jonges M. Middle East respiratory syndrome coronavirus (MERS-CoV) RNA and neutralising antibodies in milk collected according to local customs from dromedary camels, Qatar, April 2014. *Euro Surveill.* 2014;19(23). https://doi.org/10.2807/1560-7917.es2014.19.23.20829 [in eng].
43. Reusken CB, Haagmans BL, Müller MA. Middle East respiratory syndrome coronavirus neutralising serum antibodies in dromedary camels: a comparative serological study. *Lancet Infect Dis.* 2013;13(10):859–866 [in eng] https://doi.org/10.1016/s1473-3099(13)70164-6.
44. Reusken CB, Messadi L, Feyisa A. Geographic distribution of MERS coronavirus among dromedary camels, Africa. *Emerg Infect Dis.* 2014;20(8):1370–1374 [in eng] https://doi.org/10.3201/eid2008.140590.
45. Meyer B, Müller MA, Corman VM. Antibodies against MERS coronavirus in dromedary camels, United Arab Emirates, 2003 and 2013. *Emerg Infect Dis.* 2014;20(4):552–559 [in eng] https://doi.org/10.3201/eid2004.131746.
46. Müller MA, Corman VM, Jores J. MERS coronavirus neutralizing antibodies in camels, Eastern Africa, 1983-1997. *Emerg Infect Dis.* 2014;20(12):2093–2095 [in eng] https://doi.org/10.3201/eid2012.141026.
47. Müller MA, Meyer B, Corman VM. Presence of Middle East respiratory syndrome coronavirus antibodies in Saudi Arabia: a nationwide, cross-sectional, serological study. *Lancet Infect Dis.* 2015;15(5):559–564 [in eng] https://doi.org/10.1016/s1473-3099(15)70090-3.
48. Corman VM, Jores J, Meyer B. Antibodies against MERS coronavirus in dromedary camels, Kenya, 1992-2013. *Emerg Infect Dis.* 2014;20(8):1319–1322 [in eng] https://doi.org/10.3201/eid2008.140596.
49. Hemida MG, Perera RA, Al Jassim RA. Seroepidemiology of Middle East respiratory syndrome (MERS) coronavirus in Saudi Arabia (1993) and Australia (2014) and characterisation of assay specificity. *Euro Surveill.* 2014;19(23). https://doi.org/10.2807/1560-7917.es2014.19.23.20828 [in eng].
50. Adney DR, van Doremalen N, Brown VR. Replication and shedding of MERS-CoV in upper respiratory tract of inoculated dromedary camels. *Emerg Infect Dis.* 2014;20(12):1999–2005 [in eng] https://doi.org/10.3201/eid2012.141280.
51. Hemida MG, Chu DK, Poon LL. MERS coronavirus in dromedary camel herd, Saudi Arabia. *Emerg Infect Dis.* 2014;20(7):1231–1234 [in eng] https://doi.org/10.3201/eid2007.140571.
52. Mohran KA, Farag EA, Reusken CB. The sample of choice for detecting Middle East respiratory syndrome coronavirus in asymptomatic dromedary camels using real-time reversetranscription polymerase chain reaction. *Rev Sci Tech.* 2016;35(3):905–911 [in eng] 10.20506/rst.35.3.2578.
53. Memish ZA, Cotten M, Meyer B. Human infection with MERS coronavirus after exposure to infected camels, Saudi Arabia, 2013. *Emerg Infect Dis.* 2014;20(6):1012–1015 [in eng] https://doi.org/10.3201/eid2006.140402.
54. Azhar EI, El-Kafrawy SA, Farraj SA. Evidence for camel-to-human transmission of MERS coronavirus. *N Engl J Med.* 2014;370(26):2499–2505 [in eng] https://doi.org/10.1056/NEJMoa1401505.

55. Reusken CB, Farag EA, Haagmans BL. Occupational exposure to dromedaries and risk for MERS-CoV infection, Qatar, 2013-2014. *Emerg Infect Dis.* 2015;21(8):1422–1425 [in eng] https://doi.org/10.3201/eid2108.150481.
56. Corman VM, Ithete NL, Richards LR. Rooting the phylogenetic tree of Middle East respiratory syndrome coronavirus by characterization of a conspecific virus from an African bat. *J Virol.* 2014;88(19):11297–11303 [in eng] https://doi.org/10.1128/jvi.01498-14.
57. Raj VS, Farag EA, Reusken CB. Isolation of MERS coronavirus from a dromedary camel, Qatar, 2014. *Emerg Infect Dis.* 2014;20(8):1339–1342 [in eng] https://doi.org/10.3201/eid2008.140663.
58. Hemida MG, Al-Naeem A, Perera RA, Chin AW, Poon LL, Peiris M. Lack of Middle East respiratory syndrome coronavirus transmission from infected camels. *Emerg Infect Dis.* 2015;21(4):699–701 [in eng] https://doi.org/10.3201/eid2104.141949.
59. Aburizaiza AS, Mattes FM, Azhar EI. Investigation of anti-Middle East respiratory syndrome antibodies in blood donors and slaughterhouse workers in Jeddah and Makkah, Saudi Arabia, fall 2012. *J Infect Dis.* 2014;209(2):243–246 [In eng] https://doi.org/10.1093/infdis/jit589.
60. Adney DR, Brown VR, Porter SM, Bielefeldt-Ohmann H, Hartwig AE, Bowen RA. Inoculation of goats, sheep, and horses with MERS-CoV Does not result in productive viral shedding. *Viruses.* 2016;8(8). https://doi.org/10.3390/v8080230 [in eng].
61. van Boheemen S, de Graaf M, Lauber C. Genomic characterization of a newly discovered coronavirus associated with acute respiratory distress syndrome in humans. *mBio.* 2012;3(6). https://doi.org/10.1128/mBio.00473-12 [in eng].
62. Raj VS, Osterhaus AD, Fouchier RA, Haagmans BL. MERS: emergence of a novel human coronavirus. *Curr Opin Virol.* 2014;5:58–62 [in eng] https://doi.org/10.1016/j.coviro.2014.01.010.
63. Chan JF, Lau SK, To KK, Cheng VC, Woo PC, Yuen KY. Middle East respiratory syndrome coronavirus: another zoonotic betacoronavirus causing SARS-like disease. *Clin Microbiol Rev.* 2015;28(2):465–522 [in eng] https://doi.org/10.1128/cmr.00102-14.
64. Hussain I, Pervaiz N, Khan A. Evolutionary and structural analysis of SARS-CoV-2 specific evasion of host immunity. *Genes Immun.* 2020;21(6–8):409–419 [in eng] https://doi.org/10.1038/s41435-020-00120-6.
65. Raj VS, Mou H, Smits SL. Dipeptidyl peptidase 4 is a functional receptor for the emerging human coronavirus-EMC. *Nature.* 2013;495(7440):251–254 [in eng] https://doi.org/10.1038/nature12005.
66. Belouzard S, Millet JK, Licitra BN, Whittaker GR. Mechanisms of coronavirus cell entry mediated by the viral spike protein. *Viruses.* 2012;4(6):1011–1033 [in eng] https://doi.org/10.3390/v4061011.
67. Xia S, Liu Q, Wang Q. Middle East respiratory syndrome coronavirus (MERS-CoV) entry inhibitors targeting spike protein. *Virus Res.* 2014;194:200–210 [in eng] https://doi.org/10.1016/j.virusres.2014.10.007.
68. Corman VM, Eckerle I, Bleicker T. Detection of a novel human coronavirus by real-time reverse-transcription polymerase chain reaction. *Euro Surveill.* 2012;17(39). https://doi.org/10.2807/ese.17.39.20285-en [in eng].
69. Corman VM, Müller MA, Costabel U. Assays for laboratory confirmation of novel human coronavirus (hCoV-EMC) infections. *Euro Surveill.* 2012;17(49). https://doi.org/10.2807/ese.17.49.20334-en [in eng].
70. Brasil P, Pereira JP, Moreira ME. Zika virus infection in pregnant women in Rio de Janeiro. *N Engl J Med.* 2016;375(24):2321–2334. https://doi.org/10.1056/NEJMoa1602412.
71. Corman VM, Albarrak AM, Omrani AS. Viral shedding and antibody response in 37 patients with Middle East respiratory syndrome coronavirus infection. *Clin Infect Dis.* 2016;62(4):477–483 [In eng] https://doi.org/10.1093/cid/civ951.
72. WHO. Laboratory Testing for Middle East Respiratory Syndrome Coronavirus—Revised; 2018. https://www.who.int/publications/i/item/10665-259952.
73. WHO. Revised Interim Case Definition for Reporting to WHO–Middle East Respiratory Syndrome Coronavirus (MERS-CoV). Interim case definition as of 19 February 2013; 2013. http://www.who.int/csr/disease/coronavirus_infections/case_definition_19_02_2013/en/;.
74. CDC. Middle East Respiratory Syndrome. https://www.cdc.gov/mers/hcp/diagnosis-testing/.
75. Drosten C, Muth D, Corman VM. An observational, laboratory-based study of outbreaks of Middle East respiratory syndrome coronavirus in Jeddah and Riyadh, Kingdom of Saudi Arabia, 2014. *Clin Infect Dis.* 2015;60(3):369–377 [in eng] https://doi.org/10.1093/cid/ciu812.
76. Memish ZA, Al-Tawfiq JA, Makhdoom HQ. Respiratory tract samples, viral load, and genome fraction yield in patients with Middle East respiratory syndrome. *J Infect Dis.* 2014;210(10):1590–1594 [in eng] https://doi.org/10.1093/infdis/jiu292.
77. Shalhoub S, Farahat F, Al-Jiffri A. IFN-α2a or IFN-β1a in combination with ribavirin to treat Middle East respiratory syndrome coronavirus pneumonia: a retrospective study. *J Antimicrob Chemother.* 2015;70(7):2129–2132 [in eng] https://doi.org/10.1093/jac/dkv085.
78. Shalhoub S, AlZahrani A, Simhairi R, Mushtaq A. Successful recovery of MERS CoV pneumonia in a patient with acquired immunodeficiency syndrome: a case report. *J Clin Virol.* 2015;62:69–71 [in eng] https://doi.org/10.1016/j.jcv.2014.11.030.
79. Al-Gethamy M, Corman VM, Hussain R, Al-Tawfiq JA, Drosten C, Memish ZA. A case of long-term excretion and subclinical infection with Middle East respiratory syndrome coronavirus in a healthcare worker. *Clin Infect Dis.* 2015;60(6):973–974 [in eng] https://doi.org/10.1093/cid/ciu1135.

80. Kim SY, Park SJ, Cho SY. Viral RNA in blood as Indicator of severe outcome in Middle East respiratory syndrome coronavirus infection. *Emerg Infect Dis.* 2016;22(10):1813–1816 [in eng] https://doi.org/10.3201/eid2210.160218.
81. CDC. Middle East Respiratory Syndrome (MERS). Managing MERS Cases and Contacts; 2024. https://www.cdc.gov/mers/hcp/infection-control/.
82. Memish ZA, Assiri AM, Al-Tawfiq JA. Middle East respiratory syndrome coronavirus (MERS-CoV) viral shedding in the respiratory tract: an observational analysis with infection control implications. *Int J Infect Dis.* 2014;29:307–308 [in eng] https://doi.org/10.1016/j.ijid.2014.10.002.
83. Arabi YM, Mandourah Y, Al-Hameed F, et al. Corticosteroid therapy for critically ill patients with Middle East respiratory syndrome. *Am J Respir Crit Care Med.* 2018;197(6):757–767 [in eng; PMID: 29161116] https://doi.org/10.1164/rccm.201706-1172OC. [in eng; PMID: 29161116].
84. Assiri A, Al-Tawfiq JA, Al-Rabeeah AA. Epidemiological, demographic, and clinical characteristics of 47 cases of Middle East respiratory syndrome coronavirus disease from Saudi Arabia: a descriptive study. *Lancet Infect Dis.* 2013;13(9):752–761 [in eng] https://doi.org/10.1016/s1473-3099(13)70204-4.
85. Al-Tawfiq JA, Hinedi K, Ghandour J. Middle East respiratory syndrome coronavirus: a case-control study of hospitalized patients. *Clin Infect Dis.* 2014;59(2):160–165 [in eng] https://doi.org/10.1093/cid/ciu226.
86. Al Ghamdi M, Alghamdi KM, Ghandoora Y. Treatment outcomes for patients with middle eastern respiratory syndrome coronavirus (MERS CoV) infection at a coronavirus referral center in the Kingdom of Saudi Arabia. *BMC Infect Dis.* 2016;16:174 [in eng] https://doi.org/10.1186/s12879-016-1492-4.
87. Saad M, Omrani AS, Baig K. Clinical aspects and outcomes of 70 patients with Middle East respiratory syndrome coronavirus infection: a single-center experience in Saudi Arabia. *Int J Infect Dis.* 2014;29:301–306 [in eng] https://doi.org/10.1016/j.ijid.2014.09.003.
88. Arabi YM, Al-Omari A, Mandourah Y. Critically ill patients with the Middle East respiratory syndrome: a multicenter retrospective cohort study. *Crit Care Med.* 2017;45(10):1683–1695 [in eng] https://doi.org/10.1097/ccm.0000000000002621.
89. Shalhoub S, Omrani AS. Middle East respiratory syndrome. *BMJ.* 2016;355:i5281 [in eng] https://doi.org/10.1136/bmj.i5281.
90. Arabi YM, Balkhy HH, Hayden FG. Middle East respiratory syndrome. *N Engl J Med.* 2017;376(6):584–594 [in eng] https://doi.org/10.1056/NEJMsr1408795.
91. Kim CJ, Choi WS, Jung Y. Surveillance of the Middle East respiratory syndrome (MERS) coronavirus (CoV) infection in healthcare workers after contact with confirmed MERS patients: incidence and risk factors of MERS-CoV seropositivity. *Clin Microbiol Infect.* 2016;22(10):880–886 [in eng] https://doi.org/10.1016/j.cmi.2016.07.017.
92. Ahmed AE. The predictors of 3- and 30-day mortality in 660 MERS-CoV patients. *BMC Infect Dis.* 2017;17(1):615 [in eng] https://doi.org/10.1186/s12879-017-2712-2.
93. Ahmed AE. Diagnostic delays in 537 symptomatic cases of Middle East respiratory syndrome coronavirus infection in Saudi Arabia. *Int J Infect Dis.* 2017;62:47–51 [in eng] https://doi.org/10.1016/j.ijid.2017.07.008.
94. Alraddadi BM, Watson JT, Almarashi A. Risk factors for primary Middle East respiratory syndrome coronavirus illness in humans, Saudi Arabia, 2014. *Emerg Infect Dis.* 2016;22(1):49–55 [in eng] https://doi.org/10.3201/eid2201.151340.
95. Alraddadi BM, Al-Salmi HS, Jacobs-Slifka K. Risk factors for Middle East respiratory syndrome coronavirus infection among healthcare personnel. *Emerg Infect Dis.* 2016;22(11):1915–1920 [in eng] https://doi.org/10.3201/eid2211.160920.
96. Alraddadi BM, Qushmaq I, Al-Hameed FM. Noninvasive ventilation in critically ill patients with the Middle East respiratory syndrome. *Influenza Other Respir Viruses.* 2019;13(4):382–390 [in eng] https://doi.org/10.1111/irv.12635.
97. Yang Y, Zhang L, Geng H. The structural and accessory proteins M, ORF 4a, ORF 4b, and ORF 5 of Middle East respiratory syndrome coronavirus (MERS-CoV) are potent interferon antagonists. Protein. *Cell.* 2013;4(12):951–961. (in eng). https://doi.org/10.1007/s13238-013-3096-8.
98. Hong KH, Choi JP, Hong SH. Predictors of mortality in Middle East respiratory syndrome (MERS). *Thorax.* 2018;73(3):286–289 [in eng] https://doi.org/10.1136/thoraxjnl-2016-209313.
99. Feikin DR, Alraddadi B, Qutub M. Association of Higher MERS-CoV virus load with severe disease and death, Saudi Arabia, 2014. *Emerg Infect Dis.* 2015;21(11):2029–2035 [in eng] https://doi.org/10.3201/eid2111.150764.
100. Ko JH, Müller MA, Seok H. Serologic responses of 42 MERS-coronavirus-infected patients according to the disease severity. *Diagn Microbiol Infect Dis.* 2017;89(2):106–111 [in eng] https://doi.org/10.1016/j.diagmicrobio.2017.07.006.
101. Alraddadi B, Bawareth N, Omar H. Patient characteristics infected with Middle East respiratory syndrome coronavirus infection in a tertiary hospital. *Ann Thorac Med.* 2016;11(2):128–131 [in eng] https://doi.org/10.4103/1817-1737.180027.
102. de Wilde AH, Raj VS, Oudshoorn D. MERS-coronavirus replication induces severe in vitro cytopathology and is strongly inhibited by cyclosporin A or interferon-α treatment. *J Gen Virol.* 2013;94(Pt 8):1749–1760 [in eng] https://doi.org/10.1099/vir.0.052910-0.
103. Falzarano D, de Wit E, Martellaro C, Callison J, Munster VJ, Feldmann H. Inhibition of novel β coronavirus replication by a combination of interferon-α2b and ribavirin. *Sci Rep.* 2013;3:1686 [in eng] https://doi.org/10.1038/srep01686.
104. Falzarano D, de Wit E, Rasmussen AL. Treatment with interferon-α2b and ribavirin improves out-

come in MERS-CoV-infected rhesus macaques. *Nat Med.* 2013;19(10):1313–1317 [in eng] https://doi.org/10.1038/nm.3362.

105. Hart BJ, Dyall J, Postnikova E. Interferon-β and mycophenolic acid are potent inhibitors of Middle East respiratory syndrome coronavirus in cell-based assays. *J Gen Virol.* 2014;95(Pt 3):571–577 [in eng] https://doi.org/10.1099/vir.0.061911-0.
106. Al-Tawfiq JA, Momattin H, Dib J, Memish ZA. Ribavirin and interferon therapy in patients infected with the Middle East respiratory syndrome coronavirus: an observational study. *Int J Infect Dis.* 2014;20:42–46 [in eng] https://doi.org/10.1016/j.ijid.2013.12.003.
107. Omrani AS, Saad MM, Baig K. Ribavirin and interferon alfa-2a for severe Middle East respiratory syndrome coronavirus infection: a retrospective cohort study. *Lancet Infect Dis.* 2014;14(11):1090–1095 [in eng] https://doi.org/10.1016/s1473-3099(14)70920-x.
108. Arabi YM, Shalhoub S, Mandourah Y. Ribavirin and interferon therapy for critically ill patients with Middle East respiratory syndrome: a multicenter observational study. *Clin Infect Dis.* 2020;70(9):1837–1844 [in eng] https://doi.org/10.1093/cid/ciz544.
109. Arabi YM, Asiri AY, Assiri AM. Interferon Beta-1b and Lopinavir-ritonavir for Middle East respiratory syndrome. *N Engl J Med.* 2020;383(17):1645–1656 [in eng] https://doi.org/10.1056/NEJMoa2015294.
110. Arabi YM, Alothman A, Balkhy HH. Treatment of Middle East respiratory syndrome with a combination of lopinavir-ritonavir and interferon-β1b (MIRACLE trial): study protocol for a randomized controlled trial. *Trials.* 2018;19(1):81 [in eng] https://doi.org/10.1186/s13063-017-2427-0.
111. Lu L, Liu Q, Zhu Y. Structure-based discovery of Middle East respiratory syndrome coronavirus fusion inhibitor. *Nat Commun.* 2014;5:3067 [in eng] https://doi.org/10.1038/ncomms4067.
112. Channappanavar R, Lu L, Xia S. Protective effect of intranasal regimens containing peptidic Middle East respiratory syndrome coronavirus fusion inhibitor against MERS-CoV infection. *J Infect Dis.* 2015;212(12):1894–1903 [in eng] https://doi.org/10.1093/infdis/jiv325.
113. Sheahan TP, Sims AC, Graham RL. Broad-spectrum antiviral GS-5734 inhibits both epidemic and zoonotic coronaviruses. *Sci Transl Med.* 2017;9(396) [in eng] https://doi.org/10.1126/scitranslmed.aal3653.
114. Luke T, Wu H, Zhao J. Human polyclonal immunoglobulin G from transchromosomic bovines inhibits MERS-CoV in vivo. *Sci Transl Med.* 2016;8(326):326ra21 [in eng] https://doi.org/10.1126/scitranslmed.aaf1061.
115. John H, Beigel JV, Kumar P. Safety and tolerability of a novel, polyclonal human anti-MERS coronavirus antibody produced from transchromosomic cattle: a phase 1 randomised, double-blind, single-dose-escalation study. *Lancet Infect Dis.* 2018;391.
116. Yuan Y, Cao D, Zhang Y. Cryo-EM structures of MERS-CoV and SARS-CoV spike glycoproteins reveal the dynamic receptor binding domains. *Nat Commun.* 2017;8:15092 [in eng] https://doi.org/10.1038/ncomms15092.
117. Al-Amri SS, Abbas AT, Siddiq LA. Immunogenicity of candidate MERS-CoV DNA vaccines based on the spike protein. *Sci Rep.* 2017;7:44875 [in eng] https://doi.org/10.1038/srep44875.
118. Hashem AM, Algaissi A, Agrawal AS. A highly immunogenic, protective, and safe adenovirus-based vaccine expressing Middle East respiratory syndrome coronavirus S1-CD40L fusion protein in a transgenic human dipeptidyl peptidase 4 mouse model. *J Infect Dis.* 2019;220(10):1558–1567 [in eng] https://doi.org/10.1093/infdis/jiz137.
119. Bosaeed M, Balkhy HH, Almaziad S. Safety and immunogenicity of ChAdOx1 MERS vaccine candidate in healthy middle eastern adults (MERS002): an open-label, non-randomised, dose-escalation, phase 1b trial. *Lancet Microbe.* 2022;3(1):e11–e20 [in eng] https://doi.org/10.1016/s2666-5247(21)00193-2.
120. Folegatti PM, Bittaye M, Flaxman A. Safety and immunogenicity of a candidate Middle East respiratory syndrome coronavirus viral-vectored vaccine: a dose-escalation, open-label, non-randomised, uncontrolled, phase 1 trial. *Lancet Infect Dis.* 2020;20(7):816–826 [in eng] https://doi.org/10.1016/s1473-3099(20)30160-2.
121. Modjarrad K, Roberts CC, Mills KT. Safety and immunogenicity of an anti-Middle East respiratory syndrome coronavirus DNA vaccine: a phase 1, open-label, single-arm, dose-escalation trial. *Lancet Infect Dis.* 2019;19(9):1013–1022 [in eng] https://doi.org/10.1016/s1473-3099(19)30266-x.
122. Haagmans BL, van den Brand JM, Raj VS. An orthopoxvirus-based vaccine reduces virus excretion after MERS-CoV infection in dromedary camels. *Science.* 2016;351(6268):77–81 [in eng] https://doi.org/10.1126/science.aad1283.
123. Koch T, Dahlke C, Fathi A. Safety and immunogenicity of a modified vaccinia virus Ankara vector vaccine candidate for Middle East respiratory syndrome: an open-label, phase 1 trial. *Lancet Infect Dis.* 2020;20(7):827–838 [in eng] https://doi.org/10.1016/s1473-3099(20)30248-6.
124. Aleanizy FS, Mohmed N, Alqahtani FY, El Hadi Mohamed RA. Outbreak of Middle East respiratory syndrome coronavirus in Saudi Arabia: a retrospective study. *BMC Infect Dis.* 2017;17(1):23 [in eng] https://doi.org/10.1186/s12879-016-2137-3.
125. MOH. Infection Prevention and Control Guidelines for the Middle East Respiratory Syndrome Coronavirus (MERS-CoV) Infection; 2015. https://www.moh.gov.sa/Documents/2015%20update.pdf.
126. Madani TA, Althaqafi AO, Alraddadi BM. Infection prevention and control guidelines for patients with Middle East Respiratory Syndrome Coronavirus (MERS-CoV) infection. *Saudi Med J.* 2014;35(8):897–913. PMID: 25129197.
127. Saudi MOH. Middle East Respiratory Syndrome Coronavirus; Guidelines for Healthcare Professionals; 2018. https://www.moh.gov.sa/ccc/healthp/regulations/documents/mers-cov%20guidelines%20for%20healthcare%20professionals%20-%20may%202018%20-%20v5.1%20%281%29.pdf.

128. Benkouiten S, Charrel R, Belhouchat K. Respiratory viruses and bacteria among pilgrims during the 2013 Hajj. *Emerg Infect Dis.* 2014;20(11):1821–1827 [in eng] https://doi.org/10.3201/eid2011.140600.
129. Saudi MOH. Middle East Respiratory Syndrome-FAQs; 2022. https://www.moh.gov.sa/en/CCC/FAQs/Corona/Pages/default.aspx.
130. Memish ZA, Assiri A, Turkestani A. Mass gathering and globalization of respiratory pathogens during the 2013 Hajj. *Clin Microbiol Infect.* 2015;21(6):571.e1–571.e8 [in eng] https://doi.org/10.1016/j.cmi.2015.02.008.
131. Memish ZA, Almasri M, Assirri A. Environmental sampling for respiratory pathogens in Jeddah airport during the 2013 hajj season. *Am J Infect Control.* 2014;42(12):1266–1269 [in eng] https://doi.org/10.1016/j.ajic.2014.07.027.
132. WHO. WHO/Health Topics/Middle East Respiratory Syndrome Coronavirus (MERS CoV); 2024. https://www.who.int/health-topics/middle-east-respiratory-syndrome-coronavirus-mers#tab=tab_1.

CHAPTER 12

SARS-CoV-2

DANIEL N. MAXWELL
Infectious Diseases and Critical Care, UT Southwestern, Dallas VA Medical Center, Dallas, TX, United States

INTRODUCTION

In 2020, the coronavirus (COVID-19) pandemic began, and its ongoing effects have become the lens through which many of the principles in this book will be viewed. The ethical challenges in patient care and the moral injuries to the healthcare and public health sectors cannot be underestimated. It is tempting to recapitulate the specific successes and failures seen during the pandemic, including in surveillance, prevention, communication, prophylaxis, and treatment of infection. However, these topics are discussed in depth in their respective chapters of this book. This chapter will instead focus on (1) the pathogen of SARS-CoV-2, (2) its origins and spread, (3) its signs, symptoms, and the disease it causes, and (4) lessons learned or relearned.

THE EPIDEMIC AND THE PANDEMIC

As of January 2024, the World Health Organization (WHO) reports over 774,075,242 COVID-19 cases and almost 7,012,986 deaths worldwide, likely an underestimate.[1] The rapidity with which the virus, SAR-CoV-2, was transmitted globally was a remarkable feature that surprised many. A cluster of human cases of pneumonia of an unknown cause was reported in mid-December 2019 in Wuhan, China.[2] On December 31, 2019, the China office of the World Health Organization (WHO) reported 27 cases connected to the Huanan Seafood Wholesale Market, a wet market in Wuhan (Fig. 1).[3,4] Simultaneously, several healthcare facilities in Hubei province identified clusters of patients with severe pneumonia of an unknown cause.[5] Most presented with fever and cough, and severe cases developed dyspnea and rapidly progressive diffuse bilateral lung infiltrates (called ground glass opacities) and respiratory failure.[5] By January 5, 2020, the genetic sequence of the pathogen[6] identified a novel coronavirus was published,[3] and within the week the full genome sequence was released and available in the Global Initiative on Sharing All Influenza Data (GISAID) database[7] for use by international scientific teams.[8] Despite the rapidity of notifying public health authorities, this same week Thai authorities reported a COVID-19 case was reported in a traveler from Wuhan. Family and nosocomial clusters and cases in individuals without a connection to Wuhan were reported, confirming human-to-human transmission. Before the end of January, infections were identified in 19 countries, recognized in all provinces in China, much of Asia, Europe, North America, and the Middle East.[9,10] This rapid spread was facilitated by air travel from the major transportation hub of Wuhan and by viral shedding among infected individuals prior to their developing symptoms (Fig. 1). Still, many speculate the transmission had been ongoing before the first identified cluster and may have been facilitated by superspreading events.[11,12]

Chinese health imposed a citywide lockdown by January 23 to halt transmission and prevent additional cases. Within 1 week (January 30, 2020), the WHO declared a public health emergency of international concern. Cases continued to be identified at a truly explosive pace, which led to serious pressures on healthcare systems, leading the WHO to raise the risk assessment to "very high," denoting the worldwide impact. Officially, the virus was named SARS-CoV-2 in mid-February based on the phylogenetic information. Finally, on March 11, 2020, the WHO declared a pandemic. By August 2020, over 20 million cases of COVID-19 and close to 750,000 deaths were reported.

Ultimately, 425 cases were identified in the Wuhan market investigation, and 55% were linked to the market.[13] Most cases were men (56%) with a median age of 59. Important epidemiologic parameters emerged from the outbreak; an incubation period of 5.2 days (95% CI 4.1–7 days) with a 12.5-day distribution, serial interval of 7.5 days (95% CI 5.3–19 days), and case doubling

Viral Outbreaks, Biosecurity, and Preparing for Mass Casualty Infectious Diseases Events
https://doi.org/10.1016/B978-0-323-54841-0.00026-3

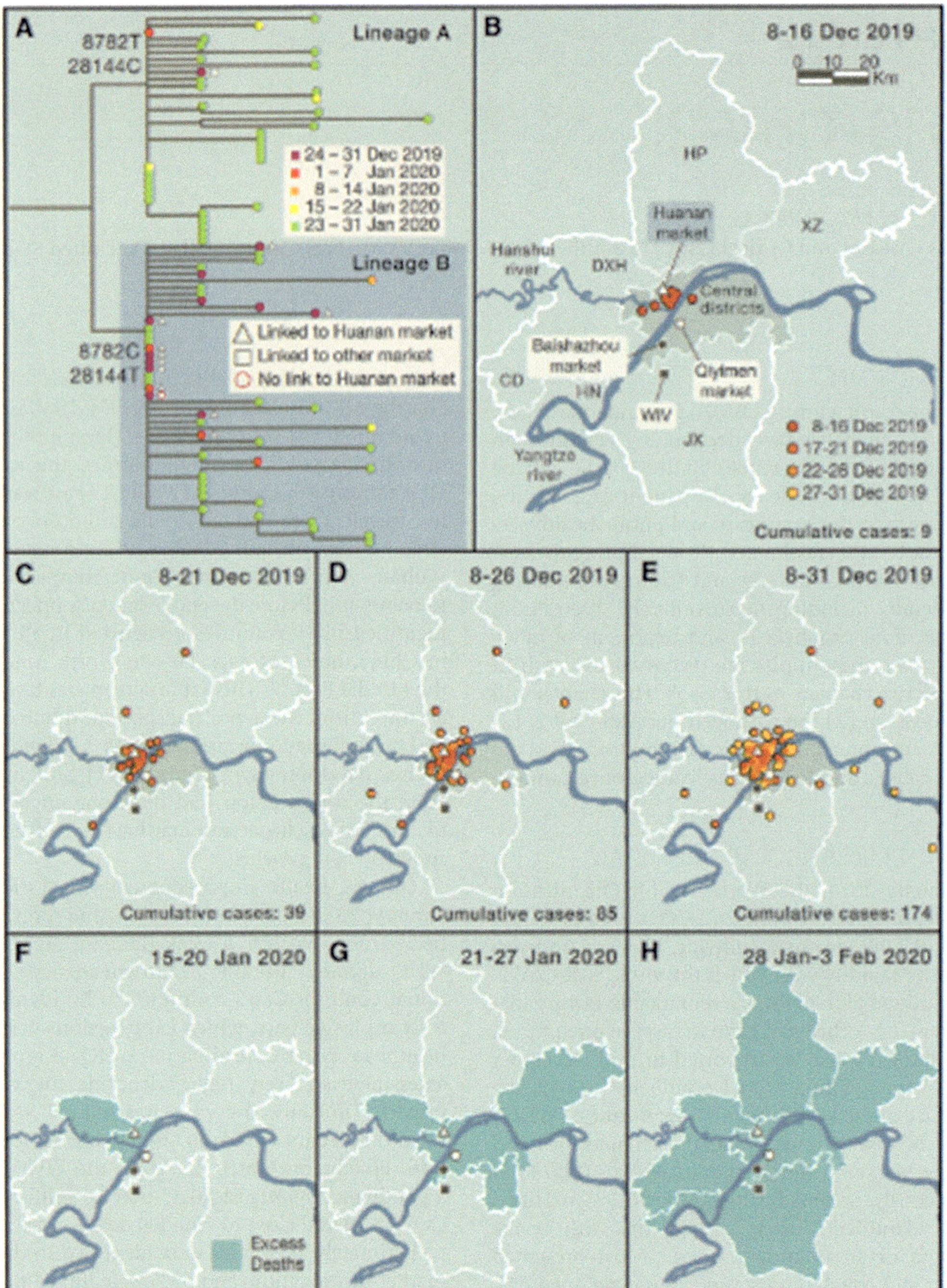

FIG. 1 SARS-CoV-2 phylogeny and early spread. Panel (A) shows the phylogeny of the early SARS-CoV-2 viruses from the Wuhan market outbreak prior to the declaration of a pandemic. The color coding of dots reveals the evolution of the virus over time with *red dots* being the earliest identified strains (December 2019), *yellow* representing strains in mid-January 2020, and *green* being those identified late in January. Panels (B–E) use the color coding to demonstrate weeks in December 2019, with red representing the second week in December. *Orange and paler orange* represent the later weeks of December with mustard representing the last days of December. Panel (B) demonstrates the locations of the Huanan Market, several other markets, and the Wuhan Institute of Virology. Panels (C–E) visualize geospatially the spread of SARS-CoV-2 infection during December 2019 in Wuhan. Panels (F–H) show excess mortality geospatially with each panel representing a week from mid-January 2020 to early February 2020. (Used with permission Holmes EC, Goldstein SA, Rasmussen AL, et al. The origins of SARS-CoV-2: a critical review. *Cell*. 2021;184(19):4848–4856.)

every 7.4 days. These parameters are comparable to other novel coronaviruses, SARS-CoV-1 and MERS-CoV. The basic reproductive number (R_0) was estimated as 2.2 (95% CI 1.4–3.9). The source of the outbreak has yet to be identified and the complexities investigators encountered illustrate the challenge. For instance, over 923 environmental samples and 457 samples from 18 animal species were collected in January 2020 from sources in the market including stray animals, frozen meats, and fish tanks.[14] SARS-CoV-2 virus was identified by PCR in 73 of 466 (16%) environmental samples, and three samples grew virus. Sequencing demonstrated 99.99%–100% homology between a human HCoV-19/Wuhan/IVDC-HB-01/2019 isolate and environmental samples.

THE SARS-COV-2 VIRUS: STRUCTURE, GENOME, CELL ENTRY, AND REPLICATION

The Severe Acute Respiratory Syndrome Coronavirus 2 (SARS-CoV-2) is a novel positive sense, single-stranded RNA virus in the *Coronaviridiae* of the subgenus *Sarbecovirus* or Beta-coronavirus (Beta-CoV sublineage B) and is closely related to the Severe Acute Respiratory Syndrome Coronavirus (SARS-CoV-1) virus described in the 2003 global outbreak (fig. 5, Chapter 1). It is also in the family of the MERS-CoV virus, which continues to cause the Middle East Respiratory Syndrome, a respiratory illness described in 2013. Based on phylogenetic analyses, the SARS-CoV-2 genome is clustered near the SARS-CoV-1 and related coronaviruses found in bats (subgenus *Sarbecovirus*, see fig. 5, Chapter 1). Importantly, both the SARS-CoV-1 and SARS-CoV-2 clades are grouped with several horseshoe bat isolates (RaTG13, RmYN02, ZC45, and ZXC21), which are phylogenetically related, yet all the betacoronaviruses are unique.

Viral Structure

The virus is spherical with an external surface covered by the surface "spike" or S proteins (Fig. 2). The name *coronavirus* was given in the 1960s to reference the appearance of the entire virion under electron microscopy "recalling the solar corona," yet the S unit trimer itself resembles a crown.[15,16] The outer membrane also contains the membrane and envelope proteins, M and E proteins, which with the S protein facilitate viral entry and assembly.[17] Within the virion is the ribonucleoprotein (RNP) complex made of the N protein and the viral genome. In addition, 16 nonstructural proteins (Nsps 1–16) are present and, once cleaved by viral proteases, perform various functions; these cleaved Nsps aid in genome replication, transcription, and RNA transport. All these building blocks of the SARS-CoV-2 virus are encoded in the viral genome for future replication. The S protein is essential to the cell entry of SARS-CoV-2 in that it mediates the fusion between the viral and human cellular membranes. The S protein is

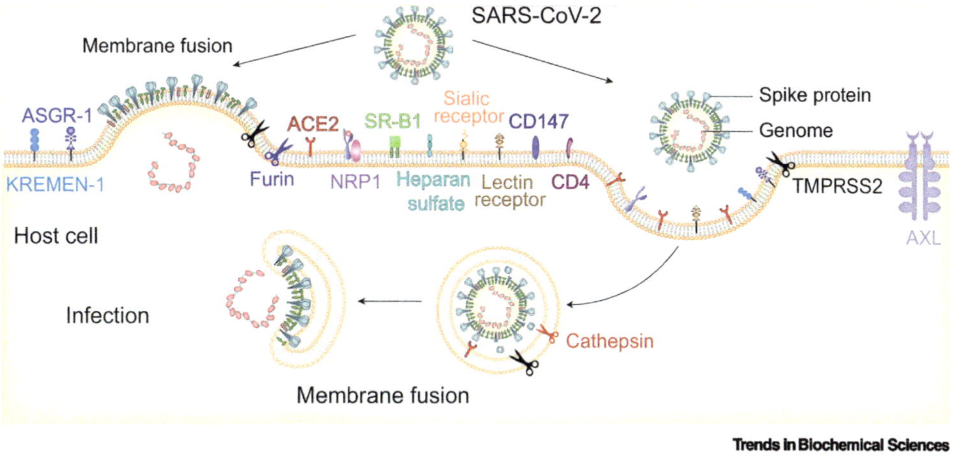

FIG. 2 Viral structure and entry of SARS-CoV-2. This schematic diagram of the SARS-CoV-2 demonstrates the cellular surface and complex process by which the virus fuses and enters the cell with the ACE-2 receptor being critical in the process. Two forms of cellular entry, depending on the availability of binding sites, are possible either via the membrane fusion (*left*) or the endosome and clathrin-mediated endocytosis (*right*). (Used with permission Peng R, Wu LA, Wang Q, Qi J, Gao GF. Cell entry by SARS-CoV-2. *Trends Biochem Sci*. 2021;46(10):848–860.)

a trimeric protein including two key subunits, S1 and S2, and has a flexible stalk that enables the virus to bind to cell receptors, which in the human host is the angiotensin-converting enzyme 2 (ACE2).[17] This binding site is crucial for interspecies transmission and is also used by the SARS-CoV-1.

Viral Genome

The genome of the virus is organized with six functional open reading frames (ORFs), replicase (ORF1a/ORF1b), spike (S), envelop (E), membrane (M), and nucleocapsid (N), which encode for various proteins.[16,18,19] The organization and any of the proteins between the SARS-CoV-1 and SARS-CoV-2 viruses are similar, yet there are some important differences.[8] The S protein houses the receptor binding domain (RBD) in the SARS viruses and is larger in SARS-CoV-2 than in SARS-CoV-1. Additionally, the SARS-CoV-2 "S protein" houses four amino acid residues (Arg-Arg-Ala-Arg), inserted at the junction of the S1 and S2 subunits, and constitutes this protein.[16] This insertion generates an S1-S2 cleavage site that can be used by furin and other proteases. The furin cleavage site is not observed in the other subgenus *Sarbecovirus* viruses and may be a recent development.[16]

The virus shares 79% of its genome with SARS-CoV-1, the etiologic agent of SARS, and 50% of its genome with the MERS-CoV virus, the two other novel human coronaviruses that have emerged this century.[8]

Viral Cell Entry: The ACE2 Receptor Is the Main Facilitator of Entry via Two Pathways

Like SARS-CoV-1, the S protein of SARS-CoV-2 binds to ACE2 with an affinity at least as tightly as SARS-CoV-1 and uses the ACE2 receptor to enter cells.[18,20,21] Notably, this binding affinity differs depending on the SARS-CoV-2 variant in question.[22] However, the organotropism of SARS-CoV-2 correlates imperfectly with the distribution of ACE2 receptors. For example, a postmortem immunohistochemical staining and immunofluorescence for SARS-CoV-2 S protein shows presence of this antigen in pneumocytes, parts of the bronchioles and trachea, as well as areas outside of the respiratory tract such as the vascular tissue of the heart and brain, the small intestine (but not the large intestine), and the distal and collecting tubules of the kidneys (but not the proximal tubules).[23] However, ACE2 expression as determined by transcriptomics is highest in the small intestine, the colon and duodenum to a lesser degree, and the kidneys, with lung expression less than in the liver.[24] Though some enrichment in type II pneumocytes is present, it is not overwhelming. This explains the SARS-CoV-2 viruses' ability to infect and replicate in intestinal epithelium yet does not explain the predominant respiratory disease associated with COVID-19.[25]

Several other mechanisms help explain the respiratory predominance of COVID-19. First, type II pneumocytes represent only about 5% of pneumocytes yet are critical for surfactant production and generation of new type I pneumocytes.[26] Second, extrapulmonary diseases such as endothelial or myocardial injury can result in pulmonary symptoms.[25,27,28] Third, the complexity of SARS-CoV-2 cell entry is becoming increasingly evident. Multiple potential alternate receptors (AXL, KREMEN1, ASGL1, CD147), coreceptors (heparan sulfate, sialic acid, lectin receptors, neuropilin-1, CD4), and cofactors, most of which serve in proteolysis (furin, PC-1, trypsin, matriptase, cathepsins, TMPRSS2), may be involved in SARS-CoV-2 pathogenesis.[16,17,29]

These cofactors can play crucial roles, with PC-1, trypsin, and matriptase possibly contributing to the S1/S2 cleavage.[30] Cathepsin and TMPRSS2, an endothelial surface protein, are two cofactors that contribute to SARS-CoV-2 cell entry (Fig. 2). In the presence of TMPRSS2, SARS-CoV-2 can enter the cell surface, utilizing the TMPRSS2 as a cofactor to cleave S2′. If the virus does not encounter this cofactor, it can still infect cells via clathrin-mediated endocytosis. After acidification of the endosome, cathepsins can then perform this S2′ cleavage.[17,30,31]

Intracellular Replication and Two Current Targets for Oral Therapy

Targeting intracellular replication has been the focus of the currently available antivirals for SARS-CoV-2. Two oral therapies for the treatment of COVID-19 in outpatients are recommended in the United States and by WHO.[32,33] Once SARS-CoV-2 viral RNA has entered the host cell, four structural proteins mentioned above and two polyproteins, pp1a and pp1ab, play key roles. The polyproteins pp1a and pp1ab are cleaved by the Mpro or 3CL proteases, an essential step for viral gene expression and replication.[34,35] Nirmatrelvir is an antiviral that, when boosted with ritonavir, becomes an effective treatment against SARS-CoV-2 (see Chapter 25).[35,36] Its mechanism of action is to inhibit Mpro. If the machinery of viral replication continues unabated, the viral RNA-dependent RNA polymerase (RdRp) is an additional target by another antiviral, molnupiravir, a prodrug for a ribonucleoside analog. It is incorporated by RdRp into the viral genome, inducing mutagenesis.[35,37,38]

ORIGINS AND SPREAD

Origins

The precise origins of SARS-CoV-2 are disputed, but there are some antecedent lessons from two other coronaviruses: MERS-CoV and SARS-CoV-1. The genomes of these viruses and the nature of the viruses, including their hosts, have considerable similarities. Bats are the natural hosts of betacoronaviruses, and for both SARS-CoV-1 and MERS-CoV, an intermediary host was identified. To date, an intermediary host for SARS-CoV-2 has not been identified.

In 2012, three people who had cleaned bat feces from an abandoned copper mine in Tongguan in Mojiang County, China, died from pneumonia of unknown etiology. A years-long investigation that included sampling local fauna for possible viruses was undertaken and yielded 293 coronaviruses.RaTG13 was identified in a bat, *Rhinolophus affinis*, and at the time was the closest of known coronaviruses to the SARS-CoV-2.[39,40] Though 96.1% similar, RaTG13 and SARS-CoV-2 differ crucially in their receptor binding domains (RBDs).[41] As the COVID-19 pandemic unfolded, similar coronaviruses have been identified throughout Southeast Asia.[42] In February 2022, the discovery of BANAL-52, a *Sarbecovirus* found in Laotian bats with 96.8% overlap in the genome, was more closely related to SARS-CoV-2 than RatG13.[43] Significantly, BANAL-52 has an RBD much more similar to SARS-CoV-2 than RatG13, differing by only one or two residues.[43] These differences between SARS-CoV-2 and other *Sarbecoviridae* remain unexplained[44,45] and the WHO states that "further studies [are] needed to follow up on several gaps in our knowledge."[46] Overall, a general scientific consensus initially coalesced around natural origins with the WHO investigative group concluding that it was "extremely unlikely" that the origin of the virus was related to a laboratory incident.[47] However, recent information has questioned these findings. The WHO considers the findings to date preliminary and views their role as to recommend further investigation, not to determine the origins of SARS-CoV-2. At this point in time, the exact spillover event or events remain unknown, and intermediate hosts for SARS-CoV-2 have not been identified. The issue has been further complicated by accusations of geopolitically motivated publication biases. The gaps in knowledge have impeded the public health community's ability to eliminate or neutralize the source (s).[48–51] Despite these barriers, investigation into potential hosts have identified bat (RaTG13 and RmYN02) and pangolin betacoronaviruses similar to SARS-CoV-1 circulate in the wild and have demonstrated that the virus does cause symptoms in cats, ferrets, mink, and white tail deer.[52] Conversely, ducks, chickens, pigs, and dogs either do not develop infection or are asymptomatic. More recently, inconclusive evidence linking *Nyctereutes procyonoidesi* (racoon dogs) to a natural cause of the outbreak has been put forward.[53]

While frustrating, it is not surprising that, despite intense efforts to fully understand the viral origins of SARS-CoV-2, it will take time to fill in the current gaps in knowledge. Consider that despite its recognition in the 1970s, understanding the origin of the Ebola virus is an ongoing effort, and a decade separates the outbreak of SARS and the discovery of SARS-like viruses in bats (see Chapter 10), a critical link in connecting the source in the wild to human infection. Given all this, the challenges in fully elucidating the origins of SARS-CoV-2 are not surprising. So, while the origins of SARS-CoV-2 are still being investigated and better understood, these words from Thucydides as he described the challenges of writing about the Athenian Plague over two millennia ago can serve as a template for the rest of our discussion about SARS-CoV-2:

"All speculation as to its origin and its causes, if causes can be found adequate to produce so great a disturbance, I leave to other writers, whether lay or professional; for myself, I shall simply set down its nature, and explain the symptoms by which perhaps it may be recognized by the student, if it should ever break out again. This I can the better do, as I had the disease myself, and watched its operation in the case of others.[54]*"*

COVID-19, ITS PATHOGENESIS IN ORGAN SYSTEMS, AND OTHER SARS-COV-2 DISEASES

COVID-19

The SARS-CoV-2 virus is primarily transmitted by respiratory secretions from human-to-human contact. While the primary transmission may be through larger droplets, aerosols play an important role, especially in certain settings. Approximately 50% of transmission occurs from asymptomatic or pauci-symptomatic individuals, in whom symptoms have not yet developed.[55] In general, transmission is linked to proximity to the case and is affected by ventilation, force of exhalation, and other factors. Viable virus has been isolated from aerosols for up to 3 h and surfaces for 72 h.[55] While the virus contaminates environmental surfaces, transmission from fomites has not been documented, although transmission is associated with poor hand hygiene and there is some evidence in support of the possibility of a small degree of fomite transmission in theory.[56] Lastly, although the virus has been found in various body fluids,[57] to date sexual and bloodborne transmission have not been documented.[55,58]

The spectrum of COVID-19 illness varies from asymptomatic to hypoxic respiratory failure and depends on factors such as the specific variant, presence of comorbid illnesses, and host immunity.[59] Based on early studies, approximately 20% of individuals remain asymptomatic, 60%–65% develop mild symptoms and do not require medical care, 12% develop more severe disease with dyspnea and hypoxia, and 4%–5% develop severe disease and require critical care. COVID-19 causes an influenza-like illness with fever, myalgias, and fatigue being common.[3,4,60,61] Symptoms typically appear 5 days after infection, with a range of 1–14 days, and the exact latency to symptoms is determined by a combination of variables including host factors, inoculum, and variant.[8] Almost all individuals develop symptoms within 12 days of exposure. In general, individuals are most infectious 2–3 days before symptom onset. Aside from the typical symptoms mentioned already, others include headache, diarrhea, anorexia (loss of appetite), anosmia (loss of sense of smell), and odynophagia (throat pain, especially on swallowing).[8,60,62]

Initial descriptions of the syndrome as a febrile respiratory illness defined COVID-19 and have become familiar to clinicians and much of the public.[5,62–65] Like other novel coronaviruses, COVID-19 produces a biphasic illness with an initial viral phase and, in a smaller portion of patients, progression to a subsequent inflammatory phase. The viral phase usually has a sudden onset and is typically characterized by fever (70%–90%), nonproductive cough (60%–85%), dyspnea (15%–45%), and myalgias (15%–44%) lasting roughly seven to 10 days. Nausea, vomiting, or diarrhea occur in 15%–40% of symptomatic individuals. Other symptoms such as fatigue (~40%), anosmia (3%), and headache (25%) are reported in a smaller portion of patients during this viral phase. After this initial viral phase, some patients progress to the inflammatory phase. This inflammatory phase is when viral replication is no longer the dominant driver of pathophysiology but rather systemic inflammation and its consequences. It is during this phase that diffuse alveolar damage seen in the lungs can progress to acute respiratory distress syndrome, respiratory failure, and death.[8,25,66,67] Severity of illness, complications, and prolonged illness is more common in those over 60 years old, the immunocompromised, those with preexisting illnesses such as cardiovascular or metabolic diseases, and those who are pregnant.[59]

As variants emerged and as the numbers of those vaccinated and those recovering from illness increased, serious illness requiring hospitalization became less frequent and was decoupled from COVID-19 incidence. This was observed with the Omicron and subsequent variants in both highly vaccinated and less highly vaccinated populations worldwide.[68,69] The global case fatality rate as reported to the WHO peaked at 7.23% in late April 2020 and declined to 2.2% by the end of the same year, with similar trends noted regionally.[70,71] This decline has proven durable thus far.[72]

Pulmonary Disease

The primary organ site affected by severe SARS-CoV-2 infection is the lung. In the initial case series of 41 patients, although cough was noted in 76% and dyspnea in 55%, all 41 patients had pneumonia with abnormal findings on chest CT scans.[60] A review of autopsies among patients who died from COVID-19 and respiratory failure demonstrated exudative diffuse alveolar damage (DAD) and massive capillary congestion.[73] DAD is characterized in general by hyaline membrane deposition, impairing gas exchange, which is similar to the DAD found in COVID-19 patients.[74] Along with the DAD and capillary congestion, microthrombi were found despite the use of anticoagulants, and pulmonary emboli were found in four of the 21 patients. Apart from thrombotic complications, superimposed bronchopneumonia was noted in almost half of cases ($n = 10/21$).[73] A subsequent review of several postmortem studies bore these results out, with three primary patterns of pathology emerging that often coincided or overlapped with each other: classic progressive DAD, superimposed bronchopneumonia, and tissue thrombosis (Fig. 3).[75]

Endothelial Damage and Coagulopathy

Thrombotic and coagulopathic complications in the lung associated with COVID-19 are themselves the result of several interacting processes, and endothelial dysfunction as a contributing cause was understood to play a role in its pathogenesis. Specifically, a nearly three-fold increase in the release of von Willebrand factor (VWF) is described,[28,76] which leads to adhesion of leukocytes and platelets to vessel walls. More recently, the roles of hypercoagulability and the hyperinflammatory immune response that are sometimes seen with COVID-19 are hypothesized as other major contributors to COVID-associated coagulopathy.[77] These complications are of particular importance because they affect not only the lung and blood vessels directly but can also result in neurologic dysfunction because of relative cerebral ischemia (Fig. 4).

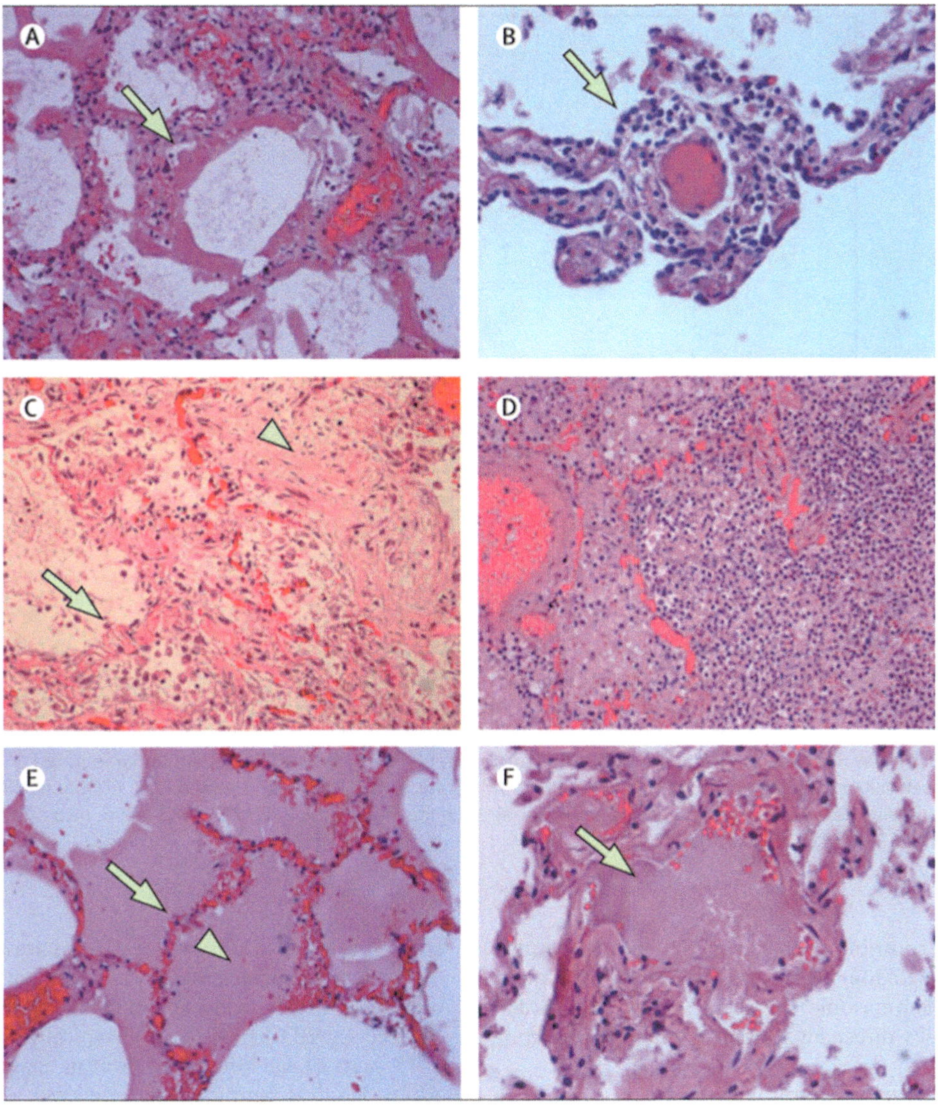

FIG. 3 Histopathologic findings in the lungs affected by COVID-19. (A) DAD with hyaline membranes (*arrow*) and alveolar wall congestion. (B) Lymphocytic infiltrate around a vessel. (C) Organizing DAD with hyaline remnants (*arrow*) and myofibroblasts (*arrowhead*). (D) Neutrophilic infiltration in bronchopneumonia. (E) Pulmonary cardiogenic edema with intra-alveolar fluid (*arrowhead*) and congested alveolar walls (*arrow*). (F) Thrombus (*arrow*) with subsequent vessel swelling. (Used with permission Milross L, Majo J, Cooper N, et al. Post-mortem lung tissue: the fossil record of the pathophysiology and immunopathology of severe COVID-19. *Lancet Respir Med*. 2022;10(1):95–106. https://doi.org/10.1016/S2213-2600(21)00408-2.)

Cardiovascular Disease

From the first months of the epidemic, cardiac injury was recognized in a portion of patients with COVID-19.[78] The initial reports suggested that 20% of hospitalized patients had cardiac injury and suggested that its presence was associated with worse outcomes. Subsequent studies find the rates of myocardial injury in COVID-19 as high as 28%.[79] The mechanism of cardiac injury is not yet fully understood and could include the previously mentioned coagulopathy and vasculopathy. In addition, the physiologic strain on the heart due to the pulmonary disease that COVID-19 can

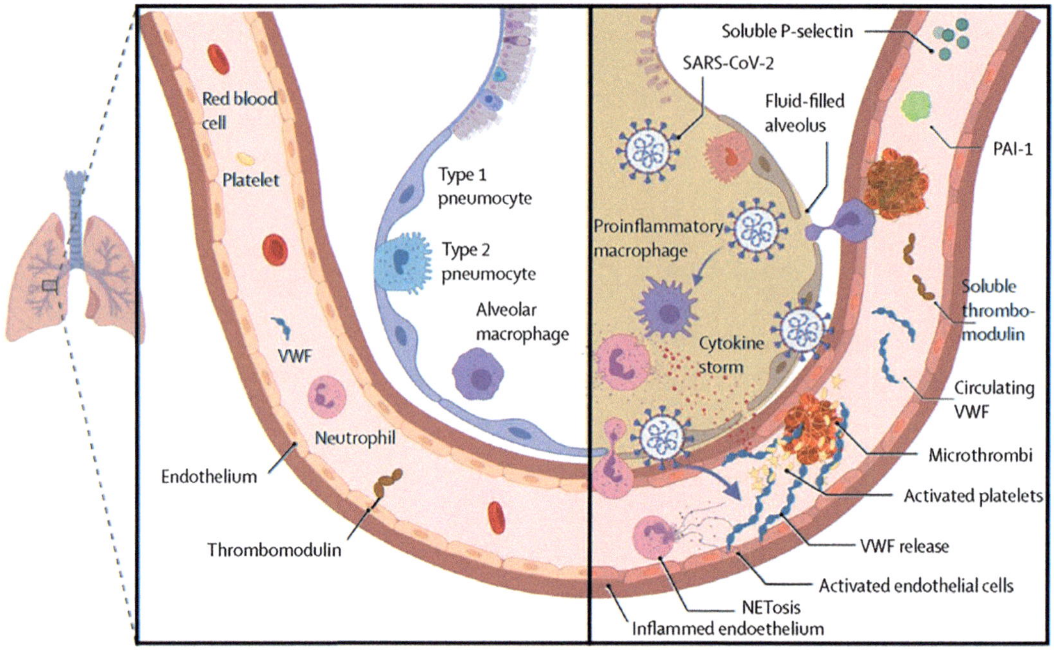

FIG. 4 Endothelial effects and coagulopathy caused by SARS-CoV-2. On the *left*, a healthy, air-filled alveolus is surrounded by its accompanying vasculature. The endothelium releases VWF and thrombomodulin appropriately, achieving a balanced coagulation cascade. On the *right*, the dysfunctional endothelium releases inappropriate VWF, and as a result, platelets and neutrophils are tethered to the vessel wall, resulting in microthrombi. (O'Sullivan JM, Gonagle DM, Ward SE, Preston RJS, O'Donnell JS. Endothelial cells orchestrate COVID-19 coagulopathy. *Lancet Haematol*. 2020;7(8):e553–e555. https://doi.org/10.1016/S2352-3026(20)30215-5.)

cause may contribute, along with systemic inflammation from cytokine release and even further activation of the inflammasome.[80] Others suggest that SARS-CoV-2 causes direct myocardial damage by infecting myocytes.[81]

The risk may be prolonged and last more than 30 days after SARS-CoV-2 infection, as patients have a significantly increased risk of several cardiovascular complications/diseases during the first year after their acute illness.[82] The risk of myocarditis after acute COVID-19 infection is 1500 per million and more than 10 times the risk after vaccination (106/million).[83] Hence the harm/benefit analysis by many medical and public health organizations has favored vaccination in most situations.[66]

Multisystem inflammatory syndrome in children **(MIS-C)**, Multisystem inflammatory syndrome in adults **(MIS-A)**.

Children often have asymptomatic or mild COVID-19 infections, which are rarely followed by an entity known as Multisystem inflammatory syndrome (MIS-C) and is characterized by hyperinflammation[84,85] which occurs 2–4 weeks after a usually mild or unrecognized COVID-19 infection. It typically affects those 5–13 years of age but ranges from neonates to young adults. Clinical symptoms include fever, conjunctival injection, vomiting, abdominal pain, rash, diarrhea, and can lead to shock. Cardiac dysfunction occurs in over 30% of patients, and treatment is typically with corticosteroids and/or intravenous immune globulin.[84,85] Though MIS-C typically follows a COVID-19 infection, there are rare reports of a similar syndrome after vaccination.[86] However, SARS-CoV-2 vaccination protects against MIS-C and reduces its likelihood by 91%.[87] Specifically, one group estimated the rate of MIS-C to be 2.9 per million following vaccinations, yet 20 times higher or 113 per million following COVID-19 infection.[88] Lastly, 185 of 382 children with a diagnosis of MIS-C who were vaccine-eligiblewere vaccinated and no serious adverse events were reported.[89] Fortunately, and perhaps as immunity develops, the incidence of MIS-C is declining over time.[90]

MIS-C is 26 times more common than a similar syndrome in adults, MIS-A.[91] One caveat is that quantifying the incidence of MIS-C is difficult as it can be hard to distinguish from COVID-19, long COVID or PASC, and other sequelae.[92] The CDC has a working definition of MIS-A that includes many of the same features as MIS-C, including lab evidence of both inflammation and recent SARS-CoV-2 infection, as well as clinical features including fever, cardiac manifestations, conjunctival injection, and rash.[93]

Neurologic Disease

Coagulopathy is also a major contributor to the neurologic sequelae, cerebrovascular events, and dysfunction seen with COVID-19. A review of 100 autopsies found that 58% of the brains had widespread microthrombi and microinfarcts. However, there are additional and less understood mechanisms by which SARS-CoV-2 and COVID-19 can cause neurologic dysfunction, leading to headaches, sleep disturbances, and delirium.[77] One notable reported consequence of COVID-19 is "COVID fog," which is marked by symptoms such as decreased memory, attention, and processing speed, which is similar to side effects of certain chemotherapeutic regimens.[94] A possible pathophysiologic link is due to elevated neurotoxic cytokines and reactive microglia. Similar to what is seen with influenza infection but less long-lasting is one cytokine, CCL11, which remains elevated in an animal model for 7 weeks after infection and has been associated with cognitive decline (Fig. 5).[94,95]

"Long COVID," or Postacute Sequalae of COVID-19 (PASC)

This long-lasting neurocognitive impairment is the second most common lingering symptom after COVID-19, following fatigue, and both affect almost one-third of patients, even 6–12 months after acute infection.[96,97] Long COVID, also called postacute sequelae of COVID-19 (PASC), is the syndrome manifested by chronic fatigue, chest discomfort, dyspnea, smell or taste changes, myalgic encephalomyelitis, postural orthostatic tachycardia, and others that persist after the resolution of the acute disease and lead to significant morbidity among affected individuals.[98] The pathophysiology is not fully described by several hypotheses including immune dysregulation, disruption of the microbiota, autoimmunity, viral persistence, and endothelial abnormalities.[98,99] While some risk factors for developing this syndrome have been identified, such as reinfection, high SARS-CoV-2 RNA copy numbers in the serum, presence of certain autoantibodies, and diabetes mellitus type 2, predicting who will suffer from PASC is still not reliably possible.[100,101] Vaccination has been shown to be protective and reduces the risk of developing long COVID up to 40%. Treatment for PASC remains primarily symptomatic and supportive, as no clearly effective treatments for PASC are yet known.[98] There is ongoing debate about whether the administration of antiviral medications such as nirmatrelvir-ritonavir reduces the risk of PASC. Some high-quality studies suggest no difference in overall risk but with a reduction in brain fog and chest tightness,[102] while others reviews conclude a significant reduction in PASC risk with early antivirals.[103,104]

Prevention, Treatment, and Vaccination

The litany of potential consequences of SARS-CoV-2 infection led to an understandable desire for prevention and treatment, some of which are covered in other chapters in this book and are so not reduplicated here. Public health and healthcare-based prevention, diagnosis, and treatment of COVID-19, and vaccination are all discussed in later chapters in this text. Regarding COVID-19 vaccines specifically, the optimal form and frequency of vaccination remain to be determined.

LESSONS LEARNED

Whether individually or collectively, medically or personally, indeed, in almost any conceivable sense, we all likely have lessons learned from the SARS-CoV-2 pandemic of 2019–22. Some of these are *sui generis* and cannot be universalized to any meaningful degree. Many, however, are worth remembering as we go forward. These lessons are encapsulated in several chapters elsewhere in this text and will not be belabored here, with only two exceptions.

First, there is a value in humility. As desperately as we may want immediate answers and treatments in times of uncertainty and pandemic, if we do not have them, then we should not proffer them. Corticosteroids were largely avoided for the first months of the pandemic based on experience with other coronaviruses, especially SARS.[105,106] To the credit of some authors, they recommended against corticosteroids only if used outside of clinical trials. Well-designed randomized clinical trials carried the day, and we discovered one of the most effective (and cost-effective) treatments for severe COVID-19.[107] The converse of this lesson is not to offer treatments without sound evidence. For navigating

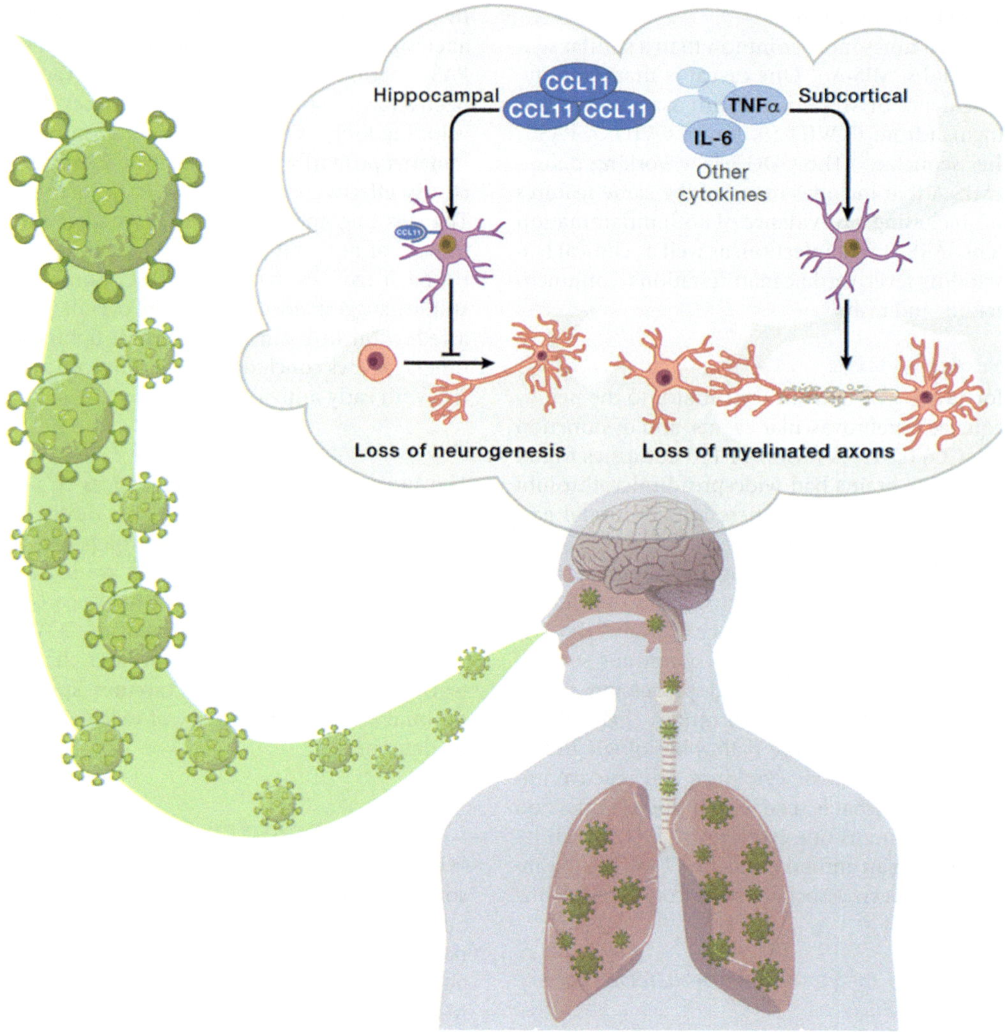

FIG. 5 Mechanism of SARS-CoV-2 neurotoxicity. Once SARS-CoV-2 enters the body and establishes a successful infectious cycle, it affects microglia in different regions of the brain through different cytokines. In the hippocampus, CCL11 drives loss of neurogenesis. In the subcortex, a different milieu of cytokines drives demyelination via the microglia. (Kao J, Frankland PW. COVID fog demystified. *Cell.* 2022;185(14):2391–2393.)

the Scylla and Charybdis of over- and undertreatment, quality clinical evidence is your surest guide. Use it if it exists, create it if it does not, and "first do no harm" during the wait.

Second, we should not rest on whatever laurels we may have from navigating this pandemic. This aphorism still holds true: before disaster strikes, any preparations may be deemed to be too much. After disaster strikes, they will be deemed too little.

REFERENCES

1. WHO. WHO Coronavirus (COVID-19) Dashboard. https://covid19.who.int/. Published 2023. Accessed April 16, 2023.
2. WHO. COVID-19—China https://www.who.int/emergencies/disease-outbreak-news/item/2020-DON229. Published 2020. Accessed March 3, 2022.
3. Wu F, Zhao S, Yu B, et al. A new coronavirus associated with human respiratory disease in China. *Nature.* 2020;579(7798):265–269.

4. Zhu N, Zhang D, Wang W, et al. A novel coronavirus from patients with pneumonia in China, 2019. *N Engl J Med.* 2020;382(8):727–733.
5. Guan W-J, Ni Z-Y, Hu Y, et al. Clinical characteristics of coronavirus disease 2019 in China. *N Engl J Med.* 2020;382(18):1708–1720.
6. Wu F., Zhao S., Yu B., et al. Severe Acute Respiratory Syndrome Coronavirus 2 Isolate Wuhan-Hu-1, Complete Genome. https://www.ncbi.nlm.nih.gov/nuccore/MN908947. Published 2020. Accessed November 21, 2021.
7. GISAID. GISAID. https://gisaid.org/. Published 2023. Accessed 2 June, 2023.
8. Hu B, Guo H, Zhou P, Shi Z-L. Characteristics of SARS-CoV-2 and COVID-19. *Nat Rev Microbiol.* 2021;19(3):141–154.
9. WHO. Novel Coronavirus(2019-nCoV) Situation Report—11; 2020.
10. Holshue ML, Debolt C, Lindquist S, et al. First case of 2019 novel coronavirus in the United States. *N Engl J Med.* 2020;382(10):929–936.
11. Reis J, Faou AL, Buguet A, Sandner G, Spencer P. Covid-19: early cases and disease spread. *Ann Glob Health.* 2022;88(1):83.
12. Kang D, Choi H, Kim JH, Choi J. Spatial epidemic dynamics of the COVID-19 outbreak in China. *Int J Infect Dis.* 2020;94:96–102.
13. Li Q, Guan X, Wu P, et al. Early transmission dynamics in wuhan, china, of novel coronavirus–infected pneumonia. *N Engl J Med.* 2020;382(13):1199–1207.
14. Liu WJ, Liu P, Lei W, et al. Surveillance of SARS-CoV-2 at the Huanan seafood market. *Nature.* 2024;631:402–408.
15. Almeida JDBD, Cunningham CH, Hamre D, et al. Virology: coronaviruses. *Nature.* 1968;220:650.
16. Jackson CB, Farzan M, Chen B, Choe H. Mechanisms of SARS-CoV-2 entry into cells. *Nat Rev Mol Cell Biol.* 2022;23(1):3–20.
17. Peng R, Wu LA, Wang Q, Qi J, Gao GF. Cell entry by SARS-CoV-2. *Trends Biochem Sci.* 2021;46(10):848–860.
18. Walls AC, Park Y-J, Tortorici MA, Wall A, McGuire AT, Veesler D. Structure, function, and antigenicity of the SARS-CoV-2 spike glycoprotein. *Cell.* 2020;181(2):281–292.e286.
19. Jamison DA, Anand Narayanan S, Trovão NS, et al. A comprehensive SARS-CoV-2 and COVID-19 review, part 1: intracellular overdrive for SARS-CoV-2 infection. *Eur J Hum Genet.* 2022;30(8):889–898.
20. Hoffmann M, Kleine-Weber H, Schroeder S, et al. SARS-CoV-2 cell entry depends on ACE2 and TMPRSS2 and is blocked by a clinically proven protease inhibitor. *Cell.* 2020;181(2):271–280.e278.
21. Nguyen HL, Lan PD, Thai NQ, Nissley DA, O'Brien EP, Li MS. Does SARS-CoV-2 bind to human ACE2 more strongly than does SARS-CoV? *J Phys Chem B.* 2020;124(34):7336–7347.
22. Han Y, Wang Z, Wei Z, Schapiro I, Li J. Binding affinity and mechanisms of SARS-CoV-2 variants. *Comput Struct Biotechnol J.* 2021;19:4184–4191.
23. Liu J, Li Y, Liu Q, et al. SARS-CoV-2 cell tropism and multiorgan infection. *Cell Discov.* 2021;7(1):17.
24. Hikmet F, Méar L, Edvinsson Å, Micke P, Uhlén M, Lindskog C. The protein expression profile of ACE2 in human tissues. *Mol Syst Biol.* 2020;16(7), e9610.
25. Osuchowski MF, Winkler MS, Skirecki T, et al. The COVID-19 puzzle: deciphering pathophysiology and phenotypes of a new disease entity. *Lancet Respir Med.* 2021;9(6):622–642.
26. Salamanna F, Maglio M, Landini MP, Fini M. Body localization of ACE-2: on the trail of the keyhole of SARS-CoV-2. *Front Med (Lausanne).* 2020;7, 594495.
27. Ramos-Casals M, Brito-Zerón P, Mariette X. Systemic and organ-specific immune-related manifestations of COVID-19. *Nat Rev Rheumatol.* 2021.
28. O'Sullivan JM, Gonagle DM, Ward SE, Preston RJS, O'Donnell JS. Endothelial cells orchestrate COVID-19 coagulopathy. *Lancet Haematol.* 2020;7(8):e553–e555.
29. Cantuti-Castelvetri L, Ojha R, Pedro LD, et al. Neuropilin-1 facilitates SARS-CoV-2 cell entry and infectivity. *Science.* 2020;370(6518):856–860.
30. Jaimes JA, Millet JK, Whittaker GR. Proteolytic cleavage of the SARS-CoV-2 spike protein and the role of the novel S1/S2 site. *iScience.* 2020;23(6), 101212.
31. Zang R, Castro MFG, McCune BT, et al. TMPRSS2 and TMPRSS4 promote SARS-CoV-2 infection of human small intestinal enterocytes. *Sci Immunol.* 2020;5(47), eabc3582.
32. Health NIo. Table 2a. In: NIH, ed. *Therapeutic Management of Nonhospitalized Adults With COVID-19*; 2022. United States.
33. WHO. Therapeutics and COVID-19: Living Guideline. https://www.who.int/publications/i/item/WHO-2019-nCoV-therapeutics-2022.4. Published 2022. Updated 14 July 2022. Accessed September 14, 2022.
34. Owen DR, Allerton CMN, Anderson AS, et al. An oral SARS-CoV-2 M(pro) inhibitor clinical candidate for the treatment of COVID-19. *Science.* 2021;374(6575):1586–1593.
35. Saravolatz LD, Depcinski S, Sharma M. Molnupiravir and nirmatrelvir-ritonavir: oral coronavirus disease 2019 antiviral drugs. *Clin Infect Dis.* 2023;76(1):165–171. https://doi.org/10.1093/cid/ciac180.
36. Hammond J, Leister-Tebbe H, Gardner A, et al. Oral nirmatrelvir for high-risk, nonhospitalized adults with Covid-19. *N Engl J Med.* 2022;386(15):1397–1408.
37. Jayk Bernal A, Gomes da Silva MM, Musungaie DB, et al. Molnupiravir for oral treatment of Covid-19 in nonhospitalized patients. *N Engl J Med.* 2021;386(6):509–520.
38. Tian L, Pang Z, Li M, et al. Molnupiravir and its antiviral activity against COVID-19. *Front Immunol.* 2022;13, 855496.
39. Wu Z, Yang L, Yang F, et al. Novel Henipa-like virus, Mojiang paramyxovirus, in rats, China, 2012. *Emerg Infect Dis.* 2014;20(6):1064–1066.
40. Zhou P, Yang X-L, Wang X-G, et al. Addendum: a pneumonia outbreak associated with a new coronavirus of probable bat origin. *Nature.* 2020;588:E6. https://doi.org/10.1038/s41586-020-2951-z.

41. Andersen KG, Rambaut A, Lipkin WI, Holmes EC, Garry RF. The proximal origin of SARS-CoV-2. *Nat Med.* 2020;26(4):450–452.
42. Wacharapluesadee S, Tan CW, Maneeorn P, et al. Evidence for SARS-CoV-2 related coronaviruses circulating in bats and pangolins in Southeast Asia. *Nat Commun.* 2021;12:972. https://doi.org/10.1038/s41467-021-21240-1.
43. Temmam S, Vongphayloth K, Baquero E, et al. Bat coronaviruses related to SARS-CoV-2 and infectious for human cells. *Nature.* 2022;604(7905):330–336.
44. Wrobel AG, Benton DJ, Xu P, et al. SARS-CoV-2 and bat RaTG13 spike glycoprotein structures inform on virus evolution and furin-cleavage effects. *Nat Struct Mol Biol.* 2020;27(8):763–767.
45. Chan YA, Zhan SH. The emergence of the spike furin cleavage site in SARS-CoV-2. *Mol Biol Evol.* 2022;39(1), msab327. https://doi.org/10.1093/molbev/msab327.
46. WHO. WHO Scientific Advisory Group for the Origins of Novel Pathogens (SAGO): Preliminary Report, 9 June 2022. World Health Organization; 2022:44.
47. WHO. WHO-Convened Global Study of Origins of SARS-CoV-2: China PART. Joint WHO-China study; 2021.
48. Wu ZHY, Wang Y, Liu B, et al. A Comprehensive Survey of Bat Sarbecoviruses Across China for the Origin Tracing of SARS-CoV and SARS-CoV-2. Research Squate; 2022.
49. Zhou H, Ji J, Chen X, et al. Identification of novel bat coronaviruses sheds light on the evolutionary origins of SARS-CoV-2 and related viruses. *Cell.* 2021;184(17):4380–4391.e4314.
50. Wu Z, Jin Q, Wu G, et al. SARS-CoV-2's origin should be investigated worldwide for pandemic prevention. *Lancet.* 2021;398(10308):1299–1303.
51. Worobey M, Levy JI, Malpica Serrano L, et al. The Huanan seafood wholesale market in Wuhan was the early epicenter of the COVID-19 pandemic. *Science.* 2022;377(6609):951–959.
52. Hale VL, Dennis PM, McBride DS, et al. SARS-CoV-2 infection in free-ranging white-tailed deer. *Nature.* 2022;602(7897):481–486.
53. Mallapati S. COVID-origins study links raccoon dogs to Wuhan market: what scientists think. Nature. https://www.nature.com/articles/d41586-023-00827-2. Published 2023. Updated March 22, 2023. Accessed April 5, 2023.
54. Crawley R. History of the Peloponnesian War Done into English by Richard Crawley. Limited: JM Dent & Sons; 1914.
55. Meyerowitz EA, Richterman A, Gandhi RT, Sax PE. Transmission of SARS-CoV-2: a review of viral, host, and environmental factors. *Ann Intern Med.* 2021;174(1):69–79.
56. Short KR, Cowling BJ. Assessing the potential for fomite transmission of SARS-CoV-2. *Lancet Microbe.* 2023;4(6):e380–e381.
57. Calvet GA, Kara E, Gonsalves L, et al. Viral shedding of SARS-CoV-2 in body fluids associated with sexual activity: a systematic review and meta-analysis. *BMJ Open.* 2024;14(2), e073084.
58. Ng SC, Chu AWH, Chan WM, et al. Re-examine the transfusion transmitted risk of SARS-CoV-2 virus during a major COVID-19 outbreak in 2022. *Transfus Med.* 2023;33(4):315–319.
59. Meyerowitz EA, Scott J, Richterman A, Male V, Cevik M. Clinical course and management of COVID-19 in the era of widespread population immunity. *Nat Rev Microbiol.* 2024;22(2):75–88.
60. Huang C, Wang Y, Li X, et al. Clinical features of patients infected with 2019 novel coronavirus in Wuhan, China. *Lancet.* 2020;395(10223):497–506.
61. Carvalho T, Krammer F, Iwasaki A. The first 12 months of COVID-19: a timeline of immunological insights. *Nat Rev Immunol.* 2021;21(4):245–256.
62. Vetter P, Vu DL, L'Huillier AG, Schibler M, Kaiser L, Jacquerioz F. Clinical features of covid-19. *BMJ.* 2020;369, m1470.
63. Al Demour S, Ababneh MA, Al-Taher RN, et al. Knowledge, practice, and attitude toward COVID-19 among physicians in Jordan and Palestine: cross-sectional study. *Int J Gen Med.* 2021;14:77–87.
64. Jaber RM, Mafrachi B, Al-Ani A, Shkara M. Awareness and perception of COVID-19 among the general population: a middle eastern survey. *PLoS One.* 2021;16(4), e0250461.
65. Liu Y, Wang D, Xu H, et al. A snapshot of public knowledge of novel coronavirus disease 2019: a web-based national survey. *BMC Public Health.* 2021;21(1):471.
66. Corrao G, Franchi M, Cereda D, et al. Increased risk of myocarditis and pericarditis and reduced likelihood of severe clinical outcomes associated with COVID-19 vaccination: a cohort study in Lombardy, Italy. *BMC Infect Dis.* 2022;22(1).
67. Wu Z, McGoogan JM. Characteristics of and important lessons from the coronavirus disease 2019 (COVID-19) outbreak in China: summary of a report of 72 314 cases from the Chinese Center for Disease Control and Prevention. *JAMA.* 2020;323(13):1239–1242.
68. Lewnard JA, Hong VX, Patel MM, Kahn R, Lipsitch M, Tartof SY. Clinical outcomes associated with SARS-CoV-2 Omicron (B.1.1.529) variant and BA.1/BA.1.1 or BA.2 subvariant infection in Southern California. *Nat Med.* 2022;28:1933–1943. https://doi.org/10.1038/s41591-022-01887-z.
69. Madhi SA, Kwatra G, Myers JE, et al. Population immunity and Covid-19 severity with Omicron variant in South Africa. *N Engl J Med.* 2022;386(14):1314–1326.
70. Hasan MN, Haider N, Stigler FL, et al. The global case-fatality rate of COVID-19 has been declining since may 2020. *Am J Trop Med Hyg.* 2021;104(6):2176–2184.
71. Cheng C, Zhou H, Weiss JC, Lipton ZC. Unpacking the drop in COVID-19 case fatality rates: a study of national and Florida line-level data. *AMIA Annu Symp Proc.* 2021;2021:285–294.

72. Edouard Mathieu H.R., L. Rodés-Guirao, C. Appel, D. Gavrilov, C. Giattino, J. Hasell, B. Macdonald, S. Dattani, D. Beltekian, E. Ortiz-Ospina, M. Roser. Mortality Risk of COVID-19. https://ourworldindata.org/mortality-risk-covid. Published 2023. Updated April 5, 2023. Accessed April 5, 2023.
73. Menter T, Haslbauer JD, Nienhold R, et al. Postmortem examination of COVID-19 patients reveals diffuse alveolar damage with severe capillary congestion and variegated findings in lungs and other organs suggesting vascular dysfunction. *Histopathology.* 2020;77(2):198–209.
74. Konopka KE, Nguyen T, Jentzen JM, et al. Diffuse alveolar damage (DAD) resulting from coronavirus disease 2019 infection is morphologically indistinguishable from other causes of DAD. *Histopathology.* 2020;77(4):570–578.
75. Milross L, Majo J, Cooper N, et al. Post-mortem lung tissue: the fossil record of the pathophysiology and immunopathology of severe COVID-19. *Lancet Respir Med.* 2022;10(1):95–106.
76. Goshua G, Pine AB, Meizlish ML, et al. Endotheliopathy in COVID-19-associated coagulopathy: evidence from a single-Centre, cross-sectional study. *Lancet Haematol.* 2020;7(8):e575–e582.
77. Conway EM, Mackman N, Warren RQ, et al. Understanding COVID-19-associated coagulopathy. *Nat Rev Immunol.* 2022;22(10):639–649.
78. Shi S, Qin M, Shen B, et al. Association of cardiac injury with mortality in hospitalized patients with COVID-19 in Wuhan, China. *JAMA Cardiol.* 2020;5(7):802.
79. Guo T, Fan Y, Chen M, et al. Cardiovascular implications of fatal outcomes of patients with coronavirus disease 2019 (COVID-19). *JAMA Cardiol.* 2020;5(7):811.
80. Hanley B, Naresh KN, Roufosse C, et al. Histopathological findings and viral tropism in UK patients with severe fatal COVID-19: a post-mortem study. *Lancet Microbe.* 2020;1(6):e245–e253.
81. Nishiga M, Wang DW, Han Y, Lewis DB, Wu JC. COVID-19 and cardiovascular disease: from basic mechanisms to clinical perspectives. *Nat Rev Cardiol.* 2020;17(9):543–558.
82. Xie Y, Xu E, Bowe B, Al-Aly Z. Long-term cardiovascular outcomes of COVID-19. *Nat Med.* 2022;28(3):583–590.
83. Heidecker B, Dagan N, Balicer R, et al. Myocarditis following COVID–19 vaccine: incidence, presentation, diagnosis, pathophysiology, therapy, and outcomes put into perspective. A clinical consensus document supported by the Heart Failure Association of the European Society of Cardiolo. *Eur J Heart Fail.* 2022;24(11):2000–2018.
84. Feldstein LR, Tenforde MW, Friedman KG, et al. Characteristics and outcomes of US children and adolescents with multisystem inflammatory syndrome in children (MIS-C) compared with severe acute COVID-19. *JAMA.* 2021;325(11):1074.
85. Molloy EJ, Nakra N, Gale C, Dimitriades VR, Lakshminrusimha S. Multisystem inflammatory syndrome in children (MIS-C) and neonates (MIS-N) associated with COVID-19: optimizing definition and management. *Pediatr Res.* 2023;93(6):1499–1508.
86. Wangu Z, Swartz H, Doherty M. Multisystem inflammatory syndrome in children (MIS-C) possibly secondary to COVID-19 mRNA vaccination. *BMJ Case Rep.* 2022;15(3), e247176.
87. Zambrano LDNM, Olson SM, et al. Effectiveness of BNT162b2 (Pfizer-BioNTech) mRNA vaccination against multisystem inflammatory syndrome in children among persons aged 12–18 years—United States, July–December 2021. *MMWR Morb Mortal Wkly Rep.* 2022;71:52–58.
88. Ouldali N, Bagheri H, Salvo F, et al. Hyper inflammatory syndrome following COVID-19 mRNA vaccine in children: a national post-authorization pharmacovigilance study. *Lancet Reg Health Eur.* 2022;17, 100393.
89. Elias MD, Truong DT, Oster ME, et al. Examination of adverse reactions after COVID-19 vaccination among patients with a history of multisystem inflammatory syndrome in children. *JAMA Netw Open.* 2023;6(1), e2248987.
90. McCrindle BW, Harahsheh AS, Handoko R, et al. SARS-CoV-2 variants and multisystem inflammatory syndrome in children. *N Engl J Med.* 2023;388(17):1624–1626.
91. Belay ED, Godfred Cato S, Rao AK, et al. Multisystem inflammatory syndrome in adults after severe acute respiratory syndrome coronavirus 2 (SARS-CoV-2) infection and coronavirus disease 2019 (COVID-19) vaccination. *Clin Infect Dis.* 2021;75(1):e741–e748.
92. Patel P, Decuir J, Abrams J, Campbell AP, Godfred-Cato S, Belay ED. Clinical characteristics of multisystem inflammatory syndrome in adults. *JAMA Netw Open.* 2021;4(9), e2126456.
93. CDC. Multisystem Inflammatory Syndrome in Adults (MIS-A) Case Definition and Information for Healthcare Providers. https://www.cdc.gov/mis/mis-a/hcp.html. Published 2023. Accessed June 6th, 2023.
94. Kao J, Frankland PW. COVID fog demystified. *Cell.* 2022;185(14):2391–2393.
95. Fernández-Castañeda A, Lu P, Geraghty AC, et al. Mild respiratory COVID can cause multi-lineage neural cell and myelin dysregulation. *Cell.* 2022;185(14):2452–2468. e2416.
96. Peter RS, Nieters A, Kräusslich H-G, et al. Post-acute sequelae of covid-19 six to 12 months after infection: population based study. *BMJ.* 2022;379, e071050.
97. Proal AD, VanElzakker MB. Long COVID or post-acute sequelae of COVID-19 (PASC): an overview of biological factors that may contribute to persistent symptoms. *Front Microbiol.* 2021;12, 698169.
98. Davis HE, McCorkell L, Vogel JM, Topol EJ. Long COVID: major findings, mechanisms and recommendations. *Nat Rev Microbiol.* 2023;21(3):133–146.
99. Narayanan SA, Jamison DA, Guarnieri JW, et al. A comprehensive SARS-CoV-2 and COVID-19 review, part 2: host extracellular to systemic effects of SARS-CoV-2 infection. *Eur J Hum Genet.* 2024;32(1):10–20.

100. Su Y, Yuan D, Chen DG, et al. Multiple early factors anticipate post-acute COVID-19 sequelae. *Cell.* 2022;185(5):881–895.e820.
101. Bowe B, Xie Y, Al-Aly Z. Acute and postacute sequelae associated with SARS-CoV-2 reinfection. *Nat Med.* 2022;28(11):2398–2405.
102. Congdon S, Narrowe Z, Yone N, et al. Nirmatrelvir/ritonavir and risk of long COVID symptoms: a retrospective cohort study. *Sci Rep.* 2023;13:19688. https://doi.org/10.1038/s41598-023-46912-4.
103. Choi YJ, Seo YB, Seo J-W, et al. Effectiveness of antiviral therapy on long COVID: a systematic review and meta-analysis. *J Clin Med.* 2023;12(23):7375.
104. Jiang J, Li Y, Jiang Q, Jiang Y, Qin H, Li Y. Early use of oral antiviral drugs and the risk of post COVID-19 syndrome: a systematic review and network meta-analysis. *J Infect.* 2024;89(2), 106190.
105. Tang C, Wang Y, Lv H, Guan Z, Gu J. Caution against corticosteroid-based COVID-19 treatment. *Lancet.* 2020;395(10239):1759–1760.
106. Russell CD, Millar JE, Baillie JK. Clinical evidence does not support corticosteroid treatment for 2019-nCoV lung injury. *Lancet.* 2020;395(10223):473–475.
107. Group; TRC. Dexamethasone in hospitalized patients with Covid-19. *N Engl J Med.* 2021;384(8):693–704.

CHAPTER 13

The Age of Synthetic Biology: Changing Biosecurity Risks

GIGI KWIK GRONVALL[a,b]
[a]Johns Hopkins Bloomberg School of Public Health, Department of Environmental Health and Engineering, Baltimore, MD, United States • [b]Johns Hopkins Center for Health Security, Baltimore, MD, United States

INTRODUCTION

Synthetic biology is a relatively new scientific discipline that aims to make biology easier to engineer, and more useful.[1] Groundbreaking and newsworthy synthetic biology techniques such as CRISPR (Clustered Regularly Interspaced Short Palindromic Repeat), which can be used to "find and replace" sections of genetic material, make living organisms more amenable to genetic manipulation. Synthetic biology is already being used for a variety of applications in medicine, environmental sensing, environmental remediation, and biomanufacturing, as well as to make detergents, adhesives, and flavorings.[2] In 2016, the World Economic Forum listed synthetic biology as one of its top 10 emerging technologies.[3] But despite the numerous beneficial medical, industrial, and basic research advances that may be made with synthetic biology, it is vulnerable to misuse: synthetic biology may be exploited for harm to increase the range and types of biological weapons that can be developed.

It is important to note that developing a biological weapon does not require synthetic biology or any new biotechnologies. Biological weapons were made without these techniques and can still be made without advanced biotechnologies. Countering biological weapons made using traditional microbiological techniques would present a major challenge for public health and national security, as other chapters in this volume make clear.

Nonetheless, synthetic biology poses additional problems for biodefense. The first problem is that by using synthetic biology techniques, a pathogen can be made "from scratch" in a laboratory, instead of requiring an actor to acquire a pathogen sample from another laboratory or from the environment. As the regulatory structure for biosecurity and laboratory management is largely based on access controls, the use of synthetic biology could allow a nefarious actor to sidestep these controls. A second problem that synthetic biology poses for biosecurity is its accessibility: the tools of synthetic biology are making the tools for biological weapons development more accessible and with ever-lowering costs.

Ideally, regulatory and governance policies would be put into place that would prevent biosecurity threats from emerging from the use of synthetic biology. The application of norms, guidance, regulations, and requirements can indeed be applied to detect and deter misuse, making biological weapons development and use more difficult to achieve without detection. However, given the dual-use nature of synthetic biology, just as in other areas of biology, preventing the misuse of this field in its entirety is not feasible. Though synthetic biology has the potential to lower barriers to biological weapons development, there are also reasons for hope: in addition to the dual-use qualities, synthetic biology has great potential to speed the medical response to biological weapons use, such as the faster development of drugs, vaccines, and other medical countermeasures.

This chapter describes the security risks of synthetic biology, potential mitigation strategies so that the benefits of synthetic biology and related fields may be realized, and steps that have already been taken to diminish biosecurity threats.

MAKING PATHOGENS "FROM SCRATCH"

Pathogen samples found in laboratory collections almost always are derived from other existing laboratory samples or from an environmental or clinical source.

Viral Outbreaks, Biosecurity, and Preparing for Mass Casualty Infectious Diseases Events
https://doi.org/10.1016/B978-0-323-54841-0.00005-6

For example, a scientist performing research on Ebola virus in a BSL-4 laboratory may use an Ebola Kikwit strain, named for the town where it was clinically isolated during the 1995 Ebola outbreak in Zaire (now the Democratic Republic of the Congo). Every sample comes from somewhere. Even the *Bacillus anthracis* strain used in the 2001 anthrax letter attacks originally came from a sample taken from an infected cow in Texas.[4]

The requirement for starting with an existing sample to acquire a pathogen has made it possible to institute regulatory biosecurity controls, intended to prevent access to samples of dangerous pathogens by people who should not have them. For a researcher to start laboratory work on Ebola virus in the United States, for example, they would likely need to acquire a sample from another Ebola researcher. In the United States, as well as in many other countries, the ability to acquire such a pathogen sample has numerous restrictions, as Ebola is a regulated pathogen under the Select Agent Rule (and is also on the Australia Group List).[5–7]

Multiple levels of clearance are required to access a select agent in the United States. An individual researcher needs to have passed an SRA, or security risk assessment, which is an electronic records check performed by the Federal Bureau of Investigation (FBI). The research facility where the work is to be done needs to be cleared by the Center for Disease Control and Prevention (CDC) or the US Department of Agriculture/Animal and Plant Health Inspection Service (APHIS). All transfers of pathogen samples from one laboratory to another require documentation.

The select agent regulations were never absolute restrictions, able to stop all access to dangerous pathogens by people who meant to do harm. The regulations could not stop an individual from acquiring a pathogen from an ongoing outbreak, for example, or finding another environmental source to acquire a pathogen, or accessing a laboratory in a country that does not limit access to certain pathogens. As there are reported clinical cases of almost all of the pathogens on the Select Agent list, every year, somewhere in the world, there are multiple opportunities to find almost all of the pathogens on the Select Agent list in the natural world.[8] Yet, the select agent regulations, as well as complementary regulations found in other nations, did make it much more difficult to acquire pathogens that may be of concern from other laboratories.

Synthetic biology has been changing the requirement to start with an existing sample, however. In 2002, a *Science* magazine article was published by researchers at the State University of New York (SUNY) at Stony Brook, which demonstrated the creation of an infectious poliovirus using mail-ordered DNA segments.[9] The researchers chemically strung together 60 base-pair pieces of DNA to build DNA molecules encoding the ~7500 base-pair virus. Once the DNA was transcribed into RNA and translated into proteins, the researchers had an infectious poliovirus. The technical challenges in developing the poliovirus were not trivial; it took 3 years to perform the polio work.[10]

The publication of chemically synthesized poliovirus caused alarm among policymakers, particularly when it became widely known that the genetic information for poliovirus, as with most other viruses, is available on the Internet through the National Center for Biotechnology Information (NCBI) databases. As gene synthesis technology is broadly and globally accessible, and the genetic sequence information for a variety of pathogens is also broadly and globally accessible, there would be little to prevent or deter a nefarious actor from making other pathogens from scratch.

Two years after the poliovirus work was published, researchers at the J. Craig Venter Institute (JCVI) synthesized and "booted up" a similarly sized bacteriophage.[11] Instead of 3 years, however, it took the JCVI researchers just 2 weeks to accomplish this task, demonstrating that the technical barriers toward making viruses from their genetic information were becoming less onerous.

Additional synthesis projects proceeded at a quick pace. In 2005, the 1918 "Spanish" influenza virus was reconstructed.[12] Other influenza viruses were synthesized for the development of a flu vaccine.[13] Eventually, all viruses were thought to be available to be synthesized and booted up. For many scientists, it was thus not a surprise when Canadian researchers synthesized and booted up an orthopoxvirus, the causative agent of horsepox.[14] The biosecurity implications of synthesizing a virus that is a close cousin to another orthopoxvirus, *variola major*, the causative agent of smallpox disease, caused controversy in the biosecurity field.[15–17] Smallpox is eradicated and is only known to be found in two secure laboratories, one in Atlanta (at the CDC) and one in Russia. Smallpox was a devastating disease, killing 30% of those who were infected. The United States has stockpiles of vaccines in case they are ever returned. In fact, creating a smallpox vaccine was one of the stated reasons for horsepox synthesis, as there is some evidence that the original smallpox vaccine used by Jenner may have been horsepox virus or horsepox virus-like.[18]

While all viruses can be synthesized and booted up to make infectious viruses, it is not as feasible to synthesize other organisms from scratch, at least not yet. In a major breakthrough in 2010, J. Craig Venter and colleagues published that they had synthesized an entire bacterial genome and booted it up.[19–21] It took 15 years and $40 M to achieve this goal.[22] They followed up this feat in 2016 with a modified version of their synthetic organism, which has a pared-down "minimal" genome that nonetheless has all the genes essential for life.[19]

Yeast has also been the focus of synthesis projects, and as a eukaryote, it has an even more complex genome than the bacterial cell that was the focus of the JCVI work. In 2014, a team of researchers produced a fully functional chromosome from *Saccharomyces cerevisiae* or baker's yeast.[23] There is a project, "Synthetic Yeast 2.0" or "Sc2.0," to design an entire yeast genome.[24] Once it is completed, there will be possibilities to research how transposons evolve and spread, as well as to understand how gene deletions and rearrangements affect viability.

An even more ambitious project is underway, now: Genome Project-write (GP-write), which aims to engineer human cell lines and other organisms of public health and agricultural significance.[25] The organizers aim to reduce the costs of engineering and testing large genomes more than 1000-fold.[25]

The malicious use of synthetic biology and modern laboratory techniques to develop a pathogen from scratch is currently limited to the synthesis and booting up of viruses. It will likely remain out of reach for some time to synthesize and boot up whole bacteria. However, it has been possible to modify bacteria for some time, and making bacteria antibiotic-resistant, for example, has been possible for decades.[26,27] Synthetic biology will make that process easier.

CONTROLS ON THE SYNTHESIS AND BOOTING UP OF PATHOGENS

In 2006, a reporter from The Guardian, in the United Kingdom, placed an online order to a gene synthesis company.[28,29] The order was for a relatively small 78-base-pair piece of DNA, but the sequence matched the sequence for *variola major*, the causative agent of smallpox disease. The reporter had ordered the DNA piece to be delivered to a residential address, not a research institution or biotechnology company, and had also made up a company name for the order. Despite these red flags, the company made the DNA and shipped it to the reporter. The complete smallpox virus is 52,000 base pairs, so the 78-base-pair piece was not of any significance, and there was no danger to the public. Nonetheless, the point was made that DNA and gene synthesis companies could unwittingly provide gene synthesis services for potentially nefarious actors. When the reporter broke the story, the DNA synthesis company had to admit that there was no routine screening of their orders to detect people ordering the DNA of regulated pathogens, and there was no customer screening performed, which could have flagged that reporter's order, using a fake company name, as suspicious.

Steps were immediately taken to make gene synthesis more secure. The Alfred P. Sloan Foundation funded the creation of the first sequence screening software; using this software, a gene synthesis company could screen the sequences of the orders they received and could be alerted if the sequence matched a regulated pathogen.[30] A consortium of gene synthesis companies banded together to share approaches and commit to screening.[31]

In 2010, the US Department of Health and Human Services issued guidance for the industry. The guidance petitions suppliers of double-stranded DNA to screen the sequences of their customer orders to look for prohibited matches.[32] In addition to screening sequences, the Department of Health and Human Services (HHS) guidance called for enhanced customer screening to ensure compliance with US trade restrictions and export controls. Should sequence screening determine that a customer has requested genetic material that is only legally available to those with clearance to work with select agents, for example, then the customer must provide documentation to the gene synthesis company that they are compliant with select agent regulations.

Some synthesis companies banded together to form codes of conduct and to agree to screen their orders. One such group, the International Gene Synthesis Consortium, exists to this day and claims that their membership of 11 DNA providers consists of 80% of the gene synthesis market.[31] It is an international group, consisting of companies in the United States, Europe, Korea, and China. While the details have not been released to the public, in 2018, the International Gene Synthesis Consrtium (IGSC) announced that they have updated their "Harmonized Screening Protocol" so that companies may identify potentially illegal requests and institute customer screening to "ensure that synthetic gene orders are only provided to validated end-users, not distributors or resellers." The screening protocol consists at least of the US Select Agent list, as well as the Australia Group List agents, the US Commerce Control List, and regulated European sequences.[33]

There are limits to the controls on gene synthesis. Nefarious actors could get around the screening performed by many gene synthesis companies by either selecting a company that does not perform screening, by ordering only oligonucleotide pieces (the screening guidance states that companies should screen double-stranded pieces longer than 200 base pairs, for example, but it is possible to string together much smaller pieces), or by making the DNA using relatively commonly acquired laboratory equipment.[34] While commercial suppliers tend to produce more reliable products than individual efforts at gene synthesis, it is possible to make genes (and viruses) without their services.

There is also the question of reporting. In the United States, if there is a suspicious gene synthesis order requested, companies are aware that they can report this to the FBI. There have been considerable efforts to spread the word about a "see something, say something" campaign for reporting bioterrorism or biosecurity issues to the FBI. In many other countries, it is not nearly as clear-cut whether or how to report suspicious orders.[35,36]

Companies that perform screening are currently at a disadvantage, as the costs for synthesis are continuing to drop, but the costs for screening (which requires human judgment for particularly problematic sequences) remain constant and may increase.[37] Sequence screening is becoming a bigger portion of the company's bottom line. This has led to concerns that more companies will drop screening from their business practices.

There are few potential biosecurity controls that are possible to institute on gene synthesis, so it is worth supporting screening so long as it could be effective as a deterrent. Some activities to support companies that perform sequence screening are already underway, such as developing a refined database that the gene synthesis companies could use for their screening.[38] Others have suggested that the screening be funded by governments, or that diplomatic pressure be exerted on those countries that do not either support screening or have a mechanism whereby potentially suspicious orders may be reported.[38]

THE AGE OF SYNTHETIC BIOLOGY

While the ability to make pathogens versus acquiring them from another source may now be the greatest potential area for misuse in synthetic biology, there are additional causes for security concerns as synthetic biology and related biotechnologies advance. One is that the application of the "design, build, test" cycle—an engineering stalwart—is now more possible in biology and can be misused. Many different designs can be designed and tested in parallel. Factors contributing to this include increased powers of computational modeling and much-decreased costs for DNA synthesis.

The ability to test many different possibilities at once is currently more likely to be misused than the design of a novel pathogen. Nonetheless, the idea that an entirely novel pathogen could be designed with new effects, or that a pathogen could be designed to target either one individual, has captured the imagination of policymakers. In 2012, an article appeared in the Atlantic magazine that described one such potential weapon that would be designed to target just one person: the US president.[39] Building upon ongoing research into developing individually tailored cancer therapies, the idea was that a weapon could be designed that would affect just one person. Such an endeavor would not be easy or likely in the immediate future, due to the amount of research funding and time required. Even with CRISPR to help in manipulating portions of the pathogen genome, there would be numerous technical challenges involved in such an effort, and an individually tailored weapon would require a great deal of research, development, and testing. Testing and refining would be complicated for a designed pathogen that has only one lethal target. Also, delivering a weapon with these characteristics would be a major research and development effort as well. In the *Atlantic* article scenario, the assassination virus would spread naturally among a group to its intended target—but this would be of uncertain statistical likelihood.

Given the complexity of an individual assassination effort using a pathogen, any concerns about an entirely novel biological weapon that does not have a great deal of similarity to an existent disease are outside of the realm of a nonstate actor group, or an individual bad actor. Perhaps nation-states that can afford to commit large amounts of resources would invest in such an effort. But at this time there are certainly many easier paths to "success" with a simpler, less novel, biological weapon.

DETERMINING WHETHER NEW ADVANCES RAISE BIOSECURITY CONCERNS—THE IMPERIALE REPORT

If this chapter were to provide a list of all the new advances in synthetic biology that have the potential to raise biosecurity concerns or to be misused, that list would almost certainly be quickly out of date. The pace and progress of synthetic biology guarantee that such a list would quickly be replaced with other potentially concerning items, as well as potentially new insights that may mitigate concerns. For example, in recent years there has been a great deal of biosecurity concern about gene drives—a mechanism of nonmendelian inheritance that can spread a gene quickly throughout a population. The idea of quickly manipulating a population of mosquitoes could lead to another method for the control of diseases like malaria and dengue, but misuse could be broadly affecting.[40] Further research is revealing that gene drives may be more complicated to introduce, for positive or negative reasons, due to natural resistance.[41]

Synthetic biology and other biotechnological advances will continue to generally raise biosecurity concerns for the foreseeable future. Unfortunately, in the last several years, specific biosecurity concerns have often been driven by events such as a published paper, or a remark by a scientist at a conference—these events can objectively distort how much a piece of scientific information is truly lowering barriers to biological weapons development. Given the volume of information that is published in the scientific literature and the rapid development of biotechnology, it became clear that a process was needed to carefully evaluate whether a particular scientific advance posed a particular biosecurity concern. The US Department of Defense, in particular, wanted a process to determine what, specifically, to be concerned about, and why.

To this end, the US DoD Chemical and Biological Defense Program funded a National Academies of Sciences, Engineering, and Medicine to appoint a committee to "address the changing nature of the biodefense threat in the age of synthetic biology."[42] The committee recently published its proposed framework to identify potential biodefense vulnerabilities posed by synthetic biology. The framework was intended to be used as a tool to aid analysts who are, for example, analyzing biotechnologies in order to evaluate how much concern they should have about those biotechnologies; to understand how different biotechnologies relate to each other in raising biosecurity concerns; to identify key bottlenecks or barriers that, if addressed or removed, would change the level of biosecurity concern for the entire technology; and for horizon scanning or future threat analyses, to project how biosecurity concerns may change over time. The framework does not address information about the *intent* of an actor to use biological weapons and does not require the use of intelligence information, which may be an important part of some biosecurity analyses.

The framework can be used by an analyst to examine a new technology, assess the capability for misuse, and assess the capability for mitigation of a potential weapon. To assess the capability of malicious use, the analyst would need to consider the **use of the technology**, including its *ease of use* (if a technology is not relatively challenging to use, it is more likely to be used), the *rate of development of the technology* (which may signal that technology may become more of a biosecurity concern in the immediate future), the *barriers to use* (these could be technological barriers, such as the inability to predict function from sequence), *synergy with other technologies*, and *cost*. The analyst would also need to consider the potential for a technology to be **used as a weapon**. Such considerations include the capacity for *production and delivery* of the technology, the *scope of casualties* if used as a weapon, the *predictability of result* (describing the degree that a malicious actor could be confident that if a technology would be used to develop a weapon that it were the intended result), the *testing* required, as well as the *fidelity* of the technology, which is another way of expressing whether it is predictable and reliable. The framework also addresses the **attributes of actors** as well, such as their *access to expertise*, *access to resources*, and whether the technology has *organizational footprint requirements*.

Any attack using a new technology would depend upon both the actor being able to use it in the development of a weapon as well as the target's capability to either deter, detect, or respond to the attack—these are **mitigation factors**. The report lists some of the *deterrence and prevention* capabilities, asking, for example, "Can the use of the technology be controlled or prevented through regulation or other means?" and "Is the technology geographically centralized, or widely distributed?" Other factors include the *capability to recognize an attack* as well as the capability for *attribution or consequence management*. By analyzing these aspects that contribute to biosecurity risks, an analyst can make a judgment about whether a piece of research is lowering barriers to biological weapons development or use.

CONCLUSION

Synthetic biology and other related biotechnologies have the potential to lower barriers to biological weapons development. Using synthetic biology, an actor could acquire pathogens without starting with an existing sample. It is also possible to test many parallel approaches to designing new functions into existing pathogens, given that the costs of DNA synthesis continue to drop. While early nonsynthetic biology paths to biological weapons development are still possible, these new issues add to existing biosecurity concerns.

REFERENCES

1. Synthetic Biology Project. *What Is Synthetic Biology?* Woodrow Wilson International Center for Scholars; 2013 [Accessed January 31, 2018].
2. Doudna JA, Charpentier E, Genome editing. The new frontier of genome engineering with CRISPR-Cas9. *Science.* 2014;346(6213), 1258096.
3. World Economic Forum. These Are the Top 10 Emerging Technologies of 2016; 2016. https://www.weforum.org/agenda/2016/06/top-10-emerging-technologies-2016/.
4. Broad WJ. Geographic gaffe misguides anthrax inquiry. *N Y Times.* 2002;(January 30).
5. Uniting and Strengthening America by Providing Appropriate Tools Required to Intercept and Obstruct Terrorism (USA PATRIOT ACT) Act of 2001, §Sec. 817. Expansion of the Biological Weapons Statute; 2001.
6. Federal Select Agent Program. Select Agents and Toxins List; 2018. http://www.selectagents.gov/SelectAgentsandToxinsList.html. Accessed January 31, 2018.
7. The Australia Group. Common Control Lists; 2017. http://www.australiagroup.net/en/controllists.html. Accessed 31 January 2018.
8. Rambhia KJ, Ribner AS, Gronvall GK. Everywhere you look: select agent pathogens. *Biosecur Bioterror.* 2011;9(1):69–71.
9. Cello J, Paul AV, Wimmer E. Chemical synthesis of poliovirus cDNA: generation of infectious virus in the absence of natural template. *Science.* 2002;297(5583):1016–1018.
10. Wimmer E. The test-tube synthesis of a chemical called poliovirus. The simple synthesis of a virus has far-reaching societal implications. *EMBO Rep.* 2006;7:3–S9. Spec. No. (S3).
11. Smith HO, Hutchison 3rd CA, Pfannkoch C, Venter JC. Generating a synthetic genome by whole genome assembly: phiX174 bacteriophage from synthetic oligonucleotides. *Proc Natl Acad Sci USA.* 2003;100(26):15440–15445.
12. Tumpey TM, Basler CF, Aguilar PV, et al. Characterization of the reconstructed 1918 Spanish influenza pandemic virus. *Science.* 2005;310(5745):77–80.
13. Dormitzer PR, Suphaphiphat P, Gibson DG, et al. Synthetic generation of influenza vaccine viruses for rapid response to pandemics. *Sci Transl Med.* 2013;5(185):185ra168.
14. Noyce RS, Lederman S, Evans DH. Construction of an infectious horsepox virus vaccine from chemically synthesized DNA fragments. *PLoS One.* 2018;13(1), e0188453.
15. Koblentz GD. The de novo synthesis of horsepox virus: implications for biosecurity and recommendations for preventing the reemergence of smallpox. *Health Secur.* 2017;15(6):620–628.
16. Inglesby T. Important questions global health and science leaders should be asking in the wake of horsepox synthesis. *The Bifurcated Needle.* 2017;2017.
17. DiEuliis D, Berger K, Gronvall G. Biosecurity implications for the synthesis of horsepox, an orthopoxvirus. *Health Secur.* 2017.
18. Schrick L, Tausch SH, Dabrowski PW, Damaso CR, Esparza J, Nitsche A. An early American smallpox vaccine based on horsepox. *N Engl J Med.* 2017;377(15):1491–1492.
19. Hutchison CA, Chuang R-Y, Noskov VN, et al. Design and synthesis of a minimal bacterial genome. *Science.* 2016;351(6280).
20. Venter JC, Gibson D. How we created the first synthetic cell. *Wall Street J.* 2010;(May 26). Opinion.
21. J. Craig Venter Institute. First Self-Replicating Synthetic Bacterial Cell Frequently Asked Questions; 2010. http://www.jcvi.org/cms/research/projects/first-self-replicating-synthetic-bacterial-cell/faq. Accessed 31 January 2018.
22. Pollack A. His corporate strategy: the scientific method. *N Y Times.* 2010;(September 5):BU1.
23. Annaluru N, Muller H, Mitchell LA, et al. Total synthesis of a functional designer eukaryotic chromosome. *Science.* 2014;344(6179):55–58.
24. Synthetic Yeast 2.0. http://syntheticyeast.org/. Accessed January 31, 2018.
25. GP-Write. http://engineeringbiologycenter.org/gp-write-consortium/. Accessed January 31, 2018.
26. Athamna A, Athamna M, Abu-Rashed N, Medlej B, Bast DJ, Rubinstein E. Selection of *Bacillus anthracis* isolates resistant to antibiotics. *J Antimicrob Chemother.* 2004;54(2):424–428.
27. Brook I, Elliott TB, Pryor 2nd HI, et al. In vitro resistance of *Bacillus anthracis* sterne to doxycycline, macrolides and quinolones. *Int J Antimicrob Agents.* 2001;18(6):559–562.
28. Randerson J. Did anyone order smallpox? *Guardian Weekly.* 2006.
29. Randerson J. Revealed: the lax laws that could allow assembly of deadly virus DNA. *The Guardian.* 2006;(June 13). Science.
30. Jones R, Craic Computing LLC. Sequence screening. In: Garfinkel MS, Endy D, Epstein GL, Friedman RM, eds. *Working Papers for Synthetic Genomics: Risks and Benefits for Science and Society*; 2005.
31. International Gene Synthesis Consortium (ICSC). Harmonized Screening Protocol: Gene Sequence & Customer Screening to Promote Biosecurity; 2009.
32. US Department of Health and Human Services. Screening framework guidance for providers of synthetic double-stranded DNA. *Fed Regist.* 2010;75(197):62820–62832.
33. International Gene Synthesis Consortium. International Gene Synthesis Consortium Updates Screening Protocols for Synthetic DNA Products and Service. January 31; 2018.
34. Gibson DG. Enzymatic assembly of overlapping DNA fragments. *Methods Enzymol.* 2011;498:349–361.
35. Kwinn L, ed. FBI connects science and security communities. *Sci Saf Secur Quart.* 2012;2:1–5.
36. Lempinen EW. FBI, AAAS Collaborate on Ambitious Outreach to Biotech Researchers and DIY Biologists. April 1; 2011.
37. Carter SR, Friedman RM. DNA Synthesis and Biosecurity: Lessons Learned and Options for the Future. J. Craig Venter Institute; 2015.
38. DiEuliis D, Carter SR, Gronvall GK. Options for synthetic DNA order screening. *mSphere.* 2017;2(4). e00319-00317. Revisited.

39 Hessel A, Goodman M, Kotler S. Hacking the president's DNA. *The Atlantic*. 2012;2012.
40. Oye KA, Esvelt K, Appleton E, et al. Regulating gene drives. *Science*. 2014;345(6197):626–628.
41. Champer J, Reeves R, Oh SY, et al. Novel CRISPR/Cas9 gene drive constructs reveal insights into mechanisms of resistance allele formation and drive efficiency in genetically diverse populations. *PLoS Genet*. 2017;13(7), e1006796.
42. National Academies of Sciences E, Medicine. A Proposed Framework for Identifying Potential Biodefense Vulnerabilities Posed by Synthetic Biology: Interim Report; 2017.

CHAPTER 14

Preparing for Viral Outbreaks and Bioterrorism: The Public Health Perspective

MARY M.K. FOOTE[a] • MITCHELL STRIPLING[b]
[a]NYC Department of Health and Mental Hygiene, Long Island City, NY, United States • [b]NYC Preparedness & Recovery Institute, New York, NY, United States

INTRODUCTION

Many of you may be familiar with the story of John Snow, the "father of modern epidemiology," and the Broad Street pump. In the 1850s, London was in the middle of one of the largest cholera epidemics in its history. John Snow, an anesthesiologist by training, had been studying recent cholera outbreaks and had developed a working hypothesis that the disease was spread by some sort of contamination in the water supply that enabled it to spread from person to person. This hypothesis was contrary to the prevailing theory at the time that many diseases were spread through "miasma," or contaminated, foul-smelling air.

In August 1854, a particularly severe outbreak exploded in the Soho neighborhood. Dr. Snow and a local priest named Henry Whitehead conducted an intensive case investigation and utilized their findings to develop a map of the district with dots representing individual cholera cases. Through this mapping, he was able to identify a strong association between cholera risk and proximity to a specific water pump located on Broad Street.

That is the most famous part of the story, but not the most important. For our purposes, we want to highlight *what happened to stop the outbreak and prepare for the next one.*

First, Snow took his findings to town officials. As an emergency measure, they removed the handle from the Broad Street well, and cholera cases dropped precipitously. However, as Snow himself admitted, many residents had fled the neighborhood, and cases were already on the decline. Did removing the handle prevent future cases? Now, we know that it almost certainly did prevent future cases, but town officials did not believe it had an effect. A few weeks later, they put the pump handle back on.

So, Snow tried again. In his *Grand Experiment,* later the same year, he studied the association of cholera cases with the use of water from two private companies that serviced the district and drew from two distinct areas of the River Thames. One firm, the Southwark and Vauxhall Water Company, drew water from a downstream area of the Thames that was polluted by sewage. Another firm, Lambeth Water Company, had recently moved its intake facilities to a location upstream of the sewers. Using statistical methods, Snow showed that Southwark customers were much more likely to develop cholera compared to Lambeth customers. These epidemiological methods introduced a scientific approach to outbreak investigation and containment, which would go on to revolutionize public health.[1]

But the private water companies objected to his findings, and the scientific community and town officials remained skeptical. An expert committee of clinicians was formed, which rejected Snow's findings. Good science did not win, and it would be more than a decade before the idea that cholera was caused by a waterborne pathogen was considered true. The water system remained contaminated for another quarter century.[2]

Since that initial failure, the field of public health has evolved its ability to control infectious diseases on a population level. Standing on Snow's shoulders, Edwin Chadwick and many other scientists of the day led a revolution to improve water quality and sanitation. By the later part of the 19th century, local and state jurisdictions in the United States began establishing health

Viral Outbreaks, Biosecurity, and Preparing for Mass Casualty Infectious Diseases Events
https://doi.org/10.1016/B978-0-323-54841-0.00023-8

departments to oversee the implementation of controls such as sanitation, quarantine, and vaccination that reduced the risk of environmental and infectious hazards. Later, that same public health infrastructure was essential in using antibiotics to control infectious diseases of public health concern such as tuberculosis and sexually transmitted infections.[3] As a result, since the 20th century, public health can take credit for significant improvements in mortality and life expectancy around the world.

But we should remember the story of Jon Snow as an early example of the modern public health response, and not just because he revolutionized epidemiology. The initial failure to permanently change policy in London led to long-term lessons in how boards of health—and, later, health departments—approached acute infectious disease outbreaks. In the Broad Street example, finding the pump was not enough. The city government needed to be convinced to take action, the population needed to understand the threat, and the private companies involved needed to institute changes based on some regulatory authority. In 1855 London, these things did not happen. But, with the benefit of hindsight, we have been learning from these lessons ever since. Public health during an infectious disease emergency response is not just about science or even clinical medicine. Rather, it must connect an increasingly complex web of systems and make sure they all work together to heal the sick and protect the healthy. A good public health emergency response must make sure that good science wins and that everyone can benefit from it.

THE ROLE OF PUBLIC HEALTH TODAY

Throughout the 20th century, the scope of public health services continued to expand. Our advancing understanding of infectious diseases, their causes, and their treatments led to the expanded role of public health. Gradually, public health's mandate has grown to address chronic diseases, injury prevention, maternal and child health, and more. As a result, the field struggled to define itself as the scope of services grew to include a broad spectrum of clinical and socioeconomic interventions.[4] In a 1988 report entitled *The Future of Public Health*, the Institute of Medicine (IOM) defined public health as "What we as a society do collectively to assure the conditions in which people can be healthy." The report also attempted to define the core functions of public health as assessment, policy development, and assurance.[5] Subsequently, IOM convened the Core Public Health Functions Steering Committee to refine the vision and mission for public health in the United States. In 1994, this committee released a policy statement on *Public Health in America*, which further articulated the expectations for what public health should be prepared to do, including:

- Preventing epidemics and the spread of disease
- Protecting against environmental hazards
- Preventing injuries
- Promoting and encouraging healthy behaviors
- Responding to disasters and assisting communities in recovery
- Assuring the quality and accessibility of health services

The last part of the *Public Health in America* statement defines how these activities are carried out through the "Ten Essential Services of Public Health." These services form a systemic, comprehensive core for public health across the United States (Fig. 1).[6,7]

Now in the 21st century, factors such as rapidly advancing technology, population growth, urbanization, globalization, environmental disruption, civil disorder, and ease of travel provide pathogens with opportunities to infect new hosts and spread more widely. Combating these emerging infectious disease threats will take a new understanding of both the behavior of infection and how to plan for and respond to large-scale outbreaks. To do this right will take a cooperative, collaborative approach based around these core public health functions and the core epidemiological principles John Snow advocated for back in London.

To better understand the role of public health in mitigating these risks, it is helpful to understand the structure and historical functions of public health and how these roles have evolved in the modern age. This chapter will focus on the US context, but it is important to understand that similar structures have been implemented in most developed countries and increasingly in lesser-resourced countries as well. While our examples are specific to the United States, the same principles are applicable across the globe.

PUBLIC HEALTH RESPONSE STRUCTURES

Governmental organizations exist on the international, national, state, and local levels that help coordinate and oversee these public health activities. They each have unique roles in ensuring the health and safety of the public (Table 1).

Nationally, in the United States (U.S.), there are several public health agencies (such as the CDC, the Food and Drug Administration, and the National Institutes of Health) that develop guidance, coordinate funding,

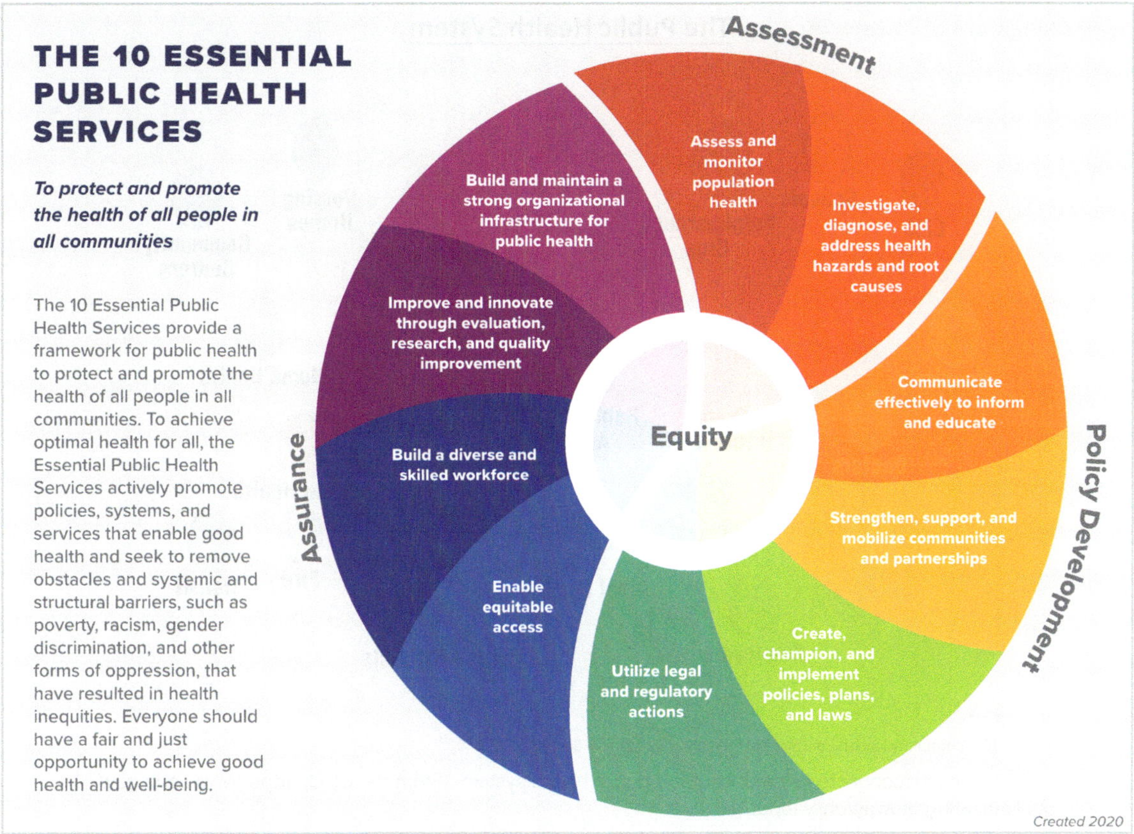

FIG. 1 The 10 essential services of public health. (From the CDC; https://www.cdc.gov/public-health-gateway/php/about/index.html.)

TABLE 1
Examples of Governmental Public Health Institutions

International	World Health Organization (WHO) European Centre for Disease Prevention and Control (ECDC)
National	Centers for Disease Control and Prevention (U.S.) Ministries of Health, e.g., Public Health Agency, Canada and Santé Publique, France.
State	State and Territorial Health Departments —Centralized, decentralized, mixed
Local	City and County Health Departments

research, and promote the implementation of public health interventions that are carried out on the state and local levels. Similar structures exist in other counties. It is important to note that these governmental agencies do not exist in isolation; they are instead part of a much larger system. A public health system can be described as "all public, private, and voluntary entities that contribute to the delivery of essential public health services within a jurisdiction (Fig. 2)." This means that public health systems extend well beyond a single national, state, or local agency. Other components of the system can include healthcare providers, public safety agencies, human service and charity organizations, education and youth development organizations, recreation and arts-related organizations, economic and philanthropic organizations, and environmental agencies/organizations.

All these entities play a role in the traditional functions of public health to ensure the well-being of a

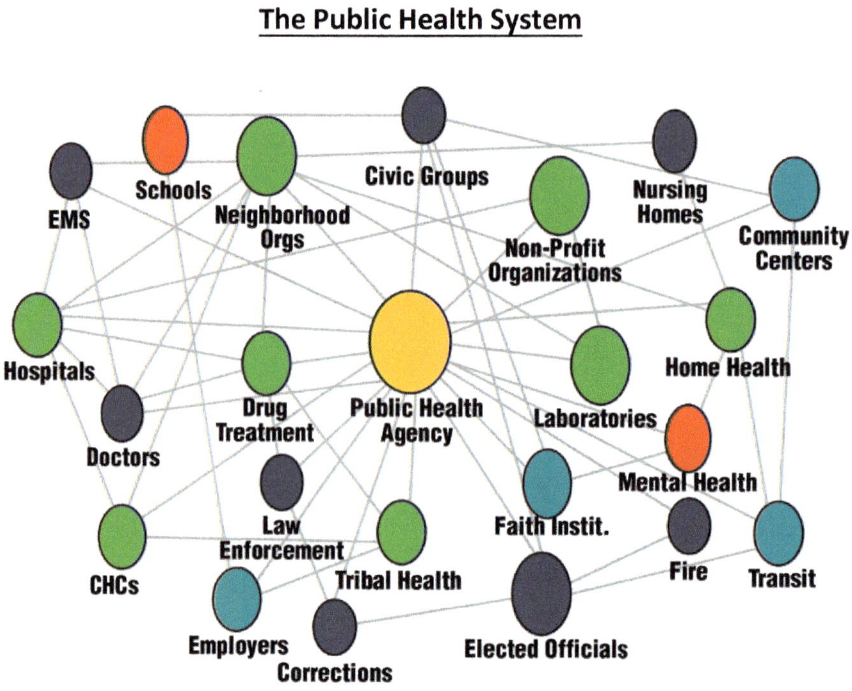

CHC, Community Health Centers; EMS, Emergency Medical Services

FIG. 2 The interconnected elements of the public health system. (From the CDC; https://www.cdc.gov/public-health-gateway/php/about/.)

community. The public health system now covers such diverse areas as chronic diseases, maternal and child health, behavioral health, and more. After the events of September 11, 2001, in the United States and the subsequent anthrax attacks the following month, bioterrorism and public health preparedness became a new and significant focus for the public health system. Although pandemics, epidemics, and even bioterrorism had existed for thousands of years, it was at this point that the formal, legal idea of a "public health emergency" was born.

What is a Public Health Emergency?

The official definition for a public health emergency is "an occurrence or imminent threat of an illness or health condition, caused by bioterrorism, epidemic or pandemic disease, or [a] novel and highly fatal infectious agent or biological toxin that poses a substantial risk of a significant number of human fatalities or incidents of permanent or long-term disability."[8]

Imagine a typical day in a hospital—in the emergency room, clinics, or lab. Each shift, the work is dedicated to the care of patients with their own symptoms, care, and treatment. One day, though, you encounter a set of symptoms that do not line up with normal narratives. Like the various diseases and agents encountered in this textbook, these symptoms are novel, even threatening. This illness may have few treatment options or startlingly high rates of infection. In short, it carries broad implications for health beyond just this individual patient. It presents a threat to your community, your city, or even the world. At that moment, you could be encountering a *public health emergency*.

Before the turn of the 21st century, the CDC and WHO worked together to codify this term and create specific emergency powers based on it, though that progress was accelerated by the 2001 anthrax attacks. By the US statute, the federal Secretary of Health can declare a public health emergency under Section 319 of the Public Health Service (PHS) Act when:

(a) a disease or disorder presents a public health emergency (PHE); or
(b) a public health emergency, including significant outbreaks of infectious disease or bioterrorist attacks, otherwise exists.

This statute gives more latitude than the CDC/WHO definition over what, exactly, a public health emergency entails.[9] That latitude has been utilized by the federal government, which has declared public health emergencies for hurricanes like Katrina, Sandy, and Maria, as well as for infectious diseases like H1N1, Zika, and SARS-CoV-2 (the virus that causes COVID-19) and broader issues such as the United States' opioid crisis. It is important to understand that this authority is separate from a presidential "disaster declaration" [Federal Emergency Management Agency (FEMA); https://www.fema.gov/disaster], although both processes may be used to respond to a disaster (both were utilized during the 2017 hurricane season, for example).[10]

Federally, the declaration of a public health emergency gives the Secretary of Health and Human Services the ability to waive certain Medicaid/Medicare requirements, adjust grant deadlines, deploy personnel, and provide direct funding to impacted areas. The CDC has developed a crisis-funding vehicle that is tied to these declarations and can be used to rapidly send money to impacted jurisdictions outside of the federal appropriations process. Still, many events considered "public health emergencies" at the local level (based on the WHO/CDC definitions) may never warrant a federal declaration.

How Does a Public Health Emergency Response Work?

When you encounter a public health emergency, your job as a healthcare worker suddenly shifts. In an instant, your role in the public health system becomes startlingly concrete. You become an active part of a new set of capabilities within a global system designed to detect and counter these high-risk threats. For this system to function well against biological threats, healthcare institutions and the medical professionals within them need to act in ways that our privatized system does not usually allow. Each institution needs to function within a unified whole, working in transparent collaboration with other healthcare institutions, local partners, and government entities, to respond effectively to the sorts of deadly agents that are more and more a part of global life.

Public health emergencies and the incident command system

In the context of an emergency, it is helpful to think of the public health system as a collection of institutions and systems working at various scales, from local all the way up to global, each of which needs to be managed in ways that help them connect easily. In 2007, the US Department of Health and Human Services developed a Medical Surge Capacity and Capability framework that delineated the full scope of a health and medical response in a series of six organizational tiers, all of which would be needed to address a serious infectious disease outbreak in your community.[11] Within the United States, the major tiers are represented in Table 2. A seventh tier of international structures (such as the WHO Emergency Framework and the United Nations) exists as well.

It is the amount and complexity of these tiers that makes something called the Incident Command System (or ICS) such an important part of a response. At a basic level, ICS is a set of structures and practices based on military antecedents that were codified by the Fire Service in response to wildland fires in the

TABLE 2
Tiers of a Unified Health and Medical Response and Their Relevant Components

Tier one	Individual Healthcare Organization	Hospitals Nursing Homes Adult Care Facilities Clinics
Tier two	Healthcare Coalition	Geographic Coalitions Healthcare Networks
Tier three	Local Jurisdiction	Medical Coordination Center City/County Public Health Agency Local Emergency Management
Tier four	State	State Health Agency State Emergency Management
Tier five	Interstate/interprovincial	State-to-state resource agreements such as the Emergency Management Assistance Compact (EMAC)
Tier six	Federal/National	HHS Response Assets
Tier seven	International	World Health Organization Nongovernmental Organizations

Adapted From Barbera J, Macintyre A. *Medical Surge Capacity and Capability: A Management System for Integrating Medical and Health Resources During Large-Scale Emergencies*. U.S. Department of Health and Human Services; 2007 and Medical Surge Capacity and Capabilities Handbook (ASPR). https://www.phe.gov/Preparedness/planning/mscc.

1970s and then adapted across the field of emergency management. Currently, the federal Department of Homeland Security uses a framework called the National Incident Management System (NIMS), which mandates the use of ICS as a coordinating structure for most emergency incidents, including infectious diseases. With ICS, your healthcare organization can connect in a standard way to all the tiers with as little confusion as possible.

Utilizing ICS involves a standardized, functional organization chart, coupled with a standardized set of project management practices to support five basic emergency functions that cover common issues in an emergency: command, operations, logistics, planning, and administrative/finance (Fig. 3). These are designed to streamline bureaucracy back to only what is essential in an emergency based on decades of response experience. This organizational structure is designed to be scalable because it is based around necessary functions rather than specific content. For example, some incidents will only need an Incident Commander and an Operations Section, perhaps, or no Public Information Officer at all.

Use of ICS in an infectious disease response

Many clinicians feel that a command-and-control model based on military structures is not relevant for their work, whether or not it is mandated. After all, why change your organization chart the moment an emergency occurs? This is a fair question; ICS is no magic pill. Some theorists have argued that it destroys the consensus model that drives most public health decision-making with an inappropriately militaristic organization.[13] However, a brief thumbnail of ICS and NIMS history in the context of infectious disease response will help show its importance.

As we have seen, infectious disease responses have improved greatly since the 19th century. However, even the tragic 1918 pandemic did not trigger large-scale preplanning for these diseases. That did not happen

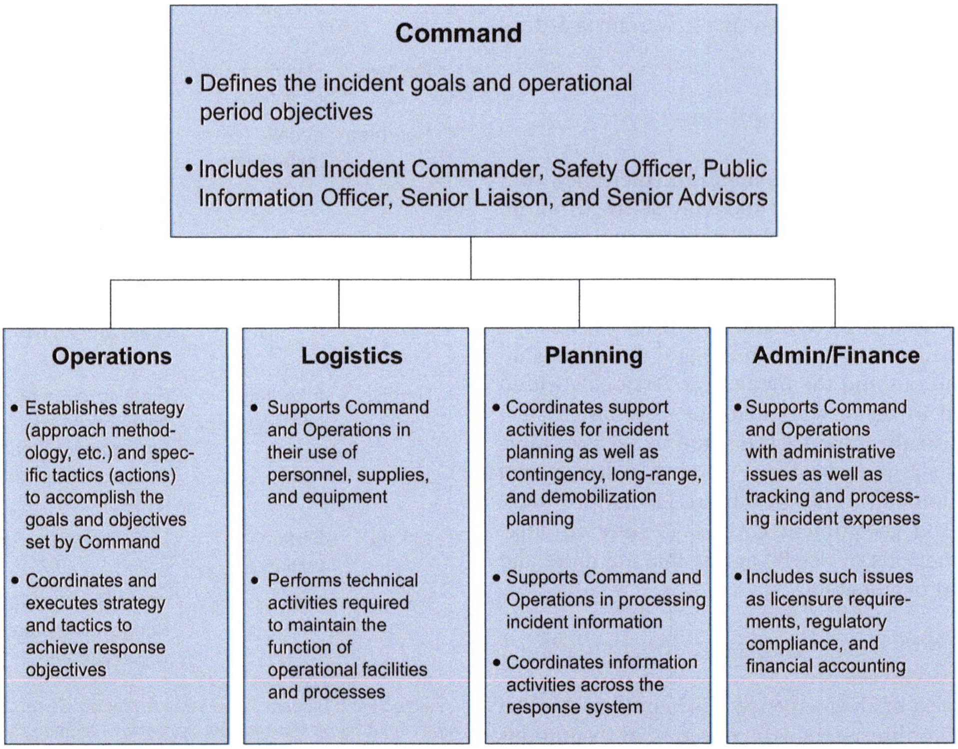

FIG. 3 The five basic functions of the incident command system.[12] (From the Administration for Strategic Preparedness and Response (ASPR); https://aspr.hhs.gov/HealthCareReadiness/guidance/MSCC/.)

until 1976, after a novel swine-origin influenza virus emerged and its subsequent vaccination campaign caused a fiasco through confirmed association with Guillain-Barre syndrome. In the 1980s and 1990s, CDC and its partners prepared for infectious disease (through the lens of pandemics) with a very specific focus: surveillance, vaccines, communication, and emergency medical services.[14]

At the same time, another type of disaster preparation was driving the national discussion. During the latter half of the 21st century, the field we think of as "emergency management" came into being through a focus on civil defense planning, hurricane response, and other noninfectious emergencies. In the 1980s, this field developed a set of structures based around common missions that came to be known as Emergency Support Functions (or ESFs), with "Public Health and Medical Services" as number eight in a list of 15. Some other ESF examples are transportation (#1) and mass care, housing, and human services (#6).[15] The high-level concept demanded that all emergencies could be addressed in an "all hazards" fashion using these core functions, all coordinated via the principles of ICS. After 9/11 and the 2001 anthrax attacks, these two models crashed headlong into each other.

CDC's outbreak response model was forced by these events to "operate at an unprecedented scale and tempo" and to rapidly adapt its emergency response operations, according to Tom Frieden, former head of the organization.[16] There was initially no central hub for the response in the form of an Emergency Operations Center, for example, and the agency had to link its investigation efforts with those of the FBI in unanticipated ways.[17,18] At the same time, the emergency management "all hazards" structures used by FEMA could not account for the central focus on human health and the specialties inherent in medical response needed for a coherent anthrax response. In this case, having Public Health as one ESF among 15 was not sufficient. Since health and healthcare essentially determined the entire response, it should be thought of as something like "first among equals" for an infectious disease response.[19] Over time, the CDC developed its own incident command structure with health officials in the lead that utilized all-hazards principles in the service of good epidemiology and good medicine.

When the first bioterrorism funds were allocated in 2002, they required jurisdictions to utilize ICS. However, that money could not be used for other kinds of infectious disease planning—including pandemic planning, which was still isolated. The massive logistical and coordination challenges of SARS in 2003 (which demanded complex quarantine housing and security planning) and the specter of a global pandemic driven by the H5N1 Avian Flu emergence in 2004 (which required preparedness in large-scale bird culling, for instance) convinced authorities that the operational complexities of infectious disease response were on par with those of a coastal storm. Infectious disease responses were no longer just about good epidemiology and good medicine; modern threats meant it had to become about good transportation, good housing, good law enforcement—good everything. It needed the same powers of coordination utilized by ESF for major disasters but in service to public health oversight. It was time to fully blend these two planning streams.

Legislatively, this effort began with the 2006 Pandemic and All-Hazards Preparedness Act (PAHPA), which triggered a 2007 Homeland Security Presidential Directive (#21) on Public Health and Medical Preparedness (HSPD 21). This established a national health security strategy, essentially making infectious disease response part of the homeland security enterprise. These advances have given public health strong new tools to fight catastrophic infectious disease outbreaks—better logistics, new security partnerships, and upgraded supply chains. At the center of this enterprise, however, the question remains the same: What are the best science-based decisions we can make to investigate a disease and safeguard the public's health? To be effective, everything else—this entirely new set of structures—must exist solely to answer this question and execute that answer.

For further information, go to the FEMA Emergency Management Institute for training resources on the US National Incident Management System and Incident Command Structures (https://training.fema.gov/ndemu/schools/emergency-management-institute/). In addition, the WHO's Public Health Emergency Operations Centre Network (EOC-NET) has developed resources and training for developing and managing a public health emergency operations center utilizing an emergency management model (who.int/groups/eoc-net).

Healthcare response

At the end of the day, healthcare institutions and coalitions (Tiers 1 and 2 from Table 2) should utilize some version of ICS. This creates three major advantages:[13]

- **Unified decision-making** - ICS breaks down siloes within and between institutions to help them work and plan together.
- **More efficient administration and procurement** - Streamlined procedures reduce bureaucracy for issues like purchasing.
- **Operational standardization and flexibility** - A standard set of positions and processes allows different health institutions to interact with each other, even if they are organized radically differently.

For the purposes of this chapter, the last point here is the most important, because it drives the structures that connect each healthcare institution to the higher tiers of the broader public health response.

The hospital incident command system (HICS). To make ICS happen, your institution probably utilizes some version of the Hospital Incident Command System (HICS) (see Chapter 19 for additional details). Developed by the California Emergency Medical Services Authority, this model adapts ICS around general hospital and healthcare departments. The Hospital Incident Management Team described by HICS is similar to the ICS model mentioned previously but gives recommended operational areas and specialists based on the healthcare setting.[20]

In the context of infectious disease responses, here are a few pieces of this coordinating structure to pay attention to (Fig. 4):

First, in HICS, all patient care is collapsed together into one operational group, the "Medical Care Branch," next to other groups like "Infrastructure" and "Business Continuity." That might seem odd; should not more of the emergency organization chart reflect the primary mission of the hospital? But HICS is much more focused on getting support and resources to these clinical areas than managing them. The central idea is that the providers are trusted; the job of the organization is

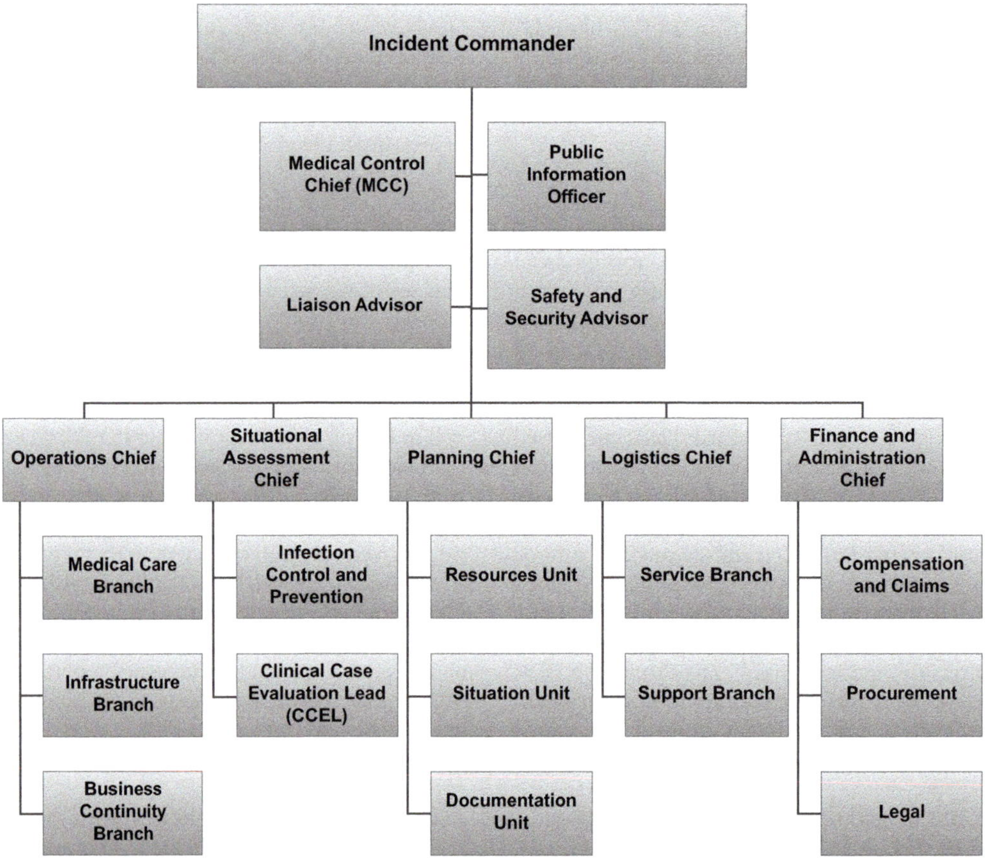

FIG. 4 Example of a hospital incident command structure adapted for epidemic and pandemic respiratory illness to include critical infection prevention and control resources.[21]

merely to get them the resources they need. Also, one unified Medical Care Branch makes sure all patient care providers collaborate and follow the same guidance, whether they are inpatient, outpatient, or even behavioral health.

Second, take a look at the "Medical-Control Chief" (or Medical Specialist) position. Reporting to the Incident Commander means that it must be a fairly important position. And it is—especially in a public health response like an infectious disease emergency. As guidance arrives from multiple sources, these specialists are charged with reviewing and synthesizing it for dissemination throughout the hospital's response groups. During an infectious disease response, this role would also be responsible for coordinating and advising the Incident Commander on decisions regarding standards of care, allocation of scarce resources, triage and admission criteria, and physician staffing.

Finally, the traditional HICS structure can be expanded to include additional functions that would be needed for a highly infectious respiratory disease outbreak, such as COVID-19 or a pandemic influenza. For example, in Fig. 4, a Situational Assessment Chief would be added to oversee activities around infection prevention and control, triage planning, case investigation, and containment strategies. This role would most likely be filled by a hospital epidemiologist or his/her designee and would be responsible for decisions pertaining to prevention, control, and containment of infected or infectious patients and healthcare personnel in close collaboration with the health department.

These simple and flexible coordinating structures exist to help your hospital manage an infectious disease emergency. There is a lot more to learn about HICS; you can find the *Hospital Incident Command System (HICS) Guidebook* at https://emsa.ca.gov/disaster-medical-services-division-hospital-incident-command-system/, and the California Hospital Association Hospital Preparedness Program has other great materials to help you delve deeper (https://www.calhospitalprepare.org/). NETEC also offers a course on HICS Considerations for Special Pathogens Activations (courses.netec.org/courses/hics-roles-and-responsibilities-considerations-for-special-pathogens-activations).

Healthcare coalitions

During an emergency, individual healthcare facilities (Tier 1) may become connected through a larger coordinating entity that can provide information and support in the form of a healthcare network or coalition (Tier 2). Coalitions are described as a group of individual healthcare facilities and response organizations—such as acute care hospitals, emergency medical service (EMS) providers, emergency management agencies, public health agencies, and more—working in a specified geographic area that has partnered to respond to emergencies or disasters in a coordinated manner. The purpose of a local healthcare coalition is to address resource needs, information sharing, and managing surge (i.e., patient load) issues between healthcare institutions. Coalitions should ideally include facilities beyond hospitals such as nursing homes, community health centers, and behavioral health facilities in order to develop the broadest possible patient surge capacity for the most severe emergency situations.[11]

Jurisdiction response

One key benefit of HICS is that it is designed to connect your institution and coalition with the wider health system response during an emergency. In particular, your jurisdiction (Tier 3 in Table 2) has two key structures relevant to you during an infectious disease emergency: public health incident command (which leads the healthcare system response) and the health and medical ESF (which coordinates the healthcare system elements and links them to other partners). Both deserve a bit of explanation.

Public health incident command. When an infectious disease outbreak becomes large enough, the lead public health agency in a jurisdiction will mobilize its own ICS response. In some cases, the local or state health department exercises sole command during these incidents. In other cases, the health department may share command with other agencies, such as a police or fire department, who might have more day-to-day experience managing large-scale emergencies. Regardless, during a public health emergency, the health department will be working through jurisdictional ICS and ESF structures (described earlier).

Your hospital or coalition may be asked for various kinds of support via this command structure. For instance, health department staff may be located at your facility for active disease surveillance or outbreak investigations. Exposed healthcare personnel may need to be monitored for symptoms or excluded from work to help keep them and their patients safe. Countermeasures may need to be distributed. Regardless of the task, working in conjunction with the public health command element is the best way to quickly address the infectious disease incident.

Health and medical emergency support function. During an emergency, emergency support functions (ESF) can provide a structure to group resources and capabilities into functional areas that may be needed during a response. Your hospital or coalition is likely connected to the larger incident command structure and other needed partners via a health and medical Emergency Support Function (ESF #8), which allows public and private partners to jointly handle issues in their areas of expertise. Locally, this is the key hub where your organization connects to a vast set of public health, emergency medical, logistical, and public safety operations and resources.[15,22]

For example, a pandemic due to a novel respiratory virus would require an extensive and prolonged coordinated response. The ESF #8 could be utilized to support the healthcare system's capacity to care for a potentially large influx of severely ill patients and other concerned but mildly ill patients who could overwhelm clinics and emergency departments. This support may include coordinating ambulance services, providing clinical or infection control guidance, and ensuring adequate space, staff, and supplies for providing clinical care. The ESF is also a connection point to federal actions. For instance, the Strategic National Stockpile (SNS)—which we will describe later—might be mobilized to supplement dwindling local supplies of personal protective equipment (PPE) and medications, or the EPA may generate new guidelines for the management of infectious waste. In addition, your hospital's requests for nonmedical assets such as environmental decontamination, victim identification, or family assistance could be processed through the ESF.

Fundamental to this, the ESF likely contains a small group of senior leaders to weigh in on key policy decisions—such as scarce resource allocation, large-scale public health interventions (like school closures), and changes to usually accepted standards of care (i.e., crisis standards of care). In New York City (NYC), for example, the NYC Health Care Coalition provides a structure that enables leadership of local response agencies and healthcare delivery systems to identify, prioritize, and address policy concerns that arise during a public health emergency. Working together, often with input from local stakeholders, this group of leaders can quickly work through difficult decisions during times of crisis, which can then be executed cleanly through ESF relationships.

State and federal response

The final three tiers defined by the *Medical Surge Capacity and Capability* handbook relate to state response (Tier 4), interstate regional support (Tier 5), and federal response (Tier 6). From a local healthcare perspective, it is helpful to treat them as one combined system.

Similar to local jurisdictions, most state emergency management systems utilize the Emergency Support Function framework (ESF). This means that your jurisdiction's Health & Medical ESF has a corresponding state-level Health & Medical ESF (generally managed by the state's health department), which, in turn, connects to the federal Health & Medical ESF, which is managed by the US Department of Health and Human Services (HHS).

In most instances, state ESFs provide strong support to local jurisdictions. To preserve local control, most of the state support relies on your jurisdiction requesting it directly. Federal agencies, in turn, cannot come in unless requested via a state or territory. State support includes helping multiple localities to collaborate. For instance, a state can assist with moving/diverting patients or staff to facilities in nearby jurisdictions. States can provide additional healthcare and support staff through medical volunteer programs like the Medical Reserve Corps (MRC; https://aspr.hhs.gov/MRC/Pages/index.aspx) or the Emergency System for Advance Registration of Volunteer Health Professionals (ESAR-VHP; https://aspr.hhs.gov/ESAR-VHP/).[23,24] Moreover, states can often provide important crisis waivers on state healthcare regulations to help local jurisdictions deal with the extreme distress caused by public health emergencies (Fig. 10).

The federal government also has a role to play. Often, the idea that a local public health emergency may have a federal component seems distant. However, the federal health and medical ESF can provide significant support to local jurisdictions, including substantial logistical aid, medical assets, and waivers on federal regulation. In fact, HHS produced a menu of available assets called the *Response and Recovery Resources Compendium*, which contains hundreds of different teams and resources that may be requested during a public health emergency.[25] Examples include the Disaster Medical Assistance Teams (DMATs), each of which contains 24–48 clinical professionals who can deploy within 12h; and the Public Health Service's Applied Public Health Teams, containing 47 Public Health Officers also deployable within 12h.

To understand how these requests might work, let us look at an example. During the 2014 Ebola outbreak, many healthcare facilities attempted to procure Powered Air-Purifying Respirators (PAPRs) for their clinicians who might be called on to perform procedures on patients at high risk for Ebola. This created supply chain shortages for PAPRs across the country. Many facilities put in requests through their local ESF. When the local ESF could not help, the PAPR request then went to each state's ESF and then to the federal ESF. Federal HHS created a workgroup to prioritize sourcing for these PAPRs to assist with supply distribution to those facilities throughout the country most likely to see Ebola patients. Subsequently, frontline facilities near ports of entry were able to secure the equipment they needed and, in short order, more supplies were available. This process may have caused frustration in a number of healthcare facilities that just wanted their equipment—but it shows the system working.

Of course, states can provide support to other states as well. The Emergency Management Assistance Compact (EMAC) was ratified by Congress in 1996 as a way for states to provide any type of mutual aid to each other in times of need (based on a governor's emergency declaration). Many public health emergency needs can be supplied state-to-state, with no federal involvement, via this EMAC process, which addresses issues such as liability and reciprocal medical certification. In past emergencies, ambulance teams, mortuary technicians, environmental health personnel, and clinical teams have all been provided to support healthcare facilities via EMAC. During the COVID-19 response in 2020, EMAC facilitated the sharing of scarce resources, such as ventilators and PPE, and licensed healthcare providers were able to provide telehealth services across state lines.

International response

In rare cases, an infectious disease can pose a threat to multiple countries, thus requiring an international response (Tier 7 in Table 2). The International Health Regulations (IHR[26]; https://www.who.int/publications/i/item/9789241580496) provide a legal framework for the global detection and management of public health emergencies and outline the processes for declaring a public health emergency of international concern (PHEIC), which is defined as "an extraordinary event which is determined to constitute a public health risk to other States through the international spread of disease and to potentially require a coordinated international response." The first PHEIC was declared in 2009 in response to the H1N1 "swine flu" pandemic and has subsequently been declared in response to polio (2014), Ebola (2014, 2019), Zika virus (2016), COVID-19 (2020), and mpox (2022, 2024).[27]

Subsequently, the Global Health Security Agenda (GHSA) was established in 2014 in order to support member states in implementing the required infectious disease prevention, detection, and response capabilities outlined in the IHR. One of the key recommendations is for all countries to establish or strengthen Public Health Emergency Operations Centers (EOC) in order to strengthen communications and coordination for more effective domestic and international responses. This can be implemented by other entities, such as nongovernmental organizations as well. While an EOC refers to a physical location or virtual space in which public health emergency management personnel can assemble to coordinate operational information and resources, a public health EOC should also "aim to integrate traditional public health services into an emergency management model utilizing an ICS or similar management structure."[28]

In parallel with the aforementioned activities, the World Health Organization (WHO) developed an Emergency Response Framework in 2013. This framework established a three-level "grading" process for public health incidents, with Grade 3 reserved for major responses that require coordination across the WHO. During the 2014–2015 West African Ebola response, the WHO recognized a "need for more effective international collaboration on health security and pandemic preparedness" and released an updated edition of this framework in 2024. This edition embedded the principles of incident management described in this chapter into global infectious disease responses by creating an incident management system for international health response.[29]

In addition, the WHO is designated as the lead organization for the Global Health Cluster, an entity established by the United Nations Inter-Agency Standing Committee to improve humanitarian response through partnerships. The Global Health Cluster is one of 11 clusters oriented around different subject areas, similar to the US-based ESFs described earlier. A health cluster can be established for any major emergency, and the WHO can work via the health cluster to establish and execute broad health policies with cluster stakeholders such as local agencies, nongovernmental organizations (NGOs), and private partners.[30]

To learn more about training opportunities for international health professionals, see the CDC's Public Health Emergency Management Fellowship program (https://www.cdc.gov/fellowships/php/about/). For additional training and education resources on the IHR and the GHSA, please refer to the Health Security Learning Platform (WHO; https://extranet.who.int/hslp/).[31,32]

The public health system in a public health emergency

This collection of systems across these six tiers (from Table 2) and onto the global level can be dizzying, and that is without spending time on private partnerships or global resources, both of which can be helpful.

For our purposes, though, this breakdown shows the breadth and depth of the networks involved in public health response.

The secret to a successful infectious disease response across the tiers of the public health system depends on the benefits provided by ICS: All these tiers, and the institutions within them, need to work in one connected, aligned fashion in order to achieve the best possible health outcomes. However hard it is, the thousands of facilities, medical professions, agencies, and organizations must act as one coherent entity to save the most lives.

PUBLIC HEALTH PREPAREDNESS FOR INFECTIOUS DISEASE EMERGENCIES AND BIOTERRORISM EVENTS

The best way for a unified public health system to respond together is to prepare together. That means that healthcare facilities and networks should engage with their public health partners while preparing for an infectious disease outbreak. In fact, all partners throughout the seven response tiers (including local, state, and national stakeholders) should prepare together. Separate preparedness work done in isolation is much less effective and can even be counterproductive, since it leads to misaligned priorities and, usually, conflicting plans. In the following section, we lay out a basic method to prepare for infectious disease emergencies in ways that unify players and help them make progressive improvements in their capabilities.

Federal Support and Coordination

As described earlier, the federal government has provided significant support for public health and medical emergency preparedness since the 2001 anthrax bioterrorism attacks, though the amounts have decreased over the past two decades.[33,34] There are two major goals for this funding: to increase local response capacity and to provide a more unified approach to these responses between all the major players. Despite improvements in local preparedness and response capacity, these issues of multiple involved federal programs and declining funding have made a fully unified approach difficult.

On the public health side, the CDC provides resources through a mechanism called the Public Health Emergency Preparedness (or PHEP) cooperative agreement (https://www.cdc.gov/readiness/php/phep/index.html). This program has provided more than $12 billion to public health departments across the nation since 2002. The goal of the funding is to make local public health departments ready to manage multiple types of emergencies, including infectious disease outbreaks. Since 2011, this funding has been tied to guidance linked to fifteen public health capabilities.[35,36]

On the healthcare system side, the most significant federal program supporting public health planning and coordination is the Hospital Preparedness Program (HPP; https://aspr.hhs.gov/HealthCareReadiness/HPP/Pages/default.aspx). The HPP program was first established in 2002 in response to 9/11 and the anthrax bioterrorism attacks to support hospital preparedness for such events.[37] In 2004, post-SARS, the emphasis of the program shifted from bioterrorism to a more general focus on large public health emergencies. Since then, the program has evolved from a sole focus on hospitals to a more inclusive view of the healthcare delivery system. HPP aims to integrate diverse groups of healthcare partners within a jurisdiction into healthcare coalitions that work together on healthcare system preparedness and response (Fig. 5).[38]

Later, following the 2014 Ebola outbreak, HPP helped establish a nationwide treatment network for Ebola and other infectious diseases and supported the creation of the National Emerging Special Pathogens Training and Education Center (https://netec.org/) to ensure our nation's healthcare system had a structure in place to respond to viral hemorrhagic fevers and other high-consequence infectious diseases.

A separate funding stream, the Urban Area Security Initiative (UASI), provides resources to high-risk urban areas primarily for law enforcement and first responder entities. However, it has also provided certain public health and medical resources, generally with a focus on equipment, technical supplies, and bioterrorism-focused training.

All three of these grant programs (CDC's PHEP, HPP, and DHS's UASI) support public health preparedness by funding work toward certain capabilities. Unfortunately, the capabilities tied to each program are somewhat different and are not fully coordinated at the federal level.[a]

These federal inconsistencies are relevant to local healthcare staff because they make it difficult for state and local health authorities to provide a unified, consistent preparedness approach. Nevertheless, this is an

[a] In March 2025, the U.S. Secretary of Health and Human Services announced that ASPR and the SNS will be reorganized under the Centers for Disease Control and Prevention (CDC). Certain centers within ASPR, such as BARDA, may also be impacted by the reorganization. https://www.hhs.gov/press-room/hhs-restructuring-doge-fact-sheet.html.

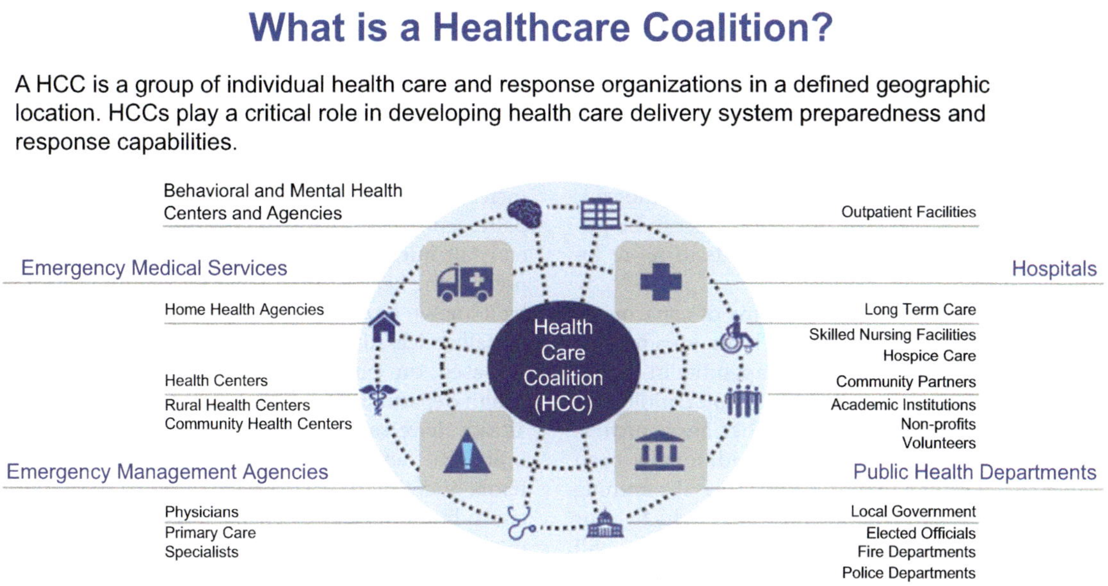

FIG. 5 What is a healthcare coalition? (From ASPR; https://aspr.hhs.gov/HealthCareReadiness/HPP/.)

important mandate, and your local health authority should be clearly managing a health and medical preparedness cycle within your jurisdiction with all partners. Let us look in depth at what that should entail.

The Preparedness Cycle

Whenever we are not actively engaged in emergency response, we should be preparing for the next event. But its routine nature does not mean preparedness is unstructured—far from it. It is a highly organized, ongoing quality improvement process. FEMA, in fact, defines preparedness as "a continuous cycle of planning, organizing, training, equipping, exercising, evaluating, and taking corrective action in an effort to ensure effective coordination during incident response." Through this cycle, we try and improve our ability to enact all the capabilities we need for an infectious disease response, described later (Fig. 6).[39,40]

Analysis and prioritization

Our first preparedness step is not formally part of the preparedness cycle. However, the vast nature of the health and medical enterprise makes it a necessity. It should be obvious from the start that preparing for "all hazards" simultaneously is not possible. It is not even possible to focus on everything required in an infectious disease response all at once. There are two main methods to focus the work on the highest priority capabilities: *risk assessment* and *capacity assessment*.

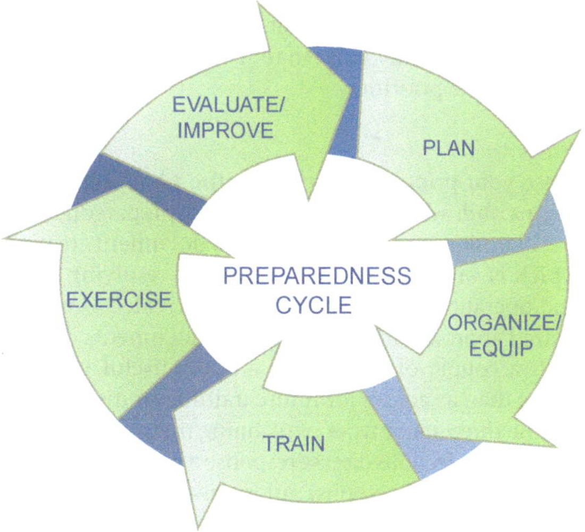

FIG. 6 The preparedness cycle. (From: FEMA; http://www.coehsem.com/emergency-management-cycle/.)

Per CDC and the Administration for Strategic Preparedness and Response (ASPR) rules tied to the funding mentioned previously, both healthcare facilities and jurisdictions are required to perform various types of risk assessment, which look at potential hazards and their accompanying vulnerabilities to those hazards. These assessments generally provide ranked lists of hazards (such as a pandemic or bioterrorist attack) to healthcare facilities, which have some utility for planning. The process is far more useful, however, when these hazards are tied to the capabilities needed to respond effectively. For example, by identifying that specialized infection control methods are needed to control outbreaks of severe respiratory pathogens, then building infection control capabilities can be prioritized. This sort of prioritization leads to more focused planning.

The same argument is true in terms of capacity assessment. It should be clear that both jurisdictions and healthcare systems have more capability in certain areas, based on resource allocation. Epidemiological capacity is often robust, whereas other areas such as infectious waste management have traditionally been considered less central to health authorities. Examining the resources—staff, equipment, time—which your systems have put into these various capabilities will give a clear idea of which are likely to succeed in an emergency.

The major preparedness goal here is for jurisdictional health authorities to work with their healthcare partners to choose a set of joint preparedness priorities. Working together on similar issues, you will accomplish exponentially more than if each facility or agency sets separate priorities.

Planning

Once your priorities are chosen, the planning process begins and, with it, FEMA's standard preparedness cycle. Planning is often thought of as document creation, which is wrong. Planning is the art of resolving policy and operational problems in order to create a workable, shared approach to a response. The documents created, with a couple of exceptions, are less useful in themselves than as guides for future training or discussions.

The three major types of planning that are most effective for an infectious disease response are capability-based all-hazards plans, response guides, and checklists.

The capability-based all-hazards plan. Although it is not feasible to plan for every possible scenario, a well-developed "all-hazards" response plan that covers functions and responsibilities common to all emergencies allows for a common framework of understanding from which all involved partners can build. Additionally, establishing a baseline plan is the first crucial step in the improvement cycle and informs stakeholder training and exercises, which will then allow us to identify planning gaps and potential challenges that need to be addressed.

Public health planning occurs on all levels of the healthcare system with an emphasis on support and coordination with individual facilities, healthcare networks, and healthcare coalitions. Infectious disease emergencies should be an integral element of any "all-hazards" plan. As part of this process, there is an increasing recognition for the need to move away from pathogen-specific plans and instead utilize a more general "all infectious hazards" approach that can better prepare the healthcare system for any infectious threat, be it known or unknown, naturally occurring or intentionally released.[41]

Based on previous infectious disease responses, health departments and healthcare entities are likely to already have several existing plans such as pandemic influenza, anthrax/bioterrorism, or more recently, Ebola and COVID-19. The next step would be to begin to build out more general strategies and protocols that address types of infectious hazards instead of specific diseases. For example, instead of focusing on an Ebola-specific plan, it is possible to look at the general capabilities and common considerations that are required for a response to other pathogens with similar characteristics (e.g., high transmissibility through close person-to-person contact with high mortality) that might require a similar healthcare response, such as other hemorrhagic fever viruses. Pathogen characteristics such as mode of transmission (respiratory vs. contact, etc.), ease of transmissibility, pathogenicity, and treatability, along with operational needs such as special infection control precautions, waste management, or lab biosafety procedures, are all considerations that can be included in infectious disease plans (Table 3).

Since public health agencies generally lead the healthcare system response during an infectious disease emergency, their planning includes many additional elements in partnership with internal and external partners to ensure a coordinated jurisdictional response. This includes ensuring that community members and community-based organizations have a voice in the planning process. Whenever possible, planning partners are engaged throughout the process to provide subject matter expertise and feedback. Planning with stakeholders also promotes shared ownership of the processes, which is essential to ensuring buy-in prior to an actual emergency.

Response guides. These capability-driven plans are likely to be fairly generic and technical. Once general agreement on the infectious disease approach is achieved, it is helpful to create brief, high-level response guides for various pathogen categories

TABLE 3
Examples of Elements to Consider in an "All Infectious Hazards" Response Plan

- Incident Command Structure and activation triggers
- Organizational roles and responsibilities
- Roles of coordinating partners
  - Local, state, federal
- Surveillance, reporting, and investigation
  - Case finding, contact tracing, and monitoring
  - Public health reporting
  - Isolation and quarantine
- Clinical and support activities
- Laboratory testing and coordination
- Situational awareness
  - Data collection and management
  - Analysis
  - Information sharing
- Communication and engagement
  - Internal
  - External partners
  - Public/patients
- Patient movement/load balancing and tracking (transport and transfers)
- Stockpile mobilization and medical countermeasure distribution
- Resource management
  - Space (e.g., airborne isolation capacity, intensive care, alternate care sites)
  - Staff (e.g., absenteeism, medical reserve corps, rapid credentialing)
  - Supplies (e.g., personal protective equipment, medications)
- Environmental interventions (e.g., disinfection, waste management, remediation)
- Responder safety and security
  - Mental health support
  - Infection control guidance
  - Personal protective equipment
  - Medical countermeasures
  - Laboratory biosafety
  - Just-in-time training
- Crisis standards of care
- Legal preparedness and regulatory relief
- Decedent management

(e.g., pandemic influenza or influenza-like illness) that can be used to guide decision-making. These documents, which range from four to eight pages, should focus on the context of the response, its clinical features, and the high-level decisions that may be required. An example of a threat response guide outline used by the New York City Health Department can be found in Table 4. Such guides can also be useful in the healthcare setting to provide a quick reference overview to relevant staff.

TABLE 4
Threat Response Guide Sections

Threat Response Guides are brief summaries used to guide leadership decision-making in the first hours of an infectious disease outbreak or other emergency.

1. Understand the health problem
   - Clinical features
   - Public health and mental health features
2. Understand the city's response
   - Citywide impacts
   - Review of city plan
   - Jurisdictional responsibilities
3. Make key decisions
   - Conduct immediate notifications
   - Address major issues/policy questions
   - Direct initial response objectives
   - Media talking points
4. Activate incident command system
   - Mobilize ICS response structure
   - Assign immediate ICS tasks
5. Request support from city, state, and federal agencies
   - Likely support requests
6. Debrief and transition with relief shift
   - Meeting agenda with incoming leadership
7. Review tactical information
   - Staffing assignments/capacity
   - Laboratory timelines/capacity
   - Mass prophylaxis availability
8. Key terms and acronyms

Response guides or the equivalent serve a number of purposes: they provide a quick briefing to leadership who have likely been less involved in preparedness activities; they distill the most important decisions as a way to focus discussions; and they provide key information on roles and responsibilities to keep your organization from reinventing the wheel.

Checklists. Staff on the front lines who are performing emergency work that they do not usually do in their day-to-day duties should have checklists. Unlike response guides, which are meant to give context and grounding, checklists are a memory aid tool. They are meant to remind already-trained staff of detailed steps they need to accomplish to ensure proper completion of a task and to reduce errors. The checklists used by biocontainment units for donning and doffing personal protective equipment (PPE) are good examples of the use of checklists (see Resources and Tools section, and for New York City, see examples at https://www.nychealthandhospitals.org/institute-for-disease-and-disaster-management/tools-and-resources/).[42]

Job action sheets are a kind of checklist built around actions that would need to be taken by someone in a specific role, rather than a specific procedure. They are often helpful when staff are responding in new positions due to the nature of the incident. Staff assigned to a specific role should be trained on and familiar with the actions they are expected to perform as outlined in the job action sheets. (See examples in the Resource section; a suite of HICS job action sheets is available at https://emsa.ca.gov/hospital-incident-command-system-job-action-sheets-2014/.[43])

Organizing and equipping

In many organizations, planning moves directly to training, which misses the crucial *organizing and equipping* step in FEMA's formal preparedness cycle. To *organize*, an institution should take the capabilities they have planned for and assign them clearly to ICS groups or bureaucratic units. This includes an analysis of the knowledge, skills, and abilities needed to perform those capabilities, an accompanying analysis of available staff, and then clear role assignments for staff into appropriate functions. For example, an *Employee Health and Safety Officer* can perform most safety functions. However, in some infectious disease incidents, more technical infection prevention and control practices may need to be conducted. Hypothetically, specialists in these areas can be preassigned as surges to an ICS Safety function to ensure that enough staff are in place to keep hospital workers safe.

To *equip*, an institution follows a similar pathway based on space, system, or inventory needs. Do they have adequate surge locations? Is there sufficient airborne isolation room capacity? Are intensive care units equipped to handle the increased burden of a high-morbidity, highly infectious agent? Are there adequate oxygen supplies, respirators, and masks on hand to get your institution through a national supply shortage? Ideally, space, systems, and supplies should be assigned to their relevant ICS groups and clearly inventoried so that they can be rapidly deployed during an incident.

Both organizing and equipping are critical to make the conceptual ideas of the planning process concrete, possible to execute, and widely known throughout your organization. We cannot emphasize enough the importance of having clear, transparent emergency roles for every member of your institution.

Training

No matter how well-developed a plan might be, it is useless if no one is aware of its contents. Training provides responding entities and personnel with the knowledge, skills, and abilities needed to fulfill their roles during a specific emergency situation. The CDC (https://www.cdc.gov/orr/publications-resources/index.html), ASPR (https://asprtracie.hhs.gov/), and other organizations have developed extensive resources for planning and training staff on incidence response for biological events and other emergencies, and some, such as NETEC, offer in-person as well as online courses (https://netec.org/education-training/).[44,45]

In terms of preparing the healthcare system for an infectious disease emergency, all staff or other stakeholders should receive training on jurisdictional, agency, or facility incident command structures that outline generally expected roles during an emergency response. Then, job-specific training can be delivered as needed based on expected roles and responsibilities during an outbreak or other infectious disease event. For example, to recognize and respond to a potential infectious threat, frontline healthcare staff in emergency rooms, urgent care centers, etc. should be trained on how to screen patients for potential infectious diseases of public health concern and what infection control measures should be taken to mitigate risk to other patients and staff (e.g., offering a mask and placing in isolation) (Fig. 7).

To minimize the training burden to staff, the prioritization should be based on the highest-risk threats and strengthening core competencies, such as infection control, that would be needed regardless of the pathogen. In addition, many components of emergency preparedness can be incorporated into other routine training activities. It is also important to consider the optimal frequency and methods for delivering training activities, whether didactic or interactive and whether in-person or virtual (online modules, etc.). Certain topics may require in-person training with hands-on practice (e.g., personal protective equipment), while many may not. However, demonstration of knowledge, understanding, and/or competency should be incorporated into training whenever possible. The checklists (or "job action sheets") developed during the planning process can be utilized during training to serve as quick reference guides to help familiarize staff with their expected actions, especially when they are not part of everyday operations.

In the event when the risk for a certain infectious disease is increased, such as when there is an ongoing outbreak, just-in-time training can be utilized to refresh staff and other responding entities' skills and to improve competency in carrying out expected duties. Once staff have been trained and are familiarized with their role in response, the next step would be to practice via drills and exercises.

Exercises

Exercises are interactive events that test and validate plans and reinforce training activities. Well-planned exercises enable organizations to identify organizational strengths

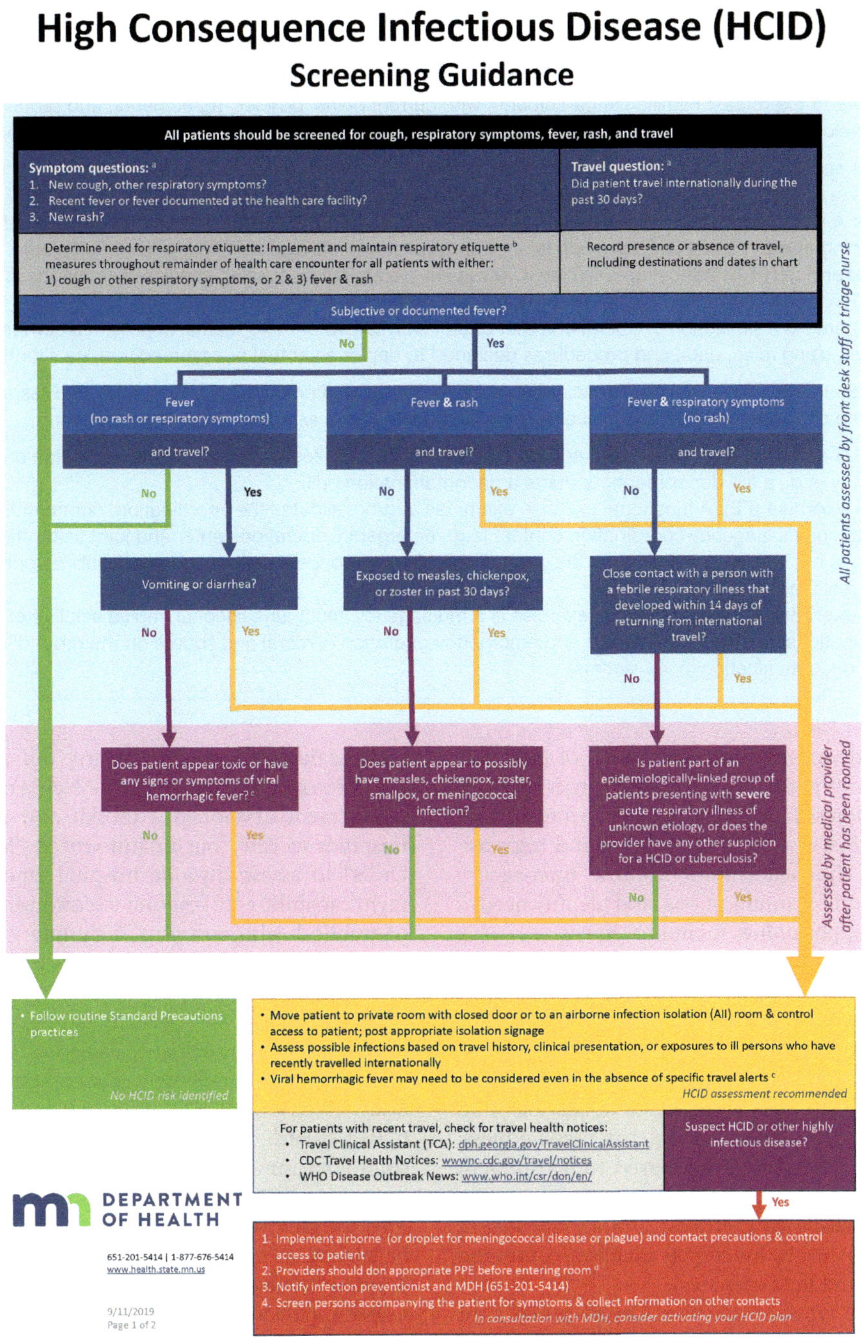

FIG. 7 Sample infectious diseases screening algorithm for emergency department staff. (From the Minnesota Department of Health; https://www.health.state.mn.us/diseases/hcid/.)

TABLE 5
Different Types of Exercises Based on the Homeland Security Exercise and Evaluation Program

Discussion-based exercises: Familiarize participants with current plans, policies, agreements, and procedures, or may be used to develop new plans, policies, agreements, and procedures. Discussion-based exercises include the following:

- **Seminar:** A seminar is an informal discussion designed to orient participants to new or updated plans, policies, or procedures (e.g., a seminar to review a new evacuation standard operating procedure).
- **Workshop:** A workshop resembles a seminar but is facilitated to build specific products, such as a draft plan or policy (e.g., a training and exercise plan workshop is used to develop a multiyear training and exercise plan).
- **Tabletop exercise (TTX):** A tabletop exercise involves key personnel discussing simulated scenarios in an informal setting. TTXs can be used to assess plans, policies, and procedures.
- **Games:** A game is a simulation of operations that often involves two or more teams, usually in a competitive environment, using rules, data, and procedures designed to depict an actual or assumed real-life situation.

Operations-based exercises: Validate plans, policies, agreements, and procedures, clarify roles and responsibilities, and identify resource gaps in an operational environment. Operations-based exercises include the following:

- **Drill:** A drill is a coordinated, supervised activity usually employed to test a single, specific operation or function within a single entity (e.g., a fire department conducts a decontamination drill).
- **Functional exercise (FE):** A functional exercise examines and/or validates the coordination, command, and control between various multiagency coordination centers (e.g., emergency operation center and joint field office). A functional exercise does not involve any "boots on the ground" (i.e., first responders or emergency officials responding to an incident in real time).
- **Full-scale exercises (FSE):** A full-scale exercise is a multiagency, multi-jurisdictional, multidiscipline exercise involving functional (e.g., joint field office and emergency operation centers) and "boots on the ground" response (e.g., firefighters decontaminating mock victims).

and can provide an objective assessment of gaps and shortfalls within plans, policies, and procedures to identify and address planning gaps prior to a real-world incident. Exercises also help clarify roles and responsibilities among different entities, improve inter-agency coordination and communications, and identify needed resources and opportunities for improvement.

One of the most utilized exercise frameworks for public health and healthcare system preparedness is the Homeland Security Exercise and Evaluation Program (HSEEP). Table 5 outlines different types of emergency preparedness exercises, which can broadly be combined into two major groups that test different aspects of an organization and/or systems' emergency preparedness: *discussion-based exercises* (often referred to by different names, including tabletop or desktop exercises, workshops or seminar-based exercises) and *operation-based exercises* (such as drills, functional exercises/command post exercises, and field exercises).[46]

Any of these types of exercises can be utilized for infectious disease preparedness planning. For example, NETEC has developed a suite of exercise templates for hospitals and healthcare coalitions based on viral hemorrhagic fevers, highly pathogenic airborne pathogens, and others available in English, French, and Spanish (repository.netecweb.org/exhibits/show/exercise-templates/exercises). Public health agencies often partner with healthcare facilities to carry out joint preparedness exercises. For example, the New York City Health Department developed a toolkit and partnered with hospitals to carry out unannounced "Mystery Patient Drills" to assess citywide hospital emergency department capabilities to respond to communicable diseases of public health concerns including measles, MERS-CoV, and SARS (on.nyc.gov/IDPrep).[47]

Evaluation and improvement

During an exercise, qualitative and quantitative data can be captured using an exercise evaluation guide. Operations-based exercises can also allow you to capture objective measures such as staff adherence to expected infection control measures and time required to perform expected actions (e.g., time from entry to mask patient and isolate). After the exercise or real-world event, participants should be invited to give feedback and share lessons learned during a "hot wash." These sessions afford an opportunity to assess staff familiarity with protocols and allow them to give feedback on how to improve processes.

All these elements are then documented, analyzed, and presented in an "after-action report," which includes recommended corrective actions. Designed to be specific, measureable, achievable, relevant with a timeframe for completion (SMART), after-action reports with corrective actions help organizations eval-

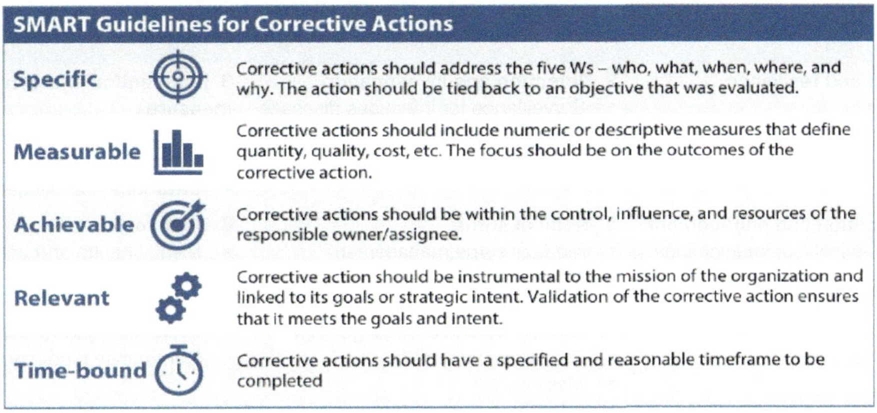

FIG. 8 An improvement plan should include corrective actions using the SMART guidelines. (From FEMA preptoolkit.fema.gov/web/hseep-resources/improvement-planning.)

uate their infectious disease capabilities and assess progress toward meeting them in a low-risk way. An effective corrective action program develops improvement plans after each exercise or real event that are dynamic documents, giving clear ownership to corrective actions, which are then continually monitored and implemented to improve preparedness (Fig. 8).

The last piece of the preparedness cycle is the most important and yet often the most ignored. That fact is that an institution can spend vast amounts of money, staff time, and political capital going through the motions of preparedness without anything to show for it. On the infectious disease front, there are dozens of examples of lessons from prior outbreaks that have simply not been learned or have even been unlearned over subsequent years. Developing an improvement plan with timelines and responsible parties can assist in mitigating gaps and applying lessons learned from the exercise and planning cycle, but this plan must be built on a basis of trust and mutual accountability with all partners.

By working together with partners throughout this preparedness process, holding each other accountable, making the work progressive from year to year, and ensuring that stakeholders are fully engaged, hospital systems and their public health partners can prevent some of these problems in the future. Template improvement plans and other HSEEP resources can be found at preptoolkit.fema.gov/web/hseep-resources.

THE ROLE OF PUBLIC HEALTH IN INFECTIOUS DISEASE RESPONSES

The emergency response capacity of public health has rapidly evolved over the last decade as the field has confronted a new range of global hazards. It is no longer enough to think of public health as a collection of epidemiologists or lab technicians. Instead, local/state health departments and their partners will use the structures described earlier to execute a wide range of capabilities. These capabilities have been described in various ways, such as with the CDC's 2011 Preparedness Capability Guidance Document (updated in 2018) and in summary reviews such as *The Common Ground Preparedness Framework*.[48] This chapter unifies various sources with the practical experience of the authors through multiple infectious disease emergencies to propose a comprehensive model, which involves six domains, or types of capabilities (Table 6).

Remember that during an infectious disease-related emergency, healthcare partners can play a key role in many of these actions. For example, most hospitals now work with social service organizations within their catchment area or could provide medical staff to partner facilities if needed. That is why it is so key to understand the whole picture of the public health response, even if it seems unrelated to the routine responsibilities of patient care. That said, some capabilities will be treated in much more depth than others to focus on the most relevant areas.

Domain One: Prevention and Resilience

Many core public health activities help prevent infectious disease outbreaks. Maintaining food and water supply safety, vector control activities, and immunization programs are all routine functions that keep the public safe every day. However, there are several additional programs and activities that are focused specifically on preventing more severe, catastrophic biological events or mitigating their impacts.

TABLE 6
An Overview of Health and Medical Capabilities Required for an Infectious Diseases Response

1. Prevention and resilience • Regulation • Prevention/immunization • Environmental systems • Resilience	**2. Detection and investigation** • Surveillance for infectious diseases • Laboratory testing • Outbreak investigation	**3. Intervention and control measures** • Mass vaccination and prophylaxis • Nonpharmaceutical interventions • Environmental mitigation
4. Communication and engagement • Provider/Clinical Communications • Public/Risk Communication • Community Outreach and Engagement	**5. Medical surge** • Medical surge management • Medical materiel management and distribution • Medical volunteer management • Fatality management • Mass care	**6. Recovery** • Mental health and behavioral health • Demobilization • Evaluation and learning • Community recovery

Regulation

As part of public health's mandate to protect the health and safety of a population, government agencies can mandate or enforce health laws and regulations.[49] Some examples include mandatory reporting for infectious diseases of public health concern, biosafety regulations in laboratories, and healthcare quality regulations meant to reduce or prevent healthcare-associated infections. At the facility level, these regulations can seem onerous. Sometimes, there may be a temptation to ignore them or circumvent them. However, these regulations provide a baseline framework that prevents infectious diseases wholesale or helps detect them quickly; they should be respected.

Prevention/immunization (see Chapter 20 for additional details)

The primary factor that prevents large-scale outbreaks remains our capacity to maintain high immunization rates for critical illnesses such as measles and pertussis and to rapidly administer vaccines for novel infections such as COVID-19 and Ebola where needed. High immunization rates give the population what is called *herd immunity*—essentially enough protection that outbreaks should be rare even among the small percent of residents that remain unvaccinated. Over the years, public health has expanded its prevention activities well beyond just immunization to include screening and treatment (e.g., tuberculosis, sexually transmitted infections), insurance provision, nutrition, maternal/child health, chronic disease, and other areas. Some of these preventative activities have come under fire from groups such as the anti-vaccination movement. These forces should be fought by the entire health and medical system; there is no better partner than healthcare providers to make sure these prevention messages are heard clearly around the world.

Environmental systems

When we think of diseases, we often think of transmission between humans. But many other pathways can create or spread disease, often based around various environmental factors. For example, most known, new, or emerging infectious disease threats are zoonotic in origin. Zoonoses are responsible for an estimated more than 2 billion human illnesses and 2 million human deaths annually.[50,51] As these pathways (e.g., water, insect vectors) have impacted health, public health agencies have built preventative environmental health systems. Food inspections, water testing, air quality, and vector control are other key parts of the public health portfolio, and together they are responsible for preventing thousands of illnesses each year. Often, these preventive measures function so well that they are not even thought of as disease prevention measures. But incidents like the Flint water crisis, the various *E. coli* outbreaks, or the spread of Zika through mosquitoes make clear that the connection between environmental health and a surge of patients at your hospital is just one system failure away.

Resilience

The idea of resilience developed in the fields of engineering and environmental ecology. It pertains to the ability of a system to both continue to function while under stress and to recover that function if it is lost due to a crisis. In public health terms, a community is more resilient if it has strong social services, local preventative health activities, and civic engagement. Other factors, such as public transportation systems, access to quality healthcare, and the presence of strong social relationships, influence community resilience as well.[52]

Communities that are more resilient before a public health emergency are more likely to survive the public health emergency with less illness and lower mortality. Underserved and traditionally marginalized communities are often less resilient due to a lack of investment and limited access to many services. The investments that health agencies make in prevention activities, healthy homes, healthy living (such as smoking prevention), and ensuring access to healthcare coverage all tend to increase the resilience of local communities and can be considered an important element in preventing local outbreaks from becoming more widespread emergencies.

More and more, hospitals and clinics find themselves on the front lines of these issues, sometimes unwillingly. Studies have found that hospitals become havens during huge infectious disease outbreaks; people go to hospitals for information when they do not trust other sources, for information about family members, or for psychosocial assistance.[53] On the other hand, facilities that are deeply embedded in their communities can expect assistance when they are overwhelmed: the community can come to their aid to help triage, disseminate messaging, and ferry people to alternative care sites.[54]

The message here and throughout the Prevention and Resilience Domain is that strengthening connections to the community, supporting preventative health activities and social services, and advocating for improved public infrastructure are critical to mitigating infectious disease outbreaks.

Domain Two: Detection and Investigation

Once a pathogen gains a foothold, the primary tool that can keep a small cluster from becoming an outbreak and, in turn, can keep an outbreak from becoming an epidemic is strong disease detection followed by a rapid, competent public health investigation. This includes identifying, characterizing, and transparently reporting threats at the earliest possible moment using strong epidemiological practices.

Surveillance for infectious diseases (see Chapter 16 for additional information)

It is important to remember that there is no substitute for an astute clinician who identifies and reports an unusual or emerging infectious disease threat. This clinical judgment is at the root of public health surveillance, which monitors patterns of disease in order to detect epidemics/outbreaks, measures changes in infectious agents, and assesses the effectiveness of interventions and control efforts.[55] Some disease surveillance is done on the international level (e.g., novel influenza, polio), but the majority of surveillance work in the United States is done on the state and local levels through notifiable disease surveillance programs. Most national surveillance programs receive reports through state and local health departments and focus on diseases that can affect multiple jurisdictions (e.g. multistate) during an outbreak, such as foodborne illness or influenza.[31,56]

Through these systems, healthcare providers, hospitals, and laboratories are required to report cases of specified diseases to the local health department (LHD), which is usually responsible for case investigation and action. For routine infectious diseases, surveillance is often done passively, meaning that healthcare facilities, providers, and labs must contact their health department when they see an infection that is unusual or on a list of notifiable conditions. Passive surveillance systems can utilize electronic health records, lab reporting, and vital records (e.g., birth and death certificates) or may require healthcare facilities or providers to phone or electronically report diseases as they are suspected or diagnosed.[55,57]

When more detailed data is needed, such as in the event of an outbreak, active surveillance can be utilized. This is much more resource-intensive as it requires health department staff to be in direct contact with a healthcare provider to investigate potential cases, collect epidemiologic information, and look for additional cases. An example of active surveillance is when a patient is reported as having active pulmonary tuberculosis. This would trigger a series of actions by public health to identify the relevant history and risk factors that may have exposed the patient to tuberculosis and would prompt an intensive contact investigation among potentially exposed persons to ensure they are notified, tested, and treated if needed.

For some types of infectious diseases, a sentinel surveillance system can focus on healthcare facilities or other reporting sites that have a higher likelihood of encountering a specific disease condition. Facilities can be selected to represent a specific geographic area or to capture a specific reporting or population subgroup. This allows you to collect information about what is going on in a specific subgroup to inform on trends that might be occurring at a population level. This information can be combined with population-level surveillance systems to guide decision-making in a response. One example of this is the use of sentinel surveillance in specialty clinics that treat sexually transmitted infections to monitor gonorrheal infections and to detect changes in antibiotic resistance.[58]

Other more specialized types of public health surveillance systems monitor for specific types of threats. For example, monitoring for bioterrorism events utilizes multiple systems in addition to traditional passive surveillance methods since many clinicians may not have the familiarity with such rare syndromes in order to recognize and report.[8] One example is the Department of Homeland Security's BioWatch program (https://www.dhs.gov/biowatch-program) provides air monitoring, analysis, notification procedures, and risk assessments to jurisdictions throughout the United States in order to provide early detection of a biologic attack.[59]

Syndromic surveillance is a newer system that focuses on a set of symptoms (e.g., fever and diarrhea), rather than a physician-diagnosed or laboratory-confirmed infection, that could signal a sufficient probability of a case or an outbreak of a particular disease to warrant further public health response. Data is most often obtained from hospital emergency department electronic medical record systems (e.g., chief complaints and diagnosis codes [see Figs. 1 and 2 and Table 1]). Additional health data can be obtained from other sources, such as urgent care centers or pharmacies. More recently, internet search terms and social media posts have also been included as part of these systems.[60] While many syndromic surveillance programs have been set up to recognize specific constellation of symptoms that could be suggestive of an agent of bioterrorism, they are also used to monitor additional syndromes that could be indicative of naturally occurring outbreaks.[61,62] For example, in early 2020, when testing for SARS-CoV-2 was limited, New York City and other jurisdictions were largely reliant on syndromic surveillance data for influenza-like illness to track the spread of COVID-19 in the population.

Healthcare staff should understand the variety and types of surveillance since they give such different resolutions of an infectious disease and clues to its severity. Passive surveillance or syndromic surveillance is standard. When active surveillance is employed or sentinel sites are established, that is a trigger that attention must be paid to what is happening. Bioterrorism monitoring systems like BioWatch provide early warning but carry risks unless their results are tied to clinical judgment or context.

Laboratory capacity and diagnostics (see Chapter 21 for additional information)

The public health laboratory (PHL) system has always been an essential tool for ongoing public health surveillance and disease control.[63] In partnership with the CDC and other federal agencies, state and local public health laboratories often provide essential diagnostic services for infectious diseases of public health importance such as tuberculosis, measles, HIV, or sexually transmitted infections such as syphilis. They can also provide reference services for laboratories to perform additional testing to further characterize disease agents of public health importance, such as with *Candida auris* or novel multidrug-resistant bacterial strains (e.g., carbapenem-resistant *Enterobacteriaceae*). In the outbreak setting, such as with tuberculosis or Legionnaire's Disease, the CDC (along with other federal and state/local PHLs) can perform specialized genetic testing such as whole genome sequencing to identify additional associated cases or even identify the source of an outbreak.[64,65] For example, the CDC's PulseNet program utilizes a database of DNA fingerprints of bacteria from patients to find clusters of disease that might represent unrecognized outbreaks and has been instrumental in identifying specific contaminated food sources.[66,67]

The anthrax attacks of 2001, the H1N1 influenza pandemic of 2009, the Ebola outbreaks in 2014 and the global mpox outbreaks in 2022 (Clade 2b) and 2024 (Clade 1) served to highlight the essential role of the PHLs in responding to infectious disease-related emergencies.[29] To support outbreak detection, response, and surveillance for uncommon, high-risk infectious diseases or potential bioterrorism agents (such as Ebola virus, *Yersinia pestis*, and novel strains of influenza A), public health labs coordinate or perform specialized testing. Additionally, the Laboratory Response Network maintains a national laboratory network of frontline (sentinel), reference, and national laboratories in order to rapidly detect and perform necessary testing for suspected agents of bioterrorism.[68]

The CDC is also often responsible for developing diagnostic testing capabilities for newly emerging pathogens, which, if needed, can then be offered through PHLs or commercial laboratories if a larger amount of testing is needed. For example, when Zika virus was found to be circulating in the Americas, initial diagnostic testing was developed and performed by the CDC, which then worked with select state and local public health labs to develop capacity for specialized Zika testing, including Zika RNA nucleic acid amplification testing (NAAT), serology, and other specialized testing. Public health labs then performed or coordinated a majority of Zika testing until commercial tests were available, and they continue to offer specialized Zika testing in special situations such as suspected congenital Zika infections.[69]

Many hospitals and most healthcare networks now have their own sophisticated lab capacity or substantial private contracting. In an infectious disease emergency, your local public health lab will set up a process of requesting, accessioning, testing, and reporting specimens. That lab, via the health department, will have to create and require a new set of procedures overnight. This will create new paperwork and, likely, headaches for hospital staff just when they need it least. However, it is impossible to overstate the importance of this process. Hospital lab staff should be ready to assist with reporting and can often help by offering to collect and test additional samples on suspected patients to provide more context to the outbreak.

Outbreak investigation

An *outbreak* or an *epidemic* is the occurrence of more cases of disease than expected in a given area or among a specific group of people over a particular period of time; the term epidemic is often applied to outbreak situations involving larger numbers of people over a wide geographic area; a pandemic refers to an epidemic occurring worldwide, or over a very wide area, crossing international boundaries and affecting a substantial portion of the population. In the event of an infectious disease outbreak or other biologic event, public health needs to respond rapidly and effectively to control or mitigate the risk (Table 7). Once a potential cluster, outbreak, or incident is identified through surveillance or disease reporting, the decision can be made to investigate based on:

- Severity of illness
- Transmissibility
- Ongoing illness/exposure
- Public concern

A public health investigation is performed to verify that the individual with the reported condition fulfills defined criteria, to determine the potential source and risk for spread of the infection/agent to others, and to implement necessary preventive and control measures. Outbreak investigations are generally initiated by local or state health departments, but federal agencies, such as CDC or FDA, may be invited to assist with the efforts.[15,70]

TABLE 7
Epidemiologic Steps of an Outbreak Investigation

1. Prepare for fieldwork
2. Establish the existence of an outbreak
3. Verify the diagnosis
4. Construct a working case definition
5. Find cases systematically and record information
6. Perform descriptive epidemiology
7. Develop hypotheses
8. Evaluate hypotheses epidemiologically
9. As necessary, reconsider, refine, and reevaluate hypotheses
10. Compare and reconcile with laboratory and/or environmental studies
11. Implement control and prevention measures
12. Initiate or maintain surveillance
13. Communicate findings

Source: https://www.cdc.gov/csels/dsepd/ss1978/SS1978.pdf; see Chapter 17 for additional details and examples of epidemic curves (Figs. 1–3). And for further training and resources on outbreak investigation and response, see the CDC's self-study courses at cdc.gov/csels/dsepd/ and the Outbreak Response Training Program (SHEA/CDC) at learningce.shea-online.org/content/sheacdc-outbreak-response-training-program-ortp.

One of the crucial initial steps in an investigation is to develop a clear *case definition,* which is a set of standard criteria for classifying whether a person has a particular infection, syndrome, or other health condition. A case definition usually includes a combination of specific symptoms, epidemiologic risk factors (e.g., time, place, and person), and diagnostic evidence (when testing is available). The use of a common case definition allows for standardization when investigating cases during an ongoing outbreak. This is especially useful when cases are being reported across multiple jurisdictions. Case definitions also help to give clarity to healthcare partners who might be involved in screening, testing, and reporting cases.

Early in an outbreak, or if a diagnosis is rare or uncertain, case definitions might start out with broader criteria or may include different categories such as confirmed, probable, or possible. Confirmed cases generally require laboratory validation. Probable cases meet specific symptom and epidemiologic criteria but lack laboratory confirmation. Possible cases meet fewer symptom criteria or have an atypical presentation. The CDC's Patient under Investigation (PUI) Guidance and Case Definition Guidance for MERS-CoV is an example of such categorization.[71] In addition, for some emerging or highly pathogenic diseases, testing may only be available through federal or public health laboratories, which have limited capacity. In these instances, case definitions can be used as criteria to evaluate the need for testing.

Based on initial investigation findings and continuing risk, public health officials may try to identify additional cases more proactively. To enhance these efforts, messaging can be distributed to healthcare providers, facilities, laboratories, or the public, describing the situation, symptoms, and risk factors with a request to report similar cases. As noted earlier, they may also implement active surveillance (or case finding) by telephoning, chart reviews, or visiting the facilities to collect information on any additional cases. Guidance may be provided to healthcare partners outlining procedures to protect, detect, and respond to patients with specific high-risk infectious diseases of public health concern. Such guidance will often include recommendations on infection control, patient isolation, and other relevant information to protect healthcare staff and patients.

Additional methods for case finding include contact tracing, which is the identification of relevant contacts of an infected person with a communicable disease of public health concern (e.g., tuberculosis, measles). Contacts may need to be made aware of the potential exposure, screened for symptoms, offered testing, and advised on what to do if they become ill. Some may be asked to monitor their symptoms for a certain period of time and report to public health authorities if they get sick. These interventions can be vital in containing an outbreak, though further measures may need to be taken to stop the chain of transmission.

Throughout an outbreak investigation and response, public health officials will be performing ongoing risk assessments by analyzing information such as epi curves, case definitions, morbidity and mortality rates, and public reaction (see Chapter 17 for additional information and Figs. 1–3 for examples of epidemic curves). These public health risk assessments create a readable portrait of investigation efforts and should be used to communicate information about severity, transmissibility, risk factors, and community impact to the public.

Recent public health work has increasingly focused on an important element for these risk assessments through its focus on the elimination of health disparities. Health disparities are defined in the *American Journal of Public Health* as "systematic, plausibly avoidable health differences according to race/ethnicity, skin color, religion, or nationality; socioeconomic resources or position (reflected by, e.g., income, wealth, education, or occupation); gender, sexual orientation, gender identity; age, geography, disability, illness, political or other affiliation; or other characteristics associated with discrimination or marginalization."[72] Many of these health disparities are *structural*–that is, they are enforced by embedded institutions of society. The most nefarious cause of these disparities is likely *structural racism,* defined as a set of "mutually reinforcing inequitable systems (in housing, education, employment, earnings, benefits, credit, media, healthcare, criminal justice, and so on) that in turn reinforce discriminatory beliefs, values, and distribution of resources, which together affect the risk of adverse health outcomes."[73]

The history of disaster research clearly shows that historically marginalized communities suffer worse impacts from crises. While health disparities were not traditionally a focus in the epidemiological analysis of outbreaks, studies done during more recent pandemics, including mpox, COVID-19, H1N1, and HIV, have demonstrated the importance of this work in illuminating stark disparities in outcomes among certain high-risk groups and allowed for a more equitable distribution of resources and targeted public health interventions. Any epidemiological reports should include analyses of the underlying structural disparities at play in the impact area and take those into consideration when designing interventions. To speak plainly, we know certain communities will probably suffer more and will need higher levels of intervention to counter their lower baseline level of health services.[74]

As both active players in these investigations and primary users of their findings, healthcare staff should be familiar with investigatory reports, with an eye to their patient populations. What do the impacted groups have in common? What does it mean for our neighborhood? Will our level of disease expand or contract over the next few days? Outbreaks are not monolithic, and each healthcare facility should be able to understand and process investigatory results for its own purposes.

Domain Three: Intervention and Control Measures

As the severity or intensity of the infectious disease outbreak increases, so does the necessity for various types of public health interventions. These should be used strategically. They are powerful but, as with all emergency measures, can provoke unanticipated consequences in the form of public backlash or unintended discrimination. There are three broad categories of public health interventions in these scenarios: medical countermeasures (such as prophylactic antimicrobials and vaccines), nonpharmaceutical interventions (such as school closures or quarantine), and environmental measures (such as decontamination).

Medical countermeasures

For certain infectious disease emergencies, the most critical control measure is the ability to rapidly distribute medications for treatment or prevention purposes. In a pandemic, the rapid development and distribution of the right vaccine are at the forefront of most providers' minds. After an aerosolized anthrax attack, what is more important than prophylactic antibiotics?

The federal government has devoted substantial resources to this topic. In 1999, Congress authorized the CDC to create the Strategic National Stockpile (SNS; https://aspr.hhs.gov/SNS/Pages/default.aspx). The SNS manages medications, vaccines, personal protective equipment (PPE), and other medical products (e.g., ventilators) that can be quickly deployed to shore up state and local supplies during emergencies or to provide countermeasures that are not commercially available (e.g. smallpox vaccine). Requests would be made by impacted states and processed by the ESF structure described earlier.[75–77]

The SNS has been utilized for anthrax attacks, foodborne hepatitis A, encephalitis, and H1N1 influenza, to name a few scenarios. During the COVID-19 response in 2020, the SNS played a critical role in supplying PPE, ventilators, and other supplies to all 50 states and US territories, though serious gaps in preparedness were revealed that will need to be addressed to ensure readiness for future pandemics. It also has capabilities well beyond these scenarios, though they are not fully public. Certainly, it contains enough anthrax vaccine to respond to aerosolized anthrax attacks in three cities and enough smallpox vaccine to inoculate every resident of the United States. It also contains chemical antidotes and antitoxins for agents such as botulinum.

In 2006, ASPR created an oversight group called the Public Health Emergency Medical Countermeasures Enterprise (PHEMCE) to unify federal work around medical countermeasures. PHEMCE coordinates the contents of the SNS, for example. It also manages the research portfolio of the Biomedical Advanced Research and Development Authority (BARDA; https://medicalcountermeasures.gov/barda), the wing of the government that researches and develops pharmaceuticals like countermeasures when little private incentive exists for their manufacture.[b] PHEMCE maintains a host of other governmental partnerships, as well. One such partner is the FDA, which can extend the shelf life of drugs based on scientific recommendations, can grant Emergency Use Authorizations (EUAs) to use investigational drugs and vaccines as medical countermeasures, and is critical to the process of monitoring adverse events from countermeasures. EUAs, in particular, are a powerful tool that give health authorities the ability to find and use experimental or nonapproved pharmaceuticals during public health emergencies.[78] This power was used successfully to treat Ebola patients during the 2014 (and subsequent) outbreaks and allowed for historically rapid development and deployment of COVID-19 vaccines, for example.

As robust as these federal assets are, it is still often the job of state and local health departments to get the right medications into the hands of the public. At the point of dispensing (POD), local staff establish a high-throughput pop-up facility with the sole purpose of screening and then distributing proper medication to the entire community. In one example, CDC guidance says that every jurisdiction must complete these antibiotic distribution operations within 48h after an aerosolized anthrax attack. PODs are not the only way to distribute medical countermeasures, of course.[79] Many hospitals can receive certain countermeasures during emergencies to distribute to staff and patients, as we saw during the initial COVID-19 vaccine distribution. Of larger impact, pharmacies can distribute high volumes of medications from locations that residents already know. Finally, the US Postal Service has plans to deliver medical countermeasures house to house in certain locations, in conjunction with local authorities.[80]

Your hospital may receive emergency countermeasures in certain situations, but not in others. You should check with your local public health agency to determine what scenarios are most likely. There are important considerations to be thought through in either case. If you receive countermeasures, will you give them to all staff, a subset of them who may be at risk, or none at all? Who should receive masks, and what type? If you do not receive them, do you know where the distribution sites in your neighborhood are supposed to be? This is important since many residents may come to the hospital to receive medication by mistake.

Whether or not your hospital is involved in distribution, an emergency in which the vast majority of the population is suddenly given one or more new medications will certainly affect your clinical practice.

Nonpharmaceutical interventions

Not all infectious disease emergencies will have ready medical countermeasures. In these cases, your jurisdiction may have to make a set of difficult judgment calls to control the spread of disease. How much should the population be tracked or restricted to slow the spread of disease? The answer is that the jurisdiction should utilize the lowest level of restriction that is still effective. What that level is will be different for different types of infectious agents, as we will see.

Active monitoring. In the event of an outbreak of a novel highly virulent and/or high-consequence pathogen, identified contacts (or other at-risk persons) may require close monitoring by public health authorities to identify the onset of symptoms early enough to prevent the spread of disease by infectious individuals. *Active monitoring* consists of direct contact—by phone, digitally, or in-person—with public health officials or a designee at least once a day to assess for symptoms and address any needs. More frequent monitoring (e.g., twice a day) can reduce the interval between the onset of symptoms and the institution of precautions (see Chapter 6, Fig. 2 for an example of a symptom diary).

[b] In March 2025, the U.S. Secretary of Health and Human Services announced that the Administration for Strategic Preparedness and Response (ASPR), which oversees the HPP cooperative agreement, will be incorporated into the Centers for Disease Control and Prevention (CDC). The impacts to the PHEP and HPP programs is yet to be determined. https://www.hhs.gov/press-room/hhs-restructuring-doge-fact-sheet.html.

If a fever or other sign of potential infection is detected, then the contact can be referred for medical evaluation, and additional infection control measures may be implemented. These processes are especially important to monitor potentially exposed healthcare workers who are not only prone to higher-risk exposures but also run the risk of exposing vulnerable patients and other staff members to infection.

Active monitoring can be undertaken voluntarily or, if needed, by legal mandate. The implementation of active monitoring should not be taken lightly, as it is incredibly resource-intensive and may not be effective in reducing the spread of every pathogen.[81] Considerations include epidemiologic features including the transmissibility and severity of the pathogen, the potential size of an outbreak, and the relationship between the time of symptom onset and infectiousness. Other issues, such as stigmatization of exposed contacts, should be proactively addressed by public health, community, and healthcare partners. Despite these challenges, active monitoring has the advantage of mitigating the risk to a community with fewer restrictions on individual liberties compared to quarantine when implemented appropriately.[82,83]

Movement restrictions. With some novel infectious diseases, persons with high-risk exposures (e.g., healthcare workers caring for an Ebola patient with a breach in PPE) may require restrictions on movement or activity in addition to monitoring. Recent examples include MERS-CoV and Ebola, where an exposed individual was unlikely to be infectious unless they developed symptoms.[84,85] In those cases, only the higher-risk exposure categories were recommended to have restrictions placed on their movement or travel. With some conditions, such as pulmonary tuberculosis or measles, federal agencies (CDC, Department of Homeland Security) can implement travel restrictions to protect travelers and the public from communicable diseases that are considered a public health threat. These restrictions can include being placed on a "do not board list" and "border lookout alert."

In extreme cases when there is a known outbreak outside of a country or jurisdiction and a significant threat of imported cases, travel and border restrictions may be considered by local, state, or federal authorities. Such actions should be carefully evaluated based on their effectiveness and potential economic and social impacts.

Quarantine. For certain asymptomatic contacts who may be infected, *quarantine* can be considered. Quarantine is the imposed isolation of these asymptomatic, high-risk case contacts to prevent the spread of infection to others. It is only appropriate for diseases where the time between the initial infection and infectiousness (the latent period) is substantially shorter than the time between the initial infection and symptom onset (the incubation period).[86] In other words, in situations when infected individuals could transmit disease for a substantial time before they show symptoms (as in COVID-19 but not Ebola). Certain other factors need to be in place to make quarantine a truly useful control measure, including an environment sophisticated enough to effectively manage its practicalities, proof that most contacts are being traced (otherwise a few quarantined individuals have no real efficacy), and an inability to immediately isolate monitored contacts once they show symptoms.

Even with these factors in place, quarantine should be treated carefully. Part of this pertains to civil liberties concerns. It is always dangerous for the government to use anything that looks like imprisonment to help the population. Quarantine can easily be overused, and extended quarantines can even lead to contacts breaking out because of the perception of imprisonment.

Further, quarantine can be expensive and difficult to scale up. Even with a few quarantined individuals, whether they are in their own residence or in a group setting like a hotel, logistical needs are considerable. Why? Since they are isolated, the point is to limit outside contact. However, people under quarantine still need food, toiletries, medication, and mail delivery. Plus, depending on the pathogen, these individuals may need constant security. Partly, that may be to keep them from infecting others, but it will primarily be to protect them from the attention of the media and all the methods they may use to get access (i.e., drones).

Generally, robust active monitoring (possibly through virtual means) coupled with rapid transition into isolation at symptom onset is likely to be more useful. Still, the more that infectiousness precedes symptom onset, the more that quarantine may need to be considered in areas with sophisticated contact tracing.

Community mitigation measures. Community mitigation measures are changes to social behaviors that people and communities can take to slow the spread of highly infectious respiratory viruses and lessen the impact of an epidemic. These actions include personal protective measures for everyday use (e.g., wearing a mask, staying home when ill, covering coughs and sneezes, and washing hands often) and community-wide measures aimed at reducing opportunities for exposure (e.g., coordinated closures and dismissals of childcare

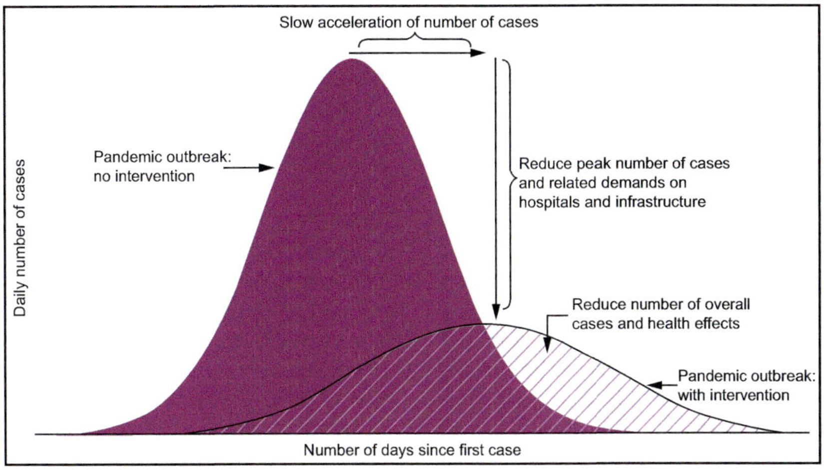

FIG. 9 Goals of community mitigation for pandemic influenza. (Source: CDC. Community Mitigation Guidelines to Prevent Pandemic Influenza — United States, 2017. cdc.gov/mmwr/volumes/66/rr/rr6601a1.htm.)

facilities and schools and canceling mass gatherings). Community mitigation measures are essential when there is widespread community transmission and no effective pharmaceutical treatment options or effective vaccines are available, such as in the early phase of a pandemic (Fig. 9).[87]

Many of these measures would be guided by local, state, or federal public health officials based on risk assessments and surveillance data. Some, such as home isolation or personal PPE usage, might be based on voluntary compliance, while others, such as school closures and prohibitions of mass gatherings, may need to be mandated through public health orders. The success of these strategies depends not only on the efficacy of the measures themselves but also on the epidemiologic characteristics of the disease, the timing of implementation, and the willingness of the community and healthcare partners to comply. Ultimately, the goal of such measures is not to prevent an outbreak altogether but to mitigate the impact.

In addition to traditional community mitigation strategies and medical countermeasures, public health agencies have been utilizing additional interventions to support the community and healthcare system in the event of a pandemic or other infectious disease emergency. For example, during recent COVID-19, Ebola, and Zika virus responses, many health departments/ministries of health established dedicated *call centers* or provided dedicated 24–7 on-call access to respond to questions, provide technical assistance, or arrange testing. Call centers and digital applications have also been used to provide medical triage, connections to care, and even medication prescriptions during a pandemic, starting in 2009 during the H1N1 pandemic when the Minnesota Department of Health implemented a statewide flu line (MN FluLine) and more recently with the use of telehealth for COVID antiviral access.[88–90] These and other interventions can allow public health and other organizations to improve access to countermeasure medications and decrease the demand for in-person clinical evaluation for less severely ill patients, which could in turn reduce the surge of patients at healthcare facilities and reduce healthcare-associated transmission of infection.[91] The trajectory of an outbreak/pandemic and ultimately the overall impact can be measured in several ways, including using mathematical models, as described in Chapter 18.

For further resources on establishing a medical triage line, see ASTHOs Flu on Call Toolkit (https://www.naccho.org/blog/articles/flu-on-call-increasing-access-to-care-and-treatment-during-pandemic-influenza) and the CDC's Algorithm to Assist in Medical Office Telephone Evaluation of Patients with Possible Influenza.

(https://www.cdc.gov/flu/hcp/testing-methods/office-evaluation.html; https://www.cste.org/page/FluOnCall; https://bioethics.miami.edu/_assets/pdf/education/public-health-ethics/pandemic-resources/pandemic-influenza-triage-tools.pdf).

Environmental mitigation

The connections between infectious disease and the environment are growing. Examples include the new wave of zoonotic diseases due to human encroachment into wildlife habitats, the connection of pathogens like

Legionella to urban infrastructure (in that case cooling towers), or the risk of environmental contamination from a disease vector, as with anthrax spores. In these cases, public health can drive a number of mitigation efforts that have implications for the infectious disease response.

As one example, zoonotic incidents (such as avian influenza) have led to widespread culling of bird flocks and/or the management of bird carcasses as a disease control measure. Integrated pest management is a robust field that contains interventions to cover all types of vector-borne disease, whether the vector is a mosquito or a rodent. Integrated pest management techniques range from standing water removal and rodenticide to the targeted application of pesticides from backpacks, trucks, and helicopters. For food and waterborne diseases, similar controls are available, from halting food distribution to inspection and cleaning of water facilities.

For agents such as anthrax that remain viable for extended periods outside the human body, environmental remediation to prevent future disease will be a major part of the infectious disease response. Remember that the cleanup from the 2001 anthrax attacks took 2 years and cost hundreds of millions of dollars for only a few buildings![92] Today, sophisticated environmental remediation plans are in place in which authorities will have to determine a level of acceptable cleanliness for the environment (never an easy choice) and then partner with large-scale private contractors to speed cleanup as much as possible.

For viral hemorrhagic fevers and other agents that produce substantial biologic waste, these decisions will play out at smaller scales in both healthcare and community settings. During the 2014 Ebola outbreak, establishing one standard environmental cleanup protocol was quite difficult; many guidance documents were created, from the CDC's guidance for commercial passenger aircraft to OSHA's guidance for nonhealthcare workplaces. Within healthcare facilities, the situation was even more complex. Special cleaning of patient locations was required, along with intensified guidance to healthcare facilities on issues like waste packaging and the use of autoclaves.

Environmental mitigation efforts can cause confusion and alarm; healthcare partners can help by supporting these efforts and explaining that they often prevent other, more restrictive control measures, not to mention further disease. Within healthcare facilities, environmental services and waste management should be key focus. The CDC's guidance on that subject during Ebola was complicated, fast-moving, and required hospitals to rapidly implement new protocols.[93] Additionally, many hospitals use contract staff for waste management who are harder to surge and may have specific employment rules that prevent them from dealing with certain categories of waste. Looking into these environmental mitigation issues now will prevent much stress during a response.

Domain Four: Communication and Engagement

Public health entities rightly focus on the scientific aspects of an infectious disease outbreak. But with experience, we have learned how important it is to tell the story of epidemic response well and to give the public clear actions to take through our risk communication. The public health system must educate, counter fears, and control rumors at the same time it builds an evidence-based investigation and implements control measures. In this age of misinformation, building a foundation of trust and credibility over time is essential because all the nonpharmacological interventions aforementioned will only be effective if there is understanding and buy-in by the community.[87,94] There are three main wings of this strategy: provider communication, public risk communication, and community outreach/engagement.

Provider communications

The first foundation of public health communications is getting appropriate, actionable information to healthcare providers. The most basic method for this is via Health Alert Networks (HAN; https://emergency.cdc.gov/han/index.asp), where the CDC and health departments can send out multiple types of messaging, including general updates, new alerts, and advisory recommendations in order to provide timely clinical, emergency-driven guidance meant for providers throughout the healthcare system.

All fifty states and many large cities are connected to the HAN system, and the health alerts that health departments send via this system can reach the providers for much of the population—though not 100%—which remains the ultimate goal. To be most effective, health alerts need to be brief, to the point, with clear recommendations, and should be quickly distributed to get information about the infectious disease to the front lines of the healthcare system where it is most needed.

Still, public health communication to providers should go far beyond health alerts. Providers of different types utilize different kinds of information sources.[95] During infectious disease emergencies, therefore, public health will use multiple outreach and education methods, including conference calls, webinars, grand rounds, town halls, publications, detailing campaigns, and clinical presentations given by health department employees or Medical Reserve Corps (MRC) volunteers. We will often partner with professional associations and organizations to develop messaging for specific groups. In addition, the CDC has a program called Clinician Outreach and Communication Activity (COCA; https://emergency.cdc.gov/coca/), which provides evidence-based health information on emerging health threats and collaborates with clinicians to develop better communication networks before, during, and after public health emergency.[96] There should always be efforts to gather feedback and questions from providers in order to improve these communications. After all, healthcare providers are the primary point of contact with the public in these difficult situations.

In infectious disease emergencies, healthcare facilities and networks have a responsibility to ensure that all their providers use the latest clinical guidance. This may seem impossible when there is a constant flow of new information, but recall that one of the key features of the HIC structure is the "Medical-Technical Specialist" position. By giving staff the specific responsibility of reviewing, summarizing, and disseminating guidance across the organization, your hospital stands a much better chance of cohesively providing care in a fast-moving outbreak.

Risk communication (see Chapter 27 for additional details)

One challenge with public health communications to the public and the broader healthcare community is that messaging can be overly technical or confusing. Unfortunately, it is a mistake that many health leaders fall into. Because of the psychology of humans in crisis, technical jargon can create real barriers with the public. Empathy carries more weight than numbers. The science of risk communication is too vast to do more than touch on here, though both the CDC's Crisis and Emergency Risk Communication (CERC) manual (https://www.cdc.gov/cerc/php/about/) and the work of Peter Sandman (https://www.psandman.com/index-intro.htm) provide strong introductions. The basic point is that during emergencies the public's perception of risk is based on a combination of the actual hazard and the outrage it inspires. Outrage gets more intense the less trust the public has in their government to handle the hazard, how little control they have, and the amount of dread the hazard causes (bioterrorist attacks create more dread than influenza, for example).

Managing this outrage means following a few core principles. The CDC highlights its risk communication principles as: *Be First, Be Right, Be Credible, Express Empathy, Promote Action, and Show Respect.*[97] The last three may be more important because they focus on the receiving end of your messaging and speak to the human side of outrage management, which needs warmth, caring, and a clear call to action; these allow people to feel that they have some control, especially in a situation where information keeps changing over time.

In the end, a public health response will need to use various modes of messaging, and multiple strategies are needed to reach different audiences—press conferences, radio and television announcements, social media, and community partnerships to name a few. However, if you are interacting with the public the core principles are the same: Pay attention to the grievances being raised, repeat them back to make sure you understand, validate the aspects of those grievances that have merit, and do not try to rebut anything that does not have merit. All you will do is inflame the outrage. Even if you are right, it will not help anything. Respond respectfully and your message is more likely to get through.

For those interested in going deeper into these issues, Sandman put together a collection of materials for infectious disease risk communication, including his summary of communication lessons from Ebola and COVID-19 (http://www.psandman.com/index-infec.htm).[98,99] One of his main points is that the most effective method of communication is face-to-face persuasion. Public health officials, no matter how they try, will never have the face-to-face impact on patients which healthcare providers may take for granted. During an infectious disease emergency, if every healthcare institution could use every patient encounter to impart key public health lessons and ask each patient to pass those lessons on, our risk communication work would become much simpler. The Crisis & Emergency Risk Communication (CERC)|CDC program offers trainings and additional resources to help you communicate more effectively during an emergency (https://emergency.cdc.gov/cerc/index.asp).

Community outreach and engagement

Often, during an outbreak, impacted communities need more direct, face-to-face interaction in order to help the residents take needed actions to improve their health outcomes. Maybe people in an area where an outbreak is occurring are not seeking care the way they should or, even more importantly, maybe they do not have access to the kind of care they need. Regardless, public health will mount community outreach campaigns to find at-risk people and make sure they are connected to care and services.

This work takes two main forms: *Community Outreach* and *Community Engagement*. A group called *Nexus Community Partners* has built a useful set of tools for distinguishing between the two (https://nexuscp.org/wp-content/uploads/2023/08/CEAssessmentTool_10.14.21.pdf).[100] Generally, health agencies use community outreach strategies. They may send teams into affected areas to hand out flyers, speak to community groups, or even distribute resources in clinical settings. This is helpful and does tend to motivate a community to take some action.

However, outreach is not as effective as true community engagement, which relies on ongoing, trusted relationships with partners within impacted communities. Using community engagement, health agencies listen to community members, integrate them into planning, and allow them real input into the activities of the public health response. This is true even though community members may give recommendations that counter standard public health practice, or express grievances about the healthcare response. The fact is that having community groups as strong allies can vastly improve the reach and efficacy of public health communications. Making them full partners cements that alliance which, in turn, helps the impacted community lead the effort to change behaviors in their community.

A notable example that demonstrated the value of engaging the community was seen during the West African Ebola epidemic in 2014–2015. It was recognized that one of the significant contributors to disease transmission was unsafe burial practices. In response, a cemetery and burial practices assessment was conducted in Sierra Leone which included interviews with community members to assess barriers to implementation and how practices could be changed to ensure them that safe burials were also dignified and culturally acceptable. This led to cemetery improvements and the development of a national standard operating procedure (SOP) on safe, dignified medical burials along with a national social mobilization effort called the "Safe Burials Save Lives" campaign which engaged the support from local political and religious leaders to educate community members on the risks of unsafe burials and the reasoning behind the changes. With continued input from local stakeholders, significant progress was made to decrease the risk of transmission from decedents.[101,102]

A more recent example that reinforces the value of community engagement was seen during the COVID-19 vaccine rollout in New York City. Early in 2021, NYC neighborhoods with the highest COVID-19 infection and fatality rates were found to have some of the lowest vaccination rates. In response, the NYC Health Department developed a provider and community engagement unit to reduce disparities in vaccination rates through three approaches:

1. Investment in marginalized neighborhoods: contracting with community-based organizations and federally qualified health centers that served the target communities to develop culturally appropriate education and outreach materials and to build out vaccination capacity.
2. Tailored community and provider engagement: developed bidirectional communication pathways with community stakeholders to create tailored approaches to address concerns and engaged in provider detailing campaigns to ensure providers had the information and resources they needed.
3. Collective impact approach to track and respond to inequities: tracked vaccination rates by age, race, and place to inform a data-driven approach to identify neighborhoods with the lowest vaccination rates and then used a cross-sector collaborative approach to close vaccination gaps.

These efforts helped dramatically increase the percentage of adults vaccinated for COVID-19 in the targeted communities and all but closed the vaccination rate gap between marginalized and nonmarginalized neighborhoods by the end of 2021.[103]

Please go to the Community Health Improvement Navigator (CDC) to find tools for successful community health engagement efforts (cdc.gov/chinav/tools/) and the WHO (who.int/publications/i/item/9789240010529; who.int/publications/i/item/risk-communication-and-community-engagement-(-rcce)-considerations) for manuals on community engagement for health promotion and Ebola risk communication.[104,105]

Domain Five: Medical Surge

Part of the importance of creating a unified system for the infectious disease response is to make sure the community's healthcare services can scale appropriately to meet the needs of the emergency, such as during an influenza pandemic or bioterrorism attack when there may be an excess demand for medical care, supplies, or specialized equipment. The major capabilities within this domain include medical surge management, patient load balancing, medical materiel management & distribution, medical volunteer management, and fatality management, but it is easiest to think of this as "space, staff, stuff, and systems." Standardized request processes are in place in most jurisdictions to provide healthcare facilities with needed staff and resources, though generally these should be triaged first through coalition partnerships.

In terms of standard medical surge or medical materiel management, this chapter has already covered how to make these requests via ESF and some of the resources available (such as DMATs). Regardless, the role of public health is to coordinate closely with the healthcare system to understand what they need and to help them get it in a timely manner. Still, the other capabilities have a few instructive points.

Medical surge management

There may be times when an emergency overwhelms the coalition's collective resources. The public health system can support the healthcare delivery system's transition to contingency and crisis care with the goal of promoting a timely return to conventional standards of care as soon as possible. Some actions that may be required include implementing legal protections and regulatory relief, providing surge space, facilitating information sharing, coordinating transfers through a Medical Operations Coordination Cell, and developing crisis standards of care protocols (Fig. 10). The COVID-19 pandemic left us with many lessons learned, including a better understanding of how structural racism and inequalities led to disproportionate impacts on certain historically marginalized communities. Incorporating these lessons into medical surge planning will require ongoing effort and coordinated engagement between local, state, and regional stakeholders.[106,107]

Medical volunteer management

Over the last decade, most jurisdictions have built out strong Medical Reserve Corps (MRC) programs, which we described briefly earlier. These contain thousands of licensed health volunteers, from physicians to nurses to technicians of various kinds. They are trained professionals who are locally licensed and indemnified by federal protections due to their membership in the program. A broader federal program called the Emergency System for Advance Registration of Volunteer Health Professionals (ESAR-VHP).

can also provide volunteers via state request. Both programs are important and healthcare providers reading this chapter are encouraged to sign up with one or both. Building a partnership with your local MRC chapter now can reduce concern about utilizing these licensed volunteers during an outbreak when your staff and system are strained.

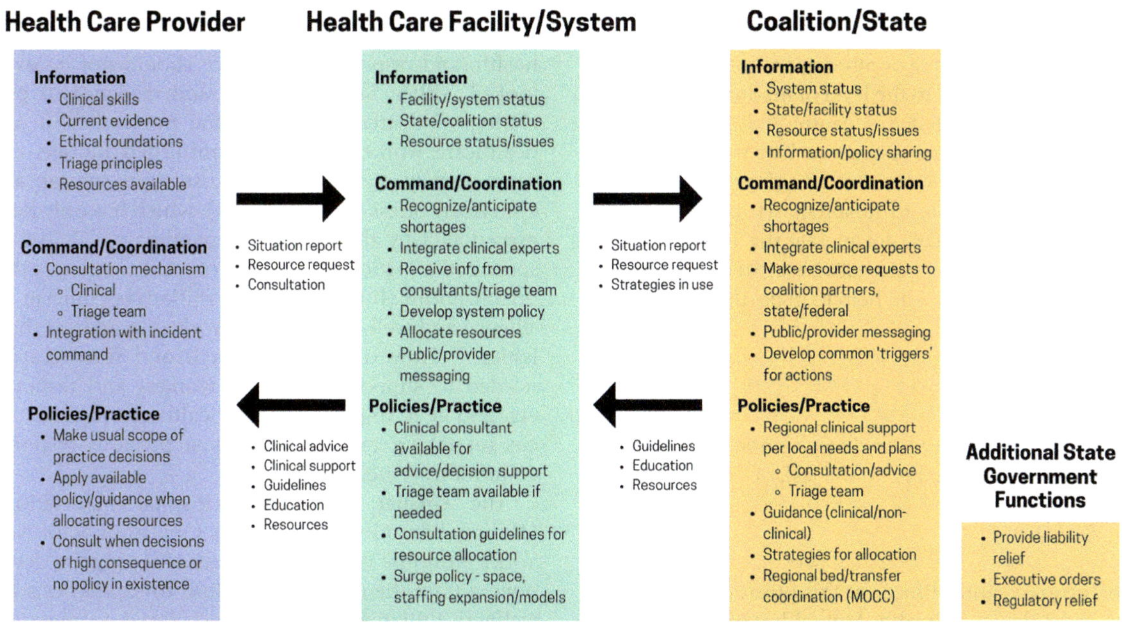

FIG. 10 Key domains and requirements for managing medical surge in crisis standards of care. (From Hick JL, Hanfling D, Wynia MK, Toner E. Crisis standards of care and COVID-19: what did we learn? How Do we ensure equity? What should we do? *NAM Perspect*. 2021;2021 https://doi.org/10.31478/202108e, https://nam.edu/crisis-standards-of-care-and-covid-19-what-did-we-learn-how-do-we-ensure-equity-what-should-we-do/.)

Fatality management

In general, hospitals have small morgue facilities, which can be easily overwhelmed in a highly pathogenic outbreak. At the same time, handling human remains is complex, requiring both technical skill and cultural understanding. Medical examiners and their staff are key members of the public health system. They can mobilize fatality management operations, including temporary morgue facilities, special precautions for infection control, long-term storage, and final disposition of remains.[108,109]

It is tragic to say, but fatality management operations are primarily for the living. In that spirit, they often involve a family assistance center, which can both provide services to grieving relatives and potentially collect important data for the public health investigation.

Mass care

In some cases of severe and widespread outbreaks, large-scale societal effects such as school closures, worker absenteeism, and transportation restrictions may create issues such as food, water, and fuel shortages, or even possible blackouts.[110] These issues create the need for a mass care capability to mitigate these effects as much as possible. Interventions in this environment have included sheltering operations, emergency food distribution, and the rapid creation of virtual education environments to keep students on track.

The success of these or other operations can stand in a direct relationship to the level of medical surge capacity that might be needed. Meaning that if the community can put mass care systems such as these into place, hospitals can focus on acute care. If not, members of the public will come to hospitals with issues created by the loss of services, not merely the infection itself. Therefore, it is in the hospital's best interest to support mass care operations and help to make them as successful as possible.

Domain Six: Recovery (see Chapter 28 for additional discussion)

At the end of an infectious disease emergency, the public health response takes on the task of normalizing the community.

Mental and behavioral health

The primary clinical focus at this point pivots to mental and behavioral health. Mental health is, of course, a concern throughout an epidemic.[111,112] Work during the 2014 Ebola epidemic, for example, showed that fear behaviors powered viral transmission in various ways, including escape from clinical wards and concealing sick family members.[113] We have seen with COVID-19 that pandemics lead to a myriad of negative mental health and substance use impacts that have disproportionately affected certain populations, including communities of color, young adults, and children—populations that have historically experienced increased barriers to care.[114] Fear behaviors, trauma responses, and exacerbations of underlying mental and behavioral health conditions are expected during epidemics and should be addressed throughout the response.

Just as important, however, are the long-term consequences that epidemic exposure can have in a small subset of the population. Research on the HIV/AIDS pandemic in Africa shows that children who lost parents show sustained social and psychological symptoms, which should be considered for ongoing public health interventions.[115] At a minimum, the ending of an epidemic should prompt a comprehensive population-based mental health needs assessment, with a concurrent set of action plans to address these lingering mental health symptoms. Within hospitals, patients seeking mental or behavioral healthcare will continue over time, forming a long tail that lingers after the wave(s) of infection has passed.

The mental health needs of the healthcare, public health, and responder workforce should not be overlooked, either. Studies have found evidence of psychological distress in responding public health and healthcare workers, such as diminished morale, elevated anxiety, elevated alcohol use, work refusal, and even Acute Stress Disorder (ASD), which has only been exacerbated by the COVID-19 pandemic.[116–118] In response, the National Academy of Medicine and other organizations (https://nam.edu/initiatives/clinician-resilience-and-well-being/) have worked to address these issues.[119] However, more research and resources are needed to support healthcare workers and responders, and it is imperative that healthcare facilities focus on taking care of their most precious response commodity—their staff.

The Greater New York Hospital Association's Healing, Education, Resilience & Opportunity for New York's Frontline Workforce (HERO-NY) program developed a train-the-trainer curriculum to expand existing wellness initiatives that can be tailored to meet the mental health and wellness needs of frontline healthcare workers during a response (gnyha.org/program/hero-ny/).

Demobilization and evaluation

Beyond the mental health focus, the public health system will be moving staff/assets back to their normal operating environments, working with healthcare system to normalize clinical operations, and pushing the jurisdiction to learn important lessons. Hospitals at this point will be participating in jurisdictional evaluations, as well as their own internal self-assessments, following the principles described in our evaluation section mentioned previously. Reimbursement and inventory reconciliation take substantial time after events like these, and healthcare facilities should be prepared for the required staff resources. Continuity of Operations Planning (COOP) work done before the outbreak will provide dividends during this recovery period, as it gives clear procedures for restoring normal operations.

The California Hospital Association (CHA) has strong tools for healthcare facilities in this area, which can be found here: https://www.calhospitalprepare.org/continuity-planning.

The capability model

Taken together, these capabilities represent more than three dozen specific functions that are critical to prevent, detect, and respond to infectious disease emergencies. This could easily get overwhelming. Therefore, the public health system must carefully balance the needs and priorities of the various capabilities throughout an infectious disease response. Before it occurs, prevention and early detection is the key. Once an outbreak or biologic event is detected, the investigation is most critical. As conclusions about the outbreak can be drawn, appropriate control measures come to the fore, followed by strong risk communication to help the public understand the situation. Through all of this, the system is working to provide the healthcare system with the needed resources to continue caring for their patients. As the wave crests, the public health system can turn to recovery, over time guiding impacted communities back to a place of strength and security.

CONCLUSION

In the event of an infectious disease emergency, public health is pivotal to the coordination, communication, and collaboration during a response. In fact, on every page of this chapter, we have emphasized relationships and collaboration. Essentially, we are advocating that all public health and healthcare entities create a unified approach that provides a single response and mutual accountability. Taken together, these ideas could address many of the major lessons learned from the last decade of infectious disease responses.

For the public, this single-response idea is crucial since it eliminates major sources of concern, such as different organizations giving different guidance. For responders, it could alleviate the massive duplication and chaos of the multiple interlocking response siloes that sometimes occur in large epidemics.

In addition, a unified approach provides mutual accountability to strengthen the everyday practices that improve our ability to prevent, detect, and respond to novel infectious disease events as a system. Basic competencies around infection control, surveillance/screening, training, exercises, and assessment are the bread and butter of this work. However, institutional will and investment are needed to make sure the healthcare system and providers are well equipped to understand and apply these practices in their day-to-day work as well as during an outbreak—when the stakes of getting them wrong are high.

At the end of the day, modern public health builds this unified approach (improving on what Jon Snow was able to do on Broad Street) by:

- Creating an integrated group of closely related partners—the "public health system"—that unites government, healthcare, and organizations together in one entity to respond to an infectious disease emergency.
- Using a standard set of structures and practices—based on the Incident Command System—to manage public health emergencies across the public health system.
- Building up health and medical capabilities that move beyond traditional epidemiologic investigation so that the public health system can address the downstream effects of an infectious disease emergency and support the needs of the entire community.
- Preparing the public health system consistently, over time, through planning, organizing, equipping, training, exercising, and evaluating.

We live in an age when local outbreaks can turn into global threats in the blink of an eye. But if we work together, we have an immense capacity to respond to these threats, too. With the partnerships and plans that we have discussed in place, the global public health system to which you belong can respond to infectious disease emergencies in ways that John Snow could never dream of.

REFERENCES

1. Koch T, Denike K. Rethinking John Snow's South London study: a Bayesian evaluation and recalculation. *Soc Sci Med.* 2006;63(1):271–283. https://doi.org/10.1016/j.socscimed.2005.12.006.
2. Johnson S. The Ghost Map: The Story of London's Most Terrifying Epidemic—and How it Changed Science, Cities, and the Modern World. Riverhead Books; 2006.
3. Centers for Disease Control and Prevention. Ten great public health achievements- -United States, 1900–1999. *MMWR Morb Mortal Wkly Rep.* 1999;48(12):241–243.
4. Frieden TR. A framework for public health action: the health impact pyramid. *Am J Public Health.* 2010;100(4):590–595. https://doi.org/10.2105/AJPH.2009.185652.
5. Institute of Medicine. The Future of Public Health. The National Academies Press; 2002. https://doi.org/10.17226/1091.
6. Public Health in America Statement. Public Health Functions Steering Committee; 1994.
7. *The Public Health System & the 10 Essential Public Health Services*. Centers for Disease Control. Updated September 9, 2020. https://www.cdc.gov/public-health-gateway/php/about/index.html. Accessed 14 April 2025.
8. Gostin LO, Sapsin JW, Teret SP, et al. The model state emergency health powers act: planning for and response to bioterrorism and naturally occurring infectious diseases. *JAMA.* 2002;288(5):622–628.
9. *A Public Health Emergency Declaration*. ASPR. https://aspr.hhs.gov/legal/PHE/Pages/Public-Health-Emergency-Declaration.aspx. Accessed 16 May 2023.
10. *How a Disaster Gets Declared*. FEMA. https://www.fema.gov/disaster/how-declared. Accessed 16 May 2023.
11. Barbera J, Macintyre A. Medical Surge Capacity and Capability: A Management System for Integrating Medical and Health Resources during Large-Scale Emergencies. U.S. Department of Health and Human Services; 2007. https://aspr.hhs.gov/HealthCareReadiness/guidance/MSCC/. Accessed 14 April 2025.
12. Emergency Management and the Incident Command System. Administration for Strategic Preparedness and Response (ASPR). https://www.phe.gov/Preparedness/planning/mscc/handbook/chapter1/Pages/emergency-management.aspx. Accessed 14 April 2025.
13. Waugh WL. Mechanisms for collaboration in emergency management: ICS, NIMS, and the problem with command and control. In: O'Leary R, ed. *The Collaborative Public Manager: New Ideas for the Twenty-First Century.* Georgetown University Press; 2009:157–175.
14. Iskander J, Strikas RA, Gensheimer KF, Cox NJ, Redd SC. Pandemic influenza planning, United States, 1978-2008. *Emerg Infect Dis.* 2013;19(6):879–885. https://doi.org/10.3201/eid1906.121478.
15. Federal Emergency Management Agency (FEMA). National Response Framework, Fourth Edition. Homeland Security U.S. Department of Homeland Security; 2019. Accessed 14 April 2025 https://www.fema.gov/emergency-managers/national-preparedness/frameworks/response. Accessed 14 April 2025.
16. Redd SC, Frieden TR. CDC's evolving approach to emergency response. *Health Secur.* 2017;15(1):41–52. https://doi.org/10.1089/hs.2017.0006.
17. Levi J, Segal LM, Lang A. Remembering 9/11 and Anthrax: Public Health's Vital Role in National Defense. Trust for America's Health; 2011. Issue report http://resource.nlm.nih.gov/101569591. Accessed 16 May 2023.
18. Roos R, Schnirring L. Public Health Leaders Cite Lessons of 2001 Anthrax Attacks. July 2018. Center for Infectious Disease Research and Policy (CIDRAP); 2011. September 1, 2011 https://www.cidrap.umn.edu/anthrax/public-health-leaders-cite-lessons-2001-anthrax-attacks. September 1, 2011.
19. Katona P, Sullivan JP, Intriligator MD. Global biosecurity: threats and responses. In: *Contemporary Security.* 1st ed. Routledge; 2011.
20. California Emergency Medical Services Authority. *Hospital Incident Command System—Forms.* https://emsa.ca.gov/hospital-incident-command-system-forms-2014/. Accessed 14 April 2025.
21. Daugherty EL, Carlson AL, Perl TM. Planning for the inevitable: preparing for epidemic and pandemic respiratory illness in the shadow of H1N1 influenza. *Clin Infect Dis.* 2010;50(8):1145–1154. https://doi.org/10.1086/651272.
22. Emergency Support *Function #8 – Public Health and Medical Services Annex.* Department of Homeland Security. https://www.fema.gov/sites/default/files/2020-07/fema_ESF_8_Public-Health-Medical.pdf. Accessed 14 April 2025.
23. Frasca DR. The medical reserve corps as part of the federal medical and public health response in disaster settings. *Biosecur Bioterror.* 2010;8(3):265–271. https://doi.org/10.1089/bsp.2010.0006.
24. *The Emergency System for Advance Registration of Volunteer Health Professionals (ESAR-VHP)*. Administration for Strategic Preparedness and Response. https://aspr.hhs.gov/ESAR-VHP/. Accessed 14 April 2025.
25. HHS Response and *Recovery Resources Compendium*. U.S. Department of Health and Human Services; 2015. Accessed 14 April 2025. https://asprwgpublic.hhs.gov/ASPR/hhscapabilities/Pages/default.aspx.
26. International Health Regulations. World Health Organization; 2005. https://www.who.int/health-topics/international-health-regulations.
27. Centers for Disease Control and Prevention, International Health Regulations (IHR); 2025. https://www.cdc.gov/global-health/topics-programs/ihr.html. Accessed 14 April 2025.
28. World Health Organization. Framework for a Public Health Emergency Operations Centre; 2015. Accessed 15 April 2025 https://www.who.int/publications/i/item/framework-for-a-public-health-emergency-operations-centre.
29. World Health Organization. Emergency Response Framework (ERF), Edition 2.1; 2024. Accessed 14 April 2025 https://www.who.int/publications/i/item/9789240058064.
30. World Health Organization. *The Cluster System.* https://healthcluster.who.int/. Accessed 16 May 2023.

31. Joint External Evaluation Tool: International Health Regulations. 3rd ed. Geneva: World Health Organization; 2005. 2022 https://www.who.int/publications/i/item/9789240051980.
32. *Health Security Learning Platform*. World Health Organization. https://extranet.who.int/hslp/. Accessed 1 May 2023.
33. Watson CR, Watson M, Sell TK. Public health preparedness funding: key programs and trends from 2001 to 2017. *Am J Public Health*. 2017;107(S2):S165–S167. https://doi.org/10.2105/AJPH.2017.303963.
34. Trust for America's Health (TFAH). The Impact of Chronic Underfunding on America's Public Health System 2024: Trends, Risks, and Recommendations. https://www.tfah.org/report-details/funding-2024/. Accessed 14 April 2025.
35. Centers for Disease Control and Prevention (CDC). Public Health Emergency Preparedness and Response Capabilities*: National Standards for State, Local, Tribal, and Territorial Public Health*. U.S. Department of Health and Human Services; 2018. Accessed 14 April 2024 https://stacks.cdc.gov/view/cdc/60062. Accessed 14 April 2024.
36. Public Health Emergency Preparedness and Response Capabilities. Centers for Disease Control and Prevention (CDC). https://www.cdc.gov/readiness/php/capabilities/. Accessed 14 April 2025.
37. ASPR. From Hospitals to Healthcare Coalitions. U.S. Department of Health and Human Services (ASPR); 2009. Accessed 15 July 2018 https://aspr.hhs.gov/HealthCareReadiness/guidance/Documents/hpp-healthcare-coalitions.pdf. Accessed 15 July 2018.
38. Toner E. Healthcare preparedness: saving lives. *Health Secur.* 2017;15(1):8–11. https://doi.org/10.1089/hs.2016.0090.
39. *National Preparedness Cycle: National Incident Management System (NIMS)*. Center of Excellence for Homeland Security. http://www.coehsem.com/emergency-management-cycle/. Accessed 16 May 2023.
40. U.S. Department of Homeland Security. *NIMS: Frequently Asked Questions*. U.S. Department of Health and Human Services. Accessed July 2018. https://www.fema.gov/pdf/emergency/nims/nimsfaqs.pdf.
41. *Prioritizing Diseases for Research and Development in Emergency Contexts.* World Health Organization. https://www.who.int/activities/prioritizing-diseases-for-research-and-development-in-emergency-contexts. Accessed 16 May 2023.
42. *NYC Health+Hospitals Institute for Disease and Disaster Management—Tools and Resources*. New York City Health+Hospitals. https://www.nychealthandhospitals.org/institute-for-disease-and-disaster-management/tools-and-resources/. Accessed 1 May 2023.
43. Hospital Incident Command System (HICS). Job Action Sheets; 2014. California EMS Authority https://emsa.ca.gov/hospital-incident-command-system-job-action-sheets-2014/. Accessed 1 May 2023.
44. Office of Public Health Preparedness and Response (CDC). *Education, Training, and Planning Resources. Centers for Disease Control and Prevention.* https://www.cdc.gov/orr/publications-resources/index.html. Accessed 14 April 2025.
45. *Technical Resources, Assistance Center, and Information Exchange (TRACIE) ASPR.* https://asprtracie.hhs.gov/. Accessed July 2018.
46. *Homeland Security Exercise and Evaluation Program.* Department of Homeland Security. https://www.fema.gov/emergency-managers/national-preparedness/exercises/hseep. Accessed May 16, 2023.
47. Foote MMK, Styles TS, Quinn CL. Assessment of hospital emergency department response to potentially infectious diseases using unannounced mystery patient drills - New York city, 2016. *MMWR Morb Mortal Wkly Rep.* 2017;66(36):945–949. https://doi.org/10.15585/mmwr.mm6636a2.
48. Gibson PJ, Theadore F, Jellison JB. The common ground preparedness framework: a comprehensive description of public health emergency preparedness. *Am J Public Health.* 2012;102(4):633–642. https://doi.org/10.2105/AJPH.2011.300546.
49. Frieden TR. Government's role in protecting health and safety. *N Engl J Med.* 2013;368(20):1857–1859. https://doi.org/10.1056/NEJMp1303819.
50. Woolhouse ME, Gowtage-Sequeria S. Host range and emerging and reemerging pathogens. *Emerg Infect Dis.* 2005;11(12):1842–1847. https://doi.org/10.3201/eid1112.050997.
51. Gebreyes WA, Dupouy-Camet J, Newport MJ, et al. The global one health paradigm: challenges and opportunities for tackling infectious diseases at the human, animal, and environment interface in low-resource settings. *PLoS Negl Trop Dis.* 2014;8(11), e3257. https://doi.org/10.1371/journal.pntd.0003257.
52. Morton MJ, Lurie N. Community resilience and public health practice. *Am J Public Health.* 2013;103(7):1158–1160. https://doi.org/10.2105/AJPH.2013.301354.
53. Paturas JL, Smith D, Smith S, Albanese J. Collective response to public health emergencies and large-scale disasters: putting hospitals at the core of community resilience. *J Bus Contin Emer Plan.* 2010;4(3):286–295.
54. Forum on Medical and Public Health Preparedness for Catastrophic Events; Board on Health Sciences Policy; Institute of Medicine. Public health surge capacity and community resilience. In: *Regional Disaster Response Coordination to Support Health Outcomes: Summary of a Workshop Series.* National Academies Press; 2015.
55. Lee LM, Teutsch SM, Thacker SB, St. Louis ME. Principles and Practice of Public Health Surveillance. 3rd ed. Oxford University Press; 2010.
56. *National Notifiable Diseases Surveillance System (NNDSS).* Centers for Disease Control and Prevention. cdc.gov/nndss/. Accessed May 16, 2023.
57. German RR, Lee LM, Horan JM, et al. Updated guidelines for evaluating public health surveillance systems: recommendations from the guidelines working group. *MMWR Recomm Rep.* 2001;50(RR-13):1–35. quiz CE1-7.

58. Quilter LAS, St. Cyr SB, Hong J, et al. Antimicrobial susceptibility of urogenital and Extragenital Neisseria gonorrhoeae isolates among men who have sex with men: strengthening the US response to resistant gonorrhea and enhanced gonococcal isolate surveillance project, 2018 to 2019. *Sex Transm Dis.* 2021;48(12S):S111–S117. https://doi.org/10.1097/olq.0000000000001548.
59. National Academies of Sciences E, Medicine. Strategies for Effective Improvements to the BioWatch System: Proceedings of a Workshop. The National Academies Press; 2018:222.
60. Pei S, Kandula S, Yang W, Shaman J. Forecasting the spatial transmission of influenza in the United States. *Proc Natl Acad Sci U S A.* 2018;115(11):2752–2757. https://doi.org/10.1073/pnas.1708856115.
61. Henning KJ. What is syndromic surveillance? *MMWR Suppl.* 2004;53:5–11.
62. *National Syndromic Surveillance Program (NSSP).* Centers for Disease Control and Prevention. https://www.cdc.gov/nssp/index.html. Accessed May 16, 2023.
63. The Association of Public Health Laboratories (APHL). The Core Functions of Public Health Laboratories, Version 4.0; 2024. https://www.aphl.org/aboutAPHL/publications/Documents/PHL-Core-Functions.pdf. Accessed 14 April 2025.
64. Fitzhenry R, Weiss D, Cimini D, et al. Legionnaires' disease outbreaks and cooling towers, New York City, New York, USA. *Emerg Infect Dis.* 2017;23(11). https://doi.org/10.3201/eid2311.161584.
65. Witt-Kushner J, Astles JR, Ridderhof JC, et al. Core functions and capabilities of state public health laboratories: a report of the Association of Public Health Laboratories. *MMWR Recomm Rep.* 2002;51(RR-14):1–8.
66. Announcement: 20th Anniversary of PulseNet: the National Molecular Subtyping Network for Foodborne Disease Surveillance - United States, 2016. *MMWR Morb Mortal Wkly Rep.* 2016;65(24):636. https://doi.org/10.15585/mmwr.mm6524a5.
67. Swaminathan B, Barrett TJ, Hunter SB, Tauxe RV, Force CDCPT. PulseNet: the molecular subtyping network for foodborne bacterial disease surveillance, United States. *Emerg Infect Dis.* 2001;7(3):382–389. https://doi.org/10.3201/eid0703.010303.
68. Centers for Disease Control and Prevention (CDC). *The Laboratory Response Network Partners in Preparedness.* https://emergency.cdc.gov/lrn/index.asp. Accessed July 2018.
69. Centers for Disease Control and Prevention (CDC). Testing Guidance for Zika Virus. U.S. Department of Health and Human Services; 2018. https://www.cdc.gov/zika/hc-providers/testing-guidance.html.
70. Dicker RC, Coronado F, Koo D, Parrish RG. Principles of Epidemiology in Public Health Practice. 3rd ed. Centers for Disease Control and Prevention; 2012. https://archive.cdc.gov/www_cdc_gov/csels/dsepd/ss1978/index.html.
71. Centers for Disease Control and Prevention (CDC). Diagnostic Testing for MERS and Testing Criteria. https://www.cdc.gov/mers/hcp/diagnosis-testing/index.html. Accessed 14 April 2025.
72. Braveman PA, Kumanyika S, Fielding J, et al. Health disparities and health equity: the issue is justice. *Am J Public Health.* 2011;101(Suppl 1):S149–S155. https://doi.org/10.2105/AJPH.2010.300062.
73. Bailey ZD, Krieger N, Agenor M, Graves J, Linos N, Bassett MT. Structural racism and health inequities in the USA: evidence and interventions. *Lancet.* 2017;389(10077):1453–1463. https://doi.org/10.1016/S0140-6736(17)30569-X.
74. Bolin B, Kurtz LC. Race, class, ethnicity, and disaster vulnerability. In: Rodríguez H, Donner W, Trainor JE, eds. *Handbook of Disaster Research.* Cham: Springer; 2018. chap 181–203. Accessed August 2018 https://link.springer.com/book/10.1007/978-3-319-63254-4#toc.
75. Center for the Strategic National Stockpile. U.S. Department of Health and Human Services. https://aspr.hhs.gov/sns. Accessed 14 April 2025.
76. Sun L. Inside the Secret U.S. Stockpile Meant to Save Us All in a Bioterror Attack. The Washington Post; 2018.
77. Gottron F, Wyatt TR. The Strategic National Stockpile: Overview and Issues for Congress; 2023:2023. https://crsreports.congress.gov/product/pdf/R/R47400.
78. *Emergency Use Authorization.* U.S. Food and Drug Administration. https://www.fda.gov/emergency-preparedness-and-response/mcm-legal-regulatory-and-policy-framework/emergency-use-authorization. Accessed May 1, 2023.
79. The Association of State and Territorial Health Officials (ASTHO) and the National Association of County and City Health Officials (NACCHO). Extended Medical Countermeasure Distribution and Dispensing Considerations for Anthrax Incidents; 2017. https://www.naccho.org/blog/articles/anticipating-anthrax-new-tools-designed-to-enhance-long-term-medical-countermeasure-distribution.
80. Committee on Prepositioned Medical Countermeasures for the Public. Prepositioning Antibiotics for Anthrax. National Academies Press; 2011.
81. Reich NG, Lessler J, Varma JK, Vora NM. Quantifying the risk and cost of active monitoring for infectious diseases. *Sci Rep.* 2018;8(1):1093. https://doi.org/10.1038/s41598-018-19406-x.
82. Fraser C, Riley S, Anderson RM, Ferguson NM. Factors that make an infectious disease outbreak controllable. *Proc Natl Acad Sci U S A.* 2004;101(16):6146–6151. https://doi.org/10.1073/pnas.0307506101.
83. Peak CM, Childs LM, Grad YH, Buckee CO. Comparing nonpharmaceutical interventions for containing emerging epidemics. *Proc Natl Acad Sci U S A.* 2017;114(15):4023–4028. https://doi.org/10.1073/pnas.1616438114.
84. Managing MERS Cases and Contacts. Centers for Disease Control and Prevention (CDC); 2024. https://www.cdc.gov/mers/php/contact-tracing/index.html. Accessed 14 April 2025.

85. Public Health Management of People with Suspected or Confirmed VHF or High-Risk Exposures. Centers for Disease Control and Prevention (CDC); 2024. https://www.cdc.gov/viral-hemorrhagic-fevers/php/public-health-strategy/people-with-suspected-or-confirmed-vhf-or-high-risk.html. Accessed 14 April 2025.
86. Fraser C, Riley S, Anderson RM, Ferguson NM. Factors that make an infectious disease outbreak controllable. *Proc Natl Acad Sci.* 2004;101(16):6146–6151.
87. Qualls N, Levitt A, Kanade N, et al. Community mitigation guidelines to prevent pandemic influenza - United States, 2017. *MMWR Recomm Rep.* 2017;66(1):1–34. https://doi.org/10.15585/mmwr.rr6601a1.
88. Spaulding AB, Radi D, Macleod H, et al. Satisfaction and public health cost of a statewide influenza nurse triage line in response to pandemic H1N1 influenza. *PloS One.* 2013;8(1), e50492. https://doi.org/10.1371/journal.pone.0050492.
89. Jacobs-Wingo J, Ezeoke I, Saffa A, et al. Using a call center to coordinate Zika virus testing-new York City, 2016. *J Emerg Manag.* 2016;14(6):391–395. https://doi.org/10.5055/jem.2016.0303.
90. Dasari S, Kurian S, Bastani R, et al. Streamlining test-to-treat: a novel care delivery model for Covid-19 Oral antiviral access to close the equity divide in Los Angeles County. *NEJM Catalyst.* 2023;4(3). https://doi.org/10.1056/CAT.22.0328. CAT.22.0328.
91. Kristal R, Rowell M, Kress M, et al. A phone call away: New York's hotline and public health in the rapidly changing COVID-19 pandemic. *Health Aff (Millwood).* 2020;39(8):1431–1436. https://doi.org/10.1377/hlthaff.2020.00902.
92. Franco C, Bouri N. Environmental decontamination following a large-scale bioterrorism attack: federal progress and remaining gaps. *Biosecur Bioterror.* 2010;8(2):107–117.
93. Centers for Disease Control and Prevention. *Handling VHF-Associated Waste.* Centers for Disease Control and Prevention (CDC). https://www.cdc.gov/viral-hemorrhagic-fevers/hcp/infection-control/handling-vhf-associated-waste.html. Accessed 14 April 2025.
94. Seale H, Dyer CEF, Abdi I, et al. Improving the impact of non-pharmaceutical interventions during COVID-19: examining the factors that influence engagement and the impact on individuals. *BMC Infect Dis.* 2020;20(1):607. https://doi.org/10.1186/s12879-020-05340-9.
95. Quinn C, Poirot E, Sanders Kim A, et al. Variations in healthcare provider use of public health and other information sources by provider type and practice setting during new York City's response to the emerging threat of Zika virus disease, 2016. *Health Secur.* 2018;16(4):252–261. https://doi.org/10.1089/hs.2018.0026.
96. *Clinician Outreach and Communication Activity (COCA).* Centers for Disease Control and Prevention (CDC). https://emergency.cdc.gov/coca/index.asp. Accessed May 18, 2023.
97. *Crisis + Emergency Risk Communication (CERC) Manual.* Centers for Disease Control and Prevention. https://emergency.cdc.gov/cerc/manual/index.asp. Accessed 16 May 2023.
98. Sandman PM. When the Next Shoe Drops — Ebola Crisis Communication Lessons from October. Center for Infectious Disease Research and Policy (CIDRAP); 2014. Accessed July 2018 http://www.cidrap.umn.edu/news-perspective/2014/12/commentary-when-next-shoe-drops-ebola-crisis-communication-lessons-october.
99. Sandman PM. Pandemic Flu and Other Infectious Diseases. https://www.psandman.com/index-infec.htm. Accessed 16 May 2023.
100. Nexus Community Engagement Institute. https://nexuscp.org/program/nexus-community-engagement-institute/. Accessed 14 April 2025.
101. Nielsen CF, Kidd S, Sillah AR, et al. Improving burial practices and cemetery management during an Ebola virus disease epidemic - Sierra Leone, 2014. *MMWR Morb Mortal Wkly Rep.* 2015;64(1):20–27.
102. Nuriddin A, Jalloh MF, Meyer E, et al. Trust, fear, stigma and disruptions: community perceptions and experiences during periods of low but ongoing transmission of Ebola virus disease in Sierra Leone, 2015. *BMJ Glob Health.* 2018;3(2), e000410. https://doi.org/10.1136/bmjgh-2017-000410.
103. Ige O, Watkins J, Pham-Singer H, Dresser M, Maru D, Morse M. Embedding health equity in a public health emergency response: New York City's Covid-19 vaccination experience. *Catalyst.* 2023;4(2). https://doi.org/10.1056/CAT.22.0425. non-issue content.
104. Community Engagement: A Health Promotion Guide for Universal Health Coverage in the Hands of the People. World health Organization; 2020. https://www.who.int/publications/i/item/9789240010529.
105. Risk Communication and Community Engagement (RCCE) Considerations: Ebola Response in the Democratic Republic of the Congo. World Health Organization; 2018. https://www.afro.who.int/publications/risk-communication-and-community-engagement-rcce-considerations-ebola-response.
106. Hick JL, Hanfling D, Wynia MK, Toner E. Crisis standards of care and COVID-19: What did we learn? How do we ensure equity? What should we do? *NAM Perspect.* 2021;2021. https://doi.org/10.31478/202108e.
107. Cleveland Manchanda E, Couillard C, Sivashanker K. Inequity in crisis standards of care. *N Engl J Med.* 2020;383(4), e16. https://doi.org/10.1056/NEJMp2011359.
108. Decedent Management during Disasters. In: *The Exchange.* ASPR TRACIE; 2022. Issue 16 https://files.asprtracie.hhs.gov/documents/aspr-tracie-the-exchange-issue-16.pdf.
109. Forum on Medical and Public Health Preparedness for Catastrophic Events. Medical Surge Capacity: Workshop Summary. National Academies Press (US); 2010. https://nap.nationalacademies.org/catalog/12798/medical-surge-capacity-workshop-summary.

110. Kelley N, Osterholm M. Pandemic Influenza, Electricity, and the Coal Supply Chain: Addressing Crucial Preparedness Gaps in the United States. Center for Infectious Disease Research and Policy, University of Minnesota; 2008.
111. Shultz JM, Baingana F, Neria Y. The 2014 Ebola outbreak and mental health: current status and recommended response. *JAMA.* 2015;313(6):567–568. https://doi.org/10.1001/jama.2014.17934.
112. Earls F, Raviola GJ, Carlson M. Promoting child and adolescent mental health in the context of the HIV/AIDS pandemic with a focus on sub-Saharan Africa. *J Child Psychol Psychiatry.* 2008;49(3):295–312. https://doi.org/10.1111/j.1469-7610.2007.01864.x.
113. Shultz JM, Cooper JL, Baingana F, et al. The role of fear-related behaviors in the 2013-2016 West Africa Ebola virus disease outbreak. *Curr Psychiatry Rep.* 2016;18(11):104. https://doi.org/10.1007/s11920-016-0741-y.
114. Panchal N, Saunders H, Rudowitz R, Cox C. The Implications of COVID-19 for Mental Health and Substance Use; 2023. https://www.kff.org/coronavirus-covid-19/issue-brief/the-implications-of-covid-19-for-mental-health-and-substance-use/.
115. Institute of Medicine (US) Committee on Envisioning a Strategy for the Long-Term Burden of HIV/AIDS: African Needs and U.S. Interests. The burden of HIV/AIDS: implications for African states and societies. In: *Preparing for the Future of HIV/AIDS in Africa: A Shared Responsibility.* National Academies Press (US); 2011.
116. Benedek DM, Fullerton C, Ursano RJ. First responders: mental health consequences of natural and human-made disasters for public health and public safety workers. *Annu Rev Public Health.* 2007;28:55–68. https://doi.org/10.1146/annurev.publhealth.28.021406.144037.
117. Bryant-Genevier J, Rao CY, Lopes-Cardozo B, et al. Symptoms of depression, anxiety, post-traumatic stress disorder, and suicidal ideation among state, tribal, local, and territorial public health workers during the COVID-19 pandemic - United States, march-April 2021. *MMWR Morb Mortal Wkly Rep.* 2021;70(48):1680–1685. https://doi.org/10.15585/mmwr.mm7048a6.
118. Raposa ME, Mullin G, Murray RM, et al. Assessing the mental health impact of the COVID-19 pandemic on US fire-based emergency medical services responders: a tale of two samples (the RAPID study i). *J Occup Environ Med.* 2023;65(4):e184–e194. https://doi.org/10.1097/jom.0000000000002745.
119. National Aademy of Medicine. *Action Collaborative on Clinician Well-Being and Resilience.* https://nam.edu/initiatives/clinician-resilience-and-well-being/. Accessed 1 May 2023.

CHAPTER 15

Prevention in Healthcare and Public Health

HEATHER L. YOUNG[a,b] • GRACE ELLEN MARX[b] • BERNADETTE ALBANESE[c,d] • CONNIE S. PRICE[a,b]

[a]Division of Infectious Diseases, Denver Health Medical Center, Denver, CO, United States • [b]University of Colorado School of Medicine, Denver, CO, United States • [c]Department of Epidemiology, Colorado School of Public Health, Aurora, CO, United States • [d]University of Colorado Denver, Greenwood Village, CO, United States

INTRODUCTION

Highly infectious pathogens have the potential to spread quickly and cause significant morbidity and mortality. For the purposes of this chapter, measles, pandemic influenza, and the coronaviruses—namely, Middle East Respiratory Syndrome (MERS), severe acute respiratory syndrome (SARS), and Severe Acute Respiratory Syndrome Coronavirus 2 (SARS-CoV-2)—are defined as highly infectious pathogens. Class A bioterrorism agents are organisms that pose a risk to national security because they can be easily disseminated or transmitted from person to person; may result in high mortality rates; may cause public panic or social disruption; and require special action for public health preparedness.[1] They include anthrax (*Bacillus anthracis*), botulism (*Clostridium botulinum*, rarely *Clostridium butyricum* or *Clostridium baratti*), plague (*Yersinia pestis*), smallpox, tularemia (*Francisella tularensis*), and viral hemorrhagic fevers (Ebola, Marburg, Lassa, and Machupo). Prevention of transmission and outbreaks due to these pathogens requires prompt identification of the infected person(s), recognition of the mechanism and route of exposure, knowledge of the pathogen's incubation and contagiousness period, and implementation of control measures to interrupt transmission.

This chapter provides an overview of the early recognition of disease outbreaks due to highly infectious pathogens and bioterrorism agents; strategies to prevent further person-to-person spread; and steps to effectively improve readiness for effective and coordinated response to these potential threats. A critical component of outbreak prevention of highly infectious pathogens is a robust public health system that can rapidly detect single cases of infection or clusters of disease through surveillance programs and leverage emergency preparedness protocols to support a coordinated and effective response.

IDENTIFYING CASES OR CLUSTERS

A single case or cluster of a highly infectious infection can begin with the reporting by an astute clinician or by public health surveillance.[2] A clinician may recognize clinical symptoms and signs that are compatible with a pathogen of concern, although the presentation of many of these conditions overlaps with other more common infections. Public health surveillance may identify single cases or unusual clusters of syndromes or infections. The latter is identified through either mandatory reporting of notifiable conditions from laboratories performing diagnostic testing or by clinician reports. Regional poison control centers may also identify clusters of persons with similar symptoms being reported by the lay public, emergency departments, or other clinicians that might suggest a bioterrorism event. Many states have set up methods to use the electronic medical record to identify individuals presenting with syndromes or a constellation of symptoms that mimic the infection, such as influenza (influenza-like illness), or that would be seen by an agent that could be associated with a bioterrorism event. The following section

Viral Outbreaks, Biosecurity, and Preparing for Mass Casualty Infectious Diseases Events
https://doi.org/10.1016/B978-0-323-54841-0.00010-X

addresses how outbreaks of highly infectious pathogens, pathogens of consequence, emerging infections, and bioterrorism agents might be identified.

Clinicians and Their Role

Identification of persons with clinical syndromes that are compatible with disease due to highly infectious pathogens or bioterrorism agents is the first step in both appropriate clinical care of the individual patient and the prevention of further cases. Recent examples highlight how important clinicians are in the recognition and the reporting to public health of patients with syndromes and signs of agents of high consequence. For example, astute clinicians recognized and reported the 2001 case of inhalational anthrax in Florida, the first case of Mpox in the Western hemisphere in 2003, and in 2014, the first US-acquired case of Ebola.[3–5] Vigilant clinicians who recognize potentially uncommon infections facilitate rapid diagnosis of the patient and protect both healthcare personnel and members of the community.

Recognition of certain pathogens as the etiologic agent is easier in some circumstances than others. Some physical examination signs, such as the pustular rash associated with smallpox, could be pathognomonic for the organism, while common symptoms such as nausea, fever, myalgia, and gastrointestinal symptoms that accompany viral hemorrhagic fevers might be more difficult to diagnose in the absence of an established outbreak or defined exposure. Similarly, severe community-acquired pneumonia might be indistinguishable from highly infectious pathogens and bioterrorism agents, making it difficult to identify these in a timely manner.[6] When a disease caused by a highly infectious pathogen is not endemic in the United States, the probability of a case occurring is very low unless the patient provides a history of exposure in another country, illustrating the importance of a thorough travel history. While the clinical presentation of these pathogens is described in detail in Chapters 1–11 of this book, clinical syndromes are typically associated with highly infectious pathogens and bioterrorism agents (Table 1). Of note, these syndromes are commonly used for syndromic surveillance, which is commonly automated from data gathered in emergency departments (see Chapter 14).

Researchers in Connecticut reviewed 4558 unexplained infectious deaths and found 133 (2.9%) to be possibly consistent with anthrax and 6 (0.13%) to be consistent with tularemia.[8] None were consistent with smallpox or botulism. No deaths had anthrax or tularemia listed in the differential diagnosis, and only 53% had minimal work-up criteria for these possible bioterrorism agents. Hence, a minority of clinicians have bioterrorism agents at the forefront of their clinical decision-making.

Resources are available to clinicians to maintain their awareness of highly infectious pathogens and

TABLE 1
Selected Clinical Syndromes[a]: Highly Infectious and Viral Pathogens Associated With Class A Bioterrorism Agents and Pandemics[6,7]

Clinical Syndrome	Highly Infectious Pathogen or Class A Bioterrorism Agent
Pustular rash	Smallpox, Mpox (see Chapter 6)
Necrotic eschar or cutaneous ulcer	*B. anthracis* (cutaneous anthrax) (see Chapter 2) *F. tularensis* (ulceroglandular tularemia) (see Chapter 3)
Severe pneumonia	*Y. pestis* (pneumonic plague) (see Chapter 4) *F. tularensis* (pulmonary tularemia) (see Chapter 3) *B. anthracis* (inhalational anthrax) (see Chapter 2) SARS-CoV (SARS) (see Chapter 9) MERS-CoV (MERS) (see Chapter 10) SARS-CoV-2 (COVID-19) (see Chapter 11) Influenza (pandemic) (see Chapters 7 and 8)
Gastroenteritis	Viral hemorrhagic fever(s) (see Chapter 5)
Flaccid paralysis	*C. botulinum*
Erythematous maculopapular rash	Measles
Influenza-like illness or COVID-like illness	Influenza, avian influenza, SARS, and SARS-CoV-2

[a]These syndromes are used for syndromic surveillance methods (see Chapter 14 for additional detail).

bioterrorism agents. Some professional societies offer training at national meetings, and review articles to guide practice are available.[6,7,9,10] The Centers for Disease Control and Prevention (CDC) and other international public health agencies have published continuing education activities for preparedness and response to biological or chemical terrorism.[11]

Once a disease outbreak is established in a region of the world, clinicians can quickly find information on the CDC's Travel Notices website, the World Health Organization, or other public health agency websites.[12a,12b] However, clinicians must have a heightened index of suspicion and awareness to access these resources. State, provincial, and local public health agencies also provide information to clinicians using Health Alerts or other means of communication if there is a situation that has the potential to impact persons traveling to or returning from an affected region. ProMED, run by the International Society for Infectious Diseases, is a reliable and often early source of information about emerging infectious disease clusters internationally.[12c] Promising alternatives include leveraging electronic health record systems to screen and identify patients who report a possible travel-related exposure and/or symptoms consistent with a highly infectious viral pathogen. Such systems have been widely deployed in healthcare systems and could provide timely prompts to providers who might not have initially considered a highly infectious pathogen. This said, these systems are not fail-proof, hence reinforcing the need for obtaining a thorough history that includes travel.[12c]

Confirming the Diagnosis (See Chapter 17 for Additional Details)

When a clinician suspects a highly infectious viral pathogen or bioterrorism agent, it is essential to promptly report the suspect case to infection prevention within the hospital, the hospital laboratory, and the public health authorities and work collaboratively to confirm the diagnosis. It is important to care for the patient and obtain appropriate testing to rule in and out the other potential causes of the patient's clinical syndrome. The decision to undergo specific laboratory testing should be based on the index of suspicion, exposure history, and presenting signs and symptoms. Laboratory commonly requires specific samples, using specific containers, and testing can be highly specialized depending on the pathogen of interest (Table 2). As new technology emerges, additional testing modalities may be available for diagnosis.

TABLE 2
Laboratory Tests Used to Diagnose Highly Infectious Pathogens or Class A Bioterrorism Agents[13–15] (See Chapter 17 and Table 5 for Further Detail)

Highly Infectious Pathogen or Class A Bioterrorism Agent	Laboratory Test(s)
Anthrax (cutaneous), *B. anthracis* (see Chapter 2)	Wound and blood culture,[a] skin lesion exudate PCR, serology, tissue biopsy immunohistochemistry
Anthrax (pulmonary), *B. anthracis* (see Chapter 2)	Pleural fluid cultures, blood, and cerebrospinal fluid or PCR, serology
Botulism, *C. botulinum*	Wound, stool, or gastric contents culture, serum for botulinum toxin
Influenza A, B, or Avian A strains (see Chapters 7 and 8)	Respiratory specimen PCR, cultures may be done in rare instances in reference laboratories, whole genome sequencing
Measles	Serum IgM, culture or PCR from throat or nasopharyngeal swab
MERS-CoV (see Chapter 10)	Respiratory specimen PCR, whole genome sequencing
Plague, *Y. pestis* (see Chapter 4)	Cultured lymph node aspirate, blood, respiratory secretions,[a] PCR in clinically appropriate specimens, acute and convalescent serum IgM
SARS (see Chapter 9)	Respiratory specimen PCR

(Continued)

TABLE 2
Laboratory Tests Used to Diagnose Highly Infectious Pathogens or Class A Bioterrorism Agents (See Chapter 17 and Table 5 for Further Detail)—cont'd

Highly Infectious Pathogen or Class A Bioterrorism Agent	Laboratory Test(s)
COVID-19 (SARS-CoV-2; see Chapter 11)	Respiratory specimen PCR, whole genome sequencing
Smallpox (see Chapter 6)	Orthopox PCR from vesicle, confirmation at reference laboratory[a,b]
Tularemia, *F. tularensis* (see Chapter 3)	Culture or PCR from tissue specimen, skin lesion swab or scraping, lymph node aspirate, pharyngeal swab, sputum specimen, gastric aspirate, or blood,[a] serology
Viral hemorrhagic fever (see Chapter 5)	Serum or whole blood PCR,[a,b] serology,[a] tissue biopsy immunohistochemistry[a]

[a]Clinicians must alert the laboratory in advance so appropriate safety procedures are put into place for specimen handling.
[b]Consult reference laboratory guidance (see Chapter 17 for additional details).

Many laboratories, particularly small community hospital laboratories, may not have the equipment, supplies, or tests readily available. Reference laboratories, including state public health laboratories and the CDC, generally process these tests and provide results to clinicians. Hence, clinicians and commercial laboratory personnel must understand where specialized testing is offered and the expected turnaround times. Providers should communicate with these reference laboratories in advance of specimen collection to determine which specimens should be collected to optimize diagnostic testing.

Surveillance (See Chapter 14 for Additional Details)

Public health authorities utilize two major types of surveillance for emerging and/or pathogens of high consequence (see Chapters 13 and 14 for additional details). One is when a patient is suspected of having an infection due to a highly infectious pathogen or bioterrorism agent that is identified. This notifiable condition requires notifying public health officials promptly, something required by public health authorities worldwide.[16] Reporting novel or emerging organisms and unusual syndromes is equally important. Infectious pathogens such as hantavirus,[17] Legionnaire's disease,[18] and *Pneumocystis jirovecii* pneumonia as an AIDS-defining illness,[19,20] and SARS were discovered as a result of correlating reports of similar clinical syndromes with epidemiologic risk factors. In these cases, astute clinicians recognized an unusual cluster of severe unexplained pneumonia and reported it to public health officials, launching an extensive collaborative investigation that ultimately led to the discovery of these novel conditions. Second is syndromic surveillance, which provides public health authorities with a timelier mechanism to look for potential events before a diagnosis is confirmed. This early warning system can be used for events such as influenza activity, to identify norovirus outbreaks or other events. In this case, medical facilities voluntarily send de-identified information including the chief complaint, diagnosis (International Classification of Diseases (ICD-) 9 or ICD-10 codes), and patient characteristics from patient visits to emergency rooms. Local or regional public health departments or aggregators receive and concatenate these data. In both cases, public health authorities have analytic tools that identify patterns of illness that can provide forewarning to the medical community.

Because delay in reporting of suspect cases of disease could result in unnecessary delay in implementing outbreak prevention and control measures both surveillance strategies are employed. Once a cluster of illnesses has been identified, a case definition is developed. Case definitions generally include criteria for clinical features, laboratory diagnostic results, and epidemiologic links to other known or suspected cases.[21]

While public health agencies are responsible for thoroughly investigating cases and exposures once the case has been reported. The knowledge of public health authorities about the epidemiology of the pathogen will serve the lead role to:

1. determine how and where the exposure occurred
2. guide public health mitigation measures
3. investigate if other cases are suspected

4. conduct contact tracing to identify other potentially exposed persons
5. assess whether postexposure prophylaxis is indicated.

Initially, public health authorities must determine if the case of the highly infectious pathogen is a single case or if there is a cluster of cases that occurred during a similar time period or geographic region.

Cases are defined to facilitate active surveillance in order to ascertain cases and to collect important epidemiologic data. Active case finding is particularly important in settings where passive surveillance is likely to be incomplete, such as in settings where social stigma of disease is high or public health reporting infrastructure is weak. The strategy of actively identifying cases is used to identify cases within the population identified as most at-risk. Active surveillance requires the use of multiple potential data sources including searching laboratory records and logs, testing of individuals that surrounded the case, or going house-to-house. This case-finding strategy was extensively employed in areas with known Ebola cases during the Ebola outbreak in West Africa in 2014–15.[22]

Identification of a case of infection due to a highly infectious pathogen or bioterrorism agent is the essential first step in the prevention of future cases. Astute clinicians are often the first to consider these pathogens as a cause of a patient's clinical syndrome, perform diagnostic testing, and notify public health officials. Public health authorities are then tasked with investigating cases, determining the risk to other community members, performing surveillance for additional cases, implementing control measures, and communicating findings to the public and to community stakeholders.

PREVENTION AND CONTROL

Data Analysis/Interpretation

Once it has been determined that an infectious pathogen is affecting a community, timely intervention to prevent additional cases is of paramount importance. Epidemic (*"epi"*) curves are a useful tool to visualize and describe the pathogen or syndrome's frequency over time, even if the exact pathogen has not been identified (Figs. 1–3). Using both epidemic curves and the known properties of highly infectious pathogens, epidemiologists determine the appropriate preventive actions and assess the response to these actions, which may include patient isolation, quarantine or testing after potential exposure, physical separation (physical [social] distancing), vaccination, and postexposure prophylaxis.

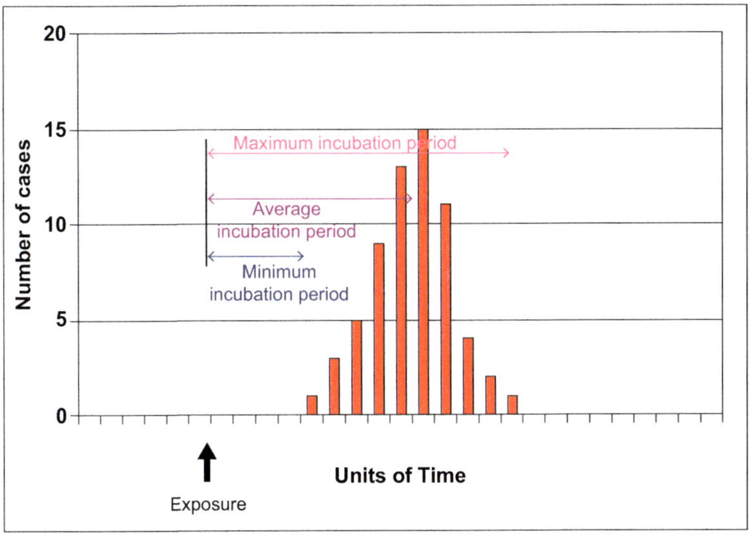

FIG. 1 Example epidemic curve of a point-source outbreak with no propagation.[23] A point source occurs after a single exposure such as a meal or a release of an infectious agent. The *red vertical bars* represent the number of cases and the time when symptoms/signs developed from the exposure. The maximum *(pink)*, average *(purple)*, and minimum *(blue)* incubation periods are estimated by determining the time from the exposure to developing symptoms in those who develop symptoms most quickly (minimum) or those whose symptoms have a later onset (maximum). (From Epidemic Curves. http://www.med.uottawa.ca/sim/data/public_health_epidemic_curves_e.htm.)

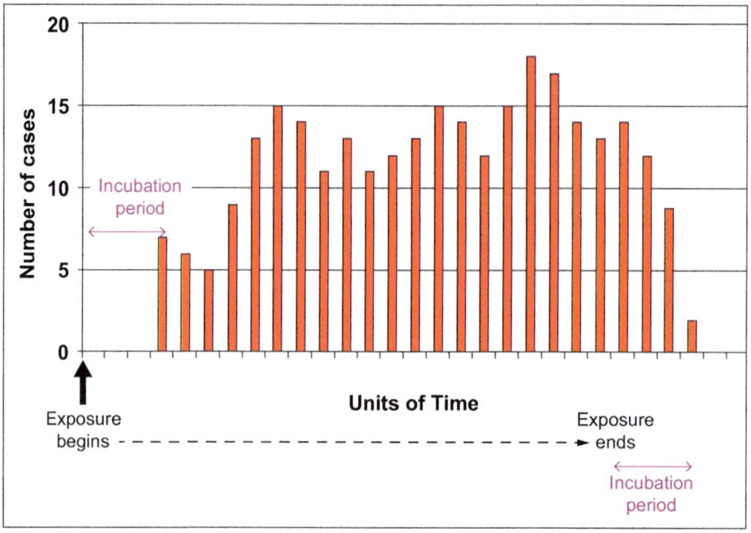

FIG. 2 Example epidemic curve of a continuous common source outbreak.[23] A continuous common source occurs when the exposure may continue over days, such as when a water source is contaminated with an infectious agent. The *red vertical bars* represent the number of cases and the time when symptoms/signs developed from the exposure. The incubation period is estimated by calculating the time from when the exposure begins to the development of symptoms or when the exposure ends to the last individuals developing symptoms/signs of infection *(purple)*. This is demonstrated with the *horizontal arrows*. (From Epidemic Curves. http://www.med.uottawa.ca/sim/data/public_health_epidemic_curves_e.htm.)

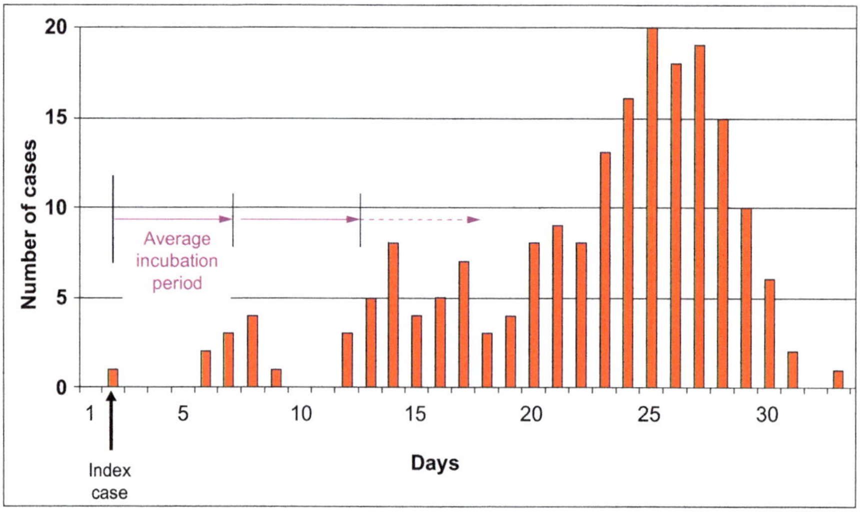

FIG. 3 Example epidemic curve of a propagated outbreak.[23] A propagated outbreak occurs when multiple individuals are exposed to an index case who then expose multiple other individuals. These exposures to nonimmune individuals continue until the exposure's ongoing transmission is stopped. The *red vertical bars* represent the number of cases and the time when symptoms/signs developed from the exposure. The average incubation period is estimated by calculating the time from when the exposure occurred to the meantime of symptom development and is illustrated by the *horizontal arrows (purple)*. The *vertical black lines* indicate the exposure for each generation of cases. (From Epidemic Curves. http://www.med.uottawa.ca/sim/data/public_health_epidemic_curves_e.htm.)

Epidemic Curves

An epidemic curve is a visual display called a histogram of the number of identified cases meeting a definition over time (see Chapter 18 for more detail). The illness in question onset dates are recorded along the *X*-axis, and the number of cases by unit of time is recorded on the *Y*-axis. Epidemic curves are used to describe the trajectory and course of an outbreak or the distribution of cases over time, the magnitude of the outbreak, the potential pattern of transmission, and the time period of exposure. They are a critical tool for an outbreak investigation (see Table 8, Chapter 13). Specific patterns of the curves can help characterize whether cases were exposed by a single point source or by person-to-person. In addition, the pathogen's incubation period can be inferred by the outbreak's temporal distribution. Through the use of the epidemic curve, the properties of unknown agents can be compared to those of well-described pathogens and may be used to guide early mitigation measures.

In a *point-source outbreak,* individuals are exposed to a single or common (infectious) source of the agent, and the exposure generally occurs in a relatively short period of time.[24] Consequently, a point-source outbreak has an epidemic curve that shows a rapid increase in cases followed by a slower decline in case count, with most illness onset dates or times occurring during one incubation period (Fig. 1). In the figure, the case distribution is tightly clustered over a relatively short unit of time, with a defined peak. In many point-source outbreaks, there is little to no secondary spread of disease.

Point-source outbreaks are best illustrated by foodborne outbreaks. In 1993, an outbreak of gastrointestinal disease after a catered lunch at two associate daycare facilities was investigated by the Lord Fairfax Health District in Virginia. The illness was both rapid in onset (median incubation period of 2 h) and resolution (median duration of 4 h).[25] Based upon interviews, consumption of fried rice served at the lunches was commonly reported, and *Bacillus cereus* was isolated from this food item.[25] Similarly, a bioterrorism event involving *Bacillus anthracis* spores would also be best characterized by a point-source outbreak epidemic curve.

A *continuous common source outbreak* is similar to a point-source outbreak, but the exposure continues over a longer period of time, and cases do not all occur within the span of a single incubation period (Fig. 2).[24] Foodborne illness outbreaks, such as the 2011 *Listeria* outbreak related to contaminated cantaloupes, can have an epidemic curve such as in Fig. 2, particularly if individuals are exposed to the contaminated product over a prolonged period of time.[26]

In contrast, a *propagated outbreak* is caused by person-to-person spread of an infectious pathogen. Without a common source of exposure, the epidemic curve is typically characterized by starting with an index case and then developing into an epidemic as secondary cases occur when contacts of the index case become infected; those newly infected people then serve as sources of transmission that propagate the outbreak. The epidemic curve of a propagated outbreak is characterized by progressively taller peaks, initially separated by one incubation period, but tending to later merge into waves with increasing case count in each generation, followed by a gradual decline as the outbreak wanes (Fig. 3).[24] Smallpox and measles are spread person-to-person through aerosolized particles and are most contagious during the incubation phase when patients lack the characteristic rash and instead exhibit vague constitutional symptoms. Both are highly infectious to those who have not been vaccinated, and cases are propagated as each infectious case exposes other susceptible persons, and the epidemic curve shape of both would be that consistent with a propagated outbreak.

Epidemiologists use epidemic curve information, in part, to determine how to determine who may be at risk of developing disease from a highly infectious pathogen and the response to any implemented mitigation measures. The definition of close contact varies by the pathogen of interest and by the mechanism of transmission. In the next several sections, we discuss the infection control methods used to prevent subsequent transmission of a highly infectious pathogen to healthcare personnel (HCP) and the public. By paying careful attention to each of these populations, the risk of secondary and ongoing transmission can be substantially reduced.

Mitigation Strategies

Isolation, quarantine, and physical (social) distancing

Isolation and quarantine are frequent interventions implemented early during a disease or outbreak investigation to reduce the likelihood of exposure and transmission. Isolation separates the individual with the infection or who is infectious from individuals who are not exposed or ill. Quarantine, on the other hand, separates and restricts the movement of individuals who have been exposed to an infectious agent and may be incubating the infection so that they do not expose others to the contagion. Isolation and quarantine are applied during the investigation of single cases, clusters, or outbreaks of a given infection. Physical (previously called social) distancing is a public health strategy to minimize transmission risk where people practice a physical separation of generally 6 ft or two meters from each other. This strategy is generally implemented for respiratory infections in the settings of pandemics and was used during influenza and the COVID-19 pandemic. All three mitigation methods are pathogen-specific and consider the mechanism of transmission and the incubation period of the disease.

Isolation can be implemented at home where the "case" is separated from the caregivers. However, in healthcare settings it is implemented using transmission-based precautions, effectively separating a patient with a communicable infection and his/her potentially contaminated environment from other susceptible individuals, primarily the healthcare personnel and visitors. While the patient is isolated, healthcare personnel wear personal protective equipment (PPE) to protect them from acquiring these pathogens (see Chapter 25 for additional details). The type of equipment required by personnel and the recommendations for the environment and room recommended are categorized by the most important transmission mechanism(s) for the pathogen being considered. These transmission-based precautions include contact precautions, droplet precautions, and airborne precautions (Table 3). With some pathogens, transmission occurs via several mechanisms, and a combination of precautions will be required. Contact precautions are utilized for pathogens that are spread via direct contact with the patient or their environment. Commonly employed to prevent transmission among patients with infections caused by antimicrobial-resistant pathogens such as methicillin-resistant *Staphylococcus aureus* and vancomycin-resistant *Enterococcus*, carbapenem-resistant gram-negative enterobacteraciae, and *C. difficile* or viral illnesses such as varicella or variola (Smallpox). Contact precautions require HCPs and visitors to use PPE including single-use gowns and gloves when entering a patient room. It is also employed for highly infectious pathogens that can spread in part by direct contact, including varicella, smallpox, SARS, MERS, and those that cause viral hemorrhagic fevers.

Droplet and airborne precautions are used for pathogens that can travel through air to infect others. Influenza, meningococcus, pertussis, and SARS-CoV-2 are common infections that can be transmitted via suspended droplets—larger droplets that are not transmitted more than 6 ft or 2 m. HCPs who enter the patient room suspected of having or being infected with one of these diseases must wear an appropriate medical mask. In some cases, pathogens may require additional precautions as, for example, they contaminate the environment, as is the case with respiratory syncytial virus. In this case, both droplet and contact precautions are required to be implemented. Airborne precautions are used for pathogens that are aerosolized, generally smaller, and may remain suspended over greater distances, such as *M. tuberculosis*, varicella, and measles. Airborne precautions require the use of a respirator that filters the air and provides more protection for the wearer. Examples include an N95 respirator (P3 or equivalent) or powered air-purifying respirator (PAPR). In addition, patients should be put into a negative pressure room or, if not available, a room that is well ventilated to prevent the airborne particles from traveling to other patients throughout the facility. Recent data demonstrate that the line between droplet and airborne is fine and that in some settings, such as the use of aerosol-generating procedures, pathogens that are transmitted by droplets can be aerosolized (e.g., influenza, SARS-CoV-2, SARS, MERS-CoV). In settings where aerosol-generating procedures are undertaken, respirators are commonly recommended.[28b]

The toll of high-consequence pathogens remains unacceptable given the current understanding of transmission of these pathogens and modern infection prevention techniques. Healthcare personnel accounted for up to one-eighth of Ebola cases, one-quarter of SARS cases, and one-half of MERS cases.[29a] Data from the CDC show that in the United States alone, 6% of hospitalized patients with COVID-19 were healthcare personnel.[29b] These data, the lessons from outbreaks, and the demonstration that PPE decreases transmission and protects healthcare personnel demonstrate that healthcare personnel must be provided with appropriate PPE and trained in its use. Observational studies demonstrate that healthcare personnel often contaminate themselves as they remove their PPE.[30,31] For this reason, referral hospitals, such as the CDC's regional Ebola treatment and assessment network hospitals, the National Centre for Infectious Diseases in Singapore, and the Infectious Diseases Center at the Princess Margaret Hospital in Hong Kong that specialize in the care of patients with high-consequence pathogens, may be desired for the care of these patients (see Chapter 26 for further details). These facilities are regularly visited by members of the regulators and perform structured drills on a number of highly infectious pathogens to ensure competence. Their staff members receive intense initial and ongoing training regarding appropriate PPE and how and when it should be worn.

These facilities may not be available in all areas or in the setting of a pandemic; specialized facilities

TABLE 3
Recommended Transmission-Based Precautions for Highly Infectious Pathogens and Category A Bioterrorism Agents[27,28a]

Highly Infectious Pathogens and Class A Bioterrorism Agents	Transmission-Based Precautions	Comments
Anthrax (cutaneous) *B. anthracis* (see Chapter 2)	Standard precautions	Contact precautions may be used if there is a large amount of uncontained secretions
Anthrax (inhalation) *B. anthracis* (see Chapter 2)	Standard precautions	Not transmitted from person to person
Botulism *C. botulinum*	Standard precautions	Not transmitted from person to person
Influenza (see Chapter 7)	Droplet precautions[a]	Duration of precautions: generally 5 days from onset of symptoms
Influenza A, Avian (see Chapter 8)	Droplet (WHO) or Airborne (CDC) precautions[a]	Limited data for the duration of precautions. Hospitalized patients are commonly critically ill and isolated for the duration of hospitalization[b]
Measles	Airborne	Duration of precautions: generally 4 days after the onset of rash
MERS (see Chapter 10) MERS-CoV-1	Droplet (WHO) or Airborne (CDC) and Contact precautions[a]	Duration of precautions: approximately 10 days after the resolution of fever or longer if respiratory symptoms persist[b]
Plague (pneumonic) *Y. pestis* (see Chapter 4)	Droplet precautions	Duration of precautions: generally 48 h after effective treatment begins
SARS (see Chapter 9) SARS-CoV-1	Droplet (WHO and HC) or Airborne (CDC) and Contact precautions[a]	Duration of precautions: approximately 10 days after the resolution of fever or longer if respiratory symptoms persist[b]
COVID-19 (see Chapter 11) SARS-CoV-2	Droplet (HC, WHO) or Airborne (CDC) and Contact precautions	Duration of precautions: approximately 10 days after symptom onset and may need to be longer if respiratory symptoms persist, immune suppression is present, or critical illness is present
Smallpox (see Chapter 6)	Airborne and Contact precautions	Duration of precautions: approximately 3–4 weeks, or until all scabs have crusted and separated
Tularemia *F. tularensis* (see Chapter 3)	Standard precautions	Not transmitted from person to person
Viral hemorrhagic fevers (see Chapter 5)	Airborne, or Droplet and Contact precautions[a,c]	Duration of precautions depends on the pathogen; Impermeable and fluid-resistant gown, double gloves, shoe covers, apron, face shield

WHO, World Health Organization; *CDC*, Centers for Disease Prevention and Control; Health Canada.
[a]WHO, CDC, and HC recommend airborne precautions when performing procedures that generate aerosols.
[b]Duration of precautions may be extended in patients who are immunocompromised or critically ill, as they may shed live viruses for longer periods of time.
[c]Droplet/airborne includes face shield to cover.

cannot accommodate all patients. In such cases, healthcare patients may be cohorted. Patients with the same infectious agent on a particular unit and dedicating and cohorting willing staff members to treat patients with the condition.[32] Cohorting allows strategic use of limited healthcare personnel, assures that they are trained in appropriate PPE, and minimizes transmission risk to other patients throughout a hospital.

Quarantine separates and restricts the movement of people who were exposed to a contagious organism from varicella virus to SARS-CoV-2. The goals of quarantine are twofold: to minimize secondary transmission and to ensure potentially infected people have rapid access to appropriate medical care if they become ill. In the hospital, patients who have been potentially exposed to a known infection may be placed into quarantine with appropriate contact and/or droplet/airborne precautions until a confirmatory test results or the incubation period passes. However, the use of quarantine in the community is considerably more complex. Home quarantine requires having the individual carefully monitor for symptoms of the disease and promptly report the illness to public health authorities. In many cases, public health authorities will actively call individuals to determine if symptoms have developed. Sometimes quarantine also includes a restriction of movement outside the home or work environment if potential exposure must be minimized if the individual becomes symptomatic and contagious. For example, in a case of imported Lassa fever to Germany in 2016, the recommendations of either observation with temperature measurement, general interdiction of work, home quarantine, quarantine in hospital, or high-level isolation in hospital were based on risk assessment of the contacts and their exposure.[33] Additionally, quarantine recommendations vary depending on whether transmission is possible during the asymptomatic incubation period. For example, smallpox and SARS-CoV-2 are transmissible before symptom onset; consequently, close contacts might be placed in quarantine for the entire incubation period. On the other hand, SARS-CoV was not transmissible until a case developed a fever, so the quarantine period could be determined by when the case developed symptoms.

It is important to consider how community members who are either isolated or quarantined at home can access medical care without risking transmission to others. The ideal situation is for these individuals to be in close contact with public health officials, who have transportation available to move individuals when symptoms develop, and predetermined healthcare facilities prepared to encounter patients, limiting the risk of transmission to transportation or medical personnel.

Physical distancing is a public health tool generally reserved for a large, community-wide epidemic or a pandemic when extraordinary measures are required to control disease spread. Physical distancing employs methods that increase the distance between individuals and reduce the likelihood of transmitting infectious pathogens via close contact by limiting personal interaction. Examples of physical distancing strategies include canceling large community events (concerts, movies, etc.) and school classes, shutting down or limiting mass transit, or closing "nonessential" businesses, schools, or community settings (houses of worship, senior centers, etc.). National, state, and local laws provide public health agencies with the authority to apply mitigation measures, including physical distancing measures, in the proper context and situation. This strategy was used during the 2010 H1N1 pandemic and more extensively during 2019–21 to contain the SARS-CoV-2 pandemic.

Isolation, quarantine, and physical distancing, while important to limit transmission of contagions, are not without negative consequences. When hospitalized patients are isolated, healthcare personnel spend less time in patient rooms; patients report higher levels of depression and anxiety and lower satisfaction with care; and adverse events are more common.[34] In the community, isolation, quarantine, and physical distancing can exacerbate social stigma and insecurity, decay trust in public health and government authority, increase psychological stress, and restrict access to basic physical and medical needs, as was documented during the 2014–15 West African Ebola Virus Disease (EVD)[35] and more recently during the SARS-CoV-2 pandemic of 2019–23.

Vaccination (See Chapter 20 for More Detailed Information)

For individuals at high risk of being exposed to and infected by bioterrorism agents or other highly infectious pathogens, vaccination provides protection in advance of (or early after) an exposure. Effective vaccines are available for measles, influenza, SARS-CoV-2, smallpox, and anthrax, among others. Measles, influenza, and SARS-CoV-2 vaccinations are widely available and strongly recommended for all community members, including those in healthcare (Table 4). Information about the anthrax vaccine, which is currently licensed for those who work in laboratories with *B. anthracis*, with occupational exposure to animals or animal products, and select military personnel (see Chapter 2).[38]

Smallpox has long been eradicated, with no known cases of naturally occurring smallpox since 1977. This

TABLE 4
Vaccinations Recommended for Healthcare Personnel (HCP)[36,37,a]

Pathogen/*Group Targeted*	Vaccine Recommendation	Test for Immunity
Hepatitis B/*All personnel working in a healthcare setting or with potential exposure to bloodborne pathogens (BBP)*	Three-dose series with the second and third doses following the first by 1 and 6 months, respectively, or two-dose series of recombinant adjuvant with doses separated by 4 weeks	Serum, hepatitis B surface antibody (anti-HBs) 1–2 months after final dose
Influenza (see Chapters 7 and 20)/*All personnel*	One dose annually	None
Measles, mumps/*All personnel*	If born in 1957 or later, two doses of MMR separated by at least 28 days If born before 1957, check for immunity; two doses of MMR separated by at least 28 days if not immune	Serum, measles IgG Serum, mumps IgG
Meningococcus/*Microbiology laboratory workers*	One dose of conjugate vaccine (A, C, WY135) for those routinely exposed to isolates with *N. meningitidis* (e.g., laboratory workers)	None
Rubella/*All personnel*	If born in 1957 or later, one dose of MMR If born before 1957, check for immunity; one dose of MMR if not immune	Serum, rubella IgG
SARS-CoV-2/*All personnel*	Recommendations vary by age and comorbid illnesses and may depend upon manufacturer.	None
Tetanus, diphtheria, pertussis/ *All personnel*	One-time Tdap; with Td boosters every 10 years afterwards. Pregnant HCPs should get Tdap with each pregnancy	None
Varicella/*All personnel*	Two doses of varicella vaccine separated by at least 28 days if not immune	Serum, varicella zoster virus IgG

Other vaccines may be recommended based on the geographic area where working or potential exposures (e.g., yellow fever vaccine).
[a]The most recent ACIP guidelines for healthcare personnel, which are the basis for this table, were published in 2011 as an update to the 1997 guidelines. Healthcare personnel include physicians, nurses, advanced practice providers, emergency medical personnel, dental professionals, medical, dental, and nursing students, laboratory, radiology, and phlebotomy technicians and students, physical, occupational, and speech therapists and students, environmental services workers, pharmacists, hospital volunteers, and administrative staff.

success was due to a successful international vaccination campaign. The CDC would release the vaccine in the event of a bioterrorist smallpox attack. Some persons have been vaccinated through the military or because they were a part of Smallpox Response Teams that were formed after the 9/11 attacks in the United States. Researchers who perform laboratory work with variola, the virus that causes smallpox, are recommended to be vaccinated. However, the vaccine does not always provide lifelong immunity, and people who have been vaccinated previously may need revaccination in a smallpox emergency.

POSTEXPOSURE PROPHYLAXIS

Postexposure prophylaxis (PEP) is a pharmaceutical intervention (usually in the form of an antibiotic/antiviral and/or vaccine) that can prevent disease if given within a specific timeframe after exposure to a highly infectious pathogen. PEP is available for certain highly infectious pathogens and bioterrorism agents (see Chapter 19, Table 1). The decision to implement PEP is based on the transmission risk to contacts and susceptibility to infection, timing of exposure, and potential for adverse effects from PEP. For example, PEP to prevent measles entails vaccination with the measles, mumps, and rubella (MMR) vaccine or immune globulin (IG). For nonimmune contacts, MMR vaccine can be administered within 72 h of exposure and IG within 6 days. Contacts who are immune (e.g., appropriately vaccinated) to measles or persons who have contraindications to receiving an MMR vaccine or immune globulin would not be eligible for PEP.

Apart from consideration of individual factors, logistical and community factors also influence whether

PEP is offered during an individual case investigation or outbreak. In the event of an outbreak due to a novel agent or an outbreak of unprecedented scope, PEP might be initially unavailable or of insufficient quantity to protect the population at risk. Under these circumstances, additional risk assessment and stratification of eligible contacts might be necessary to determine for whom PEP should be prioritized. Some individual factors, such as occupation or role in the community (i.e., provision of essential services or outbreak control support), might also be considered. For example, grocery workers and HCPs might be prioritized to receive PEP, with availability extending to the general public as more PEP products become available. Each situation is likely to be highly individualized, based on the pathogen of concern and PEP availability.

Recognizing the threat of inadequate supplies of PEP during an outbreak, federal, state, and local governmental agencies stockpile PEP in preparation for a possible bioterrorist event or outbreak. In the United States, mostly as a response to the 2001 anthrax attacks, the Strategic National Stockpile of pharmaceuticals is maintained in strategic areas of the country to enable rapid prevention and treatment in the event of a bioterrorist event. However, stockpiling can be expensive, particularly as antibiotics expire. In Israel, in an effort to reduce the expense of a stockpile, research has been done to demonstrate that pharmaceuticals can be extended beyond manufacturer-ascribed shelf life, as long as regulation standards are met.[39]

Communication (See Chapter 22 for Additional Detail)

To enable a coordinated and effective response, up-to-date information should be shared with stakeholders during an outbreak of a highly infectious pathogen or bioterrorist attack. Public health agencies often release updates through Health Alert Network (HAN) in the United States and other mechanisms outside the United States to target stakeholders, including public information officers; federal, state, territorial, and local public health practitioners; clinicians; healthcare facilities; and public health laboratories. These messages provide vital, time-sensitive information for a specific situation and can convey the need for immediate action.

Depending on the pathogen of interest, it can also be necessary to share information with the general public during an outbreak investigation and response. Transparent communication with the public is helpful to provide relevant information, engage with the community to build trust, and accurately convey risk. Public communication might also improve passive and active surveillance by increasing public awareness and prompting ill persons to seek medical care. Resources for effective communication include the World Health Organization's Effective Media Communication during Public Health Emergencies handbook.[40]

Misinformation can be extremely dangerous in the outbreak setting, particularly when the public lacks trust in the information that is being disseminated by public health authorities. In a cross-sectional study, researchers found that up to 55% of Twitter entries from Guinea, Liberia, and Nigeria that used the terms "Ebola" and "prevention OR cure" contained medical misinformation during the 2014 Ebola outbreak.[41] The World Health Organization (WHO) also reported that certain products or practices marketed on social media to prevent and cure Ebola, such as drinking large quantities of salt water, were in fact harmful and resulted in some avoidable deaths.[42]

Secondary prevention of disease due to highly infectious pathogens and bioterrorism agents necessitates a multifaceted approach. Epidemic curves can provide a model for anticipated risk to a community, and various preventive strategies are needed to address close contacts of established cases, HCPs, and the general public. These messages must be carefully crafted so that HCPs and the general public have confidence in public health agencies and follow mitigation recommendations.

PLANNING (SEE CHAPTERS 13 AND 24)

While highly infectious pathogen outbreaks and bioterrorism events are fortunately uncommon occurrences, preparation for these events takes immense resources. This section of the chapter will address how individuals can sharpen their skills, how hospitals can plan for and mitigate potential HCP shortages, and how paramedics, hospitals, and public health agencies can prepare for effective collaboration for future outbreaks.

Individuals

The Society for Healthcare Epidemiology of America and CDC published an Outbreak Response Training Program designed for hospital epidemiologists and infection preventionists to provide training that enhances skills, knowledge, and tools to provide effective leadership during both facility-level outbreaks and large-scale public health emergencies (https://learningce.shea-online.org/content/sheacdc-outbreak-response-training-program-ortp).[43] A number of additional resources can be accessed through the CDC's Emergency Preparedness and Response website (see Resources for additional information; https://emergency.cdc.gov/).[44]

Healthcare Facilities

Not all paramedics and HCPs are willing and able to provide care for cases or outbreaks of highly infectious pathogens or bioterrorism agents, yet retention of skilled paramedics and HCPs is essential to caring for patients in these situations. Surveys suggest that HCPs are more likely to work in outbreak conditions if they:

1. believe their work makes a positive impact
2. feel safe both during transportation to and during the work day
3. receive assistance with child, elder, and pet care
4. have assurance that their loved ones and themselves will not be harmed by their decision to care for those affected by a bioterrorism or large-scale infectious disease event.[45–49]

Healthcare facilities have an obligation to ensure that HCPs are up to date with recommended vaccines (Table 4). A survey of over 1500 emergency medical services (EMS) workers revealed that 96% would probably or definitely report to work in the event of an influenza pandemic, but only 59% had received an influenza vaccine in the preceding 12 months.[47] While these EMS workers reported largely being willing to work through dangerous or contagious conditions, they may put themselves into harm's way without appropriate pre-employment and annual vaccinations.

Further surveys have been performed to determine if legal protections, such as ensuring priority to healthcare for HCPs and their families, granting mental health services, and guaranteeing access to appropriate PPE, would make public health workers more likely to respond to emergencies. Sixty to eighty-three percent of public health workers agreed that a guarantee of at least one of these protections would improve their willingness to work under outbreak conditions, with the most important being access to appropriate PPE.[50]

Collaboration

Finally, the importance of collaborations between paramedics, healthcare facilities, and public health agencies cannot be understated. Laboratories report pathogens of concern via mandatory reporting requirements, and clinicians are also encouraged to report concerning or unusual clinical syndromes to public health entities. In turn, public health utilizes HAN updates to request assistance with case findings and to communicate information about novel infections and risk factors to clinicians and healthcare facilities.

As a result of the 2014–15 West African Ebola Virus Disease (EVD) outbreak, the relationships between many paramedics, healthcare facilities, and public health entities were strengthened. At that time, local public health divisions monitored individuals for symptoms of EVD for 21 days after returning from Liberia, Sierra Leone, and Guinea. If an individual developed symptoms concerning EVD, conference calls involving stakeholders from first responders, healthcare facilities, public health, and media were rapidly assembled. The infrastructure created by the Ebola response and strengthened by the SARS-CoV-2 pandemic must be actively preserved to prevent future outbreaks of highly infectious pathogens.

CONCLUSION

Disease due to highly infectious pathogens, emerging pathogens, and agents associated with bioterrorism is a very real threat to the public, healthcare systems, and public health in our increasingly connected world. The worldwide recent experience with COVID-19 highlights the importance of prompt identification of a potential agent of high consequence, implementation of appropriate infection prevention and control measures in healthcare, communication within the facility, to the public health authorities and to the public to combat misinformation, and the continual preparedness needed to ensure an effective and coordinated response. Ingraining the planning into our healthcare systems will prepare us for improved, nimble, and integrated responses when the next outbreak of highly infectious pathogens arrives.

DISCLOSURES

None to report.

REFERENCES

1. Bioterrorism Agents/Diseases. Emergency Preparedness and Response; 2017. https://emergency.cdc.gov/agent/agentlist-category.asp.
2. Dato V, Wagner MM, Fapohunda A. How outbreaks of infectious disease are detected: a review of surveillance systems and outbreaks. *Public Health Rep.* 2004;119(5):464–471.
3. Bush LM, Abrams BH, Beall A, Johnson CC. Index case of fatal inhalational anthrax due to bioterrorism in the United States. *N Engl J Med.* 2001;345(22):1607–1610. https://doi.org/10.1056/NEJMoa012948. Epub 2001 Nov. 8 11704685.
4. Ligon BL. Monkeypox: a review of the history and emergence in the Western hemisphere. *Semin Pediatr Infect Dis.* 2004;15(4):280–287. https://doi.org/10.1053/j.spid.2004.09.001. 15494953. PMCID: PMC7129998.

5. Liddell AM, Davey Jr RT, Mehta AK, et al. Characteristics and clinical management of a cluster of 3 patients with Ebola virus disease, including the first domestically acquired cases in the United States. *Ann Intern Med.* 2015;163(2):81–90. https://doi.org/10.7326/M15-0530. 25961438. PMCID: PMC4724427.
6. Dattwyler RJ. Community-acquired pneumonia in the age of bio-terrorism. *Allergy Asthma Proc.* 2005;26(3):191–194.
7. Cunha BA. Anthrax, tularemia, plague, Ebola or smallpox as agents of bioterrorism: recognition in the emergency room. *Clin Microbiol Infect.* 2002;8(8):489–503.
8. Palumbo JP, Meek JI, Fazio DM, Turner SB, Hadler JL, Sofair AN. Unexplained deaths in Connecticut, 2002-2003: failure to consider category a bioterrorism agents in differential diagnoses. *Disaster Med Public Health Prep.* 2008;2(2):87–94.
9. McGovern TW, Christopher GW, Eitzen EM. Cutaneous manifestations of biological warfare and related threat agents. *Arch Dermatol.* 1999;135(3):311–322.
10. Kman NE, Nelson RN. Infectious agents of bioterrorism: a review for emergency physicians. *Emerg Med Clin North Am.* 2008;26(2):517–547. x–xi.
11. Biological and chemical terrorism: strategic plan for preparedness and response. Recommendations of the CDC Strategic Planning Workgroup. *MMWR.* 2000;49(RR-4):1–14.
12. (a) Travel Health Notices. 2021. https://wwwnc.cdc.gov/travel/notices. Accessed 16 November 2021. (b) https://www.who.int/emergencies/disease-outbreak-news. (c) https://promedmail.org/.
13. Botulism. https://www.cdc.gov/botulism/health-professional.html.
14. Plague. https://www.cdc.gov/plague/healthcare/clinicians.html.
15. Smallpox. https://www.cdc.gov/smallpox/clinicians/diagnosis-evaluation.html.
16. National Notifiable Conditions; 2018. https://wwwn.cdc.gov/nndss/conditions/notifiable/2018/.
17. Centers for Disease Control and Prevention. Update: hantavirus disease—United States. *MMWR.* 1993;42(31):612–614.
18. Fraser DW, Tsai TR, Orenstein W, et al. Legionnaires' disease: description of an epidemic of pneumonia. *New Engl J Med.* 1977;297(22):1189–1197.
19. Gottlieb MS, Schroff R, Schanker HM, et al. *Pneumocystis carinii* pneumonia and mucosal candidiasis in previously healthy homosexual men: evidence of a new acquired cellular immunodeficiency. *New Engl J Med.* 1981;305(24):1425–1431.
20. Masur H, Michelis MA, Greene JB, et al. An outbreak of community-acquired *Pneumocystis carinii* pneumonia: initial manifestation of cellular immune dysfunction. *New Engl J Med.* 1981;305(24):1431–1438.
21. Outbreak Case Definitions. https://www.cdc.gov/urdo/downloads/casedefinitions.pdf.
22. Stehling-Ariza T, Rosewell A, Moiba SA, et al. The impact of active surveillance and health education on an Ebola virus disease cluster—Kono District, Sierra Leone, 2014-2015. *BMC Infect Dis.* 2016;16(1):611.
23. Epidemic Curves. http://www.med.uottawa.ca/sim/data/public_health_epidemic_curves_e.htm.
24. Using an Epi Curve to Determine Mode of Spread. https://www.cdc.gov/training/quicklearns/epimode/.
25. Centers for Disease Control and Prevention. *Bacillus cereus* food poisoning associated with fried rice at two child day care centers—Virginia, 1993. *MMWR.* 1994;43(10):177–178.
26. Multistate outbreak of listeriosis linked to whole canteloupes from Jensen Farms, Colorado. *Epi Curves.* 2012. https://www.cdc.gov/listeria/outbreaks/cantaloupes-jensen-farms/epi.html.
27. Guidance on personal protective equipment (PPE) to be used by healthcare workers during management of patients with confirmed Ebola or persons under investigation (PUIs) for Ebola who are clinically unstable or have bleeding, vomiting, or diarrhea in U.S. Hospitals, including procedures for donning and doffing PPE. https://www.cdc.gov/vhf/ebola/healthcare-us/ppe/guidance.html. Accessed 19 December 2017.
28. (a) Siegel JD, Rhinehart E, Jackson M, Chiarello L, Health Care Infection Control Practices Advisory Committee. Guideline for isolation precautions: preventing transmission of infectious agents in health care settings. *Am J Infect Control.* 2007;35(10 Suppl 2):S65–164. (b) Chan VW, Ng HH, Rahman L, et al. Transmission of severe acute respiratory syndrome coronavirus 1 and severe acute respiratory syndrome coronavirus 2 during aerosol-generating procedures in critical care: a systematic review and meta-analysis of observational studies. *Crit Care Med.* 2021;49(7):1159–1168. https://doi.org/10.1097/CCM.0000000000004965. 33749225.
29. (a) Suwantarat N, Apisarnthanarak A. Risks to healthcare workers with emerging diseases: lessons from MERS-CoV, Ebola, SARS, and avian flu. *Curr Opin Infect Dis.* 2015;28(4):349–361. (b) Kambhampati AK, O'Halloran AC, Whitaker M, et al. COVID-19-associated hospitalizations among health care personnel—COVID-NET, 13 states, March 1–May 31, 2020. *MMWR Morb Mortal Wkly Rep.* 2020;69:1576–1583. https://doi.org/10.15585/mmwr.mm6943e3.
30. Casanova LM, Teal LJ, Sickbert-Bennett EE, et al. Assessment of self-contamination during removal of personal protective equipment for ebola patient care. *Infect Control Hosp Epidemiol.* 2016;37(10):1156–1161.
31. Verbeek JH, Ijaz S, Mischke C, et al. Personal protective equipment for preventing highly infectious diseases due to exposure to contaminated body fluids in healthcare staff. *Cochrane Database Syst Rev.* 2016;4, CD011621.
32. Facility Guidance for Control of Carbapenem-Resistant Enterobacteriaceae (CRE); 2015. https://www.cdc.gov/hai/pdfs/cre/cre-guidance-508.pdf. Accessed 3 January 2018.

33. Lehmann C, Kochanek M, Abdulla D, et al. Control measures following a case of imported Lassa fever from Togo, North Rhine Westphalia, Germany, 2016. *Euro Surveill.* 2017;22(39).
34. Abad C, Fearday A, Safdar N. Adverse effects of isolation in hospitalised patients: a systematic review. *J Hosp Infect.* 2010;76(2):97–102.
35. Pellecchia U, Crestani R, Decroo T, Van den Bergh R, Al-Kourdi Y. Social consequences of Ebola containment measures in Liberia. *PLoS One.* 2015;10(12), e0143036.
36. Recommended Vaccines for Healthcare Workers. https://www.cdc.gov/vaccines/adults/rec-vac/hcw.html.
37. McLean HQ, Fiebelkorn AP, Temte JL, Wallace GS, Centers for Disease Control and Prevention. Prevention of measles, rubella, congenital rubella syndrome, and mumps, 2013: summary recommendations of the Advisory Committee on Immunization Practices (ACIP). *MMWR Recomm Rep.* 2013;62(RR-04):1–34.
38. Anthrax (Bacillus Anthracis). http://sfcdcp.org/anthrax.html. Accessed 1 January 2018.
39. Bodas M, Yuval L, Zadok R, et al. Shelf-life extension program (SLEP) as a significant contributor to Strategic National Stockpile Maintenance: the Israeli experience with ciprofloxacin. *Biosecur Bioterror.* 2012;10(2):182–187.
40. Effective Media Communication During Public Health Emergencies: A WHO Handbook; 2005. http://apps.who.int/iris/bitstream/10665/43511/1/WHO_CDS_2005.31_eng.pdf?ua=1.
41. Oyeyemi SO, Gabarron E, Wynn R. Ebola, Twitter, and misinformation: a dangerous combination? *BMJ.* 2014;349, g6178.
42. Ebola: Experimental Therapies and Rumoured Remedies; 2014. http://www.who.int/mediacentre/news/ebola/15-august-2014/en. Accessed 10 December 2017.
43. CDC/SHEA Outbreak Response Training Program (ORTP); 2017. http://ortp.shea-online.org/. Accessed 5 December 2017.
44. Preparation and Planning. Emergency Preparedness and Response. https://emergency.cdc.gov/planning/index.asp.
45. Devnani M. Factors associated with the willingness of health care personnel to work during an influenza public health emergency: an integrative review. *Prehosp Disaster Med.* 2012;27(6):551–566.
46. Errett NA, Barnett DJ, Thompson CB, et al. Assessment of medical reserve corps volunteers' emergency response willingness using a threat- and efficacy-based model. *Biosecur Bioterror.* 2013;11(1):29–40.
47. Barnett DJ, Levine R, Thompson CB, et al. Gauging U.S. Emergency Medical Services workers' willingness to respond to pandemic influenza using a threat- and efficacy-based assessment framework. *PLoS One.* 2010;5(3):e9856.
48. Barnett DJ, Balicer RD, Thompson CB, et al. Assessment of local public health workers' willingness to respond to pandemic influenza through application of the extended parallel process model. *PLoS One.* 2009;4(7), e6365.
49. Oh N, Hong N, Ryu DH, Bae SG, Kam S, Kim KY. Exploring nursing intention, stress, and professionalism in response to infectious disease emergencies: the experience of local public hospital nurses during the 2015 MERS outbreak in South Korea. *Asian Nurs Res.* 2017;11(3):230–236.
50. Rutkow L, Vernick JS, Thompson CB, Piltch-Loeb R, Barnett DJ. Legal protections to promote response willingness among the local public health workforce. *Disaster Med Public Health Prep.* 2015;9(2):98–102.

CHAPTER 16

Surveillance Strategies

SHERI LEWIS • SHRADDHA PATEL
Johns Hopkins University Applied Physics Laboratory, Laurel, MD, United States

INTRODUCTION

Disease surveillance was defined by Langmuir in 1963 as "the continued watchfulness over the distribution and trends of incidence through the systematic collection, consolidation, and evaluation of morbidity and mortality reports and other relevant data," with the "... regular dissemination of the basic data and interpretations to all who have contributed and to all others who need to know."[1] Thacker expanded and refined this definition in 1988 when he wrote, "Public health surveillance is the ongoing systematic collection, management, analysis, and interpretation of outcome-specific data for use in the planning, implementation, and evaluation of public health practice."[2] This linking of public health surveillance with the evaluation of public health practice emphasizes its primary purpose—to direct the expenditure of limited public health resources in a manner that yields the greatest return on investment.[3,4] These surveillance activities are the backbone of assessing health in any population and a necessary step in order to understand what interventions need to be made or to determine and measure the outcome of a particular action. Of course, the detection of major epidemics, such as SARS-CoV-2 (COVID-19), influenza, Severe Acute Respiratory Syndrome (SARS), Middle East Respiratory Syndrome (MERS), Ebola, and the like, is what most people immediately think of today when discussing the uses of public health surveillance. While surveillance activities markedly shifted toward the COVID-19 pandemic as it unfolded and detecting emerging infectious diseases remains a critical surveillance function, there will always remain the need for routine surveillance activities, such as understanding baseline illness from endemic diseases and injury in a given community, identifying potential exposures in a given population, or determining the presence of seasonal illnesses such as influenza and allergies, just to name a few.[4]

While there are many instances throughout history that constitute examples of public health surveillance, starting with John Snow's mapping of cholera cases in 1854,[5] this chapter will focus on surveillance strategies and tools that are commonly used today. These strategies and tools can be applied in many settings, to include hospitals and public health agencies at various levels of government. When combined with advances in information technology, the growing availability of both health-related and "nontraditional" data, and enhanced analytical methods, new surveillance strategies have enabled improved public health situational awareness.

Surveillance can be deemed either active or passive. Active surveillance, by definition, is when the individuals performing public health surveillance are actively seeking out cases of a particular disease or condition. Often this involves public health staff actively contacting healthcare providers, laboratories, senior living facilities, schools, and the like to find out whether they may have encountered or treated individuals with certain disease conditions. For example, when COVID-19 is diagnosed in a given individual, epidemiologists or trained contact tracers will spend time performing contact tracing to actively search for others who may have been exposed to the diagnosed individual(s). Contact tracing is the identification and diagnosis of people who may have come into contact with an infected person. Another example of active surveillance, or "active monitoring," occurs when a man has been diagnosed with prostate cancer. He may be monitored closely, more so than his undiagnosed peers, to determine if he needs to move into a treatment phase. Active surveillance, whether in the context of public health or clinical care, is resource intensive and requires dedicated personnel.[6]

In contrast to active surveillance, passive surveillance is where particular criteria, or a known case

Viral Outbreaks, Biosecurity, and Preparing for Mass Casualty Infectious Diseases Events
https://doi.org/10.1016/B978-0-323-54841-0.00012-3

definition, triggers an individual, such as a clinician or epidemiologist, to initiate a particular disease reporting action based upon meeting the predefined criteria. Building off the COVID-19 example provided above, when an individual is diagnosed with COVID-19, which is a notifiable condition, a manual or automated reporting process to the health department is initiated by the clinician or laboratory. This process submits a case report to the health department, which will then begin a period of active surveillance.[6] Of the two types of surveillance described, passive surveillance is the more common type of surveillance as it is not as labor-intensive, and therefore, less expensive to maintain over long periods of time. Passive surveillance is the type of surveillance that will be referenced throughout this chapter.

BACKGROUND

When we take time to review the role of public health officials and infection control practitioners (ICPs), we see that they conduct various activities to prevent, detect, investigate, observe, and report illness, injury, and disease among defined populations across diverse environments. Until the advent of automated disease surveillance systems, the health departments and ICPs performed many of these activities manually, and everyone relied on the astute care provider, epidemiologist, or ICP to identify unusual occurrences of disease. Most public health actions were reactionary in nature, as opposed to proactive, because data were tabulated retrospectively at predefined intervals, such as weekly or monthly. For example, health departments commonly investigate foodborne illnesses that originate from certain events or restaurants. These investigative activities are typically delayed and happen after a disease is diagnosed in individuals within the community. The development and implementation of disease surveillance systems with automated data feeds, anomaly detection capabilities, and intuitive visualizations allow system end users to monitor community illnesses as they unfold prospectively. As a result, public health officials can be less reactionary and leverage real-time or near-real-time data to make timelier decisions to slow or stop the spread of disease and make more efficient use of limited resources.[7]

The reporting of notifiable conditions is a common type of passive surveillance. Here, a predefined list of infectious disease conditions, such as human immunodeficiency virus (HIV), measles, and rabies, are required to be reported to the local health department whenever they are encountered in clinical practice. In the United States, the Centers for Disease Control and Prevention (CDC) maintains the National Notifiable Disease Surveillance System (NNDSS), though states can add clinical conditions to this list. This reporting is mandated by law and initiated at the local jurisdictional level with local health departments working with their hospitals, laboratories, clinicians, and other partners.[8] Given its passive nature, the limitation of this type of surveillance is the reliance on healthcare providers and laboratories for reporting, thereby introducing uncertainty as to whether all cases have truly been identified. Notifiable disease lists change over time and vary depending upon where you are in the world, but no matter where, the reliability of that data relies heavily on the diligence of reporting.

Once the occurrence of a disease or condition has been confirmed, to determine if that finding is typical or as expected, epidemiologists look to understand the baseline occurrence of that disease or condition in that population. Baseline values can be accessed from historic data accumulated over time or population-based surveys that periodically query the public to gain a better understanding of particular health trends, behaviors, and conditions. The National Health and Nutrition Examination Survey (NHANES) performed by the US Centers for Disease Control and Prevention (CDC) is such a survey. NHANES is an intensive set of interviews combined with physical examinations that requires teams of individuals to travel throughout the United States to understand the nutritional and physical health of the population.[9] Similarly, most local health departments will perform either written or phone-based surveys through calls to randomly selected members of the community to gain an understanding of their health behaviors and overall wellbeing. While these types of surveys still play an important role in understanding the overall health of a population, the advent of automated systems has enabled timelier collection, analysis, and visualization of data, which in turn provides meaningful information to decision makers across institutions—hospitals, schools, local/state/federal governments—far sooner than data collected by labor-intensive traditional methods. Additionally, while suited for studying chronic conditions, baseline studies are not as effective for understanding the onset, progression, or impact of an infectious disease, such as COVID-19, an antimicrobial-resistant organism or influenza, within a given community.

Seeing opportunities to improve traditional surveillance methodologies, the CDC began promoting enhanced surveillance activities through their 1998 plan entitled *Preventing Emerging Infectious Disease: A Strategy for the 21st Century, Overview of the Updated CDC Plan.*[10] Goals and objectives put forth by health officials fell into four categories. The CDC-proposed objectives for improved surveillance included:

1. Strengthening infectious disease surveillance and response.
2. Improving methods for gathering and evaluating surveillance data.
3. Ensuring the use of surveillance data to improve public health practice and medical treatment.
4. Strengthening global capacity to monitor and respond to emerging infectious diseases.[10]

Two decades, numerous disease outbreaks, and a pandemic later, these four objectives remain relevant and true today. Thus, these objectives will serve as the organizing framework for this chapter.

STRENGTHENING INFECTIOUS DISEASE SURVEILLANCE AND RESPONSE

Syndromic Surveillance

Around the time that the CDC outlined their surveillance objectives for the 21st century, early research was underway in what has come to be known as *syndromic surveillance*. In contrast to the traditional method of monitoring diagnosed diseases or conditions, the initial goal of this particular surveillance strategy was to monitor trends of disease by grouping various prediagnostic conditions into syndromes or groups of signs and symptoms. The hope was to gain a time advantage in the progression of an outbreak by detecting clusters of individuals with similar symptoms early and, through earlier intervention, reduce the impact on the community. In 2000, the CDC issued their strategic plan for preparedness and response as it related to biological and chemical terrorism.[11] This was due, in part, to increased terrorist incidents in the United States and elsewhere involving bacterial pathogens, nerve gas, and lethal toxins, which exposed vulnerabilities in the existing surveillance and response capabilities. As part of the strategic plan, the CDC announced its intention to add illness and injury from biological or chemical attacks into the existing US disease surveillance systems, but they also identified the need to develop new methods to detect, evaluate, and report suspicious events. In view of this, the original focus of syndromic surveillance was early detection of an outbreak in the event of an intentional release of a biological agent.[12] The syndromic surveillance initiative spanned the healthcare continuum to include physicians, hospital emergency departments, poison control centers, and other facilities that interacted with patients.[11]

The development of enhanced surveillance capabilities accelerated greatly as a result of the attacks on the World Trade Center and the Pentagon on September 11, 2001, and the anthrax letters that followed in the fall of that same year. While previous efforts had been made to conduct surveillance via "drop-in" surveillance systems during large events, they could only be sustained for short periods of time—typically for a few weeks pre and postevent—due to the labor resources needed to manually collect and analyze the data. Such drop-in systems typically consisted of manual inspection of Emergency Department (ED) patient triage logs for a predefined period of time before, during, and after an event, such as a political convention, major sporting event, or any other mass gathering. Given the urgency from terrorist threats, many jurisdictions, including jurisdictions in the National Capital Region (NCR), urgently implemented what could be considered a drop-in system following September 11 and tirelessly conducted much of the processing for those systems manually for over a year. In addition to the early syndromic surveillance initiatives in NCR regions, others stood up throughout the United States. The general characteristics of these efforts were very similar in that Emergency Department (ED) chief complaints, discharge diagnoses, or both were assigned into mutually exclusive syndrome groups. The health department would tally information received via faxed logbooks and would assign ED visits into the syndrome groups based on an agreed-upon syndrome assignment matrix (Fig. 1) every 24 h. The manual data collection, syndrome assignment, and data tallying were labor-intensive. Data analysis was also cumbersome because of the multiple manual data collection and collating processes.[13] For these reasons, it became clear that manual systems were not going to be sustainable long-term.

Innovative groups across the country began to develop automated syndromic surveillance systems to provide a faster alternative. However, in the early stages, they too encountered challenges, not the smallest of which was the significant cultural change those systems introduced to the public health surveillance workflow. Initially, many of these systems were developed by local health departments or "home grown"; however, with time, many converged around a few systems that leveraged locally accessible data and minimally burdensome processes to identify illness within their communities early.[7] Today, syndromic surveillance has greatly evolved and is referred to by some as "electronic disease surveillance" in recognition of the many other uses of these systems beyond syndrome-based monitoring.

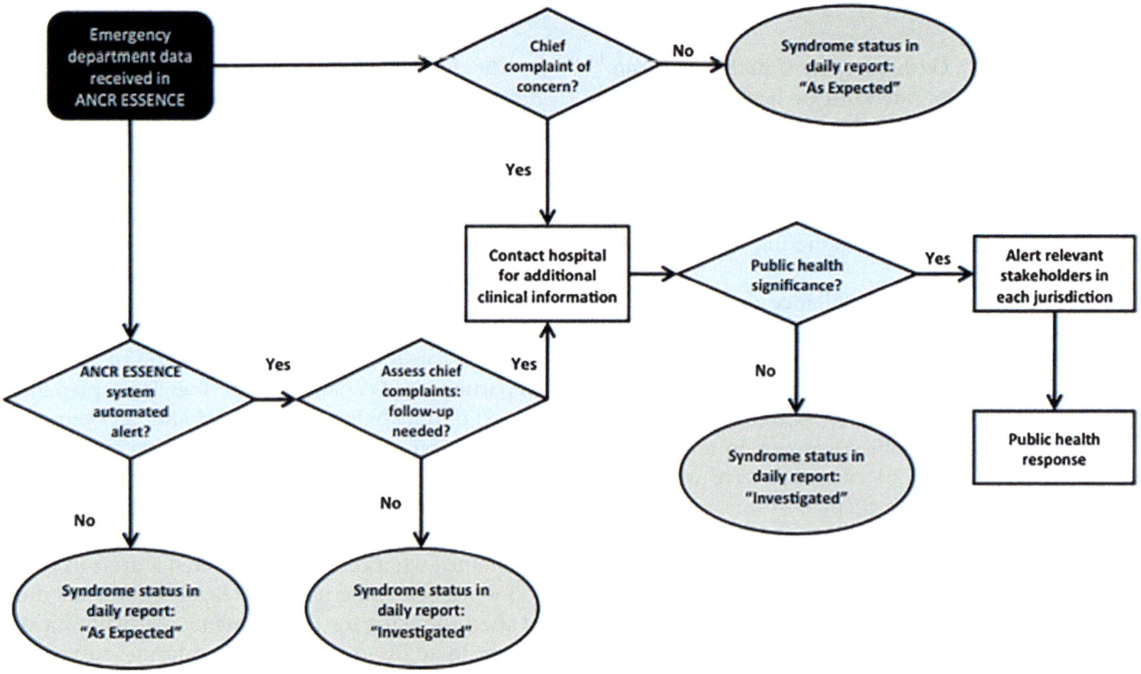

FIG. 1 National Capital Region's emergency department algorithm for syndrome assignment.[1]

Case Studies

NATIONAL ELECTRONIC DISEASE SURVEILLANCE SYSTEM

In 1999, as a result of interest from the public health community, the CDC implemented the National Electronic Disease Surveillance System (NEDSS) as a surveillance tool to collect and manage surveillance data. This system serves to facilitate data and information sharing from clinical and laboratory information systems to public health and is a primary source of data for the previously mentioned NNDSS. NEDSS serves to connect the healthcare system to health departments and, in turn, to connect health departments to the CDC.[8]

HEALTHMAP

HealthMap, a free website and mobile app, was founded in 2006 by a multidisciplinary group at Boston Children's Hospital and uses informal, publicly available internet sources to monitor potential emerging public health threats. Automated data sources used by HealthMap include online news reports, information from the field, published reports by organizations such as the World Health Organization (WHO) and the CDC, and curated discussions, such as ProMed Mail. These data are mapped and allow the end user to visually see activity on a map and mouse over various data points to obtain additional information. This system has a diverse user community in various parts of the world.[14] During the COVID-19 pandemic, HealthMap maintained a global map of COVID-19 cases using data exclusively collected from publicly available sources, including government reports and news media.[15]

ESSENCE

The Electronic Surveillance System for the Early Notification of Community-based Epidemics (ESSENCE) is widely used by numerous state and local public health departments throughout the United States, the US Department of Defense, and is the analytical tool within the CDC National Syndromic Surveillance Program (NSSP). Civilian ESSENCE was developed by the Johns Hopkins Applied Physics Laboratory (JHU/APL). ESSENCE is a data-type, agnostic, secure web-based tool that provides users analysis and visualization capability. Its features allow users with maximum flexibility to manipulate data and conduct detailed analyses using various inherent analytics. Public health agencies use its features and functionality to gain detailed insight into the health of their communities for ongoing situational awareness and decision-making.[16,17]

ESSENCE is used to conduct surveillance on various conditions that are of interest to public health. ESSENCE has been used to monitor novel and emerging infectious diseases, chronic illnesses, and other public health conditions such as mental and behavioral health disorders and environmental exposures. System enhancements across 20 plus years driven by user feedback have resulted in a system with numerous customizable features aimed to meet a range of public health electronic surveillance needs.[18]

IMPROVING METHODS FOR GATHERING AND EVALUATING SURVEILLANCE DATA

In most of the developed world, availability of data is not a particular challenge. Often, there is more data available in those regions than can be used effectively. The challenge lies with assessing and characterizing new, potentially useful data sources to maximize their effectiveness for surveillance. Often it is assumed that more data means better information; however, this is not always true. To maximize benefits while minimizing the waste of computing and manpower resources needed for storing, maintaining, and analyzing large volumes, it is better to first fully understand the utility of various data sources and data elements for public health surveillance. When public health resources are scarce, only data sources proven to add value to the surveillance task at hand should be selected. The value of various data sources is sometimes determined through extensive research and data characterization, and other times obtained from subject matter expertise gained from direct knowledge of the data: how it originates, its quality and reliability, and its relevance to the disease or condition of interest. Data sources in electronic surveillance systems can vary based upon ease of availability but often include ED chief complaints, over-the-counter pharmaceuticals, school absenteeism, emergency medical services (EMS), and calls received by poison control call centers, just to name a few (Table 1). Fortunately,

TABLE 1
Sample Data Sources and Associated Data Elements for Electronic Disease Surveillance

Data Source	Sample Data Elements
Emergency department chief complaints	Geography system (region/zip code)
	Facility/facility location
	Date/time
	Chief complaint
	Age/race/sex
	Disposition
	Discharge diagnosis
	Zipcode of residence
	Clinical impression
	Triage notes
	Temperature
	Pulse oximetry
	Recent travel
Clinic data	Geography system (region/zip code)
	Facility/facility location
	Date/time
	Chief complaint
	Age/race/gender
Emergency medical services	Patient location
	Scene/situation
	Date/time
	Age/race/gender
	Agency
	Date/time

(Continued)

TABLE 1
Sample Data Sources and Associated Data Elements for Electronic Disease Surveillance—cont'd

Data Source	Sample Data Elements
	Medical history
	Exam
	Injury
	Procedure
	Medications
	Disposition
	Outcome
Reportable diseases data	Geography system (county/zip code)
	Date/time
	Age/race/gender
	Data provider
	Reportable disease
	Diagnosis status
	Occupation
	Day care associated
	Outbreak status
	Follow-up status
Death records data	Geography system (county/zip code)
	Age/race/gender
	Death group (cause of death)
	Place of death
	Injury
	Pregnancy
Poison control call center	Caller site
	Call type
	Agent of exposure
	Exposure site
	Date/time
	Substance (major/minor category)
	Substance description
	Geography system (region/zip code)
	Clinical effect
	Call center ID
	Age group
	Status
	Patient species

TABLE 1
Sample Data Sources and Associated Data Elements for Electronic Disease Surveillance—cont'd

Data Source	Sample Data Elements
Over-the-counter medication sales	Geography system (store/region)
	Date/time
	OTC category (intended treatment use)
	OTC type (mode of administration)
	OTC target user (adult/child)
School absenteeism	Geography system (school/region/zip code)
	School type
	School day type
	% absent
Air quality data	Geography system (county/state)
	Date/time
	Air quality parameter/measurement
	Air quality station
	Reporting agency
Prescription medications data	Geography system (patient county/zip)
	Geography system (clinic county/zip)
	Drug class
	Drug name
	Age group (adult/pediatric)
	Sex
Airline travel data	Flight
	Arrival city
	Zip code
	Sex
	Ebola affected countries visited
	Jurisdiction
	Risk category
	Traveler status
	Monitoring type

there are many academic researchers who are continuing to characterize new and evolving data sources and sharing knowledge gained with the public health community and other researchers. Much of this information is shared across online communities of practice (CoP) that curate and catalog the best information and analytic methods. For example, the NSSP CoP engages individuals with expertise in areas relevant to public health surveillance to share their knowledge, supports training of individuals new to syndromic surveillance, and encourages ongoing information among state and local public health practitioners. The Council of State and Territorial Epidemiologists (CSTE) Surveillance/Informatics Steering Committee, which includes researchers, epidemiologists, public health officials, and the like, is continually looking for new ways to improve public health surveillance through data, analytic methods, and visualization tools.[19]

In addition to emerging trends in infectious disease, public health professionals use their surveillance systems to monitor other conditions that impact public health, including injury, chronic diseases, reportable conditions, and events of public health significance during mass gatherings. Given their unique nature, use of the surveillance system in each case may potentially require a modified data review process. Such is the case for surveillance during presidential Inaugurations (Fig. 1) in the NCR, where health departments collaboratively monitor conditions across the region. Additionally, as public health crises such as the COVID-19 pandemic and opioid abuse and overdose epidemic happen, surveillance practitioners share "best practices" among their peers, to include data query strings for new case definitions, optimal visualizations, and nuances to be aware of when interpreting analytic findings.[20]

Efficient evaluation of surveillance data requires analytics. Analytics allow users to process large volumes of data quickly and make available actionable information for decision makers. The best analytics enable users to sift through data and highlight anomalous patterns or areas of concern they should focus on. Public health specialists, epidemiologists, and ICPs, whether in facilities or within local or state health agencies, are often asked to perform more tasks in less time. Therefore, individuals are becoming increasingly reliant on analytical and visualization tools in surveillance systems to gain value from the increasing amount of multivariate and disparate data. Even with a single source such as ED data, it is often necessary to conduct analysis by a group of facilities, a particular health region, or a political subdivision.[21,22]

Data Analysis and Visualization

A challenge faced during the development of any electronic surveillance system lies in how to effectively analyze and present the results for an end user whose education and experience may vary from novice to a trained epidemiologist. In addition to data availability, the global variability of the workforce, both with respect to public health training as well as hands-on experience with technology, often influences the methodologies most used for analysis and visualization. While it is outside the scope of this chapter to elaborate deeply on statistical methodologies, it is important to note that there are numerous statistical methods employed with public health data depending upon the environment one is working in.[23] Important considerations in this area include:

- Evolving data streams
- Sparse or vanishing baselines
- Non-Gaussian distribution of time-series data
- Robustness of data dropouts[24]

It is important to note statistical alerting methods in surveillance systems detect statistical anomalies, which may or may not be related to public health events. Confirmation of a health event following a statistical alert requires definitive evidence that is not immediately available to most system users. This evidence is typically in the form of laboratory confirmation, which may not be available for many days. Additionally, in the absence of linked data sources, when confirmatory laboratory data is available, that information may not be linked to an individual patient encounter within a surveillance system. Therefore, while there are gains in timeliness by using prediagnostic data such as chief complaints, if linked diagnosis data is unavailable, there is a loss in specificity. This has led to debate over the years regarding high consequence decision-making by health officials based upon prediagnostic chief complaints versus clinical diagnoses. While there is still no agreement on this matter, many recognize that there is still value in prediagnostic data in the absence of confirmatory or definitive diagnosis data because that data can point to critical health trends within a given population early.[23] In disease surveillance systems that use prediagnostic data, an alert is signaled when the output of an algorithm crosses a threshold that is statistically aberrant, or too far from expected values to be plausible from random variation alone. The statistical alerts, especially in combination with other evidence, are useful to prompt investigation to rule out true health events. However, as pointed out before, statistical alerts themselves do not necessarily mean a public health event and can be generated because of other data-quality associated causes, including batched data reports, data drops, and changes in provider chief complaints recording or diagnosis coding practices.[23]

Different individuals process information differently; therefore, equally important to the analysis of surveillance data is how the information is presented to the end user. End users have specific preferences for how they interact with a surveillance system. Providing multiple ways for the user to interact with the underlying data will enable usability, and less flexibility will present a barrier to adoption.[25]

USE OF SURVEILLANCE DATA TO IMPROVE PUBLIC HEALTH PRACTICE AND MEDICAL TREATMENT

Many in the public health community believe that simply identifying problems by conducting surveillance without taking action to mitigate them is immoral.

However, as has been previously stated, public health resources are finite and may not always permit action.[7]

Many electronic surveillance system end users are faced with the challenge of when to initiate an investigation based upon the information from the system. This decision process is also driven by many factors, to include the time of year, geography, and age distribution of cases, and whether the enhanced surveillance activities are due to a mass gathering or specific concern, to name but a few. In the case of short-term enhanced surveillance activities, many health departments have enacted decision trees to aid in decision-making, since often, individuals whose daily tasking does not include monitoring the surveillance system may be called upon to serve in that capacity (Fig. 2).

In general, through effective and efficient approaches, many goals of surveillance can, in fact, be achieved. With COVID-19, public health specialists use electronic disease surveillance to monitor inflection points in the pandemic to gauge the impending impact on hospital bed utilization and other healthcare resources.[26] They use this information for community public health messaging and planning resource distribution. In 2016, when Zika was identified in the United States, the health officials were quickly able to target a particular geographic area for heightened vector control measures, thereby allowing the county to better utilize their resources. Similarly, during seasonal influenza, many hospitals implement their seasonal infection control protocols when surveillance indicates heightened respiratory or influenza-like illness.

This capability to monitor and community health trends, while seemingly simple in the age of digital data, is unfortunately not ubiquitous throughout the world due to the absence of data and various other resource constraints.[27] As a result, many are starting to discuss the concept of *precision public health*, which is reliant on the use of data to guide specific public health interventions—with surveillance being just one important aspect of precision. It has been suggested that in order to achieve precision, everyone, to include the developing world, must (1) register births and deaths, (2) track disease, (3) incorporate laboratory analyses, and (4) train more people.[27] Ensuring sound surveillance strategies, to include reliant data collection and analytic methods, in both the developed and developing world will no doubt further the goal of implementing timely interventions no matter where a disease outbreak occurs.

To aid with precision public health is the concept of predictive analytics. When data are routinely collected and population-based surveillance is in place, the question then turns to whether one can predict the new outbreak of an endemic disease. For example, if health authorities could predict there would be an upward trend in COVID-19 or an outbreak of Zika in a particular region, they would be able to tune their public health response accordingly. If resources are constrained, they could minimize expenditure by only focusing interventions on that specific area where an increase in case counts or the outbreak will likely occur.[22]

STRENGTHENING GLOBAL CAPACITY TO MONITOR AND RESPOND TO EMERGING INFECTIOUS DISEASE

Nations have long utilized health as a diplomatic tool. Improving the overall health of a given population has far-reaching effects on the economy and overall stability of that population, whether it is as small as a village or as large as an entire country. Through the efforts of many government agencies, some of whom have been tackling this problem long before the recently introduced Global Health Security Agenda (GHSA), in concert with partner countries and international organizations, the face of global health diplomacy is slowly changing. The US government, for example, now more than ever, is strongly committed to global health diplomacy as a means to improve not only health but also global economic and political stability. They believe, as do all public health professionals, that a "public health emergency anywhere is a public health emergency everywhere."[22]

One event people are particularly fearful of is a pandemic of a novel, naturally occurring disease originating overseas. This fear is understandable since these types of diseases represent the unknown, and these fears are not unfounded, as infectious diseases know no geographic boundaries, and globalization has connected people and parts of the world more than in any other time in our history. Indeed, this fear was realized beginning in late 2019, when a cluster of patients in Wuhan, China, began to experience symptoms of an atypical pneumonia-like illness. This was the beginning of the global pandemic caused by SARS-CoV-2, a novel coronavirus the world had never seen before. As of September 2022, there have been approximately 614 million cases of COVID-19 and 6.5 million deaths, according to the WHO Coronavirus (COVID) dashboard.[28]

The World Health Organization (WHO) does set requirements for member countries to report certain diseases. Prior to the SARS outbreak in 2003, the WHO International Health Regulations (IHR) required member countries to report only outbreaks of cholera, yellow fever, and plague. As illustrated by the SARS outbreak, a

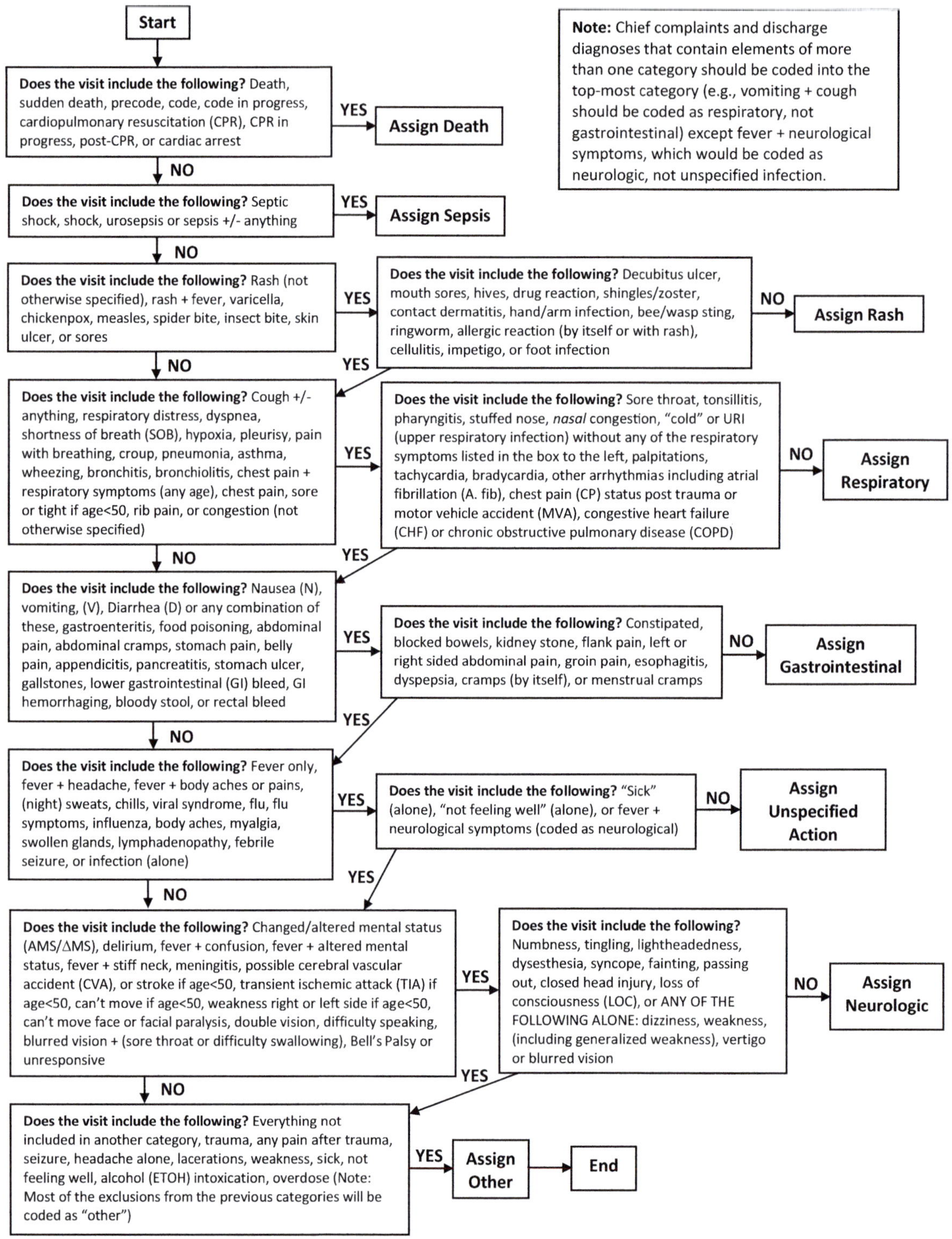

FIG. 2 National Capital Region ESSENCE data review process during enhanced surveillance for mass gatherings.

disease that was first identified in China and Hong Kong and quickly spread to the United States and Canada, the IHR did not adequately address the growing threat of emerging diseases in a globalized world. Not only did health authorities have to deal with challenging decisions related to slowing the spread of disease through closing certain venues, but few jurisdictions had a way to easily assess the health of their population. As a result, in 2005, new IHR were adopted by the WHO. The new IHR, commonly referenced as IHR 2005, requires member countries to report any disease that may constitute a public health emergency of international concern (PHEIC).[29] While this may seem like a daunting task, the IHR has provided a tool to enable public health practitioners to determine how to identify a PHEIC (Fig. 3).[30] Additionally, the IHR stipulates, albeit at a high level, that countries must improve their capacity to detect, assess, notify, and respond to public health threats. The new IHR went into effect in 2012, but to date, some countries are still having difficulties meeting the standards for compliance. However, recognizing the challenges faced when implementing a new system, useful tools have been developed to help system implementers think through necessary elements of the process (Fig. 4).

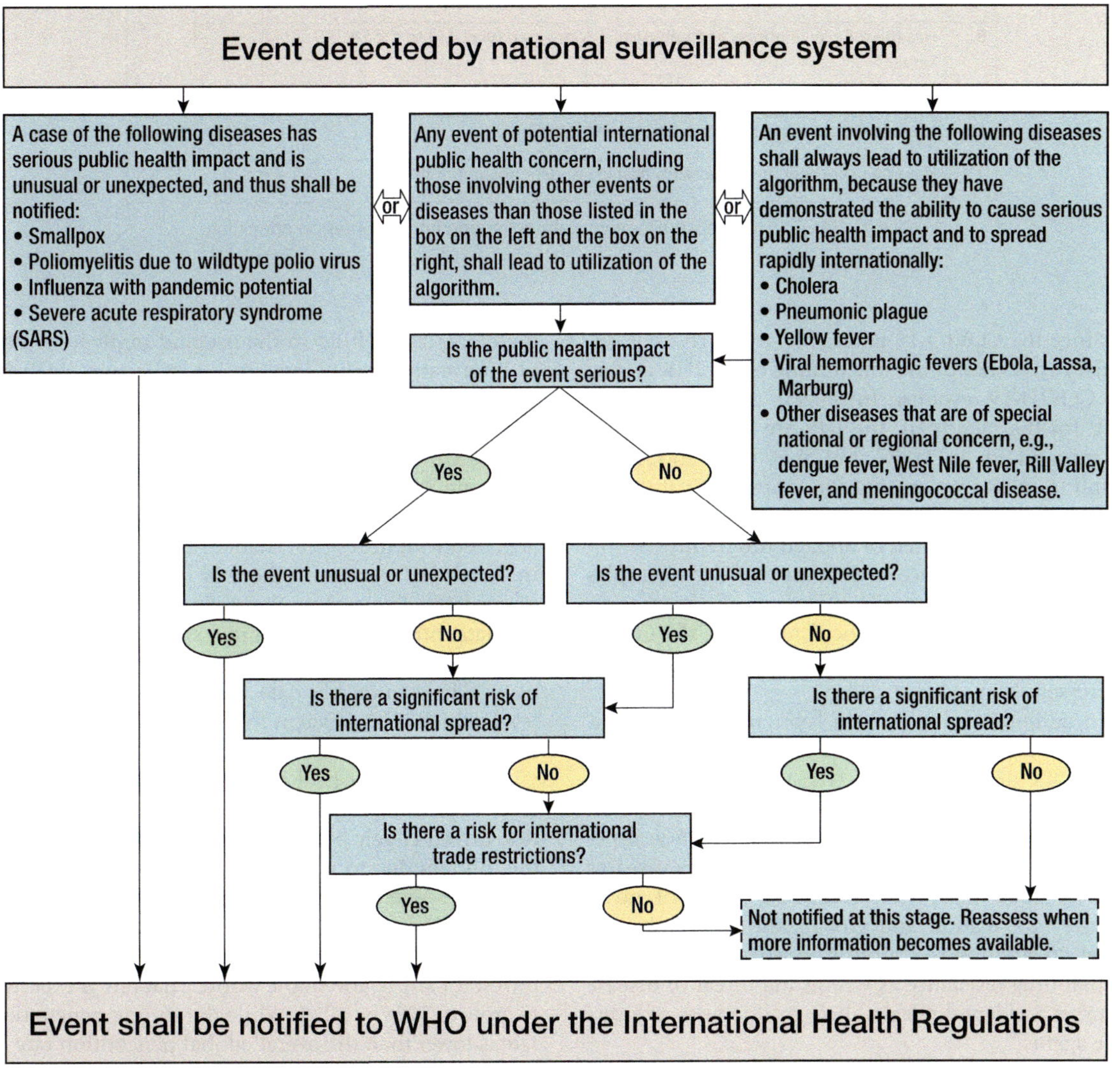

FIG. 3 WHO International Health Regulation's Annex 2 decision instrument for determination of a potential PHEIC.[27]

Directions: This tool serves as a checklist of items that should be in place prior to implementation of SAGES mCollect (an Android-based mobile data collection application).

	ITEM	Y	N
1.	Have the smartphones that will be used by the data collectors been acquired (Android version 2.3 or higher)?		
2.	Has the mCollect app been installed on each collector's smartphone?		
3.	Have the mCollect phones been distributed to each collector?		
4.	Have the data elements to be collected been identified?		
5.	Have the mCollect data entry form(s) been installed on the collector phones?		
6.	Has the mReceive smartphone been acquired?		
7.	Has the mReceive app been installed on the receiver phone?		
8.	Has the mReceive phone been physically connected (via USB) to the SAGES server?		
9.	Have all collectors been trained on using the app?		
10.	Has a technical support person been designated?		
11	Have all users been provided with training and/or documentation?		

FIG. 4 SAGES mCollect/mReceive data collection implementation checklist.

Since the COVID-19 pandemic, the WHO has engaged in a review of the functioning of the IHR during the COVID-19 response. In general, the review found that, for the most part, the IHR are appropriate and meaningful in a PHEIC, but that ways should be found to make implementation more achievable. The review also noted that some parts of the regulations may need to be updated or applied differently. For instance, the importance of sharing pathogen samples and genetic sequences, the evolution of digital technology, and the impact of social media on the uptake of public health recommendations may need to be addressed.[31]

In addition to the IHR, in February 2014, numerous countries, including the United States, committed to the aforementioned GHSA, whose goal is to accelerate progress in the prevention, detection, and response to infectious disease threats over a 5-year period. The GHSA specifically targets infectious diseases and includes the already discussed topics of novel disease propagation and globalization of trade and travel, in addition to concerns over increasing antimicrobial drug resistance as well as the threat of disease from an accidental release, theft, or illicit use of a disease agent.[30]

As was previously described as it relates to the United States, public health is often underresourced, and therefore, lags behind in the use and implementation of information technology for the collection, analysis, and visualization of public health data. Whereas industrialized nations tend to be faced with the problems associated with an abundance of data—such as data cleansing, validation, integration, and storage, to name but a few—low- and middle-income countries (LMIC) are faced with the critical challenge of data acquisition. In developed countries, there is both an abundance of available data and mechanisms to send and receive the data, but in resource-limited settings, data are still largely collected on paper, and reporting takes the form of weekly or monthly data aggregation to a regional level, which is insufficient for rapid identification of a novel disease within a community.

However, public health entities in LMIC have begun to utilize technology to assist in data collection activities, driven largely by two factors: the ubiquity of mobile phones due to more affordable smartphones and data plans, and the growing availability of Open-Source Software. For example, the mobile subscriber penetration rate in Sub-Saharan Africa in 2017 was 44%, the lowest for any region in the world. That rate is expected to grow to 52% by 2025. While the current penetration rate is lower than the overall global penetration rate of 66%, the number of mobile subscribers in Sub-Saharan Africa is expected to grow at a faster pace than the overall global rate.[32] The capacity to collect and transmit data nearly instantaneously using mobile technologies offers tremendous advantages in identifying events as they occur, even in remote, low-resource settings.[33] Open-Source Software (OSS) refers to software that is made readily available for others to use, modify, or redistribute under a licensing agreement with very few restrictions. Anyone can use the software without having to pay royalties or negotiate a license agreement. OSS is typically free to obtain, and there is no per-seat licensing cost, although implementation is not free and may require some level of skilled personnel. The proliferation of mobile technology and OSS combined has given rise to the concepts of mobile health (mHealth) and electronic health (eHealth), which describe the use of mobile initiatives and electronic processes to support healthcare. In the context of surveillance, where timely data collection is a challenge, particularly in LMIC, mobile technology and OSS can have a positive impact on driving compliance with IHR.[34]

Case Studies

DHIS2

DHIS2 (District Health Information System version 2) is a free and Open-Source Software platform for the collection, management, analysis, and use of data and information. The platform is now the national health information system in 67 countries and has become a global standard internationally. Tailored data visualizations are accessible in real-time to managers at all levels of the health system through dashboards, scorecards, pivot tables, maps, and charts. DHIS2 is typically used as a national health information system for data management and analysis purposes, for health program monitoring and evaluation, as facility registries and service availability mapping, for logistics management, and for mobile tracking of pregnant mothers in rural communities. DHIS2 offers a number of mobile solutions, including SMS, plain HTML, and Java options for feature phones, as well as a web-based solution with offline support for smartphones. Clients can use their mobile phones for registering cases, events, and personal information tracking individuals, conducting surveys, and collecting aggregate data. DHIS2 has gained a strong foothold in Africa, with several countries now using DHIS2 as a national level system, with the inclusion of mobile technology enabling the implementation of electronic disease surveillance and response (eIDSR).[35,36]

SAGES

SAGES (*Suite for Automated Global Electronic BioSurveillance*) is a suite of open-source tools intended for electronic disease surveillance in resource-limited environments. SAGES supports mobile data collection using Wi-Fi or SMS and customizable data entry forms, spatial and temporal analysis and visualization with dynamic dashboards, and anomaly (outbreak) detection algorithms that are optimized for LMIC, whose data may be vastly different from data collected in countries such as the United States. SAGES also supports role-based access for controlled information sharing, which can enable regional information sharing. Since SAGES is data agnostic, data collection is not limited to routine disease surveillance. Data entry forms can be customized, for example, to respond to a pandemic outbreak or other type of emergency. The SAGES toolkit is built upon existing and widely known open-source projects such as Open Data Kit and Rapid Android.[37,38]

USHAHIDI

Ushahidi is a web-based platform that enables crowd sourcing of disease information by citizen journalists.[39] In 2008, this system was used to map incidents of violence during the Kenyan elections. The Web platform was wildly popular because safe havens were pointed out and lives were saved from the widespread violence. Ushahidi was also used during the response to the earthquake in Haiti in 2010 to locate survivors and pinpoint possible clusters of disease. People in Haiti were able to upload geo-referenced data that described where there were possible survivors or cases of cholera. Such information was used by the coordinating agencies on the ground to allocate emergency support and medicines.[33]

THE FUTURE OF SURVEILLANCE

The public health community has been agile and adapted to less than ideal infrastructure for electronic surveillance activities over the course of the last two decades. Even with limited resources, they have been able to successfully shift the culture of their field. Automated data feeds and automated data processing mean that epidemiologists are no longer waiting to learn about outbreaks but are now proactively able to look for possible increases of disease within a given population. Similarly, the advent of electronic disease surveillance has improved the overall situational awareness of infection control professionals. Today, most public health professionals will likely agree that the capabilities and technologies described herein have had a positive effect on the field of public health as a whole. They also recognize that similar shifts in surveillance practice will continue to occur as data availability and volume increase and analysis and visualization capabilities improve. This will almost certainly require continuous workforce education and refinement of processes within all levels of surveillance.

One Health

One of the next steps in effective surveillance strategies is the development of an integrated "One Health" surveillance approach. One Health is the collaborative approach to achieving optimal health outcomes recognizing the interconnection between people, animals, plants, and their shared environment. 60% of known infectious diseases in humans and over 75% of newly emerging infectious diseases are zoonotic, meaning they can pass between human and animal populations. SARS-CoV-2, the virus responsible for COVID-19, is zoonotic, and its rapid spread across the world highlighted the need for deeper understanding of the transmission of zoonoses. Establishing adequate animal disease surveillance is imperative to maintaining human health and managing emerging infectious disease threats. Surveillance activities in animal populations can serve as an important early warning of a threat in human populations and display early indicators of potential bioterrorist or natural infectious disease epidemics. Developing systems that link human and animal disease reporting will allow public and animal health professionals to swiftly identify and facilitate a response to known and emerging zoonotic diseases.[40]

Current proven and well-established human health surveillance systems and tools provide a unique opportunity in the animal health surveillance arena. Given funding constraints in both human and animal health, integrating animal data into existing systems and leveraging existing tools will limit the resources needed while still providing the same advanced capabilities and analytics that are available for human health surveillance. This will provide public health professionals the ability to potentially predict and prevent zoonotic disease transmission or spread to human populations.[41]

Expanding human health surveillance systems to incorporate animal health data also takes strides toward developing the framework for a One Health surveillance system. There are continuing challenges at both the technical and organizational level as a One Health-based surveillance system is considered. These hurdles are currently preventing integration and range from legal issues regarding data confidentiality, limitations in data sharing, funding constraints, and unclear responsibilities and structural barriers between agencies. Open communication, strategies, and established policy across sectors need to be aligned to bring One Health surveillance to the forefront of national and global health concerns.[42]

Information and Communications Technology and New Data

Information and communications technologies (ICTs) will continue to evolve and penetrate the global marketplace in years to come. While these changes will offer more opportunities for enhanced surveillance, they will continue to challenge the workforce and require them to remain agile and quickly adapt and incorporate new innovations. As previously mentioned, resource-limited settings often rely heavily on mobile phones for data collection needs until internet penetration improves. As of the end of 2020, the International Telecommunications Union (ITU) reported the number of mobile phone subscriptions as greater than the global population, while fixed (landline) subscriptions were less than one billion.[43] Similarly, more than half of households worldwide now have access to the internet.[44]

Looking ahead, technological advancement will continue to play an important role in the field of surveillance.

Additional access to ICTs also leads one to think about whether additional data sources that rely on these modalities will prove to be useful. Such data streams include social media feeds, crowdsourcing applications, etc. As was mentioned previously, social media is an increasingly popular mode of communication that holds great promise for the early detection of infectious disease. However, before data derived from social media can effectively be utilized in disease surveillance systems, work is needed to understand if and how these data are correlated with more traditional health data. While there has been research that shows there is a correlation between the health of a community and social media data, it has yet to be proven as an effective data source in an operational, prospective system. Furthermore, these types of data sources are prone to rapid change, and therefore, require sophisticated analytics with the ability to keep pace with what is trending.[45]

"Big" Data and Cloud Computing

With the rapidly changing ICT and data source landscape comes the associated challenge of storing and analyzing the data in an efficient, yet effective, manner. Big data has come to mean many different things to different groups of people. To the public health community, both in the United States and abroad, who are not accustomed to having to collect, store, analyze, and visualize large volumes of data, the advent of electronic disease surveillance systems has ushered in what they consider to be "big data." This volume of data will only continue to increase, and while it brings many opportunities, it comes with challenges in a field with suboptimal information technology (IT) resources. Combined with existing data streams, novel data streams and their associated analytic methodologies will also push the public health field. For example, the Internet of Things (IoT), which refers to the ability of everyday objects people interact with to send and receive data, combined with artificial intelligence, cloud computing, and big data analytics will enable those charged with predicting, detecting, and responding to emerging infectious disease threats to make better, more informed decisions in less time.[22,46] Another data source poised to add both precision but also analytics, visualization, and storage challenges, is the data generated through genomic sequencing. With the introduction of sequencing technologies that fit in the palm of the hand, it is envisioned that people can sequence everything—air, soil, water, humans, and animals—anywhere in the world, regardless of how austere the setting. While this capability holds great promise, there is much work to be done before its true benefit and applicability can be recognized for everyday public health practice.

With increasing volumes of data coming from a wide variety of sources comes the associated challenge of how to collect and store the data such that it can be quickly, easily, and securely served up to the end user when it is needed. Often times, whether in the United States or not, the costs of IT services are a critical impediment to developing and sustaining an electronic surveillance capability. Cloud computing is yet another term frequently used whose meaning varies depending on context. It is often used to define computing resources that run sophisticated analytics across many computers in parallel, but it can also be used to define massive storage capabilities that manage petabytes or exabytes of data. As with anything, there are numerous potential benefits and challenges cloud computing can offer. While they are efficient, flexible, and reliable, they also introduce numerous concerns, such as security and long-term costs.[46]

CONCLUSION

As has been highlighted throughout this chapter, in the last 20 years there has been significant progress in electronic surveillance systems, which have facilitated the ease with which health professionals can prevent, detect, and respond to new and emerging challenges. However, as has been evidenced throughout the COVID-19 pandemic, the field of electronic surveillance is still in its infancy and needs to continue to grow. As new data sources are identified and data volume increases, and public health surveillance needs suddenly change as with the COVID-19 pandemic, the community will continue to be faced with the need to collect, analyze, visualize, and utilize data in ways they have not yet imagined and at much faster timeframes.

While surveillance systems were born out of concern over intentional biological attacks before becoming a common tool within the workflow, the security community is yet again faced with new challenges. Synthetic biology, while often well intentioned and practiced by many trained researchers in academia as well as industry, is presently an underregulated or self-regulated activity. Many have expressed concern over the accidental release, theft, or illicit use of a synthetically engineered disease agent. These concerns, paired with the continuing challenges with the COVID-19 pandemic, underscore the need for increased surveillance capacity throughout the world.[47]

Surveillance strategies require continued research into analytic methodologies, implementation strategies, and monitoring and evaluation for continuous system improvement as the threats continue to evolve. Systems must be able to predict, detect, and provide information that can be acted upon by public health authorities. Effective surveillance strategies are but one integral part of a much larger effort to protect the global population against the threat of emerging and re-emerging infectious diseases.

ACKNOWLEDGMENTS

The chapter authors would like to acknowledge their colleagues from the Johns Hopkins University Applied Physics Laboratory, Drs. Karen Meidenbauer and Martina Siwek, and Ms. Rekha Holtry for their assistance with the preparation of this material.

DISCLOSURE STATEMENT

The authors have no financial interests to disclose.

REFERENCES

1. Langmuir AD. The surveillance of communicable diseases of national importance. *N Engl J Med.* 1963;268:182–192.
2. Thacker SB, Berkelman RL. Public health surveillance in the United States. *Epidemiol Rev.* 1988;10:164–190.
3. Thacker SB. Historical development. In: Teutsch SM, Churchill RE, eds. *Principles of Public Health Surveillance.* New York: Oxford University Press; 1994:3–17.
4. Blazes DB, Lewis SH. Introduction to electronic disease surveillance. In: Blazes DB, Lewis SH, eds. *Disease Surveillance: Technological Contributions to Global Health Security.* Florida: Taylor & Francis Group; 2016:3–10.

5. Gordis L. Epidemiology. Pennsylvania: WB Saunders Company; 1996.
6. Principles of Epidemiology in Public Health Practice. Lesson 5: Public Health Surveillance, Section 4: Identifying or Collecting Data for Surveillance; 2012. https://www.cdc.gov/ophss/csels/dsepd/ss1978/lesson5/section4.html. Accessed 27 July 2018.
7. Lewis SH, Hurt-Mullen K, Martin C, et al. Modern disease surveillance systems in public health practice. In: *Disease Surveillance: A Public Health Informatics Approach.* New Jersey: John Wiley & Sons; 2007:265–302.
8. Jajosky RA, Ward J. National, state, and local public health surveillance systems. In: M'ikanatha NM, Iskander JK, eds. *Concepts and Methods in Infectious Disease Surveillance.* UK: John Wiley & Sons; 2015:14–25.
9. National Health and Nutrition Examination Survey; 2016. https://www.cdc.gov/nchs/nhanes/participant.htm. Accessed 27 July 2018.
10. Center for Disease Control and Prevention. Preventing emerging infectious disease: a strategy for the 21st century, overview of the updated CDC plan. *MMWR.* 1998;47(RR15):1–14.
11. Khan AS, Levitt AM, Sage MJ, et al. Biological and chemical terrorism: strategic plan for preparedness and response. *MMWR.* 2000;49(RR04):1–14.
12. Henning KJ. Overview of syndromic surveillance: what is syndromic surveillance? *MMWR.* 2004;53(Suppl):5–11.
13. Begier EM, Sockwell D, Branch LM, et al. The National Capitol Region's Emergency Department syndromic surveillance system: do chief complaint and discharge diagnosis yield different results? *Emerg Infect Dis.* 2003;9(3):393–396.
14. HealthMap; 2022. http://www.healthmap.org/en/. Accessed 18 October 2022.
15. HealthMap; 2022. https://healthmap.org/covid-19/#. Accessed 18 October 2022.
16. Lombardo J, et al. A systems overview of the Electronic Surveillance System for the Early Notification of Community-Based Epidemics (ESSENCE II). *J Urban Health.* 2003;2(Suppl. 1):i32–i42.
17. Kite-Powell A, Coletta M, Smimble J. User generated SQL queries inform evaluation of NSSP ESSENCE. *OJPHI.* 2018. https://journals.uic.edu/ojs/index.php/ojphi/article/view/8914. Accessed 27 July 2018.
18. O'Connell E, et al. Innovative uses for syndromic surveillance. *Emerg Infect Dis.* 2010;16(4):669–671.
19. Council for State and Territorial Epidemiologists' Surveillance/Informatics Steering Committee; 2022. https://www.cste.org/page/SurveillanceInfo. Accessed 18 October 2022.
20. Vivolo-Kantor AM, et al. Vital signs: trends in emergency department visits for suspected opioid overdoses—United States, July 2016–September 2017. *MMWR.* 2018;67(9):279–285.
21. Burkom HS, et al. Tradeoffs driving policy and research decisions in biosurveillance. *J Hopkins APL Tech Dig.* 2008;27(4):299–312.
22. Lewis SH, et al. Promising advances in surveillance technology for global health security. In: Blazes DB, Lewis SH, eds. *Disease Surveillance: Technological Contributions to Global Health Security.* Florida: Taylor & Francis Group; 2016:179–188.
23. Burkom HS. The role and functional components of statistical alert methods for biosurveillance. In: Blazes DB, Lewis SH, eds. *Disease Surveillance: Technological Contributions to Global Health Security.* Florida: Taylor & Francis Group; 2016:75–97.
24. Burkom HS. Analytic biosurveillance methods for resource-limited settings. *J Hopkins APL Tech Dig.* 2014;32(4):667–678.
25. Abernethy NF, Caroll LN. Effective public health data visualization. In: Blazes DB, Lewis SH, eds. *Disease Surveillance: Technological Contributions to Global Health Security.* Florida: Taylor & Francis Group; 2016:75–97.
26. Ferraro CF, Findlater L, Morbey R, et al. Describing the indirect impact of COVID-19 on healthcare utilisation using syndromic surveillance systems. *BMC Public Health.* 2021;21, 2019.
27. Dowell SF, Blazes D, Desmond-Hellman S. Four steps to precision public health. *Nature.* 2016;540:189–191.
28. WHO Coronavirus (COVID-19) Dashboard; 2022. https://covid19.who.int/. Accessed 18 October 2022.
29. International Health Regulations. Geneva, Switzerland: World Health Organization; 2005. 2008.
30. Katz R, et al. International health regulations: policy. In: Blazes DB, Lewis SH, eds. *Disease Surveillance: Technological Contributions to Global Health Security.* Florida: Taylor & Francis Group; 2016:11–28.
31. Report of the Review Committee on the Functioning of the International Health Regulations (2005) During the COVID-19 Response; 2002. https://www.who.int/publications/m/item/a74-9-who-s-work-in-health-emergencies. Accessed 18 October 2022.
32. Report of the Review Committee on the Functioning of the International Health Regulations (2005) During the COVID-19 Response; 2022. https://www.who.int/publications/m/item/a74-9-who-s-work-in-health-emergencies. Accessed 18 October 2022.
33. The Mobile Economy 2018. London, UK: GSMA Head Office; 2018.
34. Vasudevan L, Ghoshal S, Labrique AB. mHealth and its role in disease surveillance. In: Blazes DB, Lewis SH, eds. *Disease Surveillance: Technological Contributions to Global Health Security.* Florida: Taylor & Francis Group; 2016:3–10.
35. Hahn E, Blazes D, Lewis S. Understanding how the "open" of Open-Source Software (OSS) will improve global health security. *Health Security.* 2016;14(1):13–18.
36. District Health Information System, Version 2; 2018. https://www.dhis2.org/. Accessed 30 July 2018.
37. Groen P. DHIS 2. Open Health News: The Voice for the Open Health Community; 2016. http://www.openhealthnews.com/resources/dhis2-district-health-information-system-2. Accessed 31 July 2018.
38. Suite for Automated Global Electronic Biosurveillance; 2018. https://www.jhuapl.edu/sages. Accessed 30 July 2018.

39. Feighner BH, et al. SAGES overview: open-source software tools for electronic disease surveillance in resource-limited settings. *J Hopkins APL Tech Dig.* 2014;32(4):652–658.
40. Ushahidi; 2018. https://www.ushahidi.com/. Accessed 30 July 2018.
41. Mauer WA, Kaneene JB. Integrated human-animal disease surveillance. *Emerg Infect Dis.* 2005;11(9):1490–1491.
42. Jennings JM, et al. Identifying challenges to the integration of computer-based surveillance information systems in a large city health department: a case study. *Public Health Rep.* 2009;124(Suppl 2):39–48.
43. Stärk KD, et al. One Health surveillance—more than a buzz word? *Prev Vet Med.* 2015;120(1):124–130.
44. International Telecommunication Union Statistics; 2022. https://www.itu.int/en/ITU-D/Statistics/Pages/stat/default.aspx. Accessed 18 October 2022.
45. Measuring the Information Society Report 2017. Geneva, Switzerland: International Telecommunication Union; 2017.
46. Coberly JS, et al. Tweeting fever: can twitter be used to monitor the incidence of dengue-like illness in the Philippines? *J Hopkins APL Tech Dig.* 2014;32(4):667–678.
47. Loschen WA, Stewart MA, Lombardo JS. Public health applications in the cloud. *J Hopkins APL Tech Dig.* 2014;32(4):667–678.

Infectious Diseases Transmission Dynamics: Modeling of Outbreaks and Interventions

LINDSAY T. KEEGAN[a] • C. JESSICA E. METCALF[b] • LAURA B. ZEISER[c] • JUSTIN LESSLER[c,d]
[a]Department of Internal Medicine, University of Utah, Salt Lake City, UT, United States • [b]Department of Ecology and Evolutionary Biology/School of Public and International Affairs, Princeton University, Princeton, NJ, United States • [c]Department of Epidemiology, Johns Hopkins Bloomberg School of Public Health, Baltimore, MD, United States • [d]Department of Epidemiology, University of North Carolina Gillings School of Public Health, Chapel Hill, NC, United States

INTRODUCTION

Dynamic models have been part of the first-line response to emerging pathogens for decades. From the start of the HIV epidemic in the 1980s to the 2019 emergence of SARS-CoV-2, the virus responsible for the COVID-19 pandemic, models have played a critical role in understanding disease spread and mounting public health responses. This has never been truer than during the recent COVID-19 pandemic, where models not only played an important role in the public health response but were also at the forefront of the public attention as SARS-CoV-2 began to spread around the world. By relying on mechanistic assumptions, dynamical models can provide guidance in understanding and responding to emerging pathogens, even when data is limited, as is the case early in an outbreak. Although there continue to be substantial advances in disease surveillance, computational power, and modeling techniques, the same core principles have been used to assess disease threats for decades.

In this chapter, we review the basic principles of infectious disease dynamics and their application in preparing for and responding to emerging infectious threats and agents of bioterrorism. We aim to provide the basic foundations of disease dynamics needed by anyone working in preparedness and response, as well as a broad overview of research and applications in the field of infectious disease dynamics. We illustrate the use of dynamic modeling in bioterrorism preparedness and epidemic response through case studies that demonstrate the role of modeling in confronting pathogen threats. We discuss the limits of model-based approaches and attempt to provide guidance for evaluating the quality of dynamic analyses. Finally, we review new trends and opportunities in modeling infectious diseases.

THE "CLASSICAL" DYNAMIC MODELING TOOLKIT

In the context of the preparation for and response to threats posed by infectious diseases, several fundamental quantities characterize key elements of pathogen transmission and can be used to guide efforts (Fig. 1, Box 1). These quantities, and the methods for their estimation and analysis, form the "classical" dynamic modeling toolkit.[1] Three decades ago, May and Anderson[2] used mathematical models built on this toolkit to identify the key variables required to understand the likely future course of the HIV epidemic and the performance of control measures (e.g., variables such as duration of infectiousness, numbers of sexual partners per unit of time, heterogeneity in contacts). In doing so, they illuminated important priorities for HIV research and control that are still relevant 30 years later. The foundational nature and flexibility of the classical modeling toolkit mean the same basic techniques and principles remain at the forefront in planning and response for emerging pathogens and bioterrorism threats today, even as advances in theory, computational power, and data availability have led to substantial improvements in their estimation and application.

Viral Outbreaks, Biosecurity, and Preparing for Mass Casualty Infectious Diseases Events
https://doi.org/10.1016/B978-0-323-54841-0.00002-0

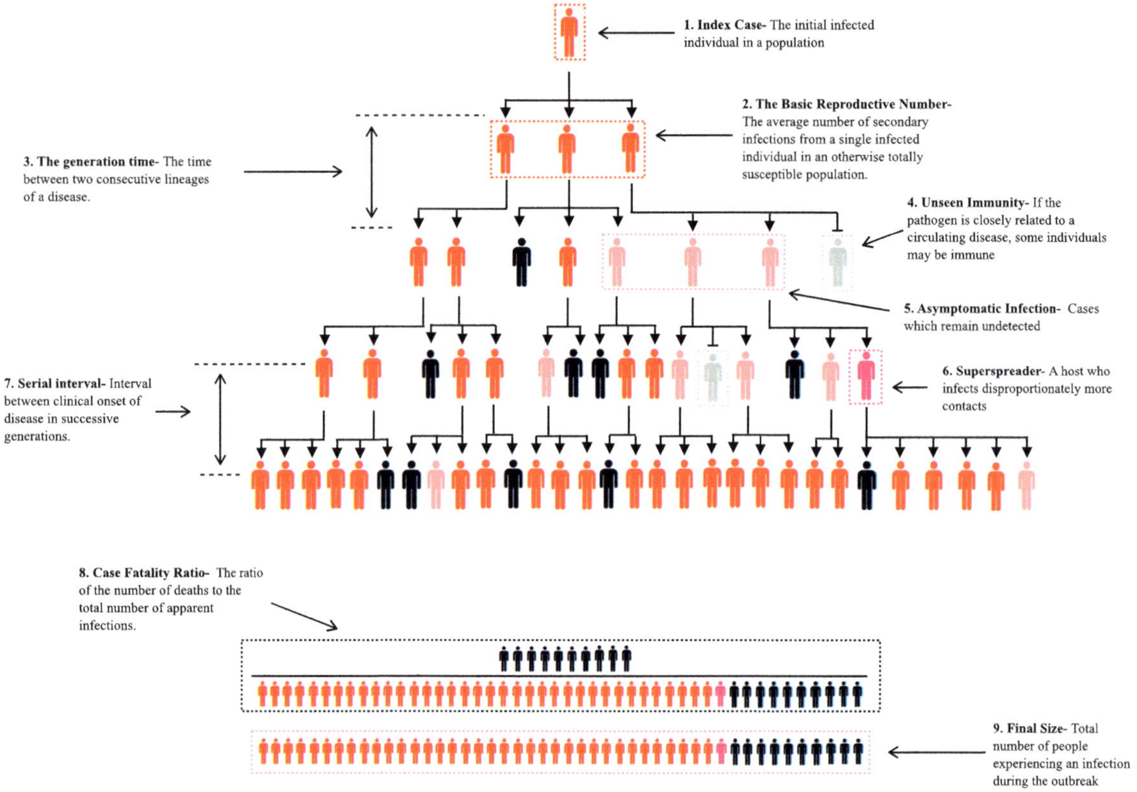

FIG. 1 *Diagram of transmission of a typical human-to-human infection.* (1) *An index case (patient zero) enters a novel population, and the pathogen begins circulating.* (2) *The basic reproductive number, R_0,* is the key to determining if a pathogen will spread in a population ($R_0 > 1$) or if it will die out ($R_0 < 1$), here $R_0 = 3$. (3) In combination with R_0,the generation time determines the speed of the epidemic. (4) In general, most models assume that all potential hosts are fully susceptible (no prior immunity). However, when the circulating pathogen is closely related to a previously circulating disease (e.g., pandemic H1N1), there may be substantial immunity. Both (5) asymptomatic infections and (6) superspreaders can have a significant effect on disease dynamics and control that can be overlooked when using average quantities such as R_0. Targeting control efforts toward these individuals can have a disproportionate impact on reducing overall disease transmission and therefore controlling the epidemic. Like (3) the generation time, (7) the serial interval also measures the time between successive generations of disease. However, unlike (3) the generation time, which is hard to observe, (7) the serial interval is fully observable. Calculating (8) the case fatality ratio and (9) the final size of the epidemic is important to determine the impact of the disease on the population. Additionally, when looking retrospectively, (9) the final size provides an alternative way to estimate the basic reproductive number.

In this section, we show how the elements of the classical modeling toolkit allow us to answer key questions about the threat posed by an infectious pathogen and can be used in planning and control.

Will a Disease Cause an Epidemic? R_0

When responding to an emergent pathogen, an early priority is determining if the pathogen will cause a significant epidemic or be confined to a small cluster of cases. A pathogen's ability to cause an epidemic is characterized by its basic reproductive number (R_0). R_0 is defined as the average number of secondary infections caused by a single infectious index (Box 2) case in a population where everyone is fully susceptible to infection (e.g., an immunologically naive population). R_0 is of particular interest in an emerging epidemic, as it provides an epidemic threshold: when R_0 is greater than one, a disease can invade and persist and has the potential to cause an epidemic or pandemic, whereas when R_0 is less than one, the disease will die out.[3,4] For example, influenza has a reproductive number of R_0 is approximately two and measles has a reproductive number of $R_0 \approx 15$. Thus, in a completely susceptible population,

BOX 1
Fundamental Quantities in Context

There are several key dynamic quantities that determine both the course of an epidemic and guide the intervention, and those should be identified quickly after pathogen emergence. These include:

The basic reproductive number (R_0): *The expected number of cases that are directly infected by a single index case in an immunologically naive population. This is a measure of the transmissibility of an emergent pathogen. When $R_0 > 1$, the pathogen can invade and spread in a population, causing a major epidemic or pandemic, whereas when $R_0 < 1$, the disease will die out. In the absence of control measures, R_0 also determines the final size of the epidemic.*

The reproductive number (R): *The expected number of secondary infections from a single infectious individual in a population with some underlying immunity.*

Generation time: *The time between successive generations of a disease, which is the time between a case becoming infected and that case causing infections.*

Serial interval: *The time between symptom onset in infector and infectee, which is approximately equal to the generation time.*

Doubling time:

Incubation period: *The time from infection to symptom onset.*

Latent period: *The time from infection to becoming infectious.*

Infectious period: *The length of time that an infected individual can transmit disease.*

Case fatality ratio: *The proportion of all cases that are fatal.*

Hospitalization rate/ Clinical attack rate: *The proportion of all cases in which manifestations of disease are severe enough to result in hospitalization, potentially affecting case detection via passive surveillance.*

Asymptomatic proportion: *The percent of infected individuals that do not develop recognizable symptoms.*

after one generation there will be an average of two influenza infections, and 15 measles infections and after three generations, there will be approximately eight influenza cases and 3375 measles infections. By contrast, MERS-CoV has been estimated to have an R_0 of 0.47 in humans; hence, infectious individuals will not (on average) be replaced with additional infections in the population, and human epidemics cannot be sustained without ongoing introductions from the animal reservoir (the likely reason why MERS-CoV has largely been confined to the Arabian peninsula).[5] However, it should be noted that transmission is a stochastic process, and R_0 may be higher in some settings than others; hence, limited epidemics are possible even when R_0 is less than one (see Section "Can we control a disease by targeting symptomatic infections?").[4]

BOX 2
Glossary of Modeling Terms

Agent-Based Model: *A class of computational models where individuals in the populations are represented as unique "agents" whose actions and interactions determine the spread of disease. In agent-based models, the actions of individuals often depend on their disease state.*

Compartmental Model: *A model that represents populations in different disease states (e.g., susceptible, infected, recovered, and immune) by a set of compartments with defined rates at which people transition between them. Populations within compartments are considered to be homogenous (i.e., there are no differences between individuals not captured by the compartment in which they currently reside).*

Deterministic Model: *A model defined by a set of mathematical equations that fully determine the behavioral system. In these models, the initial conditions of the model fully determine its subsequent behavior.*

Dynamic Model: *A model that captures the dynamic changes in disease behavior over time through a series of equations, computational simulations, or other means.*

Index Case: *The first case infected (or identified to be infected) in a population.*

Isolation: *The act of keeping individuals known to be infected with a disease separated from the larger population to prevent transmission.*

Mechanistic Model: *Any model that has specific structural or mathematical elements that attempt to capture the biological or population-level processes that drive disease spread. These contrast with purely associative statistical models.*

Quarantine: *The act of keeping individuals who have been exposed or potentially exposed to an infection isolated from the general population before they develop symptoms or are confirmed to be infected with a disease.*

Secondary Infection: *A person who is infected by another individual.*

Stochastic Model: *A model that captures the randomness in the disease process. In these models, multiple outcomes are possible from the same set of initial conditions.*

Susceptible individual: *An individual without immunity to infection.*

Since R_0 is shaped by the mechanisms underlying transmission (e.g., human contact patterns and viral aerosol dynamics), it will vary across populations and environmental conditions. Despite this, measurements of R_0 are remarkably consistent across settings for many pathogens (Table 1, Fig. 5), particularly those directly transmitted between humans. Environmental conditions have a larger impact on R_0 for vector-borne diseases such as dengue and Zika,[35,36] in many cases limiting their range.

TABLE 1
The Basic Reproductive Number and Generation Time for Multiple Diseases

Disease	R_0	Generation Time
Cholera	5.0,[6] 2.6[7] 4–15 ([8])	7.1–9.3 days,[9] 7–10 days ([8])
Dengue	1.3–6.3[10]	19–22 days,[11] 24 days[12]
Influenza	1.5–2[13]	3.6 days,[14] 2.3 days (H1N1) ,[15] 3.1 days (H3N2),[15] 2.7 day (H1N1 pdm)[13]
Malaria	1–10 Low transmission areas, 100–1000 High transmission areas,[8] 1–3000[16]	~60–120 days,[8] >200 days[16]
Measles	7.7,[17] 7.1–29.3,[18] 11–18[19]	9–17 days,[20] 12 days[21]
Rubella	2.9–7.8,[18] 3.4–5.6[22]	22 days,[22] 15–23 days[23]
SARS	2.7,[24] 1.2,[22] 2.2–3.6[25]	8.4 days[25]
Smallpox	3.2,[26] 3.5–6[27]	14–16 days,[26] 16 days,[28] 14–20 days[20]
MERS-CoV	0.47,[29] 0.8–1.3[30]	7–12 days[30]
ZIKV	1.3–1.4,[31] 4–12[32]	10–30 days[33,34]

Importantly, R_0 assumes universal susceptibility to a disease (i.e., no one in a population is immune due to previous exposure or vaccination). Transmissibility in a population where not everyone is susceptible due to preexisting immunity or active interventions is characterized by the effective reproductive number (R, sometimes simply called the reproductive number), which is the number of secondary infections caused by a single infected individual in a population with some level of immunity or protection against a disease.

While R_0 measures the fundamental potential of a pathogen in terms of causing an outbreak in a particular setting, R is a measure of the likelihood of an outbreak happening, or an epidemic continuing to grow, under current conditions in that setting. One key determinant of R is the proportion of the population that remains susceptible to a disease, as this determines the number of potentially infectious contacts that can occur. This principle leads to the simple relationship:

$$R = R_0 \times S$$

where S is the proportion of the population that remains susceptible. This relationship is key to evaluating control measures, as discussed in detail below. Variation in populations and individuals impacts these key relationships, as discussed in Section "Can we control a disease by targeting symptomatic infections?."

How Fast Will a Disease Spread? R_0 and the Generation Time

Understanding how quickly a disease will spread from person to person is especially useful in an emerging epidemic, as it provides insight into the expected number of cases in a given time, the potential geographic spread over that time, and how quickly a response must be implemented.[37] This speed of spread is dictated by the generation time of an infectious disease. The generation time is defined as the time between a case becoming infected and that case causing other infections. In combination, the reproductive number and the generation time are used to estimate how many new infections are expected over a given time period. For most diseases, it is impossible to determine the exact timing of infection under real-world conditions; hence, the generation time cannot be directly observed. Thus, the serial interval, which describes the time between symptom onset in successive generations, is usually used as a proxy for the generation time, as the two will have approximately the same distribution under a reasonable set of assumptions.

To illustrate how the combination of generation time and R_0 can be used to predict how quickly a disease will spread, we can contrast the spread of measles and influenza, two diseases with different generation times and basic reproductive numbers. Influenza has a generation time of approximately 3 days and an R_0 of two. Hence, a single case of influenza will on average generate two new cases of influenza over a period of 3 days, and the epidemic will grow by a factor of two every 3 days. Measles, on the other hand, has a much longer generation time of approximately 12 days and an R_0 of 15. A single case of measles will, therefore, on average generate 15 new cases of measles over a period of 12 days and continue to grow by a factor of 15 every 12 days. Although, on average, each incident case of measles will generate a greater number of infections than influenza, its growth will be much slower: after 12 days (4 generations of influenza and one generation of measles), there will be 16 influenza cases and 15 measles cases; and after 48 days (16 generations of influenza and 4 generations of measles), there will be 65,536 influenza cases and 50,625 measles cases.

A simple summary measure of the combined effect of R_0 and the generation time on the growth rate of an epidemic is the doubling time, that is, the time that it takes the number of cases to double. The doubling time relates to R_0 and the generation time by the formula:

$$T_d = \frac{\log 2}{\log \frac{R}{T_g}}$$

where T_d is the doubling time and T_g is the generation time. Accordingly, observation of the doubling time provides a pathway to the estimation of R_0 and the generation time.

How Large Will the Outbreak be? R_0 and the Final Epidemic Size

In addition to speed of spread, another important component of assessing disease impact is the expected final size (or expected final attack rate) of an uncontrolled epidemic. If we assume an epidemic is occurring in a well-mixed population (i.e., one where each individual in the population is equally likely to contact every other individual) without any interventions, the final size of an outbreak can be estimated from R_0[38,39] (see below). In practice, populations are usually not well mixed; hence, the final size will deviate from this simple relation. Despite some progress in characterizing patterns of mixing using novel data sources (further discussed below), the resolution of these analyses is generally insufficient to allow for the calibration of the effects of heterogeneity on final size. Alternative approaches, including leveraging statistical characterizations of the mapping between susceptible population and attack rate in particular settings,[40,41] have been deployed to adjust estimates of the final size. Even without such adjustments, the measure provides an important assessment of likely epidemic impact, giving what is likely an upper limit on the expected attack rate (though, in rare cases, it may be exceeded in small populations).

Tracking R over Time to Characterize the State of an Epidemic

As discussed above, when R is above one an epidemic will grow, and when R is below one it will decrease in size. However, it is not only whether R is above or below this critical threshold that matters, but its magnitude as well. For instance, if R is barely below one, the epidemic may persist for a long time, causing many cases, while if it is far below one, the epidemic will end rapidly. Likewise, when R is close to one, small changes in behavior or immunity may lead to changes in overall trajectory, while if R is far from one, larger changes would be needed to change the course of an outbreak.

For these reasons, the time-varying reproductive number, often denoted R_t, is often used in combination with more traditional metrics, such as case counts and hospitalization rates, to characterize the current state of an epidemic. Notably, R_t was frequently used for this purpose during the SARS-CoV-2 pandemic.[42,43] One reason R_t is useful is that it provides a summary measure about how the combination of current factors impacting transmission, including underlying immunity, inherent disease transmissibility, and control measures, are affecting disease spread. For instance, if control measures are lifted after cases drop to low levels and R_t the moves above one, this is a clear indicator that some measures may need to be reinstated to prevent a new epidemic wave. Conversely, if cases are high but R_t is below one, that is an indication that the combination of immunity and control is successfully curbing spread (though additional control measures may hasten epidemic decline and prevent cases). Another area where R_t has proven particularly useful is in assessing the likely impact of pathogen variants.[44,45] For instance, if a new variant in one part of the world leads to an increase in R_t in one part of the world through some combination of immune escape and increased intrinsic transmissibility, it can be expected to have a similar relative impact on the local R_t in other localities.

How Do We Measure R_0 and Generation Time?

Measuring R_0

Early in an epidemic, if the generation time or serial interval is known, R_0 can be estimated from the rate of epidemic growth (e.g., the doubling time of the epidemic). In other words, by assuming that the number of cases is increasing exponentially based on R_0 and the generation time, we can derive R_0 from the observed rate of growth.[46] During this early phase of the epidemic of a novel pathogen, nearly all hosts will be susceptible; hence, it is reasonable to assume that $R \approx R_0$. This assumption is likely true for many emerging infections or agents of bioterrorism, as it is unlikely that the population will have had any previous exposure or cross-immunity from other infections. If the population has previous immunity to the pathogen (perhaps from cross-reactivity with another pathogen), then the estimate obtained through this approach will reflect the reproductive number, R, rather than R_0. However, to some extent this distinction is academic, as in these settings R will also be the most relevant quantity in determining the course of the outbreak.

The exponential growth rate approach to estimating R_0 (Fig. 2A) has been used frequently in practice, including for pandemic H1N1, Ebola, and Zika,[13,47–49] and remains a linchpin in epidemic analysis. Nevertheless,

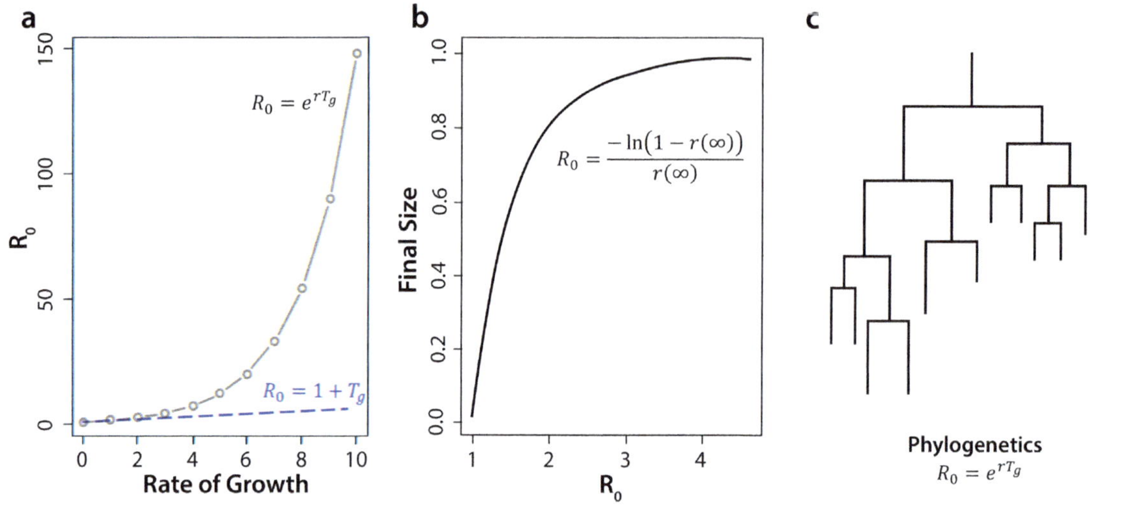

FIG. 2 Diagram of three ways to estimate R_0. The basic reproductive number can be estimated from three main sources. Panel (A) shows the curves for the two equations used to estimate the reproductive number from the initial exponential growth phase of an epidemic, which can be approximated linearly with the equation $R_0 = 1 + rT_g$, or from the equation $R_0 = e^{rT_g}$. Panel (B) shows the relationship between the final size of an epidemic and the basic reproductive number; by rearranging the final size equation in terms of R_0, we find that $R_0 = \frac{-\ln(1-r(\infty))}{r(\infty)}$. And Panel (C) illustrates estimating the reproductive number from phylogenetic distances between cases.

some factors present challenges to this approach, including a frequent subexponential growth phase early in an epidemic and an exponential growth phase that suggests an R_0 inconsistent with the final size of the epidemic.[50] In response, researchers have explored alternate methods for estimating R_0 from the initial rate of epidemic growth based on similar principles but accounting for the empirical deviations from exponential growth seen in practice.[51,52]

A second method for estimating R_0 is based on the final attack rate of an epidemic. By rearranging the final size equation (Fig. 2B), we see that R_0 can be estimated by the relation:

$$R_0 = \frac{-\ln(1-r(\infty))}{r(\infty)}$$

where $r(\infty)$ is the final attack rate. As this calculation requires knowledge of the final number of infected individuals in a complete, un-intervened upon epidemic, it may appear to be of limited utility in the context of emerging infections. However, in practice, it is often useful if there have been prior comparable epidemics or early outbreaks in closed populations. For example, when Zika virus (ZIKV) invaded the Americas in 2015, data on the American outbreak were limited both because many ZIKV infections are mild, asymptomatic, or cause non-specific symptoms, and because the ZIKV epidemic was not initially recognized as an important public health threat.[53] However, data from earlier outbreaks on Yap Island in 2007 and in French Polynesia in 2013–14 allowed for early estimates of R_0, including those derived from serology-based estimates of the final size of the outbreak.[31,53]

A third approach to estimating R_0 is to use the phylogenetic relationship between viral isolates (Fig. 2C, see Section Phylodynamics). This approach is based on the same principles as the exponential growth approach, but in this case, the rate of epidemic growth is estimated based on time-resolved phylogenetic trees and coalescent theory,[54] rather than growth in observed cases.

Another alternate approach to evaluating R_0 involves reasoning from core principles, which has been particularly useful for infections where features of the transmission process are measurable. For example, the transmission process for sexually transmitted infections is captured by the product of the average probability that a contact between an infected and susceptible individual results in a new infection (β), the duration of infectiousness (D), and the average rate at which new sexual partners are acquired (c), from which $R_0 = \beta cD$.[2] The distributions of c and D may be directly observed, opening the way to bounding the likely scope of R_0. However, it should be noted that this approach is still left with the difficult problem of estimating β, which may be as hard as estimating R_0 itself, and incorrect assumptions can lead to large errors in projection.

Measuring the generation time

For most infectious diseases, the time of infection is unobservable; hence, the generation time is impossible to measure directly. For this reason, the serial interval—the time between symptom onset in the infector and infectee—is generally measured instead. Assuming that the incubation periods of cases are independent given the timing of infection, the serial interval is an unbiased estimate of the generation time.

In practice, the serial interval can also be difficult to measure. Early in an epidemic, infector/infectee pairs can sometimes be identified, allowing the serial interval to be estimated directly (Fig. 3A).[13] Even when infection events cannot be directly identified, data on case clusters or series of infections in households can be used to estimate, or at least bound, the serial interval (Fig. 3B).[30,46] In the latter case, it is often assumed that all subsequent cases in a household were infected by the person who first developed symptoms in the household (i.e., the index case).

An alternative approach to estimating the generation time is to fit epidemic models to epidemic curves (Fig. 3C) and thus simultaneously estimate transmission parameters (e.g., R_0, providing another approach beyond those listed above) and the generation time.[55] Refinements of this approach include likelihood-based approaches that incorporate mechanistic aspects of the transmission process from epidemic theory[56] and "data augmentation" techniques that use Markov-Chain Monte Carlo methods to integrate over the possible transmission trees that could have led to the epidemic.[5] All methods are comparatively data intensive, which is one of the reasons the generation time is one of the key sources of uncertainty early in an epidemic of an emerging pathogen.

Measuring R over time

Like estimating R_0, there are several ways to estimate R_t. Many of the widely-used approaches are adaptations of a method presented by Wallinga and Teunis,[57] which estimates the reproductive number at each time step of incidence, generally this is per day, using case incidence data and the distribution of the serial interval. Conceptually, this method estimates case likely symptom onset times as infected by cases observed on a particular day and uses the ratio of cases observed on those future days to the cases observed on the day of interest to estimate R_t. In its precise mathematical form, this is calculated by:

$$p_{ij} = \frac{N_i w(t_i - t_j)}{\Sigma_{i \neq k} N_i w(t_i - t_j)}.$$

where p_{ij} is the probability that case i with onset at time and t_i was infected by case j with onset at time t_j. The effective reproductive number for case j is $R_j = \Sigma_i p_{ij}$ and is averaged as $R_t = \frac{1}{N_t} \Sigma_{\{t_j = t\}} R_j$. However, like R_0 estimates,

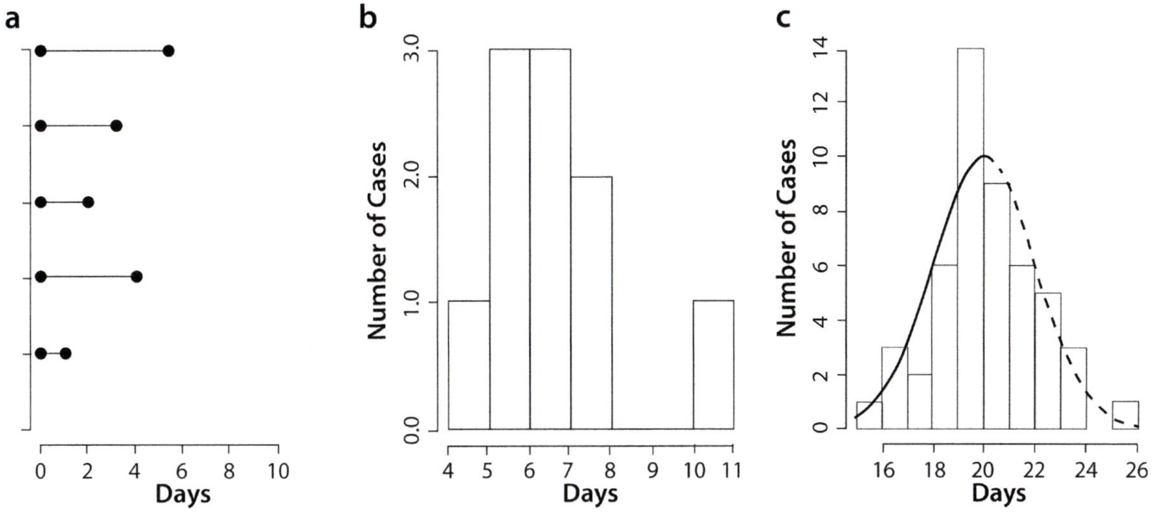

FIG. 3 Diagram of the three ways to estimate the generation time. Panel (A) shows how generation time can be directly estimated when pairs of cases (points) are known to be linked (*horizontal lines*) and where the timing of the onset of infection for both members of each pair is known (*x* axis); panel (B) shows data typical of a household outbreak, where the time of infection of the primary case in the household is known and timing of infection of secondary cases in the household is then tracked (*x* axis), and it is assumed that the primary infectee is responsible for the bulk of secondary infections; and panel (C) shows how the generation time can be estimated by fitting an epidemic model to population-level incidence data.

estimates of R_t are heavily dependent on the generation time estimate, and because R_t compares the growth rate over a time window, estimates of R_t are inherently right-censored. Adaptations of this method have been implemented in several widely-used statistical packages (e.g., EpiEstim[58]).

Another approach, presented by White and Pageno[59] and others, uses maximum likelihood to estimate the daily reproductive number, using a sequence of consecutive incident cases, and a generation time distribution. This method assumes that the number of cases produced each day is Poisson distributed with the expected value of R_t. However, this approach assumes that the first case is included in the estimates, as the reproductive number will be overestimated. If this is not the case, secondary cases will be assigned to too few index cases.

How Strong Does an Intervention Need to Be to Stop Spread?

In responding to, or preparing for an outbreak, we not only want to know how serious the epidemic might be, but we also want to gain insight into what needs to be done to stop or mitigate spread. Here too, R_0 is key to our understanding. Epidemic theory tells us that a disease will begin to die out once R falls below one, as cases will no longer replace themselves in the population.[4] Hence, any intervention that reduces transmission by a factor of $1/R_0$ or more will cause a reduction in incidence that will eventually lead to the elimination of the pathogen (although the stronger the intervention, the faster it will work). Applications of this principle depend on understanding how effective an intervention is at reducing R, which may be difficult to determine (see below).

Although likely of limited utility in the context of emerging infections and agents of bioterrorism (with smallpox as a notable exception), vaccines provide the canonical example of this approach. Based on R_0 we can calculate the "critical vaccination threshold," defined as the proportion of the population that must be *successfully* vaccinated to prevent a disease from spreading widely in a population. Based on the principle that a population will be protected when R falls below one, we can show that the critical vaccination threshold, V_c, is equal to $1-1/R_0$. Thus, for influenza, the ($R_0=2$) $V_c=0.5$, and for measles, the ($R_0=15$) $V_c=0.93$.

The critical vaccination threshold is a special case of the more general concept of "herd immunity," which is sometimes used synonymously. Herd immunity describes the extent of indirect protection that susceptible individuals in a population receive from the immunity of others in the population and begins to manifest even before the critical vaccination threshold is reached,[60] and can continue to accumulate at higher levels of protection.

The same principle can be used to estimate the ability of prophylactic chemotherapy to control an outbreak. For instance, if we presume that prophylactic use of oseltamivir reduces the risk of influenza infection by 50%[61] and that the R_0 of an emerging influenza is 1.5, we would have to administer antivirals to two-thirds ($2\times[1-1/1.5]$) of the population in order to prevent the spread of the disease. Of course, unlike vaccination, in the case of prophylactic drugs, the protective effects go away as soon as the intervention is stopped.

The ability of interventions that shorten an individual's infectious period, such as treatment or isolation of symptomatic cases, to interrupt transmission can be similarly analyzed. Assuming the probability of transmission is constant throughout the infectious period, such interventions will reduce R by the same fraction that they reduce the average infectious period. For instance, if, by treating infection, we reduce the time of viral shedding by an average of 1/3, we would also reduce R_0 by 1/3. However, the performance of such "case-based" interventions depends on our ability to identify cases before they transmit (see below).

Behavior changes and physical distancing measures such as school closure also reduce R_0 by reducing the probability of an infectious contact.[62] Here, the reduction in R_0 is equivalent to the reduction in the expected rate of infectious contacts. Therefore, if half of infectious contacts occurred in schools, closing schools would reduce R by 50%, though such analyses are complicated by the fact that these contacts might be replaced with equally infectious contacts elsewhere. In practice, it is harder to know how effective social distancing measures will be, and estimates of their impact often must be based on models that range in complexity from simple compartmental models that can be run in an Excel spreadsheet (e.g.,[63]) to complex agent-based models that attempt to capture the behavior of everyone in a population (e.g.,[64]), as illustrated in the case studies later in this chapter.

Can We Control a Disease by Targeting Symptomatic Infections?

When analyzing the effectiveness of interventions that rely on identifying and directly intervening on cases (case-based interventions), properties of an infectious disease's natural history become central. Of particular interest are when and if people develop symptoms in the course of their infections (the incubation period and asymptomatic ratio) and the timing and length of infectiousness (the latent and infectious periods).

Case-based interventions can be divided into two categories: interventions that focus on limiting the number of secondary cases caused by individuals who have already become symptomatic and those that attempt to intervene on possible secondary cases before they become symptomatic. Examples of the former include isolation of symptomatic cases and treatment with drugs aimed at shortening the infectious period, while the latter is exemplified by the quarantine or prophylactic treatment of contacts of known symptomatic cases (or other individuals with a high probability of being infected). Whether targeting symptomatic infections will work depends on the proportion of infections that occur before symptom onset (or from asymptomatic infections), which Fraser and colleagues denote Θ.[65] For diseases such as HIV, where the latent period is much shorter than the incubation period, Θ is high; by contrast, Θ will be low for diseases such as smallpox, where it is exceedingly rare for a case to cause an infection prior to developing symptoms. The combination of Θ and R_0 determines the possible success of case-based interventions (Fig. 4). When Θ is high, cases cannot be identified before transmission, so isolation or treatment are doomed to fail. Likewise, if R_0 is high, the sheer number of cases will overwhelm the ability of interventions to work. As a limit, if $\theta \times R_0 > 1$ even the most efficient possible intervention based on targeting symptomatic cases cannot effectively stop an epidemic.

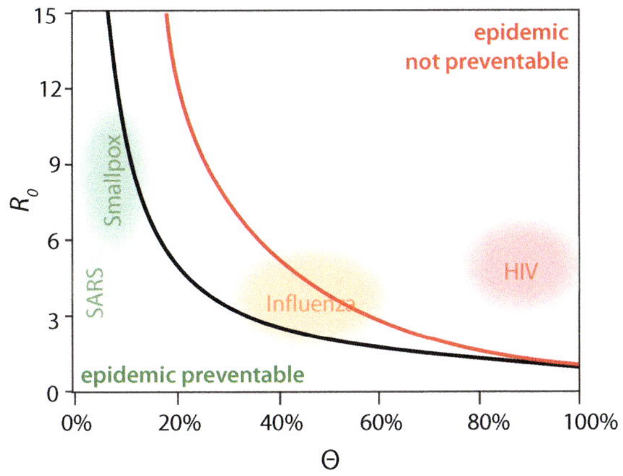

FIG. 4 Potential performance of maximally effective (100%) case-based interventions, with example diseases shown across a range of theta, or the proportion of cases that occur before symptom onset (*x* axis) and R_0 (*y* axis). Curves represent the performance of isolation alone (*black*) and isolation plus quarantine (*red*). For diseases lying in the area below the curve, an outbreak can be prevented using interventions based on symptomatic cases, while those lying above the curve cannot be controlled using these methods alone. (Adapted from Fraser C, Riley S, Anderson RM, Ferguson NM. Factors that make an infectious disease outbreak controllable. *Proc Natl Acad Sci U S A*. 2004;101:6146–6151.)

Quarantine or prophylactic treatment of potentially infected contacts can improve the efficiency of case-based interventions, though their effectiveness will also be determined by aspects of the disease's natural history.[65,66] In particular, the length of the incubation period and infectious period have a strong impact on both the feasibility of quarantine and its added value over strategies that target symptomatic cases, with quarantine providing the most benefits for diseases with a rapid course and/or infectiousness proceeding symptom onset.[66] When available, prophylactic treatment has similar properties to quarantine in terms of the additional benefits provided, and settings for effective use.

A less intensive approach to following up potentially infected individuals is "active monitoring," where those at high risk of infection are contacted on a regular basis (usually daily) to determine if they are showing symptoms of illness. Notably, this approach was used in the United States to monitor for Ebola virus infections in those returning from West Africa during the 2014–16 epidemic.[67] The relative benefits of active monitoring vs quarantine depend on the same factors that determine the benefits of quarantine mentioned above.[66] The optimal length, performance, and cost effectiveness of active monitoring approaches are defined by the serial interval and the frequency and cost of false positives (non-cases identified as possible cases) and false negatives (cases that develop symptoms outside of the monitoring period).[67]

Two of the key references cited above have companion web tools that can be used by practitioners to help decide the best way to approach disease control in an emergent epidemic.[66,67] These are available at: http://iddynamics.jhsph.edu/apps/shiny/activemonitr/ and https://coreypeak.shinyapps.io/InteractiveQuarantine.

How Do Differences Between People and Populations Impact Epidemics?

Individual-level heterogeneity

When estimating R_0, we work in average quantities, assuming the *average* number of secondary infections from an *average* infected individual. However, heterogeneity exists between individuals and settings that can affect infectious disease dynamics. For example, R_0 estimates for severe acute respiratory syndrome (SARS) range from 1.2 to 3.6. However, some individuals caused upwards of 33 secondary infections through what are termed "super-spreading events." This heterogeneity in transmission has important implications for pathogen spread, but also the success of control measures, with it being particularly important to identify settings and individuals prone to super-spreading events. For infections like SARS, with numerous, well-documented super-spreading events, individually targeted control is far more effective than population-wide control measures. Lloyd-Smith et al.[68] showed that the efficacy of control could be improved by up to threefold if half of all control efforts focused on the 20% of individuals associated with the most infectious transmission events compared to random control efforts. Importantly, these individual-level heterogeneities are masked by population-level analyses such as the estimation of R_0, which rely on average quantities; hence, more detailed epidemiologic analysis is needed for their estimation (Fig. 5).

Population structure

The classical calculation and applications of R_0 assume a well-mixed population of individuals. Most populations are structured in ways that modulate mixing: subsets of individuals may be more or less likely to encounter each other. Heterogeneities associated with super-spreading events provide one extreme example of differences in contacts across individuals within populations that might be obscured in population-level analyses and have important implications for both patterns of spread and the impact of control efforts (see above). Another very common aspect of populations that may structure contact (and thus R_0) is assortative mixing (i.e., individuals being more likely to contact those with similar characteristics) whether by age,[69] behaviors,[70,71] household structure[72]), or other factors. These heterogeneities can lead to deviations in the course of epidemics from classic epidemic theory (e.g., increasing speed of spread while reducing final attack size,[72] driving the distribution of disease and adverse outcomes,[69] and influencing the most effective way to target interventions.[73]

Projection of pathogen dynamics or inference into core parameters such as R_0 that ignore such underlying heterogeneities will be biased. For HIV, for example, assuming homogeneous mixing yields estimates of $R_0 = 4$, whereas deriving R_0 from a structured social network yields estimates of $R_0 = 22$.[70] Similarly, for vaccination behavior, individuals who are unvaccinated may cluster spatially, leaving pockets of individuals vulnerable to disease outbreaks that an assumption of homogeneity would miss.[71] Yet, heterogeneity in mixing may be hard to quantify, for example, where it involves stigmatized behaviors. Further, even where measurable heterogeneity exists (e.g., in contact over age), what we can measure (e.g., time spent in conversation) is generally only a proxy for transmission.

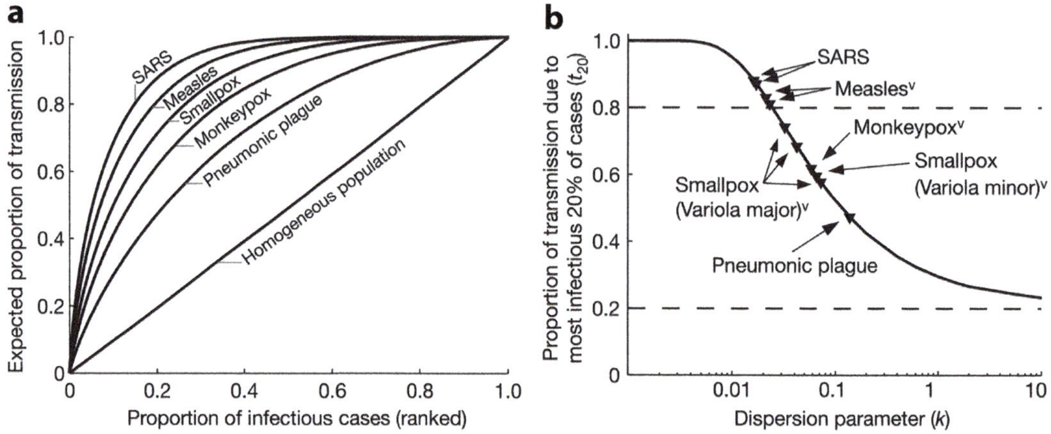

FIG. 5 (A) Expected proportion of all transmission that can be attributed to a given proportion of infectious cases. When all individuals are the same (i.e., a homogeneous population), the relationship is linear. For these five directly transmitted infections, the line is concave, a result of variation in the number of contacts an individual has. (B) Proportion of all transmission that can be expected from the top 20% most infectious cases shown for 10 outbreaks or surveillance data sets (*triangles*). The *top dashed line* shows the proportions expected under the "80/20 rule," and the *bottom dashed line* shows the proportion expected when all individuals are the same (homogeneity). The superscript "v" indicates a partially vaccinated population. (Reprint from Lloyd-Smith JO, Schreiber SJ, Kopp PE, Getz WM. Superspreading and the effect of individual variation on disease emergence. *Nature*. 2005;438:355.)

Inferential tools are required to evaluate the degree to which measured heterogeneity translates into infectious disease outcomes in situations where relative timing of cases is rarely available.[74] However, known sources of heterogeneity, such as age-assortative social mixing, household structure, and geographic clustering, are known to exist in nearly every setting; hence, it should be understood that deviations from classical dynamics are expected.

CASE STUDIES IN PREPAREDNESS

Smallpox

Smallpox was an acute, highly contagious disease caused by the *Variola* virus (see Chapter 6 for more detail). Before smallpox was officially declared eradicated in 1980,[75] this devastating disease caused infected individuals to develop fever and a progressive, disfiguring maculopapular rash, and death occurred in 30%–35% of cases.[76] Although the last known natural infection occurred in 1977, small quantities of smallpox virus still exist in research laboratories in the United States and Russia. The severity of smallpox, coupled with the fact that the smallpox vaccine has not been in use in the United States since 1972, makes use of the smallpox virus as an agent of bioterrorism a credible concern: the interruption of smallpox vaccination programs combined with an absence of natural infection means that susceptibility to smallpox is likely to characterize the bulk of both the US and the global population, and an outbreak could potentially be devastating.[77]

The key public health question that modeling can help address is the best strategy to contain a smallpox outbreak. Would isolation of cases be sufficient? Is tracing and vaccination of contacts likely to be helpful? What are the costs and benefits of mass vaccination? Side-effects associated with the smallpox vaccine make this a question requiring particular care.[78,79] Framing models to address these questions requires detailed understanding of the natural history of the infection. Estimates of R_0 vary widely, ranging from as low as 1.5 to as high as 20[27,77,80,81]; details of generation time, heterogeneity in transmission, and timing of symptoms relative to infectiousness are indicated by previous outbreaks,[78,79] and variability and uncertainty in these estimates make exploring their impact on model outcomes (i.e., "sensitivity analysis") essential.[78,79] Given the nuance of intervention strategies that are of interest in evaluating the outcome of the use of smallpox as a bioterrorism agent, appropriate modeling also requires some detail on human mobility and connectivity, including aspects such as connectivity of health care workers. Given this necessary level of detail, agent-based or individual models were broadly deployed to tackle this question.[78,79] For example, an individual based simulation combined with extensive sensitivity analysis indicated that case isolation and contact tracing with vaccination would be sufficient to halt ongoing transmission following release in the United Kingdom.[78,79]

Anthrax

Anthrax, a disease caused by the bacteria *Bacillus anthracis*, affects domestic and wild animals worldwide (see Chapter 2 for more detail). Historically, anthrax in humans was caused by close contact with animals or animal products,[82] and modern industrial hygiene has dramatically reduced the number of cases in the United States. People or animals can become infected with anthrax by inhaling or ingesting spores, or if spores get into a cut or scrape, and subsequent infection can occur in one of four forms: cutaneous, gastrointestinal, inhalation, or injection. The deadliest form of anthrax infection is inhalation anthrax, which has a 50%–80% mortality rate with treatment.[82] Infection of this kind usually develops within 1 week of exposure but can take up to 2 months; symptoms include fever, chest pains, and shortness of breath.

While natural infection with anthrax is rare, nearly 20 countries have developed anthrax into a bioterrorism weapon.[83] The first confirmed outbreak associated with the intentional release of anthrax in the United States occurred in October 2001, first affecting a journalist in Florida.[82] Shortly afterwards, a letter containing anthrax spores was mailed to a US Senator, resulting in five cases of inhalational anthrax among postal workers in a Washington, DC, postal center.[83] The outbreak did not spread further: although anthrax is a devastating disease, acquiring infection requires direct contact with anthrax spores, infection does not occur from coming into contact with a person who is currently infected with anthrax.[84] Because person-to-person transmission does not occur (i.e., $R_0 = 0$), models of anthrax focus on the number exposed in a single bioterrorism event and the natural history of infection rather than the dynamic properties that are a focus of classical dynamic models.

While the dynamics of an anthrax attack would not be driven by the transmission parameters captured in the classical modeling toolkit, there are important aspects of disease dynamics that are important to capture. Hence, models of anthrax transmission aim to understand how anthrax may spread when aerosolized[85] or when letters containing anthrax spores are sent through the mail system.[86] These models show that even a relatively small volume of anthrax spores might quickly distribute lethal doses. Further, where anthrax is sent through the mail system, cross-contamination of letters is likely and has the potential to result in many deaths in individuals not directly targeted by an attack. The impact of an attack depends not only on the number exposed but also on the dose of anthrax inhaled. Dose–response models aim to quantify the relationship between the probability of infection in the host (response) and the magnitude of the exposure (dose).[87] Together, these models provide key insights into the dynamics of anthrax transmission across a population and how to target control efforts.

Antibiotic prophylaxis is the primary tool for combating an anthrax attack. A statistical model of the 2001 outbreak[88] estimated that antibiotic prophylaxis following the attack prevented half of the possible deaths. However, the potential adverse consequences of widespread antibiotic use raised the question of the optimum duration of antibiotic prophylaxis. Use of a competing risk model[89] showed that the optimal duration of antibiotic prophylaxis depends on the exposure dose, with the highest exposure doses requiring greater than 4 months of antibiotic prophylaxis, whereas 60 days of antibiotic prophylaxis is sufficient for lower exposure doses.

Models have also been used to examine how antibiotics should be stockpiled, stored, and dispensed.[90] These models show that the most effective response to an outbreak is local stockpiling of antibiotics. In particular, a doubling of the local stockpile with higher dispensing capacity significantly reduced the cost per life year gained.[90–92]

Pandemic Influenza

Influenza is a highly transmissible, rapidly mutating respiratory virus spread by droplets created when infected individuals talk, cough, or sneeze (see Chapters 7 and 8 for more detail). Though influenza typically undergoes frequent antigenic mutations that cause yearly epidemics, influenza antigens occasionally experience more rapid and drastic changes that result in the emergence of novel strains (an occurrence known as antigenic shift). Although pandemics are rare, only four have occurred since 1918, they can cause significant morbidity and mortality. Most notably, the 1918 influenza pandemic caused over 300,000 deaths in the United States[93] and over 20 million worldwide, compared to 12,000–56,000 deaths in the US during a typical influenza season.[94] Consequently, pandemic preparedness has been the focus of most influenza modeling efforts.[a]

In 2003, a resurgence of highly pathogenic H5N1 influenza in domestic poultry and associated infections of humans raised concerns of a nascent 1918 influenza pandemic.[97] Human infections with this virus had occurred before (in 1997), and the increasing frequency of such infections raised concerns that the virus could mutate and have sustained transmission in human hosts—a particularly frightening prospect given that the observed case fatality ratio for H5N1 is ~60%.[98] Because of the inherent lack of epidemiologic data, dynamic models were the primary tool for planning the response to a potential pandemic of a novel avian influenza strain.[64,99–101] As vaccines would likely be unavailable for many months following initial person-to-person spread, modeling efforts focused on assessing the effectiveness of physical distancing measures, travel restrictions, and prophylactic use of antiviral drugs.

Initial modeling efforts aimed to see whether, if infections were detected early enough, a nascent pandemic in southeast Asia (the location of most H5N1 cases at the time) could be contained. Using structured stochastic simulation models[100] and geographically explicit agent-based models[64] of Thailand, two groups independently showed that one to three million courses of antiviral prophylaxis and treatment combined with physical distancing, quarantine, and other non-pharmaceutical interventions (NPIs) could halt an emerging pandemic so long as R_0 was less than 1.6–1.8. As the precise properties of an emerging influenza virus were unknown, each group considered a range of values for critical quantities such as the serial interval, asymptomatic ratio, and reproductive number, informed by previous pandemics, and performed extensive sensitivity analyses.

Critically, this exercise showed that early detection (i.e., within the first 20 days of an outbreak) was likely needed for successful containment.[64,100] Hence, detection of less pathogenic strains was unlikely to occur quickly enough to be contained, and even containment of highly pathogenic influenza was far from assured. Models of mitigation strategies applied in the United States when a strain was uncontained were, therefore,

[a]It is of note that while the primary focus of influenza research has been on natural emergence of pandemic strains, recent "gain-of-function" experiments in ferrets that led to an airborne version of the highly pathogenic H5N1 virus[95,96] raise concern that influenza could also be used as an agent of bioterrorism.

performed.[99,101] These studies suggested that border and travel restrictions might slightly delay, but would do little to dampen, an epidemic. However, other strategies showed promise. School closures could reduce peak attack rates by as much as 40% but would be unlikely to lessen the final size of the epidemic.[101] Quarantine and isolation of exposed or infected individuals could be effective, and targeted use of antivirals in the households of infected individuals could reduce clinical attack rates by as much as half. Likewise, widespread use of even a weakly efficacious vaccine could substantially reduce the impact of an influenza pandemic.[99]

This and subsequent work illustrate the critical role that highly detailed agent-based models can play in preparing for hypothetical disease threats, for which any empirical data from an emergence event would come too late to be of use. Based in part on this work, several countries, including the United States and the United Kingdom, began keeping a strategic stockpile of antiviral drugs to combat an emerging flu pandemic (though some have questioned this decision based on concerns about drug efficacy[102]). This work also helped guide the response in 2009, when an H1N1 pandemic did occur (see below).

CASE STUDIES IN EPIDEMIC RESPONSE

This section illustrates how mathematical models can inform efforts to understand transmission patterns of infectious disease and to control their spread, using examples from infectious diseases emerging during the past decade. In the past decade, there have been several viral emergence events where mathematical modeling was used to inform the public health response, including the 2009 pandemic of novel H1N1 influenza, the emergence of Middle East Respiratory Syndrome-associated coronavirus (MERS-CoV) in the Arabian peninsula, the Ebola virus outbreak in West Africa, and the epidemic of ZIKV in the Americas. These infections differ in terms of key transmission features.

Pandemic H1N1 (2009)

In April 2009, a novel H1N1 influenza strain first emerged in Mexico before rapidly spreading worldwide (see Chapter 7 for more detail). By mid-June, the WHO raised the pandemic alert to the highest level, phase 6,[103] declaring the first pandemic of the 21st century. The novel H1N1 influenza (H1N1pdm) stain had been circulating in the swine population before crossing into the human population.[104] Although, like seasonal influenza, the lack of previous exposure to the virus or a similar virus (immunity) and the impact on otherwise healthy individuals made this influenza strain's pandemic potential a much more serious threat.[105]

The emergence of H1N1pdm raised serious concerns about the potential for a devastating global pandemic, particularly given that this was the same strain that caused the deadly 1918 influenza pandemic. The size, severity, and transmissibility of this new epidemic were initially unclear; hence, resolving these uncertainties was a critical goal of the first dynamic models fit to the event.[55] This early work attempted to triangulate these key quantities using three primary sources of information: pathogen genetics, observation of a "complete" outbreak in some settings, and patterns of incidence in international travelers. These analyses suggested H1N1pdm emerged in humans around January 12, 2009 (95% credible interval [CrI]: November 3, 2008 to March 2, 2009) and had infected 23,000 (range: 6000 to 32,000) people in Mexico by late April 2009.[55] The case fatality ratio was estimated to be 0.4% (range: 0.3%–1.8%).

Assuming that the generation time was like seasonal influenza, R_0 was estimated between 1.31 and 1.42 based on the rate of exponential growth,[55] consistent with what was seen in previous pandemics. Qualitatively similar results were obtained from sophisticated Bayesian estimation methods ($R_0 = 1.40$, 95% CrI: 1.15 to 1.90), estimates based on pathogen genetics (1.22, 95% CrI: 1.05 to 1.60), and a model allowing for heterogeneous and age-dependent mixing ($R_0 = 1.58$, 95% CI: 1.34–2.04).[55] Detailed analysis of a locally completed outbreak also provided an early, independent estimate of the mean generation time (Tg = 1.91 days, 95% CI: 1.30–2.71 days).[55]

As the epidemic progressed, analyses of data from the United States, Canada, the United Kingdom, and the European Union found an upper bound on the case fatality ratio ranging from 0.20% to 0.68%, though there were suggestions of case fatality rates as high as 1.2% (95% CI: 1.0%–1.5%) in Mexico.[106,107] Using data from households and schools in the United States, the lower bound of R_0 was estimated to be around 1.3 to 1.7 and the upper bound as high as 2.1.[106] Using maximum likelihood methods on data from Mexico, R_0 was estimated to be 2.3 (95% CI: 2.1–2.5), and the generation time was estimated to be Tg = 3.2 days (95% CI: 3.0 days to 3.5 days).[106] In a study on influenza-like illness in a New York high school, the within-school reproductive number of H1N1pdm was estimated to be 3.3 (95% CI, 3.0–3.6), and the secondary attack rate in households with at least one confirmed case was 17.7% (95% CI, 14.1–21.8), implying a probability of household transmission of 0.14 (95% CI, 0.11–0.18).[13]

Pandemic H1N1 2009 influenza highlights the critical ways that the assumptions of a priori modeling of emergency events can be wrong. Prior to 2009, pandemic preparedness activities had largely focused on the highly pathogenic H5N1 avian influenza, assumed emergence would most likely occur in southeast Asia, that the new strain would be a different subtype than the currently circulating strain, and it would be highly pathogenic.[64,100,101] The 2009 influenza pandemic did not meet any of these expectations, though these previous modeling efforts still played an important role in informing new work that helped guide the response to the 2009 H1N1 pandemic.

MERS-CoV

The novel coronavirus, MERS-CoV, was first identified in 2012 in patients from, or having recently visited, the Arabian peninsula (see Chapter 10 for more detail).[108,109] Early identification of a cluster of household transmission proved the virus could be transmitted between humans,[108] prompting concerns that the virus could spark a global pandemic. Additional clusters of hospital[110] and family[111] transmission in Saudi Arabia throughout 2013 further fueled these concerns, and a large uptick in cases in late spring 2014 caused great concern about global spread, particularly given the number of people who travel to Saudi Arabia for the Hajj.[112] However, the 2014 epidemic receded, and as of late 2017, sustained circulation of MERS-CoV has remained largely confined to the Arabian Peninsula; though the evolution of the virus during ongoing infections of humans raises concerns that it may someday evolve into a pandemic threat.

Early analyses focused on characterizing the dynamic properties of MERS-CoV, including R_0 and the generation time, to determine its pandemic potential. Analysis of an early hospital cluster provided early estimates of the median incubation period (5.2 days; 95% CI, 1.9–14.7) and serial interval (7.6 days; 95% CI 2.5–23.1).[110] A review of the overall epidemic provided additional estimates for these epidemiologic measures and the first estimates of R_0, the CFR, and the asymptomatic ratio for MERS-CoV. Cauchemez et al. analyzed the size of clusters of MERS-CoV transmission (particularly travel-related cases) and phylogenetic data from seven early sequences to estimate that the CFR was around 20% (95% CI, 7–42) and that the R_0 among secondary cases was 0.63 (95% CI, 0.47–0.85).[30] They did find evidence for a higher R_0 among cluster index cases (1.25 or 0.83 depending on the assumptions used), perhaps due to bias toward detecting clusters with at least one secondary case. A contemporaneous analysis by Chowell et al. based on fitting stochastic models to final outbreak size found similar results, estimating an overall R_0 of 0.45 (95% CI, 0.29–0.61) and an R_0 for index cases of 0.88 (95% CI, 0.58–1.20).[113] These early results suggested that MERS-CoV did not transmit efficiently enough for sustained transmission; hence, it was not an immediate pandemic threat, and highlighted the likely importance of the (then unknown) camel reservoir in sustaining transmission.

Additional concern about the MERS-CoV threat was sparked by a substantial increase in case reports in Saudi Arabia in spring 2014 and a large multi-hospital associated outbreak in South Korea in 2015. A particular worry in the former case was the potential for a large outbreak during the Hajj, as incidence had been concentrated in areas frequented by pilgrims. However, analysis showed that the long generation time made a substantial outbreak among pilgrims unlikely,[112] though exported cases were a concern. The 2014 epidemic also allowed a more detailed analysis of MERS-CoV dynamics, which largely confirmed previous results: data augmentation techniques suggested R_0 was around 0.45 (95% CI: 0.33–0.58) and the mean serial interval was 6.8 (95% CI: 6.0–7.8).[5] Likewise, statistical models aimed at estimating the hidden burden of MERS-CoV showed about 20% (22%, 95% CI, 18–25) of those infected with MERS-CoV died and that around 50% went unobserved,[114] and illustrated the substantial heterogeneity by age in the probability of developing clinical symptoms or death. The 2015 MERS-CoV outbreak in South Korea is the largest to date outside of the Arabian peninsula (186 cases) and had similar disease dynamics to previous outbreaks, though perhaps a slightly longer serial interval (CFR of 21%, mean serial interval 12.6 days).[115] Kucharski et al. analyzed this outbreak in light of previous estimates of R_0 and showed that the size was not inconsistent with these previous estimates,[29] thereby illustrating an important point: While an $R_0 < 1$ precludes sustained epidemic or pandemic spread, it is still possible to have outbreaks of a size that require a significant (and expensive) public health response.

Ebola Virus

In March 2014, when the World Health Organization was first notified of an outbreak in Guinea, the *Ebola virus* was thought to be a fairly well-characterized threat, of greatest concern in a limited area in East Africa, with little potential for spread (see Chapter 5 for more detail). The international community was slow to respond to its emergence in West Africa, and tragically, the subsequent rate and scale of spread proved much greater than had seemed plausible based on previous experience with this pathogen.[116] The foundation for modeling this outbreak was based on analysis of cases reported up to September 2014, which indicated an incubation period of ~11 days, a serial interval of ~15 days, and a R_0 between 1.4 and 2.3; all of which was in line with previous estimates.[117] In retrospect, a likely failure of surveillance to detect early cases allowed for explosive growth of the epidemic in a context of mobile populations, dysfunctional health systems, and local customs that enhanced spread.[118]

Despite the scale of this outbreak, extremely pessimistic forecasts generated early during the outbreak far outstripped the case numbers observed.[63] This was partially a result of the impact of control efforts (indeed, model projections encompassing control efforts were much more in line with observed patterns). A mismatch also emerged because of hard-to-anticipate behavioral changes, which likely slowed the speed of transmission. Despite these challenges and uncertainties, forecasts from early models likely proved important for galvanizing the international community during the first phases of the Ebola outbreak. Modeling also played an extensive role in strategic comparisons of implemented mitigation strategies. By building mechanistic model framings of different interventions, researchers were able to compare the impact of case isolation, contact tracing with quarantine, and sanitary funeral practices,[119] to the impact of travel bans and exit and entry screening at airports.[120] In addition, such models quantified the degree to which bed capacity was sufficient to meet the needs at individual phases of the epidemic,[121] all of which contributed to informing public health and other policy decisions.

Beginning with the early days of the Ebola outbreak and in tandem with deploying the "classic" dynamical modeling toolset (applied to case counts, etc.), viral genetic sequences were analyzed. This revealed that the outbreak represented a single spillover event (rather than several introductions into the population) and shed light on the degree of mixing across the three primarily affected countries.[122] As transmission and cases declined, the public health focus shifted to developing a more nuanced understanding of sporadic outbreaks. Increasingly tractable approaches to data collection (e.g., real-time, portable genome sequencing approaches[123]) provided data of sufficient resolution to evaluate Ebola virus re-introduction patterns, as well as cluster size over the course of the epidemic,[124] proving a valuable alternative window onto the transmission dynamics.

As the prospects for the development of an Ebola vaccine became more likely, even as case numbers were falling, mathematical models were used to evaluate how vaccine trials could be most effectively deployed.[125]

Zika Virus

Zika virus (ZIKV), a flavivirus transmitted primarily by *Aedes* mosquitoes, was long considered a relatively innocuous pathogen because of its generally asymptomatic or mild infections. However, in 2015 the virus became cause for greater concern[126] when a correlation between ZIKV infection and congenital defects was observed in Brazil. Additionally, concerning was the correlation between ZIKV and Guillain-Barre Syndrome (GBS), a severe neurological condition, initially observed in the French Polynesian Islands in 2012–13.[127] The seemingly sudden appearance and rapid spread of highly detrimental complications related to infection with ZIKV necessitated prompt action to control the spread of the virus, develop surveillance systems to monitor infections, and protect pregnant women from infection. However, due to the asymptomatic to mildly symptomatic presentation and the similarity to other widespread flaviviruses, including dengue and chikungunya, many cases of ZIKV had gone unrecognized. Consequently, the clinical and epidemiological data required to implement interventions were sparse. In this context, quantitative models became essential for improving understanding of the pathogenesis and transmission dynamics of ZIKV.

In the investigation of ZIKV, epidemiologic and dynamical models were used to quantify the risk of GBS and microcephaly among those infected, to forecast the speed at which the epidemic would evolve, and to predict the areas at risk of ZIKV introduction. To estimate the risk of GBS among people infected with ZIKV, it was necessary to calculate the total number of people infected (i.e., ZIKV incidence), but such a calculation was complicated by two factors: first, ZIKV cases can be difficult to diagnose and identify, and second, at the time, serological tests were not specific enough to distinguish ZIKV from dengue virus. Models were used to adjust estimates of ZIKV incidence by making assumptions about the proportion of cases reported, which allowed investigators to calculate the risk of developing GBS upon infection with ZIKV. For the 2015 outbreak in the Americas, models estimated the risk of GBS ranged from 1 to 8 cases per 10,000 infections, yet uncertainties remained regarding inter-country variation in risk.[31,128]

In addition to the difficulties involved in calculating the risk of GBS, calculating the risk of microcephaly was difficult because, prior to the ZIKV epidemic, no standard definition of microcephaly existed and tools for diagnosing the condition were limited.[129] Further, early prospectively collected data showed that the risk of developing fetal abnormalities among pregnant women with laboratory-confirmed ZIKV infections was 29%. However, a small sample of only 42 pregnancies was studied to make this determination. Further prospective studies of microcephaly among infants would take time, as women needed to be followed throughout their entire pregnancy. Modelers, then, turned to retrospective data to build models that related the timing and magnitude of the ZIKV epidemic to the stage of the pregnancy. These models demonstrated that the risk of ZIKV-related microcephaly was highest when maternal infection occurred early in pregnancy.[130] However, models were not able to determine the uncertainty around estimates of microcephaly risk because estimates ranged from 14% to 100% for those exposed in the first trimester.[131]

Once it was clear that a novel pathogen was spreading throughout Brazil, the imperative was to determine its reproductive number, the rate at which it would spread, and how many people would ultimately become infected over the course of the epidemic. Based on the previous ZIKV epidemics in Yap and French Polynesia, epidemiologists and modelers calculated the basic reproductive number and generation time of ZIKV and estimated R_0 ranged from 1.3 to 1.4 in Martinique[31] and 4–12 in Yap[32] (Fig. 6). The serial interval, used as a proxy for generation time, was calculated at 10–30 days.[33,132] These differences between models are likely due to a few factors: true variation in spread between locations, differences in model assumptions, and differences in estimation methods. Validation of and variability for both the estimated R_0 and generation time between models was difficult because data were limited.

Finally, models were used during the ZIKV epidemic to predict which countries might see the emergence of the virus, which was important to inform preparedness, prevention, and control efforts. To emerge, viruses require both the proper environment and introduction into that

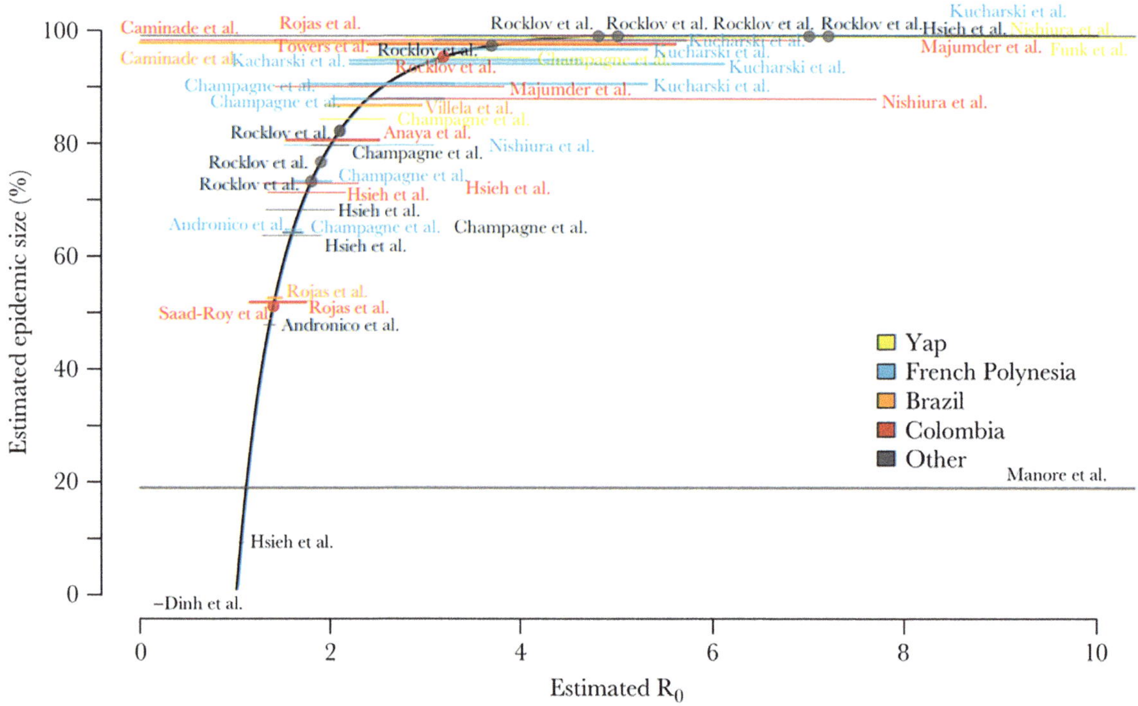

FIG. 6 R_0 estimates for different locations and theoretical epidemic size. Location-specific R_0 estimates are shown superimposed on the theoretical relationship between R_0 and the final epidemic size (for homogeneous populations). The *horizontal lines* show the reported range or 95% confidence interval of estimates when reported and are placed vertically corresponding to the epidemic size associated with the mean or median estimate. *Thick lines* represent national-level estimates, *thin lines* represent estimates for subnational areas (e.g., states or cities), and points represent estimates for which only point estimates were reported. (Reprint from Keegan, LT, Lessler J, Johansson MA. Quantifying Zika: advancing the epidemiology of Zika with quantitative models. *J Infect Dis*. 2024.)

environment. Hence, researchers used niche models to identify environments appropriate for an introduction and to calculate R_0 depending upon other characteristics such as temperature and population density. These models were subsequently used to estimate the geographic distribution of ZIKV, and most models concluded that ZIKV would not spread beyond the geographical distributions of dengue and chikungunya.[35,133,134]

SARS-CoV-2 Pandemic

In late 2019, a cluster of pneumonia cases was reported in Wuhan, China (see Chapter 11 for more detail). By early January, the Chinese Center for Disease Control and Prevention had isolated a novel coronavirus from the throat swab of a hospitalized patient. Clinical evidence of severe outcomes, including morbidity and mortality associated with Acute Respiratory Distress Syndrome, emerged[135] alongside evidence for human-to-human transmission associated with familial and nosocomial clusters.[135,136] Illness due to the virus was rapidly detected in other parts of the world.[137] Models leveraging contact tracing data[138] and those examining growth in case numbers[139,140] rapidly provided primary estimates of core pathogen parameters, including the R_0 and the generation time. While early data demonstrated the strong association between age and poor outcomes,[139] the existence of asymptomatic transmission complicated calculations of the case fatality ratio. Modeling based on data from travelers and serologic surveys began to fill gaps, although it also contributed to some confusion in epidemiologic measurement. Prior to the availability of effective vaccines, NPIs were the primary strategies to mitigate transmission, and models explored the potential of various control measures (e.g., contact tracing,[141] lockdowns[142]) while simultaneously evaluating their impact in reducing transmission of cases and over time.[143] Finally, models were used to explore expectations for the longer term, contingent on uncertainty around characteristics of the duration of immunity, clinical features, and transmission characteristics.[144] This included understanding vaccine deployment and prospects for reaching the critical vaccination threshold to generate adequate herd immunity .[145] Modeling also focused on the future of COVID-19 as it moves from the pandemic to the endemic stage.[146]

CHALLENGES OF MODEL-BASED APPROACHES

Models of emergent pathogens can help researchers forecast the course of epidemics, investigate transmission mechanisms, and evaluate control options. The future of global biosecurity relies on our ability to confront the threat of emerging pathogens. While mechanistic models continue to play an important role in minimizing this threat, there are limitations and drawbacks to the traditional approach (Box 3).

Capturing Medium-Term Trends

Overall, mechanistic models are successful in predicting short-term incidence and capturing longer-term trends. Our ability to forecast over both timescales has been rapidly improving with the availability of new data-streams, including more detailed climate data and better disease surveillance systems that shorten the time between an incident case and the report of that case, as well as more powerful computational resources, which have allowed us to do more computationally intensive forecasting efforts. While this has improved short- and long-term forecasts, medium-term forecasting efforts still struggle to accurately forecast disease incidence, as they require unattainably detailed data on biological, ecological, and social systems. Below we detail several reasons medium-term forecasting is challenging.

Variability in susceptibility

After a disease moves beyond the initial exponential growth period, a multitude of factors affect the incidence and thus our ability to forecast it. First, as a disease invades and spreads through a population, it begins to use up the available pool of susceptible hosts. During the initial exponential growth period, we can assume this does not affect the ability of the disease to spread because there are relatively few immune individuals compared to the total population. However, when forecasting at the medium- and long-term, it becomes important to address the depletion of susceptible hosts.

The pattern of regularly using up the available susceptible population during an epidemic and then burning out until more susceptible individuals are added has been shown to result in epidemic cycles and has been well documented for vaccine-preventable diseases (prior to the introduction of a vaccine) and in influenza.[147,148] When producing long-term forecasts, including information on susceptibility can inform multi-annual patterns of disease incidence; however, the impact on susceptibility is less clear for medium-term time scales.[148]

Even in a pandemic, estimates of immunity can be highly uncertain, leading to different conclusions about the epidemic trajectory and basic underlying epidemiologic quantities. For example, in the spring and summer of 2020, some scientists hypothesized that

BOX 3
Checklist for Evaluating Models of Infectious Disease

What is the purpose of the model?

Theoretical or Strategic Models

This class of models is used to understand how a scenerio works under a set of specified assumptions to gain insight into a theoretical or hypothetical disease system and understand the impacts of specified control measures.

Appropriate model types: Any model type, agent based or deterministic models are common

- ☐ Are the assumptions and model structure clearly stated?
- ☐ Do parameters have clear sources based in the literature (or data)?
- ☐ Is there a sensitivity analysis and/or reasonable uncertainity to parameters and model structure?
- ☐ Are the results plausible given the real world contitions (e.g. not more cases than the total population)?
- ☐ Are the results appropriately presented as hypothetical or assumption driven (i.e. don't claim to provide an actual number of cases to a specific time and place)?

Inferential Models

This class of models is a useful tool to understand the properties of a specific population or epidemic event and can be used to derive parameter and understand fundamental components of the biology of a given infectious agent.

Appropriate model types: Stochastic compartmental or a hybrid of statistical and mechanistic models

- ☐ Are the assumptions and model structure clearly stated?
- ☐ Is actual data from the setting being examined?
- ☐ Is there minimal use of "prior" parameters from the literature and are those parameters from good sources?
- ☐ Is there statistically grounded calculations of confindence intervals, credible intervals, or other measures of uncertainty?
- ☐ Is there a sensitivity analysis and/or reasonable uncertainity to parameters and model structure?
- ☐ Is there an appropriate alignment of source data and the scope of the conclusions made?

Predictive or Forecasting Models

This class of models is used to predict or forecast future trends of a specific disease or epidemic event in a given location or set of locations and can be used to plan an epidemic response.

Appropriate model types: Stochastic compartmental, statistical forecasting (ARIMA), ensamble techniques (Bayesian model averaging)

- ☐ Are the assumptions and model structure clearly stated?
- ☐ Is actual data being used, whenever possible?
  - ☐ Does it have the ability to update the prediction or forecast with new data?
- ☐ Does it capture both statistical process and parameter uncertainity for either statistically grounded techniques or scenerio-based analyses?
- ☐ Are prior parameters based on literature values whenever possible?
- ☐ Is the forecast specificity and extent well aligned with the data and underlying techniques used?
- ☐ Are the results discussed in the context of plausibility and relation to known pathogens?

cross-reactive cellular immunity translated into higher underlying levels of protection against COVID-19 and "herd immunity" might be near.[149,150] SARS-CoV-2 serosurveys with different methods, study designs, and assumptions led to significantly different estimates of population seroprevalence, which led to variable estimates of the infection fatality ratio.[151–154] This demonstrates the challenges in estimating susceptibility to a novel infection, which is critical for modeling efforts, and while modeling may seem straightforward, highly variable results arise. The coupling of asymptomatic or pauci-symptomatic infections, imperfect tests, different populations, and varied study design can obfuscate the true susceptibility of a population, further complicating modeling efforts.

Variability due to interventions

In addition to the overall pool of available susceptible individuals changing over time, variations in infectious contacts arise. In the face of an emerging pathogen, behavior changes occur that can alter the progression of an epidemic. These behavior changes happen either with or without an official directive and affect transmission at the local and regional scale. At the local scale, these changes include social distancing, wearing protective masks, and increased uptake of vaccination, while at the regional scale, they include variation in mobility.[155] At the local scale (i.e., individual scale), behavior changes are well documented for sexually transmitted infections, including HIV. Multiple studies have shown that increased knowledge of HIV, including knowing a person with HIV/AIDS and having knowledge of how the virus is spread, makes people more likely to use a condom.[156] This pattern of individual behavioral change in response to an epidemic was also clear during the Ebola epidemic in 2014. In response to the ongoing Ebola epidemic, particularly as people became aware of the epidemic, they began to change their behavior, including changing burial practices.[157] These changes likely changed the outcome of the epidemic and may have contributed to the mismatch between actual case counts and the pessimistic forecasts of the 2014 West African Ebola outbreak.[158]

Even without formal directives, individual behavioral changes have the potential to alter the course of an epidemic in ways that make forecasting models difficult to implement and test. For example, during the 2009 H1N1 influenza pandemic, individuals and groups began changing interpersonal behaviors in the interest of avoiding infection. One notable example of these behavioral changes occurred during the onset of the epidemic when the University of Buffalo. discouraged handshaking and provided hand sanitizer dispensers at their 2009 graduation ceremony, which was held 4 days before the Centers of Disease Control and Prevention (CDC) issued a formal directive on behavioral changes to curb influenza transmission.[159]

Another challenge for medium-term forecasting is that transmission dynamics change over time because interventions are implemented, and these changes can be difficult to capture. At the onset of an epidemic, most models do not account for control measures or account for them as a fixed reduction in transmission. Prevention and control efforts tend to change the course of an epidemic in ways that are often unaccounted for by models, and therefore when comparing an epidemic forecast to the outcome of an epidemic, models may be inaccurate.

This phenomenon was starkly illustrated early in the 2020 SARS-CoV-2 pandemic when initial models of SARS-CoV-2 struggled to capture the complex dynamics that resulted from the combination of rapidly evolving formal public health control measures and individual behavior changes. Policies, which could change weekly, were implemented at varying spatial scales, including down to the city level, making it nearly impossible to accurately keep track of which measures were implemented at any time, much less project into the future. This reality was in stark contrast to early models that assumed strict and uniform measures would remain in place until the pandemic was resolved (e.g., [160]). Indeed, the nature of the response and individual behavior change has made it difficult to retrospectively estimate the impact of interventions, as these tended to be so strongly correlated in space and time that it is difficult to disentangle the impact of individual control measures.[161]

Environmental variability

Another challenge to medium-term forecasting is the impact of environmental variation on transmission. When looking over a sufficiently small-time horizon, environmental variability may be negligible, and when looking over a sufficiently large time horizon, environmental variability may converge to seasonal averages, however, in the medium term, environmental factors may play a larger role in disease transmission, particularly for vector-borne diseases.

For vector-borne diseases such as malaria, dengue, and ZIKV, environmental variation plays a critical role in the mosquito life cycle and therefore the overall disease. Take malaria for example, where temperature has been shown to have a non-linear effect on transmission by impacting both the vector and the parasite.[162] Temperatures between 22°C and 35°C promote malaria transmission. Below 22°C and above 35°C, transmission is unstable and becomes unsuitable. Of note, mosquitoes can escape the extreme temperatures by resting in occupied houses, where temperatures can be more moderate than outside, further complicating the effect of temperature on transmission (Fig. 7).[162,163]

For directly transmitted diseases such as cholera or influenza, climate also plays a key role in transmission. For cholera, a disease that can spread through contaminated water, environmental variability has a significant impact on transmission. One of the ways in which environmental variability affects cholera transmission is through rainfall. It has been shown that an increase in local rainfall was correlated with an increase in cholera incidence 4–7 days later.[164] On a regional scale, there is evidence of a relationship between the El Niño/Southern Oscillation (ENSO) and cholera prevalence in the Pacific basin and Africa.[165,166] For influenza, an airborne virus, temperature, and relative humidity (RH) have strong roles in influencing seasonal patterns of transmission.[167] Influenza transmission is most efficient under dry, cold conditions (5°C and 20%–35% RH), perhaps because of the improved stability of aerosolized droplets, which may account for the improved transmission in these conditions.[167]

For existing diseases or emerging pathogens that are closely related to existing diseases (e.g., pandemic H1N1, which is closely related to seasonal influenza, or ZIKV, which is related to other flaviviruses such as

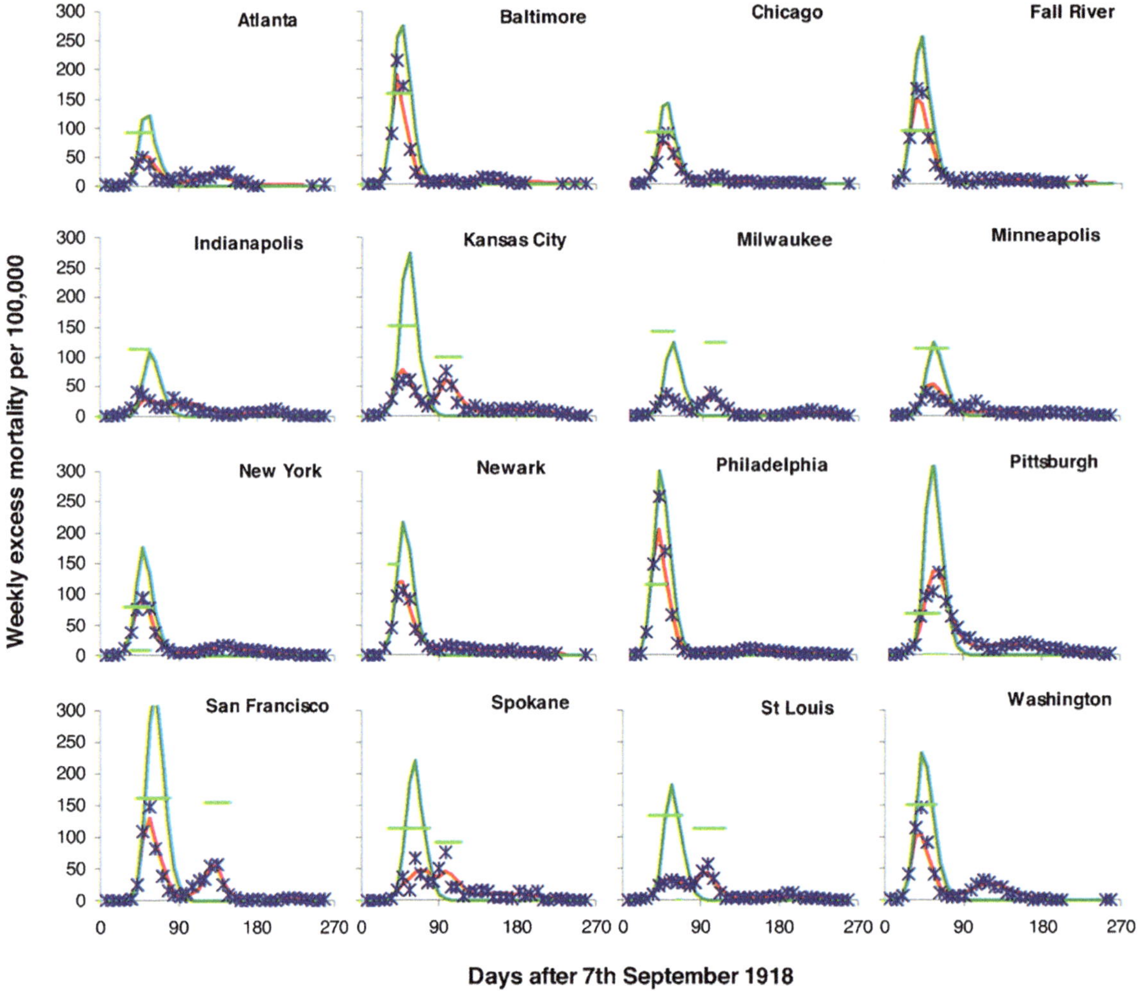

FIG. 7 Weekly excess mortality (per 100,000) resulting from the 1918 pandemic in 16 United States cities (*blue points*) compared to model fits with (*red curves*) and without (*dark-green curves*) control efforts implemented. The effectiveness and period of implementation of control measures are shown as *light-green horizontal lines*, where the *horizontal position* indicates the start date, the horizontal length indicates the duration of interventions, and the *vertical position* indicates estimated effectiveness. The top of the vertical axis is 100% effective, whereas the bottom is 0% effective. (Reprint from Bootsma MCJ, Ferguson NM. The effect of public health measures on the 1918 influenza pandemic in U.S. cities. *Proc Natl Acad Sci U S A*. 2007;104:7588–7593.)

dengue), we can make assumptions about the influence of environment on these pathogens. While environmental variability is incredibly important for existing infectious diseases, for truly novel emerging threats, the effect of environment on transmission is entirely unknown, and our ability to model transmission dynamics is, therefore, complicated. Indeed, as was the case for SARS-CoV-2, the availability of susceptible hosts proved to be a much stronger driver of transmission than the environmental variability, which may be a feature of transmission of pandemic pathogens compared to endemic pathogens.[168]

Modeling Catch 22: Limited Data

Mechanistic models are often most useful early in an epidemic when data are limited. The "catch-22" of these models is that they are only as good as the data they rely upon, and the lack of data is precisely what makes mechanistic models essential in responding to emergent threats. It has been shown both through modeling exercises and through past experience that, for interventions to be successful, they must be implemented early in an epidemic.[64,169] While this is when models are most useful, it is also when they are the most difficult to generate, due to the unavailability of data. In these situations, we must be careful to evaluate models in the context of their limitations and pitfalls.

During the early phase of an emerging pathogen, the potential for high-impact publications coupled with the desire to have a meaningful impact on the public health response can result in an explosion of modeling studies. This is exemplified by the two most recent disease epidemics: Ebola and ZIKV. Since 2014, a search of "PubMed" yields over 300 results for "mathematical model Ebola," and since 2015, a similar "PubMed" search for ZIKV yields over 150 results. These publications rely on data and methods that are of varying quality and do not attempt to provide cohesive intervention strategies.

When data are limited, one solution is to increase reliance on our understanding of biological mechanisms. An example of this is work on the response of malaria to climate change. Models attempting to predict the range of malaria in the face of climate change rely on laboratory studies of temperature tolerance of mosquitoes.[170] However, models that rely too heavily on biological assumptions, particularly complex models, have the potential to be wrong, sometimes spectacularly wrong. For example, models that attempted to forecast the spread of ZIKV outside of Central and South America that relied too heavily on mechanistic assumptions of vector ecology and the role of sexual transmission projected that ZIKV would spread rampantly throughout temperate regions of the United States.[133,171] These predictions were in contrast with both previous experience and with the course of the epidemic thus far. Consequently, special care must be taken when interpreting results that rely heavily on biological mechanisms, especially if the results deviate from prior experience.

Communicating Uncertainty and Assumptions

Capturing and communicating uncertainty are major challenges in modeling emergent pathogens. Since the classical dynamic modeling toolkit relies heavily on systems of ordinary differential equations, statistical uncertainty is often neglected. Including appropriate uncertainties that arise from limited data or from chance events in the epidemic process (i.e., "process" uncertainty) must be deliberately included. Recently, the best work has moved to take advantage of a variety of methods and computational resources to include appropriate uncertainties and account for knowledge gaps. When conducting or evaluating modeling work, epidemiologists must carefully evaluate if appropriate uncertainty was included.

Communicating the results of modeling work is equally challenging. When explaining results outside of the scientific community (e.g., to media or to laypersons), the focus is often on the direct results of the model, neglecting more likely outcomes. In the midst of the 2014 Ebola epidemic, researchers at the CDC projected that by early 2015, in the absence of intervention, more than half a million people would become infected with Ebola in Sierra Leone and Liberia.[63] These projections proved to be an order of magnitude higher than the actual case counts. However, when looking at the projections that included prevention and control measures (for example, increasing the use of specialized Ebola treatment units), the projections much more closely matched the true number of cases. Yet the media focus was entirely on the failure of the projections without considering whether control measures were implemented and how effectively the implementation was. This resulted in the forecasting effort appearing as if it were a complete failure.[172] In addition to a focus on extreme events, nuance, including differences between forecasting incidence and planning scenarios, is often missed, resulting in a further exaggeration of potential outcomes. This was the case with planning exercises early in the influenza H1N1pdm epidemic. Scenario-based analyses that considered multiple potential courses for the pandemic,[173] each with its own uncertainties, were covered in the media with an almost exclusive focus on the worst-case scenarios, once again leading to a sense that the models had been overly pessimistic. While not directly part of the modeling process itself, successfully capturing and communicating these uncertainties is essential to effective use of models in guiding policy and practice.

Communicating uncertainty during the COVID-19 pandemic has had a new set of associated challenges. As the world shut down to decrease transmission, models were thrust into the public and media spotlight, and for the first time, the general public began to regularly consume model projections. As models became headlines, many media outlets sensationalized their results, reporting the highest or lowest values from the confidence bounds in the headlines, sometimes intentionally shifting these to form a political narrative. Unfortunately, the uncertainty in those estimates is either not communicated or buried deep in the article or report. Beyond intentional cherry picking of results, communicating the multitude of model types, their best uses, assumptions, and limitations to a new set of model consumers with limited attention, amid responding to the pandemic, was a significant challenge. Consequently, the purpose and assumptions of many models were not well communicated. As a result, decisionmakers received pressure from their constituents based often on misunderstandings of models and their results. Further, traditional peer-reviewed publication channels failed to keep up with the fast-paced and evolving nature of the COVID-19 pandemic. By the time articles were peer reviewed, the information contained therein was often no longer novel or relevant. Scientists scrambled to identify novel ways to communicate results; however, most of these channels did not include a peer review process, which may have fueled further misinformation. Thus, the usual scientific vetting process was not completed before results were shared. While this allowed for the rapid dissemination of critical results necessary to respond to the pandemic, it also resulted in the dissemination of results that were not well founded, further complicating the implications of modeling findings to media outlets and the general public.

TRENDS AND OPPORTUNITIES IN MODELING INFECTIOUS DISEASE

The "classical" dynamical modeling toolkit has played an important role in recent pathogen emergence events, providing both mechanistic insight and forecasts of incidence when data are limited and strategic planning is urgent. Increased affordability of whole-genome sequencing, the widespread availability of large, high-resolution data sets of key landscape scale variables, and the increasing availability of high-performance computing resources provide opportunities to expand and improve our ability to model emerging pathogens. The ability of mathematical models of infectious diseases to synthesize multiple data sources in the context of existing biological knowledge generates a variety of novel opportunities in a public health landscape increasingly enriched with diverse data-streams.

Phylodynamics

Phylodynamics is the study of how immunology, epidemiology, and evolutionary biology interact and shape the genetic makeup of pathogen populations, as captured in phylogenetic trees.[174] The analytical foundation of the field is a set of tools allowing construction of phylogenetic trees from sequence data. The central insight is that properties of phylogenetic trees can be interpreted in terms of the characteristics of pathogen populations, from their growth to their population structure to the degree of immune escape. Hence, these phylogenies can be used to make inferences on disease dynamics.

For rapidly evolving RNA viruses (as have dominated most recent emergence events), the assumption that random sampling of sequences dominates their evolution (equivalent to assuming that selection pressure plays a minor role relative to mutation) opens the way to defining a "molecular clock" characterizing the rate of sequence change. From this clock, the time to the most recent common ancestor (MRCA) that connects two sequences can be inferred. An array of powerful software is available to extend such analyses across populations of sequences to construct phylogenetic trees (e.g., BEAST, www.beast2.org) using tools such as the coalescent model, which provides a framework for estimating the probability of multiple lineages converging at a common ancestor (e.g., a coalescent event) while stepping back in time and accounting for changes in population size.[175] Inference into the timing of coalescent events (available as pathogen genetic divergence is expected to map onto time as described by the molecular clock) should inform the timing of the MRCA of each population of sequences.[176] A very recent MRCA across all human infections might suggest recent emergence and potentially a spillover event, whereas a distant MRCA could suggest a phase of hidden circulation. Similar logic can be applied to identifying recent introductions into a geographic population. Both conclusions might be at odds with or could enhance what is known from classical data streams, e.g., incidence. For example, during the 2015 ZIKV epidemic, phylodynamic methods were used to determine when ZIKV was introduced into Brazil. Although the first case of ZIKV was not confirmed until May of 2015, phylodynamic models estimated that ZIKV was introduced much earlier, in January 2014.[177] Phylodynamic methods indicated that the Ebola viral spillover event underlying the 2014 outbreak occurred between December 2013 and February 2014 and further identified the location, confirming epidemiologic studies.[178] Further refinements to leverage sequence data to explore spatial patterns of spread have been developed,[179] alongside increasingly integration and visualization tools deployed to analyze the wide availability of sequence data (e.g., www.nextstrain.org[180]).

The time to coalescent events and structure of the tree also provide information on the speeds at which pathogen populations grow (Fig. 2C), which can be formalized to obtain estimates of R_0 and other epidemiologic parameters by overlaying a mechanistic process of pathogen survival, such as a susceptible-infected-recovered (SIR) or other infectious disease life history, onto the model framing tree construction.[54,181] For instance, this latter approach was used to analyze sequence data from the Ebola outbreak,[182] yielding estimates for R_0, incubation period, and infectious periods consistent with other approaches. While phylodynamic methods inevitably have their own set of biases and limitations, these are different from the biases that affect estimates based on case data and therefore provide an independent method to corroborate results and strengthen inference into the features of core pathogens.

Big Data Revolution

The term "big data" generally refers to large and complex data sets that can reveal relationships that might be unobservable in smaller datasets and may be best analyzed with alternative techniques to traditional statistical analysis (although the exact scaling required to be "big" is not clearly defined[183]). Like many other fields, epidemiology has benefited from the recent "big data" revolution. Amidst the expanding pool of datasets generated through automated data collection, a number are relevant to pathogen emergence. High-resolution (sub-kilometer) satellite-based measurements, for example, of land surface temperature or vegetation index, are widely available, with fine spatial resolution and ever-expanding and finely resolved time horizons. Such variables are particularly relevant to vector-borne pathogens. Machine learning techniques have been used to combine such satellite-derived data with existing information on vector and pathogen occurrence to predict pathogen potential range (e.g.,[134] for ZIKV) or outbreak characteristics. For example, Perkins et al.[35] used measures of land surface temperatures combined with mechanistic model framing to forecast the likely occurrence of ZIKV in childbearing women. This analysis also leveraged another increasingly widely-used big-data-derived product: highly resolved maps of human demography (100×100 m) obtained by using machine learning to disaggregate national census data using satellite imagery and other geostatistical data streams.[184] Such high-resolution population data is a prerequisite for many disease models, which depend on knowing the population at risk. Without novel big data-based approaches, this type of information would often be unavailable in resource-poor settings where disease burdens are the highest.

The increasing availability of human mobility data, such as air-travel data[185] or mobile phone-call records[186] also yields unprecedented temporal and spatial resolution onto another aspect of human demography of relevance for pathogen emergence and is likely to be otherwise poorly detailed in resource-poor settings. For example, mobile-phone-derived human mobility has been combined with a highly spatially resolved simple epidemic model to map routes of parasite dispersal[187] and focus control efforts.[188] While mobile phone data yield unprecedented spatial and temporal resolution, like all data sources, they have their limitations. There are biases in terms of who owns the phones, the possibility that an individual owns multiple sim cards, and the spatial and temporal accuracy is determined by the density of mobile phone towers and individual calling behaviors.[189]

Overall, big-data-based approaches are of particular utility in resource-poor settings, where the burden of infection may be high, but traditional data streams, from surveillance to censuses, are likely to be sparse. Importantly, incorporating these types of data into existing disease modeling frameworks requires an understanding of the spatial, population, and temporal biases in these types of data.

Computing Resources

The advancement of either phylodynamic or "big data" techniques would not have been possible without the increased availability of affordable, high-performance computing resources. This widespread availability has allowed for the implementation of novel statistical and mathematical techniques that were previously prohibitively computationally intensive. By allowing more complex models to be run, advancements in computational power have improved the rigor of models of emergent pathogens.[190] With sufficient computing power, essentially any probabilistic model can be fit to data. More specifically, advancements in computing power have allowed researchers to integrate across multiple transmission models and combine multiple representations of transmission processes with statistical inference to appropriately quantify uncertainty.

Increase in computing power and resources has made it possible to fit nearly any probabilistic model. This allows researchers to combine complex representations of the transmission process with statistical inference techniques to estimate key parameters while appropriately accounting for uncertainty.[190] This has been aided by the increased availability of state-of-the-art fitting methods including particle filters (i.e., Maximum likelihood via iterated filtering, MIF[191]), Kalman filtering (i.e., extended Kalman filtering,[192] and Bayesian Markov chain Monte Carlo (i.e., just another

Gibbs sampler, JAGS.[193] This has led to a clear improvement in forecasting established pathogens and may prove useful in forecasting emergent threats. Continued advances in computing power may allow agent-based approaches to utilize a robust statistical framework through similar techniques, a goal that has proved elusive due to the challenges of conducting large numbers of complex simulations.

Real-Time Modeling

Since time is of the essence when responding to an emerging threat, researchers have been working toward the promise of updating model results in "real-time." Google Flu Trends is an example of using "big data" to try to predict influenza in near real-time,[194] and it illustrates one of the major limiting factors in producing real-time disease models: data flow. Google Flu Trends used search queries and historical influenza data to provide estimates of influenza burden weeks before the official CDC influenza data were released. Prior to developing real-time models, improvements in data flow and improvements in how data are processed by models are required, as once data are updated in a timely fashion, models must be sensibly adjusted to that new data.

A major hurdle that has yet to be overcome is how to assess the performance of real-time model forecasts during the event being forecasted. While forecasts are an integral tool in guiding an epidemic response, rarely are forecasts evaluated during or, though more common, after an epidemic. As we move toward updating models in real time, standards for evaluating performance will be important in making reliable forecasts. Currently, work is being done to outline best practices and methods for evaluating mathematical models of infectious diseases in real time.[195]

Immunologic Landscape

A key unknown early on during pathogen emergence or even as an outbreak progresses is defining who is susceptible to infection and who is protected or immune. Even a pathogen with a high R_0 might have very little impact if most individuals are immune (e.g., $R < 1$). Thus, calibrating this variable is of considerable public health value. However, the potential of understanding the landscape of immunity stretches beyond measuring outbreak risk for a single focal pathogen. Immune cross-reactivity is a feature of the biology of many pathogen strains (e.g., influenza[196]) and even species (e.g., the flaviviruses[197]), meaning that existing cross-immunity has the potential to shape the public health burden and trajectory associated with pathogen emergence, but also the success of vaccine deployment, where there is potential for adverse events based on existing immunity.[197,198]

Novel technology is emerging to meet the challenge of characterizing existing immunity. Important advances in multiplex serology (e.g., phage display[199] or Luminex approaches[200]) could be leveraged to develop a window onto the landscape of immunity for multiple pathogens simultaneously.[201] Technical and methodological approaches will be required to achieve the full potential of these advances. Beyond developing novel laboratory methods and the automation necessary to allow scaling of efforts to achieve representation across focal populations, analytical pipelines will be needed. Translating measures from serological assays into characterizations of individual immune status is always a challenge, especially for pathogens with complex patterns of immune escape or cross-reactivity. Development and integration of statistical and mechanistic models across a range of scales and study designs are critical.

As we are increasingly negotiating complex immunological landscapes caused by related pathogens, such immunological analyses become increasingly important. For example, interactions between dengue serotypes on the degree of immunologic response can lead to increased severity with a repeat infection.[202] Models of a recent dengue vaccine that attempted to account for the underlying immunological landscape suggested that vaccination might be acting as a first dengue exposure, and in turn could increase individual risk of complications in some settings.[203] This supposition, at the time of writing, appears to have correctly predicted findings from the field deployment of the vaccine, causing the manufacturer to change their labeling. This interaction between prior immunity to related strains and pathogenicity has also been suggested to help explain patterns of disease for ZIKV[204] and the 1918 influenza pandemic.[205]

The Crucible of COVID-19 and the Rise of Modeling Hubs

In 2020, the rapid and global spread of SARS-CoV-2 led to an unprecedented interest in infectious diseases modeling and disease dynamics, including extensive press coverage of the projections from epidemic models,[206–208] with many new researchers and individuals modeling and forecasting infectious diseases. This flurry of interest has exposed both the utility of epidemic modeling in informing public health and pandemic responses from transmissible pathogens. Likewise, it has revealed the many shortcomings of existing approaches, and the sheer number of models created has created new challenges for the field, particularly around communication and planning.

With tens to hundreds of models being created to forecast the future of the COVID-19 pandemic and project the impact of prevention and control measures, disagreements between the interpretation of various models and their findings were inevitable. These differences not only caused confusion, but they also created situations where those with a particular bias could pick and choose among the various projections to find data needed to support their positions and recommendations. However, differences between model projections often result not from scientific disagreements about epidemic dynamics (though those did occur), but rather from differing assumptions about the ongoing epidemic response. For example, in the spring of 2020, the model from the Institute of Health Metrics and Evaluation was used to support that the ongoing lockdowns were in fact evidence that the pandemic threat was receding.[209] In another example, the Imperial College London developed a model that projected the impact of a completely controlled epidemic that did not come to pass and was sometimes used as evidence that the pandemic threat was overblown, despite the fact of vigorous (if varied) attempts at pandemic control worldwide.[209]

A further issue with the intense focus on disease modeling in the SARS-CoV-2 pandemic arises from the entry of so many new players into the field, many applying novel techniques. While this proliferation has spurred innovation, these new entrants often repeat old mistakes. To best take advantage of the proliferation in interest has been a challenge for the field and has led to the creation of several modeling "hubs" that collect projections from multiple modeling teams in a single location and create ensembles summarizing the various outputs.[210] These include the COVID-19 Forecast Hub,[211] the COVID-19 Scenario Modeling Hub,[212] and the European COVID-19 Forecast Hub,[213] among others.

These hubs serve several purposes. By creating a central platform for display and a unified data format for model projections, they facilitate model comparison and (when appropriate) evaluate standard metrics. Comparison is further facilitated by ensuring submitting teams are focused on the same problem and use a shared set of assumptions, whether it be short-term forecasting or creating longer-term planning scenarios. This also provides a platform for new participants to contribute. Perhaps most importantly, by creating ensembles that summarize the results of all contributing models, the hubs allow the scientific community to provide a consensus of findings of how events might unfold and can capture the extent to which models agree or disagree. The idea of such ensemble models is not a new one, and it has long been known that ensemble models perform better in weather forecasting.[214] Evaluation of the COVID-19 Forecast Hub,[215] as well as earlier disease forecasting challenges,[216] demonstrates that even naive ensembles lead to improved disease forecasting, although their performance is not guaranteed given the complexity of the questions.[217] The SARS-CoV-2 experience with mathematical modeling revealed the need to better summarize and compare across epidemic models in the setting of an infectious disease crisis and has provided a potential solution to this challenge in the creation of the modeling hubs. The field would undoubtedly benefit from additional structure and innovation, particularly in having established platforms formed before the advent of a future crisis.

CONCLUSION

In this chapter, we present the basic principles used in dynamic models of emerging infectious diseases and agents of bioterrorism, along with recent examples of the application of such models. Further, we have attempted to give some insight into the challenges and opportunities inherent in the use of model-based approaches to forecasting epidemic trajectories and the impact of mitigation strategies in the hopes of making the reader a more discerning consumer of such analyses. The dynamics of infectious disease transmission is a critical component of understanding the epidemiology of infectious pathogens and has touched on nearly every aspect of disease research and control over recent decades. Hence, as with any brief introduction to a topic, there is important work and topics we have not covered. Notable are the 2001 outbreak of foot and mouth disease outbreak among cattle in the United Kingdom[218] and the 2003 SARS-CoV epidemic.[24] Dynamics infectious disease models played an important role in the response to both crises, and they played a critical role in driving the field and innovation in the field forward. Likewise, dynamics models have played a role in understanding and combating the ongoing emergence of antibiotic-resistant organisms[219] and in understanding how potentially emergent pathogens spread in animal populations.[220] While there are unique issues and innovations in each of these, they still build on the core principles presented herein.

It is our hope that the material presented here provides the foundation needed to critically read, evaluate, and apply core principles to the dynamic modeling literature. While we caution that the technical skills and domain knowledge needed for quality work go far beyond what is presented in this chapter, we hope that this material and the critical references cited can serve as a road map for those wishing to understand and apply dynamic mathematical models in research and practice.

DISCLOSURE STATEMENT

Disclosure of any relationship with a commercial company that has a direct financial interest in subject matter or materials discussed in article or with a company making a competing product.

The authors declare no conflicts of interest.

REFERENCES

1. Metcalf CJE, Lessler J. Opportunities and challenges in modeling emerging infectious diseases. *Science.* 2017;357:149–152.
2. May RM, Anderson RM. COMMENTARY—transmission dynamics of HIV infection. *Nature.* 1987;326:137.
3. Kermack WO, McKendrick AG. A contribution to the mathematical theory of epidemics. *Proc R Soc Lond A Math Phys Sci.* 1927;115:700–721.
4. Cummings DAT, Lessler JL. Chapter 6 Mathematical modeling: The dynamics of infection. In: Nelson KE, Williams C, eds. *Infectious Disease Epidemiology.* 3rd ed. Jones & Bartlett Learning; 2014.
5. Cauchemez S, Nouvellet P, Cori A, et al. Unraveling the drivers of MERS-CoV transmission. *Proc Natl Acad Sci U S A.* 2016;113:9081–9086.
6. Longini Jr IM, Nizam A, Ali M, Yunus M, Shenvi N, Clemens JD. Controlling endemic cholera with oral vaccines. *PLoS Med.* 2007;4, e336.
7. Chao DL, Halloran ME, Longini Jr IM. Vaccination strategies for epidemic cholera in Haiti with implications for the developing world. *Proc Natl Acad Sci U S A.* 2011;108:7081–7085.
8. Checchi F, Gayer M, Grais R, Mills EJ. Public Health in Crisis-Affected Populations. A Practical Guide for Decision-Makers. Humanitarian Practice Network; 2007. Available: http://www.who.int/entity/hac/techguidance/training/analysing_health_systems/public_health_in_crisis_affected_populations_07.pdf?ua=1.
9. Mari L, Bertuzzo E, Righetto L, et al. Modelling cholera epidemics: the role of waterways, human mobility and sanitation. *J R Soc Interface.* 2012;9:376–388.
10. Johansson MA, Hombach J, Cummings DAT. Models of the impact of dengue vaccines: a review of current research and potential approaches. *Vaccine.* 2011;29:5860–5868.
11. Hsieh Y-H, Ma S. Intervention measures, turning point, and reproduction number for dengue, Singapore, 2005. *Am J Trop Med Hyg.* 2009;80:66–71.
12. Hsieh YH, Chen C. Turning points, reproduction number, and impact of climatological events for multi-wave dengue outbreaks. *Trop Med Int Health.* 2009. Available: http://onlinelibrary.wiley.com/doi/10.1111/j.1365-3156.2009.02277.x/full.
13. Lessler J, Reich NG, Cummings DAT. New York City Department of Health and Mental Hygiene swine influenza investigation team, Nair HP, Jordan HT, et al. outbreak of 2009 pandemic influenza A (H1N1) at a new York City school. *N Engl J Med.* 2009;361:2628–2636.
14. Cowling BJ, Fang VJ, Riley S, Malik Peiris JS, Leung GM. Estimation of the serial interval of influenza. *Epidemiology.* 2009;20:344–347.
15. Carrat F, Vergu E, Ferguson NM, et al. Timelines of infection and disease in human influenza: a review of volunteer challenge studies. *Am J Epidemiol.* 2008;167:775–785.
16. Smith DL, McKenzie FE, Snow RW, Hay SI. Revisiting the basic reproductive number for malaria and its implications for malaria control. *PLoS Biol.* 2007;5, e42.
17. Mossong J, Muller CP. Estimation of the basic reproduction number of measles during an outbreak in a partially vaccinated population. *Epidemiol Infect.* 2000;124:273–278.
18. Edmunds WJ, Gay NJ, Kretzschmar M, Pebody RG, Wachmann H, ESEN Project. European Sero-epidemiology Network. The pre-vaccination epidemiology of measles, mumps and rubella in Europe: implications for modelling studies. *Epidemiol Infect.* 2000;125:635–650.
19. Anderson RM, May RM. Infectious Diseases of Humans: Dynamics and Control. Oxford: Oxford University Press; 1991:169.
20. Fine PEM. The interval between successive cases of an infectious disease. *Am J Epidemiol.* 2003;158:1039–1047.
21. Bailey N. The Mathematical Theory of Infectious Diseases and Its Applications; 1975. Available: https://www.cabdirect.org/cabdirect/abstract/19762902036.
22. Chowell G, Fenimore PW, Castillo-Garsow MA, Castillo-Chavez C. SARS outbreaks in Ontario, Hong Kong and Singapore: the role of diagnosis and isolation as a control mechanism. *J Theor Biol.* 2003;224:1–8.
23. Aycock WL, Ingalls TH. Maternal disease as a principle in the epidemiology of congenital anomalies; with a review of rubella. *Am J Med Sci.* 1946;212:366–379.
24. Riley S, Fraser C, Donnelly CA, et al. Transmission dynamics of the etiological agent of SARS in Hong Kong: impact of public health interventions. *Science.* 2003;300:1961–1966.
25. Lipsitch M, Cohen T, Cooper B, et al. Transmission dynamics and control of severe acute respiratory syndrome. *Science.* 2003;300:1966–1970.
26. Halloran ME, Longini Jr IM, Nizam A, Yang Y. Containing bioterrorist smallpox. *Science.* 2002;298:1428–1432.

27. Gani R, Leach S. Transmission potential of smallpox in contemporary populations. *Nature.* 2001;414:748–751.
28. Nishiura H, Eichner M. Infectiousness of smallpox relative to disease age: estimates based on transmission network and incubation period. *Epidemiol Infect.* 2007;135:1145–1150.
29. Kucharski AJ, Althaus CL. The role of superspreading in Middle East respiratory syndrome coronavirus (MERS-CoV) transmission. *Euro Surveill.* 2015;20:14–18.
30. Cauchemez S, Fraser C, Van Kerkhove MD, et al. Middle East respiratory syndrome coronavirus: quantification of the extent of the epidemic, surveillance biases, and transmissibility. *Lancet Infect Dis.* 2014;14:50–56.
31. Andronico A, Dorléans F, Fergé J-L, et al. Real-time assessment of health-care requirements during the Zika virus epidemic in Martinique. *Am J Epidemiol.* 2017;186:1194–1203.
32. Funk S, Kucharski AJ, Camacho A, et al. Comparative analysis of dengue and Zika outbreaks reveals differences by setting and virus. *PLoS Negl Trop Dis.* 2016;10, e0005173.
33. Ferguson NM, Cucunubá ZM, Dorigatti I, et al. Countering Zika in Latin America. *Science.* 2016;aag0219.
34. Majumder MS, Cohn E, Fish D, Brownstein JS. Estimating a feasible serial interval range for Zika fever. *Bull World Health Organ.* 2016. Available: http://www.who.int/bulletin/online_first/16-171009.pdf.
35. Perkins TA, Siraj AS, Ruktanonchai CW, Kraemer MUG, Tatem AJ. Model-based projections of Zika virus infections in childbearing women in the Americas. *Nat Microbiol.* 2016;1:16126.
36. Siraj AS, Oidtman RJ, Huber JH, et al. Temperature modulates dengue virus epidemic growth rates through its effects on reproduction numbers and generation intervals. *PLoS Negl Trop Dis.* 2017;11, e0005797.
37. Diekmann O, Heesterbeek JA, Metz JA. On the definition and the computation of the basic reproduction ratio R0 in models for infectious diseases in heterogeneous populations. *J Math Biol.* 1990;28:365–382.
38. Diekmann O, Heesterbeek JAP. Mathematical Epidemiology of Infectious Diseases: Model Building, Analysis and Interpretation. John Wiley & Sons; 2000.
39. Blumberg S, Lloyd-Smith JO. Comparing methods for estimating R0 from the size distribution of subcritical transmission chains. *Epidemics.* 2013;5:131–145.
40. Takahashi S, Metcalf CJE, Ferrari MJ, et al. Reduced vaccination and the risk of measles and other childhood infections post-Ebola. *Science.* 2015;347:1240–1242.
41. Simons E, Ferrari M, Fricks J, et al. Assessment of the 2010 global measles mortality reduction goal: results from a model of surveillance data. *Lancet.* 2012;379:2173–2178.
42. Huisman JS, Scire J, Angst DC, et al. Estimation and worldwide monitoring of the effective reproductive number of SARS-CoV-2. *ELife.* 2022;11. https://doi.org/10.7554/eLife.71345.
43. Abbott S, Hellewell J, Thompson RN, et al. Estimating the time-varying reproduction number of SARS-CoV-2 using national and subnational case counts. *Wellcome Open Res.* 2020;5:112.
44. Gozzi N, Chinazzi M, Davis JT, et al. Preliminary modeling estimates of the relative transmissibility and immune escape of the omicron SARS-CoV-2 variant of concern in South Africa. *bioRxiv.* 2022. https://doi.org/10.1101/2022.01.04.22268721.
45. Liu Y, Rocklöv J. The effective reproductive number of the omicron variant of SARS-CoV-2 is several times relative to Delta. *J Travel Med.* 2022;29. https://doi.org/10.1093/jtm/taac037.
46. Wallinga J, Lipsitch M. How generation intervals shape the relationship between growth rates and reproductive numbers. *Proc R Soc B Biol Sci.* 2007;274:599–604.
47. Chowell G, Nishiura H. Transmission dynamics and control of Ebola virus disease (EVD): a review. *BMC Med.* 2014;12:196.
48. Mills CE, Robins JM, Lipsitch M. Transmissibility of 1918 pandemic influenza. *Nature.* 2004;432:904–906.
49. Nishiura H, Kinoshita R, Mizumoto K, Yasuda Y, Nah K. Transmission potential of Zika virus infection in the South Pacific. *Int J Infect Dis.* 2016;45:95–97.
50. Viboud C, Simonsen L, Chowell G. A generalized-growth model to characterize the early ascending phase of infectious disease outbreaks. *Epidemics.* 2016;15:27–37.
51. Burghardt K, Verzijl C, Huang J, Ingram M, Song B, Hasne M-P. Testing modeling assumptions in the West Africa Ebola outbreak. *Sci Rep.* 2016;6:34598.
52. Chowell G, Viboud C, Simonsen L, Moghadas SM. Characterizing the reproduction number of epidemics with early subexponential growth dynamics. *J R Soc Interface.* 2016;13. https://doi.org/10.1098/rsif.2016.0659.
53. Duffy MR, Chen T-H, Hancock WT, et al. Zika virus outbreak on Yap Island, Federated States of Micronesia. *N Engl J Med.* 2009;360:2536–2543.
54. Volz EM, Kosakovsky Pond SL, Ward MJ, Leigh Brown AJ, Frost SDW. Phylodynamics of infectious disease epidemics. *Genetics.* 2009;183:1421–1430.
55. Fraser C, Donnelly CA, Cauchemez S, et al. Pandemic potential of a strain of influenza A (H1N1): early findings. *Science.* 2009;324:1557–1561.
56. Forsberg White L, Pagano M. A likelihood-based method for real-time estimation of the serial interval and reproductive number of an epidemic. *Stat Med.* 2008;27:2999–3016.
57. Wallinga J, Teunis P. Different epidemic curves for severe acute respiratory syndrome reveal similar impacts of control measures. *Am J Epidemiol.* 2004;160:509–516.
58. Cori A. Estimate Time Varying Reproduction Numbers from Epidemic Curves [R package EpiEstim version 2.2-4]; 2021. [cited 9 Nov 2022]. Available: https://cran.r-project.org/web/packages/EpiEstim/index.html.
59. White LF, Pagano M. Transmissibility of the influenza virus in the 1918 pandemic. *PLoS One.* 2008;3, e1498.
60. Fine PE. Herd immunity: history, theory, practice. *Epidemiol Rev.* 1993;15:265–302.

61. Jefferson T, Demicheli V, Rivetti D, Jones M, Di Pietrantonj C, Rivetti A. Antivirals for influenza in healthy adults: systematic review. *Lancet.* 2006;367:303–313.
62. Earn DJD, He D, Loeb MB, Fonseca K, Lee BE, Dushoff J. Effects of school closure on incidence of pandemic influenza in Alberta. *Canada Ann Intern Med.* 2012;156:173–181.
63. Meltzer MI, Atkins CY, Santibanez S, et al. Estimating the future number of cases in the Ebola epidemic—Liberia and Sierra Leone, 2014–2015. *MMWR Suppl.* 2014;63:1–14.
64. Ferguson NM, Cummings DAT, Cauchemez S, et al. Strategies for containing an emerging influenza pandemic in Southeast Asia. *Nature.* 2005;437:209–214.
65. Fraser C, Riley S, Anderson RM, Ferguson NM. Factors that make an infectious disease outbreak controllable. *Proc Natl Acad Sci U S A.* 2004;101:6146–6151.
66. Peak CM, Childs LM, Grad YH, Buckee CO. Comparing nonpharmaceutical interventions for containing emerging epidemics. *Proc Natl Acad Sci U S A.* 2017;114:4023–4028.
67. Reich NG, Lessler J, Varma JK, Vora NM. Quantifying the Risk and Cost of Active Monitoring for Infectious Diseases; 2017. https://doi.org/10.1101/156497.
68. Lloyd-Smith JO, Schreiber SJ, Kopp PE, Getz WM. Superspreading and the effect of individual variation on disease emergence. *Nature.* 2005;438:355.
69. Mossong J, Hens N, Jit M, et al. Social contacts and mixing patterns relevant to the spread of infectious diseases. *PLoS Med.* 2008;5, e74.
70. Williams BG, Dye C. Dynamics and control of infections on social networks of population types. *Epidemics.* 2017. https://doi.org/10.1016/j.epidem.2017.10.002.
71. Lieu TA, Ray GT, Klein NP, Chung C, Kulldorff M. Geographic clusters in underimmunization and vaccine refusal. *Pediatrics.* 2015;135:280–289.
72. Pellis L, Ball F, Trapman P. Reproduction numbers for epidemic models with households and other social structures. I. Definition and calculation of R0. *Math Biosci.* 2012;235:85–97.
73. Cauchemez S, Valleron A-J, Boëlle P-Y, Flahault A, Ferguson NM. Estimating the impact of school closure on influenza transmission from sentinel data. *Nature.* 2008;452:750–754.
74. Goeyvaerts N, Hens N, Ogunjimi B, et al. Estimating infectious disease parameters from data on social contacts and serological status. *J R Stat Soc Ser C Appl Stat.* 2010;59:255–277.
75. History of Smallpox | Smallpox | CDC. 2017 [cited 4 Jan 2018]. Available: https://www.cdc.gov/smallpox/history/history.html.
76. Ogden HG. CDC and the Smallpox Crusade; 1987. Available: https://stacks.cdc.gov/view/cdc/21534.
77. Henderson DA, Inglesby TV, Bartlett JG, et al. Smallpox as a biological weapon: medical and public health management. *JAMA.* 1999;281:2127–2137.
78. Cooper B. Poxy models and rash decisions. *Proc Natl Acad Sci U S A.* 2006;103(33):12221–12222.
79. Riley S, Ferguson NM. Smallpox transmission and control: spatial dynamics in Great Britain. *Proc Natl Acad Sci U S A.* 2006;103:12637–12642.
80. O'Toole T. Smallpox: an attack scenario. *Emerg Infect Dis.* 1999;5:540–546.
81. Henderson DA. Bioterrorism as a public health threat. *Emerg Infect Dis.* 1998;4:488–492.
82. Jernigan JA, Stephens DS, Ashford DA, et al. Bioterrorism-related inhalational anthrax: the first 10 cases reported in the United States. *Emerg Infect Dis.* 2001;7:933–944.
83. Mayer TA, Bersoff-Matcha S, Murphy C, et al. Clinical presentation of inhalational anthrax following bioterrorism exposure: report of 2 surviving patients. *JAMA.* 2001;286:2549–2553.
84. How People Are Infected | Anthrax | CDC. [cited 4 Jan 2018]. Available: https://www.cdc.gov/anthrax/basics/how-people-are-infected.html.
85. Reshetin VP, Regens JL. Simulation modeling of anthrax spore dispersion in a bioterrorism incident. *Risk Anal.* 2003;23. Available: http://onlinelibrary.wiley.com/doi/10.1111/j.0272-4332.2003.00387.x/full.
86. Webb GF, Blaser MJ. Mailborne transmission of anthrax: modeling and implications. *Proc Natl Acad Sci U S A.* 2002;99:7027–7032.
87. Gutting BW, Channel SR, Berger AE, et al. Mathematically modeling inhalational Anthrax successive advances in modeling applied to updated data help in estimating risks from inhalational anthrax[no title]. *Microbe Wash DC.* 2008;3(2):3.
88. Brookmeyer R, Blades N. Statistical models and bioterrorism. *J Am Stat Assoc.* 2003;98:781–788.
89. Brookmeyer R, Johnson E, Bollinger R. Modeling the optimum duration of antibiotic prophylaxis in an anthrax outbreak. *Proc Natl Acad Sci U S A.* 2003;100:10129–10132.
90. Bravata DM, Zaric GS, Holty J-EC, et al. Reducing mortality from anthrax bioterrorism: strategies for stockpiling and dispensing medical and pharmaceutical supplies. *Biosecur Bioterror.* 2006;4:244–262.
91. Zaric GS, Bravata DM, Cleophas Holty J-E, McDonald KM, Owens DK, Brandeau ML. Modeling the logistics of response to anthrax bioterrorism. *Med Decis Making.* 2008;28:332–350.
92. Hupert N, Mushlin AI, Callahan MA. Modeling the public health response to bioterrorism: using discrete event simulation to design antibiotic distribution centers. *Med Decis Making.* 2002;22:S17–S25.
93. Murray CJL, Lopez AD, Chin B, Feehan D, Hill KH. Estimation of potential global pandemic influenza mortality on the basis of vital registry data from the 1918–20 pandemic: a quantitative analysis. *Lancet.* 2006;368:2211–2218.
94. Estimating Seasonal Influenza-Associated Deaths in the United States | Seasonal Influenza (Flu) | CDC; 2017. [cited 29 Dec 2017]. Available: https://www.cdc.gov/flu/about/disease/us_flu-related_deaths.htm.
95. Herfst S, Schrauwen EJA, Linster M, et al. Airborne transmission of influenza A/H5N1 virus between ferrets. *Science.* 2012;336:1534–1541.

96. Imai M, Watanabe T, Hatta M, et al. Experimental adaptation of an influenza H5 HA confers respiratory droplet transmission to a reassortant H5 HA/H1N1 virus in ferrets. *Nature.* 2012;486:420–428.
97. Guan Y, Poon LLM, Cheung CY, et al. H5N1 influenza: a protean pandemic threat. *Proc Natl Acad Sci U S A.* 2004;101:8156–8161.
98. Li FCK, Choi BCK, Sly T, Pak AWP. Finding the real case-fatality rate of H5N1 avian influenza. *J Epidemiol Community Health.* 2008;62:555–559.
99. Germann TC, Kadau K, Longini Jr IM, Macken CA. Mitigation strategies for pandemic influenza in the United States. *Proc Natl Acad Sci U S A.* 2006;103:5935–5940.
100. Longini Jr IM, Nizam A, Xu S, et al. Containing pandemic influenza at the source. *Science.* 2005;309:1083–1087.
101. Ferguson NM, Cummings DAT, Fraser C, Cajka JC, Cooley PC, Burke DS. Strategies for mitigating an influenza pandemic. *Nature.* 2006;442:448–452.
102. Jefferson T, Jones M, Doshi P, Spencer EA, Onakpoya I, Heneghan CJ. Oseltamivir for influenza in adults and children: systematic review of clinical study reports and summary of regulatory comments. *BMJ.* 2014;348, g2545.
103. Zarocostas J. World Health Organization declares A (H1N1) influenza pandemic. *BMJ.* 2009;338, b2425.
104. Munster VJ, de Wit E, van den Brand JMA, et al. Pathogenesis and transmission of swine-origin 2009 A(H1N1) influenza virus in ferrets. *Science.* 2009;325:481–483.
105. How Is Pandemic Flu Different From Seasonal Flu? | Pandemic Influenza (Flu) | CDC; 7 Apr 2017. [cited 3 Jan 2018]. Available: https://www.cdc.gov/flu/pandemic-resources/basics/about.html.
106. Yang Y, Sugimoto JD, Halloran ME, et al. The transmissibility and control of pandemic influenza A (H1N1) virus. *Science.* 2009;326:729–733.
107. Garske T, Legrand J, Donnelly CA, et al. Assessing the severity of the novel influenza A/H1N1 pandemic. *BMJ.* 2009;339, b2840.
108. Centers for Disease Control and Prevention (CDC). Update: severe respiratory illness associated with a novel coronavirus—worldwide, 2012-2013. *MMWR Morb Mortal Wkly Rep.* 2013;62:194–195.
109. [No title]. [cited 13 Dec 2017]. Available: http://www.emro.who.int/images/stories/csr/documents/epi_monitor__issue_no__39.coronavirus.pdf.
110. Assiri A, McGeer A, Perl TM, et al. Hospital outbreak of Middle East respiratory syndrome coronavirus. *N Engl J Med.* 2013;369:407–416.
111. Memish ZA, Zumla AI, Al-Hakeem RF, Al-Rabeeah AA, Stephens GM. Family cluster of Middle East respiratory syndrome coronavirus infections. *N Engl J Med.* 2013;368:2487–2494.
112. Lessler J, Rodriguez-Barraquer I, Cummings DAT, et al. Estimating potential incidence of MERS-CoV associated with hajj pilgrims to Saudi Arabia, 2014. *PLoS Curr.* 2014;6. https://doi.org/10.1371/currents.outbreaks.c5c9c9abd636164a9b6fd4dbda974369.
113. Chowell G, Blumberg S, Simonsen L, Miller MA, Viboud C. Synthesizing data and models for the spread of MERS-CoV, 2013: key role of index cases and hospital transmission. *Epidemics.* 2014;9:40–51.
114. Lessler J, Salje H, Van Kerkhove MD, et al. Estimating the severity and subclinical burden of Middle East respiratory syndrome coronavirus infection in the Kingdom of Saudi Arabia. *Am J Epidemiol.* 2016;183:657–663.
115. Cowling BJ, Park M, Fang VJ, Wu P, Leung GM, Wu JT. Preliminary epidemiological assessment of MERS-CoV outbreak in South Korea, May to June 2015. *Eurosurveillance.* 2015;20. https://doi.org/10.2807/1560-7917.ES2015.20.25.21163.
116. Piot P. Ebola's perfect storm. *Science.* 2014;345:1221.
117. WHO Ebola Response Team. Ebola virus disease in West Africa—the first 9 months of the epidemic and forward projections. *N Engl J Med.* 2014;371:1481–1495.
118. Farrar JJ, Piot P. The Ebola emergency—immediate action, ongoing strategy. *N Engl J Med.* 2014;371(16):1545–1546.
119. Pandey A, Atkins KE, Medlock J, et al. Strategies for containing Ebola in West Africa. *Science.* 2014;346:991–995.
120. Read JM, Diggle PJ, Chirombo J, Solomon T, Baylis M. Effectiveness of screening for Ebola at airports. *Lancet.* 2015;23–24.
121. Camacho A, Kucharski A, Aki-Sawyerr Y, et al. Temporal changes in Ebola transmission in Sierra Leone and implications for control requirements: a real-time modelling study. *PLoS Curr.* 2015;7. https://doi.org/10.1371/currents.outbreaks.406ae55e83ec0b5193e30856b9235ed2.
122. Simon-Loriere E, Faye O, Faye O, et al. Distinct lineages of Ebola virus in Guinea during the 2014 west African epidemic. *Nature.* 2015;524:102–104.
123. Quick J, Loman NJ, Duraffour S, et al. Real-time, portable genome sequencing for Ebola surveillance. *Nature.* 2016;530:228–232.
124. Dudas G, Carvalho LM, Bedford T, et al. Virus genomes reveal factors that spread and sustained the Ebola epidemic. *Nature.* 2017;544:309–315.
125. Camacho A, Eggo RM, Funk S, Watson CH, Kucharski AJ, Edmunds WJ. Estimating the probability of demonstrating vaccine efficacy in the declining Ebola epidemic: a Bayesian modelling approach. *BMJ Open.* 2015;5, e009346.
126. Chan MK. WHO Director-General Summarizes the Outcome of the Emergency Committee Regarding Clusters of Microcephaly and Guillain-Barré Syndrome. Geneva: World Health Organization; 2016.
127. Oehler E, Watrin L, Larre P, et al. Zika virus infection complicated by Guillain-Barré syndrome—case report, French Polynesia, December 2013. *Eurosurveillance.* 2014;19:20720.
128. Alfaro-Murillo JA, Parpia AS, Fitzpatrick MC, et al. A cost-effectiveness tool for informing policies on Zika virus control. *PLoS Negl Trop Dis.* 2016;10, e0004743.
129. de Oliveira WK. Increase in reported prevalence of microcephaly in infants born to women living in areas with confirmed Zika virus transmission during the first trimester of .... *MMWR Morb Mortal Wkly Rep.*

2016. Available: https://espanol.cdc.gov/enes/mmwr/volumes/65/wr/mm6509e2.htm?s_cid=mm6509e2.htm_w&mobile=nocontent.
130. Cauchemez S, Besnard M, Bompard P, et al. Association between Zika virus and microcephaly in French Polynesia, 2013–15: a retrospective study. *Lancet.* 2016;387:2125–2132.
131. Nishiura H, Mizumoto K, Rock KS, Yasuda Y, Kinoshita R, Miyamatsu Y. A theoretical estimate of the risk of microcephaly during pregnancy with Zika virus infection. *Epidemics.* 2016;15:66–70.
132. Majumder MS, Santillana M, Mekaru SR, McGinnis DP, Khan K, Brownstein JS. Utilizing nontraditional data sources for near real-time estimation of transmission dynamics during the 2015-2016 Colombian Zika virus disease outbreak. *JMIR Public Health Surveill.* 2016;2, e30.
133. Bogoch II, Brady OJ, Kraemer MUG, et al. Anticipating the international spread of Zika virus from Brazil. *Lancet.* 2016;387:335–336.
134. Messina JP, Kraemer MU, Brady OJ, et al. Mapping global environmental suitability for Zika virus. *Elife.* 2016;5. https://doi.org/10.7554/eLife.15272.
135. Chen N, Zhou M, Dong X, et al. Epidemiological and clinical characteristics of 99 cases of 2019 novel coronavirus pneumonia in Wuhan, China: a descriptive study. *Lancet.* 2020;395:507–513.
136. Chan J.F.-W., Yuan S., Kok K.-H., To KK-W, Chu H., Yang J., et al. A familial cluster of pneumonia associated with the 2019 novel coronavirus indicating person-to-person transmission: a study of a family cluster. Lancet 2020;395: 514–523.
137. Fisher D, Heymann D. Q&A: the novel coronavirus outbreak causing COVID-19. *BMC Med.* 2020;18:57.
138. Bi Q, Wu Y, Mei S, et al. Epidemiology and transmission of COVID-19 in 391 cases and 1286 of their close contacts in Shenzhen, China: a retrospective cohort study. *Lancet Infect Dis.* 2020;20:911–919.
139. Li Q, Guan X, Wu P, et al. Early transmission dynamics in Wuhan, China, of novel coronavirus-infected pneumonia. *N Engl J Med.* 2020;382:1199–1207.
140. Read JM, Bridgen JRE, Cummings DAT, Ho A, Jewell CP. Novel coronavirus 2019-nCoV (COVID-19): early estimation of epidemiological parameters and epidemic size estimates. *Philos Trans R Soc Lond B Biol Sci.* 2021;376:20200265.
141. Grantz KH, Lee EC, D'Agostino McGowan L, et al. Maximizing and evaluating the impact of test-trace-isolate programs: a modeling study. *PLoS Med.* 2021;18, e1003585.
142. Report 9—Impact of Non-Pharmaceutical Interventions (NPIs) to Reduce COVID-19 Mortality and Healthcare Demand. In: Imperial College London [Internet]. [cited 8 Sep 2022]. Available: https://www.imperial.ac.uk/mrc-global-infectious-disease-analysis/covid-19/report-9-impact-of-npis-on-covid-19/.
143. Hsiang S, Allen D, Annan-Phan S, et al. The effect of large-scale anti-contagion policies on the COVID-19 pandemic. *Nature.* 2020;584:262–267.
144. Saad-Roy CM, Wagner CE, Baker RE, et al. Immune life history, vaccination, and the dynamics of SARS-CoV-2 over the next 5 years. *Science.* 2020;370:811–818.
145. Makhoul M, Ayoub HH, Chemaitelly H, et al. Epidemiological impact of SARS-CoV-2 vaccination: mathematical modeling analyses. *Vaccines (Basel).* 2020;8. https://doi.org/10.3390/vaccines8040668.
146. Beams AB, Bateman R, Adler FR. Will SARS-CoV-2 become just another seasonal coronavirus? *Viruses.* 2021;13. https://doi.org/10.3390/v13050854.
147. Earn DJ, Rohani P, Bolker BM, Grenfell BT. A simple model for complex dynamical transitions in epidemics. *Science.* 2000;287:667–670.
148. Keeling MJ, Rohani P. Modeling infectious diseases in humans and animals. Princeton University Press; 2011.
149. Doshi P. Covid-19: do many people have pre-existing immunity? *BMJ.* 2020;370, m3563.
150. Le Bert N, Tan AT, Kunasegaran K, et al. SARS-CoV-2-specific T cell immunity in cases of COVID-19 and SARS, and uninfected controls. *Nature.* 2020;584:457–462.
151. Ioannidis JPA. Infection fatality rate of COVID-19 inferred from seroprevalence data. *Bull World Health Organ.* 2021;99:19–33F.
152. Bendavid E, Mulaney B, Sood N, et al. COVID-19 antibody seroprevalence in Santa Clara County, California. *Int J Epidemiol.* 2021;50:410–419.
153. Pathela P, Crawley A, Weiss D, et al. Seroprevalence of severe acute respiratory syndrome coronavirus 2 following the largest initial epidemic wave in the United States: findings from new York City, 13 May to 21 July 2020. *J Infect Dis.* 2021;224:196–206.
154. Samore MH, Looney A, Orleans B, et al. Probability-based estimates of severe acute respiratory syndrome coronavirus 2 Seroprevalence and detection fraction, Utah, USA. *Emerg Infect Dis.* 2021;27:2786–2794.
155. Funk S, Gilad E, Watkins C, Jansen VAA. The spread of awareness and its impact on epidemic outbreaks. *Proc Natl Acad Sci U S A.* 2009;106:6872–6877.
156. Gregson S, Zhuwau T, Anderson RM, Chandiwana SK. Is there evidence for behaviour change in response to AIDS in rural Zimbabwe? *Soc Sci Med.* 1998;46:321–330.
157. Sharareh N., Sabounchi N.S., Sayama H., MacDonald R. The Ebola Crisis and the Corresponding Public Behavior: A System Dynamics ApproachVaccine Hesitancy CollectionPLOS Science Reddit AMAHealthMap EbolaNew Twitter. PLoS Curr. November 3, 2016November 5, 2016November 7, 2016August 7, 2017 [cited 14 Dec 2017]. https://doi.org/10.1371/currents.outbreaks.23badd9821870a002fa86bef6893c01d.
158. Camacho A, Kucharski AJ, Funk S, Breman J, Piot P, Edmunds WJ. Potential for large outbreaks of Ebola virus disease. *Epidemics.* 2014;9:70–78.
159. Kiviniemi MT, Ram PK, Kozlowski LT, Smith KM. Perceptions of and willingness to engage in public health precautions to prevent 2009 H1N1 influenza transmission. *BMC Public Health.* 2011;11:152.

160. IHME COVID-19 health service utilization forecasting team, CJL M. Forecasting COVID-19 impact on hospital bed-days, ICU-days, ventilator-days and deaths by US state in the next 4 months. *bioRxiv.* 2020. https://doi.org/10.1101/2020.03.27.20043752. medRxiv.
161. Yang B, Huang AT, Garcia-Carreras B, et al. Effect of specific non-pharmaceutical intervention policies on SARS-CoV-2 transmission in the counties of the United States. *Nat Commun.* 2021;12:3560.
162. Shanks GD, Hay SI, Omumbo JA, Snow RW. Malaria in Kenya's western highlands. *Emerg Infect Dis.* 2005;11:1425–1432.
163. Lunde TM, Bayoh MN, Lindtjørn B. How malaria models relate temperature to malaria transmission. *Parasit Vectors.* 2013;6:20.
164. Eisenberg MC, Kujbida G, Tuite AR, Fisman DN, Tien JH. Examining rainfall and cholera dynamics in Haiti using statistical and dynamic modeling approaches. *Epidemics.* 2013;5:197–207.
165. Rodo X, Pascual M, Fuchs G, Faruque ASG. ENSO and cholera: a nonstationary link related to climate change? *Proc Natl Acad Sci U S A.* 2002;99:12901–12906.
166. Moore SM, Azman AS, Zaitchik BF, et al. El Niño and the shifting geography of cholera in Africa. *Proc Natl Acad Sci U S A.* 2017;114:4436–4441.
167. Lowen AC, Steel J. Roles of humidity and temperature in shaping influenza seasonality. *J Virol.* 2014;88:7692–7695.
168. Shaman J, Goldstein E, Lipsitch M. Absolute humidity and pandemic versus epidemic influenza. *Am J Epidemiol.* 2011;173:127–135.
169. Aylward B, Barboza P, Bawo L. al. Ebola virus disease in West Africa-the first 9 months of the epidemic and forward projections. *N Engl J Med.* 2014;371(16).
170. Mordecai EA, Paaijmans KP, Johnson LR, et al. Optimal temperature for malaria transmission is dramatically lower than previously predicted. *Ecol Lett.* 2013;16:22–30.
171. Shacham E, Nelson EJ, Hoft DF, Schootman M, Garza A. Potential high-risk areas for Zika virus transmission in the contiguous United States. *Am J Public Health.* 2017;107:724–731.
172. Stobbe M. CDC's overblown estimate of Ebola outbreak draws criticism. In: *The Seattle Times [Internet]*; 2015. [cited 14 Dec 2017]. Available: https://www.seattletimes.com/nation-world/cdcs-overblown-estimate-of-ebola-outbreak-draws-criticism/.
173. Swine Flu Could Infect Half of U.S., Panel Estimates. The Washington Post; 2009. Available: http://www.washingtonpost.com/wp-dyn/content/article/2009/08/24/AR2009082401733.html. Accessed 13 Dec 2017.
174. Grenfell BT, Pybus OG, Gog JR, et al. Unifying the epidemiological and evolutionary dynamics of pathogens. *Science.* 2004;303:327–332.
175. Drummond AJ, Nicholls GK, Rodrigo AG, Solomon W. Estimating mutation parameters, population history and genealogy simultaneously from temporally spaced sequence data. *Genetics.* 2002;161:1307–1320.
176. Volz EM, Koelle K, Bedford T. Viral phylodynamics. *PLoS Comput Biol.* 2013;9, e1002947.
177. Faria NR, Quick J, Claro IM, et al. Establishment and cryptic transmission of Zika virus in Brazil and the Americas. *Nature.* 2017;546:406–410.
178. Grubaugh ND, Ladner JT, Kraemer MUG, et al. Genomic epidemiology reveals multiple introductions of Zika virus into the United States. *Nature.* 2017;546:401–405.
179. Lemey P, Rambaut A, Drummond AJ, Suchard MA. Bayesian phylogeography finds its roots. *PLoS Comput Biol.* 2009;5, e1000520.
180. Hadfield J, Megill C, Bell SM, et al. Nextstrain: Real-Time Tracking of Pathogen Evolution; 2017. https://doi.org/10.1101/224048.
181. Stack JC, Welch JD, Ferrari MJ, Shapiro BU, Grenfell BT. Protocols for sampling viral sequences to study epidemic dynamics. *J R Soc Interface.* 2010;7:1119–1127.
182. Stadler T, Kühnert D, Rasmussen DA, du Plessis L. Insights into the early epidemic spread of ebola in Sierra Leone provided by viral sequence data. *PLoS Curr.* 2014;6. https://doi.org/10.1371/currents.outbreaks.02bc6d927ecee7bbd33532ec8ba6a25f.
183. Bansal S, Chowell G, Simonsen L, Vespignani A, Viboud C. Big data for infectious disease surveillance and modeling. *J Infect Dis.* 2016;214:S375–S379.
184. Tatem AJ. WorldPop, open data for spatial demography. *Sci Data.* 2017;4, 170004.
185. Mao L, Wu X, Huang Z, Tatem AJ. Modeling monthly flows of global air travel passengers: an open-access data resource. *J Transp Geogr.* 2015;48:52–60.
186. Deville P, Linard C, Martin S, et al. Dynamic population mapping using mobile phone data. *Proc Natl Acad Sci U S A.* 2014;111:15888–15893.
187. Wesolowski A, Eagle N, Tatem AJ, et al. Quantifying the impact of human mobility on malaria. *Science.* 2012;338:267–270.
188. Tatem AJ, Huang Z, Narib C, et al. Integrating rapid risk mapping and mobile phone call record data for strategic malaria elimination planning. *Malar J.* 2014;13:52.
189. Wesolowski A, Buckee CO, Engø-Monsen K, Metcalf CJE. Connecting mobility to infectious diseases: the promise and limits of mobile phone data. *J Infect Dis.* 2016;214:S414–S420.
190. Yang W, Karspeck A, Shaman J. Comparison of filtering methods for the modeling and retrospective forecasting of influenza epidemics. *PLoS Comput Biol.* 2014;10, e1003583.
191. Ionides EL, Bhadra A, Atchadé Y, King A. Iterated filtering. *Ann Stat.* 2011;39:1776–1802.
192. Chen S, Fricks J, Ferrari MJ. Tracking measles infection through non-linear state space models. *J R Stat Soc.* 2012. Available: http://onlinelibrary.wiley.com/doi/10.1111/j.1467-9876.2011.01001.x/full.
193. Depaoli S, Clifton JP, Cobb PR. Just another Gibbs sampler (JAGS): flexible software for MCMC implementation. *J Educ Behav Stat.* 2016;41:628–649.

194. Carneiro HA, Mylonakis E. Google trends: a web-based tool for real-time surveillance of disease outbreaks. *Clin Infect Dis.* 2009;49:1557–1564.
195. Funk S, Camacho A, Kucharski AJ, Lowe R, Eggo RM, et al. Assessing the performance of real-time epidemic forecasts: a case study of Ebola in the Western Area region of Sierra Leone, 2014-15. *PLoS Comput Biol.* 2019;15(2), e1006785. Available: https://doi.org/10.1371/journal.pcbi.1006785.
196. Smith DJ. Mapping the antigenic and genetic evolution of influenza virus. *Science.* 2004;305:371–376.
197. Balmaseda A, Stettler K, Medialdea-Carrera R, et al. Antibody-based assay discriminates Zika virus infection from other flaviviruses. *Proc Natl Acad Sci U S A.* 2017;114:8384–8389.
198. Martínez-Vega RA, Carrasquila G, Luna E, Ramos-Castañeda J. ADE and dengue vaccination. *Vaccine.* 2017;35:3910–3912.
199. Xu GJ, Kula T, Xu Q, et al. Viral immunology. Comprehensive serological profiling of human populations using a synthetic human virome. *Science.* 2015;348:aaa0698.
200. Anderson S, Wakeley P, Wibberley G, Webster K, Sawyer J. Development and evaluation of a Luminex multiplex serology assay to detect antibodies to bovine herpes virus 1, parainfluenza 3 virus, bovine viral diarrhoea virus, and bovine respiratory syncytial virus, with comparison to existing ELISA detection methods. *J Immunol Methods.* 2011;366:79–88.
201. Metcalf CJE, Farrar J, Cutts FT, et al. Use of serological surveys to generate key insights into the changing global landscape of infectious disease. *Lancet.* 2016;388:728–730.
202. Ferguson N, Anderson R, Gupta S. The effect of antibody-dependent enhancement on the transmission dynamics and persistence of multiple-strain pathogens. *Proc Natl Acad Sci U S A.* 1999;96:790–794.
203. Ferguson NM, Rodríguez-Barraquer I, Dorigatti I, Mier-Y-Teran-Romero L, Laydon DJ, Cummings DAT. Benefits and risks of the Sanofi-Pasteur dengue vaccine: modeling optimal deployment. *Science.* 2016;353:1033–1036.
204. Priyamvada L, Quicke KM, Hudson WH, et al. Human antibody responses after dengue virus infection are highly cross-reactive to Zika virus. *Proc Natl Acad Sci U S A.* 2016;113:7852–7857.
205. Shanks GD, Brundage JF. Pathogenic responses among young adults during the 1918 influenza pandemic. *Emerg Infect Dis.* 2012;18:201–207.
206. Levenson H., Azad A. Expert explains why estimated US deaths have doubled. Cesk Neurol Neurochir. Available: https://www.cnn.com/videos/us/2020/05/04/christopher-murray-coronavirus-death-model-tsr-vpx.cnn.
207. Glanz J, Leatherby L, Bloch M, et al. Coronavirus could overwhelm U.S. without urgent action, estimates say. *The New York Times.* 2020. Available: https://www.nytimes.com/interactive/2020/03/20/us/coronavirus-model-us-outbreak.html. Accessed 9 Sep 2022.
208. Pflanzer LR. A Report That Helped Convince Trump to Take Coronavirus Seriously Projected That 2.2 Million People Could Die in the US If We Don't Act. Business Insider; 2020. Available: https://www.businessinsider.com/coronavirus-uk-report-projects-2-million-deaths-without-action-2020-3. Accessed 9 Sep 2022.
209. Aizenman N. 5 Key Facts Not Explained in White House COVID-19 Projections. NPR. 2020. Available: https://www.npr.org/sections/health-shots/2020/04/01/824744490/5-key-facts-the-white-house-isnt-saying-about-their-covid-19-projections. Accessed 9 Sep 2022.
210. Reich NG, Lessler J, Funk S, et al. Collaborative hubs: making the most of predictive epidemic modeling. *Am J Public Health.* 2022;112:839–842.
211. Home—COVID 19 forecast hub. [cited 9 Sep 2022]. Available: https://covid19forecasthub.org/.
212. Home—COVID 19 scenario model hub. [cited 9 Sep 2022]. Available: https://covid19scenariomodelinghub.org/.
213. European Covid-19 Forecast Hub. [cited 9 Sep 2022]. Available: https://covid19forecasthub.eu/.
214. Hemri S, Scheuerer M, Pappenberger F, Bogner K, Haiden T. Trends in the predictive performance of raw ensemble weather forecasts. *Geophys Res Lett.* 2014;41:9197–9205.
215. Cramer EY, Ray EL, Lopez VK, et al. Evaluation of individual and ensemble probabilistic forecasts of COVID-19 mortality in the United States. *Proc Natl Acad Sci U S A.* 2022;119, e2113561119.
216. Johansson MA, Apfeldorf KM, Dobson S, et al. An open challenge to advance probabilistic forecasting for dengue epidemics. *Proc Natl Acad Sci U S A.* 2019;116:24268–24274.
217. Pinson P. On the Predictability of COVID-19. International Institute of Forecasters [Internet]; 2021. [cited 9 Sep 2022]. Available: https://forecasters.org/blog/2021/09/28/on-the-predictability-of-covid-19/.
218. Keeling MJ, Woolhouse ME, Shaw DJ, et al. Dynamics of the 2001 UK foot and mouth epidemic: stochastic dispersal in a heterogeneous landscape. *Science.* 2001;294:813–817.
219. Cooper B, Lipsitch M. The analysis of hospital infection data using hidden Markov models. *Biostatistics.* 2004;5:223–237.
220. Pulliam JRC, Epstein JH, Dushoff J, et al. Agricultural intensification, priming for persistence and the emergence of Nipah virus: a lethal bat-borne zoonosis. *J R Soc Interface.* 2012;9:89–101.

CHAPTER 18

Risks and Challenges for First Responders Managing Patients Infected With or Exposed to High-Consequence Infectious Diseases

AL LULLA[a] • FAROUKH MEHKRI[a] • ANDREW CHOU[b] • RONNA G. MILLER[c,*] • S. MARSHAL ISAACS[a]
[a]Division of Emergency Services, Disaster, and Global Health, Department of Emergency Medicine, UT Southwestern, Dallas, TX, United States • [b]Department of Surgery and Perioperative Care, UT Austin Dell Medical School/Austin-Travis County EMS, Austin, TX, United States • [c]Formerly, Emergency Medicine at UT Southwestern, Dallas, TX, United States

INTRODUCTION

First responders in emergency medical services (EMS), law enforcement, and fire protection represent a critical aspect in both the management of the individual patient and the broader effect of an epidemic outbreak on the general health of the public. The prehospital setting is a unique environment with significant challenges, especially in the setting of infectious diseases. This chapter describes the unique risks and challenges for EMS clinicians and other first responders providing prehospital evaluation, care, and transport of patients with high-consequence infectious diseases. This includes a brief history of the impact of prior outbreaks on first responders, considerations for emergency preparedness on a regional and national level, first responder safety, and management of possible occupational and off-duty exposures to transmissible pathogens.

THE IMPACT OF INFECTIOUS DISEASE IN THE PREHOSPITAL SETTING

The role of EMS and first responders can be traced back to the American Civil War era, where medical officers tended to soldiers who were wounded on the battlefield. However, it was not until the unprecedented influenza pandemic of 1918, which claimed the lives of at least 50 million people worldwide, that the significance of prehospital care for patients exposed to or suffering from infectious diseases was recognized.[1] Various American Red Cross chapters across the United States lent their ambulances and trucks to cities to assist in the transport of symptomatic patients to hospital wards or houses for convalescence. The deceased were also transported for burial. In addition to management of those persons afflicted with the virus, the motor corps had a much more widespread effect on combating the outbreak through the dissemination of masks (at the time often made of surgical dressings), gowns, and medications, as well as transport of volunteers.[2] The critical role of prehospital care was further demonstrated in subsequent infectious disease cases, outbreaks, and pandemics, including those caused by influenza, Severe Acute Respiratory Syndrome (SARS), Middle East Respiratory Syndrome (MERS), Ebola, and SARS-CoV-2 (COVID-19).

As a core component of the general public's emergency medical safety net, EMS and other first responders answer 9-1-1 requests for evaluation, stabilization, and resuscitation of critically ill patients, as well as triage and transport of patients to appropriate destination facilities. Unlike a hospital-based environment, which offers a greater degree of control, personal protection from possible exposure, and diagnostic and treatment options, the prehospital environment, on the other hand, is unpredictable and requires medical decision-making and treatment often with limited information. Furthermore, this environment often

*Currently, Independent Consultant.

Viral Outbreaks, Biosecurity, and Preparing for Mass Casualty Infectious Diseases Events
https://doi.org/10.1016/B978-0-323-54841-0.00016-0

requires evaluation and treatment in small enclosed spaces, potentially exacerbating the exposure and transmission of infectious disease.[3] Given these conditions and the lack of adequate information, first responders are at high risk of exposure to infectious disease and serving as a vector in the spread of disease. This effect is only compounded by evidence suggestive of overall inadequate infection prevention practices and resources in the prehospital environment.[4]

In addition to the clinical management of these patients, first responders are tasked with identification of patients who may have a contagious infectious disease, often with limited available information and a lack of diagnostic testing, and are responsible for coordination with local, regional, and national agencies as well as healthcare receiving facilities. Early prehospital identification of possible infectious disease carriers is critical in terms of public health disease mitigation and containment efforts.

NATURALLY OCCURRING INFECTIOUS DISEASE OUTBREAKS/PANDEMICS

Infections transmitted by both respiratory secretions and blood, including tuberculosis, meningococcal infections, HIV, viral hepatitis, and respiratory viruses (viral respiratory infections—VRIs), have long been included during initial and ongoing EMS education and training because they may lead to EMS occupational exposure.[5]

The global SARS-CoV-2 pandemic represents the most recent and dramatic example of a novel, high-consequence infectious disease requiring reinforcement of care principles and ongoing development of new expert guidance for EMS clinicians and other first responders.[6] Other, less significant outbreaks and pandemics have impacted EMS response and management. For example, EMS clinicians were the "tip of the spear" for the US index case during the 2014 Ebola outbreak that impacted Dallas, Texas, and other areas of the United States.[7,8] In 2019, more than 1200 US cases of measles—the most since 1992—may have placed unvaccinated EMS clinicians and other first responders at potential risk, especially in jurisdictions with case clusters among large groups of unvaccinated individuals.[9] This risk was likely compounded because measles had been declared eliminated from the United States in 2000, thereby necessitating booster vaccinations and other mitigation measures for frontline personnel who may not have had vaccine-induced immunity.

Each of these *naturally occurring* outbreaks presented its own risks and challenges for first responders, based on the mode(s) and ease of person-to-person transmission, the availability (or lack thereof) of vaccines and therapeutics, as well as other factors. These recent historical examples highlighted the need for source control and workforce protection [including personal protective equipment (PPE)], vaccination, and other preventive measures. Additionally, the implementation of robust screening protocols will minimize the risk of inadvertent disease transmission through infected EMS clinicians.

In addition, *intentional release* of bioterrorism agents, including viruses (such as smallpox or viral hemorrhagic fevers) and bacteria (such as Anthrax, plague, or tularemia), also presents a potential risk to first responders and is discussed in more detail below.[10] There is no "one size fits all" EMS clinical or workplace safety protocol for all communicable infectious diseases. EMS medical directors, agency/system administrators, and Designated Infection Control Officers (DICOs) have learned from previous outbreaks and must exercise due diligence for currently circulating agents while planning ahead for the next high-consequence infectious disease outbreaks, epidemics, or pandemic situations, whether naturally occurring or intentional.[11]

BIOTERRORISM

Terrorism is the "unlawful use of force against people in order to cause fear, intimidate, coerce government, or affect the civilian population or any segment thereof in the furtherance of political or social objectives."[12] The category of "CBRNE" terrorism and counterterrorism deals with threats that involve chemical, biological, radiological, nuclear, and explosives (CBRNE).[13] Unfortunately, first responders (FRs), many of whom may be EMS providers, will always be among the first individuals to arrive at these incidents, and thus it is of paramount importance to have a basic understanding of biological terrorism and potential agents, as well as the best practices required to maintain scene safety and protect frontline workers engaged in this form of asymmetrical warfare.[14] Providers must be prepared to do what is necessary to protect themselves and patients in the event of a bioterrorism attack. Indeed, Admiral Stansfield Turner, former Director, Central Intelligence Agency, has asserted "only bioweapons and nuclear weapons have the potential to bring the United States past the point of non-recovery."[15]

Among the most challenging aspects of any response to bioterrorism is the initial phase; unless authorities have been alerted by terrorist organizations or prior intelligence indicates an attack is underway, there will already be casualties or exposed/infected patients prior to identification of the infectious agent. Attacks of biological nature can be indolent and difficult to detect. For example, some agents may be aerosolized or impregnated into a municipal water supply, making detection extremely difficult, if not impossible.[14]

Therefore, it is essential for the appropriate authorities to recognize clusters of individuals showing similar symptoms. If a concerning biological agent is identified, it is essential that FRs be alerted as soon as possible. Likely FRs have already transported patients who were victims of the initial attack and that they themselves may have become exposed. Once contact tracing begins, FRs may need to be isolated if deemed appropriate by public health officials and possibly vaccinated, and/or administered antidotes and/or chemoprophylaxis.[16]

At the "street" level, FRs must keep in close contact with other teammates and units and consider the potential for bioterrorism, especially in high-threat—high-risk cities and events. The potential for these attacks exists anywhere, but large ports of entry (such as Miami, FL), capital cities (such as Austin, Texas), large metropolitan subway systems (such as the New York City Metro Transit Authority), and cities of political importance (such as Washington, DC) are high-risk targets. Large national special security events (NSSEs) are another potential target to consider. First responders at these locations and events in particular should be vigilant at entry and exit points, noting suspicious packages and activities, uncredentialed or unusual individuals, and being in constant communication with the event security to help identify any potential concerns. Indoctrinating the right mindset, constantly engaging in "what if" scenarios, and educating oneself and one's team are the first steps to combating bioterrorist events.

Agents of bioterrorism have been classified into three categories based on level of risk to national security and other factors.[17] A comprehensive review of many of these biological agents and their treatments is found in Chapters 3–13. Still, a brief review with examples behooves this discussion.

Category A: these include agents such as Anthrax, Botulinum toxin, *Yersinia pestis* (plague), and viral hemorrhagic fevers (such as Ebola). These agents are extremely dangerous/deadly with high casualty potential and can be easily disseminated via close contact through airborne, respiratory, and/or interpersonal contact. These are the high priority agents for agencies such as FEMA, CDC, and DHS. These require the highest level of handling, isolation, response, action, and coordination.[17]

Category B: these include agents such as *Vibrio cholerae*, hemorrhagic *E. coli* O157:H7, and Ricin toxin (from castor beans). These agents have moderate morbidity but lower fatality rates. They can cause public panic, are easily disseminated, but are generally less virulent and require special surveillance and diagnostic capacity by the CDC.[17]

Category C: these agents are high priority for awareness as they include emerging pathogens that could be engineered for mass exposure in the future because of their accessibility, ability to be disseminated, and ability to cause high morbidity and mortality.[17]

Recommended best practices regarding preparation for such agents and EMS include, but are not limited to:

Agencies should develop response plans for these potential man-made disasters and asymmetric threats.

EMS agencies should contact their local health departments and neighboring EMS departments for assistance, as well as federal agencies and free online resources.

- Recommendations for the use of appropriate body substance isolation and personal protective equipment should be clearly written and available.[18]
- A public health emergency readiness and acute phase (first 24 h) response should be designed and initiated.[19]
- Guidance for local first responders on how to approach suspicious packages, threats, letters, and so on should be available.
- The nearest national stockpile location and identification of the appropriate channels to obtain appropriate antidotes must be delineated.[20]
- Utilization of the epidemic information exchange and a secure online communications network connecting the CDC with state and local health departments, poison control centers, and other public health professionals can be utilized.[21]
- Rules and regulations to help contain spread and conduct quarantine and isolation procedures should be reviewed and understood by local officials.[22]
- Tabletop planning exercises should be held on a regular basis to ensure key stakeholders are current in their understanding of these critical issues.

EMERGENCY PREPAREDNESS AND MULTIJURISDICTIONAL RESPONSE

In widespread infectious disease outbreaks, such as in the case of pandemic influenza and the COVID-19 pandemic, immediate and long-term effects can have a crippling impact on the healthcare system, national economy, transportation system, and infrastructure. Overloading the healthcare system can lead to significant shortages of medical supplies, therapeutics, and even primary care. Worker absenteeism because of disease exposure or the need to care for family members can further exacerbate economic and social disruption.[23]

EMS and first responder agencies, along with emergency (911) public safety answering points (PSAPs), play a critical role as the point of access for those requesting emergency services. In 2007, the US Department of Transportation and the National Highway Traffic Safety Administration (NHTSA) released "EMS Pandemic Influenza Guidelines for Statewide Adoption," stressing the importance of a national strategy for pandemic influenza and the importance of both EMS and 911 PSAP integration into the National Response Plan, which has subsequently been replaced by the National Response Framework. While historically the National Response Plan was coordinated with the federal government to include terrorist attacks, natural disasters, and other emergencies, the plan also forms the basis for the federal pandemic response, ensuring close coordination with state and local agencies.[24]

A key component of the federal response to pandemics and high-consequence infectious disease outbreaks is the National Incident Management System (NIMS). Central to the mission of NIMS is the concept of coordinated response and mutual aid between both local and state jurisdictions, along with federal agencies, to allow for a unified approach to incident management and appropriate resource allocation. In order for there to be a successful deployment of the National Response Framework and NIMS, preestablished delegations of leadership and authority and outlines of individual responsibilities are critical.[25,26]

In addition to unified command and a robust incident management system, specific local and state plans for high-consequence infectious disease events or outbreaks should extensively utilize training and educational programs during the prepandemic preparedness phase. These exercises should focus on principles in accordance with the central concepts of NIMS. Adequate training and deliberate practice for the prevention, management, and response toward high-consequence infectious diseases allows for both the assessment and improvement of performance prior to a widespread infectious disease event.[23]

A systems-based approach is essential to a coordinated and sustainable response effort. The National Response Framework calls for a reliable process for the gathering and disseminating of information, including treatment protocols and clinical standards, between state, local, and tribal EMS agencies as well as larger state and federal entities. This systems-based approach should also include a public information and media plan as part of an incident command system in order to maintain an avenue to deliver important information and instructions to the public.[23]

EMS systems at the local and regional level play an important role in surveillance prior to and during an outbreak. Aggregation of patient information, signs and symptoms, geographic identifiers as part of real-time EMS operations, and 911 data collection can play a critical role in both the surveillance and mitigation efforts during a pandemic.[23]

FIRST RESPONDER DISPATCH CONSIDERATIONS

As with most prehospital encounters, EMS personnel are often first notified of a high-consequence infectious disease incident via a public safety answering point, generally a 911 answering and dispatch location. While the true nature or severity of the incident can be difficult to determine at an early stage, multiple considerations related to dispatch protocols and policy can help promote optimal resource utilization, first responder safety, as well as appropriate patient care.[27]

Many 911 callers are unaware of any exposure to a highly infectious disease agent and may in fact be "second- or third-party callers" who are unfamiliar with the specific circumstances surrounding the exposure. In such circumstances, dispatch providers must rely on alternative factors to facilitate an appropriate response. These may include using permanent flags within the dispatch system for addresses known to handle infectious disease agents (i.e., bioweapon laboratories or Centers for Disease Control research facilities), asking the caller to provide additional information regarding symptoms suggestive of an infectious disease (e.g., recent travel, multiple sick individuals, profuse vomiting, diarrhea, etc.), or even using a universal screening questionnaire in the event of a widespread outbreak. In some instances, particularly for highly transmissible infectious diseases that require mandatory reporting to the local health department, communication between 911 dispatch field crews, medical control, and local health authorities may enable the community to flag addresses for individuals who are known to be infected. This matrixed response can be a valuable tool to ensure that FRs are adequately prepared for and respond to an infectious risk. However, given patient privacy and HIPAA concerns, this strategy may potentially only be available for those diseases that require mandatory reporting under local, state, or federal regulations.

For incidents where a known infectious agent is endemic, dispatch plays an integral role in ensuring scene safety and making sure that appropriate resources are deployed. Initially, dispatch can notify first responder crews of the infectious disease concerns so that they can don the appropriate personal protective equipment. For high-consequence agents, such as measles or Ebola, special response units such as Hazardous Materials (HAZMAT) can even be recruited given their specialized training and equipment, including the use of self-contained breathing apparatus and Level A personal protective equipment (the highest level of protection). In these situations, dispatch may also instruct responding crews to "stage" (that is, to wait in a prepared state) a safe distance away until scene safety has been established.[28]

Some dispatch centers may also be equipped with the capability to employ an outbreak/epidemic protocol as part of a large-scale, prolonged response plan. These protocols are typically implemented to help prevent or respond to the emergency response capacity being overwhelmed by extreme call volume, hospital emergency department overload, as well as staffing shortages due to provider or family illness. The protocol may also allow for a modified response matrix, including only providing telephone instructions without dispatching an EMS unit, providing evaluation or treatment on-scene without transport to a local hospital, or even transport to alternate destinations besides the hospital. Due to the existing perception in most communities that calling 911 will always result in first responder dispatch and hospital transport for medical complaints, implementation of a modified response matrix may require collaboration between community leaders, legal experts, health care authorities, and even the media.[29]

EMS/FIRST RESPONDER PERSONAL PROTECTIVE EQUIPMENT CONSIDERATIONS

With any unknown potentially deadly agent, the standard mantra of safety should always be followed by rescuers and considered nonnegotiable:

1. Always secure the scene before attending to victims so as not to become victims themselves.
2. Use PPE for first responders (FRs) in the midst of an outbreak.
3. Begin with a standard set of PPE and precautions to broadly protect against any potential infectious or biologically dangerous agents *rather than* attempt to protect for specific agents. The recommendations for specific PPE will be dictated by the clinical care that is required as well as the patients' presenting signs and symptoms. Protocols, policies, and guidelines—by themselves—do not suffice. They need to be accompanied by education, training, and equipment fit testing.[30]

For an example of PPE considerations for first responders, please see Fig. 1: UT Southwestern/Parkland BioTel COVID-19 EMS PPE Guidance.

Among the most common and important recommendations are "good hand hygiene, gloves, and adding eye protection and masks for patients with respiratory symptoms and during airway interventions, and gowns for potential splash exposures."[31] It is of pivotal importance early in the recognition of a potential outbreak to clearly set guidelines for FRs regarding on- and off-duty PPE rules and requirements. During the COVID-19 epidemic, FRs and health care personnel were more likely to become exposed secondary to community spread than through the workplace.[32] As such, the authors note that without strong, clear recommendations from leadership who lead by example, the waxing and waning behavior of FRs and laxity with PPE (hand washing, sharing meals, close proximity, and mask wearing) can be a significant detriment to their ability to function as well as a liability during a pandemic wherein the skilled workers are the most valuable resource.

Initially, during patient care evaluations, FRs should assess patients from a distance as much as possible. A minimum of 6–10 ft from the patient should be allowed, when possible, to minimize airborne exposure. FRs should then re-evaluate if their current PPE suffices or if additional measures should be considered. Additional PPE considerations can include impermeable gowns, N95 or similar respirators, eye shields, face shields, and even Personal Air Purifying Respirators (PAPRs). One of the most important practices in any viral outbreak is good hand washing with soap and water or hand sanitizers if soap and water are unavailable. First responders must be diligent about regular, frequent hand washing, remembering to avoid touching their faces and personal items while performing patient care, and removing PPE.[33]

When donning and doffing PPE, it is of utmost importance for the provider to remain vigilant and not be careless with the recommended procedure. There are many recommended systems designed to ensure appropriate donning and doffing of PPE, and readers are referred to their own occupational health and safety officers for specific steps for particular PPE types. In general, some steps should be remembered and universal. A checklist is useful to help FRs doff alertly, ensuring all necessary and recommended items are available and utilized. In some settings, such as with a suspected viral hemorrhagic fever case, a "buddy" can be used to assure doffing is done correctly. Once patient care is complete,

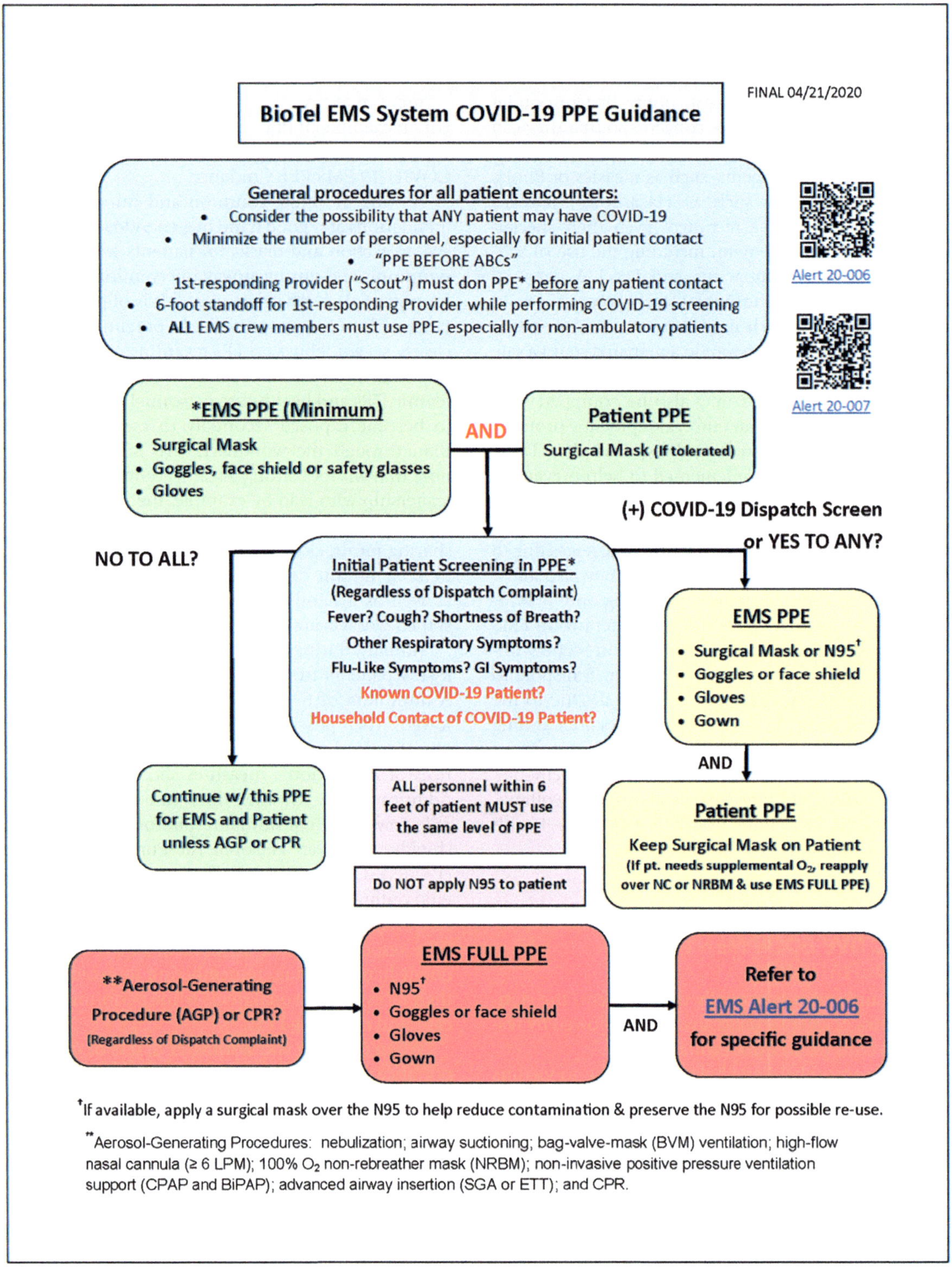

FIG. 1 UT Southwestern Medical Center/Parkland Health BioTel COVID-19 EMS PPE Guidance.
Legend: BioTel is the unified EMS system and communications center that is comprised of 13 city EMS agencies in and around Dallas, Texas, who all function under the same medical direction, policies, and protocols for patient care and transport. *EMS*, emergency medical service; *PPE*, personal protective equipment; *pt*, patient; *O_2*, oxygen; *N95*, N95 respirator or equivalent; *GI*, gastrointestinal; *AGP*, aerosol-generating procedure; *ETT*, endotracheal tube; *SGA*, supraglottic airway; *CPR*, cardiopulmonary resuscitation.

PPE must be removed in an appropriate location that will prevent secondary contamination of providers and others. Whenever possible, impermeable biohazard bags and bins should be used to store used PPE until destroyed.[31]

Decontamination and disinfection of equipment and apparatus is of paramount importance when considering both first responder and patient safety. An "ounce of prevention is worth a pound of cure" as regards mitigating exposure through attention to this important matter. Patients with any suspected respiratory infections should be immediately given a surgical mask to wear (source control) and tissues to collect nasal secretions. When possible, the windows of the transporting apparatus should be open while ensuring that ventilator exhaust fans are constantly running, and providers should be instructed to spend the minimum amount of time necessary to care for the patient when in a confined space with a symptomatic patient. Hospital-grade EPA-registered disinfectants should be used as soon as possible to decontaminate highly used surfaces and equipment. When possible, disposable equipment should be used, being removed from the apparatus following completion of the patient encounter. When or if this is not possible, hospital-grade EPA-registered disinfectants should be used on equipment prior to responding to the next patient.[31]

Occupational Health, Infection Prevention, Operations, and Risk Management departments should be closely involved with ensuring the necessary education and training of staff on PPE use. All FRs should have initial training and continuing educational refresher training on evidence-based practices for PPE usage. It is imperative, especially in times of resource constraint, to ensure that employees are competent in the use of PPE.[31,34,35] Training can be accomplished at any agency headquarters, typically in the training areas where other skills and new equipment are introduced. Alternatively, training can be accomplished at the station level. It is best to choose a senior leader in the organization who is already embedded in the operations, risk management, and/or occupational health departments to oversee the training. Prior to training, the newest research, best practices, and expert recommendations should be reviewed. During any novel infectious agent outbreak, it is common for new information to become available and for new policies and recommendations to be issued by local state and/or federal agencies. As a result, it is critical to inform staff of potential changes so as to not lose trust or cause confusion.[36] Many agencies elect to use a system of "EMS alerts" or a similar platform to disseminate time-sensitive issues that are either new or a refresher. Further core concepts can be introduced as part of a continuing education program for EMS providers.

Certain responsibilities are best left to regulatory entities (e.g., Occupational Safety and Health Administration) and to the employer during an infectious disease outbreak. It is important for employers to be aware of their responsibilities as well. Workers who feel safe and respected by their agencies are more likely to show up for work in the midst of a pandemic. It is imperative therefore that agencies reinforce their concern and support for first responders from the top down. Employers are expected to provide two important tangibles during any infectious disease outbreak: equipment and training. In addition to ensuring adequate supplies of gloves, gowns, respiratory masks, and eye shields, employers should provide visual, verbal, and audio cues that may increase compliance and should empower their staff to speak up and remind one another about safe best practices. For outbreaks that have respiratory concerns, "employers must establish a respiratory protection program that is compliant with OSHA's Respiratory Protection Standard, 29 CFR 1910.134". OSHA consultation can assist with understanding respiratory protection requirements. The Occupational Safety and Health Act of 1970 mandates that employers provide a safe work environment for employees. OSHA exists to help promote these conditions and provide resources and education to ensure this occurs. Individual departments and organizations can reach out to OSHA to receive confidential advice as well as on-site consultation.[34]

First responders must be aware of department updates regarding outbreaks in the response jurisdiction. Any discussion of the more practical and tangible considerations for first responders and PPE requirements must begin with the concept of source control. Prior to transporting any patient who may have been exposed to or is infected with a highly contagious agent, first responders should, after they protect themselves, provide PPE equipment to the patient to limit their ability to spread the infection. In addition, the transport vehicle(s) for the patient(s) should be kept protected as much as possible, limiting the patient's touching of handlebars, side rails, equipment, etc. First responders must ensure that the receiving hospital has been alerted to an incoming high-risk patient, especially if droplet or airborne precautions have been initiated. Finally, healthcare personnel must obtain reliable contact information, including, when possible, addresses as well as any known close contacts of the source patient(s) so that contact tracing and isolation may begin.[31]

Standard precautions always begin even before the FRs arrive on scene. Patients are told to gather their medications and belongings, cover their nose and mouth, if necessary, based on complaints, open locked doors, and make others aware of incoming EMS personnel. Typically, this process is initiated by emergency dispatchers. In addition, providers should be alerted by dispatch as to the nature of the call so that they can make a safe and measured approach with a distanced initial assessment. Standard precautions also include proper work uniforms, closed-toe shoes, gloves, masks, face shields, gowns, and other appropriate items as previously mentioned. When making transport decisions, providers should ensure that the receiving hospital is alerted and has the capability to take the patient. After transport, the unit and all reusable medical equipment should be disinfected utilizing an EPA-registered hospital disinfectant.[31]

Contact precautions are critically important when managing patients releasing body secretions due to contagious agents that can be easily transmitted by touch. While pathogen specific examples include Norovirus, *Clostridiodes difficile*, and methicillin-resistant *Staphylococcus aureus*, FR should think about syndromes associated with these pathogens, such as diarrhea. When evaluating a patient, the FR should ask: Is there a risk that the diarrhea is infectious? EMS providers should inquire specifically about infections that are prevalent in the community, if the patient has ever contracted them in the past, or if certain members of the household have recently developed similar illnesses. Medications such as antiemetics should be considered if the patient has significant vomiting that could worsen the spread of the outbreak (such as with Norovirus).[31]

Droplet precautions must be taken for diseases with known transmission through coughing, sneezing, and mucosal involvement. These include highly contagious pathogens like *Neisseria meningitidis*, Influenza, Group A Streptococcus, Rhinovirus, and Pertussis. Such precautions assist in preventing the inhalation of large respiratory droplets from the patient by providers. In addition, first responders should utilize disposable surgical masks (respirators are not required in the above-mentioned illnesses) and eye/face shields. It is also essential to provide the patient with a surgical mask and encourage hand hygiene and cough etiquette practices. When possible, the provider should maintain a precautionary distance from the patient, remembering to minimize airway interventions that may cause worsening respiratory spray through coughing, sneezing, or gagging. During transport, first responders should continue PPE use, should have exhaust fans engaged, and (if possible) have the windows open in the transporting vehicle.[31,37]

Airborne precautions are imperative when considering diseases such as measles, tuberculosis, and varicella. The goal of airborne precautions is to avoid inhalation of the smaller, aerosolized infectious pathogens. In addition, first responders must be provided with disposable fit-tested N95, P3, or other respirators. When supply chain challenges limit access to disposable N95 respirators, alternatives include elastomeric half-face respirators and powered air purifying respirators (PAPRs) with full hoods and HEPA filters. The latter may be especially important for personnel with facial hair, poor respiratory fit, or other factors making disposable respirators impractical. If invasive airway management of a critically ill patient is required for a patient who is known or suspected to have aerosolized pathogens, then rapid sequence induction (RSI) with a paralytic is recommended to minimize aerosolization, and a bag-valve mask (BVM) with HEPA filter addition should be used to ventilate the patient. First responders must notify the receiving facility of the need for airborne precautions upon arrival.[31]

Special Respiratory Precautions (SRPs) are utilized when there is a high index of suspicion gathered from historical data, federal, state, and local public health alerts, and dispatch algorithms. SRPs may be utilized for diseases that include MERS, smallpox, and the all too familiar SARS-CoV-2. Such patients have the potential to be infectious through airborne droplets for longer time periods and over farther distances. In addition to standard historical questions, 911 call-takers and first responders may inquire about travel to endemic areas and the potential for high-risk exposures. In addition to the previously mentioned PPE, first responders should additionally consider long gowns down to the mid-calf area, double gloving, boot/shoe covers, and disposable or cleanable face shields/goggles, especially if aerosol-generating procedures (AGP's) are necessary. Finally, providers should minimize the number of personnel and family members in close contact with the patient, and they should be present for the least amount of time required.[31,38]

Ebola Virus Disease/Viral Hemorrhagic Fever Precautions (EVD/VHF) include, as the name suggests, Ebola, Marburg, Crimean-Congo Hemorrhagic Fever, and other such hemorrhagic contagious infections. In addition to all previous PPE discussed, first responders should utilize impermeable barriers and respiratory protection. Public safety officers should request that others stay clear of the patient in order to minimize contact. If the responding agency has special transport vehicles available to transport such patients, they should be dispatched along with experienced, highly trained personnel familiar with the care protocols required for these patients. Documentation and charting in these specific circumstances should be either verbal or delayed until after patient transport and decontamination. For patient transport, the most direct safe route should be taken to the appropriate receiving hospital, with appropriate notification of the destination facility while en route. Upon arriving at the hospital, the most direct route should be taken to an appropriate isolation room. EVD/VHF patients will likely be managed in a multidisciplinary approach, with ongoing surveillance of the first responders and healthcare personnel involved. Public information or communication professionals should advise on any media inquiries.[31,39,40]

PATIENT ASSESSMENT AND TREATMENT

Once appropriate personal protective precautions have been established, EMS personnel must turn their attention to patient assessment and treatment. One of the primary general modifications to routine care involves minimizing the number of clinicians providing direct patient care to lessen the opportunity for exposure. In addition, patient assessment and initial management should ideally occur at the site where the patient is found in order to prevent potential contamination of multiple locations, unless the scene is considered unsafe or remaining on scene would pose a serious risk of patient deterioration or infectious risk to the public. In such cases, expedited movement to the patient compartment of the transporting ambulance is prudent.

EMS clinicians generally follow their standard treatment guidelines and protocols in accordance with local or state medical direction. However, in the case of highly infectious agents, certain treatment modifications may be considered. For bloodborne diseases, intravenous access should be obtained only if necessary for immediate stabilization and treatment. When intravenous access is necessary, it should be performed prior to transport or only while the vehicle is not in motion in order to minimize the risk for needlestick injury. In addition, extra care should be taken to ensure that contaminated sharps are disposed of properly.

The highest potential need for treatment modification comes into play in the event of highly infectious respiratory infections, particularly those that can be transmitted by airborne particles (as opposed to droplets). Importantly, in some settings, pathogens that are traditionally transmitted by droplets may be aerosolized, especially when aerosol-generating procedures are used. For these pathogens and those airborne-transmissible diseases, the bulk of the effort lies in minimizing the use of aerosol-generating procedures for those patients with critical needs, as well as optimizing the location in which necessary aerosol-generating procedures are performed. With the realization that even spontaneous speech or coughing can be aerosol-generating in some circumstances, a critical first step is that a protective barrier of some sort, such as a face mask, should be placed over the patient's nose and mouth, assuming it does not significantly interfere with respiration or patient care.[41]

Although there is insufficient evidence to compile a definitive list of aerosol-generating procedures (AGP), there are certainly a number of prehospital procedures that can be reliably assumed to pose a significant risk of aerosol generation. These include, but are not limited to, cardiopulmonary resuscitation (chest compressions), endotracheal intubation, manual BVM ventilation, use of supraglottic airway devices, airway suctioning, as well as noninvasive ventilation such as continuous positive airway pressure (CPAP) and (bilevel positive airway pressure) BiPAP.[42,43a] Recent data show that nebulizer treatments could also generate infectious aerosols, and alternatives to nebulizer treatments, such as the use of handheld inhalers or even intramuscular medication injection, may be considered in the appropriate patient population.[43b,43c] The use of high-flow oxygen may also pose an aerosol risk, although there is insufficient evidence to quantify the specific flow rate at which oxygen delivery may generate aerosols.[43d] However, as a standard precaution, the placement of a facemask over a nasal cannula or nonrebreather mask may help to mitigate this risk.

In true epidemic or pandemic situations, EMS clinicians may also be authorized to use modified termination-of-resuscitation protocols for patients in cardiac arrest. Standard termination-of-resuscitation protocols have been a component of prehospital care since the early 2000s and generally apply to patients who meet a very specific set of criteria, including but not limited to (1) arrest not witnessed by EMS personnel, (2) no shockable rhythm, and (3) no return of spontaneous circulation.[44] Specific local protocols often dictate the minimum duration of resuscitation efforts as well as the minimum interventions that must be performed prior to field termination. In epidemic or pandemic situations, particularly with EMS and hospital systems at or overcapacity with concurrent staffing shortages caused by illness, the termination-of-resuscitation protocols may be broadened to include other patients for whom continued resuscitation and transport to the hospital are deemed to be futile, in accordance with the best available evidence for the infectious disease processes. In extreme circumstances, resuscitation may even be withheld, or EMS personnel may not even be dispatched. These methods, while drastic, could potentially allow for more effective utilization of scarce resources, minimize the risk of infecting critically needed healthcare personnel, and eliminate the standard risks associated with EMS transport, such as traffic accidents. However, the ethical, legal, and moral considerations associated with these changes in practice require implementing community standards, the involvement of content experts, and careful discussion and consultation prior to implementation.

TRANSPORT—RISK REDUCTION FOR PERSONNEL, PATIENTS, AND PASSENGERS

Caring for and transporting patients with communicable infectious diseases may understandably evoke hesitation and emotional distress for EMS clinicians.[45] Rebmann et al. in January 2020, shortly before the global SARS-CoV-2 pandemic, similarly reported a survey of 433 EMS clinicians in which being *requested* versus being *required* to work during a hypothetical influenza pandemic resulted in significantly lower willingness to work, due in part to a lack of pandemic training.[46] Hence, the planning and preparedness for out-of-hospital care can be looked at with fresh ideas to further develop protocols, processes, and practices that will keep communities safe.

Thus, in addition to the modified patient care guidelines already discussed, EMS patient transport procedures may also be modified using the best available and evidence-based science in order to optimize EMS clinician and patient safety and confidence. As with on-scene care, source control for the patient and appropriate levels of PPE for personnel play a vital role. In addition to PPE, Lowe et al. in 2015 described two additional, critical components for EMS transport of patients infected with Ebola virus and similar agents: ambulance preparation and environmental decontamination.[47] For infectious agents with known or potential droplet and/or airborne spread (such as SARS-CoV-2), aerosol-generating procedures should ideally be performed outdoors prior to initiating transport.[48] Best practices also include the same three critical steps described by Lowe et al., as well as:

- Maximize ventilation by establishing settings in the patient compartment (and cab) that provide for maximal air flow.
- Open windows and vents, if possible.
- Minimize the number of personnel providing patient compartment care before initiating and during transport.
- Do not permit family members to accompany the patient, especially in the patient compartment (at least for adult patients).
- Notify prearrival online medical control (OLMC) or the hospital directly.
    - o EMS clinicians may need to modify patient handoff procedures to accommodate Emergency Department protocols.
- Implement robust personnel, apparatus, and equipment disinfection and decontamination procedures prior to returning the apparatus to service.

High-quality and ongoing education and training on the modified protocols for all personnel, ideally with case-based scenarios and ideally with simulation, should be provided before implementation. Adopting modified protocols/guidelines without educating FR and such training is a recipe for failure. Direct involvement of EMS medical directors, experienced training officers, and subject matter experts can enhance acceptance and buy-in from "street-level" personnel who may be skeptical of the proposed changes and the data supporting those changes.

During the time when the most stringent SARS-CoV-2 mitigation procedures were implemented, EMS call volumes initially dropped significantly in many regions across the United States for complex and multifactorial reasons. Yet, the initial decline did not eliminate the need to plan for local/regional EMS call volume surges in the face of extensive community spread, especially in vulnerable populations who developed severe clinical illness. Hence, agency/system level surge plans should be established in collaboration with other local/regional EMS agencies and their medical directors, public health experts, hospitals and healthcare facilities, and online medical control (OLMC) for equitable patient triage and transport decision-making to minimize strain on individual receiving hospitals and maximize the effective utilization of emergency services.

The SARS-CoV-2 pandemic also drove unprecedented consideration for even more extreme crisis standards of care for EMS patient transport in the event that local hospitals lacked both emergency department and inpatient capacity.[49] For example, during periods of extreme widespread community disease transmission and limited hospital resources, many EMS agencies/systems developed algorithms to permit prehospital triage of carefully selected, mildly ill patients for nontransport, reserving emergency ambulance transport only for those patients meeting certain high-risk physiologic criteria and/or certain social determinants that would affect their outcomes (Fig. 2A and B).[50]

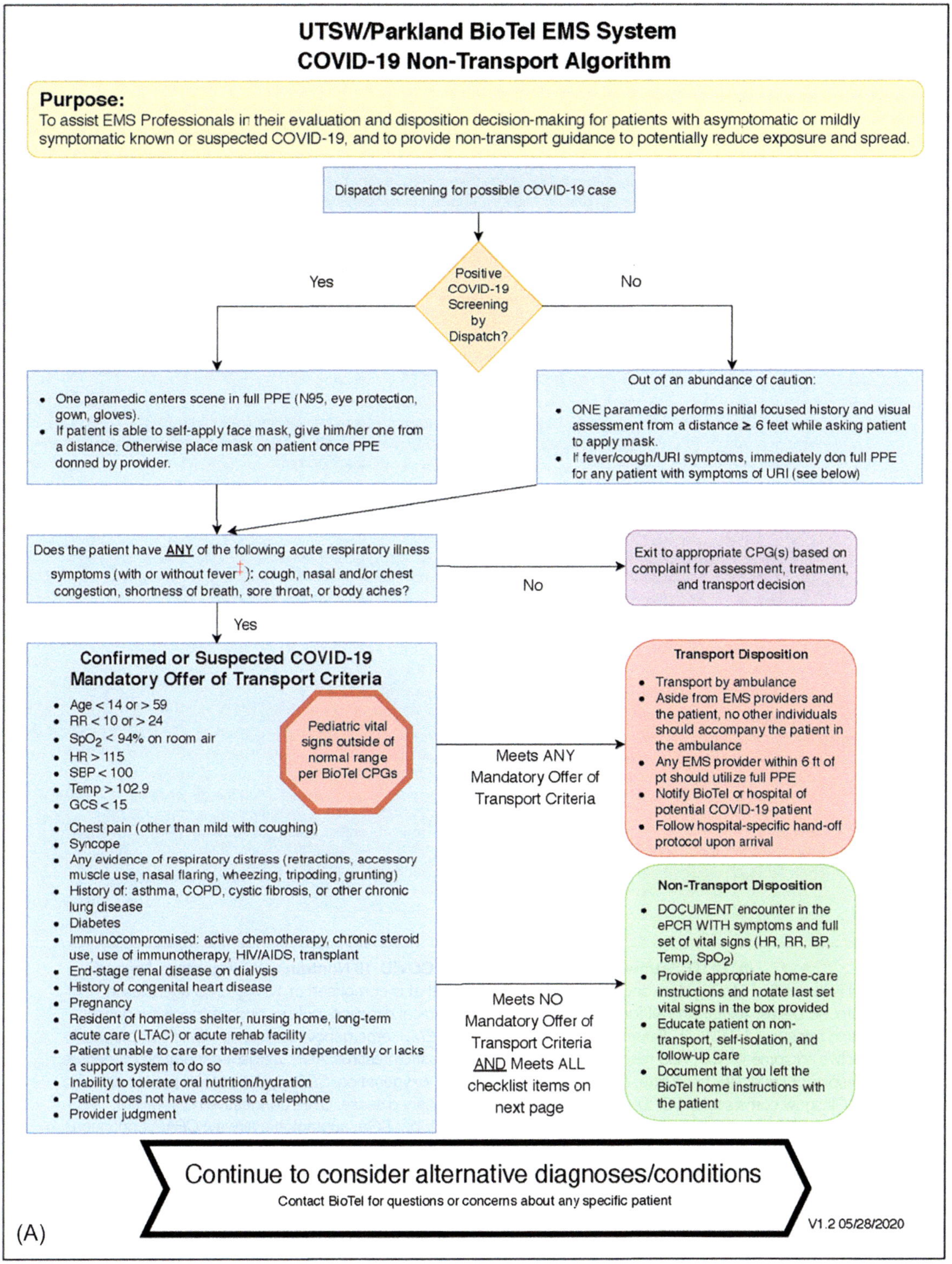

FIG. 2 See the legend in next page.

(Continued)

UTSW/Parkland BioTel EMS System
COVID-19 Non-Transport Algorithm

EMS Checklist: The patient may be left at home if ALL the following are met:

- The patient meets the inclusion criteria and appears to ONLY have symptoms of a mild acute respiratory illness
- The patient meets NO Mandatory Offer of Transport Criteria (you must ASK to rule out each of the criteria)
- The patient is fully alert and oriented at their baseline and can understand the home instructions
- The patient is NOT obviously suffering from an exacerbation of a chronic illness, such as COPD, CHF, asthma, etc.
- The patient is able to care for themselves or has appropriate and available caregivers at home
- The patient has resources and access to food, telephone, and/or other basic necessities
- The patient understands they should contact 911 again if their symptoms worsen

Clinical Pearls

- PPE
  - Upon first contact, provide a surgical mask to the patient to limit spread of their respiratory droplets
  - Wear appropriate PPE at all times during the encounter, taking care to doff appropriately and avoid contamination
  - Use meticulous hand hygiene (soap & water preferred) after any patient contact
- Assessment:
  - ONE single provider should perform the assessment in full PPE (N95, eye protection, gloves, and gown)
  - ‡Fever may be subjective or confirmed (defined as ≥100°F), but it is not always present in patients with COVID-19
    - A patient can have COVID-19 without a fever
    - In the absence of upper/lower respiratory symptoms, strongly consider other sources of fever, such as pneumonia, abdominal pain, GI symptoms, indwelling lines and drains, or skin/wound complaints.
  - Recommended exam (and documentation) includes:
    - Full set of vital signs (HR, RR, BP, Temp, and SpO2)
    - Mental status
    - Neurological
    - HEENT
    - Heart
    - Lungs
    - Skin
- COVID-19
  - Considered a droplet-precaution viral disease
  - Droplets can easily aerosolize by coughing, sneezing, etc
  - Aerosol generating procedures (AGPs) may aerosolize droplets which may remain in the air for several hours, making appropriate PPE prior to assessment very important. AGPs include: nebulization, suctioning, BVM ventilation, high-flow nasal cannula (≥6 LPM); **100% O2 non-rebreather mask; CPAP and BiPAP; advanced airway insertion (SGA or ETT); and CPR.**

V1.2 05/28/2020

(B)

FIG. 2, CONT'D **(A, B) UT Southwestern/Parkland BioTel COVID-19 Nontransport Algorithm.** Legend: BioTel is the unified EMS system and communications center that is comprised of 13 city EMS agencies in and around Dallas, Texas, who all function under the same medical direction, polices and protocols for patient care and transport. *UTSW*, UT Southwestern Medical Center; *EMS*, emergency medical service; *PPE*, personal protective equipment; *N95*, N95 respirator or equivalent; *GI*, gastrointestinal; *AGP*, aerosol-generating procedure; *RR*, respiratory rate; *HR*, heart rate; *BP*, blood pressure; *SpO_2*, oxygenation; *SBP*, systolic blood pressure; *GCS*, Glasgow coma scale; *COPD*, chronic obstructive pulmonary disease; *CHF*, congestive heart failure; *HEENT*, head, eyes, ears, nose and throat; *ETT*, endotracheal tube; *SGA*, supraglottic airway; *CPAP*, continuous positive airway pressure; *BIPAP*, bilevel positive airway pressure; *LPM*, liters per minute; *CPR*, cardiopulmonary resuscitation; *911*, emergency number to contact law enforcement and ambulances in the United States.

Such guidelines must consider the ethics of EMS-initiated nontransport, striking a delicate balance between public expectations and perceptions, and the reality of rationing scarce local healthcare resources. These guidelines must be developed in consultation with local infectious diseases and public health experts based on the best available science and local home health equipment and laboratory resources. Several conditions should be met before implementation:

- Prior approval by stakeholders, such as municipal, legal, and EMS agency leaders.
- Focused training and education for first responders to assist with buy-in, including live "Town Halls" to encourage personnel to ask questions and voice concerns.
- An information "packet" or flyer to be left with the patient, explaining why transport was not offered, including home-care instructions (based on CDC or other authoritative guidelines) and what to do to seek assistance if the patient's clinical condition worsens:
    - o This should be available in different languages and be culturally appropriate and based on local demographics.

MANAGEMENT OF POSSIBLE PERSONNEL EXPOSURES

Management of EMS clinicians' occupational and off-duty exposures during viral outbreaks, epidemics, or pandemics mirrors that for other healthcare professionals, as described in Chapters 2–11, 13, 15, 19, and 24.[50]

Protocols for screening, testing, tracing, isolation/quarantine, treatment, and return to work will likely evolve over time as experience and data accumulate. They should be based on the best available science, be adapted quickly as new data emerge, and should account for the need to balance individual, agency, and community safety with the very real need to maintain minimum staffing levels for FRs who are critical frontline public safety workers. Fortunately, the SARS-CoV-2 pandemic has led to the publication (and frequent updating) of detailed guidance documents and other resources from the CDC, WHO, and OSHA tailored to EMS personnel, firefighters, and other first responders.[51,52] These resources will also be invaluable starting points for guidance during future infectious disease outbreaks, epidemics, or mass casualty events. Agency/system protocols and procedures should strive to build and maintain resilience for personnel subjected to stress and other mental health issues during an outbreak or pandemic.

Direct, hands-on involvement by EMS medical directors can be extremely valuable and facilitate communication and can include: "Town Halls," small group and individual outreach; frequent, focused EMS "Alerts" and memos; and use of social media and other platforms to provide access to credible, authoritative information sources.[50] For example, to combat vaccine hesitancy during the SARS-CoV-2 pandemic, many EMS medical directors used their own vaccination "selfies" or public/filmed vaccination as a means to encourage vaccine acceptance.

Such communication techniques when vaccines, prophylactic measures, or other-directed prevention modalities are or become available for the outbreak agent can be key to enhancing acceptance and further protecting a key element of the response.

Considerations unique to fire service-based EMS personnel who typically work 24-h shifts include the operational feasibility of nearly 24-h-a-day masking; physical distancing in cramped living and sleeping quarters; and shared cooking duties and meals. Longstanding firehouse/EMS station behaviors and practices for these activities that have increased comradery and improved teamwork may need to be significantly modified under extenuating pandemic conditions. Finally, first responders must make EMS responses and transports within the close quarters of emergency vehicles and must provide patient care to often critically ill patients in the undifferentiated prehospital setting. Coupled with the physical demands of PPE donning and doffing, as well as the pervasive duty to complete vehicle/equipment disinfection and decontamination, this can lead to fatigue, stress, and burnout. Outbreaks, and especially pandemics, are unique disasters in that they can go on for long periods of time, minimizing the ability for recovery. Furthermore, when the pathogen is communicable and associated with high morbidity and mortality, as was the case with SARS-CoV-2, emotional stress and burnout can be further exacerbated. In these circumstances, in addition to resources available from public health agencies, the EMS physicians can be particularly helpful and should play a vital role supporting their personnel and their communities during emergencies, including infectious disease outbreaks and pandemics.[50]

CONCLUSION

EMS professionals play a key role in the planning, response, and mitigation phases of responding to individual or multiple patients during outbreaks of high-consequence infectious diseases. There are many risks and challenges to be addressed by EMS systems so that patient care may be optimized, morbidity and mortality lessened, and the impact on the community and disruption of daily life is minimized. As Hans Zinsser (1878–1940), a renowned American bacteriologist and epidemiologist, said, "Infectious disease is one of the few adventures left in the world. The dragons are all dead, and the lance grows rusty in the chimney corner."

ACKNOWLEDGMENTS

The authors wish to acknowledge all the brave and dedicated EMS professionals throughout the world, particularly those in the UTSW/Parkland BioTel EMS System who worked and fought valiantly during the COVID-19 pandemic to ensure that those suffering from this infection as well as all other "routine" emergencies received appropriate and compassionate emergency care. We recognize and honor those who gave their lives or whose health was impacted in service of their communities. We also wish to thank Dr. Raymond Fowler for his thoughtful review of this chapter.

REFERENCES

1. Goniewicz M. Effect of military conflicts on the formation of emergency medical services systems worldwide. *Acad Emerg Med.* 2013;20(5):507–513.
2. Jones MM. The American Red Cross and local response to the 1918 influenza pandemic: a four-city case study. *Public Health Rep.* 2010;125(Suppl. 3):92–104.
3. Centers for Disease Control and Prevention. First Responders: Interim Recommendations for Emergency Medical Services (EMS) Systems and 911 Public Safety Answering Points/Emergency Communication Centers (PSAP/ECCs) in the United States During the Coronavirus Disease (COVID-19) Pandemic. Updated July 15, 2020. https://www.cdc.gov/coronavirus/2019-ncov/hcp/guidance-for-ems.html. Accessed May 10, 2021.
4. Thomas B, O'Meara P, Spelten E. Everyday dangers—the impact infectious disease has on the health of paramedics: a scoping review. *Prehosp Disaster Med.* 2017;32(2):217–223.
5. El Sayed M, Kue R, McNeil C, Dyer KS. A descriptive analysis of occupational health exposures in an urban emergency medical services system: 2007-2009. *Prehosp Emerg Care.* 2011;15(4):506–510.
6. What Firefighters and EMS Providers Need to Know About COVID-19. Centers for Disease Control and Prevention; 2020. Updated November 6, 2020. https://www.cdc.gov/coronavirus/2019-ncov/community/organizations/firefighter-EMS.html. Accessed May 5, 2021; COVID-19 Information for the Workplace. National Institute for Occupational Safety and Health (NIOSH). Reviewed July 20, 2020. Accessed May 5, 2021.
7. McCoy CE, Loftipour S, Chakravarthy B, et al. Emergency medical services public health implications and interim guidance for the Ebola virus in the United States. *West J Emerg Med.* 2014;XV(7):723–727. https://doi.org/10.5811/westjem.2014.10.24155.
8. Bell BP, Damon IK, Jernigan DB, et al. Overview, control strategies, and lessons learned in the CDC response to the 2014-2016 Ebola epidemic. *CDC Morb Mortal Wkly Rep.* 2016;65(3):4–11.
9. Patel M, Lee AD, Clemmons NS, et al. National update on measles cases and outbreaks—United States, January 1–October 1, 2019. *CDC Morb Mortal Wkly Rep.* 2019;68(40):893–896.
10. Bioterrorism Agents/Diseases. Centers for Disease Control and Prevention; 2018. Reviewed April 4, 2018. https://emergency.cdc.gov/agent/agentlist-category.asp. Accessed May 5, 2021.
11. National Association for Public Safety Infection Control Officers (NAPSICO). https://www.napsico.org/. Accessed May 5, 2021.
12. Terrorism 2002/2005. Federal Bureau of Investigation; 2005. https://www.fbi.gov/stats-services/publications/terrorism-2002-2005.
13. Chemical Biological, Radiological and Nuclear Terrorism. United Nations Office of Counter Terrorism; 2021. https://www.un.org/counterterrorism/cct/chemical-biological-radiological. Accessed 12 June 2021.
14. Bioterrorism Awareness for EMS. EMS World; 2004. https://www.emsworld.com/article/10324787/bioterrorism-awareness-ems.
15. Center for Health Security, Johns Hopkins. FEMA's Role in Managing Bioterrorist Attacks | Testimony Before Senate. Johns Hopkins Center for Health Security; 2001. https://www.centerforhealthsecurity.org/our-work/publications/femas-role-in-managing-bioterrorist-attacks.
16. Center for Health Security J FEMA's Role in Managing Bioterrorist Attacks | Testimony Before Senate. Johns Hopkins Center for Health Security. https://www.centerforhealthsecurity.org/our-work/publications/femas-role-in-managing-bioterrorist-attacks. Published 2001.
17. CDC. Bioterrorism Agents/Diseases (by Category) | Emergency Preparedness & Response; 2021. Emergency.cdc.gov. https://emergency.cdc.gov/agent/agentlist-category.asp.
18. National Institute for Occupational Safety and Health (NIOSH). Respirators and Protective Clothing for Protection Against Biological Agents; 2009. https://www.cdc.gov/niosh/docs/2009-132/default.html. Accessed June 12, 2021.
19. Public Health Emergency—Strategic National Stockpile; 2021. Phe.gov. https://www.phe.gov/about/sns/Pages/default.aspx.
20. Suspicious Package Biothreat; 2021. Emergency.cdc.gov https://emergency.cdc.gov/planning/pdf/suspicious-package-biothreat.pdf.
21. CDC. Epidemic Information Exchange; 2018. Emergency.cdc.gov. https://emergency.cdc.gov/epix/.
22. Title 42—The Public Health and Welfare Chapter 6A—Public Health Service Subchapter II—General Powers and Duties; 2011. Govinfo.gov. https://www.govinfo.gov/app/details/USCODE-2010-title42/USCODE-2010-title42-chap6A-subchapII-partG-sec264.
23. EMS Pandemic Influenza Guidelines for Statewide Adoption; 2007. https://www.ems.gov/pdf/preparedness/Resources/Pandemic_Influenza_Guidelines.pdf. Accessed June 14, 2021.
24. National Response Framework; 2019. https://www.fema.gov/sites/default/files/2020-04/NRF_FINALApproved_2011028.pdf. Accessed June 14, 2021.
25. National Incident Management System; 2017. http://www.fema.gov/sites/default/files/2020-07/fema_nims_doctrine-2017.pdf. Accessed June 14, 2021.
26. Farcas A, Ko J, Chan J, Malik S, Nono L, Chiampas G. Use of incident command system for disaster preparedness: a

model for an emergency department covid-19 response. *Disaster Med Public Health Prep Published online.* 2020;1–6.
27. Clawson JJ. EMS dispatch. *Emerg Med Serv.* 2015;94–112.
28. Blackwell T, Brennan K, DeAtley C, Yee A. Medical support for hazardous materials response. *Emerg Med Serv.* 2015;321–333.
29. Pandemic/Epidemic/Outbreak (Surveillance or Triage); 2021. https://cdn.emergencydispatch.org/iaed/pdf/NAE_Pandemic_v13-3.pdf.
30. Cash RE, Rivard MK, Camargo CA, et al. Emergency medical services personnel awareness and training about personal protective equipment during the COVID-19 pandemic. *Prehosp Emerg Care.* 2021. https://doi.org/10.1080/10903127.2020.1853858. Accessed May 5, 2021.
31. EMS Infectious Disease Playbook; 2017. Ems.gov https://www.ems.gov/pdf/ASPR-EMS-Infectious-Disease-Playbook-June-2017.pdf. Accessed 14 June 2021.
32. Jacob J, Baker J, Fridkin S, et al. Risk factors associated with SARS-CoV-2 seropositivity among US Health Care Personnel. *JAMA Netw Open.* 2021;4(3): e211283. https://doi.org/10.1001/jamanetworkopen.2021.1283.
33. Hand Washing: Proper Technique, Antibacterial Soap, Hand Sanitizers and More. Cleveland Clinic; 2021. https://my.clevelandclinic.org/health/articles/17474-hand-washing. Accessed 14 June 2021.
34. Protecting Workers During a Pandemic. Occupational Safety and Health Administration; 2014. https://www.osha.gov/sites/default/files/publications/OSHAFS-3747.pdf. Accessed June 14, 2021.
35. Designing an Effective PPE Program: OSH Answers. Canadian Centre for Occupational Health & Safety; 1997. https://wwwccohsca/oshanswers/prevention/ppe/designinhtml. Accessed June 14, 2021.
36. Lemon S. Ethical and Legal Considerations in Mitigating Pandemic Disease. Washington, DC: National Academies Press; 2007.
37. Transmission-Based Precautions | Basics | Infection Control. CDC; 2016. Cdcgov. https://wwwcdcgov/infectioncontrol/basics/transmission-based-precautionshtml. Accessed June 14, 2021.
38. Healthcare Workers. Centers for Disease Control and Prevention; 2020. https://www.cdc.gov/coronavirus/2019-ncov/hcp/guidance-for-ems.html. Accessed 14 June 2021.
39. Shoemaker T, Choi M. Viral Hemorrhagic Fevers—Chapter 4–2020 Yellow Book | Travelers' Health. CDC; 2019. https://wwwnc.cdc.gov/travel/yellowbook/2020/travel-related-infectious-diseases/viral-hemorrhagic-fevers. Accessed 14 June 2021.
40. Viral Hemorrhagic Fevers (VHFs). United States Department of Labor a; 2021. https://www.osha.gov/vhf. Accessed June 14, 2021.
41. Asadi S, Wexler AS, Cappa CD, Barreda S, Bouvier NM, Ristenpart WD. Aerosol emission and superemission during human speech increase with voice loudness. *Sci Rep.* 2019;9(1).
42. Tran K, Cimon K, Severn M, Pessoa-Silva CL, Conly J. Aerosol generating procedures and risk of transmission of acute respiratory infections to healthcare workers: a systematic review. *PloS One.* 2012;7(4): e35797. https://doi.org/10.1371/journal.pone.0035797.
43. (a) Clinical Questions About COVID-19: Questions and Answers. CDC. Centers for Disease Control and Prevention; 2021. https://www.cdc.gov/coronavirus/2019-ncov/hcp/faq.html. Updated 2021-06-11T05:06:31Z. (b) Heinzerling A, Stuckey MJ, Scheuer T, et al. Transmission of COVID-19 to Health Care Personnel during exposures to a hospitalized patient—Solano County, California, February 2020. *MMWR Morb Mortal Wkly Rep.* 2020;69(15):472–476. https://doi.org/10.15585/mmwr.mm6915e5. (c) Cummings DAT, Radonovich LJ, Gorse GJ, et al. Risk factors for healthcare personnel infection with endemic coronaviruses (HKU1, OC43, NL63, 229E): results from the respiratory protection effectiveness clinical trial (ResPECT). *Clin Infect Dis.* 2020; ciaa900. https://doi.org/10.1093/cid/ciaa900. (d) Haymet A, Bassi GL, Fraser JF. Airborne spread of SARS-CoV-2 while using high-flow nasal cannula oxygen therapy: myth or reality? *Intensive Care Med.* 2020;46(12):2248–2251. https://doi.org/10.1007/s00134-020-06314-w.
44. Physici NAOE. Termination of resuscitation in non-traumatic cardiopulmonary arrest. *Prehosp Emerg Care.* 2011;15(4):542.
45. Alexander AB, Master MM, Warren K. Caring for infectious disease in the prehospital setting: a qualitative analysis of EMS providers experiences and suggestions for improvement. *Prehosp Emerg Care.* 2020;24(1):77–84. https://doi.org/10.1080/10903127.2019.1601313.
46. Rebmann T, Charney RL, Loux TM, et al. Emergency medical services personnel's pandemic influenza training received and willingness to work during a future pandemic. *Prehosp Emerg Care.* 2020;24(5):601–609. https://doi.org/10.1080/10903127.2019.1701158.
47. Lowe JJ, Jelden KC, Schenarts PJ, et al. Considerations for safe EMS transport of patients infected with Ebola virus. *Prehosp Emerg Care.* 2015;19(2):179–183. https://doi.org/10.3109/10903127.2014.983661.
48. Jackson T, Deibert D, Wyatt G, et al. Classification of aerosol-generating procedures: a rapid systematic review. *BMJ Open Respir Res.* 2020;7:e000730 1–9. https://doi.org/10.1136/bmjresp-2020-000730.
49. Leider JP, DeBruin D, Reynolds N, et al. Ethical guidance for disaster response, specifically around crisis standards of care: a systematic review. *Am J Public Health.* 2017;107: e1–e9. https://doi.org/10.2105/AJPH.2017.303882.
50. Cabañas JG, Williams JG, Gallagher JM, Brice JH. COVID-19 pandemic: the role of EMS physicians in a community response effort. *Prehosp Emerg Care.* 2021;25(1): 8–15. https://doi.org/10.1080/10903127.2020.1838676.
51. Infection Control Guidance for Healthcare Professionals About Coronavirus (COVID-19). Centers for Disease Control and Prevention; 2020. Updated June 3, 2020. https://www.cdc.gov/coronavirus/2019-ncov/hcp/infection-control.html. Accessed May 5, 2021; Protecting Workers: Guidance on Mitigating and Preventing the Spread of COVID-19 in the Workplace. Occupational

Safety and Health Administration (OSHA). Updated: January 29, 2021. https://www.osha.gov/coronavirus/safework. Accessed May 5, 2021.

52. First Responders—Interim Recommendations for Emergency Medical Services (EMS) Systems and 911 Public Safety Answering Points/Emergency Communication Centers (PSAP/ECCs) in the United States During the Coronavirus Disease (COVID-19) Pandemic. Centers for Disease Control and Prevention; 2020. Updated July 15, 2020. https://www.cdc.gov/coronavirus/2019-ncov/hcp/guidance-for-ems.html. Infection Control Guidance for Healthcare Professionals about Coronavirus (COVID-19). Centers for Disease Control and Prevention. Updated June 3, 2020. https://www.cdc.gov/coronavirus/2019-ncov/hcp/infection-control.html. Accessed May 5, 2021.

CHAPTER 19

Healthcare Preparedness for Infectious Diseases Mass Casualty Events, Including Bioterrorism, Viral Outbreaks and Pandemics

MADHURI M. SOPIRALA[a,b] • LAURA BUFORD[a]
[a]Infection Prevention, Parkland Health, Dallas, TX, United States • [b]Division of Infectious Diseases and Geographic Medicine, Department of Internal Medicine, University of Texas Southwestern Medical Center, Dallas, TX, United States

Mother nature is the greatest bioterrorist of them all, with no financial limitations or ethical compunctions.

MICHAEL T. OSTERHOLM[1]

While most of the natural disasters that affect humans have a man-made component in some shape or form, one can easily imagine the destruction that a deliberate, well-organized, and well-thought-out bioterrorism event can cause in its wake. Even those with poor imagination do not have to look further than Hollywood, where the silver screen artfully depicts the horrid effects of such an event.[2] Man-made disasters can also be unintentional, resulting from either innocent laboratory accidents such as accidental injection or mucous membrane exposure to contaminated materials or bites from research animals, or they can be a result of unintentional release during an otherwise unlawful or criminal act. Natural disasters, however, are the most commonly occurring infectious disease events. They can range from small-scale outbreaks, which are brief with limited consequences or with limited capability to cause damage, to pandemics that can result in large-scale loss of human life and have a significant economic impact. COVID-19 demonstrated how a pandemic can cause (1) fear among the public and healthcare personnel (HCP), (2) put enormous pressure on healthcare systems, (3) cause front-line worker staffing shortages, (4) Disrupt critical supply chains, and (5) significantly impact regional and national economics. Many biological agents that cause natural disasters have the potential to be bioengineered (see Chapter 12), which could lead to more devastation than would have occurred with natural emergence.

Recall the panic caused by the West African-based Ebola Virus Disease (EVD) outbreak in 2014–15.[3] A total of 11 people were treated in the United States.[3,4] Two HCPs were infected after exposure to cases cared for in the United States and recovered fully. Seven additional HCPs were infected while volunteering in the EVD-affected West African countries. While the toll of HCP was significant in West Africa, in the United States, two of 11 (18%) died during this epidemic in their EVD. The Centers for Disease Control and Prevention (CDC) launched a massive public health response ranging from establishing a system to screen and follow all travelers returning from Ebola-affected countries and to define levels of care and tiers for hospitals to plan for should potential and confirmed EVD patients present. Approximately 29,000 persons were monitored between October 2014 and December 2015.[3] Among the tiers developed for hospital readiness were hospitals that assessed patients, hospitals with resources to treat patients, and front-line hospitals that identified, triaged, and isolated persons under investigation and transferred them to an assessment or treatment hospital with more expertise and resources.[3,5] In other words, front-line hospitals were only expected to triage and isolate patients, which would be followed by a "quick" transfer to a higher-tier institution. Assessment

Viral Outbreaks, Biosecurity, and Preparing for Mass Casualty Infectious Diseases Events
https://doi.org/10.1016/B978-0-323-54841-0.00001-9

hospitals were expected to care for a patient for up to 5 days until an Ebola diagnosis was either confirmed or ruled out.[5] Some assessment hospitals had up to three rooms designated to care for persons of interest and 55 hospitals were designated as treatment facilities that provided facilities and care for patients with high-consequence pathogens yet required extensive preparations.[5] While the CDC's efforts were heroic, the planning and execution of the plan, including training and providing resources, took several months during the active outbreak, leading to widespread concern about the risk to the public. One of the challenges the CDC encountered was a lack of adequately trained staff at healthcare facilities to provide the complex care needed by EVD-infected patients, including those who knew how to use the necessary personal protective equipment (PPE) required for these patients, who were experts in EVD patient management, and facilities that had identified dedicated space appropriate for the care of such patients.[5]

Now imagine a scenario where the Ebola virus is genetically engineered to be more transmissible or more virulent and then released in a planned bioterrorist event. In the worst-case scenario, a much higher number of patients would flood healthcare facilities, including front-line hospitals. In this scenario, there likely would not be adequate time or resources to transport patients to assessment and treatment hospitals. Higher-tier hospitals may not have room or the requisite staffing to accept patients from the front-line hospitals because of the influx of patients they are simultaneously experiencing. Hence, all hospitals would be expected to take care of these patients. A valid question to ask is, "Are our hospitals and our healthcare facilities prepared for such an event?"

While the tenets of preparedness are similar between a bioterrorism event and cases of pathogens of high consequence or with pandemic potential, the response may require different strategies and the deployment of resources. In general, a bioterrorism event occurs after a single exposure, so the influx of patients and potential exposure will occur over a defined time period. The pressure on the healthcare system will be intense, but its anticipated duration will be shorter. That said, there are agents such as smallpox that are transmissible from person to person and could propagate, or EVD, where containment of the source may take weeks, or a pandemic where ongoing transmission occurs. The pressure on the healthcare system may not be as intense, but it will persist for an extended period, leading to HCP fatigue and a continuous demand for equipment, resources, and supplies.

CURRENT STATE OF US HOSPITAL/ HEALTHCARE SYSTEM PREPAREDNESS

In a bioterrorist attack or large-scale infectious disease mass casualty event, federal, state, and local officials realized that front-line hospitals and their emergency departments may not have the capability to receive and treat a mass influx of patients. The TOPOFF, the abbreviated name for the Top Officials Exercise, was a national exercise that ran from 2000 to 2009 and was a congressionally mandated biennial cycle of planning events, national exercises, and seminars to "strengthen the United States' capacity to prevent, prepare for, respond to, and recover from large-scale terrorist attacks."[6,7] The TOPOFF 2000 conducted exercise testing using a bioterrorism scenario using *Yersinia pestis*, the causative agent of pneumonic plague, being released at a public event in a single location in one city.[8,9] The third day following the release, 500 persons reported symptoms, and the number grew to 800 cases and over 100 deaths by the end of the day. Antibiotic and ventilator shortages started to occur on the first day and became worse in the succeeding 2 days. Moving antibiotics from the stockpile delivery points to the hospitals and persons needing treatment and prophylaxis proved to be difficult. Medical care was not sustainable due to inadequate hospital staffing and space (i.e., beds), equipment (i.e., ventilators), and medication shortages. Isolation capabilities were severely impacted, hindering the ability to prevent transmission to hospital staff.[8,9] One week after the release, an estimated 3700 plague cases in multiple cities and countries including England and Japan were recorded. In this scenario, between 950 and 2000 deaths occurred, and patients arrived at hospitals at 10 times the normal volumes.

In the year 2000, Congress passed the Public Health Improvement Act, which directed the United States General Accounting Office (GAO) to examine hospital preparedness for a bioterrorist attack.[9] As tasked by Congress, GAO surveyed over 2000 urban hospitals, and 73% of those responded. The GAO survey included information about planning activities, staff training, hospital resources, and capacity for response. Their findings were not unexpected and clearly demonstrated the absence of adequate hospital preparedness in the United States. While most hospitals participated in basic planning and coordination activities for bioterrorism response, they lacked all the necessary medical equipment, trained hospital staff, and appropriate quarantine or isolation spaces to manage large volumes of patients. While they had reported having provided some level of training to the hospital staff on the identification and diagnosis of most common biological agents likely to be used in an attack, only a few hospitals had conducted drills or exercises with a bioterrorism scenario. Some did not have an emergency response plan for bioterrorism, and if they did, the plan lacked key components.[9] Though the Federal Government increased funding to enhance hospital preparedness in the aftermath of this report, the gaps remained. In testimony before the House of Representatives Committee on Government Reform, the GAO rightfully stated that many of the capabilities required for responding to a large-scale bioterrorism event are the same as those required for hospital response to naturally occurring large-scale infectious disease disasters, such as those that occurred with Severe Acute Respiratory Syndrome (SARS).[10] The report confirmed that building dual-use infrastructure improves our capacity to respond to all infectious disease hazards, and the lack of developing such infrastructure and resources could possibly lead to an inability to effectively respond in a devastating pandemic.[10] Almost 20 years later, that prediction correctly identified vulnerabilities that became evident as COVID-19 emerged. While this describes the state of preparedness in the United States, similar gaps likely exist worldwide, and the SARS-CoV-2 pandemic demonstrated that such gaps are a universal challenge.

HEALTHCARE PREPAREDNESS FOR BIOTERRORISM OR LARGE-SCALE INFECTIOUS DISEASE EVENTS

Disaster Preparedness Plan for Emerging Infectious Diseases or Mass Casualty Events

While this chapter focuses on acute care hospitals, the principles of preparedness are the same across the spectrum of healthcare, even if the facility infrastructure and resources are different. Preparedness activities can be tailored to a specific site, but all require planning. Clinic personnel, for example, will need to be able to recognize syndromes and be alert for unusual events even if they do not care for these patients. Their preparedness approach may focus on case recognition, yet it also needs to include keeping other patients and staff safe. Likewise, smaller, critical access hospitals may not care for a patient infected with a high-consequence pathogen, but they need to prepare for case recognition, stabilization, and initial treatment until a transfer can be executed.

All hospitals and most healthcare facilities must have a disaster preparedness plan, which should include responses to infectious disease events.[11–16] Such a plan is ideally made after a thorough multidisciplinary risk assessment examining knowledge, education, and infrastructure, including building space, and staffing capabilities (Table 1). Because of the complexity

TABLE 1
Elements of Policy/Protocol for Bioterrorism and Pandemic Showing All-Hazards Approach With Minimal Differences in Hospital Procedures Between Bioterrorism and Pandemic

Introduction
o Primary objective is to provide guidance in responding to an influx of a high number of patients either infected with, suspected to be infected with, or exposed to a contagion. The goal is to provide safe care while containing the contagion and preventing transmission among patients and healthcare personnel
Procedures: (for both bioterrorism and pandemic unless otherwise indicated)
Decision to Activate
o Identifying an unusually high influx of patients with sepsis or respiratory illness
o Demonstration of a larger epidemic than would be expected in a given community
o Identification of multiple patients with similar but unusual symptoms at the facility's triage locations
o Identification of an infectious agent or disease that is either geographically or seasonally unusual
Bioterrorism
o Recognition or suspicion of a highly infectious agent known to be associated with biological warfare
o Notification from law enforcement of a biological attack
Pandemic
o Declaration of a pandemic or an impending pandemic by public health officials
Prior to Activation
o Leadership of the incident command center, including the incident commander, the associate incident commander/s, and the hospital epidemiologist, should agree that activation is needed

(Continued)

TABLE 1
Elements of Policy/Protocol for Bioterrorism and Pandemic Showing All-Hazards Approach With Minimal Differences in Hospital Procedures Between Bioterrorism and Pandemic—cont'd

Communication
- Activate incident command center
- Notify clinical leaders and appropriate local and regional health authorities
- Notify staff utilizing appropriate avenues, such as town hall updates, to keep them informed
- Plan for updates at regular and frequent intervals
- Publicize critical information to staff and the public

Bioterrorism
- Notify appropriate law enforcement officials

Authority
- Direction and oversight of healthcare facility activities is provided by the incident commander, associate incident commander, other leaders in the incident command center, and hospital epidemiologist

Education
- Educate staff on the recognition, diagnosis, and reporting of an event

Security
- Limit access and egress of hospital/health facility entrances

Bioterrorism
- Provide security at main entrances that remain open

Triage
- Identify site/s and designate staffing

Infection Prevention and Control
- Ensure adequate hand hygiene stations and personal protective equipment (PPE) supplies
- Evaluate if masking of healthcare personnel is needed at entry points
- Implement strict standard precautions especially while the nature of transmission is unknown
- Manage patient placement to cohort as applicable
- Assess patient placement location to find the most appropriate space in the facility with proper ventilation, isolation capabilities, etc.
- Supervise/support/implement syndromic surveillance and case finding
- Manage healthcare personnel staffing in the selected areas of interest as applicable based on immune status, vaccine status, etc.
- Implement strategies to maintain a healthy workforce such as providing vaccines, preexposure, and postexposure prophylaxis, etc.
- Engage pharmacy and therapeutics committee to manage antibiotics and other critical drugs
- Publish guidance for management of patients
- Assess the need to close nonessential hospital functions

Facilities/Environmental Services
- Create negative pressure in the areas of interest as applicable
- Erect temporary walls to create physical separation between affected patients and healthcare staff or other patients

Supplies and Equipment
- Ensure adequate supplies and equipment are available and reach out to other hospitals and public health for interhospital collaboration as needed
- Assure adequate supplies of personal protective equipment

Pharmacy
- Secure appropriate antimicrobial agents/vaccines/prophylactic agents
- Distribute medications/vaccinations per recommendations
- Monitor supplies

Laboratory
- Develop guidance for collection and transport of samples/specimens
- Provide laboratory staff with adequate PPE to handle specimens safely
- Obtain testing capabilities for the emerging pathogen as applicable and when feasible

TABLE 1
Elements of Policy/Protocol for Bioterrorism and Pandemic Showing All-Hazards Approach With Minimal Differences in Hospital Procedures Between Bioterrorism and Pandemic—cont'd

Occupational Health
o Provide respirator fitness testing to healthcare personnel as applicable
o Administer vaccines/prophylactic medications to healthcare personnel
o Assess healthcare worker exposures and monitor exposed healthcare workers for symptoms during the incubation period
Public Affairs, Media, and Communication to Patients and Families
o Institutional representatives should collaborate with subject matter experts prior to media briefings
o Timely communication to patient and family members
Ethics Professionals
o Guide clinicians and healthcare personnel with implementing critical care standards, development of strategies to use medications, vaccines, equipment (i.e., ventilators), and space (i.e., intensive care units) in short supply
Responsibilities
o Assign individual departmental responsibilities
o Reassign staff to needed areas depending on the need
Potential Appendices
o Definitions
o Isolation and other infection prevention and control procedures
o Patient treatment and prophylaxis guidelines
o Transportation routes
o Cleaning and disinfection recommendations
o Waste management routes
o Frequently asked questions about the disease

of the responses, especially for pandemic planning or large-scale infectious disease mass casualty events, it is key to engage stakeholders to anticipate and identify the impact of the altered care, patient flow, limited resources, or other issues that would occur in such an event. The approach needs to be scalable and should address the nuances associated with various agents, such as those that are transmitted via airborne routes versus those that are not transmissible. Plans should include procedures for

1. Educating providers to facilitate prompt identification and diagnosis of the disease.
2. Notifying and communicating with key departments (e.g., emergency, critical care), hospital administration, laboratory, security, infection prevention and public health authorities.
3. Implementing quarantine and isolation to limit transmission.
4. Securing the facility and maintaining biocontainment areas.
5. Supporting an incident command structure, its authority and hierarchy.
6. Providing for a command center.
7. Identifying space to increase capacity and mechanisms to augment staffing during sudden influxes.
8. Evacuating staff and patients.
9. Maintaining an adequate supply chain.
10. Educating and training to assure appropriate donning, doffing and use of PPE.
11. Developing alternate care sites.
12. Providing ethical care.
13. Supporting ongoing internal and external communications and media relations. Importantly, when developing a policy or plan for the management of patients exposed to or infected with agents of high consequence, a pandemic, or a bioterrorism event, the responsibilities and accountability should be clearly delineated. Such structure reinforces the quality of the response, builds trust among responders, and provides support to institutional and public health leadership.

HOSPITAL/HEALTH SYSTEM INCIDENT COMMAND CENTER

When inappropriately managed, disasters lead to chaos. Conceptual frameworks outlining healthcare bioterrorism and/or pandemic preparedness demonstrate that a set of diverse response functions are required

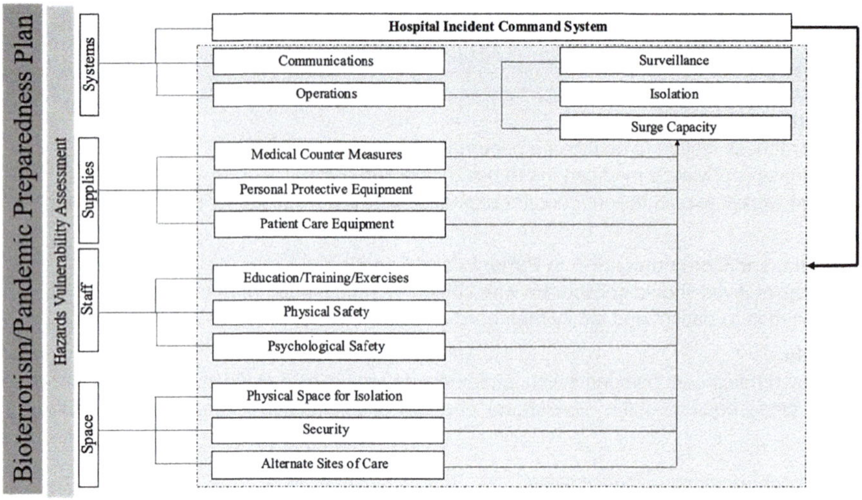

FIG. 1 Framework for incident command for hospitals/health systems.

for and from each separate health system/hospital areas[17] (Fig. 1). Organizing a response, whether for bioterrorism or a prolonged large mass casualty infectious disease event, is best coordinated with an "all-hazards approach." This model is designed to prevent disruption to institutions, facilitate response to events, and enhance recovery from unexpected events, including bioterrorism or a pandemic. This approach facilitates a comprehensive and structured process to minimize risks to clinical operations and to the facility and its infrastructure. All these responses will need to be integrated by one Hospital Incident Command Center [(HICC), Fig. 1] that is generally organized into functions that protect various institutional elements (the facility, the personnel, the supplies, and the systems).[15,18] The HICC, with a commander at the helm, coordinates the response using a common language and continuously assesses the situation to assure flexibility and fluidity in the response. Each identified area has a set of operational and logistical responsibilities that support the hospital or health system. Understanding the infectious agent, its characteristics, and its mechanism of transmission facilitates the response. Still, given the dynamic nature of outbreaks, flexibility and agility in this response are required.[19] The HICC model places four to five individuals under the commander, usually called chiefs or officers, who are responsible for aspects of protecting the institution and its mission. The responsibilities for the different areas the chiefs oversee may vary by institution. For example, a chief may have responsibility for maintaining the physical space, such as ensuring security is in place, there is isolation capacity, ventilation is appropriate, and alternative sites of care are available, and another chief may be responsible for personnel and ensure that necessary education and training is implemented, and resources for HCP and patient emotional support and equipment for physical safety are organized. Logistics and availability for supplies, including patient care equipment, medications, and personal protective equipment, may be the responsibility of another chief. Operations that are integral to supporting the facility, such as communications and environmental services, require a fourth chief. Some frameworks include a finance chief who tracks the financial impact of the institutional needs and assumes responsibility for claims, compensation, and billing, all important in the recovery phase.

The incident command center should be comprised of experts from multiple disciplines so that a well-thought-out and coordinated response can be launched. Emergency management experts, hospital epidemiologists, infection prevention experts, nurses with key skills, infectious diseases, emergency, critical care, and occupational health physicians and providers, engineers, facilities, maintenance, environmental services and security staff, mental health providers, ethicists, pharmacists, and hospital administrators should be included among others in the multidisciplinary team. The structure provides the flexibility needed and the expertise required during events such as a bioterrorism or pandemic event, when it may become necessary to decontaminate the victims or hospital staff, particularly during the early phase of an event. In other scenarios, there may be a mass influx of victims requiring critical care support or a persistent and steady stream of victims that require persistent care and tax the system over long periods of time. Hence, the commander has the authority to activate necessary resources, such as the hazardous material (HazMat) personnel that can perform complex functions related to hazardous material management, obtain additional beds or staffing, or procure other resources to protect the institution and its mission of patient care.[15,20]

Challenges: While strong, level-headed leaders serve as incident commanders, they will be faced with the enormous task of managing hospital/health system resources in the setting of extreme hardship. Limited medical equipment available in hospitals may not meet the demand during a disaster despite a well-functioning HICC and may require the allocation of limited resources.[21,22] Recently, the use of modeling (see Chapter 18) has been used to predict the trajectory of outbreaks and facilitate healthcare planning. Another important challenge that the incident command center will face is that hospital staff may refuse or be unable to work. Staff may be concerned about their own safety, not have childcare, have underlying medical conditions, or have other reasons for not working further, stretching resources. This will further cripple an already stretched system and could lead to further pressures on healthcare resources with devastating consequences. TOPOFF 2000 exercise demonstrated a significant degree of panic among HCPs could occur during a bioterrorism attack.[6,7] Similar concerns, from worried well to panic, have been witnessed during other natural disasters and pandemics. For example, during COVID-19, there was palpable anxiety among HCPs, especially in the early days, which dictated the way hospitals functioned and altered the standards of care for a significant period of time.[23] A survey in 2010 revealed that among 586 emergency medical service workers, 12% would not voluntarily report to work.[24] A more recent meta-analysis found that among HCPs, their willingness to work increased when they (1) perceived their personal safety was improved by access to vaccines, PPE, and implementation of other mitigation strategies; (2) were aware of the risks associated with a pandemic and had clinical and role-specific knowledge of those risks; (3) had received pandemic response training; and (4) had confidence in their own personal skills.[25]

Recommendations: The HICC needs to anticipate these challenges and plan. Because hospital preparedness is very closely tied to public health preparedness, public health authorities, political leaders, and emergency management experts need to collaborate to avert shortages and should anticipate needs in advance rather than scrambling for resources amid the event. To reassure HCPs, mitigate worry, and minimize miscommunication, it is extremely important for the HICC to have strong, frequent, and repetitive communication using multiple media platforms for HCPs. Likewise, relationships with external media that complement the internal efforts can reassure the public and quell panic and misinformation so that both the hospital personnel and the public are well informed of the current state of the epidemic/event, the dynamic nature of the event, how things may change, and all the existing efforts that are being put forth to protect safety.

SECURITY

Security is important during a bioterrorism or equivalent event to maintain patient flow, facilitate patient care, and protect both patients and staff.[26–28] Once entry points are designated and to ensure processes are followed, security personnel should be posted at entries and triage points, outside isolation units, and in emergency departments. Entrances that cannot be supervised should be closed. Even during pandemics, with increased patient influx, there will be increased traffic, and the deployment of security personnel is essential in ensuring ambulances can transport and unload patients in emergency departments. Hospitals and healthcare facilities may become targets themselves during a bioterrorist attack in the form of terrorists entering the building intending harm.[26] Furthermore, those exposed, potentially exposed, and worried well could use emergency departments to obtain prophylaxis and reassurance, leading to further crowd control challenges. Long waits, perceived delays in care, and other experiences can inflame frustration, leading to violence. Finally, security personnel may need to monitor human movement into the hospital campus and aid with evacuations if needed.

Challenges: Hospital security staff may be stretched too thin because of all the areas that require monitoring during a bioterrorism attack. These critical personnel, themselves, may get exposed to infected individuals; hence, need to be educated and protected.

Recommendations: Closing selected entrances and routing all patients through selected entry points and triage areas will help maintain the security staff workforce. Staff can be protected and reassured when hospitals have protocols in place for prompt recognition of patients presenting with syndromes consistent with bioterrorism or infectious disease events that could lead to mass casualty situations to minimize staff exposures, including those to security personnel, and to enhance the safety of other patients.

RECOGNITION, DIAGNOSIS, AND REPORTING OF AN EVENT

The first and most crucial step in response to a bioterrorism attack or event with mass casualty potential is recognizing an unusual event or attack. This responsibility often rests on the shoulders of clinicians. Bioterrorism events are usually covertly evolving over several days depending on the agent before they are recognized.[16] Pandemic events may evolve slowly, and commonly, public health authorities will designate the event. Naturally occurring pandemics and bioterrorism events have many overlapping characteristics, making an all-hazards approach that much more effective and easily interpretable across institutions.[29] Commonly, the symptoms are nonspecific and mimic many common infections, whether a bioterrorism event or an event of high consequence. Initial suspicion may arise when a series of cases or unusual patterns of disease are noticed by the front-line staff, especially emergency physicians or primary care doctors. Pathologists or laboratory personnel may identify an unusual organism in the culture. Therefore, it is important to train hospital staff on how to recognize and respond to various biological agents, especially agents of high consequence that pose a risk to national security. All-hazards approaches are based on the concept that most disaster events, whether natural events such as pandemics or bioterrorism events, have common disaster-response functions and should be triggered by such an event.[29] An outbreak of unusual infection, of a disease that presents in a geographic region or during a seasonal not normally expected, or with unusual epidemiologic features (atypical age distribution among outbreak cases, a new route of transmission for a typical pathogen, or an atypical presentation) that make it more transmissible or virulent should prompt clinicians to think of the possibility of intentional use of an infectious agent.[30] These suspicions of a biological attack or an outbreak should be promptly reported to the hospital's infection prevention and control (IPC) and to public health authorities who can investigate and provide information that may lead to the activation of a hospital disaster event.

Laboratory personnel should be immediately notified to prevent personnel exposures, to assure that appropriate supplemental testing can be undertaken if needed, and to store samples for further investigation. In addition, the laboratory personnel can provide guidance on the best site(s) to sample, any necessary precautions when obtaining a sample, and the type of sample(s) to obtain (see Chapter 17 for additional details). They will identify procedures for the safe handling and transport of specimens within the hospital or outside laboratories or public health laboratories. They also may have additional reporting responsibilities to the public health laboratories. All these laboratory procedures should be detailed in the institutional bioterrorism and pandemic preparedness plans/policies.[26] In addition to safety issues and diagnostic responsibilities, supply planning, and constraints become important considerations. Depending on the biological agent, a hospital may need additional supplies such as blood culture bottles, PCR reagents, equipment including continuous-monitoring blood culture machines, level II Biological Safety Cabinets, and additional trained laboratory staff to support the increased numbers of specimens.[26,31,32]

The CDC categorizes various biological agents with the potential to be used for bioterrorism into three groups. Category A consists of the highest priority agents that pose a risk to national security because they can be easily disseminated or transmitted from person to person, result in high mortality, cause public panic, and lead to social disruption. They would also require special action for public health response.[33] These include *Bacillus anthracis*, *Clostridium botulinum* toxin, *Y. pestis*, *Variola major*, *Francisella tularensis*, filoviruses (Ebola, Marburg), and arenaviruses (Lassa, Machupo).[33] Diseases caused by these agents, signs of an attack, and the type of hospital resources needed for each agent in the event of bioterrorism are listed in Table 2. Category B includes agents that are moderately easy to disseminate, have a lower mortality rate, and require specific enhancements to diagnostic capacity and disease surveillance. These include *Brucella* species, Epsilon toxin of *Clostridium perfringens*, *Salmonella* species, *Escherichia coli* O157:H7, *Shigella*, *Burkholderia mallei*, *Burkholderia pseudomallei*, *Chlamydia psittaci*, *Coxiella burnetii*, Ricin toxin from *Ricinus communis* (castor beans), Staphylococcal enterotoxin B, *Rickettsia prowazekii*, alphaviruses, such as Eastern equine encephalitis, Venezuelan equine encephalitis, and Western equine encephalitis, *Vibrio cholera*, and *Cryptosporidium parvum*.[33] Category C agents that are easily available and can result in wider dissemination and high mortality if bioengineered in the future. These include emerging infectious diseases such as the Nipah virus and Hantavirus.[33] Not included in the list but equally likely to lead to human illness, morbidity, mortality, the health system, and economic disruption are the agents that have pandemic potential listed in Table 3.

TABLE 2

Hospital/Health System Preparedness Elements for Pathogens of High Consequence in a Potential Bioterrorism Event[19]

Infections Caused by High-Consequence Pathogens (Agents)	ELEMENTS OF HOSPITAL/HEALTH SYSTEM PREPAREDNESS						
	RECOGNITION OF A PATHOGEN OF HIGH CONSEQUENCE		CONTROL MEASURES		MEDICAL COUNTERMEASURES		
	Clinical Features	**Clues of Potential Bioterrorism**	**Isolation**	**Person-Person Transmission**	**Treatment**	**Postexposure Prophylaxis**	**Vaccine**
Inhalation anthrax (*Bacillus anthracis*)	Respiratory distress with fever and shock	Sudden influx of many persons with severe flu-like symptoms	Standard (add contact for cutaneous anthrax and for gastrointestinal-al anthrax if diarrhea is not controlled)	No—inhalational anthrax. Yes—cutaneous anthrax	Ciprofloxacin or doxycycline or penicillin (if susceptible)	Ciprofloxacin or amoxicillin (if susceptible) or doxycycline	Yes
Pneumonic plague (*Yersinia pestis*)	Fever, headache, weakness, and a rapidly developing pneumonia with shortness of breath, chest pain, cough	Sudden influx of many persons with acute, rapidly developing pneumonia	Droplet precautions until 48h of effective therapy	Yes	Gentamicin or doxycycline or ciprofloxacin	Doxycycline or ciprofloxacin	No
Tularemia (*Francisella tularensis*)	Fever, headache, chills and rigors, lymphadenopathy, generalized body aches, coryza, sore throat, and pulse-temperature dissociation	Sudden influx of many persons with acute, nonspecific febrile illness	Standard precautions	No	Gentamicin or doxycycline or ciprofloxacin	Doxycycline or ciprofloxacin	Yes
Smallpox (*Variola major*)	Fever, malaise, headache, and rash that goes through several stages (macular, papular, pustular, crusting) in centrifugal distribution	Patients with febrile rash consistent with smallpox	Airborne and contact precautions	Yes	Supportive care	Vaccinia IgG	Yes

(Continued)

TABLE 2
Hospital/Health System Preparedness Elements for Pathogens of High Consequence in a Potential Bioterrorism Event—cont'd

	ELEMENTS OF HOSPITAL/HEALTH SYSTEM PREPAREDNESS						
	RECOGNITION OF A PATHOGEN OF HIGH CONSEQUENCE		CONTROL MEASURES		MEDICAL COUNTERMEASURES		
Infections Caused by High-Consequence Pathogens (Agents)	**Clinical Features**	**Clues of Potential Bioterrorism**	**Isolation**	**Person-Person Transmission**	**Treatment**	**Postexposure Prophylaxis**	**Vaccine**
Botulism (*Clostridium botulinum* toxin)	Nausea, vomiting, diarrhea, ptosis, blurred vision or diplopia, dry mouth, sore throat, and dysphagia, descending paralysis, respiratory failure	Sudden influx of many persons with difficulty breathing or descending paralysis	Standard precautions	No	Botulism antitoxin from CDC	None	Yes
Hemorrhagic fever—filoviruses (Marburg, Ebola)	Fever, malaise, myalgia, maculopapular rash, pharyngitis, hematemesis, melena, bleeding; shock	Sudden influx of patients with symptoms consistent with hemorrhagic fever	Standard, contact and droplet; use of eye protection; Add airborne precautions during aerosol generating procedures	Yes	None	None	Only available for *Zaire Ebolavirus*
Hemorrhagic fever—arenaviruses (Lassa, Machupo)	Fever, malaise, myalgia, headache, nausea, vomiting, pharyngitis, cough, retrosternal pain, bleeding,shock, aseptic meningitis, coma	Sudden influx of patients with symptoms consistent with hemorrhagic fever	Standard, contact and droplet; use of eye protection; Add airborne precautions during aerosol generating procedures	Yes	Ribavirin—some benefit	None	No

TABLE 3
Hospital/Health System Preparedness Elements for Infections That Are Likely to Cause Future Pandemics

Infections That are Likely to Cause Future Pandemics	ELEMENTS OF HOSPITAL/HEALTH SYSTEM PREPAREDNESS						
			CONTROL MEASURES		MEDICAL COUNTERMEASURES		
	Clinical Features	Clues of an Outbreak	Isolation	Person-Person Transmission	Treatment	Chemoprophylaxis	Vaccine
Highly pathogenic H5N1 avian influenza[34]	High fever and cough, lower respiratory tract illness (shortness of breath, viral pneumonia), diarrhea, abdominal pain, and vomiting	Sudden influx of many persons with severe flu-like symptoms in the setting of a public health alert	Standard and airborne (add contact for diarrhea); might include contact precautions depending on the transmission pattern of the emerging pandemic influenza strain	Yes	Antiviral medications depending on the circulating strain and resistance pattern	Antiviral medications should be reserved for treatment to prevent development of resistance	Yes, but there will be a few months delay in production
Severe acute respiratory syndrome (SARS)-CoV[35]	Influenza-like syndrome with rigors, fatigue and high fever, nausea, vomiting, diarrhea, atypical pneumonia, hypoxia	Influx of patients with pneumonia with a clear history of exposure either to a SARS patient(s) or to a setting in which SARS-CoV transmission is occurring	Standard, contact and airborne precautions	Yes	None	None	No
Middle East respiratory syndrome (MERS)-CoV[36]	Severe respiratory illness, including fever, cough, and shortness of breath, acute respiratory distress syndrome (ARDS), refractory hypoxemia and extrapulmonary complications such as acute kidney injury, hepatic inflammation, and septic shock	Influx of symptomatic patients who traveled from affected areas or were in contact with persons who traveled from affected areas	Standard, contact and airborne precautions	Yes	None	None	No

Challenges: Capturing the imagination and sustaining the interest of clinicians about a potential future bioterrorism event or an emerging infection with pandemic potential when they are focused on the real, everyday existential threats in healthcare can be challenging. Albeit rare, these events can be devastating when they occur.

Recommendations: Given the risks to the public, health systems, and economic stability, providers need to be educated, trained, and frequently updated about the potential of a naturally occurring or planned event.

EDUCATION, TRAINING, AND EXERCISES

Hospital staff education, training, and exercise on biological hazards is a key part of the response.[13,37–39] Education should include agent recognition and diagnosis for at least CDC category A biological agents and agents with pandemic potential, signs of a bioterrorism attack, types and indications for PPE, patient and staff safety, infection prevention and control policies and procedures such as isolation and quarantine, decontamination, management of patient influx, including incident command structure, plans for triage, prophylaxis and treatment, fatality management, critical incident stress management, and risk communication. Education can be enhanced when supplemented by training around potential events. In addition, just-in-time training to reinforce concepts should occur during events to assure that concepts and needed skills are fresh and to remind and reassure HCPs. In both cases, supplemental, simple guidance documents can be generated (Table 4) and include basic definitions of cases and exposures, isolation and precaution recommendations, patient placement instructions, and communication instructions, and they can be available both on paper and electronically. Periodic education may be required when a new pathogen emerges and is transmitted, putting the public at risk. Education is best provided using multimodal means to enhance theoretical knowledge with lectures, town halls, videos, posters, emails, and websites. Simulation training is best used to enhance technical skills or processes that involve multiple HCPs.[40] Hands-on training should occur at least to a group of preidentified staff with different skill sets and jobs as part of ongoing preparedness planning. Several groups have demonstrated that the simulation training is critical to optimize workflow, develop new care processes, procure supplies and equipment, manage staffing, and provide consistent and equitable patient care.[41–43] Recent studies advocate for the use of training and simulation as more effective in identifying potential problems with preparedness plans, engaging HCP in the process, and reinforcing best practices.[42] Regular exercises and drills help hospitals identify system weaknesses, assess staff knowledge, and promote needed skill development. Regional exercises that include public health authorities, first responders, and other groups that will collaborate in these events can also identify gaps that can be addressed to assure a well-coordinated response in such an event. Simulation activities can be developed to train individuals in the use of PPE and doing tasks while wearing PPE.[40,44] These exercises will prepare both the facility and staff for both a bioterrorism response and also naturally occurring infectious disease epidemics or pandemics. As noted previously during an event, just-in-time training can reinforce important safety considerations and provide reminders to staff about changes in medical care processes or how to use certain equipment, including PPE. Of note, some experts suggest competency requirements to assure that training was successful in teaching best practices.

Challenges: Ongoing education, training, and exercises take time and resources. Facilities may not be motivated to conduct hands-on training and exercises when there is no immediate looming threat. Mandates from national and regional governmental agencies and regulatory bodies may provide motivation for drills, especially when associated with financial incentives or disincentives that are tied to preparedness for emerging pathogens and mass casualty infectious disease events. While countries like Israel have trained for such events, no such detailed mandates exist from many Western countries to shape bioterrorism or pandemic planning. Some regulatory agencies, such as the Joint Commission, have developed standards (e.g., EM.15.01.01 and EM.16.01.01) that address education, training, and conducting exercises to test hospitals' emergency operations plans and response procedures, but these are very general in nature.[45]

Recommendations: To assure a prepared workforce that can recognize high-consequence pathogens and is trained in the use of PPE and other protective measures, healthcare institutions should create and execute annual biological hazard education and training for providers and other hospital staff, especially those on the front lines.

TABLE 4
Example of a Checklist for Triaging a Patient With Suspected Ebola Virus Disease in a Healthcare Setting

Triage Checklist for Electronic Medical Record (EMR) or Manual Use for Ebola Virus Disease (EVD)	
Patient Name: ______	
Medical Record Number: ______	
Date: ______	
Patient presents with:	
Primary Symptoms	**Secondary Symptoms**
Fever ≥100.4°F, nausea, vomiting, diarrhea, severe abdominal pain, bleeding (gums, nose, in stool)	Muscle pain, weakness, headache, cough
If patient is symptomatic, proceed with the following:	
□ Did the patient travel to an area with known cases of or an area of high risk for EVD in the past 21 days? (Add name(s) of specific country or area with known cases)	
□ Did they have close contact with someone who had travelled to a high-risk area?	
If **NO** to travel or contact with person who travelled, proceed with routine triage/assessment.	
If **YES**, proceed with the following:	
At this time, staff should don personal protective equipment (PPE) – mask, gown, and gloves.	
□ Did patient have direct contact, contact with body fluids, or was in the same room for several hours with a person with EBV without proper PPE (all skin and clothing covered, including shoes)?	
□ Did the patient handle bats, rodents, primates, or raw bush meat?	
□ If **YES** to either of the two questions above:	
• Immediately place patient into a designated private room and contact Infection Prevention (IP).	
• IP will notify Disaster/Emergency Management to assemble trained care team.	
• IP will communicate with public health authority.	
• Set up area surrounding designated room for PPE donning and doffing areas, soiled waste areas, and establish a traffic flow.	
• IP will notify public health (local, regional, or state health department) to determine any transfer required for further care of the patient if applicable.	
□ If **NO** to either of the two questions above:	
• Proceed with routine triage/assessment. Contact IP to notify public health for monitoring of patient for 21 days.	

COORDINATION AND COMMUNICATION INTERNALLY AND WITH PUBLIC HEALTH AUTHORITIES (SEE CHAPTER 13 FOR ADDITIONAL DETAILS)

During both a bioterrorism event and a mass casualty event such as a pandemic, communication is crucial. Disaster communications internally and externally need to be carefully crafted to avoid mixed messages and to minimize confusion. Communication includes alerting public health officials to a significant event that will put the health and safety of the population at risk but also that might require political and law enforcement action to access needed resources. In addition to reporting a case or potential event to the public health authority, hospitals may need additional support, including additional medications, supplies, and medical equipment from strategic national stockpiles, or may need help with additional personnel to support staffing. Regional authorities (state or provincial health agencies), national agencies (CDC), or international agencies (World Health Organization, WHO) may lend their scientific expertise and may offer "boots-on-ground" help to implement mitigation strategies and curb the epidemic.[46] These agencies can also provide additional information, such as surveillance data and mathematical model estimations, that can help predict the trajectory of the outbreak and facilitate resource needs and planning. Therefore, it is extremely important to keep in constant touch with public health authorities and have bidirectional communication mechanisms. Individuals from different disciplines should be designated as the leads for various communications. For example, in most healthcare settings, infection prevention and control communicate with the public health authorities, but the public information officer is the liaison with the media. Likewise, emergency management and disaster authorities may primarily communicate about staffing, equipment, and supply needs. Credibility in the communication content and who delivers the information during an infectious disease disaster, whether natural or man-made, by relying on operational and content experts aids with public health messaging and with building trust with the external community.

To facilitate the multiple activities involved in these complex responses, identify internal departments or key personnel, including leadership, appropriate clinicians, and front-line workers who need to be notified when an event is suspected. Such details can be defined in policies and can facilitate the institutional response. Furthermore, redundant communications are essential to assure that critical information is disseminated in a timely fashion. This should be coordinated with information provided to the public and ideally implemented through the incident command framework, which can use a multimodal strategy. Use of detailed tools, specific algorithms, and checklists can and should be used to reinforce messages communicated and decrease confusion. These tools can be modified to support messaging as it evolves throughout the progression of the event.

Challenges: Coordination and communication during an infectious diseases disaster must be both horizontal (between the local public health departments within a region and across the state/province) and vertical (between the public health department and the CDC, European CDC [ECDC], WHO, health care providers, and other agencies) to be effective.[47] Public health departments themselves become overwhelmed and may be slow to respond, resulting in delayed vertical communications. In anticipation of a bioterrorism attack, a GAO report that assessed the coordination and preparedness of the country noted inadequacies in public health infrastructure that continue to exist and were witnessed during the COVID-19 pandemic.[48] TOPOFF 2000 exercise for a pneumonic plague event revealed that public health authorities were overwhelmed and functions like moving antibiotics from the national stockpile delivery points to the hospitals were difficult to execute.[6,7] This led to improving the public health infrastructure and integrating healthcare into preparedness to better support front-line hospitals and the public.

Recommendations: Coordination within the hospital between different departments is also a challenge, so establishing a structure for the incident command center within the preparedness plan and defining its functions, including methods of communication, will help address these challenges. Gaps identified in both vertical and horizontal communications during exercises and drills can be solved before a real event.

LEADERSHIP

While HICC may manage the health system response with its access to resources, supportive institutional leadership within healthcare organizations is required. Strong, proactive, and prepared leadership creates trust in health systems during large-scale mass casualty events.[49] One case study used the COVID-19 pandemic planning experience to empower HICC further and to transform healthcare subsequently from the lessons learned.[50] Leaders followed the Kotter eight-stage framework for organizational change to enhance surge capacity for COVID-19 and to improve vaccination rates. The Kotter framework required creating a sense of urgency, forming a powerful guiding coalition, creating and communicating a vision, empowering others to act and manage the vision, planning and creating short-term "wins," consolidating the improvements, facilitating changes, and then implementing new approaches. The approach helped them lead the nation in vaccination, led to a lower death rate, and implemented strategies like telemedicine in the long term.

Challenges: Leaders may have competing priorities that are more existential threats affecting day-to-day operations; therefore, they may be less motivated to support the health care system in an infectious disease disaster preparedness, whether for a bioterrorism event or a pandemic. They may also find it difficult to allocate funds to this purpose with those other competing priorities.

Recommendations: Educate and engage leadership as soon as an issue arises and keep them apprised of emerging pathogens and potential challenges with staffing, medical care, patients, and HCP safety is key. Build coalitions between disaster planning, nursing, medical, disaster planning, and other personnel to determine and apprise leadership of institutional risks to enhance planning. Reminders of potential global threats may capture leadership's sustained interest and help them prioritize pandemic and bioterrorism preparedness.

COMMUNICATIONS AND MEDIA RELATIONS (SEE CHAPTER 22 FOR ADDITIONAL DETAILS)

Timely and credible communication about an incident, the agent if known, the disease it causes, symptoms to watch for, diagnostic methods, precautions to be taken, including any postexposure prophylaxis, and control and preventive efforts implemented by hospital and public health authorities is important. Given the content expertise of healthcare facilities and their providers, aggressive communications can minimize misinformation and prevent miscommunication from unofficial sources.[19,27,51] Essential and factual information sharing will help limit unnecessary patient surges stemming from worry (worried well). Communication with the public media ensures accurate information reaches the public in a timely fashion.[27]

The HICC coordinates communication to ensure that the messaging is consistent and timely. For external communication, HICC should identify institutional spokespersons who can communicate effectively using the basic tenets of risk communication, which are being accurate and credible, being the first to tell the story, and being compassionate in messaging. Internal communication is also best managed by respected leaders and content experts who understand the mission of the institution but can also address the basic fears and concerns of the staff. Communication may need to be daily, providing previously discussed and new information as additional HCPs enter the environment. The topics will change as the situation evolves and should address emerging concerns. Finally, communication must continue into the recovery phase of an event with planning for critical incidence stress debriefings with culturally sensitive strategies and potentially multiple languages. Recovery may occur over a prolonged period and may need to include providing group activities and support and access to counseling and medical treatment.[52]

Challenges: While clinicians may suspect a potential event, communication strategies need to be modulated and appropriate. For example, law enforcement authorities will likely announce that an event is the result of a bioterrorist attack, and public health authorities will declare a public health emergency.[30] Hospitals and their staff need to exercise caution and coordinate any such announcements to the staff and public with the appropriate law enforcement and public health agencies. Premature announcements by hospitals or their personnel could fuel misinformation and rumors.[30] Regardless of whether it is bioterrorism or a natural disaster, managing media, especially with the emergence of social media, external communication remains one of the most challenging tasks during disaster management.

Recommendations: Hence, thoughtful, prompt, and coordinated efforts to disseminate information transparently establish a legitimate source of truth that the staff, patients, and the public can rely upon. Updating the staff and public during a rapidly moving scenario is an important part of maintaining credibility and developing trust.

SURVEILLANCE AND SURVEILLANCE SYSTEMS (SEE CHAPTER 14 FOR ADDITIONAL DETAILS)

Early epidemic detection and case tracking facilitate prompt situational awareness, enhance decision-making about mitigation strategies, and promote an effective disaster response. Performed correctly, surveillance requires defined sources of data, a systematically applied definition, and data collation and interpretation. Surveillance data may be culled from multiple sources and used for different ends in a response. Surveillance and case-finding commonly begin with symptoms and other clinical data before a specific diagnostic test is performed or is available.[53–55] Such syndromic surveillance, looking for a constellation of symptoms, allows for prompt quarantine or isolation of exposed and infected individuals, thereby minimizing further transmission, determining high-risk groups to target for postexposure prophylaxis, treatment, and chemoprophylaxis, and other preventive strategies such as vaccination, if applicable. These data are commonly captured by the infection prevention and control (IPC) teams using various case-finding strategies. As information and diagnostics become available, surveillance may pivot to identifying potential or true cases. Regardless of surveillance strategy, cases or suspected cases should be reported to IPC verbally or via email. In addition, the IPC team may review other potential sources of data to identify cases, including reviewing microbiology records or having clinical informatics mine data available in the electronic health record to ensure case capture. Once potential cases are identified, the IPC team will apply a standardized definition generally developed by public health authorities to verify and determine whether a potential case needs further confirmation. As more information is available, definitions will be refined and generally become more precise. Laboratory techniques typically confirm the diagnosis in suspected cases, or personnel may recommend additional testing. Testing information and other data are gathered, and then the IPC team transmits key information to the local, regional, or national public health agency. In addition, these data are collected in a spreadsheet or on a "line list" that includes information about the case (name, age, medical record number, other demographic information), the case timing (date of symptom onset, exposure (if known), admission), symptom onset and symptoms, and where the person was exposed. Such information is important for institutional awareness and helps IPC develop internal mitigation strategies. While providers must notify IPC of cases, it is the role of IPC to catalog data and interface with public health authorities. Commonly, laboratories are required to also report key laboratory findings to public health agencies, providing important redundancy that enhances the robustness of surveillance data.

Challenges: The effectiveness of syndromic and disease-specific surveillance will depend on the accuracy of definitions, the data sources and information management, and the availability of resources for follow up.[55] Because of the lack of sensitivity and specificity in syndromic surveillance definitions, disease-specific surveillance data, if not appropriately verified, may suggest an event triggering predetermined response measures that will place undue burden on the system. Such false alarms can be minimized by working closely with public health authorities to establish clear case definitions and criteria for initiating investigations. These definitions will change and evolve over time. Surveillance will provide more information than just cases; it can help identify individuals who are exposed and who should receive postexposure prophylaxis, treatment, chemoprophylaxis, or vaccination as applicable.

Recommendations: In addition, as the COVID-19 pandemic demonstrated, the health sector is critical to the timely collection of data that provides internal and external situational awareness. Healthcare facilities need coordinated and, more importantly, timely data collection that is shared to support ongoing preparedness efforts and help infectious disease modeling specialists estimate important measures of epidemic growth, such as the reproductive number.[56]

PHARMACY, STOCKPILING, AND SUPPLY CHAIN

The pharmacy and their personnel are key stakeholders in any healthcare response. They are responsible for both maintaining supplies of key pharmaceuticals for patient care and also obtaining agents to be used for postexposure care of HCPs and patients. Fluids, vasopressors, certain antimicrobials, and antivirals may be quickly consumed and require replenishment. In addition, postexposure vaccination and chemoprophylaxis of the potentially exposed is important to protect HCPs and the public by reducing morbidity and mortality after a bioterrorism event or during a pandemic.[19,57,58] These early interventions can be utilized to reassure and protect HCP and, in turn, maintain the workforce, an essential component of the response effort. In rare circumstances, there may be a need to provide prophylaxis to patients who were exposed to other contagious patients. This may require strategies to prioritize the highest-risk healthcare personnel and patients when short supplies exist.[59] Administering these measures to HCPs who might have had or are likely to have an exposure could be lifesaving and could also help signal to the staff that everything at the hospital's disposal is being employed to protect them.

A hazard vulnerability analysis should be performed to identify the equipment and supplies that will be necessary to address the greatest biological agent threats.[19] Pharmaceuticals and biological agents, in addition to ventilators and hospital beds, are among the crucial items that will be in high demand during a pandemic or after a bioterrorism event.[28] Local and regional supply and the population at risk should be considered in determining the institutional approach. As was witnessed during the COVID-19 pandemic, many localities and institutions saw delays in supply distribution. On the other hand, it was the medical institutions that were able to provide much of the expertise and support needed to administer COVID-19 vaccines to large numbers of high-risk patients. These lessons and considerations should be factored into institutional (and regional) planning. Institutions may consider purchasing equipment such as disposable ventilators or stockpiling of necessary medications to use while waiting for additional supplies from local, regional, state-wide, or federal caches.

Challenges: In the event of bioterrorism or a pandemic, demand will be widespread, and hospitals will be simultaneously requesting additional supply, which will limit availability. However, most hospitals use "just-in-time" strategies to manage supplies and pharmaceuticals and do not maintain stockpiles. Stockpiling medications in anticipation of a mass infectious disease casualty event may lead to waste if they expire. Similarly, equipment such as ventilators that may be needed may quickly be depleted, which fosters ethical considerations around the best resource utilization.[19] The ability to rapidly obtain resources is critical to preventing "casualties," but the "just-in-time" practice does not necessarily support rapid deployment of these critical resources. Some supplies, equipment, and pharmaceuticals can be obtained from federal and regional stockpiles, but delays in distribution could prove devastating in situations such as a toxin exposure that require rapid intervention. In addition, healthcare facilities may be called upon to support the public health response with their resources. For example, during the COVID-19 pandemic, when the SARS-CoV-2 vaccine was released, the expertise and resources of healthcare institutions, including the ability to provide specialized temperature storage for the vaccine and knowledge of emergency use governmental waivers for pharmaceutical agents, made them ideal vaccination sites.

Recommendations: Use a combination of sources including local, regional, state-wide, and federal caches to maintain robust supply chains. Take care that not all hospitals are dependent on the same supply and equipment sources. In addition, networking with regional hospitals can help identify resources that can be shared during a crisis. That said, include plans for some stockpiling of critical supplies and equipment in hospital preparedness plans and base needs on a risk assessment. To avoid such loss, many medications and supplies can be rotated through the pharmacy or other stocks prior to expiring.

INTERHOSPITAL COLLABORATION

Information sharing between hospitals in a timely manner provides a clear picture of the status of the outbreak and needed situational awareness.[13,20] Collaborating on surge capacity can lead to sharing of resources, including equipment and supplies, protocols, and even hospital staff, including physicians, sharing of spaces, and rerouting of patients. The local public health department should lead and support such collaborations. One lesson learned from the SARS-CoV-1 outbreak in Toronto demonstrated the utility of a daily call where clinicians joined and provided status updates and collaborated on medical decision-making and rapidly coordinated research studies.[60]

Challenges: In large events, it is likely that regional hospitals are facing similar situations with increased demand for resources and are unable to share with other hospitals. In situations of widespread overcrowding, there may not be capacity to reroute patients, especially those requiring higher levels of care.

Recommendations: Hospitals may have to increase their capacity to care for patients by other means than transferring patients. Facilities may need to stop elective procedures, limit outpatient visits so that they share and repurpose staff, or utilize healthcare volunteers that may have limited training to step into the specialized tasks that these types of patients require. In addition, in situations where expanded care is needed, working with public health authorities and emergency planners to develop alternative sites of care and "pop up" hospitals in public spaces.

PHYSICAL SPACE (FACILITIES)

Hospitals and other healthcare facilities in the already overwhelmed healthcare system will quickly run out of patient rooms, waiting room space, and patient care areas in the event of a bioterrorism attack.[26,51,61] The process in an outbreak or pandemic may be more prolonged. The HICC needs to prepare to expand the facility to care for additional patients and the worried well. Cohorting of patients may be one effective early strategy to liberate space. In this case, patients with similar diagnoses or exposures can be placed together. Consideration for the suspected agent may limit the ability to cohort. For example, if the agent is spread by respiratory droplets, IPC and public health may recommend that patients need to be at least one to two meters apart. In critical care areas, patient placement may be limited by access to medical gases. Shutting down nonemergent or urgent services such as elective surgeries or routine outpatient visits can also allow for space to be repurposed and provide additional capacity in nontraditional areas. These strategies may require the facility personnel to reconfigure ventilation systems to maximize patient and HCP safety, the building of temporary walls to provide needed barriers, and the placement of additional hand hygiene stations. These requests and needs can be managed by HICC, given their access to resources.

Many bioterrorism agents, agents of high consequence, and emerging pathogens can be transmitted to other patients or staff.[33] Therefore, in these instances, care areas are ideally separated from the rest of the hospital to minimize the risk of transmission. In such cases, tents can be used for triage areas or for decontamination. Tents may also be used in open areas for testing and possibly care of affected patients. Spaces with large open areas such as gymnasiums in schools, sports arenas, and community centers can also be considered. Temporary field hospitals may be established and staffed in collaboration with other hospitals and local public health authorities.[26,51,61] Long-term care facilities, dormitories, and hotels have also been used to care for less critically ill patients and to expand capacity.[26,51,61]

Challenges: Some agents are transmitted by mechanisms that require more than just physical separation from other patients.[33] To provide safe care and protect HCPs and patients, they require additional ventilation (air exchanges/hour), such as airborne isolation with a minimum number of air exchanges, a negative pressure relationship to the corridor, and high-efficiency particle absorption filtration. This is particularly important in the emergency department. While there are several specialized infectious diseases hospitals in the world (e.g., Singapore, Norway, and Hong Kong) that are designed to care for these patients, most hospitals rarely plan for a surplus of negative airflow rooms and isolation units even as they construct new facilities. This limits the ability for many hospitals to easily support large numbers of patients requiring airborne isolation with specialized ventilation.[9] A small number of hospitals in North America and Europe have biocontainment units built to take care of patients ill with a pathogen of high consequence and have this capacity (see Chapter 26).[9] Hence, a widespread attack with large numbers of affected patients or prolonged pandemic could overwhelm a country's facilities. In this case, other healthcare facilities and hospitals would need to fill the gap and care for the affected patients for extended periods of time. Beyond the physical space, which poses one of the greatest challenges during a mass biological event, staffing for the many patients in the expanded and alternate care sites will likely be an exponential challenge.

Recommendations: In hospitals, engineers can determine if they can change the ventilation characteristics and pressure relationships to have multiple rooms or large areas under negative pressure when locations to manage patients are considered. If the number of patients needing airborne isolation exceeds, the hospital's capacity for these specialized rooms, a plan to increase this capacity using portable high-efficiency particulate air devices or other strategies is needed. Such devices can also be used in areas where patients may congregate, such as waiting areas, to enhance the ventilation.

WORKFORCE

Healthcare settings and hospitals may quickly find that they have an inadequate workforce to care for a large influx of patients, especially if they are critically ill and require more intense care.[26,51,61] During these events, HCPs work long hours, are caring for more patients than can be done safely, may have inadequate supplies to support their work, and are working in an environment with risk (infectious patients). In previous outbreaks of SARS-CoV, MERS-CoV, EVD, and SARS-CoV-2, nosocomial transmission occurred under these circumstances, which then increased the anxiety and fear among HCPs. The uncertainty associated with pandemics, changing information, large numbers of critically ill patients, and inadequate PPE supplies also drove psychological stress.[62,63]

The staffing challenges go beyond managing increased volumes of patients or increased severity of illness among patients. Staff themselves may develop infection, need to be quarantined, may develop psychological or mental health issues, or need to care for family. Work-related absences increased from 8.4% to 57.7% during previous pandemics and were highest among nursing and allied health staff.[64] Among HCPs, physicians are the most willing to work in these circumstances, and the willingness of any HCP working is enhanced by education around pandemics and pandemic response training.[25] These data highlight the importance of training all hospital staff continuously around readiness for pandemics and bioterrorism events.

Finally, HCPs are at risk of psychological strain or burnout in the settings of pandemics where they are working for long periods of time, exposed to significant patient morbidity and mortality, and living with external sources of stress. In one study, up to 50% of staff (56% nurses) reported burnout.[65] Hence the challenge may go beyond replacing HCP and may require repurposing others. Key response staff (and positions) should be identified and supported with ongoing training in anticipation of a major infectious disease event, whether it is natural or man-made. Creating a core group of knowledgeable and trained individuals for the initial response facilitates education and communication and decreases fear and anxiety among HCPs. In addition, planning for deploying alternate personnel by identifying volunteers or repurposing individuals and supporting staff by developing buddy systems where inexperienced staff, such as those from ambulatory areas or those rerouted from other nonacute care areas, are paired with and supervised by experienced staff. Volunteer HCPs should be adequately screened by hospital security prior to undergoing training and by clinical colleagues to assure they have the needed skills.[26] Protecting the front-line staff with a robust, rotating "call system" prevents burnout and stress management problems.[15]

Challenges: In addition to being exposed to individuals with pathogens of high consequence and at risk themselves of getting infected, having to care for their ill family members, up to 50% of HCPs may not show up for work for fear of getting infected.[66]

Recommendations: Robust and transparent communications that brief hospital staff continuously and provide them with current situational awareness, provide updates on process and policy changes, and remind them of ongoing preparedness plans and successes will maintain staff's confidence in the hospital/health system during a pandemic or bioterrorism event and shield the hospital/health system from additional staff retention due to fear, anxiety, or concerns about personal safety. Institutional support for mental health care, childcare, and financial stress helps staff focus on serving the hospital and health system in times of need during a pandemic or bioterrorism event. Reassuring staff by providing PPE, vaccines, and prophylaxis for themselves when appropriate and vaccines and prophylaxis for family members and offering systematic protections when altered standards of care are implemented provide reassurance to the staff and allow them to care for patients without fear of their personal safety or legal retribution.[66]

PERSONAL PROTECTIVE EQUIPMENT AND DECONTAMINATION

In addition to being concerned for physical and psychological safety during a pandemic or bioterrorist attack, hospital staff will also be concerned about their personal risk of acquiring the agent. This concern is not unreasonable, as demonstrated by recent outbreaks of pathogens of high consequence, where HCP infections accounted for up to 27% of infections with the Middle East Respiratory Syndrome coronavirus and between 2.5% and 12% of EVD.[67] During SARS-CoV-1, between 11% and 57% of cases were HCPs.

Decontamination of patients will be rarely needed, as most patients will present several days after an exposure. However, in the unusual instance where it is needed, patients and staff exposed to a biological agent should be decontaminated to reduce the biological burden on skin and mucous membranes after exposure. Decontamination areas should be established outside and downwind of a hospital.[68–71]

When there is an influx of patients after an attack or even during natural infectious disease disasters, there may be scenarios where every incoming patient will be considered infectious until triage is complete or until a provisional diagnosis is made depending on the agent or the nature of its manifestation. In these cases, PPE is critical to protect HCPs from exposure. Respiratory protection ranges from medical masks to respirators (N95 or P3), including powered air purifying respirators (PAPR), depending on the scenario. Other protective gear may include isolation gowns, gloves, eye protection, shoe covers, or protective gear covering from head-to-toe for protection against certain agents that require such protections. Several issues arise in that PPE must be available; staff must know how to don and doff correctly, and finally, staff must comply with the recommended PPE.[72] Failure at each of these steps has been associated with transmission to HCPs, as was the case with EVD and SARS-CoV-1. As mentioned above, HCPs should be trained on wearing appropriate PPE while caring for potential cases to assure their own personal safety.[73,74] Such training is critical for donning and doffing gowns and gloves with the care of EVD patients and for respiratory protection in the setting of organisms that can be aerosolized. Some PPE, such as respirators, require fit testing to assure that they appropriately seal against the skin, which renders them most effective. This activity is usually managed by occupational health.

Challenges: The COVID-19 pandemic demonstrated that our stockpiles were not adequate to support a massive infectious disease disaster, and the consequences of this shortcoming were well documented in the literature.[23] Unfortunately, we learned that this aspect of hospital preparedness goes beyond the control of individual hospitals and involves a complicated global supply chain. Solutions to ensuring that the supply chain can support the healthcare requirements will require intervention at a national level.

Recommendations: Health systems and hospitals should maintain a stockpile of PPE to assure they can protect their workforce. Hospitals must continuously train their workforce to be ready for the next event, yet the challenge is balancing competing priorities. Another important strategy is to target resources and develop a core response team of individuals that are regularly trained with plans to train additional staff just-in-time when the need arrives, which may ultimately be the most cost-effective use of resources.

WASTE MANAGEMENT AND CORPSE DISPOSAL

Human bodily secretions and waste can be infectious, and exposure to them may result in transmission to other individuals and to new infections.[75] Waste can also be hazardous, toxic, or radioactive, especially during bioterrorism events or with pathogens of high consequence. Hence, plans should be made to properly dispose to reduce potential for harm and secondary disasters.[75,76] Standard procedures should be developed during pandemics and bioterrorism events.[76] The death toll may be high during pandemics and bioterrorism events.

Challenges: Staff lacking knowledge could either be underprepared to handle human trash and corpses resulting in secondary events or they could be overly concerned due to media exposure with unverified information. Hospitals are usually underprepared with these two aspects of hospital preparedness.[76]

Recommendations: Hospitals must have a plan for proper and safe disposal of dead bodies during pandemics and bioterrorism events.[76] Hospitals must assess for morgue capacity, temporary morgue space, and additional refrigerated storage facilities.[76] Educate staff early during the process, develop protocols pertaining to the said event, and frequently engage staff with ongoing education and monitoring.

OCCUPATIONAL (EMPLOYEE) HEALTH AND MONITORING

Occupational health (also called employee health) plays a vital role in response to a pandemic or a bioterrorism event and therefore should be included in planning. Occupational health providers should receive preparedness training that could help them identify individuals presenting with a contagion. The diversity of tasks, knowledge, and exposure among HCP makes such preparations challenging. Furthermore, not all HCP possess the same risk as others after exposure.[77] The level of protection used during exposure also alters the risk posed to an individual during patient care. As evidenced during the COVID-19 pandemic, occupational health providers may be bombarded with potential HCP exposures and associated concerns. Occupational health professions play an important role in sorting out the nature of the exposure and the risk to determine needed actions such as the need for quarantine, postexposure prophylaxis, treatment, and other medical countermeasures. Crucial to a robust response, they also provide needed prevention such as vaccinations and preexposure prophylaxis as applicable with many pathogens of high consequence. Their responsibilities include contact tracing, record keeping, monitoring of exposed employees, and making decisions about return to work or for needed medical or mental health care in the short and long term. Importantly also, they need to collaborate with local, regional, state, and federal partners to ensure healthcare workers are adequately protected.

Challenges: Occupational health providers are commonly understaffed and may be stretched, especially with the increased demands during a pandemic. These providers face challenges in being able to reach employees for follow up or to make them comply with the pre or postexposure prophylaxis recommendations.

Recommendations: Healthcare institutions should have plans in place to augment their staffing with providers that can temporarily be trained and can function as occupational health providers, which can alleviate some burdens that these services face during pandemics. There may be a delay in receiving guidance from regional, state, and national public health authorities, and occupational health providers may need to fill in this gap with internal guidance to facilitate smooth operations.[78]

CRITICAL INCIDENT STRESS MANAGEMENT

These events, whether a single patient is infected with an agent of high consequence, a pandemic, or a planned release of infectious organisms, leave many invisible scars. Having witnessed or experienced tragedy, death, threatening situations, and other personal stresses can undermine the resilience of any workforce, leading to critical incident stress.[27] Critical incident stress affects the functioning of workforce members when exposed to a prolonged response, such as in a pandemic. This stress, in turn, fuels manpower losses due to illness or attrition. Given the importance of supporting the workforce, hospitals need to have a plan in place for ensuring their physical and psychological. Therefore, including mental health experts in the planning process is extremely important. Critical incident stress management trains individuals to address the effects of exposure to the highly stressful critical incidents using a range of services, including individual counseling, group debriefings, education, and other prevention and mitigation efforts.[52] A facilitated critical incident stress debriefing conducted soon after a traumatic event with groups of individuals under stress from a traumatic exposure such as a bioterrorism event supports staff recovery by providing group support and by opening doors for future counseling and treatment services if needed.[52] Such efforts help retain and return the workforce to normal activities following a critical incident.

Challenges: Staff may not admit to the critical incident stress they are experiencing due to the stigma associated with mental health issues.

Recommendations: Having transparent discussions about the possibility of critical incident stress among hospital staff, providing ongoing education about the condition, and addressing the need may encourage staff to join efforts in combating this issue.

CONCLUSION

Public health officials and hospital/health system leadership commonly do not prioritize extending resources for pandemic and bioterrorism preparedness. This perception arises from the misconception that the likelihood of either a pandemic or a well-planned, extensive bioterrorism attack is unlikely due to other safeguards that exist with national security. Furthermore, events such as EVD were far away and did not affect most hospitals, while a pandemic such as COVID-19 rarely occurs. However, one needs to realize that when these attacks do occur, the toll on human life will be devastating. Michael T. Osterholm,[1] in a prescient comment, stated that "Mother Nature is the greatest bioterrorist of them all." As was acknowledged in a GAO report over 20 years ago, the US hospitals are ill prepared for bioterrorism response.[9] It follows that healthcare systems worldwide are in general ill prepared for large outbreaks. Our recent experience with COVID-19 must open the eyes of certainly the United States and other hulking healthcare and public health systems that foresight and advanced preparations will prepare them for the future. These preparations must occur well in advance of an infectious disease disaster to avoid devastating consequences to ill-prepared healthcare systems, populations, and economies. While hospitals will need to commit to the importance of ongoing preparedness, political leaders must not only allot resources to these important hospital activities but also help hold healthcare systems and public health accountable. Resources are needed. Federal and regional (state/provincial) support that strengthens stockpiles, enhances regulations around physical space in health systems, and requires ongoing preparedness among healthcare system personnel and leaders will be critical. Given the recent morbidity, mortality, and costs of the COVID-19 pandemic, creative solutions are needed, including federal incentives to enhance the ability to prevent and respond to these devastating events.

REFERENCES

1. Osterholm MT, Olshaker M. Deadliest Enemy: Our War Against Killer Germs. 1st ed. New York: Little, Brown, and Company; 2017.
2. Pappas G, Seitaridis S, Akritidis N, Tsianos E. Infectious diseases in cinema: virus hunters and killer microbes. *Clin Infect Dis.* 2003;37(7):939–942. https://doi.org/10.1086/377740.
3. Bell BP, Damon IK, Jernigan DB, et al. Overview, control strategies, and lessons learned in the CDC response to the 2014-2016 Ebola epidemic. *MMWR Suppl.* 2016;65(3):4–11. https://doi.org/10.15585/mmwr.su6503a2. 27389903.
4. Centers for Disease Control and Prevention. Ebola Outbreak in West Africa; 2014-2016. https://wwwcdcgov/vhf/ebola/history/2014-2016-outbreak/indexhtml#_ftn2. Accessed 23 February 2023.
5. Van Beneden CA, Pietz H, Kirkcaldy RD, et al. Early identification and prevention of the spread of Ebola—United States. In: *CDC Response to the 2014–2016 Ebola Epidemic—West Africa and United States*; 2016. MMWR Suppl; 65 [Suppl. 3].
6. US Department of State. Top Officials (TOPOFF); 2001-2009. https://2001-2009.state.gov/s/ct/about/c16661.htm#:~:text=TOPOFF%20is%20a%20national%2Dlevel,of%20Mass%20Destruction%20(WMD). Accessed 23 February 2023.
7. United States Department of Justice, State and Local Domestic Preparedness Stakeholders Forum. Executive Summary on the TOPOFF Exercise: Planning Conference Final Report; 1999. May 20–21 https://www.hsdl.org/c/abstract/?docid=94. Accessed February 23, 2023.
8. Inglesby TV, Grossman R, O'Toole T. A plague on your city: observations from TOPOFF. *Clin Infect Dis.* 2001;32(3):436–445. https://doi.org/10.1086/318513. Epub 2001 Jan 29 11170952.
9. United States General Accounting Office. Report to Congressional Committees. Hospital Preparedness. Most Urban Hospitals Have Emergency Plans But Lack Certain Capacities for Bioterrorism Response; August 2003. https://www.gao.gov/assets/gao-03-924.pdf. Accessed 23 February 2023.
10. United States General Accounting Office. Testimony Before the Committee on Government Reform, House of Representatives. Bioterrorism Preparedness Efforts Have Improved Public Health Response Capacity, But Gaps Remain; April 2003. https://www.gao.gov/assets/gao-03-654t.pdf. Accessed 24 February 2023.
11. Adini B, Goldberg A, Laor D, Cohen R, Zadok R, Bar-Dayan Y. Assessing levels of hospital emergency preparedness. *Prehosp Disaster Med.* 2006;21(6):451–457.
12. Schultz CH, Mothershead JL, Field M. Bioterrorism preparedness. I: the emergency department and hospital. *Emerg Med Clin North Am.* 2002;20(2):437–455.
13. Shaikh ZHA. Practical aspects of implementation of a bioterrorism preparedness program in a hospital setting. *Infect Dis Clin.* 2006;20(2):443–453.
14. Kaji AH, Koenig KL, Lewis RJ. Current hospital disaster preparedness. *JAMA.* 2007;298(18):2188–2190.
15. Dowlati M, Seyedin H, Moslehi S. Hospital preparedness measures for biological hazards: a systematic review and meta-synthesis. *Disaster Med Public Health*

Prep. 2021;15(6):790–803. https://doi.org/10.1017/dmp.2020.132.
16. Eitzen EM. Use of biological weapons. In: Bellamy RF, Azjtchuk MC, eds. *Textbook of Military Medicine, Part I: Warfare, Weaponry, and the Casualty (Medical Aspects of Chemical and Biological Warfare)*. Washington, DC: Office of the Surgeon General, US Department of the Army; 1997:437–450.
17. Preparedness and Response: Systems, Supplies, Staff, and Space. Institute of Medicine and National Research Council. Public Health Risks of Disasters: Communication, Infrastructure, and Preparedness: Workshop Summary. Washington, DC: The National Academies Press; 2005. https://doi.org/10.17226/11201.
18. Hospital Incident Command System Guidebook. The California Emergency Medical Services Authority (EMSA); 2006. http://www.emsa.ca.gov/hics/. Accessed February 26, 2023.
19. Koenig KL, Kahn CA, Schultz CH. Medical strategies to handle mass casualties from the use of biological weapons. *Clin Lab Med.* 2006;26(2):313–327.
20. Vastag B. Experts urge bioterrorism readiness. *JAMA.* 2001;285(1):30–32.
21. Devereaux AV, Dichter JR, Christian MD, et al. Definitive care for the critically ill during a disaster: a framework for allocation of scarce resources in mass critical care: from a task force for mass critical care summit meeting, January 26-27, 2007, Chicago, IL. *Chest.* 2008;133(5 Suppl):51S–66S.
22. Rubinson L, Hick JL, Hanfling DG, et al. Definitive care for the critically ill during a disaster: a framework for optimizing critical care surge capacity: from a task force for mass critical care summit meeting, January 26-27, 2007, Chicago, IL. *Chest.* 2008;133(5 Suppl):18S–31S.
23. Sopirala MM. Predisposition of COVID-19 patients to secondary infections: set in stone or subject to change? *Curr Opin Infect Dis.* 2021;34(4):357–364.
24. Barnett DJ, Levine R, Thompson CB, et al. Gauging U.S. Emergency Medical Services workers' willingness to respond to pandemic influenza using a threat- and efficacy-based assessment framework. *PLoS One.* 2010;5(3):e9856.
25. Aoyagi Y, Beck CR, Dingwall R, Nguyen-Van-Tam JS. Healthcare workers' willingness to work during an influenza pandemic: a systematic review and meta-analysis. *Influenza Other Respir Viruses.* 2015;9(3):120–130.
26. White SR. Hospital and emergency department preparedness for biologic, chemical, and nuclear terrorism. *Clin Occup Environ Med.* 2002;2(2):405–425.
27. Scharoun K, van Caulil K, Liberman A, Bioterrorism vs. Health security-crafting a plan of preparedness. *Health Care Manag (Frederick).* 2002;21(1):74–92.
28. Bennett R. Chemical or biological terrorist attacks: an analysis of the preparedness of hospitals for managing victims affected by chemical or biological weapons of mass destruction. *Int J Environ Res Public Health.* 2006;3(1):67–75.
29. Daugherty EL, Carlson AL, Perl TM. Planning for the inevitable: preparing for epidemic and pandemic respiratory illness in the shadow of H1N1 influenza. *Clin Infect Dis.* 2010;50(8):1145–1154.
30. Centers for Disease Control and Prevention. Crisis Emergency Risk Communication. CERC: Terrorism and Bioterrorism Communication Challenges. https://emergency.cdc.gov/cerc/ppt/CERC_Terrorism%20and%20Bioterrorism%20Communication%20Challenges.pdf. Accessed February 24, 2023.
31. Shapiro DS. Surge capacity for response to bioterrorism in hospital clinical microbiology laboratories. *J Clin Microbiol.* 2003;41(12):5372–5376.
32. Gilchrist MJ. A national laboratory network for bioterrorism: evolution from a prototype network of laboratories performing routine surveillance. *Mil Med.* 2000;165(Suppl. 2):28–31.
33. Centers for Disease Control and Prevention. Bioterrorism Agents/Diseases. https://emergency.cdc.gov/agent/agentlist-category.asp. Accessed February 24, 2023.
34. Centers for Disease Control and Prevention. National Center for Immunization and Respiratory Diseases (NCIRD). H5N1 Bird Flu: Current Situation Summary. https://www.cdc.gov/flu/avianflu/avian-flu-summary.htm. Accessed 30 May 2023.
35. Centers for Disease Control and Prevention. National Center for Immunization and Respiratory Diseases, Division of Viral Diseases. Severe Acute Respiratory Syndrome (SARS). https://www.cdc.gov/sars/clinical/index.html. Accessed 30 May 2023.
36. Centers for Disease Control and Prevention. National Center for Immunization and Respiratory Diseases, Division of Viral Diseases. Middle East Respiratory Syndrome (MERS). https://www.cdc.gov/coronavirus/mers/. Accessed 30 May 2023.
37. Krajewski MJ, Sztajnkrycer M, Baez AA. Hospital disaster preparedness in the United States: new issues, new challenges. *Int J Rescue Disaster Med.* 2005;4(2):22–25.
38. Niska RW, Burt CW. Bioterrorism, and mass casualty preparedness in hospitals: United States, 2003. *Adv Data.* 2005;364:1–14.
39. Klein KR, Brandenburg DC, Atas JG, Maher A. The use of trained observers as an evaluation tool for a multi-hospital bioterrorism exercise. *Prehosp Disaster Med.* 2005;20(3):159–163.
40. Nayahangan LJ, Konge L, Russell L, Andersen S. Training, and education of healthcare workers during viral epidemics: a systematic review. *BMJ Open.* 2021;11(5):e044111.
41. Dubé M, Kaba A, Cronin T, Barnes S, Fuselli T, Grant V. COVID-19 pandemic preparation: using simulation for systems-based learning to prepare the largest healthcare workforce and system in Canada. *Adv Simul (Lond).* 2020;5:22.
42. Brydges R, Campbell DM, Beavers L, et al. Lessons learned in preparing for and responding to the early stages of the COVID-19 pandemic: one simulation's program experience adapting to the new normal. *Adv Simul (Lond).* 2020;5:8.
43. Grasselli G, Pesenti A, Cecconi M. Critical care utilization for the COVID-19 outbreak in Lombardy, Italy: early

experience and forecast during an emergency response. *JAMA*. 2020;323(16):1545–1546.
44. Watson CM, Duval-Arnould JM, McCrory MC, et al. Simulated pediatric resuscitation use for personal protective equipment adherence measurement and training during the 2009 influenza (H1N1) pandemic. *Jt Comm J Qual Patient Saf*. 2011;37(11):515–523.
45. The Joint Commission. R3 Report. New and Revised Standards in Emergency Management. https://www.jointcommission.org/-/media/tjc/documents/standards/r3-reports/final-r3-report-emergency-management.pdf. Accessed February 26, 2023.
46. Centers for Disease Control and Prevention Office of Readiness and Response. CDC Emergency Operations Center (EOC). https://www.cdc.gov/orr//eoc/eoc.htm Accessed February 26, 2023.
47. Stoto MA, et al. "REFERENCES." Learning from Experience: The Public Health Response to West Nile Virus, SARS, Monkeypox, and Hepatitis A Outbreaks in the United States. RAND Corporation; 2005:130–132. JSTOR http://www.jstor.org/stable/10.7249/tr285dhhs.17. Accessed 25 February 2023.
48. United States General Accounting Office. Testimony Before the Subcommittee on Government Efficiency, Financial Management, and Intergovernmental Relations, Committee on Government Reform, House of Representatives; October 2001. BIOTERRORISM. Hospital Preparedness. Coordination and Preparedness https://www.gao.gov/assets/gao-02-129t.pdf. Accessed 23 February 2023.
49. Ahern S, Loh E. Leadership during the COVID-19 pandemic: building and sustaining trust in times of uncertainty. *BMJ Leader*. 2021;5:266–269.
50. Crain MA, Bush AL, Hayanga H, et al. Healthcare leadership in the COVID-19 pandemic: from innovative preparation to evolutionary transformation. *J Healthc Leadersh*. 2021;13:199–207.
51. Rinnert KJ. Local perspectives on bioterrorism: an approach to terrorism preparedness: parkland health and hospital system. *Proc (Baylor Univ Med Cent)*. 2001;14(3):231–235.
52. United States Department of Labor. Occupational Safety and Health Administration. Emergency Preparedness Guides. Critical Incident Stress Guide. https://www.osha.gov/emergency-preparedness/guides/critical-incident-stress. Accessed February 24, 2023.
53. Romao VC, Martins SAM, Germano J, Cardoso FA, Cardoso S, Freitas PP. Lab-on-chip devices: gaining ground losing size. *ACS Nano*. 2017;11(11):10659–10664.
54. Buehler JW, Whitney EA, Smith D, Prietula MJ, Stanton SH, Isakov AP. Situational uses of syndromic surveillance. *Biosecur Bioterror*. 2009;7(2):165–177.
55. Buehler JW, Berkelman RL, Hartley DM, Peters CJ. Syndromic surveillance and bioterrorism-related epidemics. *Emerg Infect Dis*. 2003;9(10):1197–1204.
56. Arvisais-Anhalt S, Lehmann CU, Park JY, et al. What the coronavirus disease 2019 (COVID-19) pandemic has reinforced: the need for accurate data. *Clin Infect Dis*. 2021;72(6):920–923.
57. Katona P. Bioterrorism preparedness: a generic blueprint for health departments, hospitals, and physicians. *Infect Dis Clin Pract*. 2002;11(3):115–122.
58. Sharp TW, Brennan RJ, Keim M, Williams RJ, Eitzen E, Lillibridge S. Medical preparedness for a terrorist incident involving chemical and biological agents during the 1996 Atlanta Olympic Games. *Ann Emerg Med*. 1998;32(2):214–223.
59. Cosgrove SE, Fishman NO, Talbot TR, et al. Strategies for use of a limited influenza vaccine supply. *JAMA*. 2005;293(2):229–232.
60. Booth CM, Stewart TE. Communication in the Toronto critical care community: important lessons learned during SARS. *Crit Care*. 2003;7(6):405–406.
61. Rebmann T. Assessing hospital emergency management plans: a guide for infection preventionists. *Am J Infect Control*. 2009;37(9):708–714.
62. Asnakew S, Getasew L, Liyeh TM, et al. Prevalence of post-traumatic stress disorder on health professionals in the era of COVID-19 pandemic, Northwest Ethiopia, 2020: a multi-centered cross-sectional study. *PLoS One*. 2021;16(9).
63. d'Ettorre G, Ceccarelli G, Santinelli L, et al. Post-traumatic stress symptoms in healthcare workers dealing with the COVID-19 pandemic: a systematic review. *Int J Environ Res Public Health*. 2021;18(12):601.
64. Ip DKM, Lau EHY, Tam YH, et al. Increases in absenteeism among health care workers in Hong Kong during influenza epidemics, 2004–2009. *BMC Infect Dis*. 2015;15:586.
65. Rotenstein LS, Brown R, Sinsky C, Linzer M. The Association of Work Overload with burnout and intent to leave the job across the healthcare workforce during COVID-19. *J Gen Intern Med*. 2023;1–8 [published online ahead of print, 2023 Mar. 23].
66. Altered standards of care in mass casualty events. Rockville, MD: Agency for Healthcare Research and Quality; April 2005. Prepared by Health Systems Research Inc. Under Contract No. 290-04-0010. AHRQ Publication No. 05-0043. https://www.hsdl.org/c/view?docid=453728. Accessed February 26, 2023.
67. Suwantarat N, Apisarnthanarak A. Risks to healthcare workers with emerging diseases: lessons from MERS-CoV, Ebola, SARS, and avian flu. *Curr Opin Infect Dis*. 2015;28(4):349–361.
68. Case GG, West BM, McHugh CJ. Hospital preparedness for biological and chemical terrorism in Central New Jersey. *N J Med*. 2001;98(11):23–33.
69. Macintyre AG, Christopher GW, Eitzen Jr E, et al. Weapons of mass destruction events with contaminated casualties: effective planning for health care facilities. *JAMA*. 2000;283(2):242–249.
70. Inglesby TV, O'Toole T, Henderson DA, et al. Anthrax as a biological weapon, 2002: updated recommendations for management. *JAMA*. 2002;287(17):2236–2252.
71. Lepler L, Lucci E. Responding to and managing casualties: detection, personal protection, and decontamination. *Respir Care Clin N Am*. 2004;10(1):9–21.

72. Mumma JM, Durso FT, Casanova LM, et al. Common behaviors and faults when doffing personal protective equipment for patients with serious communicable diseases. *Clin Infect Dis.* 2019;69(Suppl. 3):S214–S220.
73. Wetter DC, Daniell WE, Treser CD. Hospital preparedness for victims of chemical or biological terrorism. *Am J Public Health.* 2001;91(5):710–716.
74. Loutfy MR, Wallington T, Rutledge T, et al. Hospital preparedness and SARS. *Emerg Infect Dis.* 2004;10(5):771–776.
75. Al-Shareef AS, Alsulimani LK, Bojan HM, et al. Evaluation of hospitals' disaster preparedness plans in the Holy City of Makkah (Mecca): a cross-sectional observation study. *Prehosp Disaster Med.* 2017;32(1):33–45.
76. Yao L, Zhang Y, Zhao C, Zhao F, Bai S. The PRISMA 2020 statement: a system review of hospital preparedness for bioterrorism events. *Int J Environ Res Public Health.* 2022;19(23):16257.
77. United States Department of Labor. Occupational Safety and Health Administration. Pandemic Influenza Preparedness and Response Guidance for Healthcare Workers and Healthcare Employers. https://www.osha.gov/sites/default/files/publications/OSHA_pandemic_health.pdf. Accessed 14 May 2023.
78. McPhaul KM. COVID-19 lessons learned: pandemic preparedness is an occupational health imperative. *Workplace Health Saf.* 2022;70(1):4–5.

CHAPTER 20

Special Care Units

RADU POSTELNICU[a] • VIKRAMJIT MUKHERJEE[a] • LAURA EVANS[b]
[a]Division of Pulmonary, Critical Care, and Sleep Medicine, New York University School of Medicine, Bellevue Hospital, New York, NY, United States • [b]Division of Pulmonary, Critical Care and Sleep Medicine, University of Washington, Seattle, WA, United States

INTRODUCTION

The global spread of emerging infectious diseases highlights the importance of hospital and health system planning for the care of hazardous infectious diseases. Historically, the emergence of epidemics has prompted the medical profession to reexamine its responsibilities to society. Providing care for patients with avian and novel influenza (i.e., H7N9), severe acute respiratory syndrome (SARS-CoV), Middle Eastern respiratory syndrome (MERS-CoV), or viral hemorrhagic fevers (VHF) while maintaining optimal safety for staff has led to the development of specialized units to care for these patients. These areas are clinical facilities specifically designed to contain pathogens of high consequence, minimize nosocomial transmission, and contribute to the successful management of outbreaks.[1a,b]

In general, these specialized care units are secure facilities with isolation processes to prevent the release of these agents. They function with standard operating procedures that support clinical care, laboratory services, waste management, communications, and interactions with the public health sector. The physical structure of these units is commonly separated into three main areas of high- and low-risk zones and the zone outside the main unit.[1c] These may be color-coded and importantly designate the types of activities, the contamination, the types of personnel, and the amount of and type of personal protective equipment (PPE) that is needed. The high-risk zone, commonly called the red zone, is the area inside the facility for patient care, laboratory work, and the disposal of all contaminated waste, disposal of sharps, organic waste, and contaminated supplies. The low-risk zone sometimes designated as yellow includes the staff changing rooms (unidirectional and one for entry and exit), office space, pharmacy, storage room for supplies, and the laundry area. The outside zone or green area is an area where no infectious material is present and may contain waiting areas and separate areas for counseling families.

Beyond these core principles, the models differ depending on whether they are established in high-, middle-, or low-income countries. For example, Ebola Treatment Units (ETUs) were developed in low-income countries and based on the experience of the Democratic Republic of the Congo (DRC) managing outbreaks of Ebola Virus Disease (EVD) and the subsequent experience of the World Health Organization (WHO), Médicins Sans Frontières (MSF), and the Centers for Disease Prevention and Control (CDC) managing EVD during the 2014 EVD outbreak in West Africa. These units may have different names in different parts of the world, yet the model ETU has between 10 and 30 beds and is designed to handle a localized outbreak or cases that are part of a larger outbreak occurring within a rural or semi-urban population and is responsible for triage, diagnosis, and treatment of EVD. [1d] In this model, the ETU is part of a comprehensive unit that also does community engagement, case finding, communication, and safe burials. Importantly, there are also much larger ETUs (e.g., >200 beds), and these larger facilities may have multiple units or wards and additional organizational and communications requirements to address patient management. The model ETU has laboratory capabilities for onsite testing for the pathogen of interest. In settings where there are no human resources or laboratory equipment and supplies, mobile laboratories can be deployed, or samples can be sent to more distant facilities.

In high-income countries, these units are commonly called biocontainment care units (BCU) or High-Level Containment Care (HLCC) and focus on the diagnosis and clinical care of the patient infected with pathogens of high consequence. Unlike ETUs, these units

Viral Outbreaks, Biosecurity, and Preparing for Mass Casualty Infectious Diseases Events
https://doi.org/10.1016/B978-0-323-54841-0.00015-9

will not be responsible for the triage of patients and will primarily focus on the complex care associated with these infections. In Europe and North America, these units are primarily located in academic medical centers because of the intensive and specialized care that is likely required in managing critically ill patients with infections caused by agents that require containment. In addition, such units may have responsibility for communication and liaison with the public health department(s) and the public. As these units are sophisticated assets, their design is notable for advanced air handling systems, which are monitored continually, their secure access, waste management systems, on-site diagnostic laboratory facilities, some radiologic services, and telemedicine capabilities (Fig. 1).[1e]

Regardless of the setting, many of the principles of care in these settings are similar. Both settings require trained staff and protocols and policies, which, while complex, are critical to safe care. The goals of these protocols are to assure that these units are properly staffed and will facilitate management of the setting; clarify the roles and responsibilities of team members; manage the movement of staff and materials in the space; and ensure consistent management of patients and their data. Provisions of safe and effective care in either a BCU or ETU require considerable investment in planning, training, and material resources.[2]

This chapter will focus on the specialized BCU units and the important components of developing a BCU team and will discuss the structure, training, and administrative concerns that must be considered when developing a response to bio-emergencies, as well as the details of designing appropriate facilities. Many of the principles discussed apply to all settings, including those where ETUs are commonly used.

STAFFING AND TEAM COMPOSITION

Healthcare personnel (HCP) and patient safety are the ultimate measures of a successful staffing model, which requires a multidisciplinary team. This ensures adequate patient care and minimizes the number of HCPs potentially exposed to these highly infectious pathogens. Because of the emotional and physical toll of caring for these patients, teams need redundancy. In addition, these teams must be readily available and reflect the anticipated clinical and critical care capabilities of the unit.[1,2] BCU teams require leadership from a physician with experience in critical care and infectious diseases, as well as a nurse leader with administrative skills. The BCU team should also include hospital administrators and educators in addition to the clinical HCP discussed later.

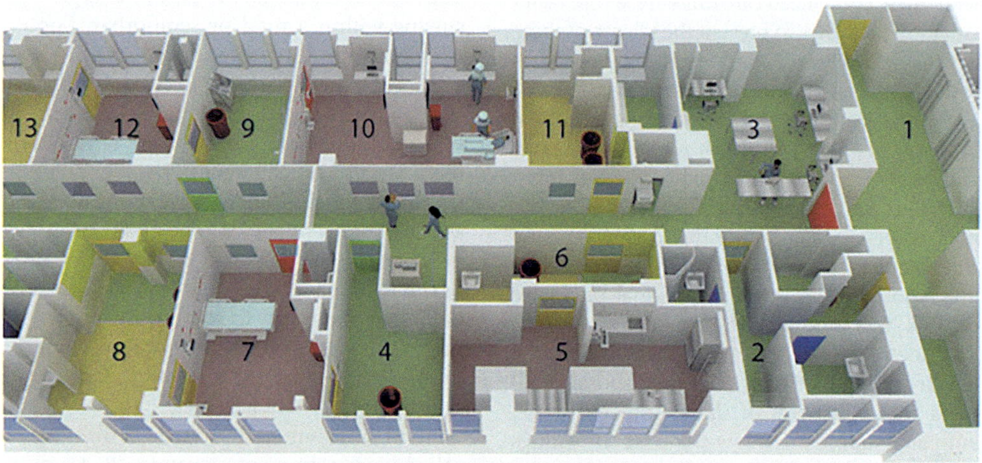

FIG. 1 Layout a model BCU. General layout of the BCU. Patient rooms and the laboratory have dedicated space for donning and doffing PPE. There is a unidirectional flow with green indicating clean space, red indicating contaminated space, and yellow indicating doffing rooms. (1) Off-unit area with dedicated elevators, locker room, changing area, and lounge for staff; (6) clean entry and exit space for staff; (7) nurse station; (8) shared donning room for laboratory and patient room; (9) laboratory; (10) doffing room for laboratory; (15, 19, 24) patient rooms and associated doffing room (17, 23, 25); (18) shared donning room for patient rooms. (Source: Garibaldi BT and Chertow DS. High-Containment Pathogen Preparation in the Intensive Care Unit. *Infect Dis Clin North Am*. 2017 Sep; 31 (7): 561–576. https://doi.org/10.1016/j.idc.2017.05.008)

Staffing Models and Considerations

Prior to developing a BCU team, a staffing model must be determined with the goal of providing adequate coverage for the patient care responsibilities while considering local cultural and institutional factors. Because of the intense training requirements, the need for well-functioning teams, and the choreographed care, a stable team best serves the BCU needs. Ultimately, to develop a functional team, members should be invested in the growth and development of the BCU, and such commitments help reduce turnover rates that would require additional recruitment, onboarding, and training. In general, medical, nursing, and other trainees, such as students and pre- and postdoctoral learners, are not ideal members of BCU teams.[1]

One of the most difficult issues is to decide whether team members should be mandated (compelled) to work in the event of a bio-emergency, or if they can self-select (volunteer) to work in these units.[2] Each model has benefits and limitations. A volunteer-based model favors the selection of individuals who are motivated to participate in bio-emergencies. This model would mobilize available staff that would be readily engaged and motivated to participate in a high impact and critical management of patients with highly hazardous communicable diseases (HHCD). Additionally, individuals who are hesitant to participate in a staffing model that mandates participation have an acceptable avenue to disengage or may choose to participate in activities that do not require them to be in the BCU.

The mandatory staffing approach is based on an expectation of duty model that utilizes the ethical principle of duty to care (see Chapter 16 for additional information). This approach has many advantages, including facilitating the timely activation of team members who are already present and on site and providing the resources to scale the response to a larger event. However, this model may create an environment where individuals refuse to participate in the BCU activities and patient care. Such refusals in supporting the institutional mandates and care delivery can affect the public's perception of the institution providing care to patients in bio-emergencies and may also impact overall team and hospital personnel morale.

Staffing the BCU

Teams that support BCUs need to be multidisciplinary and provide not only the clinical support but also the administrative and regulatory support required to care for these complex patients. Proposed staffing models exist for both ETUs and BCUs and can be adapted from the experience of others.[2b]

Provider (Medical) Team

The team leadership should include a physician trained in critical care or infectious diseases, as bio-emergencies involve HHCDs, which require extensive knowledge and management strategies that these specialties provide.[3] These providers should also have extensive experience with medical procedures used to support critically ill patients including central line placement, airway management and intubation, chest tube insertion, thoracentesis, lumbar puncture, and paracentesis. Additionally, medical consultants who can provide and support other types of care, such as hemodialysis and cardiac support, are critical resources that need to be involved in the care model and team structure. Furthermore, bio-emergencies could also potentially impact pediatric and pregnant patients, and consultants such as pediatricians and obstetricians may also be called upon to provide expertise in the BCU. For some pathogens, expertise in neurology or psychiatry may be critical to patient care. In addition, advanced care providers, including physician assistants and nurse practitioners, can serve as key providers of medical care in these settings. Once team members have been selected, appropriate onboarding and training should be performed. Our model uses the checklist in Table 1 as part of the onboarding process. Other models evaluate competencies to assure adequate training is provided.

Nursing Team

The nursing team is fundamental to the appropriate functioning of a BCU and should contain highly trained and sufficient numbers of nurses with critical care and emergency skills, educators, and those with administrative and logistical expertise. In general, those who have worked in intensive care units and emergency departments are used to working in high-pressure situations and have the experience to deliver care to potentially critically ill patients in the BCU. Nurses should have experience in monitoring cardiac, respiratory, renal, and neurological status in critically ill patients and understand the infection prevention and safety needs in order to minimize environmental contamination and effectively manage medical waste.[4] Ideally, a significant portion of nurses on each shift should have critical care expertise to provide appropriate bedside care as needed. These nursing teams require a breadth of expertise including experience with hemodialysis, pediatric and obstetric patients, and obstetric support.[4,5] Some BCUs include infection preventionists as part of the team. These individuals can provide guidance about placement issues, medical waste, cleaning, and disinfection and, in some cases, monitor the donning and doffing processes of other

TABLE 1
Physician Onboarding Activities and Checklist: Biocontainment Unit

(1) Three donning and doffing sessions within 4 weeks of initial session
(2) All MDs will have an initial in-person meeting with ICU MD, which will involve the following:
- i. Team structure in the BCU
- ii. Role of the MD, including participation in nonroutine tasks such as waste management and spill cleanup
- iii. Procedural considerations in the BCU, including:
  1. role of ultrasound
  2. challenges of central lines/intubations in PPE and how to carry out a safe procedure
  3. specimen collection
- iv. Brief overview of current pathogens of concern
  1. Include the importance of being part of this team in the context of your institution's role in disaster preparedness
- v. National Ebola Training and Education Center orientation (https://courses.netec.org/)

(3) BCU walkthrough
- i. Explain technological aspects, including teleconferencing capabilities and laboratory processes

(4) On-call schedule and responsibilities
(5) Training schedule and responsibilities
(6) Introduction to the Hospital Incident Command System and activation alert
(7) Introduction to the Department of Health and its role in the BCU.

TABLE 2
Nurse Onboarding Activities and Checklist: Biocontainment Unit

Once a nurse or float pool nurse has completed their orientation and 6 months in the critical care area (if this is where they are assigned), they are eligible to begin their donning and doffing sessions.

1. Three donning and doffing sessions
   - a. Initial session
     - i. Two to two and ½ hours
     - ii. Donning and doffing using infection prevention and control principles
     - iii. Orientation to members of the Special Pathogens Team
       1. Lab, Emergency Management, EVS, Nursing Leadership, Medical Team
     - iv. Unit orientation.
       1. Fire lane
       2. Unit, donning room, lab, patient room, guidebook, initial cart, anteroom, call light system, and activation schedule
       3. Orientation to standard operating procedures of the BCU
       4. Rules of activation
          - Give a pre-report if on the activation schedule.
          - 40-min from floor to fire lane
          - Roles and responsibilities of the nurses in various zones in receiving a patient (i.e., red versus yellow)
       5. Monitoring after an activation
          - 21 days temperature reported to the Department of Health
       6. NETEC orientation (https://courses.netec.org/)
       7. How to contact the training center or nursing
     - v. Brief overview of current pathogens of concern
       1. Include the importance of being part of this team in the context of the hospitals' role in disaster preparedness
   - b. Second donning and doffing session (to be done within 2 weeks of the initial session)
     - i. 1 to 1.5 h
     - ii. Trainer will don and doff if there is not another participant to teach the buddy system.
     - iii. Answer any questions brought up after the initial session.
   - c. Third Donning and Doffing session (to be done within 2 weeks of the second session)
     - i. Can be completed during an all-day training
     - ii. Once completed, the nurse can be placed on the Special Pathogens Activation List.

HCPs. Onboarding processes for nurses again must be structured and should follow a certain protocol and require training (Table 2).

Additional Support Staff

In addition to medical and nursing providers, laboratorians, respiratory therapists, and technicians who can provide complex medical care should be included as determined by the service needs. Additional staff that carries out specific procedures, such as respiratory therapists, laboratory technicians, and x-ray and hemodialysis technicians, should be part of the BCU team.[5] Recent experience with acute respiratory failure from viral infections such as the Middle East Respiratory Syndrome (MERS) and SARS-CoV-2 has also shown the importance of recruiting specialized providers such as perfusionists and specialized cardiovascular nurses in the event that extracorporeal membrane oxygenation (ECMO) would be required.[6] Additional members of these teams who support but may not be physically in the BCU may include ethicists, social workers, chaplains, pharmacists, and members of the institutional review board. Finally, and in order to minimize the number of individuals that enter the BCU, routine tasks that are usually performed by environmental services staff, patient care technicians, or ancillary staff should be taken over by the BCU team, which means that the nurses and physicians perform an array of tasks. One such task, of high concern, is the management of spills, particularly of bodily fluids. It is important to develop a very thorough protocol to assure the rapid and appropriate management of spills. For example, both physicians and nurses assume the responsibility of containment, as seen in an example protocol (Table 3).

STAFF TRAINING/PREPAREDNESS

While protocols outline processes and define responsibilities, training staff around these protocols is paramount to them and their colleagues' safety. The protocols in BCUs are complex and require training and reinforcement. HCPs commonly wear significant amounts of PPE when caring for these patients. Training enhances their familiarity with protocols and the equipment and allows them to practice and enhance their dexterity while in PPE. For example, studies are limited but suggest that doffing of PPE is an activity associated with contamination, and thus a structured fashion to remove PPE is thought to reduce the risk of self-contamination.[6c] Hence, training around practices, and procedures is critical and must be done repeatedly over time.[6d] Furthermore, competency around critical protocols further ensures HCP and patient safety.

TABLE 3
Example BCU Protocol: Spill Containment

Red zone (see Fig. 1)

1. Contain spill
2. Hand hygiene and change gloves
3. Notify Buddy Nurse and site manager of the spill.
4. Check PPE for any visible contamination. If there is any contamination, disinfect the area with approved disinfectant wipes.
5. Hand hygiene and change gloves

Runner nurse

1. Will obtain spill kit and 2 sets of 2 mop pads premoistened with disinfectant from the donning room and hand into Buddy Nurse
2. Will obtain any materials needed for the Buddy Nurse and the RED Zone nurse

Yellow zone/Green zone (see Fig. 1)

1. Buddy Nurse will hand in the spill kit and mop pads.
2. Buddy Nurse will observe procedure and report any breaches to the site manager.

RED zone (see Fig. 1)

1. Spill kit will be opened, and the items removed.
2. Bucket will be lined with small red bag.
3. Material used to contain the spill will be placed in the lined bucket.
4. Any of the following equipment can be used to clean up the spill:
   a. Grabbers
   b. Solidifier
   c. Squeegee
   d. Disposable underpad
   e. Approved disinfectant wipes
   f. Dustpan
5. Once the spill has been cleaned, all material, except the grabbers and the handles of the squeegee and dustpan, will be placed into the lined blue bucket.
6. Tie the small bag closed and place the lid on the spill bucket.
7. Place the bucket into the larger red bag and tie large bag closed.
8. Place the large bag in the bathroom until it is time for trash removal.
9. Hand hygiene
10. Using the premoistened mop pads, mop the area from the cleanest to the dirtiest area.
11. Place used mop pads in the red waste bin.
12. Disinfect the poles of the mop, squeegee, dustpan, and grabbers and place them in the bathroom.
13. Check PPE for any visible contamination *(please refer to SOP for Contaminant/ Breach in the BCU).*
14. Hand hygiene and change gloves

To achieve competency, training is required and competency assessment (see Resource section selected tools, including checklists and competency assessment). Complex tasks such as cardiopulmonary resuscitation where multiple individuals are involved are more complex and require defining roles and additional understanding of processes. Training may occur using many forms and modalities from in-person individualized training and didactic sessions to "train the trainer," online learning, video presentations, and simulation training sessions. Recently, investigators found that as the number of training sessions increased among BCU personnel, the participant's perceived competence in activities also increased.[6e] The National Emerging Special Pathogens Training and Education Center (NETEC) is a consortium of institutions that have expertise in the management of patients infected with agents of high consequence and that are global leaders in the management and operations of BCUs. NETEC (https://netec.org/) and its partners have developed educational and training courses, videos, and tools to manage and care for these patients, consulting services, readiness assessments, exercise templates, and tools for contingency and crisis capabilities in the management of special pathogens. These resources are free and meant to provide and facilitate the safe care of patients.

INFECTION PREVENTION AND CONTROL

The BCU must have robust infection prevention and control (IPC) practices and procedures to protect HCPs and minimize the risk of transmission of a pathogen of high consequence (see example Table 3). These practices and procedures will require cross-disciplinary work with Occupational Health Safety and Hygiene (OHSH) specialists. While there are overall umbrella IPC practices and procedures (hand hygiene, cleaning, and disinfection; reprocessing of devices; isolation; and use of barrier precautions) that will form the foundation of the BCU safety program, there is a need to address practices based on the potential risk assessment for each potential pathogen or bio-emergency that could affect patients admitted to the BCU (see chapters 13, 15, 24, and 25 for additional details). Furthermore, in partnership with OHSH, there is a need for robust protocols and approaches to assure that the HCP working in these areas have been appropriately screened for immunity, tested for respiratory protection, and recommended vaccination(s). This must include processes to assess and manage any HCP who may be inadvertently exposed to a high-consequence pathogen while working in a BCU. The portfolio of activities and protocols should be robust and comprehensive and will require training, oversight, and accountability.[1,3,7] These experts can provide guidance to manage waste, cleaning and disinfection processes, management of laboratory samples, and assure that appropriate personal protective equipment is available. Furthermore, they can assume responsibility for training of BCU staff and can develop additional competency assessments if needed (see Resources for competency tools). During activation of the BCU, IPC will implement precautions based on the pathogen the patient was potentially exposed to or infected with. In addition, they should directly observe clinical care and assist during activities such as donning and doffing of the PPE, as well as other critical steps in patient care. IPC may also play a critical role in selection of PPE (Chapter 24), occupational health for HCPs working on the unit (e.g., vaccinations, screenings), environmental and large equipment disinfection, transportation of patients to the unit, and the overall biosafety program.[1]

CLEANING AND DECONTAMINATING THE ENVIRONMENT

Delivering care for patients with HHCDs presents challenges in the safe management of waste contaminated with infectious pathogens. Decontamination of the patient area should also occur in a manner that utilizes appropriate IPC protocols and procedures. Meticulous detail in following protocol is key to assuring effective cleaning. Processes should include how to clean surfaces, equipment, especially that which will be reused, and linens. In some cases, supplemental decontamination with no-touch technology is also utilized.[7a] Medical waste generated during the care of patients with HHCD, as well as the environment where the patient was cared for, poses a significant risk to healthcare, environmental service, and waste-handling workers due to the potential contamination of surfaces, equipment, and supplies with transmissible HHCD pathogens. Medical waste and its management are two of the most challenging aspects of caring for these patients. Any object that is contaminated or is suspected to be contaminated with an HHCD should be packaged, collected, stored, and disposed of in a manner that adheres to the appropriate regulatory guidance for that waste.[8] Many units have steam sterilizers or autoclaves to augment waste management capacity within the unit.[11]

COLLABORATION WITH PUBLIC HEALTH AUTHORITIES (SEE CHAPTER 13)

Whether a BCU, ETU, or similar unit, preparing for bio-emergencies requires close collaboration with public health resources to ensure a unified response, access to expert advice, and providing special services that facilitate the response. Each unit or healthcare system should work closely with their local health department(s), emergency medical system(s), and other community and health partners to facilitate an exchange of information, develop individual response and collaboration, and ensure adequate preparedness for such emergencies. In cases involving HHCD patients in the United States, a healthcare system should collaborate and coordinate with the jurisdictional public health agency and the CDC to ensure close communication, a coordinated response, and to access additional resources that are available to healthcare facilities preparing for or responding to potential bio-emergencies. Examples in the United States include the Regional Ebola and Other Special Pathogen Treatment Center network and NETEC (https://netec.org/). As a healthcare system has developed an appropriate framework for responding to bio-emergencies, the system should look toward other national services to further expand and improve its protocols and planned responses. Most testing to diagnose HHCDs would be done outside the BCU, with preliminary testing likely carried out at a Laboratory Response Network, while confirmatory testing would be completed at the CDC.[9] Both processes involve packaging and shipping specimens, and this should be done in a highly systematic manner.[10]

DESIGNING SPECIAL CARE UNITS

The physical structure and design of these spaces are important to facilitate HCP and patient safety by engineering processes that support best practice (Fig. 1).[10b,c] Whether an ETU or BCU, several principles are key to design and offer certain advantages, making them a desirable environment for managing such patients while minimizing transmission risk to healthcare personnel and the surrounding community.[1] Ideally, these units should be constructed with materials that resist breakdown from solutions containing hypochlorite, have minimal seams, and be constructed to minimize leakage of infectious materials. They should be located away from other clinical areas in order to limit traffic and should have clear transportation routes to and from their entries and exits.[10d,e] As discussed earlier, these units should have zones that delineate the risk of contamination (i.e., high-risk (red); low-risk (yellow)); space to don and doff PPE; space for a laboratory; and unidirectional flow again to minimize the risk of cross contamination. Many include spaces to shower on exiting these units. Stations to clean hands are important. Green zones are safe zones where the chance of contamination is similar to that in other healthcare settings.

In BCU and places where resources can support additional features, air handling is of crucial importance, especially if a pathogen can be aerosolized. Appropriate ventilation helps minimize contamination and helps protect HCPs if infectious particles might be aerosolized.[11] The BCU room should be capable of being used as an Airborne Infection Isolation Room (AIIR) with special air handling and ventilation capacity, in accordance with the American Institute of Architects/FGI (AIA/FGI) standards (Table 4).[3,12–14] An example of a newly constructed BCU demonstrates some of the features of the patient rooms, laboratory space, and space for donning and doffing (Fig. 1).

TABLE 4
Air Handling Requirements in the Biocontainment Unit

Characteristic	Comments
The BCU ventilation system is independent of the other building heating, ventilation, and air conditioning system.	While this is the ideal scenario, building a separate AHU (air handling unit) is a resource-intensive project.
Each patient room should have an anteroom.	This allows for proper environmental controls as well as a staged doffing process.
Air flows and pressure gradients within the BCU run from the cleanest to the most contaminated areas; with the patient room at negative air pressure relative to adjacent areas, a suggested differential pressure gradient of more than 15 Pa between patient room and anteroom and between anteroom and the rest of the unit, and an effective ventilation rate of at least 12 air changes per hour in the patient rooms.	Rate of 6 air changes per hour is acceptable for existing infrastructures. Rate of 12 air changes per hour is recommended for new healthcare construction.
Air from the BCU is not recirculated, and exhaust air is vented 100% to the outside of the building.	Air reentry can cause rapid dissemination of virus inside a hospital building.[12]

(Continued)

TABLE 4
Air Handling Requirements in the Biocontainment Unit—cont'd

Characteristic	Comments
Exhaust air is discharged at a site and distance from the building that minimizes the risk of contamination of building occupants (e.g., by down-draught into open windows) and the community.	
HEPA filtration of exhausted air is preferable, and if there is any possible risk of reentry of exhaust air or of human exposure to exhausted air, HEPA filtration is obligatory.	
HEPA filters are appropriately protected by prefilters, housed correctly, and sited for ease of safe access for maintenance.	HEPA filters in the HVAC system successfully decrease the bioaerosol concentrations in the hospital environment.[13]
BCU ventilation systems are designed to be fail-safe, and to minimize cross contamination in the event of system failure in the unit or elsewhere on the site (e.g., built-in redundancy—BCU ventilation system with dual fans each capable of exhausting 100% air; air flow shutdown system independent of site system to protect against unwanted shutdown after alarm elsewhere on site; interlocking supply and exhaust systems so that supply fan is prevented from running if exhaust fans fail).	Under circumstances of exhaust failure, the HVAC system maximizes air flow to areas adjacent to isolation room in an effort to maintain negative pressure differential. However, transport through cracks around doors/door handles out of the BCU via airflow alone may be possible[14]
Ventilation systems incorporate current best practice performance checking tools (e.g., visual pressure check gauges, audible alarms); have a schedule for planned preventive maintenance.	

AUDIO-VISUAL CAPABILITIES AND INTERNAL COMMUNICATION

Auditory perception is often impaired because of the physical barriers imposed by PPE. Ambient noise, such as that created by the heating, ventilation, and air conditioning systems and monitors, can also play a major role in limiting auditory communication and can cause a decrease in auditory processing function, especially when conversations carry critical information.[15] Furthermore, some equipment, such as purified air respirators, can create significant background noise and reduce the HCP's visibility. In addition, visitors are commonly not allowed in these units, which can lead to the patient feeling isolated.

While efforts should be made to keep ambient noise to a bare minimum, investing in a robust telecommunications system is crucial in the design of a BCU. An efficient telecommunication system allows for many advantages: (i) Observation of the patient and their care delivery and real-time feedback; (ii) ability to provide multidisciplinary care to the patient while minimizing the number of HCPs in the room; and (iii) remote monitoring of staff behavior and safety. Less expensive options such as smartphones and tablets have been adopted to allow patient and family communication, but those have been less successful at supporting consultation with specialists and communication between the BCU teams. Hence, to facilitate care, a BCU can install a secure telehealth system that allows a 2-way talk-back intercom and provides seamless video feeds into the patient room and the anteroom. Some systems provide technology and headsets that are integrated into PPE. Other models use video streaming technology with computers on wheels. Regardless of the technology chosen, teams should also be trained in their use and be well-versed in nonverbal forms of communication.[7] Team-building exercises can be implemented to improve staff communication as well as job satisfaction.[16]

LABORATORY PROCESSING AND TESTING

Laboratory support is crucial for providing optimal patient care in a BCU. Accurate testing and timely results are important given the critical nature of these patients' illnesses (see Chapter 17). In addition, the high-risk nature of HHCDs and the potential risk associated with transporting samples and cross-contaminating equipment have led most facilities to co-locate laboratory testing in the BCU. Furthermore, because of the potentially severe consequences of occupational exposure in this setting, advanced planning around staffing, location, and types of equipment is critical in providing a safe working environment.[17] In addition to staffing, training to use the equipment with PPE is needed for laboratorians. Special consideration should be given to the following:

- *Location of testing:* Point-of-care testing inside the patient's room, and laboratory capabilities inside the BCU or within the hospital (outside the BCU) are all possible solutions. Irrespective of location, the laboratory should be equipped to safely perform basic laboratory tests (e.g., complete blood count, chemistries, arterial blood gas analyses, coagulation studies, and basic microbiology) that are required to provide care to a patient with HHCD. Additionally, these laboratories should provide testing for malaria, sepsis, and respiratory viral infections—processes that are relatively common in patients suspected of having an HHCD.[18] Point-of-care, compact, and core analyzers are commonly used across BCUs to provide required testing of patients.[17]
- *Training and staffing:* A core team of laboratory personnel should be trained in the use of institution-specific PPE and testing equipment, packaging and shipping of specimens, and HHCD-specific laboratory practices.
- Risk assessment: The CDC provides guidance on risk assessment for any laboratory that plans to test patients for Ebola and other special pathogens (Table 5).[19] The goal of this risk assessment is to identify potential hazards to those working with these pathogens, assess an individual's likelihood of exposure to the pathogen along each step in movement through the laboratory, and determine methods to mitigate the risk. The specimen's path through the laboratory should be carefully followed to determine the potential areas of risk, and then the response should examine engineering controls, presence of PPE, and equipment to minimize any exposure risk.

TABLE 5
CDC Risk Assessment Tool for Laboratory Safety When Collecting, Handling, and Testing Specimens for Ebola and Other Special Pathogens

- Evaluate the specimen management and movement through the laboratory with particular attention to high-traffic areas.
- Look for any steps where needles or other sharps are used and disposed of.
- Determine the potential for splashes, sprays, or droplet generation.
- Examine equipment for potential hazards (such as the potential for creating aerosols, sprays, and splashes of the specimen when performing testing and using equipment).
- Assure that the biological safety cabinet is certified and its operation is associated with safe work practices.
- Review decontamination procedures, including spill response, and methods for decontamination of equipment to assure they are safe and appropriate products are available.
- Assess how infectious waste is managed and disposed of, including processes to handle "sharps."
- Review the laboratory design to minimize the risk of exposure to other HCPs in the area, including evaluating the ventilation and filtration capacities.
- Develop recommended measures to minimize the risk of laboratory transmission when testing patient specimens, which may include limiting the number of staff engaged in testing, evaluating and segregating equipment used for testing, performing testing in a dedicated space, having well-developed entry and exit procedures, and having policies to monitor potentially exposed employees and to care for those who are associated with an exposure.
- Assure the laboratory has the appropriate engineering controls and safety equipment.
- Develop laboratory communication protocols.
- Identify the necessary PPE, maintain stocks, and train workers in its proper use. Assure that they can safely don and doff when using PPE.

Adapted from the CDC. *Guidance for US Hospitals and Clinical Laboratories on Performing Routine Diagnostic Testing for Patients with Suspected Ebola Disease.* https://www.cdc.gov/vhf/ebola/laboratory-personnel/safe-specimen-management.html.

CONCLUSIONS

When developing a specialized unit including a BCU, many factors need to be considered to successfully deliver care for patients infected with HHCDs. It requires a leadership structure that supports the unit goals and adequate staffing models that support patient care and protect the HCPs working in these units. These models can vary between institutions, but they need to be developed to meet the needs of individual facilities and specific emergencies. Retention and recruitment of staff committed to developing and following care protocols, infection prevention and control standards, and overall safety is critical to the success of such units. Training and retraining have emerged as an element that is a cornerstone to providing care in these units. Not every hospital or healthcare facility can develop an incredibly complex infrastructure with different design features in a specialized BCU, but healthcare facilities may be faced with these patients that will require care prior to transfer. In such cases, institutions can integrate many aspects of these units to care for these patients and to minimize the risk of spread of HHCDs. Preparedness for acceptance and care of such facilities can be assessed using a tool from NETEC (Table 6; https://docs.google.com/viewer?url=https%3A%2F%2Frepository.netecweb.org%2Ffiles%2Foriginal%2F4809eb55906643bfad1ca6a90364849e.docx&embedded=true).

TABLE 6
Health Care Facility Viral Hemorrhagic Fever (VHF) Preparedness Checklist

NETEC

Health Care Facility Viral Hemorrhagic Fever (VHF) Preparedness Checklist

Viral Hemorrhagic Fevers (VHF) are a group of diseases caused by several families of viruses. The term VHF refers to an illness that can affect multiple organ systems and can be accompanied by fever, headache, vomiting, abdominal pain, diarrhea, and hemorrhage. VHFs addressed in this document include **Crimean-Congo Hemorrhagic Fever (CCHF)**, **Ebola Virus Disease (EVD)**, **Lassa Fever**, and **Marburg Virus Disease (MVD)**.

Health care facility preparedness to care for patients with a viral hemorrhagic fever (VHF) is essential to prevent transmission to staff, other patients and our communities. To assist healthcare facilities assess and advance their VHF preparedness, the National Emerging Special Pathogens Training and Education Center (NETEC) developed the Health Care Facility Viral Hemorrhagic Fever Preparedness Checklist as a VHF planning tool. This tool will help health care facilities assess their readiness to identify, isolate, inform, and provide initial treatment for patients suspected or confirmed to have a VHF.

This checklist is intended to guide facilities through a review of their immediate care capabilities and provide resources to assist in the resolution of preparedness gaps it reveals.

For a more in-depth assessment of your special pathogen program, we recommend requesting to complete the NETEC Special Pathogen Operational Readiness Self-Assessment (SPORSA). Visit www.NETEC.org for more information.

1 | The National Emerging Special Pathogens Training and Education Center (NETEC) | netec.org

TABLE 6
Health Care Facility Viral Hemorrhagic Fever (VHF) Preparedness Checklist—cont'd

(Continued)

TABLE 6
Health Care Facility Viral Hemorrhagic Fever (VHF) Preparedness Checklist—cont'd

IDENTIFY

The first step in the VHF response framework for health care facilities is to quickly recognize and safely manage patients with a suspected or confirmed VHF to reduce transmission risk. Screening all patients upon entry to a facility for signs, symptoms, and epidemiological risk factors for VHFs will facilitate early identification of a patient at risk for having the disease.

Identify Readiness Items

#	Item	Status Yes or No	Notes
1.	There is an established process to complete periodic review of countries where VHFs are endemic or are currently experiencing VHF outbreaks.	Yes ☐ No ☐	Click here to enter facility notes.
2.	Screening for symptoms and travel history occurs at all points of patient entry to the facility including those arriving by EMS.	Yes ☐ No ☐	Click here to enter facility notes.
3.	Signage is present at all points of entry into the health system to enable patients to self-identify if their symptoms are consistent with a VHF and what next steps are (e.g., mask and notify staff).	Yes ☐ No ☐	Click here to enter facility notes.
4.	Staff who will complete patient screening have received training on the VHF "Identify" process.	Yes ☐ No ☐	Click here to enter facility notes.

Identify Resource/ Guidance

NETEC Town Hall: Preparing Frontline Health Care Workers for Ebola
https://youtu.be/Okh_Sa9cVa4

Identify Worksheet:
https://repository.netecweb.org/files/original/c1c81476c9626fd1d8f8be5fa75f9ad3.pdf

Global Outbreak Resources:
https://www.cdc.gov/outbreaks/index.html
https://dph.georgia.gov/TravelClinicalAssistant

Screening Algorithm Example:
https://repository.netecweb.org/items/show/458 [repository.netecweb.org]

3 | The National Emerging Special Pathogens Training and Education Center (NETEC) | netec.org

TABLE 6
Health Care Facility Viral Hemorrhagic Fever (VHF) Preparedness Checklist—cont'd

Identify Isolate Inform Webinar/ Course:
https://youtu.be/QkGflp7W7Cc
https://courses.netec.org/courses/identify-isolate-inform

Mystery Patient Drill Kit:
https://repository.netecweb.org/pdfs/specialpathogenmysterydrill.zip

4 | The National Emerging Special Pathogens Training and Education Center (NETEC) | netec.org

(Continued)

TABLE 6
Health Care Facility Viral Hemorrhagic Fever (VHF) Preparedness Checklist—cont'd

ISOLATE

The second step of the VHF response framework for health care facilities is to safely isolate and manage patients with a suspected or confirmed VHF to reduce transmission risk. Rapid isolation allows infection prevention and control measures to be implemented to reduce exposure to staff, visitors, and other patients.

Isolate Readiness Items

#	Item	Status Yes or No	Notes
1.	Masks are available at all points of entry for patients entering the facility to quickly apply if indicated.	Yes ☐ No ☐	Click here to enter facility notes.
2.	An isolation space has been identified and:	Yes ☐ No ☐	Click here to enter facility notes.
2a.	Staff are oriented to its location, use, and limitations.	Yes ☐ No ☐	Click here to enter facility notes.
2b.	The process for using the space has been developed and tested (e.g., moving out other patients or extra equipment, initiating negative pressure).	Yes ☐ No ☐	Click here to enter facility notes.
2c.	A written checklist has been developed to direct the preparation of the isolation space.	Yes ☐ No ☐	Click here to enter facility notes.
2d.	There is a private restroom or bedside commode available for the patient to use in accordance with facility and jurisdictional regulations for human waste management.	Yes ☐ No ☐	Click here to enter facility notes.
2e.	The isolation space is an airborne infection isolation room (AIIR) or can accommodate a portable negative pressure unit if needed and available. **	Yes ☐ No ☐	Click here to enter facility notes.
2f.	There is a process for communication to occur into and out of the room, while maintaining isolation precautions (e.g., white boards, speaker phones, call light system).	Yes ☐ No ☐	Click here to enter facility notes.
2g.	There is a process to limit the number of personnel that enter the isolation space to essential personnel.	Yes ☐ No ☐	Click here to enter facility notes.
2h.	There is a process to clearly identify, document, and follow up with all personnel that enter the isolation space.	Yes ☐ No ☐	Click here to enter facility notes.

TABLE 6
Health Care Facility Viral Hemorrhagic Fever (VHF) Preparedness Checklist—cont'd

3.	There is a written plan for the internal transfer of a patient from the point of entry into the facility to the designated isolation space. The written plan includes the following:	Yes ☐ No ☐	Click here to enter facility notes.
3a.	Ability to control the internal route to the isolation space, minimizing risk of exposure to others.	Yes ☐ No ☐	Click here to enter facility notes.
3b.	Preparing the isolation space for the patient arrival including isolation signage and delineation of zones.	Yes ☐ No ☐	Click here to enter facility notes.
3c.	Guidance on safely managing the patient until the isolation space is ready for admission (e.g., masking and maintaining 6ft distance from other patients, visitors, and staff)	Yes ☐ No ☐	Click here to enter facility notes.
3d.	Personnel who have current training to implement the plan.	Yes ☐ No ☐	Click here to enter facility notes.
4.	Staff who will work in the isolation area have been trained on special pathogen workflows and processes.	Yes ☐ No ☐	Click here to enter facility notes.

**Refer to the Isolation Worksheet in Resources for more detailed guidance*

***If there are no AIIR and portable negative pressure devices are not available, identify a private, closed-door room that the patient can be placed in while remaining masked.*

Isolation Resources/ Guidance

Isolation Worksheet:
https://repository.netecweb.org/files/original/77003e56292b75db4d90bccdea9120ca.pdf

CDC Guidance on Hospital Room Infection Control for Ebola Virus:
https://www.cdc.gov/vhf/ebola/clinicians/cleaning/hospitals.html

Containment Wrap Protocol:
https://repository.netecweb.org/files/original/b68363bffb7eec4a6189ada3a480317f.pdf

Log Sheet:
https://repository.netecweb.org/files/original/78157aefeb472e0d99e300509f72a1a.pdf

6 | The National Emerging Special Pathogens Training and Education Center (NETEC) | netec.org

(Continued)

TABLE 6
Health Care Facility Viral Hemorrhagic Fever (VHF) Preparedness Checklist—cont'd

INFORM

The third step of the VHF response framework for health care facilities is to promptly notify key partners to reduce transmission risk. Timely and efficient communication processes are essential to be able to alert internal and external stakeholders of the identification of a patient suspected to have a VHF. External stakeholders, such as a Department of Public Health, may also be needed to determine if a patient meets VHF PUI criteria.

Inform Readiness Items

#	Item	Status Yes or No	Notes
1.	Key personnel internal (e.g., Infection preventionists, health care administrator, etc.) to your facility who will provide support and/or be involved in the care of a PUI have been identified.	Yes ☐ No ☐	Click here to enter facility notes.
2.	Key partners both internal and external to your facility, such as county and state public health partners and Laboratory Response Network (LRN) partners, have been identified and staff know who to inform.	Yes ☐ No ☐	Click here to enter facility notes.
3.	Contact information for internal and external key personnel is readily accessible.	Yes ☐ No ☐	Click here to enter facility notes.
4.	Staff who will inform key personnel are knowledgeable on the process, including what information to provide.	Yes ☐ No ☐	Click here to enter facility notes.

Inform Resources/ Guidance

Inform Worksheet:
https://repository.netecweb.org/files/original/a537618495fdb8be570540cb604ca035.pdf

CDC Health Alert Network:
https://emergency.cdc.gov/han/

Health Department Directories:
https://www.cdc.gov/publichealthgateway/healthdirectories/index.html

TABLE 6
Health Care Facility Viral Hemorrhagic Fever (VHF) Preparedness Checklist—cont'd

PERSONAL PROTECTIVE EQUIPMENT (PPE)

PPE ensembles worn during the care of patients suspected or confirmed to have a VHF must provide enhanced contact and droplet protection and should consider both the condition of the patient and the risk of exposure to blood and other potentially infectious materials posed by care tasks. Complex and infrequently used PPE ensembles require additional training to ensure staff safety and may require additional personnel to assist in doffing. The use of a trained observer is recommended to ensure correct donning and safe doffing practices to reduce self-contamination.

PPE Readiness Items

#	Item	Status Yes or No	Notes
1.	The PPE ensemble has been selected based on pathogen transmission and patient condition (, e.g., wet vs dry) and includes consideration to elevate based on presumptive positive test results.	Yes ☐ No ☐	Click here to enter facility notes.
2.	Staff have received training on VHF PPE donning and doffing protocols.	Yes ☐ No ☐	Click here to enter facility notes.
3.	There is a clean space to don PPE and a separate safe space to doff PPE.	Yes ☐ No ☐	Click here to enter facility notes.
4.	There are PPE donning and doffing checklists to guide staff utilizing PPE ensembles.	Yes ☐ No ☐	Click here to enter facility notes.
5.	There is an adequate amount of appropriate PPE available to provide care for at least 1 patient for 24-48 hours. See DASH tool HERE for guidance on determining facility PPE supply needs.	Yes ☐ No ☐	Click here to enter facility notes.
6.	A trained observer is utilized to monitor activities in the isolation room and donning and doffing of PPE.	Yes ☐ No ☐	Click here to enter facility notes.

PPE Resources/ Guidance

ASPR/TRACIE Disaster Available Supplies in Hospitals (DASH) tool:
https://dashtool.org

(Continued)

TABLE 6
Health Care Facility Viral Hemorrhagic Fever (VHF) Preparedness Checklist—cont'd

CDC PPE Guidance for Ebola Virus Care:
https://www.cdc.gov/vhf/ebola/healthcare-us/ppe/guidance.html

Know Your PPE:
https://repository.netecweb.org/items/show/1053

Space Recommendations for Donning and Doffing Personal Protective Equipment (PPE) in Biocontainment Areas:
https://repository.netecweb.org/items/show/1708

Viral Hemorrhagic Fevers PPE Matrix:
https://repository.netecweb.org/files/original/8c1dda9b0654d3013ddc57a29b960ab2.pdf

9 | The National Emerging Special Pathogens Training and Education Center (NETEC) | netec.org

TABLE 6
Health Care Facility Viral Hemorrhagic Fever (VHF) Preparedness Checklist—cont'd

TREATMENT & CARE

The goal of caring for patients suspected or confirmed to have a VHF is to provide safe, effective, high-quality patient care while maintaining the safety of all personnel.

Treatment and Care Readiness Items

#	Item	Status Yes or No	Notes
1.	If a PUI arrives at your facility, personnel are familiar with internal processes and have access to resources for just-in-time-training.	Yes ☐ No ☐	Click here to enter facility notes.
2.	The care interventions that can be safely provided for patients suspected or confirmed to have VHF have been discussed and clinicians are aware of how to safely offer care including expansion of duties to reduce the number of staff (clinical and non-clinical) in the patient's room (e.g., diagnostic imaging, invasive procedures, specimen collection).	Yes ☐ No ☐	Click here to enter facility notes.
3.	There is a written plan to collaborate with employee health and/or public health to monitor personnel involved in the care of a patient with a confirmed diagnosis. (including laboratory personnel who may have handled biospecimens or EVS who may have managed environmental cleaning and disinfection).	Yes ☐ No ☐	Click here to enter facility notes.
4.	Diagnostic testing for presumptive and confirmatory pathogen identification will be conducted in coordination with the public health department.	Yes ☐ No ☐	Click here to enter facility notes.
5.	If routine clinical laboratory testing is required, either dedicated point of care devices will be used, or risk assessment of the main clinical laboratory completed to determine what tests can be safely performed.	Yes ☐ No ☐	Click here to enter facility notes.
6.	The facility has access to resources for guidance on packaging and shipment of presumed category A specimens.	Yes ☐ No ☐	Click here to enter facility notes.
7.	The facility is aware of and has identified available resources for decedent management and will seek support to conduct the process if needed.	Yes ☐ No ☐	Click here to enter facility notes.

Treatment and Care Resources/ Guidance

Treatment and Care Worksheet:
https://repository.netecweb.org/files/original/71028eadfb30cd38c0ba31e01a5fa28a.pdf

10 | The National Emerging Special Pathogens Training and Education Center (NETEC) | netec.org

(Continued)

TABLE 6
Health Care Facility Viral Hemorrhagic Fever (VHF) Preparedness Checklist—cont'd

JIT Training Resources:
https://repository.netecweb.org/exhibits/show/netec-education/justintime

Laboratory Testing for Crimean-Congo Hemorrhagic Fever:
https://repository.netecweb.org/items/show/1698

Laboratory Testing for Ebola:
https://netec.org/2022/10/11/laboratory-testing-for-ebola/

Laboratory Testing for Lassa Fever:
https://repository.netecweb.org/items/show/1667

Laboratory Testing for Marburg:
https://repository.netecweb.org/exhibits/show/netec_guides/item/1705

Laboratory Activation Checklist:
https://repository.netecweb.org/files/original/760672f218efe45fdf61c2d96991b2c2.docx

11 | The National Emerging Special Pathogens Training and Education Center (NETEC) | netec.org

TABLE 6
Health Care Facility Viral Hemorrhagic Fever (VHF) Preparedness Checklist—cont'd

WASTE MANAGEMENT AND CLEANING & DISINFECTION

Waste generated in the care of suspected or confirmed to have a viral hemorrhagic fever (VHF) is subject to procedures set forth by local, state, and federal regulations. Basic principles for spills of blood and other potentially infectious materials are outlined in the U.S. Occupational Safety and Health Administration (OSHA). Waste contaminated (or suspected to be contaminated) with certain VHFs is a Category A infectious substance regulated by the U.S. Department of Transportation Hazardous Materials Regulations (HMR; 49 CFR, Parts 171-180). Requirements in the HMR apply to any material DOT determines is capable of posing an unreasonable risk to health, safety, and property when transported in commerce. The EPA maintains lists of registered disinfectants that should be used to destroy certain pathogens. For a list of disinfectants that are effective against the VHF and analogous pathogens visit https://www.epa.gov/pesticide-registration/list-l-disinfectants-use-against-ebola-virus#check.

Waste Management and Cleaning and disinfection Items

#	Item	Status Yes or No	Notes
1.	There is a written plan for the management of waste generated during the care of a person suspected or confirmed to have a pathogen and it includes the following:	Yes ☐ No ☐	Click here to enter facility notes.
1a.	A designated secured waste holding area where waste can be separated from the department and facility's normal waste holding area.	Yes ☐ No ☐	Click here to enter facility notes.
1b.	Staff training on high-risk biohazard waste management process including proper handling of human biological waste, used and unused medical equipment, used and unused disposable supplies, patient linen and clothing, and terminal cleaning of patient room.	Yes ☐ No ☐	Click here to enter facility notes.
1c.	Secure packaging/ containment of waste to include proper closure of biohazard bags and approved hard sided transport containers.	Yes ☐ No ☐	Click here to enter facility notes.
1d.	If required, a vendor licensed to transport category A infectious substance will transport the waste for off-site inactivation.	Yes ☐ No ☐	Click here to enter facility notes.
2.	There is a written cleaning and disinfection plan for the isolation area that includes the following:	Yes ☐ No ☐	Click here to enter facility notes.
2a.	Guidance on the type of PPE to be worn when performing cleaning and disinfection in the special pathogen isolation area.	Yes ☐ No ☐	Click here to enter facility notes.

12 | The National Emerging Special Pathogens Training and Education Center (NETEC) | netec.org

(Continued)

TABLE 6
Health Care Facility Viral Hemorrhagic Fever (VHF) Preparedness Checklist—cont'd

2b.	A process to ensure an appropriate disinfectant has been selected and is available for use that is effective against the pathogen.	Yes ☐ No ☐	Click here to enter facility notes.
2c.	Detailed checklist(s) that guide staff in all steps to ensure safe and effective management of the space after the patient has been discharged or transferred.	Yes ☐ No ☐	Click here to enter facility notes.
2d.	Guidance and oversight of the cleaning and disinfection process by a special pathogens infection control expert.	Yes ☐ No ☐	Click here to enter facility notes.

Waste Management Resources/ Guidance

Managing Solid Waste Contaminated with a Category A Infectious Substance:
https://www.phmsa.dot.gov/sites/phmsa.dot.gov/files/2022-06/Cat%20A%20Waste%20Planning%20Guidance_Final_2022_06.pdf

Ebola-Associated Waste Management:
https://www.cdc.gov/vhf/ebola/clinicians/cleaning/waste-management.html

Fact Sheet. Safe Handlin, Treatment, Transport and Disposal of Ebola-Contaminated Waste:
https://www.osha.gov/sites/default/files/publications/OSHA_FS-3766.pdf

COVID-19 Waste Container Use:
https://repository.netecweb.org/files/original/7cc5c14094799b74298210150878a02f.pdf

Interim Guidance for Environmental Infection Control in Hospitals for Ebola Virus:
https://www.cdc.gov/vhf/ebola/clinicians/cleaning/hospitals.html

TABLE 6
Health Care Facility Viral Hemorrhagic Fever (VHF) Preparedness Checklist—cont'd

TRANSPORTATION

Patients suspected or confirmed to have a VHF may require transportation either to or from your facility. Having a plan in place will facilitate the movement of the patient in a manner that maintains safety for facility and transportation staff.

Transportation Readiness Items

#	Item	Status Yes or No	Notes
1.	There is a written plan to request the transfer of a patient suspected or confirmed to have a VHF that includes:	Yes ☐ No ☐	Click here to enter facility notes.
1a.	Current contact information for local and state public health authorities, an identified EMS agency that can provide ACLS and/or BLS transport as needed, and a higher tier facility that the patient can be transferred to.	Yes ☐ No ☐	Click here to enter facility notes.
1b.	Guidance on how to prepare the patient for transport (e.g., protective ensemble and premedication considerations)	Yes ☐ No ☐	Click here to enter facility notes.
2.	Your facility has identified a specific location and established processes for the transfer of patient care between EMS personnel and facility personnel.	Yes ☐ No ☐	Click here to enter facility notes.

Transportation Resources/Guidance

Example: Standard Operating Procedure (SOP) for Decontamination of an Ambulance that has Transported a Person under Investigation or Patient with Confirmed Ebola:
https://www.cdc.gov/vhf/ebola/clinicians/emergency-services/ambulance-decontamination.html

EMS Infectious Disease Playbook:
https://www.ems.gov/pdf/ASPR-EMS-Infectious-Disease-Playbook-June-2017.pdf

Example: Standard Operating Procedure (SOP) for Patient Handoff between a Health care Facility and a Transporting Ambulance:
https://www.cdc.gov/vhf/ebola/clinicians/emergency-services/patient-handoff.html

EMS biosafety: Identify, Isolate, Inform:
https://repository.netecweb.org/files/original/4e07db6e4f6caba74c3d2a461447bb24.pdf

(Continued)

TABLE 6
Health Care Facility Viral Hemorrhagic Fever (VHF) Preparedness Checklist—cont'd

Handoff Protocol Example:
https://repository.netecweb.org/files/original/ae752dc3510f6b0804fe746a752a6f58.pdf

Updated: 04/18/2023

REFERENCES

1. (a) Smith PW, Anderson AO, Christopher GW, et al. Designing a biocontainment unit to care for patients with serious communicable diseases: a consensus statement. *Biosecur Bioterror.* 2006;4(4):351–365. (b) Gleason B, Redd J, Kilmarx P, et al. Establishment of an Ebola treatment unit and laboratory - Bombali District, Sierra Leone, July 2014-January 2015. *MMWR Morb Mortal Wkly Rep.* 2015;64(39):1108–1111. https://doi.org/10.15585/mmwr.mm6439a4 [PMID: 26447483]. (c) Sterk E. Filovirus Haemorrhagic Fever Guideline. Médecins Sans Frontières, Barcelona Spain: Mimeograph; 2008. Available at: http://ebolaalert.org/wp-content/themes/ebolaalert/assets/PDFS/SOPMSFReference.pdf. (d) Muyembe-Tamfum, et al. Ebola virus outbreaks in Africa: past and present. *Onderstepoort J Vet Res.* 2012;79(22):1–8. (e) Pfäfflin F, Stegemann MS, Heim KM, et al. Preparing for patients with high-consequence infectious diseases: Example of a high-level isolation unit. *PLoS One.* 2022;17(3):e0264644. https://doi.org/10.1371/journal.pone.0264644. PMID: 35239726; PMCID: PMC8893674.
2. (a) Decker BK, Sevransky JE, Barrett K, Davey RT, Chertow DS. Preparing for critical care services to patients with Ebola. *Ann Intern Med.* 2014;161(11):831–832. (b) Frank MG, Croyle C, Beitscher A, Price C. The role of hospitalists in biocontainment units: a perspective. *J Hosp Med.* 2020;15(6):375–377. https://doi.org/10.12788/jhm.3402. PMID: 32195660.
3. Bannister B, Puro V, Fusco FM, Heptonstall J, Ippolito G, Group EW. Framework for the design and operation of high-level isolation units: consensus of the European network of infectious diseases. *Lancet Infect Dis.* 2009;9(1):45–56.
4. Johnson SS, Barranta N, Chertow D. Ebola at the National Institutes of Health: perspectives from critical care nurses. *AACN Adv Crit Care.* 2015;26(3):262–267.
5. Torabi-Parizi P, Davey Jr RT, Suffredini AF, Chertow DS. Ethical and practical considerations in providing critical care to patients with Ebola virus disease. *Chest.* 2015;147(6):1460–1466.
6. (a) Al-Dorzi HM, Aldawood AS, Khan R, et al. The critical care response to a hospital outbreak of Middle East respiratory syndrome coronavirus (MERS-CoV) infection: an observational study. *Ann Intensive Care.* 2016;6(1):101. (b) Dave S, Shah A, Galvagno S, et al. A dedicated Veno-venous extracorporeal membrane oxygenation unit during a respiratory pandemic: lessons learned from COVID-19 part I: system planning and care teams. *Membranes (Basel).* 2021;11(4):258. https://doi.org/10.3390/membranes11040258. PMID: 33918355; PMCID: PMC8065909. (c) M.F. Wong, Z. Matić, G.C. Campiglia, C.M. Zimring, J.M. Mumma, C.S. Kraft, L.M. Casanova, F.T. Durso, V.L. Walsh, P.Y. Shah, A.L. Shane, J.T. Jacob, J.R. Dubose, For the CDC prevention epicenters program, design strategies for biocontainment units to reduce risk during doffing of high-level personal protective equipment, Clin Infect Dis, 69, Supplement_3, 2019, S241–S247, https://doi.org/10.1093/cid/ciz617. (d) Verbeek JH, Ijaz S, Mischke C. Personal protective equipment for preventing highly infectious diseases due to exposure to contaminated body fluids in healthcare staff. *Cochrane Database Syst Rev.* 2016;4, CD011621. (e) Pfäfflin F, Stegemann MS, Heim KM, et al. Preparing for patients with high-consequence infectious diseases: example of a high-level isolation unit. *PloS One.* 2022;17(3), e0264644. https://doi.org/10.1371/journal.pone.0264644. PMID: 35239726; PMCID: PMC8893674.
7. (a) Garibaldi BT, Kelen GD, Brower RG, et al. The creation of a biocontainment unit at a tertiary care hospital. The Johns Hopkins medicine experience. *Ann Am Thorac Soc.* 2016;13(5):600–608. (b) Weber DJ, Rutala WA, Anderson DJ. Effectiveness of ultraviolet devices and hydrogen peroxide systems for terminal room decontamination: focus on clinical trials. *Am J Infect Control.* 2016;44:e77–e84.
8. Herstein JJ, Biddinger PD, Gibbs SG, et al. High-level isolation unit infection control procedures. *Health Secur.* 2017;15(5):519–526.
9. Jackson JC, Gordon SM, Hart RP, Hopkins RO, Ely EW. The association between delirium and cognitive decline: a review of the empirical literature. *Neuropsychol Rev.* 2004;14(2):87–98.
10. (a) Polderman KH, Ely EW, Badr AE, Girbes AR. Induced hypothermia in traumatic brain injury: considering the conflicting results of meta-analyses and moving forward. *Intensive Care Med.* 2004;30(10):1860–1864. (b) Kortepeter MG, Kwon EH, Cieslak TJ. Designing medical facilities to care for patients with highly hazardous communicable diseases. In: Hewlett AK, Murthy A, eds. *Bioemergency Planning.* Cham: Springer; 2018. https://doi.org/10.1007/978-3-319-77032-1_2. (c) Sterk E. Filovirus Haemorrhagic Fever Guideline. Médecins Sans Frontières, Barcelona Spain: Mimeograph; 2008. Available at: http://ebolaalert.org/wp-content/themes/ebolaalert/assets/PDFS/SOPMSFReference.pdf. (d) Kortepeter MG, Kwon EH, Cieslak TJ. Designing medical facilities to care for patients with highly hazardous communicable diseases. In: Hewlett A, Murthy K, A., eds. *Bioemergency Planning.* Cham: Springer; 2018. https://doi.org/10.1007/978-3-319-77032-1_2. (e) Janke C, Heim KM, Steiner F, et al. Beyond Ebola treatment units: severe infection temporary treatment units as an essential element of Ebola case management during an outbreak. *BMC Infect Dis.* 2017;17(1):124. https://doi.org/10.1186/s12879-017-2235-x. PMID: 28166739; PMCID: PMC5295220.
11. Garibaldi BT, Chertow DS. High-Containment Pathogen Preparation in the Intensive Care Unit. *Infect Dis Clin North Am.* 2017;31(3):561–576. https://doi.org/10.1016/j.idc.2017.05.008. PMID: 28779833; PMCID: PMC5568084.
12. Wehrle PF, Posch J, Richter KH, Henderson DA. An airborne outbreak of smallpox in a German hospital and its significance with respect to other recent outbreaks in Europe. *Bull World Health Organ.* 1970;43(5):669–679.

13. Mousavi MS, Hadei M, Majlesi M, et al. Investigating the effect of several factors on concentrations of bioaerosols in a well-ventilated hospital environment. *Environ Monit Assess.* 2019;191(7):407.
14. Therkorn J, Drewry Iii D, Pilholski T, et al. Impact of air-handling system exhaust failure on dissemination pattern of simulant pathogen particles in a clinical biocontainment unit. *Indoor Air.* 2019;29(1):143–155.
15. Way TJ, Long A, Weihing J, et al. Effect of noise on auditory processing in the operating room. *J Am Coll Surg.* 2013;216(5):933–938.
16. Amos MA, Hu J, Herrick CA. The impact of team building on communication and job satisfaction of nursing staff. *J Nurses Staff Dev.* 2005;21(1):10–16. quiz 7–8.
17. Herstein JJ, Iwen PC, Jelden KC, et al. U.S. high-level isolation unit clinical laboratory capabilities update. *J Clin Microbiol.* 2018;56(2):e01608–e01617.
18. Kulkarni P, Lifshitz E, Carothers B, Kidder R, Semple S, Tan C. Description of persons under investigation for Ebola virus disease—New Jersey, august 2014–may 2015. Open forum. *Infect Dis.* 2015;2(Suppl 1):LB-3.
19. Prevention CDC. Guidance for Collection, Transport and Submission of Specimens for Ebola Virus Testing. Available from: https://www.cdc.gov/vhf/ebola/laboratory-personnel/specimens.html.

CHAPTER 21

Diagnostics

KAEDE V. SULLIVAN
Department of Pathology and Laboratory Medicine, Lewis Katz School of Medicine at Temple University, Philadelphia, PA, United States

LABORATORY TESTING AND SAFETY

The laboratory identification of biological agents of bioterrorism requires collaboration between highly trained clinical, laboratory, and public health teams who work closely together to ensure efficient case assessment; procurement of patient specimens; transport of specimens to the local laboratory; initial "rule-out" testing if applicable; shipment of specimens or laboratory product (e.g., culture isolates) to a designated reference laboratory for confirmatory testing; and communication of testing results. This chapter provides an overview of the structures, procedures, and resources that are in place to ensure that critical laboratory diagnoses are generated as quickly as possible while emphasizing the safety of laboratory and nonlaboratory personnel who handle potentially hazardous infectious material.

CATEGORIES OF POTENTIAL AGENTS OF BIOTERRORISM AND INFECTIOUS DISEASES

The classification system that the Centers for Disease Control and Prevention (CDC) uses to categorize potential agents of bioterrorism considers: person-to-person transmissibility of the agent; the associated mortality rate; potential for major public health impact; potential for public panic and social disruption; and whether specific action is required for public health preparedness (Table 1).[1]

LABORATORY TESTING STRUCTURES AND RESOURCES

History of the Laboratory Response Network

In 1995, President William Clinton signed Presidential Decision Directive (PDD) 39, which described how the government would respond to threats or acts of terrorism involving nuclear, biological, or chemical materials or weapons of mass destruction. PDD-39 was classified at the time of signing. However, details about the directive were communicated to the public in a fact sheet through Presidential Decision Directive 69, which was signed by President Clinton in 1998.[2,3] In response to PDD-39, the Laboratory Response Network (LRN) was established in 1999 by the Department of Health and Human Services and the CDC to ensure swift and safe laboratory response to acts of biological terrorism. The CDC provides oversight for the LRN program and is accountable for its activities.[4] The Federal Bureau of Investigations (FBI) and the Association of Public Health Laboratories (APHL) were the founding partners of the LRN and continue to be key players.[4] More details about the legislative and organizational history related to the LRN have been published elsewhere.[5–7]

Structure of the Laboratory Response Network

The LRN consists of three levels. Sentinel laboratories generally consist of front-line hospital and commercial laboratories that perform routine diagnostic testing. They are certified by the Centers for Medicare and Medicaid Services to perform high-complexity testing under the Clinical Laboratory Improvement Amendments of 1988 (CLIA). Their role is to rapidly rule out an agent of bioterrorism and determine if human specimens and/or laboratory products (e.g., bacterial isolates) should be referred to an LRN Reference laboratory for confirmatory testing. Sentinel laboratories use the Sentinel-Level Clinical Laboratory Protocols that were developed collaboratively by the CDC, APHL, and the American Society for Microbiology (ASM) for selected CDC Category A and B agents of bioterrorism. They can be viewed online and are regularly reviewed and updated.[8,9] These protocols provide information about specimen collection when an agent

Viral Outbreaks, Biosecurity, and Preparing for Mass Casualty Infectious Diseases Events
https://doi.org/10.1016/B978-0-323-54841-0.00013-5

TABLE 1
Classification of Potential Agents of Bioterrorism

Class	Description	Disease (Agent)
A	• Can be easily disseminated or transmitted from person to person. • Result in high mortality rates and have the potential for major public health impact. • Might cause public panic and social disruption and require special action for public health preparedness.	• Anthrax (*Bacillus anthracis*) • Botulism (*Clostridium botulinum* toxin) • Plague (*Yersinia pestis)* • Smallpox (Variola major) • Tularemia (*Francisella tularensis*) • Viral hemorrhagic fevers
B	• Moderately easy to disseminate • Result in moderate morbidity rates but low mortality rates • Require specific enhancements to CDC's diagnostic capacity and enhanced disease surveillance.	• Brucellosis *(Brucella* species) • Epsilon toxin of *Clostridium perfringens*. • Food safety threats (e.g., *Salmonella* species, *Escherichia coli* 0157:H7, *Shigella*). • Glanders (*Burkholderia mallei*) • Melioidosis *(Burkholderia pseudomallei*) • Psittacosis *Chlamydia psittaci*) • Q fever (*Coxiella burnetii)* • Ricin toxin from *Ricinus communis* (castor beans) • Staphylococcal enterotoxin B • Typhus fever (*Rickettsia prowazekii*) • Viral encephalitis (alphaviruses, e.g., eastern equine encephalitis, Venezuelan equine encephalitis, and western equine encephalitis) • Water safety threats (*Vibrio cholera, Cryptosporidium parvum*)
C	• Include emerging pathogens that could be engineered for mass dissemination in the future because of availability, ease of production, and dissemination • Potential for high morbidity and mortality rates and major health impacts.	• Nipah virus • Hantavirus

Adapted from Centers for Disease Control and Prevention. Bioterrorism Agents/Diseases by Category. https://emergency.cdc.gov/agent/agentlist-category.asp. Accessed May 25, 2021 from the Centers for Disease Control and Prevention.

of bioterrorism is suspected; standardized laboratory methods to determine if an agent of bioterrorism can be ruled out in a suspicious bacterial isolate; and when to forward patient specimens or concerning bacterial isolates to a local LRN Reference Laboratory for primary testing or confirmation. The protocols also describe the safety measures required when laboratories process specimens in this situation. Most sentinel laboratories operate with Biological Safety Level (BSL) 2 containment, and do not have the equipment, infrastructure, or personnel training required for BSL-3 or BSL-4 containment, which is required for handling many of the agents listed in Table 1. The key responsibility of sentinel laboratories is therefore to identify concerning specimens and to refer them to the appropriate LRN Reference Laboratory when appropriate. Sentinel laboratories should not test environmental, animal, food, or water samples for potential agents of bioterrorism. These types of samples need to be directed to the local LRN Reference Laboratory.

LRN reference laboratories perform the next level of testing and consist of more than 150 local, state, and federal public health, military, food testing, veterinary, and environmental testing laboratories in the United States, Canada, Mexico, Australia, the United Kingdom, and South Korea. LRN reference laboratories follow BSL-3 containment procedures, and maintain the technology and expertise required to provide rapid confirmatory testing for agents of bioterrorism.[9] When a case is suspected in a clinical setting, local and/or state public health procedures are followed. In many cases, local public health officials are alerted prior to testing to assess the case history and clinical findings. If a case is deemed suspicious, the sentinel laboratory and the nearest LRN Reference Laboratory will then coordinate to ensure appropriate specimen collection and transport to the LRN Reference Laboratory, where further testing will occur.[8,9]

Finally, national laboratories, which are located at the CDC, the US Army Medical Research Institute of Infectious Diseases (USAMRIID), and the Naval Medical Research Center (NMRC), are responsible for strain characterization and maintaining the BSL-4 containment facilities required for activities involving BSL-4 agents (e.g., Ebola, Marburg, and smallpox viruses).[9]

LABORATORY-ACQUIRED INFECTIONS

Laboratory personnel handle infectious agents on a regular basis. Safety measures are implemented to reduce exposure and prevent laboratory-acquired infections (LAIs). Unfortunately, LAIs are not uncommon and are frequently reported in clinical, research, and other laboratories. In a literature review that included manuscripts from 1979 to 2015, Byers and Harding found that >3200 symptomatic LAIs and 42 deaths were reported during that period.[10]

Among the agents listed in the CDC's lists of Category A and B potential agents of bioterrorism, LAIs involving all but *Clostridium perfringens* toxin and ricin toxin have been reported in the literature.[10–13] In many cases, nonadherence to safety measures was noted when the cases were investigated. In 2002, laboratory-acquired cutaneous anthrax was reported in a worker who was processing environmental samples at a CDC laboratory that was supporting the investigation into the 2001 bioterrorist attacks in the United States. An investigation concluded that the infected worker was likely exposed through the surface of vials containing *B. anthracis* isolates, which were handled without gloves.[14]

In 2004, a fatal case of septicemic plague in a research laboratory worker with hereditary hemochromatosis involving an attenuated strain of *Yersinia pestis* was reported. The mechanism of exposure was unclear. As lung histology did not suggest inhalational plague, investigators felt that transdermal or mucosal exposure was most likely. Inconsistent use of gloves when handling *Y. pestis* was reported by co-workers of the patient, which may have put the patient at risk.[15] In 1962, Burmeister et al. described a case of pneumonic plague in which *Y. pestis* was recovered from a researcher's sputum cultures. The infection was attributed to possible inhalation of aerosols during a centrifugation procedure.[16]

Burkholderia mallei was isolated from a researcher with type 1 diabetes at USAMRIID in 2000. The patient presented initially with tender axillary adenopathy and fever, which remitted temporarily with clarithromycin therapy. He then relapsed and developed hepatic and splenic abscesses. *B. mallei* was recovered from the patient's blood and from a fine-needle aspiration biopsy of the liver abscess. Investigators noted that the patient did not consistently wear gloves when handling *B. mallei* stocks and hypothesized that the infection was acquired transdermally.[17]

A 2005 report from the Boston Public Health Commission described three cases of laboratory-acquired tularemia that involved laboratory personnel who handled the attenuated Live Vaccine Strain (LVS) of *Francisella tularensis* in BSL-2 facilities. Laboratory manipulations of the isolate included aerosolizing procedures such as vortexing and centrifugation. Genomic testing at the CDC showed that the LVS stock used by the laboratory was contaminated with the virulent, type A strain of *F. tularensis* (wild type). As a result of the investigation, the Health Commission recommended that all research involving *F. tularensis* be conducted in facilities with BSL-3 containment.[18]

Laboratory-acquired brucellosis is the most common LAI reported in the literature. Cases have been associated with sniffing culture plates, splashes of organism suspensions, aerosol generating procedures, and routine organism manipulations outside of biological safety cabinets.[19] In 2008, the CDC reported two cases of brucellosis in microbiologists who were working in two clinical laboratories. In both cases, *Brucella* was recovered in blood cultures drawn from laboratory personnel. Noting that investigators had reported that *Brucella* isolates were handled on the open bench (as opposed to using a biological safety cabinet) in the early stages of organism identification, the CDC encouraged clinicians to notify laboratories of suspected cases of *Brucella* as early as possible and for laboratory personnel to be trained to be aware of suspicious isolates early in the course of processing cultures.[19]

Finally, two laboratory-acquired infections involving SARS coronavirus were reported in Singapore and Taiwan in 2003. In the latter, a researcher who was working with SARS in a BSL-4 laboratory was exposed when he opened a waste transport chamber in a BSL-4 cabinet to clean a spill. The patient recovered without complications.[20]

LABORATORY SAFETY INFRASTRUCTURE AND PRACTICES

General Principles

To minimize the risk of LAIs, laboratories need to ensure the containment of potentially harmful biological agents. The following section is intended to be an overview of material that is described in greater detail in the CDC's Biosafety in Microbiology and Biomedical Laboratories document,[21] and its supplement, the Guidelines for Safe Work Practices in Human and Animal Medical Diagnostic Laboratories[22]; the American Society for Microbiology's Sentinel Level Clinical Laboratory Guidelines pertaining to Biological Safety[23]; as well as the Occupational Safety and Health Administration's Occupational safety and health standards.[24]

The concept of containment includes the practices, facility features, and equipment used to handle potentially infectious materials safely. Examples of safety equipment include personal protective equipment (PPE), which in turn, includes gowns, gloves, and masks, as well as goggles and face shields that protect the mucous membranes. Biological safety cabinets (BSCs) and centrifuge cups are also considered safety equipment. Because they are designed to contain droplets and/or aerosols produced by laboratory procedures and prevent exposure of the personnel performing the procedure, the term "primary barrier" is used to describe them. By contrast, "secondary barriers" encompass facility design and engineering features that provide a barrier that protects the wider community (e.g., laboratory personnel and persons outside of the laboratory). Examples of secondary barriers include autoclaves, sinks for handwashing, and restricted access of personnel entering laboratories.[21]

Biological Safety Levels

To standardize the enforcement of the practices, safety equipment, and barriers used to contain infectious agents in laboratories, the CDC has established four biological safety levels: BSL-1 through BSL-4. They are summarized in Tables 2 and 3. All laboratories need to adhere to standard microbiological practices regardless of their BSL. Additional special microbiological practices are used in BSL-2 through BSL-4 to ensure safety when handling agents that require additional containment. Key requirements are summarized in Table 3, but details can be accessed in the Biosafety in Microbiology and Biomedical Laboratories document.[21] It is important to be aware that BSL requirements are additive (i.e., a laboratory operating at BSL-3 needs to adhere to all BSL-1 and BSL-2 requirements) and that laboratory personnel need to be trained in and assessed for proficiency in all BSLs required for their activities.

BSL-1 is the lowest level of containment and is typically appropriate for teaching laboratories that use microorganisms that do not consistently cause disease in healthy adult humans. An example is *Bacillus subtilis*. BSL-1 requires standard microbiological practices and techniques, which are summarized in Table 2.[21] A BSC is not usually required. There are no facility requirements aside from a sink for handwashing and a door to control access.

BSL-2 is appropriate for most activities performed in a laboratory that involve handling microorganisms that cause human diseases of variable severity (e.g., *Staphylococcus aureus*, HIV, hepatitis B virus). With a few exceptions, BSL-2 is also appropriate for initial processing of primary human specimens (e.g., preparing culture plates) when it is uncertain if they harbor infectious agents or not. Most clinical microbiology laboratories use BSL-2 containment routinely. Because the emphasis of BSL-2 is prevention of percutaneous and mucous membrane exposures, a Class II BSC is used mainly for procedures that generate aerosols (e.g., use of a vortex or sonicator). BSL-2 requires restricted access (with self-closing doors with locking mechanisms) and monitoring of safety training and proficiency of personnel.[21]

BSL-3 is required in laboratories when handling agents that can cause serious or lethal infection and have the potential for respiratory transmission (e.g., *M. tuberculosis*). All manipulations of agents requiring BSL-3 are performed in a BSC or other containment device. Additional facility design requirements include separation of facilities from main access corridors and use of an entry airlock or anteroom. Special ventilation requirements ensure that agents are not released outside of the laboratory. BSL-3 laboratories are most commonly used in reference laboratories and a limited number of academic and commercial laboratories.[21]

Finally, BSL-4 containment is used when handling agents that are associated with high morbidity and mortality, can be transmitted via aerosols, and for which there is no treatment or vaccine. Ebola and Marburg viruses are examples. All manipulations of agents requiring BSL-3 are performed in a Class III BSC (this is called a "Cabinet Laboratory"). Alternatively, a Class I or Class II BSC can be used with the operator using a full-body, air-supplied, positive pressure personnel suit (called a "Suit Laboratory"). Additional facility design requirements include either a separate building or a completely isolated zone. Specialized procedures are required for ventilation and waste management.[21]

TABLE 2
Standard Microbiological Practices and Techniques

1. The laboratory supervisor must enforce the institutional policies that control access to the laboratory.
2. Persons must wash their hands after working with potentially hazardous materials and before leaving the laboratory.
3. Eating, drinking, smoking, handling contact lenses, applying cosmetics, and storing food for human consumption must not be permitted in laboratory areas. Food must be stored outside the laboratory area in cabinets or refrigerators designated and used for this purpose.
4. Mouth pipetting is prohibited; mechanical pipetting devices must be used.
5. Policies for the safe handling of sharps, such as needles, scalpels, pipettes, and broken glassware must be developed and implemented. Whenever practical, laboratory supervisors should adopt improved engineering and work practice controls that reduce the risk of sharps injuries. Precautions, including those listed below, must always be taken with sharp items. These include:
    1. Careful management of needles and other sharps is of primary importance. Needles must not be bent, sheared, broken, recapped, removed from disposable syringes, or otherwise manipulated by hand before disposal.
    2. Used disposable needles and syringes must be carefully placed in conveniently located puncture-resistant containers used for sharps disposal.
    3. Nondisposable sharps must be placed in a hard-walled container for transport to a processing area for decontamination, preferably by autoclaving.
    4. Broken glassware must not be handled directly. Instead, it must be removed using a brush and dustpan, tongs, or forceps. Plastic ware should be substituted for glassware whenever possible.
6. Perform all procedures to minimize the creation of splashes and/or aerosols.
7. Decontaminate work surfaces after completion of work and after any spill or splash of potentially infectious material with appropriate disinfectant.
8. Decontaminate all cultures, stocks, and other potentially infectious materials before disposal using an effective method. Depending on where the decontamination will be performed, the following methods should be used prior to transport.
    1. Materials to be decontaminated outside of the immediate laboratory must be placed in a durable, leak-proof container and secured for transport.
    2. Materials to be removed from the facility for decontamination must be packed in accordance with applicable local, state, and federal regulations.
9. A sign incorporating the universal biohazard symbol must be posted at the entrance to the laboratory when infectious agents are present. The sign may include the name of the agent(s) in use, and the name and phone number of the laboratory supervisor or other responsible personnel. Agent information should be posted in accordance with the institutional policy.
10. An effective integrated pest management program is required.
11. The laboratory supervisor must ensure that laboratory personnel receive appropriate training regarding their duties, the necessary precautions to prevent exposures, and exposure evaluation procedures. Personnel must receive annual updates or additional training when procedural or policy changes occur. Personal health status may impact an individual's susceptibility to infection, and ability to receive immunizations or prophylactic interventions. Therefore, all laboratory personnel particularly women of childbearing age should be provided with information regarding immune competence and conditions that may predispose them to infection. Individuals having these conditions should be encouraged.

Adapted from reference Centers for Disease Control and Prevention. Biosafety in Microbiological and Biomedical Laboratories. https://www.cdc.gov/labs/BMBL.html. Accessed 25 May 2021.

Biological Safety Cabinets

BSCs are designed to protect the operator (i.e., the individual manipulating infectious materials) and the environment from contamination with agents inside the BSC. In some cases, they may also protect the "product" being handled in the BSC from contamination.

There are three classes of BSC. Class I BSCs protect the operator and the environment from exposure to infectious agents but do not protect the product from contamination. Typically, the exhaust system (either an internal assembly or the building exhaust system) maintains negative pressure inside the BSC, which draws air into the BSC, away from the operator, and through a HEPA filter, which removes particulate matter. Air is then expelled. By contrast, Class II BSCs protect the operator, the environment, and

TABLE 3
Special Requirements for the Biological Safety Levels

BSL	Agents	Practices	Primary Barriers and Safety Equipment	Facilities (Secondary Barriers)
1	• Not known to consistently cause diseases in healthy adults.	Standard microbiological practices	• No primary barriers required. • PPE: laboratory coats and gloves; eye, and face protection, as needed.	• Laboratory bench and skin required.
2	• Agents associated with human disease. • Routes of transmission include percutaneous injury, ingestion, mucous membrane exposure.	BSL-1 practice plus: • Limited access • Biohazard warning signs • "Sharps" precautions • Biosafety manual defining any needed waste decontamination or medical surveillance policies	Primary barriers: • BSCs or other physical containment devices used for all open manipulations of agents • PPE: Laboratory coats, gloves, face and eye protection, as needed.	BSL-1 plus: • Autoclave available
3	• Indigenous or exotic agents that may cause serious or potentially lethal disease through the inhalation route of exposure.	BSL-2 practice plus: • Controlled access • Decontamination of all waste • Decontamination of laboratory clothing before laundering	Primary barriers: • BSCs or other physical containment devices used for all open manipulations of agents • PPE: Protective laboratory clothing, gloves, face, eye and respiratory protection, as needed.	BSL-2 plus: • Physical separation from access corridors • Self-closing double-door access • Exhausted air not recirculated • Negative airflow into the laboratory • Entry through airlock or anteroom • Hand washing sink near laboratory exit
4	• Dangerous/exotic agents that post a high individual risk of aerosol-transmitted laboratory infections that are frequently fatal, for which there are no vaccines or treatments. • Agents with a close or identical antigenic relationship to an agent requiring BSL-4 until data are available to redesignate the level • Related agents with unknown risk of transmission.	BSL-3 practice plus: • Clothing change before entering • Shower on exit • All material decontaminated on exit from the facility	Primary barriers: • All procedures conducted in Class III BSCs or Class I or II BSCs in combination with full-body, air-supplied, positive pressure suit.	BSL-3 plus: • Separate building or isolated zone • Dedicated supply and exhaust, vacuum, and decontamination systems • Other requirements outlined in the text.

BSL, biological safety level.
Adapted from reference Centers for Disease Control and Prevention. Biosafety in Microbiological and Biomedical Laboratories. https://www.cdc.gov/labs/BMBL.html. Accessed 25 May 2021.

the product. A downward flow of air into the front grille of the BSC protects both the operator and the product by directing the movement of particles entering the BSC from the room and inside the BSC away from the operator and product. Class II BSCs employ "laminar flow," that is, unidirectional movement of air at a fixed speed along parallel lines, which helps to maintain predictable particle movement. Care is needed to ensure that the grille is not obstructed and to avoid activities that disrupt the laminar flow (e.g., avoid frequent, unnecessary movement of objects in and out of the BSC; place the BSC in a location that avoids gusts of air generated from laboratory doors). Exhaust air is HEPA-filtered before circulation back into the room (class 2A) or outside of the building (class 2B).

Finally, Class III BSCs are gas-tight, fully enclosed structures. The operator manipulates objects inside the BSC through long, heavy-duty rubber gloves that are attached to BSC ports in a gas-tight fashion. Materials enter and are removed through either a double-doored autoclave or chemical dunk tank. These structures are used to allow disinfection and sterilization of materials exiting the cabinet. Both supply and exhaust air are HEPA-filtered. The exhaust system is hard ducted to the building's exhaust system; includes either two successive HEPA filters or an air incinerator; and maintains negative pressure inside the BSC. All BSCs require regular maintenance and certification by qualified professionals.[25]

Handwashing and Personal Protective Equipment

Handwashing is a critical aspect of laboratory safety and must not be overlooked. Personnel must wash their hands immediately after working with potentially hazardous materials or removing PPE, when there is contact with blood or body fluids, and before exiting the laboratory. For most agents, soap and water or alcohol-based hand rubs are equivalent and active. For organisms that produce spores, handwashing with soap and water is preferred because the additional friction is critical to the removal of the agent. Availability of a working sink is mandatory.

PPE provides a primary barrier that protects laboratory personnel from exposure to the agents they are handling. PPE requirements in each successive BSL are additive. Personnel in BSL-1 and 2 settings should follow standard precautions and wear laboratory coats or gowns. Eye and face protection (e.g., goggles, surgical mask, face shield, splash guard) are required with anticipated splashes and must be discarded or decontaminated prior to reuse. In BSL-3 settings, gowns with a solid front are required and must be decontaminated prior to laundering. Finally, requirements in BSL-4 settings vary according to the setup. In cabinet laboratories, gowns with a solid front are required, must be removed to a dirty side change room prior to a decontamination shower, and are autoclaved before reuse. Disposable gloves are worn underneath the rubber cabinet gloves to ensure protection in the event of a tear in the cabinet gloves. In a suit laboratory, operators wear standard laboratory attire (e.g., scrubs) and disposable gloves underneath a one-piece positive pressure air-supplied suit. The inner and outer attire is completely removed prior to a mandatory shower.[21]

Decontamination and Waste Management

Work surfaces are decontaminated after completion of work with an appropriate disinfectant, and all potentially infectious materials (e.g., primary specimens, culture plates) are decontaminated prior to disposal. Laboratory equipment is routinely decontaminated by trained personnel. For BSL-1 through BSL-3 laboratories, decontamination of laboratory waste should be performed in the facility, preferably within the laboratory using an autoclave, chemical disinfection, incineration, or another validated decontamination method. If materials need to be transported outside of the facility for decontamination, applicable local, state, and federal regulations need to be met. In BSL-4 facilities, laboratory waste needs to be decontaminated within the laboratory. In cabinet laboratories using a Class III BSC, double door, a pass-through autoclave decontaminates materials passing out of the Class III BSC(s). For decontamination of items that cannot be decontaminated in the autoclave, Class III cabinets also have a pass-through dunk tank, fumigation chamber, or other equivalent decontamination method available.[23,26]

Biological Risk Assessment

All laboratories should periodically perform a biological risk assessment, where all laboratory activities are evaluated for their level of risk to personnel and the containment level(s) required is assessed. The experience and skill level of personnel are also carefully considered. The product of a biological risk assessment is typically a written biosafety manual that delineates hazards that may be encountered in the laboratory, the associated risks, the practices that should be followed to reduce personnel exposure and manage accidental exposure, the required training of personnel, and a plan for monitoring personnel proficiency and ongoing risk.[21–23]

Shipping of Infectious Agents

The International Air Transport Association's (IATA) Dangerous Goods Regulations and the US Department of Transportation's United States Hazardous Materials Uniform Safety Regulations lay out regulations for the shipment of dangerous goods, which include potential agents of bioterrorism. These regulations cover classification and naming of substances being shipped; packaging requirements (to ensure the protection of carrier personnel if the package is damaged); required markings and labeling (to alert carrier personnel that the contents of the package are hazardous); and any additional documentation required. IATA and DOT regulations require that individuals involved in the shipping of dangerous goods be appropriately trained. This section provides a general overview of these regulatory requirements, and details are beyond the scope of this chapter. Useful references include a current version of IATA and DOT regulations. Comprehensive overviews are available elsewhere.[26]

Substances in IATA Division 6.2 (infectious substances) are designated as Category A or Category B. A Category A microorganism is "an infectious substance which is transported in a form that, when exposure to it occurs, is capable of causing permanent disability, life-threatening or fatal disease in otherwise healthy humans or animals." Category B microorganisms are defined as "an infectious substance which does not meet the criteria for inclusion in Category A." As an example, blood samples obtained from patients with suspected Ebola virus require Category A designation. Shipping of Category A substances has specific packing, marking, labeling, and documentation requirements, including a shipper's declaration of dangerous goods.[26]

If a sentinel laboratory recovers a possible agent of bioterrorism in culture, the local LRN Reference Laboratory must be consulted to determine if referral is appropriate. If a case involving a suspected agent of bioterrorism is identified, the local LRN Reference Laboratory should be consulted prior to specimen collection, if possible, to discuss the case. Laboratory products and/or primary specimens suspected of harboring an agent of bioterrorism or a Category A substance should not be shipped to an LRN Reference Laboratory without prior consultation.

SPECIMEN COLLECTION AND PROCESSING IN CASES INVOLVING POTENTIAL AGENTS OF BIOTERRORISM

Specimen Collection

The earlier a laboratory becomes aware that a specimen harboring a potential agent of bioterrorism may be arriving in the laboratory, the earlier appropriate safety measures can be taken. The ordering physician (usually a clinician or an anatomic pathologist performing an autopsy) must notify the clinical microbiology laboratory if such a diagnosis is suspected. Similarly, if an agent of bioterrorism is suspected, the sentinel laboratory needs to coordinate with the local LRN Reference Laboratory at the earliest opportunity to confirm what specimens are required and to discuss shipping, specimen retention, and later, specimen destruction. Early communication ensures correct specimen collection and reduces the need for repeated specimen collection events, which may increase exposure of personnel to hazardous infectious materials. Concurrent to the notification of the regional LRN Reference Laboratory, public health officials should be notified according to local and state procedures.

Details about specimen collection for detection of CDC Category A and B Potential Agents of Bioterrorism are summarized in Table 4. Additional information can be obtained from the Sentinel-Level Clinical Laboratory Protocols, the CDC's test directory, and other resources.[8,27–33]

Specimen Processing

As summarized in Tables 5 and 6, in some cases, sentinel laboratories will perform initial culturing and "rule-out" testing. The Sentinel-Level Clinical Laboratory Protocols provide guidance pertaining to the basic testing that is required to rule out potentially dangerous agents and the safety measures required.[8]

Reporting of Results

When a clinical culture meets criteria for referral to a local LRN Reference Laboratory, a report is provided to the ordering physician that a potential agent of bioterrorism cannot be ruled out and that further testing for confirmation is in process. The patient's attending physician, infection prevention, and the infectious diseases team should be notified. Positive test results should be reported to the state if they are listed on the applicable state's list of notifiable diseases. If there is confirmation of a positive test for a "Select Agent" from the CDC's "Select Agents and Toxins List," the result must be reported to

TABLE 4
IATA Category A Microorganisms (UN 2814, Infectious Substances Affecting Humans)[a]

Bacillus anthracis (cultures only)
Brucella abortus (cultures only)
Brucella melitensis (cultures only)
Brucella suis (cultures only)
Burkholderia mallei–Pseudomonas mallei–Glanders (cultures only) *Burkholderia pseudomallei–Pseudomonas pseudomallei* (cultures only) *Chlamydia psittaci*–avian strains (cultures only)
Clostridium botulinum (cultures only) *Coccidioides immitis* (cultures only) *Coxiella burnetii* (cultures only) Crimean-Congo haemorrhagic fever virus Dengue virus (cultures only)
Eastern equine encephalitis virus (cultures only) *Escherichia coli*, verotoxigenic (cultures only) Ebola virus
Flexal virus *Francisella tularensis* (cultures only)
Guanarito virus
Hantaan virus
Hantavirus causing hemorrhagic fever with renal syndrome Hendra virus Hepatitis B virus (cultures only)
Herpes B virus (cultures only)
Human immunodeficiency virus (cultures only)
Highly pathogenic avian influenza virus (cultures only) Japanese Encephalitis virus (cultures only)
Junin virus
Kyasanur Forest disease virus
Lassa virus
Machupo virus
Marburg virus
Monkeypox virus
Mycobacterium tuberculosis (cultures only)
Nipah virus
Omsk haemorrhagic fever virus
Poliovirus (cultures only)
Rabies virus (cultures only)
Rickettsia prowazekii (cultures only)
Rickettsia rickettsii (cultures only)
Rift Valley fever virus (cultures only)
Russian spring-summer encephalitis virus (cultures only) Sabia virus
Shigella dysenteriae type 1 (cultures only) Tick-borne encephalitis virus (cultures only)
Variola virus
Venezuelan equine encephalitis virus (cultures only) West Nile virus (cultures only)
Yellow fever virus (cultures only)

[a]This list is consistent with the 58th edition of the International Air Transport Association's Dangerous Goods Regulations from 2017. Laboratories should use the most up-to-date edition available.

TABLE 5
Acceptable Specimens for Detection of Category a Potential Agents of Bioterrorism and Other Emerging Pathogens

Agents	Appropriate Human Specimens[a]	Comments
Bacillus anthracis	• Skin lesion exudate • Stool • Respiratory specimens • Pleural fluid • Blood • Cerebrospinal fluid • Tissue (biopsy or autopsy)	• Contact local LRN Reference Laboratory as early as possible. • Contact public health according to local and state procedures. • Depending on the circumstances, the LRN Reference Laboratory may perform cultures and/or rapid tests (e.g., PCR) directly on patient specimens and/or bacterial isolates recovered from culture. • Refer to Sentinel-Level Clinical Laboratory Protocol "Anthrax" (*B. anthracis*, Ref. 8). • Refer to CDC's "Recommended Specimens for Microbiology and Pathology for Diagnosis of Anthrax" (Ref. 28).

(*Continued*)

TABLE 5
Acceptable Specimens for Detection of Category a Potential Agents of Bioterrorism and Other Emerging Pathogens—cont'd

Agents	Appropriate Human Specimens[a]	Comments
Clostridium botulinum toxin	• Serum • Stool • Rectal swab (acceptable if infant) • Gastric contents • Wound (if applicable)	• Due to the highly infectious nature of *C. botulinum* toxin, Sentinel Laboratories are only responsible for specimen collection and shipment and should not attempt testing. • Contact local LRN Reference Laboratory as early as possible. • Contact public health according to local and state procedures. • Botulinum toxin in serum, stool, or food (using a mouse bioassay and ELISA) or culturing *C. botulinum*, *C. butyricum*, or *C. baratii* from stool, a wound, or food. • Refer to Sentinel-Level Clinical Laboratory Protocol "Botulism" (Ref. 8). • Refer to CDC botulism testing information (Ref. 29).
Yersinia pestis	• Bubo/ulcer aspirate or swab • Blood • Tissue (e.g., liver, spleen, lung) • Respiratory specimens • Acute and convalescent serum	• Contact local LRN Reference Laboratory as early as possible. • Contact public health according to local and state procedures. • Diagnosis is confirmed through culture using direct fluorescent antibody testing and bacteriophage lysis technique. Serological testing uses passive hemagglutination technique with inhibition. • Refer to Sentinel-Level Clinical Laboratory Protocol "Plague" for details (Ref. 8). • Refer to CDC *Y. pestis* culture and identification (test code 10418) and serology information (test code 10419)[b] (see directory, Ref. 27).
Variola major	• Consult with LRN Reference Laboratory and notify public health if a case is suspected.	• Refer to Sentinel-Level Clinical Laboratory Protocol "Smallpox" (Ref. 8).
Francisella tularensis	• Swab (ulcer or conjunctival) • Tissue (ulcer or node) • Respiratory specimens • Bone marrow • Cerebrospinal fluid • Serum for acute and convalescent serology	• Contact local LRN Reference Laboratory as early as possible. • Contact public health according to local and state procedures. • Diagnosis is confirmed through culture using direct fluorescent antibody testing and biochemical techniques. Serological testing uses microagglutination techniques. • Refer to Sentinel-Level Clinical Laboratory Protocol "Tularemia" (Ref. 8). • Refer to CDC information on *F. tularensis* culture and identification (test code CDC-10313) and serology (test code CDC-10314)[b] (see directory, Ref. 27).
Agents of viral hemorrhagic fever	Consult with LRN Reference Laboratory and public health prior to specimen collection.	• Sentinel laboratories are only responsible for specimen collection and shipment and should not attempt confirmatory testing. • For Ebola virus testing, refer to "Guidance for Collection, Transport and Submission of Specimens for Ebola Virus Testing in the United States" (Ref. 30).

TABLE 5
Acceptable Specimens for Detection of Category a Potential Agents of Bioterrorism and Other Emerging Pathogens—cont'd

Agents	Appropriate Human Specimens[a]	Comments
Brucella species	• Blood culture • Bone marrow • Sterile fluid (joint, abdominal fluid) • Tissue • Serum for acute and convalescent serology	• Contact local LRN Reference Laboratory as early as possible. • Contact public health according to local and state procedures. • Depending on the circumstances, the LRN Reference Laboratory may perform cultures and/or rapid tests (e.g., PCR) directly on patient specimens and/or bacterial isolates recovered from culture. Biochemical, and phage susceptibility techniques may also be used to confirm the diagnosis in bacterial isolates. Serological testing uses microagglutination techniques. • Refer to Sentinel-Level Clinical Laboratory Protocol "Brucella" (Ref. 8). • Refer to CDC information on *Brucella* culture and identification (test code 10207), molecular detection (test code CDC-10208), and serology (test code CDC-10197)[b] (see directory, Ref. 27).
Clostridium perfringens toxin	• Stool	• Contact local LRN Reference Laboratory • Contact public health according to local and state procedures • Toxin tests are commercially available for testing of food only. The CDC has the capacity to perform culture and PCR on stool specimens but this testing is only available in the context of foodborne outbreaks and requires consultation with the Enteric Diseases Laboratory Branch. • Refer to CDC information on *C. perfringens* detection in foodborne outbreaks (test code CDC-10111)[b] in the directory in Ref. 27.
Food safety threats (e.g., *Salmonella* spp., *Shigella* spp., enterohemorrhagic *Escherichia coli)*	• Stool	• Most Sentinel-Level Clinical Laboratories have the capacity to detect these pathogens. • Local and/or state public health department procedures should be followed with respect to reporting and specimen submission to public health laboratories.
Burkholderia mallei, Burkholderia pseudomallei	• Blood culture • Bone marrow • Respiratory specimens • Tissue (spleen, liver) • Urine • Acute and convalescent serum (*B. pseudomallei*)	• Contact local LRN Reference Laboratory as early as possible. • Contact public health according to local and state procedures. • Depending on the circumstances, the LRN Reference Laboratory may perform cultures and/or rapid tests (e.g., PCR) directly on patient specimens and/or bacterial isolates recovered from culture. Biochemical techniques may be used to confirm the diagnosis in bacterial isolates. Serological testing for *B. pseudomallei* uses IHA-indirect hemagglutination techniques. • Refer to Sentinel-Level Clinical Laboratory Protocol (Ref. 8). • Refer to CDC information on *B. mallei and pseudomallei* culture and identification (test code CDC-10210), molecular detection (test code CDC-10211), and serology (test code CDC-10198)[b] (see directory, Ref. 27)

(Continued)

TABLE 5
Acceptable Specimens for Detection of Category a Potential Agents of Bioterrorism and Other Emerging Pathogens—cont'd

Agents	Appropriate Human Specimens[a]	Comments
Chlamydia psittaci	• Nasopharyngeal, oropharyngeal, other respiratory specimens • Tissue • Cerebrospinal fluid	• Contact local LRN Reference Laboratory as early as possible. • Contact public health according to local and state procedures. • Diagnostic testing options include serology and PCR. *C. psittaci* serology is available at various commercial reference laboratories. LRN Reference Laboratories and the CDC offer both. • Refer to CDC information on *C. psittaci* molecular detection (test code CDC-10153)[b] (see directory, Ref. 27).
Coxiella burnetii	• Whole blood or serum (PCR) • Acute and convalescent serum	• Due to the highly infectious nature of *C. burnetii*, Sentinel laboratories should not attempt to culture this organism. • Contact local LRN Reference Laboratory as early as possible. • Contact public health according to local and state procedures. • Diagnostic testing options include serology and PCR (whole blood, serum, tissue), which are available at various commercial reference laboratories, LRN Reference Laboratories, and the CDC. • Refer to Sentinel-Level Clinical Laboratory Protocol "*C. burnetii*" in Ref. 8. • Refer to "Diagnosis and Management of Q Fever—United States, 2013: Recommendations from CDC and the Q Fever Working Group" in Ref. 32.
Staphylococcal enterotoxin B	• Stool • Vomitus	• Contact local LRN Reference Laboratory. • Contact public health according to local and state procedures. • Toxin tests are commercially available but are only FDA-cleared for testing of food. The CDC has the capacity to perform culture and PCR on stool and vomitus but this testing is only available in the context of foodborne outbreaks and requires consultation with the Enteric Diseases Laboratory Branch. • Refer to CDC information on *Staphylococcus aureus* detection in foodborne outbreaks (test code CDC-10113)[b] in the directory in Ref. 27.
Rickettsia prowazekii	• Whole blood • Acute and convalescent serum	• Contact local LRN Reference Laboratory. • Contact public health according to local and state procedures. • Diagnostic testing options include serology (indirect fluorescent assay) and PCR (whole blood), which are available at the CDC. • Refer to CDC information on *Rickettsia* serology for Typhus group (test code CDC-10404), and *Rickettsia* molecular detection (test code CDC-10402) (see directory, Ref. 27).

TABLE 5
Acceptable Specimens for Detection of Category a Potential Agents of Bioterrorism and Other Emerging Pathogens—cont'd

Agents	Appropriate Human Specimens[a]	Comments
Agents of viral encephalitis (eastern equine encephalitis virus, Venezuelan equine encephalitis virus, western equine encephalitis virus)	• Acute and convalescent serum • Cerebrospinal fluid	• Contact local LRN Reference Laboratory • Contact public health according to local and state procedures • Diagnosis is serological and tests are available through the CDC's Arbovirus Diagnostic Laboratory in the Division of Vector-Borne Diseases.
Agents of water safety threats (e.g., *Vibrio cholera*, *Cryptosporidium parvum*)	• Stool	• Many Sentinel-Level Clinical Laboratories have the capacity to detect these pathogens. • Follow local and/or state public health departments' procedures for case reporting and specimen submission to public health laboratories.
SARS coronavirus	Consult with LRN Reference Laboratory and public health prior to specimen collection.	• The CDC offers a PCR assay. Testing requires preapproval.
MERS coronavirus	Consult with LRN Reference Laboratory and public health prior to specimen collection.	• Most state laboratories are approved to test for MERS-CoV using a PCR assay that was developed by the CDC.
Pandemic influenza	Consult with LRN Reference Laboratory and public health prior to specimen collection.	• The CDC offers a PCR assay. Testing requires preapproval.

CDC, Centers for Disease Control and Prevention; *LRN*, Laboratory Response Network; *PCR*, polymerase chain reaction.
[a]Required specimens will depend on clinical presentation. Confirm required specimens with local LRN Reference Laboratory.
[b]Refer to the CDC's Infectious Diseases Laboratories' Test Directory: https://www.cdc.gov/laboratory/specimen-submission/list.html.

TABLE 6
Rule-Out Testing for Category A and B Potential Agents of Bioterrorism[a,b]

Agents	Sentinel Clinical Laboratory Criteria for Referral to LRN Reference Laboratory[a]	BIOLOGICAL SAFETY LEVEL (BSL) REQUIRED[c-f]	
		Specimen handling	Culture manipulations for "Rule-out" Testing
Bacillus anthracis	• Colonies have ground glass appearance, edges undulate ("Medusa heads"), nonpigmented. • Nonhemolytic • Large Gram-positive rods • Catalase-positive • Nonmotile • No growth on MacConkey agar	• BSL-2	• BSL-2
Yersinia pestis	• Slow growing: Pinpoint or no colonies on sheep's blood agar at 24 h. 1–2 mm at 48 h opaque and gray/white/slight yellow. • Nonlactose fermenting on MacConkey agar. • Plump Gram-negative rods. • Oxidase, Indole, Urease-negative. • Catalase-positive.	• BSL-2 • Use biological safety cabinets, gowns, and gloves for all work	• BSL-2 • Use biological safety cabinets, gowns, and gloves for all work

(*Continued*)

TABLE 6
Rule-Out Testing for Category A and B Potential Agents of Bioterrorism—cont'd

Agents	Sentinel Clinical Laboratory Criteria for Referral to LRN Reference Laboratory[a]	BIOLOGICAL SAFETY LEVEL (BSL) REQUIRED[c-f] Specimen handling	Culture manipulations for "Rule-out" Testing
Francisella tularensis	• Scant to no growth on sheep's blood agar, no growth on MacConkey agar, gray/white colonies on chocolate agar at 48h. • Faintly staining tiny Gram-negative coccobacilli • Oxidase-negative, catalase-negative/weak positive, β-lactamase-positive.	• BSL-2 • Use biological safety cabinets, gowns, and gloves for all work.	• BSL-2 • Use biological safety cabinets, gowns, and gloves for all work.
Brucella species	• Growth on sheep's blood agar without the requirement of a Staphylococcus streak, nonhemolytic, nonpigmented on sheep's blood agar; no growth on MacConkey agar at 48h • Faintly staining tiny Gram-negative coccobacilli • Oxidase-positive, catalase-positive, urease-positive.	• BSL-2 • Use biological safety cabinets, gowns, and gloves for all work • Products of conception should be processed with BSL-3.	• BSL-2 • Use biological safety cabinets, gowns, and gloves for all work
Burkholderia mallei	• Growth on sheep's blood agar, gray translucent colonies, nonhemolytic; poor or no growth on MacConkey agar at 48h • Gram-negative coccobacilli • Oxidase-variable, catalase-positive, indole-negative, nonmotile, no growth at 42°C • Resistant to penicillin, polymyxin B, and colistin; susceptible to amoxicillin-clavulanate.	• BSL-2 • Use biological safety cabinets, gowns, and gloves for all work	• BSL-2 • Use biological safety cabinets, gowns, and gloves for all work
Burkholderia pseudomallei	• Growth on sheep's blood agar, gray nonhemolytic; growth on MacConkey agar at 48h • Gram-negative rod, may have bipolar staining • Oxidase-positive, catalase-positive, indole-negative, nonmotile, no growth at 42°C • Resistant to penicillin, polymyxin B and colistin.	• BSL-2 • Use biological safety cabinets, gowns, and gloves for all work	• BSL-2 • Use biological safety cabinets, gowns, and gloves for all work

BSL, biological safety level; *BSC*, biological safety cabinet.
[a]Refer to Sentinel-Level Clinical Laboratory Protocols (Ref. 8).
[b]Sentinel laboratories should not attempt definitive identification of isolates that cannot be ruled out as potential agents of bioterrorism. Do not use automated (e.g., BD Phoenix, Vitek 2, MicroScan, Vitek MS, Bruker CA systems) or kit-based systems on such isolates. Usage may lead to unnecessary exposure to dangerous pathogens and erroneous identifications.
[c]Standard precautions are always mandatory regardless of BSL.
[d]Refers to practices, safety equipment, and facilities for the BSL.
[e]Tape plates and ensure the contents are clearly labeled.
[f]Procedures with a high risk of aerosol production require BSL-3.

the Federal Select Agent Program.[34,35] The local LRN Reference Laboratory should be consulted about the required Select Agent reporting documentation at the time that the positive report is issued. Additional details are available at www.selectagents.gov.[34,35]

THE LABORATORY AND THE COVID-19 PANDEMIC

The world-wide COVID-19 pandemic has been the most overwhelming event that has confronted laboratories in recent memory. All laboratories (hospital-based, commercial, governmental) faced unprecedently demand for SARS-CoV-2 testing to support diagnosis in symptomatic patients; screening of asymptomatic patients prior to admission or preprocedure to facilitate decisions about inpatient placement and PPE use; testing of symptomatic HCP to ensure quarantine of those who test positive to mitigate HCP-to-patient and HCP-to-HCP transmission.

Early in the pandemic, laboratories faced regulatory challenges when implementing SARS-CoV-2 PCR testing. On February 4th, 2020, the secretary of the U.S. Department of Health and Human Services announced an emergent public health need for in vitro diagnostic tests that detect SARS-CoV-2. The secretary's announcement effectively compelled all clinical laboratories to either obtain an emergency use authorization (EUA) from the FDA for their SARS-CoV-2 test or send specimens to a laboratory that offers a test with an EUA. Many hospital laboratories chose to undergo the laborious and unfamiliar process of submitting validation data to the FDA and requesting an EUA for their test. Later, when more vendors of commercially available tests obtained EUAs for their tests, hospital laboratories were able to more easily implement SARS-CoV-2 testing in-house.

The overwhelming demand for testing caused global supply chain shortages, which led to limited availability of swabs, viral transport media, testing kits, reagents, and testing instruments. Many hospitals were forced to triage patients to ensure that the most urgent cases underwent testing.[34] Laboratories found themselves validating SARS-CoV-2 PCR testing for multiple specimen types (nasopharyngeal swab, anterior nares swab, oropharyngeal swab, nasopharyngeal wash, nasal wash, and in some cases, saliva) due to shortages in swabs.[35,36] Many laboratories also validated unconventional transport media (e.g., saline, PBS) when viral transport media became difficult to obtain.[37] Finally, novel procedures were developed to conserve reagents and laboratory supplies (e.g., respiratory specimen pooling, heat extraction, or extraction-free testing).[38–40] Because of test kit shortages, many laboratories implemented SARS-CoV-2 PCR testing on multiple platforms to meet demand.

SARS-CoV-2 antigen testing also emerged early in the pandemic as a modality of testing that offered rapid and easy administration at the bedside. Accumulating data generally suggested comparable specificity but lower sensitivity compared to molecular methods of SARS-CoV-2 testing.[41] Similarly, SARS-CoV-2 antibody (IgG and IgM) assays that detect immune response to SARS-CoV-2 nucleocapsid and spike protein have become widely available. While positive results provide evidence of natural infection and/or vaccination, the CDC has been clear that antibody testing cannot be used to accurately diagnose acute infection or determine whether an individual is immune to SARS-CoV-2.[42] Finally, as SARS-CoV-2 variants have emerged, the importance of public health-level monitoring of circulating strains through viral typing (via viral nucleic acid sequencing) has become apparent, but its role at the bedside is still under investigation.[43] As testing modalities have evolved, laboratory leaders have played an important role as advisers and educators to healthcare and infection prevention personnel and hospital leaders. Understanding the nuances related to SARS-CoV-2 testing, such as the comparative performance of different molecular SARS-CoV-2 platforms[43]; the relative sensitivity of different specimen types[35]; the impact of the timing of testing (relative to onset of symptoms) on molecular SARS-CoV-2 PCR and antigen test sensitivity[44]; and the strengths and limitations of antigen, antibody testing, and variant detection, has been crucial for hospitals as they have navigated this pandemic (Table 6).

DISCLOSURE STATEMENT

I have no disclosures.

REFERENCES

1. Centers for Disease Control and Prevention. Bioterrorism Agents/Diseases by Category. https://emergency.cdc.gov/agent/agentlist-category.asp. Accessed 25 May 2021.
2. PDD-39. https://fas.org/irp/offdocs/pdd39.htm. 1995. Accessed 25 May 2021.
3. PDD-62. https://fas.org/irp/offdocs/pdd-62.htm. 1998. Accessed 25 May 2021.
4. Centers for Disease Control and Prevention. Laboratory Response Network Partners in Preparedness. https://emergency.cdc.gov/lrn/. 2024. Accessed 25 May 2021.

5. Snyder JW. The laboratory response network: before, during, and after the 2001 anthrax incident. *Clin Micro Newsl.* 2005;27(22):171–175.
6. Craft DW, Lee PA, Rowlinson MC. Bioterrorism: a laboratory who does it? *J Clin Microbiol.* 2014;52(7):2290–2298.
7. Wagar E. Bioterrorism and the role of the clinical microbiology laboratory. *Clin Microbiol Rev.* 2016;29(1):175–189.
8. Sentinel Level Clinical Laboratory Protocols for Suspected Biological Threat Agents and Emerging Infectious Diseases. https://asm.org/Articles/Policy/Laboratory-Response-Network-LRN-Sentinel-Level-C. 2013. Accessed 25 May, 2021.
9. Centers for Disease Control and Prevention. Frequently Asked Questions About the Laboratory Response Network (LRN). https://emergency.cdc.gov/lrn/faq.asp. 2024. Accessed 25 May 2021.
10. Byers KB, Harding L. Laboratory-associated infections. In: Wooley DP, Byers KB, eds. *Biological Safety: Principles and Practices.* 5th ed. ASM Press; 2017.
11. Holzer E. Botulism caused by inhalation. *Med Klin.* 1962;57:1735–1738.
12. Rusnak JM, Kortepeter M, Ulrich R, Poli M, Boudreau E. Laboratory exposures to staphylococcal enterotoxin B. *Emerg Infect Dis.* 2004;10(9):1544–1549.
13. Kortepeter MG, Martin JW, Rusnak JM, et al. Managing potential laboratory exposure to ebola virus by using a patient biocontainment care unit. *Emerg Infect Dis.* 2008;14(6):881–887.
14. Centers for Disease Control and Prevention. Suspected cutaneous anthrax in a laboratory worker—Texas. *Morb Mortal Wkly Rep.* 2002;51(13):279–281.
15. Centers for Disease Control and Prevention. Fatal laboratory-acquired infection with an attenuated *Yersinia pestis* strain—Chicago, Illinois, 2009. *Morb Mortal Wkly Rep.* 2011;60(7):201–205.
16. Burmeister RW, Tigertt WD, Overhold EL. Laboratory-acquired pneumonic plague, report of a case and review of previous cases. *Ann Intern Med.* 1962;56(5):789–800.
17. Srinivasan A, Kraus CN, DeShazer D, et al. Glandersin a military research microbiologist, 2001. *N Engl J Med.* 2001;345(4):256–258.
18. Boston Public Health Commission. Report of Pneumonic Tularemia in Three Boston University Researchers. 2005. https://archive.org/stream/reportofpneumoni00bost/reportofpneumoni00bost_djvu.txt. Accessed 22 April 2025.
19. Centers for Disease Control and Prevention. Laboratory-acquired brucellosis—Indiana and Minnesota, 2006. *Morb Mortal Wkly Rep.* 2008;57(2):39–42.
20. Normile D. Second lab accident fuels fears about SARS. *Science.* 2004;303:26.
21. Centers for Disease Control and Prevention. Biosafety in Microbiological and Biomedical Laboratories. https://www.cdc.gov/labs/pdf/SF__19_308133-A_BMBL6_00-BOOK-WEB-final-3.pdf. 2020. Accessed 25 May 2021.
22. Centers for Disease Control and Prevention. Guidelines for safe work practices in human and animal medical diagnostic laboratories. *Morb Mortal Wkly Rep.* 2012;61(Supplement).
23. American Society for Microbiology. Sentinel Level Clinical Laboratory Guidelines for Suspected Agents of Bioterrorism and Emerging Infectious Diseases—Biological Safety; 2018. https://asm.org/ASM/media/Policy-and-Advocacy/Biosafety_Sentinel_Guideline_October_2018_FINAL.pdf. Accessed 25 May 2021.
24. Occupational Safety and Health Administration. Occupational Safety and Health Standards. Z. Toxic and Hazardous Substances. Bloodborne Pathogens. Standard No.1910.1030. https://www.osha.gov/pls/oshaweb/owadisp.show_document?p_id=10051&p_table=STANDARDS. Accessed 25 May 2021.
25. Kruse RH, Puckett WH, Richardson JH. Biological safety cabinetry. *Clin Microbiol Rev.* 1991;4(2):207–241.
26. Denys GA, Gray LD, Relich RF. Section 15: Biohazards and safety. In: Leber A, ed. *Clinical Microbiology Procedures Handbook.* 4th ed. ASM Press; 2016.
27. Centers for Disease Control and Prevention. Test Directory. https://www.cdc.gov/laboratory/specimen-submission/list.html. 2025. Accessed 25 May 2021.
28. Centers for Disease Control and Prevention. Anthrax (Collecting Samples to Send to Laboratories). 2025. https://www.cdc.gov/anthrax/php/lab-testing/?CDC_AAref_Val=https://www.cdc.gov/anthrax/lab-testing/recommended-specimens/index.html. Accessed 22 April 2025.
29. Centers for Disease Control and Prevention. Botulism (Submit a Specimen for Testing). 2024. https://www.cdc.gov/botulism/php/submit-specimen/?CDC_AAref_Val=https://www.cdc.gov/botulism/botulism-specimen.html. Accessed 22 April 2025.
30. Centers for Disease Control and Prevention. Ebola (Collection, Transport, & Submission for Ebola Virus Testing in the US). 2024. https://www.cdc.gov/ebola/hcp/communication-resources/guidance-for-collection-transport-and-submission-of-specimens-for-ebola-virus-testing-in-the-u-s.html. Accessed 22 April 2025.
31. Centers for Disease Control and Prevention. Brucellosis Reference Guide: Exposures, Testing, and Prevention. 2017. https://www.cdc.gov/brucellosis/media/pdfs/2025/02/brucellosi-reference-guide.pdf. Accessed 22 April 2025.
32. Diagnosis and Management of Q Fever—United States. Recommendations from CDC and the Q fever working group. *MMWR.* 2013;62(RR03):1–23.
33. Federal Select Agent Program. www.selectagents.gov. Accessed 12 February 2019.
34. Reporting Requirements. https://www.selectagents.gov/compliance/faq/reporting.htm. 2021. Accessed 12 February 2019.
35. Frosch D. Covid-19 testing is hampered by shortages of critical ingredient. *Wall St J.* 2020;22. https://www.wsj.com/articles/covid-19-testing-is-hampered-by-shortages-of-critical-ingredient-11600772400. Accessed 22 April 2025.
36. Lee RA, Herigon JC, Benedetti A, Pollock NR, Denkinger CM. Performance of saliva, oropharyngeal swabs, and nasal swabs for SARS-CoV-2 molecular detection: a systematic review and meta-analysis. *J Clin Microbiol.* 2021;59:e02881-20.

37. Böger B, Fachi MM, Vilhena RO, Cobre AF, Tonin FS, Pontarolo R. Systematic review and meta-analysis of the accuracy of diagnostic tests for COVID-19. *Am J Infect Control.* 2021;49(1):21–29.
38. Rodino KG, Espy MJ, Buckwalter SP, et al. Evaluation of saline, phosphate-buffered saline, and minimum essential medium as potential alternatives to viral transport media for SARS-CoV-2 testing. *J Clin Microbiol.* 2020;58:e00590-20.
39. More S, Narayanan S, Patil G, et al. Pooling of nasopharyngeal swab samples to overcome a global shortage of real-time reverse transcription-PCR COVID-19 test kits. *J Clin Microbiol.* 2021;59:e01295-20.
40. Barza R, Patel P, Sabatini L, Singh K. Use of a simplified sample processing step without RNA extraction for direct SARS-CoV-2 RT-PCR detection. *J Clin Virol.* 2020;132:104587.
41. Visseaux B, Collin G, Houhou-Fidouh N, et al. Evaluation of three extraction-free SARS-CoV-2 RT-PCR assays: a feasible alternative approach with low technical requirements. *J Virol Methods.* 2021;291:114086.
42. Centers for Disease Control and Prevention. COVID-19 (Testing for COVID-19). 2025. https://www.cdc.gov/covid/testing/index.html. Accessed 22 April 2025.
43. Centers for Disease Control and Prevention. Overview of Testing for SARS-CoV-2 (COVID-19). 2023. https://archive.cdc.gov/#/details?url=https://www.cdc.gov/coronavirus/2019-ncov/hcp/testing-overview.html. Accessed 22 April 2025.
44. Axell-House DB, Lavingia R, Rafferty M, Clark E, Amirian ES, Chiao EY. The estimation of diagnostic accuracy of tests for COVID-19: a scoping review. *J Infect.* 2020;81(5):681–697.

Protecting the Frontline and Preventing Transmission of High-Consequence Agents and Other Pathogens With Pandemic Potential in Healthcare Settings

DEEPA RAJ[a] • EMILIO HORNSEY[b] • TRISH M. PERL[a,c]
[a]Division of Infectious Diseases and Geographic Medicine, UT Southwestern Medical Center, Dallas, TX, United States • [b]UK Public Health Rapid Support Team, Public Health England, London, England, United Kingdom • [c]Peter O'Donnell Jr School of Public Health, UT Southwestern Medical Center, Dallas, TX, United States

INTRODUCTION

Healthcare facilities are critical infrastructure supporting routine care and care for those with acute medical issues. Over the past 20 years, changes in healthcare economics have led institutions to decrease in-patient capacity, minimize staffing, and utilize just-in-time supply chains. These facilities are directly affected by changes in utilization, such as infectious diseases and mass casualty events (bioterrorism and pandemics), in several ways. For example, in 1997–98, Los Angeles experienced a twofold to fourfold increase in influenza and pneumonia hospitalizations, leading to a 40% increase in Emergency Department (ED) diversions, suggesting inadequate medical capacity.[1] Previous analyses looking at the impact of pandemics or other extraordinary events on healthcare facilities report that without layered surveillance, institutions do not have adequate situational awareness to plan for patient influxes, changes in illness severity, needed equipment and supplies, including personal protective equipment (PPE) and diagnostics, and staffing.[2] In the early phases of the coronavirus infection of 2019 (COVID-19), inadequate hospital capacity and equipment and a lack of healthcare personnel (HCP) were commonly reported and degraded critical functions.[3] The demand for ventilators exceeded availability by 10-fold, global shortages of PPE were reported, testing capacity was limited, and worker shortages plagued healthcare facilities.[3] Surges of patients led to hospitals adopting crisis of care standards, operating in makeshift conditions, deviating from normal care, and suspending medical or surgical procedures, especially in the early months of the outbreak.[4] After reviewing US hospital utilization data between July 2020–July 2021 when the Delta variant (SARS-CoV-2 B.1.617.2) was circulating, CDC investigators determined that when more than 75% of Intensive Care Unit (ICU) beds were in use, over 12,000 excess deaths occurred.[4] The number of deaths increased to 80,000 if ICUs were at 100% capacity. Others have modeled the impact of pandemics on the workforce and found that by week four of a pandemic and the anticipated peak, conservatively 1.2%–2.7% of the medical workforce would be lost.[5] Most of the vacancies in the workforce (88%) were due to illness, with an additional 4% being hospitalized, and 31% were due to caring for others. One percent of the workforce would die prematurely. The 2003 severe acute respiratory syndrome (SARS) outbreak identified that HCP experienced long-term effects of chronic stress. Unfortunately, these prescient models reflect the impact of the COVID-19 pandemic in the United States, with over 1,065,200 (95% CI 909,800–1,218,000) deaths, of which 84% are directly due to SARS-CoV-2 infection.[6] Importantly, 622 (95% CI 476–769) or 43/100,000 excess deaths in physicians

Viral Outbreaks, Biosecurity, and Preparing for Mass Casualty Infectious Diseases Events
https://doi.org/10.1016/B978-0-323-54841-0.00024-X

were reported prior to the COVID-19 vaccine being available.[7] In sum, a bioterrorism event or pandemic, whether deliberate or naturally occurring, could cripple even well-prepared healthcare facilities.

Since 2001, after the September 11 terrorist attacks and subsequent dissemination of letters contaminated with anthrax spores, the United States has redoubled its efforts to address gaps and deficiencies in its emergency preparedness capabilities.[8,9] The SARS outbreak further demonstrated the difficulties in containing similar outbreaks and the challenges associated with the containment of a previously unknown infectious agent. Finally, the 2014 emergence of Ebola Virus Disease (EVD) in western Africa, where it had not previously been known to exist, led to international challenges in addition to socio-economic dysfunction and strains on the healthcare systems. These events demonstrated the capacity that bioterrorism, emerging infectious diseases, or large outbreaks have on society by causing social disruption and panic in populations and economic instability in countries. These broad effects highlight the critical need for planning and preparing a multipronged response. As part of this process, many countries developed national strategies for pandemic influenza as a model for preparedness and implementation plans designed to align with the WHO global framework.[10–13] Subsequently, in the United States, to ensure that the agencies overseeing emergency response and public health were coordinating efforts, the Department of Health and Human Services supplemented these strategic efforts with Pandemic Influenza Plan Updates, the most recent published in 2017.[14] Among the assumptions made, they estimated that 30% of the population will be infected, leading to 90,000,000 infections. Assuming that 50% of those infected will seek medical care, the additional burden to the healthcare system will depend on the severity of the virus, whether it causes moderate (i.e., a 1957-like influenza virus) or severe illness with a 1918-like influenza virus.[14] Based on models, this could lead to between 865,000 and 9,900,000 hospitalizations, 128,750 to 1,485,000 ICU admissions, and 64,875 to 745,500 persons requiring mechanical ventilation. In reviewing the response to the 2009 H1N1 pandemic, the CDC updated the preparedness and response framework developed in 2005–06 for influenza pandemics, providing more detail on the timing of decisions and actions at both a local and regional level and nationally that would be needed to slow the spread in a pandemic.[15] These plans and frameworks have increasingly recognized the role of healthcare in the response to these events. Healthcare strategies for emergency preparedness include formulating protocols for identifying and managing cases in the event of a deliberate release of a biological agent or a pandemic event, and the development of such policies is widely promoted in most healthcare facilities in the United States and Europe.

Many of these preparedness efforts have focused on the physical environment. Modeling of the SARS outbreak, as was done across 48 hospitals in Taiwan, sheds light on physical strategies that have been incorporated into planning to enhance the facility's safety and minimize nosocomial transmission.[16] Among the structural changes assessed, the investigators installing fever screening outside the ED was most important, followed by altering ED traffic, having an outbreak or pandemic management plant, mandatory temperature screening of patients and HCP, hand hygiene states, adding isolation rooms, and standardizing methods to transport patients. However, the most important of these was HCP use of prevention measures. A core focus of preparedness initiatives, therefore, must be ensuring that HCP are adequately prepared to diagnose cases, identify an etiologic agent and appropriate treatment, and institute the correct infection prevention and control (IPC) measures required to reduce further spread of disease between HCP and the many patients that could require treatment following a catastrophic infectious disease-related event.[17]

Despite the critical role HCP plays in containing an outbreak propagated by a biologic agent or a pandemic, many feel unprepared to address the potential challenges of bioterrorism or a pandemic. Following the September 2001 anthrax bioterror attacks in the United States, the US government identified critical gaps in emergency preparedness and response. This led to the creation of new laws and funding designed to address these gaps. A notable step in 2007 was the establishment of a National Strategy for Public Health and Medical Preparedness, enacted when the White House released Homeland Security Presidential Directive-21 (HSPD-21). HSPD-21 was a strategy designed to fund and improve preparedness for disaster events, including public health and bioterrorism emergencies.[18] As such programs were being rolled out, a national, cross-sectional survey was conducted in 2003. Researchers found that in this baseline period, only 43% of emergency physicians and 21% of primary care physicians felt well-prepared to participate in the public health response to a bioterrorism event.[19] Surprisingly, even after almost a decade of extensive federal interest and funding, little has changed in physician preparedness when it comes to bioterrorism events.[20] In fact, another national, cross-sectional survey conducted between October 2011 and January 2012 demonstrated that of more than 1600 responding physicians, only 34% felt prepared to handle a bioterror attack.[20] Similar research found that almost 80% of surveyed physicians have never participated in bioterrorism preparedness and response training and that 91% had only fair to poor awareness of how to identify and manage cases of bioterrorism.[21] Internationally, similar studies demonstrate the paucity of knowledge and training that exist among HCP. A nationwide cross-sectional survey among 1030 Emergency Department, laboratory, and poison control center personnel in Saudi Arabia demonstrated low mean knowledge scores about basic concepts, clinical presentations of the primary bioterrorism agents, and policies and procedures to follow in case of an event.[22] An additional study from Ghana similarly found that HCP have inadequate knowledge of the pathogens and clinical presentations, demonstrating similar challenges in lower- and middle-income countries.[23]

Historically, many outbreaks and mass casualty events related to infectious diseases are naturally occurring, and these events have had devasting impacts on the health and lives of many individuals as well as regional and worldwide economies. Because of the changing climate, increasing mobility, displacement of large populations, and human encroachment on animal habitat, the size, number, and magnitude of large infectious events are increasing. Again, HCP have been on the frontlines, yet feel unprepared to identify and support these events. While knowledge gaps are well documented in multiple studies worldwide, other factors have been identified that could inform strategies to enhance HCP willingness to work during an influenza pandemic. Among a snapshot survey of 586 emergency medical services workers in the United States, only 12% would voluntarily report to work during a pandemic.[24] Using a risk framework, these investigators determined that 52% would not work if there was a risk of transmission to their family members. However, those who were confident in their ability to protect themselves were threefold more likely to say they would report to work. A 2015 metaanalysis of 43 studies revealed that contextual factors determined the willingness to work.[16] Factors that contributed to HCP willingness to work during a pandemic did not include knowledge but did include being a nurse or physician, being male, having role-specific knowledge, and having previous pandemic response training.

The reasons behind these data are not fully understood; however, information emerging about the physical and emotional toll on HCPs from COVID-19 is emerging. A cross-sectional survey in 2400 US-based HCPs (31% physicians, 27% nurses, 13% emergency medical technicians, and 29% others) found that 29% reported symptoms or a test positive for COVID-19.[25] COVID-19 was contracted by HCPs in the ED (32%) most commonly, followed by the wards (25%) and the ICU (23%). Most notable is the psychological impact on HCP manifested by mental health issues, "burnout," and many prematurely leaving their practices. In the above survey, those HCP who reported COVID-19 were more likely to report symptoms of depression (mean difference = 0.31; 95% CI 0.16 to 0.47), anxiety (mean difference = 0.34; 95% CI 0.17 to 0.52), and burnout (mean difference = 0.54; 95% CI 0.36 to 0.71). The magnitude of the problem among this workforce is difficult to estimate. One metaanalysis found that during the COVID-19 pandemic, nurses more commonly than physicians reported[25] stress, anxiety, depression, and sleep disturbances, and overall these conditions were reported 37% (95% CI 32.87–41.22), 31.8% (95% CI 29.2–34.61), 29.4% (95% CI 27.13–31.84), and 36.9% (95% CI 33.78–40.05) of the time, respectively.[26] Another recent analysis of 161 studies that included over 341,000 HCP reported burnout in 47% (95% confidence interval [CI], 35%–60%), anxiety in 38% (95% CI, 35%–41%), depression in 34% (95% CI 30%–38%), acute stress in 30% (95% CI, 29%–31%), and posttraumatic stress disorder in 26% (95% CI, 21%–31%).[27] In contrast, another recent review found that the prevalence rates of depression, anxiety, and posttraumatic stress symptoms among HCP ranged from nine to 48% but were not increased from prepandemic levels.[28] While these data have increased interest in the well-being of HCPs and their retention, whether this will translate into improved "readiness" has yet to be seen. However, some previous gains in protecting the workforce may be important in supporting HCP as they prepare for other such infectious disease emergencies. A European systematic review found that those willing to obtain an influenza vaccination were 5.7 times more likely (OR = 5.70; 95%CI = 2.08–15.60) to receive a SARS-CoV-2 vaccination and to fear COVID-19. In fact, several studies report higher influenza vaccination rates post-COVID-19.[29] With increased access to these agents of high consequence or of naturally occurring events, the urgency of improving knowledge of biological and emerging infectious agents and identifying mechanisms to enhance HCP willingness to work is a priority. A confident and knowledgeable workforce will be best prepared to contribute to the frontline response in a biodefense, infectious disease mass casualty, or pandemic effort. Such confidence can be enhanced by a plan in a healthcare facility that outlines the principles of preparedness that can improve knowledge among HCP and promote readiness within an institution, such as the example for MERS-CoV (Table 1).

TABLE 1
Example of Principles of Preparedness for Emerging Respiratory Diseases in Healthcare Settings

BEFORE THE FIRST CASE ARRIVES	
Surveillance	▪ Institutions are responsible for tracking information about MERS-CoV (and other emerging pathogens)
Education	▪ Ensure that staff in clinical areas (i.e., emergency departments, in-patient units, surgery centers, occupational health, etc.) are aware of risk factors and updated as needed regarding case definition and screening for travel history ▪ Consider audits of outpatient triage screening and admission screening of transfer patients ▪ Provide information to care providers on precautions to be taken for patients with suspect/confirmed MERS-CoV infection
Laboratory readiness	**Establish** ▪ A notification system for laboratories regarding suspect patients ▪ A mechanism for notification and prompt delivery of specimens from suspected patients to your local or state/district health department laboratories for confirmatory testing ▪ A system for communicating results to the patient, relevant staff, and departments
Communication	▪ Draft an outline of the communication plan associated with admission of suspect/confirmed case ▪ Share communication documents to incorporate into local organization plans
Planning	▪ Develop case management that includes recommendations to minimize exposures when patients come into the healthcare system ▪ Review/update plan annually or as needed with local, state, national, or international guidance updates
Case assessment	▪ For scheduled appointments, instruct patients to notify healthcare providers if they have respiratory symptoms, follow respiratory etiquette principles, and wear a face mask ▪ Develop a strategy to triage patients at risk of MERS-CoV and other infections and to isolate promptly
CASE MANAGEMENT OF SUSPECTED OR DOCUMENTED MERS-CoV CASE	
Accommodation	▪ Identify an appropriate private room for patients under investigation (PUI). The CDC recommends an airborne isolation room; WHO does not require this ▪ Establish a timeline for the movement of the patient to an appropriate level of care and isolation if they require admission
Additional precautions	▪ Ensure that contact and droplet or airborne precautions are initiated whenever a case is suspected. Patients will require private. Place a mask on the patient and isolate them in a private room until appropriate measures can be taken ▪ Airborne precautions will be required either for all patient care, or during the performance of aerosol-generating procedures ▪ Infection prevention staff or their designee determine when precautions can be discontinued
Diagnosis	▪ Document process for confirming that patient meets case definition and requires testing ▪ Consider availability of materials to remind staff regarding how to obtain specimens using appropriate barrier precautions, per local lab requirements and procedures ▪ Document process and communications required for rapid transport and testing of relevant specimens, per local lab requirements and procedures
Communication	▪ Review health department algorithms for notification of local/state health departments ▪ Establish local protocols for notification of key staff if a patient meets criteria for a person under investigation ▪ Notify predesignated internal stakeholders as per plan (e.g., senior leadership team, occupational health, infection prevention, communications, microbiology laboratory) ▪ Draft messages/information needed for family and visitors, in collaboration with the local public health department

TABLE 1
Example of Principles of Preparedness for Emerging Respiratory Diseases in Healthcare Settings—cont'd

CASE MANAGEMENT OF SUSPECTED OR DOCUMENTED MERS-CoV CASE	
Education/training	▪ Establish mechanisms for updating institutions' knowledge regarding the status of MERS-CoV (e.g., via the CDC and WHO websites) ▪ Define what materials will be needed (e.g., FAQs for staff; email to clinical leadership; reassurance to laboratory staff who will be handling regular specimens); who will be responsible for drafting and review ▪ Define which hospital departments may provide care and/or provide diagnostic services for the patient and require information (e.g., nursing areas, respiratory therapy, physical/occupational therapy, nutrition, medical imaging, pastoral care, laboratories, pharmacy, security)
Follow-up for identification of transmission	▪ Consult with public health authorities regarding risk assessment and develop a plan for follow-up of exposed staff and visitors ▪ Define contractors and external agencies whose employees may have been exposed (e.g., first responders, home care services) and create a plan for communication/exposure investigation ▪ Report to local public health to identify and manage relevant out-of-hospital exposures ▪ Confirm WHO/CDC guidelines for follow-up for staff and patients ▪ Identify staff/patients/visitors who require follow-up

GUIDANCE FOR FOLLOW-UP OF EXPOSED HEALTHCARE PERSONNEL

Required Follow-Up

The following HCP requires follow-up:

- A HCP who provided direct clinical or personal care to or examined a symptomatic confirmed case

  OR

- A HCP in the same room at the time an aerosol-generating procedure was performed

  OR

- A HCP with more than 15 min of face-to-face contact

  AND

- Who was not wearing gown/gloves/eye protection/N95 respirator

Visitors who require follow-up:

- Visitors at the bedside of a confirmed case for more than 15 min without wearing gown/glove/face protection (i.e., not adhering to either droplet/contact or airborne/contact precautions)
- Those close contacts who may have accompanied a confirmed case (i.e., travel partners for patients from abroad)

What Follow-Up Is Required

If a person of interest develops a fever or respiratory symptoms after a definite exposure:

For those that require follow-up:

- Assess daily for respiratory symptoms for 14 days (may be active or passive for persons not present in the hospital; those working should be screened at the beginning of each work shift). Use a symptom diary
- If fever or any respiratory symptoms develop, exclude the individual from work, restrict them to home, and collect a nasopharyngeal swab for multiplex PCR and MERS-CoV testing
- Acute (as soon as convenient after exposure identified) and convalescent (day 21 after last exposure) serology for MERS-CoV antibody testing

TRANSMISSION OF ORGANISMS AND CHAIN OF INFECTION

Epidemiologists describe the "chain of infection," which is a method to describe the steps and linked circumstances that are required to acquire an infection and to pass it on to others. In each of these steps, there are interventions that can interrupt transmission and "break" the chain. This chain of events and the six links highlight why infectious agents are readily propagated in healthcare settings and further help explain why the propagation can be exponential.

1. There must be a susceptible host, which can be a person in good health receiving preventive healthcare but also those with impaired immunity, whether very young, elderly, immunocompromised, or unvaccinated.
2. There must be a portal of entry. Organisms can enter the human body via mucous membranes, including the eyes, nasopharynx, respiratory or gastrointestinal tract, or via breaks in the skin. For example, respiratory viruses such as influenza and coronaviruses are primarily acquired via the respiratory tract, and smallpox is acquired by both respiratory secretions and direct and indirect contact. Some infections require a large inoculum to cause infection, and for others, one organism may be enough. For example, norovirus causes gastroenteritis with fever, diarrhea, nausea, and vomiting, and requires a low inoculum of organisms (10–100 viral particles) to cause infection.[30] The risk of acquiring influenza is decreased from 67% to 38% in those receiving neuraminidase prophylaxis, likely because of increased inoculum needed for establishing infection and decreased duration of the sources shedding.[31]
3. Infectious pathogens need a mode of transmission. They are transmitted by several routes: direct contact with an infected surface, contaminated fomites, or inanimate objects; droplets and/or aerosols; ingestion or another vehicle (i.e., a needlestick); and by vectors. In healthcare settings, transmission occurs primarily via direct or indirect contact, by large droplets, which generally travel one to two meters, by aerosols, which are smaller droplets and can be suspended in the air for longer periods of time, or by a mixture of large and small droplets, primarily via aerosolization. The risk of transmission via exposure to blood, including a needlestick, is a concern for all pathogens, including hepatitis B, C, HIV, malaria, and pathogens of high consequence as those causing EVD or Marburg. Organisms can also be transmitted via contaminated products such as medications, fluids, disinfectants, or medical devices. While these modes of transmission are well described, they would be unlikely routes of transmission for most agents of bioterrorism or with pandemic potential, so this later route will not be discussed further.
4. An infectious agent must be present, whether a bacteria, fungus, virus, or parasite. This requires diagnosis and, at times, sophisticated testing with access to reference laboratories that have equipment and facilities to work with highly transmissible pathogens.
5. There must be an exit portal. Once the organisms have entered a susceptible host, they replicate and commonly can then infect others when individuals cough or sneeze, when in contact with their contaminated bodily secretions (e.g., blood, stool), or by touching contaminated surfaces and then touching mucous membranes. The duration of shedding in an individual and hence infectiousness also varies depending on the organism, the host, and treatments such as vaccines and antimicrobials. As an example, an individual infected with SARS-CoV-2 may shed culturable virus for up to 10 days, and the duration of shedding culturable virus is longer when they are critically ill or immunocompromised.[32] Furthermore, different variants such as the Delta (SARS-CoV-2 B.1.617.2) and Omicron (SARS-CoV-2 B.1.1.529) vary in transmissibility and shedding virus.[33] Drugs and vaccination can decrease both the transmissibility of these organisms and the duration of shedding. For example, neuraminidase inhibitors used for prophylaxis in individuals infected with influenza result in less viral shedding and a decreased duration of shedding.[31]
6. There must be a reservoir for transmission to occur. This reservoir can be poultry in the case of avian influenza viruses, small mammals such as mice, squirrels, and rabbits for *F. tularensis*, a rat (*Mastomys natalensis*) for Lassa fever, or a dromedary camel for the MERS-CoV virus. Water and soil are the reservoirs for other organisms. In healthcare settings, the reservoir can be indirect via fomite transmission.

The mechanism by which organisms are transmitted, the dose or number of organisms required, and the duration and type of exposure vary. These characteristics of the exposure potentially impact whether a person develops infection and may alter the severity of the infection. Still, the chain of infection and hence the risk of acquiring an infection affect the entire healthcare community, from patients to visitors to HCP. Contagious patients can transmit to HCP, other patients, and visitors. Contagious HCP can transmit to patients, other HCP, and visitors. Visitors can transmit to both HCPs and patients.

This chapter will describe mechanisms to interrupt transmission in healthcare settings or associated with healthcare procedures with a focus on protecting

HCP, especially when working with high-consequence pathogens and viruses with epidemic and pandemic potential. The goal in healthcare settings is to create an environment that protects patients, visitors, and HCP. Approaches to preventing transmission in healthcare settings consider how the organism is transmitted, and the duration that the host is infectious. Strategies to prevent transmission may be more aggressive in settings where the pathogen is not recognized, there is less immunity in the human population, shedding may be prolonged, and the risk of transmission is increased.

RISKS OF PATIENTS OR VISITORS ACQUIRING AN INFECTION IN HEALTHCARE

The risk of transmission to patients in healthcare settings is well described in endemic situations and with a myriad of outbreaks worldwide and in well- and less well-resourced settings.[34,35] These descriptions include acute care hospitals, EDs, outpatient, ambulatory, and alternative settings such as long-term care facilities, all of which care for vulnerable patients and those who are potentially infectious. Many of these outbreaks include examples of transmission to and from visitors and family members, although the frequency is less well documented. Nonetheless, when examining the risk in the setting of the agents under discussion, several considerations are important. Consider an influenza outbreak in a medical unit of a large hospital where the index case gives the patient in a shared room influenza.[36] Ultimately, 41% of the patients (43% had received an influenza vaccine) and 23% of HCP (36% vaccinated) developed influenza. Among the 22 HCP who developed influenza, 14 person days of leave were taken, several scheduled admissions were postponed, and emergency admissions were stopped for 11 days. In another example, 79 of 87 (88.7%) employees in a large children's hospital with pertussis were furloughed for 5 days (total 395 days) while infectious and being treated, and 622 employees received 14 days of prophylactic antimicrobials after exposure.[37] The work ethic among HCPs is defined by a huge commitment to their patients, and because of that, they commonly work while ill. Tartari et al. examined the role of presentism or HCPs who work with influenza-like symptoms and could then transmit infection to patients and other staff and found that among 522 respondents (from 49 countries), 312 (58.5%; 95% CI, 56.2–64.6) would work, sick, and in this case with influenza-like symptoms.[38] Sixty-seven (26.9%) HCP would work with fever, and most HCP (>90%) would work with minimal influenza-like symptoms. Data from early in the COVID-19 pandemic among a cohort of 66,184 patients, of which 920 tested positive for SARS-CoV-2 (1.4%), 571 tested positive while hospitalized, and 97 (10.5%) occurred after 7 days of hospitalization and were considered healthcare-associated.[39] Further, among patients, each additional day of sharing space (room, ward, unit) added 7.5 COVID-19 infections per 1000 patient days (95% CI 5.5 to 9.5/1000 susceptible patients/day), a risk that was much higher than with infections acquired in the community.[40] Similar data from the state of Minnesota demonstrated that among 5374 HCP working in acute and nonacute care (nursing homes, long-term care), 373 (6.9%) had COVID-19 within 14 days.[41] The numbers of days of work missed while isolated or ill were not provided. Beyond the staffing implications, one metaanalysis reported that 5% (95% CI 3–8) of healthcare workers developed severe disease and 0.5% (95% CI 0.02–1.3) died.[42] These examples provide insight into the transmission patterns that can exacerbate and further disrupt the healthcare setting and staffing in a setting of an outbreak or when caring for a case of a high-consequence pathogen. One only needs to amplify these examples to imagine the impact on a healthcare system in a pandemic.

RISKS TO HEALTHCARE PERSONNEL

Healthcare personnel (HCP) are a heterogenous group of individuals involved in varied ways in the healthcare system, having varied levels of risk depending on the type and duration of exposure to patients with communicable diseases regardless of the setting, whether a traditional hospital setting, long-term care or nursing home, rehabilitation facility, or other sites supporting the sick. HCP include those with direct patient care responsibilities, such as nurses, community health workers, medical assistants, physicians, respiratory, occupational, and physical therapists, environmental and dietary workers, and transporters. They include those who enter the patient room to deliver food, those who may be exposed to sterile fluids in the laboratory, and those cleaning or maintaining the environment. They may include family members who are caring for a person. The various roles expose those working in such roles to special risks, which, as noted above, pose threats to both the physical and mental health of an HCP, especially when caring for in stressful situations that include individuals with pathogens of consequence.

Transmission of infectious agents to healthcare personnel has been well documented over the years and is associated with morbidity and mortality (Table 2).

TABLE 2
Reasons for Healthcare Exposures Leading to HCP or Patient Transmissions Associated With Pathogens of High Consequence and Those Causing Outbreaks and Pandemics

Situation/Behavior	Increased Risk to Patients or HCP[a]	Examples of Infections or Pathogens Where Transmission Has Occurred
Patient with atypical symptoms[b] atypical, not recognized	Risk to both	SARS, COVID-19, influenza, smallpox, Mpox, anthrax, plague, avian influenza, VHF, *M. tuberculosis*, and other respiratory pathogens
HCP shedding with or without symptoms[b]	Risk to both	COVID-19, influenza, MERS, *M. tuberculosis*, and other respiratory pathogens
Visitors with shedding with or without respiratory symptoms	Risk to both	COVID-19, influenza, MERS, SARS, *M. tuberculosis*, and other respiratory pathogens
Patients presenting primarily with illness other than infection/injury[c]	Risk to both	COVID-19, influenza, SARS, MERS, VHF, *M. tuberculosis*, and other respiratory pathogens, *C. difficile*, MDROs
Symptoms attributed to alternate diagnosis[d]	Risk to both	COVID-19, influenza, SARS, MERS, VHF, smallpox, plague, *M. tuberculosis*, and other respiratory pathogens
Unprotected exposure, isolation precautions not implemented, delayed or prematurely removed[e]	Risk to both	COVID-19, influenza, SARS, Plague, VHF, MERS, VHF, EVD, *M. tuberculosis*, and other respiratory pathogens, *C. difficile*, MDROs
Patients with shedding and absence of symptoms	Risk to both	EVD, SARS, COVID-19, influenza, MERS, and other respiratory pathogens, *C. difficile*, MDROs
Cohorting of patients; > than one patient per room	Greater risk to patient	SARS-CoV-2, SARS, influenza, MERS, EVD, VHF, *M. tuberculosis*, and other respiratory pathogens, *C. difficile*, MDROs
Individuals (including immunocompromised) with symptoms and shedding	Risk to both	COVID-19, influenza, SARS, MERS, avian influenza, *M. tuberculosis*, and other respiratory pathogens, *C. difficile*, MDROs, Varicella (and V. zoster)
Inadequate immunity	Risk to both	COVID-19, influenza, EVD, smallpox, measles, varicella (and V. zoster)
Lack of PPE supplies	Greater risk to HCP	EVD, SARS-CoV-2, SARS
Lack of training or education about infection or use of PPE	Greater risk to HCP	EVD, MERS, SARS-CoV-2, SARS
Improper use of PPE	Greater risk to HCP	EVD, SARS, SARS-CoV-2
Lack of N95 respirator fit testing	Greater risk to HCP	Influenza, SARS, MERS, SARS-CoV-2
Deficiencies in donning PPE	Greater risk to HCP	SARS, MERS, SARS-CoV-2
Self-contamination during PPE removal	Greater risk to HCP	EVD, VHF
Use of less-than-recommended levels of protection	Greater risk to HCP	Influenza, SARS, MERS, COVID-19, EVD, VHF, *M. tuberculosis*, other respiratory pathogens, measles, varicella (and V. zoster)
Use of droplet precautions in the setting of aerosolizing procedures or aerosolization	Greater risk to HCP	SARS, MERS, COVID-19, influenza, avian influenza, VHF
Lack of training and education, including HCP choosing to utilize less-than recommended PPE	Risk to HCP	EVD, SARS-CoV-2, SARS, MERS

TABLE 2
Reasons for Healthcare Exposures Leading to HCP or Patient Transmissions Associated With Pathogens of High Consequence and Those Causing Outbreaks and Pandemics—cont'd

Situation/Behavior	Increased Risk to Patients or HCP[a]	Examples of Infections or Pathogens Where Transmission Has Occurred
Inadequate ventilation	Yes	Smallpox, COVID-19, MERS, SARS, measles, varicella (and disseminated zoster), *M. tuberculosis*
Inadequate cleaning/disinfection of the environment, equipment, or supplies	Risk to both	EBV, VHF, SARS, *C. difficile*, MDROs
Inadequate disposal of linens	Risk to patient	Smallpox, fungi (*Aspergillus*)
Overcrowding	Risk to patient	MERS, influenza, SARS, SARS-CoV-2, *C. difficile*, norovirus, MDROs
Longer duration in room	Risk to HCP	SARS, EVD, VHF
Inadequate staffing	Risk to patient	SARS-CoV-2, SARS, EVD, VHF, *C. difficile*, MDROs
Lack of scientific evidence on transmission to make appropriate PPE recommendations	Risk to both	SARS and MERS (early in outbreaks), COVID-19 (early in pandemic)

[a]*HCP*, healthcare personnel; *BT*, bioterrorism; *ID*, infectious diseases; *PPE*, personal protective equipment; *EVD*, Ebola virus disease; *VHF*, viral hemorrhagic fever; *SARS*, systemic acute respiratory syndrome (SARS-CoV-1); *MERS*, middle east respiratory syndrome (MERS-CoV); *MDRO's*, multidrug-resistant organisms.
[b]Symptoms and signs depend on infection/syndrome but would include fever, respiratory, gastrointestinal symptoms, or rash as appropriate.
[c]Examples of other illnesses or reasons to present to medical care: elective surgeries, trauma, cardiac events, gastrointestinal bleeding, stroke, etc.
[d]Examples of alternative diagnoses: noninfectious diarrhea (ulcerative colitis exacerbation, etc.); rash (disseminated herpes, varicella, varicella zoster, etc.), shortness of breath (exacerbation of chronic obstructive pulmonary disease, asthma), community-acquired bacterial pneumonias (i.e., coinfections) congestive heart failure, etc.).
[e]Isolation discontinued prematurely because of false-negative test results, incomplete testing, or continued shedding after antiviral therapy.

Such infections can incur great expense to the HCP, the institution, and society. Importantly, the extent of the consequences of this population is likely underestimated in the literature. Many HCP fail to report exposures and symptoms, delay reporting, and minimize the events that led to the infection. Some institutions will not allow reporting of these infections for fear of institutional risk or legal liability. Furthermore, many published reports examine the risks in traditional healthcare settings where risk may be lower because these settings have access to education, equipment, and resources. That may not be available during pandemics or crises brought on by bioterrorism.

Outbreaks have demonstrated the risk to HCP with common communicable diseases including varicella, *M. tuberculosis*, measles, pertussis, HIV, hepatitis B, and hepatitis C.[43] Using a German comprehensive national compensation board database, a review of HCP-acquired infections over a 5-year period revealed that 1.5 HCP/100,000 develop an infection.[44] In acute care settings, hepatitis B and C were the most common occupationally acquired infections, followed by *M. tuberculosis*. In nursing home or long-term care settings, scabies was the most likely infection acquired. A Norwegian national registry of over 14,000 workers compared seasonal influenza absenteeism to that during the 2009 Influenza A H1N1 pandemic and found that sick leave increased from 2.9% (95% CI 2.4%–4.8%) by 1.5-fold.[45] Work loss increased during the pandemic fourfold to care at home for sick children. Kuster et al. performed a metaanalysis to determine the risk among HCP. Among the 29 studies reviewed, the incidence rate ratio for acquiring influenza when compared to healthy adults was 18.7 (95% CI 15.8–22.1).[46] The rate was twice as high among unvaccinated HCPs than those who were vaccinated. A Canadian team prospectively determined the risks of HCP acquiring influenza in a cohort of HCP working in acute care hospitals during the 2009 Influenza A H1N1 pandemic and found that 13 symptomatic HCP of the 563 in the cohort (2.2%) tested positive for influenza.[47] In this cohort, the risk of influenza was highest when family members had an acute respiratory illness (adjusted odd's ratio [AOR] 6.9, 95% CI 2.2–21.8) and when performing an aerosol-generating procedure (AOR 2.0, 95% CI 1.1–3.5).

The COVID-19 pandemic has provided more profound insights into the risks to HCP, which include those associated with the organism but also some of the less tangible risks associated with mental health and well-being. Among 120, 075 participants from the UK during the early phases of the COVID-19 pandemic, the risk of severe COVID-19 or complications of the infection was significantly higher than that with other occupations (RR 7.43, 95% CI 5.52 to 10.00).[48] Overall, around 1.1%–23% of HCP developed COVID-19, and among HCP, nurses (48%), and those working outside of the ED (43%) were most commonly infected with the SARS-CoV-2 virus.[42] Although data from cross-sectional studies show that at least 2.4% of HCP are asymptomatic but are shedding virus, and the seroprevalence finds that 24.4% had evidence of infection (prevaccination availability).[49] Based on systematic reviews, the risk of severe COVID-19 infection and complications in HCP ranged from 0.7% to 10.2%, with 0%–14.4% requiring hospitalization.[50] While early studies demonstrated increased mortality, later data suggest the consequences of infection are less severe, with a lower mortality (0%–1.2%) than in the general population.[50] Other risk factors that increase the risk of infection include being black and Hispanic, older, having direct exposure to patients, performing high-risk procedures, working in certain workplace areas, not using PPE or wearing facial coverings, decreased access to PPE, or lack of knowledge about how to use PPE.[42,49,51] Studies continue to demonstrate the effectiveness of masks, although the debate between whether N95 (or P2) or medical masks are superior remains unanswered.[52–56] Importantly, transmissions occurred not only from patients but during unprotected contact with other HCP.[57,58] Subsequent studies have demonstrated that HCP who were vaccinated with one of the mRNA vaccines have a lower risk of infection, reinfection, and complications of COVID-19.[51,54,59] The risk of acquiring influenza among HCP varies by setting and job function. Researchers reviewed data from 6093 HCP during the 2009 Influenza A H1N1 pandemic and found that 49% of those who developed H1N1 influenza constituted 20% of the workforce.[60] This represented a 10%–24% increase in illness over previous years and, also, varied by phase of the pandemic. Overall, infection acquisition was highest among physicians and medical providers (6.7%), followed by security and transportation personnel (4.0%), housekeeping and food services workers (2.7%), and finally by nurses and clinical technicians (2.2%). Only 1%–1.2% of administrators and those providing counseling services developed influenza infections. At this time the ED experienced a 10%–20% increase in volumes, and HCPs working in the adult and pediatric EDs accounted for 29% and 25% of the reported influenza, respectively. Occupational health and safety personnel accounted for 14% of the infections, followed by anesthesiology with 11%, pediatrics with 5.4%, and intensive care with 4.1%.

Pathogens of high consequence with high mortality, such as the viral hemorrhagic fevers caused by the Filoviridae, EVD, and Marburg, have also affected HCPs and are spread generally through direct or indirect exposure to blood or body fluids. In the West-African EVD outbreak between 2014 and 2016, over 860 HCP were infected, which was approximately 3.9% of the total infections.[61] A comprehensive analysis of the risk to HCP with these two organisms examined 22 outbreaks that occurred between 1967 and 2017 and demonstrated that for EVD, the percent of patients who were HCPs ranged from 2% to 100%.[61] Among those HCP exposed to EVD, between 0.6% and 92% developed infection. Marburg infection is much rarer, and among the eight clusters included, between 5% and 50% of the patients were HCP's, and among HCP's exposed, 1%–10% developed infection. However, several studies from the 2014–16 West-African EVD outbreak provide more robust population-based estimates. Among HCPs exposed in Sierra Leone, Guinea, and Liberia, the percent of exposed HCPs who developed infection was between 1.4% and 8%, compared to 0.03%–0.08% in the general population. Depending on the country, the risk of developing EVD was 47–100 times higher. One cluster of infections occurred in the United States, where two of 149 HCP developed infections. Nursing and physicians, followed by laboratorians, were the most likely to become infected. Overall, five factors leading to exposures were: (1) insufficient quantities or incorrect use of PPE; (2) exposure to an unrecognized case; (3) lack of recognition of risk such as exposure to corpses; (4) inability to implement environmental controls, including adequate cleaning, cohorting patients, and infrastructure deficiencies; and (5) inadequate staffing and inadequate specialists, such as in infection prevention.

Despite these data, the risk to HCP remained, and data from the COVID-19 pandemic again demonstrates that HCP are a vulnerable population. For example, an elegant cohort of over 2035, 395 community individuals and 99, 795 HCPs in the United Kingdom and the United States found that the risk of developing COVID-19 (positive SARS-CoV-2 test) was 11-fold higher (747/100,000 HCP compared with 242/100,000; adjusted hazard ratio [HR] 11 · 61, 95% CI 10 · 93–12 · 33).[62] Risk factors for infection included reuse of or inadequate PPE, being black, Hispanic/Latinx, or Asian, and working in an acute care setting or a nursing home (adjusted HR 24.30, 95% CI 21.83–27.06; 16.24, 13.39–19.70), respectively. These authors also report that HCPs working in nursing homes (16.9%) reported inadequate PPE most frequently, whereas those working in acute care settings reported reuse of PPE most often (23.7%). Additional analyses support the risk among HCP with patient contact with a threefold higher risk of developing COVID-19 than HCP who do not have patient contact (HR 3.30, 95% CI 2.13 to 5.13) and more importantly demonstrating the increased risk among household members of HCP with direct patient contact whose risk of developing infection was increased (HR 1.79, 95% CI 1.10 to 2.91).[63] This study identified that direct patient contact, use of aerosol-generating procedures, and working in the ICU increased the risk of acquiring infection.

The fear of uncertainty with a constant stream of information, changing processes and practices, inadequate PPE, and the risk of transmitting infection to others were drivers of psychological stress and ultimately burnout. Multiple studies report high levels of depression, anxiety, and psychological distress among HCPs who cared for patients during the COVID-19 pandemic.[64] These reports are also complicated by "burnout," or the physical, mental, and moral exhaustion that occurs in the settings of pandemics or outbreaks where HCP make difficult decisions, lose patients and colleagues, and are at risk of acquiring infection themselves or giving it to their families. Up to 40% of HCP met criteria for burnout in some studies during the COVID-19 pandemic.[65] Burnout was more common than depression, and, overall, 24% of HCPs reported depression, with the rate being highest in frontline workers.[66] This should be no surprise, as between 11% and 73% of HCP report posttraumatic stress during outbreaks, and these symptoms can last up to 3 years in 10%–40%.[67] In the setting of outbreaks, depression, insomnia, and severe anxiety are reported in addition to the stress of working. However, work, individual-related factors, and organizational support can be important to modulate the impact of this consequence of a pandemic or bioterror event. To prepare for these potential consequences and to assure an adequate and healthy workforce, several factors are important to increase the willingness of HCPs to work in such settings, especially pandemics. One metaanalysis found that willingness to work was highest among males, physicians, and nurses, those with full-time employment, those who felt safe personally (adequate PPE), awareness of risk and knowledge of pandemics, training, and confidence in personal skills.[16] One important factor that impeded a willingness to work was childcare or elder care obligations.

Overall, HCP are at increased risk of developing infections of high consequence or unknown pathogens or those causing pandemics due to multiple factors including job function, types of exposures, compliance with PPE, building design, education around infections, their transmission and prevention, the use of PPE, staffing, and fatigue, among others (Table 2). Factors affecting this risk also depend on the agent and its transmissibility. The risk to the HCP extends beyond the physical illness but is associated with mental health and wellness, and the HCP stress that accompanies patient care in these settings has consequences to the health system and to society. Perhaps most concerning are the repeated examples that illustrate much of the risk could be mitigated with adequate supplies, training, and staffing.

DIAGNOSIS OF INFECTION

Beyond being responsible for providing emergency care, following a catastrophic event, HCP are responsible for identifying the etiologic agent causing an outbreak and implementing mitigation strategies to contain the initial spread of infection and minimize the impact in the healthcare setting. This requires comprehensive knowledge of the various clinical presentations of biologically significant agents, many of which are nonspecific and require confirmation via time-consuming and labor-intensive laboratory diagnoses.[17] Access to a laboratory with facilities to diagnose unusual organisms is critical, especially if large numbers of patients present simultaneously. The sheer number of patients may overwhelm HCP, a healthcare facility, and the diagnostic and supporting resources in the wake of an outbreak.[68,69] In addition, because of the many routes of transmission, time becomes of the essence to implement appropriate strategies to protect patients and the caring HCP. While many infections can be treated successfully with appropriate chemotherapy, clinical management of suspected and confirmed cases can result in nosocomial transmission, especially if an etiologic agent has not been suspected and precautions are not implemented. Outbreaks of SARS-CoV-1, MERS-CoV, SARS-CoV-2, and EVD[61] provide illustrations of nosocomial transmission to patients, HCPs, and visitors that occur prior to identification of the pathogen.

Many of the agents of high consequence cause nondescript constellations of symptoms, especially early in the process, and may include fever, cough, and malaise, all symptoms that are difficult to differentiate from a common respiratory viral pathogen. Some can cause diarrhea, nausea, and vomiting, mimicking common causes of gastroenteritis or foodborne illness. Others may present with a rash syndrome, as occurs with varicella. Identifying a potential epidemiologic link or a clustering of unusual cases or clinical presentations are the common initial factors that trigger recognition of something unusual. Hence, directed pathogen specific testing may require time for either cultures to grow, PCRs to be processed, or for the patient's symptoms to progress into a more recognized clinical syndrome. Proper identification may be further complicated due to atypical disease presentations (especially in the case of an outbreak involving an atypical host or stemming from an engineered biologic agent) or partial immunity.

Several biologic agents, such as *B. anthracis* and *Y. pestis*, can present as a nonspecific pneumonia-like illness.[70] For example, in 2001 in the United States, most of the anthrax cases presented with fever, chills, and lethargy, and several had elevated liver transaminases, infiltrates on chest X-rays, mediastinal widening, and pleural effusions. Together, these symptoms and signs indicate inhalation of anthrax spores in otherwise healthy individuals.[70,71] Inhalational anthrax typically presents in two phases: the first begins after a brief incubation period and includes low-grade fever, general malaise, and cough. After 2 or 3 days of respite, the second phase manifests with a sudden onset of severe respiratory symptoms, high-grade fever, chills, and pronounced diaphoresis.[72] In many cases, prodromal symptoms and chest radiographs are nonspecific and easily attributed to common viral respiratory infections.[73] In the absence of identifiable symptoms beyond respiratory distress, it may be difficult for HCP to immediately discern the cause of an outbreak.

Of similar concern and because of the challenge posed to diagnosis is the fact that weaponized agents can be transmitted through less common routes. For example, the majority of naturally occurring *F. tularensis* infections are transmitted to humans when skin or mucous membranes come into contact with the blood or bodily fluids of infected animals.[74] Patients infected in this manner will present with clinical syndromes typical of ulceroglandular tularemia, characterized by headache, fever, chills, malaise, painful regional lymphadenopathy, and, most notably, an ulcerated skin lesion.[74] However, the agent causing tularemia, *F. tularensis*, is likely to be aerosolized for use in bioterrorism. Inhalation of infectious aerosolized particles will cause either pneumonic tularemia, a severe, atypical, yet pneumonia that presents with nonspecific symptoms and may be fulminant, or typhoidal tularemia, characterized by fever, prostration, weight loss, and severe but nonspecific respiratory distress.[75] Three other routes of transmission produce glandular, oculoglandular, and oropharyngeal tularemia, all of which differ drastically in their clinical presentation.[74] This range of clinical presentations from the same pathogen, depending on the route of dispersal and transmission, presents yet another challenge in properly diagnosing cases that may present following a catastrophic public health event. Additional details are provided elsewhere for the clinical overview of specific organisms (Chapters 2–11) and recommendations for chemotherapy and chemoprophylaxis (Chapter 19).

Given all the challenges in diagnosing an infectious process resulting from an agent of high consequence or an unknown agent, several aids can aid the clinician or epidemiologist. First and most directly, knowledge of the syndromes in question and of any salient features can accelerate diagnosis considerably. Resources should be kept accessible when the possibility of such a disease enters the diagnostician's mind. Second, as the clinician gathers information, they must obtain a detailed history and look for unusual exposures. Third, as the technology to produce and disperse such agents has increased, so has the diagnostic technology. Multiplex and genomic testing, rapid diagnostic processes, and other tools are often available through specialty laboratories, regional centers, and governmental organizations if they are not available locally. Lastly, acts of bioterrorism or emerging infections typically result in clusters of cases. These can be temporal, spatial, or temporospatial clustering, which may heighten the clinician's suspicion of an unusual event. Hence, identification of an organism or an event requires a vigilant clinician, suspicion when various pieces of information fit or do not fit into a pattern, and critical assessment to assure that appropriate diagnostic resources are employed and public health officials notified.

BASIC INFECTION PREVENTION FOR HCP RESPONDING TO MANAGEMENT OF AN AGENT OF HIGH CONSEQUENCE OR AN INFECTIOUS DISEASE MASS CASUALTY EVENT

Many healthcare facilities mandate that, at a minimum, HCPs use standard precautions when providing patient care, regardless of the patient's diagnosis.[68] Standard precautions are a bundle of practices to prevent exposure to potentially infected material and are based upon the principle that any blood, bodily fluid, secretion, and mucous membrane may harbor infectious agents that can be transmitted from person to person (Table 3).[76] This strategy called a horizontal approach to IPC practices is designed to protect HCP, visitors, and patients alike from a broad range of nonpathogen-specific disease exposure by assuming that any exposure could harbor organisms.[77] Hand hygiene is the foundation of standard precautions and should be used universally with any interaction with patients or the environment. A group modeled nosocomial transmission among 48 hospitals, 664 patients, and 119 HCP and found that placing hand hygiene stations in the ED was one of the single most important interventions to prevent infection with the SARS-CoV-1 virus (Odds Ratio [OR] 1.07, $P = .012$).[78] In the setting of a patient with an infection that is potentially contagious or a mass infectious disease casualty event, healthcare organizations must provide adequate and ample hand hygiene stations in patient care areas, waiting rooms, and entrances to facilities to provide both safe patient care and to minimize a circle of transmission. Respiratory etiquette is an element of standard precautions that emerged after the H1N1 pandemic and the SARS and MERS outbreaks. Beyond hand hygiene, it promotes the routine education of patients, visitors, and HCPs about practices that will prevent transmission of respiratory viruses. It also includes the masking of individuals with respiratory symptoms, physically separating them from other patients, and the appropriate disposal of tissues. For example, in the initial outbreak of MERS-CoV, 21 of the 23 cases were acquired by person-to-person transmission, which occurred in three settings: hemodialysis units, intensive care units, or in-patient units.[79] Standard precautions, while advocated, were not practiced, and transmission was documented in three different health care facilities within the region. Subsequently, investigators elegantly demonstrate how MERS-CoV was transmitted within hospitals and to other hospital settings by describing three generations of infections in each setting.[80] Among the 185 cases, excluding the index case, 84% of the transmissions that occurred in these hospitals were in the setting of unrecognized infection and occurred in patients and visitors not practicing respiratory etiquette. Standard precautions can be used in other cases as well if the HCP anticipates exposure to blood, body fluid, or pathogens based on the patient's symptoms and the planned activities. The activities include patient placement and the handling, care, and disposal of needles, sharps, equipment, and linens. It also promotes the appropriate cleaning of medical equipment and medical devices. Selvaraj and colleagues summarized the Ebola and Marburg outbreaks, which described transmissions in the healthcare setting and described the sources of transmissions to HCP.[61] They found that most exposures occurred at the initial encounter, and many were due to unrecognized infection and inadequate use of standard precautions or access to appropriate PPE and hand hygiene. Additional precautions may be recommended for patient care depending on the situation, and these are always added on top of standard precautions and are based on the type of transmission pattern associated with the infective agent.

The general level of HCP compliance with standard precautions, however, is low[81]; some studies have characterized self-reported compliance with all elements of standard precautions to be as low as 31%–38%.[82] A recent rapid evidence review highlights the complexity around HCP complying with IPC[80] measures, including standard precautions.[83] Among the 56 papers included in a review, factors that improved compliance included working in the ED or the ICU, known contact with a confirmed case, and concern about the risk of acquiring infection. Noncompliance was associated with staff observation of noncompliance, among others, lack of PPE availability, inconvenience of PPE, difficulty donning PPE, discomfort wearing PPE, perceived ineffectiveness of PPE, and worries about PPE negatively impacting the quality of the HCP-patient interaction. In addition to these ever-present challenges to maintaining standard precautions, established standards of care can be further disrupted during a public health emergency.[84] For example, during the 2001 anthrax letter events in the United States, patients presenting to different EDs received radically different treatment. Some patients were released without receiving any decontamination or prophylactic treatment; others underwent decontamination procedures with 0.5% sodium hypochlorite washes followed by clinical counseling and postexposure prophylaxis, while still others underwent multiple decontamination procedures alone, without chemoprophylaxis.[85] These inconsistencies highlight the variation in case management despite similar clinical presentations and can

TABLE 3
Key Elements of Standard Precautions

Elements	Indications	Comments/Resources
Perform hand hygiene	Perform hand hygiene • Before and after any direct patient contact; between patients, whether gloves are worn • Immediately after gloves are removed • Before handling an invasive device • After touching blood or body fluids or contaminated items, whether or not gloves are worn • During patient care when going from contaminated to clean body site • After contact with inanimate objects in the immediate patient area	Hand washing: use soap[a] and water for 40–60 s, rub all surfaces, rinse hands, dry hands with a single towel, and use the towel to turn off the faucet Hand rub/alcohol[b]: apply enough product to cover all areas of the hands and rub until dry References 1. World Health Organization & WHO Patient Safety. (2009). WHO guidelines on hand hygiene in health care. World Health Organization. https://apps.who.int/iris/handle/10665/44102 2. https://www.cdc.gov/handhygiene/providers/guideline.html 3. https://www.cambridge.org/core/journals/infection-control-and-hospital-epidemiology/article/sheaidsaapic-practice-recommendation-strategies-to-prevent-healthcare-associated-infections-through-hand-hygiene-2022-update/FCD05235C79DC57F0E7F54D7EC314C2C
Use PPE[c] for a potential exposure to infectious materials	• Select PPE based on risk of contamination • Wear gloves when touching blood, bodily fluids, or mucous membranes • Wear a medical/surgical mask with goggles or a face shield if there is a risk of splashes and sprays during routine care • Wear a gown if skin or clothing will be exposed to blood or body fluids	Select appropriate PPE after making an assessment of the risk of exposure to body fluids or a contaminated environment and before contact • Clean, nonsterile gloves • Clean, nonsterile fluid resistant gown • Mask and eye protection or face shield *Gloves*: change between tasks/procedures on the same patient; remove after use before touching noncontaminated surfaces and going to another patient; perform hand hygiene after removal *Facial protection* includes eyes, nose, and mouth. Hand hygiene after removal *Gown*: change gown in between patients; remove soiled gown as soon as possible
Follow respiratory hygiene/cough etiquette	• Cover mouth and nose when coughing or sneezing • Perform hand hygiene after contact with respiratory secretions • Mask individuals with acute respiratory symptoms with or without fever • Physically separate persons with respiratory symptoms from others by 1–2 m	Educate HCPs, patients, and visitors Provide signage and visual clues Provide receptacles for disposing of tissues after use HCP should observe droplet precautions in addition to standard precautions when examining patients with acute respiratory symptoms Consider providing hand hygiene stations, tissues, and masks in common areas References https://www.cdc.gov/flu/professionals/infectioncontrol/resphygiene.htm

Ensure the patient is placed properly	• Place patients in single rooms • If single rooms are not available, cohort patients	Use single rooms when there is a risk of transmitting an infection to others
Clean and disinfect patient care equipment/ instruments and devices appropriately	• Handle soiled equipment (with blood and body secretions/excretions) to prevent skin and mucous membrane exposures, contamination of clothing, or transfer to other patients or the environment • Clean, disinfect, and reprocess reusable equipment appropriately and before use on another patient	
Clean and disinfect the environment appropriately	• Use adequate procedures for routine cleaning and disinfection of environmental and other frequently touched surfaces	
Manage and care for linens carefully	• Handle, transport, and process used linen to protect from skin and mucous membrane exposures	Prevents transfer of pathogens to other patients, the environment, and HCPs Prevents contamination of clothing
Follow safe injection practices	• Use aseptic technique to avoid contaminating a sterile site or injection equipment • Use sterile, single-use, disposable needles and syringes for each injection • Wear a surgical mask for lumbar puncture procedures	
Handle and dispose of needles and sharps properly	• Handle, clean, or dispose of needles, scalpels, and other sharp instruments/devices with care • Clean used instruments with care • Dispose of used needles and other sharp instruments with care	Avoid mucous membrane and skin exposures, contamination of Treat waste contaminated with blood and body fluids as clinical waste per local regulations

[a]Soap does not need to be antibacterial.
[b]Alcohol-based hand hygiene products include solutions, rubs, and gels.
[c]*PPE*, personal protective equipment.
Modified from https://cdn.who.int/media/docs/default-source/documents/health-topics/epr_am2_e77a9f9250-e9f7-4cc3-9e81-754f12b00c4d.pdf?sfvrsn=a568a3f9_1&download=true and CDC 2007 Guideline for Isolation Precautions https://www.cdc.gov/infectioncontrol/guidelines/isolation/index.html.

also promote distrust in healthcare recommendations. Such data argue for assuring HCP have and can access needed information quickly.

Healthcare facilities, their staff, their patients, and their inhabitants routinely encounter infectious diseases that can easily be transmitted between the susceptible patients, visitors, and HCP. This risk is exacerbated when incubating patients present with an unidentified contagious illness or before being aware of any exposure to a biological agent, whether a routine respiratory virus or an agent of high consequence.[69] One elegant prospective study calculated the relative risk of developing either an influenza-like illness or influenza over three respiratory seasons in over 21,500 patients and 2100 HCP, which depended upon whether individuals were exposed to contagious HCP or patient.[86] The risk of a patient acquiring influenza when exposed to at least one contagious HCP was 5.48 (95% CI, 2.09–14.37) higher than the nonexposed. However, when a patient was exposed to a contagious patient, that risk increased sharply to 17.96 (95% CI, 10.07–32.03) fold higher than the nonexposed. When patients were exposed to at least one contagious patient and an infected HCP, the relative risk rose yet again to 34.75 (95% CI, 17.70–68.25). HCP are also consistently at an increased risk of exposure to infectious pathogens, especially during an initial patient encounter at the outset of an outbreak.[68,85] Healthcare environments are already susceptible to increased disease transmission given overcrowding and high censuses, close cohorting of suspected and confirmed cases, and improper utilization of appropriate isolation precautions.[87] It is therefore critical that, at the very least, standard precautions are adhered to as completely as possible to reduce the possibility of nosocomial transmission at the outset of outbreaks, whether naturally occurring or due to a bioterrorism event.

BARRIER PRECAUTIONS AND OTHER INFECTION PREVENTION AND CONTROL MEASURES

The CDC designates two tiers of nonpharmacological interventions to halt transmission of infectious and contagious agents. The first is the implementation of standard precautions, which are always used in the patient care environment but should also be used in triage areas in the case of a mass casualty event (Table 3). The second is the use of appropriate transmission-based precautions (Table 4). Specific transmission-based precautions are added on top of standard precautions when additional IPC practices are required to completely interrupt disease transmission.[76] When an epidemiologically-significant infectious agent is suspected to be the cause of disease, the HCP must first determine the agent's route of transmission, then empirically institute the appropriate transmission-based measures: contact, airborne, or droplet isolation precautions.[85] For some diseases that may have multiple routes of transmission, more than one transmission-based precaution can be applied. In the event that the etiologic agent cannot quickly be confirmed, HCP can assess the patient's syndromes and, based on knowledge, determine the most appropriate type of precautions.[70] There are three categories of transmission-based precautions[88] (Table 4):

1. *Contact precautions* are designed to prevent transmission caused by direct contact with contaminated bodily fluids or direct and indirect contact from contaminated surfaces. These are recommended in the presence of diarrhea, excessive wound drainage, fecal incontinence, or other bodily fluids that suggest an increased risk for personal and environmental contamination, and therefore, disease transmission. These are also recommended for certain organisms that have a predilection to contaminate the environment, including *Clostridiodes difficile* and certain antibiotic-resistant organisms.
2. *Droplet precautions* are designed to prevent transmission caused by large (>100 μm) respiratory droplets, which can travel short distances in the air and remain suspended in the air for short periods of time, usually only a few seconds. These should be used when the patient presents with a fever, respiratory symptoms such as coughing and sneezing, influenza-like illness, or vomiting where large droplets can be propelled one to two meters. These are commonly recommended for suspected respiratory viruses, including influenza.
3. *Airborne precautions* are designed to prevent transmission caused by very small (<5 μm) respiratory particles, which can remain buoyant for up to 24–30 min and can be easily propelled through the air. These are required for patients appearing to suffer from severe respiratory or viral illness, measles-like or pox-like rash, or hemorrhagic fever where organisms are spread on these lighter particles. Note that some organisms that are typically transmitted via droplets can become aerosolized and spread via the airborne route, especially in healthcare settings where aerosol-generating procedures such as endotracheal intubation are performed.

TABLE 4
Transmission-Based Precautions

IN ADDITION TO STANDARD PRECAUTIONS, CAN APPLY			
Precaution type and rationale	*Contact* To prevent transmission of infectious agents spread by direct or indirect contact with a patient or patient's environment	*Droplet precautions* To prevent transmission of infectious agents spread by droplets (measuring >5 µm) through close mucous membrane or respiratory contact with respiratory secretions produced through coughing, sneezing, talking, or other aerosol-generating procedures	*Airborne precautions* To prevent transmission of infectious agents that are spread by airborne droplets (≤5 µm) that remain infectious and suspended in air for long periods of time and can be widely dispersed with air currents
Patient placement and considerations	Private room or cohort like patients	• Private room or cohort like patients with >1 m between beds • Place a droplet mask on the patient when s/he leaves the room • Follow cough etiquette and respiratory hygiene	• Place patients in private rooms with monitored negative pressure ventilation of 6 to 12 air exchanges per hour; an airborne infection isolation room is preferred • Place a droplet mask on the patient when the patient leaves the room • Follow cough etiquette and respiratory hygiene
HCP considerations	• Hand hygiene • Don gloves and gowns prior to entering a patient's room • Before exiting the room, doff and discard PPE that may be contaminated with pathogens	• Hand hygiene • Wear a mask (medical or surgical) when working within 1 m of the patient • Follow cough etiquette and respiratory hygiene	• Hand hygiene • Don respiratory protection (i.e., N-95 mask, PAPR, P3) required for susceptible persons must be donned prior to entering the room, and removed upon exit • Air must be discharged to the outdoors or HEPA-filtered prior to recirculation • Follow cough etiquette and respiratory hygiene
Examples of use in clinical syndromes	Diarrhea, wounds with drainage, etc.	Influenza-like illness, COVID-like illness, respiratory symptoms, etc.	Pox-like rash; measles-like rash, etc.
Examples of infections or organisms	Vancomycin-resistant enterococcus, methicillin-resistant *Staphylococcus aureus, C. difficile*; scabies, norovirus, smallpox, varicella, VHF, etc.	Influenza, pertussis, meningococcus, respiratory syncytial virus, *Yersinia pestis* pneumonia, etc.	Varicella, disseminated herpes zoster, measles, *M. tuberculosis*, novel respiratory viruses, smallpox, etc.
Other considerations	Limit patient transport to essential purposes only	Limit patient transport to essential purposes only	Use for aerosol-generating procedures and coronavirus or novel influenza virus infections Limit patient transport to essential purposes only

PPE, personal protective equipment; *PAPR*, powered air purified respirators; *N-95 and P3*, respiratory protective devices designed for efficient filtration; *VHF*, viral hemorrhagic fevers.

Adapted from Siegel JD, Rhinehart E, Jackson M, Chiarello L, Health Care Infection Control Practices Advisory C. 2007 Guideline for isolation precautions: preventing transmission of infectious agents in health care settings. *Am J Infect Control.* 2007;35(10 Suppl. 2):S65–S164. https://doi.org/10.1016/j.ajic.2007.10.007.

One caveat is worth mentioning and is described in more detail in the introduction, which is that the line between droplet and aerosol transmission has become more nuanced in modern healthcare settings where aerosol-generating procedures are used, and as we understand the dynamics of coughing, singing, and other means of projecting these particles.[89–92] Engineering studies, observational data from outbreaks, and pragmatic clinical trials have demonstrated that in these settings, organisms traditionally considered spread by droplets can be aerosolized.[92–94] These data demonstrate that additional caution is needed in the settings of respiratory viruses in particular, including influenza, SARS-CoV1, SARS-CoV-2, and endemic coronaviruses.

The effectiveness of standard precautions is enhanced with adherence to other practices that also reduce disease transmission.[95] While standard precautions alone are sufficient to significantly slow the spread of infectious organisms, especially those that are prone to transmission in healthcare environments, there is commonly a need for additional strategies to impede transmission. EVD, an infection associated with high morbidity and mortality and the potential to propagate dramatically, is an example. In 1995, an EVD outbreak erupted with more than 300 documented cases and 280 resulting deaths (case fatality rate = 88%) was ultimately interrupted when standard precautions and isolation were implemented at the epicenter of the outbreak, Kikwit General Hospital.[96] Following the initiation of standard precautions and isolation of patients, only one subsequent HCP contracted EVD, and this was associated with a known contact with a mucous membrane.

Compliance with transmission-based precautions, like with standard precautions, can be poor. In some cases, when a patient had a known diagnosis requiring application of contact-based precautions, HCP compliance with the appropriate precaution was as low as 29%.[97] Similarly, when these patients were transported from one location to another, compliance with transmission-based protocols for patients was as low as 7%.[97] Research suggests that low compliance may be due to deficiencies in HCP knowledge and indicates a need for regular training in transmission-based precautions and ongoing reinforcement.[98,99] Interestingly, a recent metaanalysis found that HCP have reasonable knowledge about standard precautions, hand hygiene, and certain organisms (*M. tuberculosis*, methicillin-resistant *Staphylococcus aureus*, MERS-CoV, and SARS-CoV-2), but have poor knowledge about modes of transmission, occupational vaccination requirements, risks associated with infections, and the practices that prevent infection, including safe needle and sharp care and the prevention of central line infections.[100] Low compliance with IPC protocols, however, can lead to active failures in transmission-based precautions and PPE use, thereby causing an increased risk of healthcare transmission.[98] HCPs who have faulty IPC practices may be more likely to contaminate their own skin and clothing, especially while donning and doffing PPE.[101] It is these types of failures that were thought to contribute to the transmission of EVD in the 2014 outbreak in West Africa.[102,103]

A unique case study is presented by a 2014 experience in an American hospital. A man traveled to Liberia during the 2014 Ebola outbreak in West Africa. Five days after returning to Dallas, Texas, the man sought medical care because of fever, abdominal pain, and headache and was diagnosed with sinusitis. He was discharged home. Three days later, he returned to the same ED with persistent fever, abdominal pain, and diarrhea and was admitted. The patient was placed in a private room, and standard, contact, and droplet precautions were initiated while awaiting EVD testing results.[104] Of the 21 HCP who were exposed to the case while he was infectious, two ICU nurses developed the disease. No ED providers developed disease. Although the ICU nurses wore recommended PPE consistent with standard, contact, and droplet precautions while caring for the patient, public health recommendations changed over he was hospitalized.[104] It is hypothesized that HCP infection resulted from an exposure that occurred in the setting of rapidly changing infection prevention practices, human error, and missteps as the HCP doffed PPE or performed high-risk procedures.[105] Nonetheless, this event highlighted the importance of strict compliance with transmission-based precautions, but also reinforced the notion that HCP must have appropriate education and training to properly implement IPC protocols.

Deviations from recommended PPE protocols are common with both the PPE recommended for contact precautions as well as the PPE used in EVD care. While deviations occur most commonly with doffing, they do occur with donning also.[101,106,107] Mumma et al. identified 19 failure modes where 41 HCP failed to appropriately follow commonly recommended doffing steps for PPE used in EVD care.[103] The step where HCP are most likely to contaminate themselves is with glove removal. PPE doffing is in general to be the greatest risk for self-contamination. IPC practices are more likely to be followed when HCP are monitored to assure appropriate steps and procedures are followed.[22] Recommended practices, which include standard and isolation precautions (Tables 3 and 4), for many pathogens are summarized for category A agents of bioterrorism and other highly contagious agents in Table 5. It also includes some additional considerations when managing patients who are suspected of such infections. Please note that these recommendations change as new information becomes available.

B. anthracis (See Chapter 2)

Because anthrax is not transmitted from person to person, **standard precautions** are the only isolation precaution required.[108] A sporicidal disinfectant should be used after any invasive procedure or autopsy.[75]

F. tularensis (See Chapter 3)

Tularemia is not transmitted from person to person. **Standard precautions** are sufficient to protect HCP, visitors, and other patients.[109] Heat and disinfectants can easily render the organism inactive.[75]

Y. pestis (See Chapter 4)

Y. pestis can be transmitted to humans via bites from infected fleas, causing bubonic and septicemic plague. These forms of disease are not transmitted from person to person unless a patient has respiratory involvement. If it can be confirmed with certainty that there are no respiratory symptoms and no secondary pneumonia, then no isolation or barrier precautions are required for these two forms of disease. In other words, **bubonic or septicemic plague require only standard precautions**.[110] Pneumonic plague, however, is extremely contagious and can be transmitted from person to person through exposure to respiratory droplets. Therefore, **pneumonic plague requires droplet precautions in addition to standard precautions**.[75] Patients should be placed in a single room until patients have been on appropriate antibiotic therapy for 24 h, after this time they can be cohorted.[75,111]

Alphaviruses

None of the viral encephalitis infections caused by alphaviruses can be transmitted from human to human, even in the case of aerosolized release. **Only standard precautions** are required.

Arenaviruses (See Chapter 5)

Lassa fever is a highly contagious infection that is transmitted to humans via direct contact with the excretions of infected rats, inhalation of dust contaminated with rat excreta, or ingestion of an infected rat.[112] Person-to-person transmission is highly likely to occur via contact with infected blood or bodily fluids, and **contact precautions in addition to standard precautions** are required to prevent disease exposure.[108] Ideally, confirmed patients should be placed in private rooms.[111]

Filoviruses (See Chapter 5)

Ebola and Marburg viruses are extremely contagious, and transmission to humans occurs when humans have direct contact with the blood and bodily fluids of infected animals or humans or consume infected animals.[113] A bioterrorism event could involve the inhalation of aerosols, or in the setting of a mass casualty event, procedures such as intubation could produce aerosols, which would be particularly deadly as both viruses require a low infective dose to cause disease in humans. Several studies have also demonstrated that nosocomial transmission can occur through the airborne route when HCP perform aerosol-generating procedures, such as intubation.[114] In addition, these patients can have copious watery diarrhea, which also increases the risk of transmission via secretions if HCP are not in appropriate PPE. Given the high pathogenicity of Ebola and Marburg virus diseases, **airborne precautions, especially with aerosol-generating procedures, contact precautions, and standard precautions, are all required.**[75] Ideally, patients should be cared for in private rooms with negative airflow that have an anteroom HCP can use to don and doff PPE and perform hand hygiene with all encounters and when doffing PPE.[111]

Variola Virus (See Chapter 6)

Smallpox is a highly contagious disease that is transmitted from person to person by respiratory droplets containing the variola virus, by direct contact with infected scabs or skin lesions,[108] and by contaminated objects such as linens. Droplets can enter through the mucous membranes, and virions can persist on fomites for up to 1 week.[111] It can be aerosolized through ventilation systems or through aerosol-generating procedures. **Airborne precautions, contact precautions, and standard precautions are** all **required** when there is a risk of exposure to smallpox.[75] Patients are placed in rooms with negative pressure and high-efficiency particulate air filters (HEPA). Their linens and waste must be placed in biohazard containers and autoclaved prior to

TABLE 5
Agents of High Consequence: Infection Prevention and Control Practices for Patient Management

	BACTERIAL AGENTS									
Important Phone Numbers: Infectious Disease Service: Infection Prevention Control: Local Health Authority:	**Anthrax (*B. antracis*)**	**Tularemia**	**Plague, Bubonic (*Yersinia pestis*)**	**Pneumonic Plague**	**Glanders**	**Brucellosis**	**Cholera**	**Q Fever**	**Influenza**	**Avian Influe Strair**
STANDARD AND TRANSMISSION-BASED PRECAUTIONS										
Standard precautions for all aspects of patient care	X	X	X	X	X	X	X	X	X	X
Contact precautions	*				X	X			X	X
Airborne precautions									C	C
Airborne precautions for aerosol-generating procedures									X	X
Droplet precautions				X					X	
Hand hygiene	X	X	X	X	X	X	X	X	X	X
PATIENT PLACEMENT										
No additional restrictions	X	X						X		
Cohort "like" patients when private rooms are unavailable			X	X			X	X	X	
Single room with ensuite toilet and washing facilities			X	X	X	X	X		X	X
Single room with negative pressure										X
Door closed at all times									X	X
PATIENT TRANSPORT										
No restrictions	X	X			X	X		X		
Limit movement to essential medical purposes only			X	X	X	X	X			X
Place a mask on the patient to minimize dispersal of droplets				X	X				X	X
MANAGEMENT OF PATIENT ENVIRONMENT										
Routine terminal cleaning of the room upon discharge and as needed		X			X		X	X	X	X
Disinfect surfaces with bleach/water sol. 1:9 (10% sol.)	X		X	X		X				C
Dedicated equipment is disinfected prior to leaving room						X			X	X
Clinical specimens, labeled as high-risk and transported to the laboratory with special procedures	X	X	X	X	X	X	X	X		X
Medical waste handled with special considerations	X									X

VIRUSES							BIOLOGICAL TOXINS				
SARS	MERS	SARS-CoV-2	Smallpox	VHF (Ebola, Marburg, Lassa, etc.)	Venez Equine Enceph	Viral Encephalitis	Botulism	Ricin	T-2 Mycotoxins	Staph, Enterotoxin B	Unknown Other Designer Pathogens
X	X	X	X	X	X	X	X	X	X	X	X
X	X	X	X	X							X
X	X	X	X	C		P					X
X	X	X	X	X							X
		C		C	X						X
X	X	X	X	X	X	X	X	X	X	X	X
							X	X	X	X	X
X		X	X	X		X					X
X	X	X	X	X	X	X					X
X	X	X	X	C							X
X	X	X	X	X							X
						X	X	X	X	X	X
X	X	X	X	X	X						X
X	X	X	X		X						X
			X		X	X	X	X	X	X	X
X	X	X	X	X							X
X	X	X	X	X							X
X	X	X	X	X	X	X	X	X	X	X	X
			X	X			X	X	X	X	X

(Continued)

TABLE 5
Agents of High Consequence: Infection Prevention and Control Practices for Patient Management—cont'd

	BACTERIAL AGENTS									
Important Phone Numbers: Infectious Disease Service: Infection Prevention Control: Local Health Authority:	**Anthrax (*B. antracis*)**	**Tularemia**	**Plague, Bubonic (*Yersinia pestis*)**	**Pneumonic Plague**	**Glanders**	**Brucellosis**	**Cholera**	**Q Fever**	**Influenza**	**Avian Influe Strain**
DISCHARGE MANAGEMENT										
No additional IPC considerations	X		X	X		X		X		
Not discharged from hospital until determined no longer infectious				X						
Prophylactic treatment of contacts (may include vaccination)				X					X	X
POSTMORTEM CARE										
Survival of viable organisms in cadavers; special considerations	X									
Follow the principles of standard precautions	X	X	X	X	X	X	X	X	X	X
Droplet precautions				X					X	
Airborne precautions										X
Use of N95 mask by all individuals entering the room										X
Contact Precautions										
Avoid autopsy except under special circumstances	X									X
Disinfect surfaces with bleach/water sol. 1:9 (10% sol.)	X		X	X						X

Standard Precautions: Prevents direct contact with all body fluids, including blood, secretions, excretions, intact skin (including rashes), and mucous membranes. Transmission-based precautions: contact, droplet or airborne (see Table 3); X = generally required; C = country-to-country variation depending on guidance; P = possible depending on host and diagnostic considerations;
* use with skin form (ulcer).
Adapted from Walter Reed Medical Center.

	VIRUSES							BIOLOGICAL TOXINS				
	SARS	MERS	SARS-CoV-2	Smallpox	VHF (Ebola, Marburg, Lassa, etc.)	Venez Equine Enceph	Viral Encephalitis	Botulism	Ricin	T-2 Mycotoxins	Staph, Enterotoxin B	Unknown Other Designer Pathogens
				X	X	X						
	X	X		X	X							X
			X	X	X							?
				X	X							
	X	X	X	X	X	X	X	X	X	X	X	X
												X
	X	X	X	X	X							X
	X	X	X	X	X							X
				X	X							X
	X	X	X	X	X						X	X
	X	X	X	X	X							X

being laundered or incinerated, as fomites can remain contaminated for long periods of time.[108] Standard hospital disinfectants can be used to clean surfaces, but rooms of confirmed smallpox patients must be aggressively cleaned following their removal.[75] Ideally, HCPs caring for these patients should be vaccinated.

CONCLUSION

The deliberate utilization of biological agents and pandemic events have been well documented throughout the course of history and have left terrible marks. Bioterrorism as well as pandemics pose continuous threats to the health and safety of the people, to healthcare systems, and to societies the world over. Along with naturally occurring threats, various biological agents have the potential to be weaponized, with many being naturally occurring and ubiquitous, as well as susceptible to genetic engineering. Modified biological agents could be more virulent, become more "fit," and then be more capable of person-to-person transmission, leading to an increase in morbidity and mortality when compared to their naturally occurring progenitors.

HCP form the first line of defense following both pandemics and bioterrorism events and must have a working knowledge of potential agents of these potential catastrophes, as they would be responsible for recognizing clinical presentation and identifying the agent of concern. In addition to having surveillance systems that provide situational awareness, they must be able to function as efficiently and effectively as possible in these trying situations. Among the priorities is to assure they feel safe, which requires implementation of the appropriate IPC protocols to manage existing cases and prevent further disease transmission, both of which would be critical if a biological agent is aerosolized for widespread dissemination with person-to-person transmission involved or when there are multiple patients that overwhelm existing resources. Clinical vigilance and a degree of suspicion could enable early recognition to mitigate more severe ramifications of a pandemic or bioterrorism event. HCP must be regularly educated and trained on the various agents that could be utilized in a biological attack or present during a pandemic, their clinical signs and symptoms, the appropriate IPC practices that should be observed as part of clinical management, and diagnostic and therapeutic options that may be available. All these steps can be articulated in a simple yet overarching approach that provides the processes needed to protect HCP, the health system, and societies (Table 1).

REFERENCES

1. Glaser CA, Gilliam S, Thompson WW, et al. Medical care capacity for influenza outbreaks. *Los Angeles Emerg Infect Dis.* 2002;8(6):569–574. https://doi.org/10.3201/eid0806.010370.
2. Ungchusak K, Sawanpanyalert P, Hanchoworakul W, et al. Lessons learned from influenza A(H1N1) pdm09 pandemic response in Thailand. *Emerg Infect Dis.* 2012;18(7):1058–1064. https://doi.org/10.3201/eid1807.110976.
3. El Bcheraoui C, Weishaar H, Pozo-Martin F, Hanefeld J. Assessing COVID-19 through the lens of health systems' preparedness: time for a change. *Glob Health.* 2020;16(1):112. https://doi.org/10.1186/s12992-020-00645-5.
4. French G, Hulse M, Nguyen D, et al. Impact of hospital strain on excess deaths during the COVID-19 pandemic—United States, July 2020-July 2021. *MMWR Morb Mortal Wkly Rep.* 2021;70(46):1613–1616. https://doi.org/10.15585/mmwr.mm7046a5.
5. Wilson N, Baker M, Crampton P, Mansoor O. The potential impact of the next influenza pandemic on a national primary care medical workforce. *Hum Resour Health.* 2005;3:7. https://doi.org/10.1186/1478-4491-3-7.
6. Lee WE, Woo Park S, Weinberger DM, et al. Direct and indirect mortality impacts of the COVID-19 pandemic in the United States, March 1, 2020 to January 1, 2022. *Elife.* 2023;12. https://doi.org/10.7554/eLife.77562.
7. Kiang MV, Carlasare LE, Thadaney Israni S, Norcini JJ, Zaman JAB, Bibbins-Domingo K. Excess mortality among US physicians during the COVID-19 pandemic. *JAMA Intern Med.* 2023;183(4):374–376. https://doi.org/10.1001/jamainternmed.2022.6308.
8. Anderson PD, Bokor G. Bioterrorism: pathogens as weapons. *J Pharm Pract.* 2012;25(5):521–529. https://doi.org/10.1177/0897190012456366.
9. O'Brien KK, Higdon ML, Halverson JJ. Recognition and management of bioterrorism infections. *Am Fam Physician.* 2003;67(9):1927–1934 [In eng].
10. World Health Organization. Pandemic Influenza Risk Management: A WHO Guide to Inform and Harmonize National and International Pandemic Preparedness and Response. Geneva, Switzerland: World Health Organization; 2017.
11. Council HS. National Strategy for Pandemic Influenza. Washington, DC: Council HS; 2005:1–12.
12. Council HS. National Strategy for Pandemic Influenza: Implementation Plan; 2006:1–227. https://www.cdc.gov/flu/pandemic-resources/pdf/pandemic-influenza-implementation.pdf.
13. COVID-19 Clinical Research Coalition. Global coalition to accelerate COVID-19 clinical research in resource-limited settings. *Lancet.* 2020;395(10233):1322–1325. https://doi.org/10.1016/S0140-6736(20)30798-4.
14. Services HH. Pandemic Influenza Plan: 2017 Update. 52. Services USDoHaH; 2017.

15. Holloway R, Rasmussen SA, Zaza S, Cox NJ, Jernigan DB. Updated preparedness and response framework for influenza pandemics. *MMWR Recomm Rep.* 2014;63(RR-06):1–18. https://www.ncbi.nlm.nih.gov/pubmed/25254666.
16. Aoyagi Y, Beck CR, Dingwall R, Nguyen-Van-Tam JS. Healthcare workers' willingness to work during an influenza pandemic: a systematic review and meta-analysis. *Influenza Other Respir Viruses.* 2015;9(3):120–130. https://doi.org/10.1111/irv.12310.
17. Rothman RE, Hsieh YH, Yang S. Communicable respiratory threats in the ED: tuberculosis, influenza, SARS, and other aerosolized infections. *Emerg Med Clin North Am.* 2006;24(4):989–1017. https://doi.org/10.1016/j.emc.2006.06.006.
18. Inglesby TV, Henderson DA. Biosecurity and bioterrorism: biodefense strategy, practice, and science. A decade in biosecurity. Introduction. *Biosecur Bioterror.* 2012;10(1):5. https://doi.org/10.1089/bsp.2012.0319.
19. Alexander GC, Larkin GL, Wynia MK. Physicians' preparedness for bioterrorism and other public health priorities. *Acad Emerg Med.* 2006;13(11):1238–1241. https://doi.org/10.1197/j.aem.2005.12.022.
20. SteelFisher GK, Blendon RJ, Brule AS, et al. Physician emergency preparedness: a National Poll of physicians. *Disaster Med Public Health Prep.* 2015;9(6):666–680. https://doi.org/10.1017/dmp.2015.114.
21. Spranger CB, Villegas D, Kazda MJ, Harris AM, Mathew S, Migala W. Assessment of physician preparedness and response capacity to bioterrorism or other public health emergency events in a major metropolitan area. *Disaster Manag Response.* 2007;5(3):82–86. https://doi.org/10.1016/j.dmr.2007.05.001.
22. Nofal A, AlFayyad I, AlJerian N, et al. Knowledge and preparedness of healthcare providers towards bioterrorism. *BMC Health Serv Res.* 2021;21(1):426. https://doi.org/10.1186/s12913-021-06442-z.
23. Atakro CA, Addo SB, Aboagye JS, et al. Nurses' and medical officers' knowledge, attitude, and preparedness toward potential bioterrorism attacks. *SAGE Open Nurs.* 2019;5. https://doi.org/10.1177/2377960819844378.2377960819844378.
24. Barnett DJ, Levine R, Thompson CB, et al. Gauging U.S. Emergency Medical Services workers' willingness to respond to pandemic influenza using a threat- and efficacy-based assessment framework. *PLoS One.* 2010;5(3), e9856. https://doi.org/10.1371/journal.pone.0009856.
25. Firew T, Sano ED, Lee JW, et al. Protecting the front line: a cross-sectional survey analysis of the occupational factors contributing to healthcare workers' infection and psychological distress during the COVID-19 pandemic in the USA. *BMJ Open.* 2020;10(10), e042752. https://doi.org/10.1136/bmjopen-2020-042752.
26. Al Maqbali M, Alsayed A, Hughes C, Hacker E, Dickens GL. Stress, anxiety, depression and sleep disturbance among healthcare professional during the COVID-19 pandemic: an umbrella review of 72 meta-analyses. *PLoS One.* 2024;19(5), e0302597. https://doi.org/10.1371/journal.pone.0302597.
27. Huang J, Huang ZT, Sun XC, Chen TT, Wu XT. Mental health status and related factors influencing healthcare workers during the COVID-19 pandemic: a systematic review and meta-analysis. *PLoS One.* 2024;19(1), e0289454. https://doi.org/10.1371/journal.pone.0289454.
28. Witteveen AB, Young SY, Cuijpers P, et al. COVID-19 and common mental health symptoms in the early phase of the pandemic: an umbrella review of the evidence. *PLoS Med.* 2023;20(4), e1004206. https://doi.org/10.1371/journal.pmed.1004206.
29. Bianchi FP, Cuscianna E, Rizzi D, et al. Impact of COVID-19 pandemic on flu vaccine uptake in healthcare workers in Europe: a systematic review and meta-analysis. *Expert Rev Vaccines.* 2023;22(1):777–784. https://doi.org/10.1080/14760584.2023.2250437.
30. Robilotti E, Deresinski S, Pinsky BA. Norovirus. *Clin Microbiol Rev.* 2015;28(1):134–164. https://doi.org/10.1128/CMR.00075-14.
31. Hayden FG, Treanor JJ, Fritz RS, et al. Use of the oral neuraminidase inhibitor oseltamivir in experimental human influenza: randomized controlled trials for prevention and treatment. *JAMA.* 1999;282(13):1240–1246. https://doi.org/10.1001/jama.282.13.1240.
32. Wolfel R, Corman VM, Guggemos W, et al. Virological assessment of hospitalized patients with COVID-2019. *Nature.* 2020;581(7809):465–469. https://doi.org/10.1038/s41586-020-2196-x.
33. Boucau J, Marino C, Regan J, et al. Duration of shedding of culturable virus in SARS-CoV-2 omicron (BA.1) infection. *N Engl J Med.* 2022;387(3):275–277. https://doi.org/10.1056/NEJMc2202092.
34. Sood G, Perl TM. Outbreaks in health care settings. *Infect Dis Clin N Am.* 2021;35(3):631–666. https://doi.org/10.1016/j.idc.2021.04.006.
35. Sydnor ER, Perl TM. Hospital epidemiology and infection control in acute-care settings. *Clin Microbiol Rev.* 2011;24(1):141–173. https://doi.org/10.1128/CMR.00027-10.
36. Sartor C, Zandotti C, Romain F, et al. Disruption of services in an internal medicine unit due to a nosocomial influenza outbreak. *Infect Control Hosp Epidemiol.* 2002;23(10):615–619. https://doi.org/10.1086/501981.
37. Christie CD, Glover AM, Willke MJ, Marx ML, Reising SF, Hutchinson NM. Containment of pertussis in the regional pediatric hospital during the Greater Cincinnati epidemic of 1993. *Infect Control Hosp Epidemiol.* 1995;16(10):556–563. https://doi.org/10.1086/647008.
38. Tartari E, Saris K, Kenters N, et al. Not sick enough to worry? "Influenza-like" symptoms and work-related behavior among healthcare workers and other professionals: results of a global survey. *PLoS One.* 2020;15(5), e0232168. https://doi.org/10.1371/journal.pone.0232168.

39. Mo Y, Eyre DW, Lumley SF, et al. Transmission of community- and hospital-acquired SARS-CoV-2 in hospital settings in the UK: a cohort study. *PLoS Med.* 2021;18(10), e1003816. https://doi.org/10.1371/journal.pmed.1003816.
40. Uyeki TM, Milton S, Hamid CA, et al. Highly pathogenic avian influenza A(H5N1) virus infection in a dairy farm worker. *N Engl J Med.* 2024. https://doi.org/10.1056/NEJMc2405371.
41. Fell A, Beaudoin A, D'Heilly P, et al. SARS-CoV-2 exposure and infection among health care personnel—Minnesota, March 6-July 11, 2020. *MMWR Morb Mortal Wkly Rep.* 2020;69(43):1605–1610. https://doi.org/10.15585/mmwr.mm6943a5.
42. Gomez-Ochoa SA, Franco OH, Rojas LZ, et al. COVID-19 in health-care workers: a living systematic review and meta-analysis of prevalence, risk factors, clinical characteristics, and outcomes. *Am J Epidemiol.* 2021;190(1):161–175. https://doi.org/10.1093/aje/kwaa191.
43. Weber DJ, Rutala WA, Schaffner W. Lessons learned: protection of healthcare workers from infectious disease risks. *Crit Care Med.* 2010;38(8 Suppl):S306–S314. https://doi.org/10.1097/CCM.0b013e3181e69ebd.
44. Nienhaus A, Kesavachandran C, Wendeler D, Haamann F, Dulon M. Infectious diseases in healthcare workers—an analysis of the standardised data set of a German compensation board. *J Occup Med Toxicol.* 2012;7(1):8. https://doi.org/10.1186/1745-6673-7-8.
45. de Blasio BF, Xue Y, Iversen B, Gran JM. Estimating influenza-related sick leave in Norway: was work absenteeism higher during the 2009 A(H1N1) pandemic compared to seasonal epidemics? *Euro Surveill.* 2012;17(33). https://www.ncbi.nlm.nih.gov/pubmed/22913978.
46. Kuster SP, Shah PS, Coleman BL, et al. Incidence of influenza in healthy adults and healthcare workers: a systematic review and meta-analysis. *PLoS One.* 2011;6(10), e26239. https://doi.org/10.1371/journal.pone.0026239.
47. Kuster SP, Coleman BL, Raboud J, et al. Risk factors for influenza among health care workers during 2009 pandemic, Toronto, Ontario. *Canada Emerg Infect Dis.* 2013;19(4):606–615. https://doi.org/10.3201/eid1904.111812.
48. Mutambudzi M, Niedwiedz C, Macdonald EB, et al. Occupation and risk of severe COVID-19: prospective cohort study of 120 075 UK Biobank participants. *Occup Environ Med.* 2020;78(5):307–314. https://doi.org/10.1136/oemed-2020-106731.
49. Shields A, Faustini SE, Perez-Toledo M, et al. SARS-CoV-2 seroprevalence and asymptomatic viral carriage in healthcare workers: a cross-sectional study. *Thorax.* 2020;75(12):1089–1094. https://doi.org/10.1136/thoraxjnl-2020-215414.
50. Chou R, Dana T, Selph S, Totten AM, Buckley DI, Fu R. Update alert 6: epidemiology of and risk factors for coronavirus infection in health care workers. *Ann Intern Med.* 2021;174(1):W18–W19. https://doi.org/10.7326/L20-1323.
51. Chou R, Dana T, Buckley DI, Selph S, Fu R, Totten AM. Update alert 11: epidemiology of and risk factors for coronavirus infection in health care workers. *Ann Intern Med.* 2022;175(8):W83–W84. https://doi.org/10.7326/L22-0235.
52. Boucau J, Uddin R, Marino C, et al. Characterization of virologic rebound following nirmatrelvir-ritonavir treatment for coronavirus disease 2019 (COVID-19). *Clin Infect Dis.* 2023;76(3):e526–e529. https://doi.org/10.1093/cid/ciac512.
53. Radonovich Jr LJ, Simberkoff MS, Bessesen MT, et al. N95 respirators vs medical masks for preventing influenza among health care personnel: a randomized clinical trial. *JAMA.* 2019;322(9):824–833. https://doi.org/10.1001/jama.2019.11645.
54. Chou R. Comparative effectiveness of mask type in preventing SARS-CoV-2 in health care workers: uncertainty persists. *Ann Intern Med.* 2022;175(12):1763–1764. https://doi.org/10.7326/M22-3219.
55. Loeb M, Bartholomew A, Hashmi M, et al. Medical masks versus N95 respirators for preventing COVID-19 among health care workers : a randomized trial. *Ann Intern Med.* 2022;175(12):1629–1638. https://doi.org/10.7326/M22-1966.
56. Kunstler B, Newton S, Hill H, et al. P2/N95 respirators & surgical masks to prevent SARS-CoV-2 infection: effectiveness & adverse effects. *Infect Dis Health.* 2022;27(2):81–95. https://doi.org/10.1016/j.idh.2022.01.001.
57. Schneider S, Piening B, Nouri-Pasovsky PA, Kruger AC, Gastmeier P, Aghdassi SJS. SARS-Coronavirus-2 cases in healthcare workers may not regularly originate from patient care: lessons from a university hospital on the underestimated risk of healthcare worker to healthcare worker transmission. *Antimicrob Resist Infect Control.* 2020;9(1):192. https://doi.org/10.1186/s13756-020-00848-w.
58. Gordon CL, Trubiano JA, Holmes NE, et al. Staff to staff transmission as a driver of healthcare worker infections with COVID-19. *Infect Dis Health.* 2021;26(4):276–283. https://doi.org/10.1016/j.idh.2021.06.003.
59. Dorr T, Haller S, Muller MF, et al. Risk of SARS-CoV-2 acquisition in health care workers according to cumulative patient exposure and preferred mask type. *JAMA Netw Open.* 2022;5(8), e2226816. https://doi.org/10.1001/jamanetworkopen.2022.26816.
60. Santos CD, Bristow RB, Vorenkamp JV. Which health care workers were most affected during the spring 2009 H1N1 pandemic? *Disaster Med Public Health Prep.* 2010;4(1):47–54. https://doi.org/10.1017/s193578930000241x.
61. Selvaraj SA, Lee KE, Harrell M, Ivanov I, Allegranzi B. Infection rates and risk factors for infection among health workers during Ebola and Marburg virus outbreaks: a systematic review. *J Infect Dis.* 2018;218(suppl_5):S679–S689. https://doi.org/10.1093/infdis/jiy435.
62. Nguyen LH, Drew DA, Graham MS, et al. Risk of COVID-19 among front-line health-care workers and the general community: a prospective cohort study.

Lancet Public Health. 2020;5(9):e475–e483. https://doi.org/10.1016/S2468-2667(20)30164-X.

63. Shah ASV, Wood R, Gribben C, et al. Risk of hospital admission with coronavirus disease 2019 in healthcare workers and their households: nationwide linkage cohort study. *BMJ.* 2020;371, m3582. https://doi.org/10.1136/bmj.m3582.
64. Chou R, Dana T, Buckley DI, Selph S, Fu R, Totten AM. Update alert: epidemiology of and risk factors for coronavirus infection in health care workers. *Ann Intern Med.* 2020;173(2):W46–W47. https://doi.org/10.7326/L20-0768.
65. Matsuo T, Kobayashi D, Taki F, et al. Prevalence of health care worker burnout during the coronavirus disease 2019 (COVID-19) pandemic in Japan. *JAMA Netw Open.* 2020;3(8), e2017271. https://doi.org/10.1001/jamanetworkopen.2020.17271.
66. Olaya B, Perez-Moreno M, Bueno-Notivol J, Gracia-Garcia P, Lasheras I, Santabarbara J. Prevalence of depression among healthcare workers during the COVID-19 outbreak: a systematic review and meta-analysis. *J Clin Med.* 2021;10(15). https://doi.org/10.3390/jcm10153406.
67. Preti E, Di Mattei V, Perego G, et al. The psychological impact of epidemic and pandemic outbreaks on healthcare workers: rapid review of the evidence. *Curr Psychiatry Rep.* 2020;22(8):43. https://doi.org/10.1007/s11920-020-01166-z.
68. Suwantarat N, Apisarnthanarak A. Risks to healthcare workers with emerging diseases: lessons from MERS-CoV, Ebola, SARS, and avian flu. *Curr Opin Infect Dis.* 2015;28(4):349–361. https://doi.org/10.1097/QCO.0000000000000183.
69. Huttunen R, Syrjänen J. Healthcare workers as vectors of infectious diseases. *Eur J Clin Microbiol Infect Dis.* 2014;33(9):1477–1488. https://doi.org/10.1007/s10096-014-2119-6.
70. Lee BY. The role of internists during epidemics, outbreaks, and bioterrorist attacks. *J Gen Intern Med.* 2007;22(1):131–136. https://doi.org/10.1007/s11606-006-0030-2.
71. Jernigan JA, Stephens DS, Ashford DA, et al. Bioterrorism-related inhalational anthrax: the first 10 cases reported in the United States. *Emerg Infect Dis.* 2001;7(6):933–944 [In eng] https://doi.org/10.3201/eid0706.010604.
72. Balali-Mood M, Moshiri M, Etemad L. Medical aspects of bio-terrorism. *Toxicon.* 2013;69:131–142. https://doi.org/10.1016/j.toxicon.2013.01.005.
73. Cunha BA. Anthrax, tularemia, plague, Ebola or smallpox as agents of bioterrorism: recognition in the emergency room. *Clin Microbiol Infect.* 2002;8(8):489–503. https://doi.org/10.1046/j.1469-0691.2002.00496.x.
74. Weant KA, Bailey AM, Fleishaker EL, Justice SB. Being prepared: bioterrorism and mass prophylaxis: part I. *Adv Emerg Nurs J.* 2014;36(3):226–238. quiz 239–40. [In eng] https://doi.org/10.1097/tme.0000000000000029.
75. Darling RG, Catlett CL, Huebner KD, Jarrett DG. Threats in bioterrorism. I: CDC category A agents. *Emerg Med Clin North Am.* 2002;20(2):273–309. https://doi.org/10.1016/s0733-8627(02)00005-6.
76. Siegel JD, Rhinehart E, Jackson M, Chiarello L. 2007 Guideline for isolation precautions: preventing transmission of infectious agents in health care settings. *Am J Infect Control.* 2007;35(10 Suppl. 2):S65–164 [In eng] https://doi.org/10.1016/j.ajic.2007.10.007. pii: S0196-6553(07)00740-7.
77. Septimus E, Weinstein RA, Perl TM, Goldmann DA, Yokoe DS. Approaches for preventing healthcare-associated infections: go long or go wide? *Infect Control Hosp Epidemiol.* 2014;35(7):797–801. https://doi.org/10.1086/676535.
78. Yen MY, Lu YC, Huang PH, Chen CM, Chen YC, Lin YE. Quantitative evaluation of infection control models in the prevention of nosocomial transmission of SARS virus to healthcare workers: implication to nosocomial viral infection control for healthcare workers. *Scand J Infect Dis.* 2010;42(6–7):510–515. https://doi.org/10.3109/00365540903582400.
79. Assiri A, McGeer A, Perl TM, et al. Hospital outbreak of Middle East respiratory syndrome coronavirus. *N Engl J Med.* 2013;369(5):407–416. https://doi.org/10.1056/NEJMoa1306742.
80. Lee SS, Wong NS. Probable transmission chains of Middle East respiratory syndrome coronavirus and the multiple generations of secondary infection in South Korea. *Int J Infect Dis.* 2015;38:65–67. https://doi.org/10.1016/j.ijid.2015.07.014.
81. Gammon J, Morgan-Samuel H, Gould D. A review of the evidence for suboptimal compliance of healthcare practitioners to standard/universal infection control precautions. *J Clin Nurs.* 2008;17(2):157–167 [In eng] https://doi.org/10.1111/j.1365-2702.2006.01852.x.
82. Michalsen A, Delclos GL, Felknor SA, et al. Compliance with universal precautions among physicians. *J Occup Environ Med.* 1997;39(2):130–137 [In eng] https://doi.org/10.1097/00043764-199702000-00010.
83. Brooks SK, Greenberg N, Wessely S, Rubin GJ. Factors affecting healthcare workers' compliance with social and behavioural infection control measures during emerging infectious disease outbreaks: rapid evidence review. *BMJ Open.* 2021;11(8), e049857. https://doi.org/10.1136/bmjopen-2021-049857.
84. Nelson C, Lurie N, Wasserman J, Zakowski S. Conceptualizing and defining public health emergency preparedness. *Am J Public Health.* 2007;97(Suppl. 1):S9–11 [In eng] https://doi.org/10.2105/ajph.2007.114496.
85. Keim M, Kaufmann AF. Principles for emergency response to bioterrorism. *Ann Emerg Med.* 1999;34(2):177–182. https://doi.org/10.1016/s0196-0644(99)70227-1.
86. Vanhems P, Voirin N, Roche S, et al. Risk of influenza-like illness in an acute health care setting during community influenza epidemics in 2004-2005, 2005-2006, and 2006-2007: a prospective study. *Arch Intern Med.* 2011;171(2):151–157. https://doi.org/10.1001/archinternmed.2010.500.

87. Fusco FM, Schilling S, De Iaco G, et al. Infection control management of patients with suspected highly infectious diseases in emergency departments: data from a survey in 41 facilities in 14 European countries. *BMC Infect Dis.* 2012;12:27 [In eng] https://doi.org/10.1186/1471-2334-12-27.
88. Siegel JD, Rhinehart E, Jackson M, Chiarello L. Health care infection control practices advisory C. 2007 guideline for isolation precautions: preventing transmission of infectious agents in health care settings. *Am J Infect Control.* 2007;35(10 Suppl. 2):S65–164. https://doi.org/10.1016/j.ajic.2007.10.007.
89. Tran K, Cimon K, Severn M, Pessoa-Silva CL, Conly J. Aerosol generating procedures and risk of transmission of acute respiratory infections to healthcare workers: a systematic review. *PLoS One.* 2012;7(4), e35797. https://doi.org/10.1371/journal.pone.0035797.
90. Noti JD, Lindsley WG, Blachere FM, et al. Detection of infectious influenza virus in cough aerosols generated in a simulated patient examination room. *Clin Infect Dis.* 2012;54(11):1569–1577. https://doi.org/10.1093/cid/cis237.
91. Weissman DN, de Perio MA, Radonovich Jr LJ. COVID-19 and risks posed to personnel during endotracheal intubation. *JAMA.* 2020;323(20):2027–2028. https://doi.org/10.1001/jama.2020.6627.
92. Leal J, Farkas B, Mastikhina L, et al. Risk of transmission of respiratory viruses during aerosol-generating medical procedures (AGMPs) revisited in the COVID-19 pandemic: a systematic review. *Antimicrob Resist Infect Control.* 2022;11(1):102. https://doi.org/10.1186/s13756-022-01133-8.
93. Bourouiba L. Turbulent gas clouds and respiratory pathogen emissions: potential implications for reducing transmission of COVID-19. *JAMA.* 2020;323(18):1837–1838. https://doi.org/10.1001/jama.2020.4756.
94. Milton DK, Fabian MP, Cowling BJ, Grantham ML, McDevitt JJ. Influenza virus aerosols in human exhaled breath: particle size, culturability, and effect of surgical masks. *PLoS Pathog.* 2013;9(3), e1003205. https://doi.org/10.1371/journal.ppat.1003205.
95. Morgan DJ, Pineles L, Shardell M, et al. The effect of contact precautions on healthcare worker activity in acute care hospitals. *Infect Control Hosp Epidemiol.* 2013;34(1):69–73. https://doi.org/10.1086/668775.
96. Khan AS, Tshioko FK, Heymann DL, et al. The reemergence of Ebola hemorrhagic fever, Democratic Republic of the Congo, 1995. *J Infect Dis.* 1999;179(Supplement_1):S76–S86. https://doi.org/10.1086/514306.
97. May L, Lung D, Harter K. An intervention to improve compliance with transmission precautions for influenza in the emergency department: successes and challenges. *J Emerg Med.* 2012;42(1):79–85. https://doi.org/10.1016/j.jemermed.2010.02.034.
98. Krein SL, Mayer J, Harrod M, et al. Identification and characterization of failures in infectious agent transmission precaution practices in hospitals: a qualitative study. *JAMA Intern Med.* 2018;178(8):1016–1057. https://doi.org/10.1001/jamainternmed.2018.1898.
99. Gershon RR, Vlahov D, Felknor SA, et al. Compliance with universal precautions among health care workers at three regional hospitals. *Am J Infect Control.* 1995;23(4):225–236 [In eng] https://doi.org/10.1016/0196-6553(95)90067-5.
100. Alhumaid S, Al Mutair A, Al Alawi Z, et al. Knowledge of infection prevention and control among healthcare workers and factors influencing compliance: a systematic review. *Antimicrob Resist Infect Control.* 2021;10(1):86. https://doi.org/10.1186/s13756-021-00957-0.
101. Tomas ME, Kundrapu S, Thota P, et al. Contamination of health care personnel during removal of personal protective equipment. *JAMA Intern Med.* 2015;175(12):1904–1910. https://doi.org/10.1001/jamainternmed.2015.4535.
102. Fischer 2nd WA, Hynes NA, Perl TM. Protecting health care workers from Ebola: personal protective equipment is critical but is not enough. *Ann Intern Med.* 2014;161(10):753–754. https://doi.org/10.7326/M14-1953.
103. Mumma JM, Durso FT, Casanova LM, et al. Common behaviors and faults when doffing personal protective equipment for patients with serious communicable diseases. *Clin Infect Dis.* 2019;69(Suppl. 3):S214–S220. https://doi.org/10.1093/cid/ciz614.
104. Chevalier MS, Chung W, Smith J, et al. Ebola virus disease cluster in the United States—Dallas County, Texas. *MMWR Morb Mortal Wkly Rep.* 2014;63(46):1087–1088 [In eng].
105. Beam E, Gibbs SG, Hewlett AL, Iwen PC, Nuss SL, Smith PW. Clinical challenges in isolation care. *Am J Nurs.* 2015;115(4):44–49 [In eng] https://doi.org/10.1097/01.Naj.0000463027.27141.32.
106. Kwon JH, Burnham CD, Reske KA, et al. Assessment of healthcare worker protocol deviations and self-contamination during personal protective equipment donning and doffing. *Infect Control Hosp Epidemiol.* 2017;38(9):1077–1083. https://doi.org/10.1017/ice.2017.121.
107. Hall S, Poller B, Bailey C, et al. Use of ultraviolet-fluorescence-based simulation in evaluation of personal protective equipment worn for first assessment and care of a patient with suspected high-consequence infectious disease. *J Hosp Infect.* 2018;99(2):218–228. https://doi.org/10.1016/j.jhin.2018.01.002.
108. Kman NE, Nelson RN. Infectious agents of bioterrorism: a review for emergency physicians. *Emerg Med Clin North Am.* 2008;26(2):517–547. x–xi [In eng] https://doi.org/10.1016/j.emc.2008.01.006.
109. Adalja AA, Toner E, Inglesby TV. Clinical management of potential bioterrorism-related conditions. *N Engl J Med.* 2015;372(10):954–962. https://doi.org/10.1056/NEJMra1409755.
110. Branda JA, Ruoff K. Bioterrorism. Clinical recognition and primary management. *Am J Clin Pathol.*

2002;117(Suppl):S116–S123 [In eng] https://doi.org/10.1309/5g7e-f5hq-3g6e-vqmb.
111. Moran GJ, Talan DA, Abrahamian FM. Biological terrorism. *Infect Dis Clin N Am.* 2008;22(1):145–187. vii. [In eng] https://doi.org/10.1016/j.idc.2007.12.003.
112. Brosh-Nissimov T. Lassa fever: another threat from West Africa. *Disaster Mil Med.* 2016;2:8 [In eng] https://doi.org/10.1186/s40696-016-0018-3.
113. Leffel EK, Reed DS. Marburg and Ebola viruses as aerosol threats. *Biosecur Bioterror.* 2004;2(3):186–191 [In eng] https://doi.org/10.1089/bsp.2004.2.186.
114. Osterholm MT, Moore KA, Kelley NS, et al. Transmission of Ebola viruses: what we know and what we do not know. *MBio.* 2015;6(2), e00137 [In eng] https://doi.org/10.1128/mBio.00137-15.

CHAPTER 23

Vaccines: Science and Public Health Applications

CHARLES-ANTOINE GUAY[a] • CAROLINE QUACH[b]
[a]Department of Medicine, Laval University, Quebec, QC, Canada • [b]Department of Microbiology, Infectiology, and Immunology, University of Montreal, Quebec, QC, Canada

INTRODUCTION

In recent years, the world has faced major challenges posed by emerging infectious diseases and pandemics. From the devastating impact of the severe acute respiratory syndrome coronavirus (SARS-CoV) outbreak to the reemerging threat from H5N1 and other avian influenza viruses or the emergence of Mpox, communities worldwide have been reminded repeatedly of the critical importance vaccines for infectious disease control and pandemic preparedness have played over the last decades.[1–3] The rapid development of several safe and effective vaccines against severe acute respiratory syndrome coronavirus 2 (SARS-CoV-2), which have contributed to contain the unprecedented COVID-19 pandemic, is the latest example of the essential role of vaccines in the ongoing fight against emerging and reemerging infectious diseases.[4]

Vaccines have long been recognized as one of the most effective public health interventions, capable of saving millions of lives and preventing widespread outbreaks. By stimulating the immune system to recognize and fight specific pathogens, vaccines offer a powerful tool in controlling infectious diseases. The development of promising new technologies such as the messenger RNA (mRNA) vaccines used against COVID-19[5,6] has allowed to generate rapid protection, despite complex challenges.

Susceptibility to infectious diseases and response to vaccines vary greatly between individuals, as highlighted by the overrepresentation of elderly individuals with comorbidities and immunocompromised individuals among deaths caused by COVID-19.[7–11] Furthermore, even less vulnerable populations can contribute significantly to the transmission of an infectious disease, and their vaccination can be essential to contain an ongoing outbreak.[12,13] Thus, decisions regarding whom to vaccinate, which vaccine to use, and when to vaccinate are crucial during an outbreak. Faced with uncertainty, policymakers and public health experts therefore need clear guidance to implement vaccination campaigns in a timely manner to help control outbreaks of emerging infectious diseases.

The objective of this chapter is to review the main concepts in the fields of immunology and public health that are useful for a better understanding of how vaccines can be a crucial tool for pandemic preparedness. It also discusses the main vaccine technologies and introduces those that are most promising for rapid deployment during an outbreak of an emerging infectious disease. Finally, it highlights the main criteria that should be used to prioritize target populations when developing a vaccination campaign against and during an epidemic.

VACCINE IMMUNOLOGY

Vaccines protect by inducing an immune response capable of rapidly controlling replicating pathogens or inactivating their virulent factors. The main effectors of the vaccine-mediated protection comprise antibodies produced by B lymphocytes capable of binding specifically a toxin or a pathogen (i.e., humoral immunity) and T lymphocytes (i.e., $CD4^+$ T-helper and cytotoxic $CD8^+$ T lymphocytes, cellular immunity).[14–16] Most vaccines trigger both humoral and cellular immunity, and both responses should be considered when identifying a correlate of protection.[17–19]

Viral Outbreaks, Biosecurity, and Preparing for Mass Casualty Infectious Diseases Events
https://doi.org/10.1016/B978-0-323-54841-0.00009-3

Innate Immunity

The human immune system consists of two main components: innate and adaptive immunity. While shaping adaptive immunity is the primary objective for most vaccines, innate immunity plays a lesser known, however essential role in the immune response to vaccines. The activation of B and T lymphocytes by specific antigen-presenting cells, such as dendritic cells, is crucial in the induction of an antigen-specific immune response after vaccination. When exposed to pathogens in tissues or at the vaccine injection site, immature dendritic cells mature and acquire specific surface receptors before migrating to secondary lymph nodes, where B and T lymphocytes will be activated. Other important components of the innate immunity include monocytes and neutrophils, which, alongside dendritic cells, produce pro-inflammatory cytokines and chemokines that, in turn, induce an essential inflammatory reaction to activate dendritic cells and trigger their migration to the draining lymph nodes. It is worth noting that one of the main mechanisms for enhanced vaccine response through adjuvants is the modulation of these crucial innate immunity pathways.[20]

In recent years, a growing body of evidence has challenged the dogma that only adaptive immunity exhibits immune memory.[21] The term "trained immunity" was introduced to describe the functional reprogramming of innate immune cells, including monocytes, macrophages, and natural killer cells, following exposure to endogenous and exogenous stimuli, whether through natural exposure or after vaccination. Trained immunity leads to an altered response, either enhancing cells' ability to mount more robust and rapid responses upon subsequent encounters with unrelated pathogens but also explaining the hypo-response following a second challenge by certain antigens (e.g., PS), and adjusting this response in time and context.[22] Mechanistically, epigenetic modifications and metabolic rewiring play pivotal roles in orchestrating this innate cellular memory, which can be maintained for extended periods without the direct involvement of adaptive immune components. However, trained immunity can be a reversible phenomenon and typically has a shorter duration than the classical adaptive immune memory.[23] Nonetheless, this novel aspect of immune memory opens new avenues for understanding and optimizing immune defenses, thereby paving the way for innovative strategies in vaccine development and disease prevention.

Adaptative Immunity

Specific and long-lasting protection against infectious diseases by the immune system requires effective adaptive immunity. Both humoral and cellular immunity mediate the adaptative immune response. B lymphocytes produce antibodies that can bind to and neutralize pathogens, while T lymphocytes play various roles, including directly killing infected cells (i.e., $CD8^+$ T lymphocytes) and coordinating immune responses (i.e., $CD4^+$ T lymphocytes). The key feature of adaptive immunity is its ability to generate immune memory, which vaccines exploit to induce long-lasting protection against a pathogen without causing the disease.[24] When the immune system encounters a specific pathogen for the first time, naïve B lymphocytes and T lymphocytes, after first being activated by specific antigen-presenting cells, and then undergoing clonal expansion and differentiation, leading to the production of effector cells that eliminate the pathogen. During this initial response, some of these cells transform into memory cells. This memory enables a swift and robust response upon subsequent encounters with the same pathogen, providing long-lasting protection.[25]

Classically, the cascade leading to the production of antigen-specific antibodies by activated B lymphocytes can be divided into two different pathways: a T-dependent response and a T-independent response.[26] The T-dependent response to vaccines represents a sophisticated and finely orchestrated immune process that underlies the generation of durable and effective immunity against pathogens. Following their activations by dendritic cells, antigen-specific $CD4^+$ T lymphocytes release a range of cytokines that are essential both to the activation of naïve B lymphocytes and to trigger clonal expansion and their differentiation in plasma cells or memory B lymphocytes.[27,28] During the proliferation of plasma cells, immunoglobulins (Ig) undergo a class switch from IgM to IgG, IgA, and IgE, which are characteristic of the secondary immune response (i.e., after exposure to a booster antigen) and gain affinity for their specific antigen.[29] This reaction occurs over a couple of weeks in a specific lymph node structure called germinal centers, such that specific IgG against vaccine antigens may only appear 10 to 14 days after vaccination.[30] This delay explains, in part, why vaccinated individuals remain susceptible in the first 2 weeks after vaccination and why cases that occur during this period are not counted in the vaccinated group in efficacy trials. Additionally, the germinal center reaction typically ends within 4 to 6 weeks, which corresponds to the peak of IgG following primary immunization.[31] This T-dependent response plays a major role in the mechanism of action of most vaccine types outside of polysaccharide (PS) vaccines (Table 1).

TABLE 1
Vaccine Types: Main Characteristics and Examples

Vaccine Type	Main Characteristics	Examples
Live attenuated	Contains weakened but live pathogens, which can replicate to stimulate a strong immune response	MMR, yellow fever, varicella (chickenpox, shingles, i.e., zostavax)
Inactivated	Contains inactivated or killed pathogens or their components	Cholera, hepatitis A, polio, rabies
Subunit	Contains only specific antigens or parts of the pathogen, which reduces the risk of adverse reactions	Hepatitis B, HPV, influenza
Polysaccharide	Contains purified polysaccharides from the pathogen, which can stimulate an immune response to the capsule of certain bacteria	Meningococcal PS, pneumococcal PS
Conjugate	Attaches pathogen antigens to a carrier molecule, enhancing the immune response, especially in infants and young children	Hib, pneumococcal conjugates
Recombinant	Uses genetic engineering techniques to produce specific pathogen antigens in a host organism, such as bacteria or yeast	Hepatitis B, shingles (i.e., shingrix)
Viral vector	Utilizes a harmless virus as a carrier to deliver genetic material that instructs cells to produce pathogen antigens, triggering an immune response	SARS-CoV-2
mRNA-based	Uses messenger RNA to provide instructions for antigen production within cells, triggering an immune response	SARS-CoV-2
DNA-based	Uses a plasmid containing pathogen DNA to provide instructions for antigen production within cells, triggering an immune response	None[a]

Abbreviations: *Hib*, *Haemophilus influenzae* type b; *HPV*, human papillomavirus; *MMR*, measles, mumps, and rubella; *PS*, polysaccharide; *SARS-CoV-2*, severe acute respiratory syndrome coronavirus 2.
[a]There are no DNA-based vaccines currently approved for human use outside of India, where a COVID-19 DNA vaccine received Emergency Use Authorization during the pandemic.

The T-independent response to vaccines allows for an effective defense against certain pathogens in the absence of T lymphocytes. PS antigens, through direct activation in the lymph nodes marginal zone, trigger signaling pathways leading to B cell activation, proliferation, and subsequent differentiation into antibody-secreting plasma cells. However, unlike the T-dependent response, the T-independent pathway typically generates a less diverse antibody repertoire with lower affinity and only partial immune memory.[32] PS vaccines are thus generally known to induce moderate titers of low-affinity antibodies and an absence of immune memory.[33–35]

Immunogenicity

Initial Phase 2 and Phase 3 clinical trials (see Chapter 24) normally include an immunogenicity outcome to evaluate a new vaccine protective response.[36,37] Immunogenicity refers to the vaccine's ability to provoke an immune response. However, immunogenicity does not necessarily imply long-term protection.[19,38] Although early vaccines protective efficacy is primarily conferred by the induction of antigen-specific antibodies, which is the main marker of immunogenicity in clinical trials, it may be insufficient for long-term protection. Cellular immunity, persistence of vaccine antibodies above protective thresholds, and maintenance of immune memory cells capable of rapid and effective reactivation with subsequent pathogen exposure must also be considered in the evaluation of the immune response to a vaccine.[39]

In fact, identifying reliable correlates of protection is a complex yet critical goal when developing a new vaccine. It serves as a surrogate marker for vaccine efficacy and can be used to guide vaccine development or identify possible waning in immunity through sero-surveillance and decrease the burden of clinical trials based on clinical efficacy, allowing for bridging with immune correlates of protection.[36,40] Moreover, correlates of protection are major tools in the context of emerging infectious diseases, as they allow for rapid assessment of vaccine efficacy against newly identified pathogens and aid in the implementation of targeted vaccination strategies.[37]

Determinants of Vaccine Response

Vaccine efficacy against COVID-19 has differed greatly, decreasing in older age groups and in immunocompromised individuals.[11,41] A similar heterogeneity in vaccine response was observed for seasonal influenza and the H1N1 pandemic strain.[42,43] Moreover, major differences in vaccine efficacy may exist between types of vaccines targeting the same pathogen.[44,45] Numerous determinants modulate both the primary vaccine antibody response and the long-term vaccine-mediated protection. One of the main determinants is the nature of the vaccine antigen and its intrinsic immunogenicity, which may differ between vaccine types. For example, live-attenuated vaccines generally induce a more sustained antibody response compared to inactivated vaccines. By closely resembling the natural infectious process, live attenuated vaccines most efficiently trigger both humoral and cellular immune responses through multiple pathogen-associated signals.[46] Conversely, nonlive vaccines mainly rely on the local activation of immune responses at their injection site, which typically results in lower peaks of antigen-specific antibodies and the need for multiple boosters to maintain long-term protection.[47,48]

By definition, a healthy immune system is needed for an efficient vaccine response. As a result, any immunosuppression may hamper vaccines' immunogenicity. For instance, a large metaanalysis found that individuals who underwent organ transplantation were 16 times less likely to seroconvert compared to immune-competent individuals after receiving COVID-19 vaccines.[41] Similar results were obtained for individuals with solid cancers, hematologic malignancies, and, to a lesser degree, immune-mediated inflammatory disorders. Most often, immunocompromised individuals will require more doses for their primary series to induce a satisfactory immune response and will need more frequent booster doses to maintain a certain level of protection.[49,50]

Age plays a crucial role in shaping the immune response to vaccination, with distinct patterns observed in the extremes of age. In early life, interference from maternal antibodies and the relative immaturity of the immune system can reduce the efficacy and duration of vaccine-induced immunity in infants and children.[51,52] For instance, responses to most PS vaccines are not elicited during the first 2 years of life because of age-dependent antigen-presenting cell function,[53,54] thus requiring PS conjugation to a protein carrier to transform the immune response into a T-dependent one, overcoming the hypo-response. Therefore, these unique characteristics must be considered when developing a vaccination schedule. It is necessary to find the right balance between an enhanced vaccine response and the risk posed by the specific infectious disease. Additionally, elderly individuals often experience immunosenescence, a gradual decline in immune function associated with aging. The hallmark features of immunosenescence include a decline in the diversity and functionality of both T and B lymphocytes, impaired antigen presentation, dysregulation of cytokine production, and a shift toward pro-inflammatory states.[55] This age-related decline can lead to reduced vaccine responses characterized by lower antibody production, and diminished cellular immune responses. Consequently, vaccines in older populations often require higher antigen doses, adjuvants, or alternative vaccination strategies, as observed with the administration of additional doses of the COVID-19 vaccines in the elderly, to overcome immunosenescence and achieve optimal protection.[11,56]

TYPES OF VACCINE

Edward Jenner's first vaccine used a whole live cowpox virus to protect against its human counterpart, smallpox.[57] Since Jenner's first vaccine, a range of vaccine types have been developed, protecting against diverse pathogens (Table 1); however, important distinctions must be made between live attenuated vaccines and nonlive vaccines.

Live Attenuated Vaccines

Live attenuated vaccines are derived from live viruses or bacteria, whose virulence has been reduced through laboratory or genetic manipulations. By closely reproducing the natural infection process, live attenuated vaccines can elicit both humoral and cellular immune responses, providing comprehensive and long-lasting immunity (see vaccine immunology above). Examples of live attenuated vaccines include the Measles, Mumps, Rubella vaccine (MMR), the varicella vaccine, the oral rotavirus and polio vaccines, the yellow fever vaccine, and the Japanese encephalitis vaccine, among others (Table 1). The immune response induced by live attenuated vaccines is achieved through the systemic recognition of antigens after the injection or mucosal exposure. They generally produce fewer local reactions and more systemic reactions than nonlive vaccines.[46,48] Systemic reactions can occur several days after exposure, reflecting the underlying immunological response that mimics the natural infection process. The vaccination schedule is also influenced by the type of vaccine. Indeed, the recommended interval between two doses of the same vaccine or between two different live-attenuated vaccines is generally 4 weeks. This timeframe allows for the induction of the immune response and, specifically, for the germinal center reaction to be completed.[30]

An important limitation to live attenuated vaccines is that they are generally contraindicated in pregnant women and in severely immunocompromised individuals. In both cases, this caution results from the possibility that the attenuated virus or bacteria used in the vaccine could cause severe systemic disease, even in its attenuated form. Additionally, the immune response elicited by live attenuated vaccines, which involves replication of the weakened pathogen in the body, may pose a theoretical risk to the developing fetus.[58] Therefore, pregnant women and immunocompromised individuals are typically advised to receive nonlive vaccines. However, there are exceptions to this general rule, such as situations where the risk of exposure to a specific disease outweighs the potential risks associated with the live attenuated vaccine. In such cases, careful evaluation by healthcare professionals should weigh the benefits and potential risks for the individual.

Nonlive Vaccines

Unlike live attenuated vaccines, nonlive vaccines do not contain live organisms and instead rely on different strategies to stimulate the immune response. There are several types of inactivated vaccines (see Table 1). Inactivated vaccines are composed of whole, inactivated pathogens or their components, such as proteins or polysaccharides. Subunit vaccines, on the other hand, consist of purified antigens derived from the pathogen. By presenting the immune system with specific components of the pathogen, nonlive vaccines trigger an immune response without causing the disease. However, in the absence of microbial replication, vaccine-induced immune response remains more limited, and several booster doses may be needed to achieve a sustained immune memory and long-lasting protection.[48] The site and route of administration are also more important than for live vaccines since vaccine response depends on the local recognition of antigens (see "Vaccine Immunology" section). As a result of this local activation of the immune system, nonlive vaccines can lead to local inflammatory reactions, at the injection site within 24 h of vaccination, including redness, warmth, and tenderness. Axillary or inguinal lymphadenopathy following injection may also occur. Nonlive vaccines can be administered concomitantly at different sites without a minimal interval, which justifies the development of combined vaccines.[59] A trend toward lower antibody responses with concomitant vaccine administration was observed in immunogenicity studies for vaccines such as COVID-19, pneumococcal, and influenza vaccines.[60–62] However, current evidence does not suggest that this lower antibody response translates into lower vaccine efficacy or effectiveness.[61,62] Although manufacturers often suggest a minimal interval of 3 weeks between primary doses of the same vaccine and a minimal interval of 4 months between priming and boosting to allow sufficient antibody response and memory cell development, we know that the longer the interval between doses, the more robust and long-lasting the immune response.[63] Extending the interval between doses enables the maturation of memory lymphocytes, resulting in a higher affinity for the antigen and a more potent immune response, ultimately enhancing the overall effectiveness of the vaccine. This important principle of vaccinology allowed the National Advisory Committee on Immunization (NACI) in Canada to recommend an extended interval between primary COVID-19 vaccine doses to maximize the number of people protected against COVID-19 at the beginning of 2021 in the context of an inadequate vaccine supply.[64] This recommendation was soon followed by other national advisory committees.[65] Another important advantage of nonlive vaccines is that they are generally considered safe and suitable for individuals with weakened immune systems, including pregnant women and immunocompromised individuals. However, in these circumstances, their effectiveness may be reduced.[66]

New Technologies

One major drawback of old technologies such as live attenuated vaccines and even inactivated vaccines is the time needed for their development.[46,48] The COVID-19 pandemic has highlighted the great potential of nucleic acid-based vaccines for pandemic preparedness, such as mRNA, DNA, and viral vector vaccines. These vaccines utilize the pathogen's genetic material, encoding specific viral proteins, to induce the host immune response. The mRNA vaccines, such as those developed against COVID-19, deliver a synthetic messenger RNA into lipid nanoparticles, which instruct cells to produce viral antigens, thereby triggering an immune response (Fig. 1).[67] Similarly, DNA vaccines introduce a plasmid containing the pathogen's genetic information into cells, stimulating the production of viral proteins, while viral DNA vector vaccines utilize harmless viruses, such as human adenoviruses, to deliver genetic material that stimulates the production of viral proteins.[68] In both cases, the production of viral proteins by cells triggers

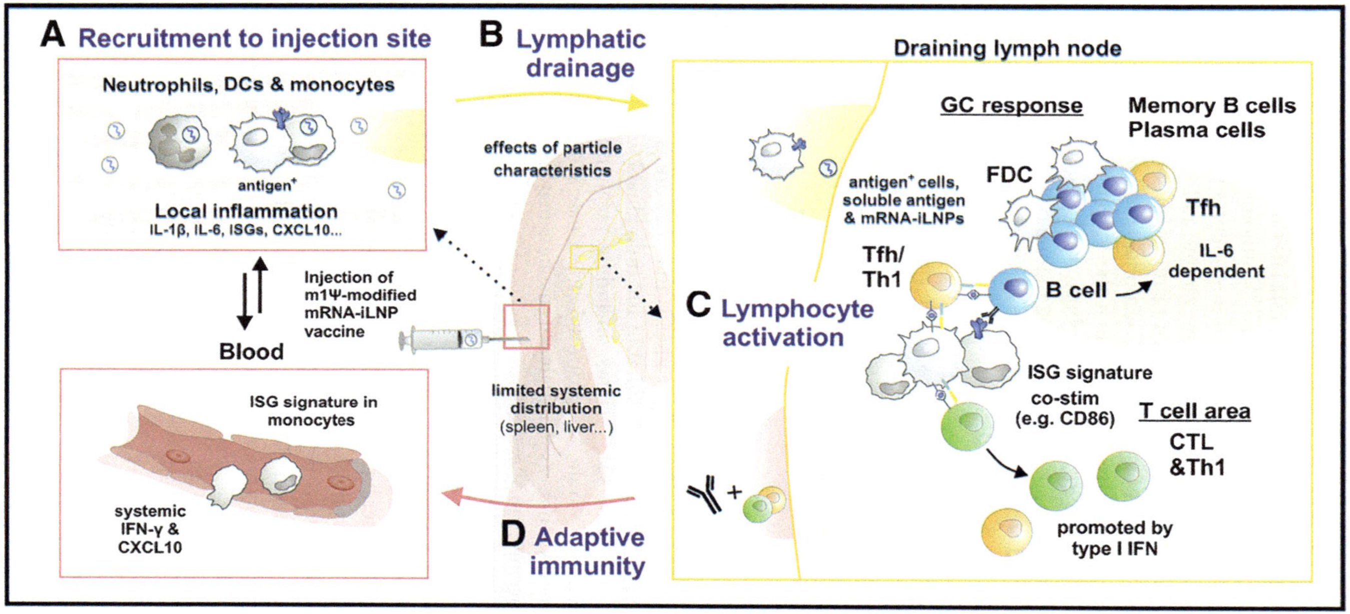

FIG. 1 Bio distribution and innate immune cell dynamics upon administration of mRNA-iLNP vaccines. (A) Intramuscular administration of nucleoside-modified mRNA-iLNP vaccines results in local inflammation, which recruits neutrophils, monocytes, and various dendritic cell (DC) subsets from the blood to the injection site by production of chemokines and other inflammatory mediators contributing to the extravasation of immune cells. (B) mRNA-iLNPs and/or antigen-expressing cells are transported to the draining lymph node. The size and surface properties of the particles can impact biodistribution, protein absorption (opsonization), and cellular uptake. (C) DCs and monocytes/macrophages contribute to antigen presentation and priming of T cells. (D) T follicular helper (Tfh) cells provide help to B cells in germinal center (GC) reactions in the presence of follicular DCs, leading to affinity maturation. In mice, an important role for iLNP-induced IL-6 was found in the induction of Tfh and GC B cell responses, while type I IFNs promoted CTL responses. Abbreviations: *m1Ψ*, N1-methylpseudouridine; *iLNP*, ionizable lipid nanoparticle; *IL*, interleukin; *IFN*, interferon; *ISG*, interferon-stimulated gene; *CXCL10*, C-X-C motif chemokine ligand 10; *CD86*, cluster of differentiation 86; *FDC*, follicular dendritic cell; *CTL*, cytotoxic T lymphocyte; *Th1*, T-helper 1. (Reprinted with permission from Verbeke R, Hogan MJ, Loré K, Pardi N. Innate immune mechanisms of mRNA vaccines. *Immunity*. 2022;55(11):1993–2005. Copyright © 2022 Elsevier Inc.)

an immune response, leading to the development of immunity against the pathogen.

One significant advantage of nucleic acid-based vaccines is their rapid development and production capacities. During a pandemic or an uncontrolled outbreak where speed is of the essence, these vaccines can be designed and manufactured in a relatively short time frame. Because nucleic acid-based vaccines do not rely on the actual pathogen's culture in laboratories, the required genetic information can be swiftly disseminated to production sites worldwide, enabling an unprecedented acceleration in vaccine development and production.[69] Additionally, their versatility allows for rapid modification to target emerging variants, such as the numerous variants that have emerged following the original SARS-CoV-2.[70] For instance, it took only a few months to adapt the two main mRNA vaccines available to provide protection against the highly contagious Omicron variant of SARS-CoV-2.[71] Nucleic acid-based vaccines are thus likely to play a crucial role in pandemic preparedness due to their unique characteristics. Despite their great success in combating viral diseases, nucleic acid-based vaccines have not yet demonstrated their efficacy against bacteria or higher-order organisms (such as malaria), where rapid development still poses a significant challenge.[72]

VACCINES AS A PUBLIC HEALTH TOOL

A comprehensive understanding of how vaccines confer immunity is crucial for designing effective control measures in response to public health emergencies, but infectious diseases epidemiology and public health notions are essential to properly guide policymaking.

Vaccine Effectiveness

Immunogenicity does not necessarily translate to vaccine effectiveness. The numerous failed attempts to find an effective vaccine against *Staphylococcus aureus* infections after promising results in Phase II trials is a good example of the latter statement.[73] Vaccine efficacy refers to the capacity of a vaccine to decrease the occurrence of a disease or its effects among those who have been vaccinated. In epidemiological terms, it quantifies the percentage decrease in disease incidence that can be attributed to vaccination.[74] Vaccine efficacy is best assessed in Phase III randomized controlled clinical trials, where one group of participants is administered the vaccine, and another placebo. Although crucial for decision-making, vaccine efficacy only represents the ability of a vaccine to prevent disease under ideal conditions.[36] Vaccine efficacy is influenced by factors such as the vaccine's immunogenicity, formulation, dosage, and administration schedule. Furthermore, it can vary across different populations, age groups, and even against different strains or variants of a pathogen. Vaccine efficacy will also vary depending on the outcomes studied. For instance, vaccine efficacy against COVID-19 was much higher and longer-lasting against severe forms of the disease (i.e., hospitalizations and deaths) than against asymptomatic or even mild infections and transmission.[75] The efficacy of a vaccine can also be influenced by the specificity of outcomes measured. For example, the vaccine efficacy of the pneumococcal polysaccharide conjugated vaccine is much higher against pneumococcal community-acquired pneumonia compared to all-cause community-acquired pneumonia.[76]

Of greater importance when one wants to evaluate the actual performance of a vaccine in a vaccinated population under real-life conditions, is vaccine effectiveness. Vaccine effectiveness depends on vaccine efficacy, host characteristics, immunization coverage, and variations in the administration of the vaccine.[36] It will also vary depending on the pathogen's circulation. Indeed, exposure to the disease is an important confounder in epidemiological studies that try to assess vaccine effectiveness and may explain disparity in vaccine effectiveness between countries during a pandemic.[74,77,78] Additionally, vaccine effectiveness encompasses both direct protection of vaccinated individuals and indirect effects, such as herd immunity, which shields unvaccinated individuals from infection. Finally, during a pandemic, vaccine effectiveness can be assessed in real-time, which enables monitoring of long-lasting immunity within a vaccinated population and facilitates the prompt identification of potential waning in immunity. This latter feature was exploited by different jurisdictions during the COVID-19 pandemic to optimize vaccine strategies and mitigate the impact of the epidemic.[79–81] The test-negative design, a modified case-control study first introduced to assess vaccine effectiveness against influenza, is a powerful tool used for monitoring vaccine effectiveness against COVID-19.[82,83] In a test-negative design study, controls are selected among individuals who test negative for a particular disease. It leverages the fact that individuals seeking medical care for symptoms consistent with the disease are more likely to undergo diagnostic testing, regardless of their vaccination status. Vaccine effectiveness against influenza measured using a test-negative design has been found to closely resemble the efficacy values obtained in randomized controlled trials.[84–86] Despite its strengths, the test-negative design also has limitations. Indeed, it assumes that the likelihood of seeking healthcare and of being tested for the disease is unrelated to vaccination status. However, there may be unmeasured factors that affect both vaccination status and testing behavior, potentially introducing cofounding in the absence of randomization.[87]

Vaccine Coverage

Vaccines have provided a rare opportunity in human history: to eradicate a specific disease through human intervention. This dream was achieved once when smallpox was officially eradicated in 1980.[88] Eradication of an infectious disease is possible when the human is the only reservoir and when adequate herd immunity is achieved. Herd immunity occurs when a significant portion of the population is immune to a specific infectious disease, either through vaccination or prior infection, thereby reducing the transmission of the pathogen within the population. Herd immunity not only protects those who have not been vaccinated, including those who are unable to be vaccinated due to medical reasons, but also helps prevent deadly outbreaks in a population even after the disease is eliminated from a territory.[89] The threshold required for herd immunity depends on the infectiousness of the disease, usually estimated by the basic reproduction number (see Chapter 17) and vaccine effectiveness.[89] It also depends on the homogeneity of transmission in the population.[90] For highly contagious diseases, such as measles, a high vaccine coverage rate, typically above 90%–95%, is necessary to achieve herd immunity. Unfortunately, even with high vaccine coverage, a breakthrough outbreak is still possible, as seen in 2014–15 with a large measles outbreak across multiple states and provinces in the United States and Canada.[91,92] Such outbreaks typically originate in, though not exclusively limited to, communities with low vaccination coverage where vaccine hesitancy is widespread. Monitoring vaccine coverage and ensuring high immunization coverage are, thus, vital in maintaining herd immunity and preventing the resurgence of vaccine-preventable diseases.

Vaccine Hesitancy

Vaccine hesitancy represents another significant challenge to public health efforts in preventing and controlling infectious diseases during and after a pandemic. Vaccine hesitancy is described as a state of indecision and uncertainty that precedes the decision of whether to receive a vaccine.[93] It is influenced by various factors, including individual beliefs, attitudes, and concerns about vaccine safety, efficacy, and need.[94] Distrust in healthcare systems or vaccine manufacturers can also contribute to vaccine hesitancy, as highlighted during the COVID-19 pandemic, and it was further amplified by the surge in misinformation.[95] Furthermore, macro-level factors, such as the political context and the public's attention to a particular vaccine, influence vaccine hesitancy.[96] The consequences of vaccine hesitancy can be far-reaching, leading to decreased vaccine coverage, increased vulnerability to outbreaks, and the potential resurgence of vaccine-preventable diseases. To increase vaccine acceptance at an individual level, healthcare providers must provide support, encouragement, and attentively consider the patient's perspective and concerns.[97] At the population level, addressing vaccine hesitancy requires a comprehensive approach that involves engaging with communities, addressing concerns through transparent communication, providing accurate information, and building trust in the safety and effectiveness of vaccines. Thus, communication strategies tailored to vaccine hesitancy need to be implemented as part of broader pandemic preparedness.

Decision-Making Framework

To guide decision-making, advisory committees such as NACI in Canada and the Advisory Committee on Immunization Practices (ACIP) in the United States have employed specific criteria for comprehensive and systematic evaluation of all relevant factors that should be considered.[98–101] These criteria include factors such as the burden of disease (i.e., infection prevalence, hospitalization rates, mortality), vaccine characteristics (i.e., vaccine efficacy and safety), acceptability, feasibility, and cost-effectiveness. Additionally, ethical considerations have gained significant importance in decision-making processes over the past decade.[101]

As such, when an infectious disease outbreak occurs, policymakers are often faced with the challenging dilemma of deciding whom to prioritize for vaccination due to limited vaccine supply. For instance, as COVID-19 vaccines became gradually available toward the end of 2020, countries had to make choices on whether to prioritize vaccination of healthcare personnel, workers in essential industries, or vulnerable individuals.[102] To ensure priority-setting that reflects the values of the population, the recommendations of the NACI in Canada were informed by several surveys conducted among the general population.[103] For example, surveys conducted after the initial prioritization guidance from NACI for COVID-19 vaccination confirmed that the most important vaccination strategy for both the general population and experts was to protect the most vulnerable individuals from severe illness and death during the period of initial vaccine scarcity.[104] These surveys thus ensured that experts' recommendations were aligned with the priorities of the general public throughout the many waves of the pandemic and the evolving availability of vaccines. Nonetheless, during a pandemic, safeguarding the integrity of the healthcare system is of utmost importance and has been acknowledged by public health authorities in recent outbreaks. As a result, healthcare personnel, as well as essential workers involved in vaccine production, are typically prioritized.[104,105] This prioritization ensures that those who are directly involved in caring for patients and maintaining critical healthcare services are protected early on, reducing the risk of healthcare system overload, and enabling them to continue providing essential care to the population.

Furthermore, ensuring equitable access to vaccines should be a critical component of global health efforts during a pandemic. This is essential to effectively mitigate ongoing transmission of the infection and reduce the potential emergence of new variants. Vaccine equity involves providing fair distribution of vaccines to address disparities and prioritize vulnerable populations. To achieve vaccine equity, proactive measures are essential, such as targeted outreach programs, community engagement, culturally sensitive communication, and removing financial and logistical barriers to access.[106] Collaboration between governments, international organizations, manufacturers, and civil society is crucial in promoting equitable vaccine distribution and mitigating the disproportionate burden of disease in marginalized populations.

Ultimately, in emergency situations such as a pandemic, the off-label use of vaccines, which refers to using a vaccine in a manner not specifically approved by regulatory agencies, can be considered as a potential solution to accelerate disease control. This approach allows for flexibility and adaptation to rapidly changing situations and knowledge, potentially increasing the number of people vaccinated and thus speeding up disease control.[107] For example, the extended interval between the primary doses of the COVID-19 vaccine, which differs from the manufacturer's recommended 3-week interval, maximized the number of people protected against COVID-19, while potentially increasing effectiveness.[108,109] However, it is important to note that recommendations for vaccine off-label use should be based on scientific evidence, expert guidance, and careful risk-benefit assessments to ensure safety and effectiveness of such an approach.

CONCLUSION

In conclusion, vaccines are indispensable tools for pandemic preparedness. They have the potential to control and prevent the spread of infectious diseases. However, their development, distribution, and administration must be guided by a thorough understanding of vaccine immunology, determinants of vaccine response, and the specific characteristics of the target population. Continued investment in vaccine research and development, along with robust public health policies, will ensure that vaccines remain effective tools in combating future pandemics and emerging infectious diseases.

REFERENCES

1. Cherry JD, Krogstad P. SARS: the first pandemic of the 21st century. *Pediatr Res.* 2004;56(1):1–5.
2. Huang P, Sun L, Li J, et al. Potential cross-species transmission of highly pathogenic avian influenza H5 subtype (HPAI H5) viruses to humans calls for the development of H5-specific and universal influenza vaccines. *Cell Discov.* 2023;9(1):58.
3. Lum FM, Torres-Ruesta A, Tay MZ, et al. Monkeypox: disease epidemiology, host immunity and clinical interventions. *Nat Rev Immunol.* 2022;22(10):597–613.
4. Hu B, Guo H, Zhou P, Shi ZL. Characteristics of SARS-CoV-2 and COVID-19. *Nat Rev Microbiol.* 2021;19(3):141–154.
5. Polack FP, Thomas SJ, Kitchin N, et al. Safety and efficacy of the BNT162b2 mRNA Covid-19 vaccine. *N Engl J Med.* 2020;383(27):2603–2615.
6. Mulligan MJ, Lyke KE, Kitchin N, et al. Phase I/II study of COVID-19 RNA vaccine BNT162b1 in adults. *Nature.* 2020;586(7830):589–593.
7. Mohammed AH, Blebil A, Dujaili J, Rasool-Hassan BA. The risk and impact of COVID-19 pandemic on immunosuppressed patients: cancer, HIV, and solid organ transplant recipients. *AIDS Rev.* 2020;22(3):151–157.
8. Ssentongo P, Heilbrunn ES, Ssentongo AE, et al. Epidemiology and outcomes of COVID-19 in HIV-infected individuals: a systematic review and meta-analysis. *Sci Rep.* 2021;11(1):6283.
9. Baden LR, El Sahly HM, Essink B, et al. Efficacy and safety of the mRNA-1273 SARS-CoV-2 vaccine. *N Engl J Med.* 2021;384(5):403–416.
10. Liu K, Chen Y, Lin R, Han K. Clinical features of COVID-19 in elderly patients: a comparison with young and middle-aged patients. *J Infect.* 2020;80(6):e14–e18.
11. Andrews N, Tessier E, Stowe J, et al. Duration of protection against mild and severe disease by Covid-19 vaccines. *N Engl J Med.* 2022;386(4):340–350.
12. Mossong J, Hens N, Jit M, et al. Social contacts and mixing patterns relevant to the spread of infectious diseases. *PLoS Med.* 2008;5(3):e74.

13. Richterman A, Meyerowitz EA, Cevik M. Indirect protection by reducing transmission: ending the pandemic with severe acute respiratory syndrome coronavirus 2 vaccination. *Open Forum Infect Dis.* 2022;9(2), ofab259.
14. Cooper NR, Nemerow GR. The role of antibody and complement in the control of viral infections. *J Invest Dermatol.* 1984;83(1 Suppl):121s–127s.
15. Cooper MD. The early history of B cells. *Nat Rev Immunol.* 2015;15(3):191–197.
16. Sakaguchi S, Wing K, Miyara M. Regulatory T cells—a brief history and perspective. *Eur J Immunol.* 2007;37(S1):S116–S123.
17. Spensieri F, Siena E, Borgogni E, et al. Early rise of blood T follicular helper cell subsets and baseline immunity as predictors of persisting late functional antibody responses to vaccination in humans. *PLoS One.* 2016;11(6):e0157066.
18. Spensieri F, Borgogni E, Zedda L, et al. Human circulating influenza-CD4+ICOS1+IL-21+T cells expand after vaccination, exert helper function, and predict antibody responses. *Proc Natl Acad Sci USA.* 2013;110(35):14330–14335.
19. Khoury DS, Schlub TE, Cromer D, et al. Correlates of protection, thresholds of protection, and immunobridging among persons with SARS-CoV-2 infection. *Emerg Infect Dis.* 2023;29(2):381–388.
20. Töpfer E, Boraschi D, Italiani P. Innate immune memory: the latest frontier of adjuvanticity. *J Immunol Res.* 2015;2015:478408.
21. Netea MG, Domínguez-Andrés J, Barreiro LB, et al. Defining trained immunity and its role in health and disease. *Nat Rev Immunol.* 2020;20(6):375–388.
22. Novakovic B, Habibi E, Wang SY, et al. β-Glucan reverses the epigenetic state of LPS-induced immunological tolerance. *Cell.* 2016;167(5):1354–1368.e14.
23. Xing Z, Afkhami S, Bavananthasivam J, et al. Innate immune memory of tissue-resident macrophages and trained innate immunity: re-vamping vaccine concept and strategies. *J Leukoc Biol.* 2020;108(3):825–834.
24. Charles A, Janeway J, Travers P, Walport M, Shlomchik MJ. Immunological memory. In: *Immunobiology: The Immune System in Health and Disease.* 5th ed. Garland Science; 2001. [Internet]. [cited 2023 Jul 12]. Available from: https://www.ncbi.nlm.nih.gov/books/NBK27158/.
25. Palm AKE, Henry C. Remembrance of things past: long-term B cell memory after infection and vaccination. *Front Immunol.* 2019;10:1787.
26. Goodnow CC, Vinuesa CG, Randall KL, Mackay F, Brink R. Control systems and decision making for antibody production. *Nat Immunol.* 2010;11(8):681–688.
27. Paus D, Phan TG, Chan TD, Gardam S, Basten A, Brink R. Antigen recognition strength regulates the choice between extrafollicular plasma cell and germinal center B cell differentiation. *J Exp Med.* 2006;203(4):1081–1091.
28. Barra NG, Gillgrass A, Ashkar AA. Effective control of viral infections by the adaptive immune system requires assistance from innate immunity. *Expert Rev Vaccines.* 2010;9(10):1143–1147.
29. Deenick EK, Hasbold J, Hodgkin PD. Decision criteria for resolving isotype switching conflicts by B cells. *Eur J Immunol.* 2005;35(10):2949–2955.
30. Mesin L, Ersching J, Victora GD. Germinal center B cell dynamics. *Immunity.* 2016;45(3):471–482.
31. Wolniak KL, Shinall SM, Waldschmidt TJ. The germinal center response. *Crit Rev Immunol.* 2004;24(1):39–65.
32. MacLennan ICM, Toellner KM, Cunningham AF, et al. Extrafollicular antibody responses. *Immunol Rev.* 2003;194:8–18.
33. O'Brien KL, Hochman M, Goldblatt D. Combined schedules of pneumococcal conjugate and polysaccharide vaccines: is hyporesponsiveness an issue? *Lancet Infect Dis.* 2007;7(9):597–606.
34. Poolman J, Borrow R. Hyporesponsiveness and its clinical implications after vaccination with polysaccharide or glycoconjugate vaccines. *Expert Rev Vaccines.* 2011;10(3):307–322.
35. González-Fernández A, Faro J, Fernández C. Immune responses to polysaccharides: lessons from humans and mice. *Vaccine.* 2008;26(3):292–300.
36. Fedson DS. Measuring protection: efficacy versus effectiveness. *Dev Biol Stand.* 1998;95:195–201.
37. Excler JL, Saville M, Berkley S, Kim JH. Vaccine development for emerging infectious diseases. *Nat Med.* 2021;27(4):591–600.
38. Plotkin SA. Correlates of protection induced by vaccination. *Clin Vaccine Immunol.* 2010;17(7):1055–1065.
39. Plotkin SA, Gilbert PB. Nomenclature for immune correlates of protection after vaccination. *Clin Infect Dis.* 2012;54(11):1615–1617.
40. Fritzell B. Bridging studies. *Dev Biol Stand.* 1998;95:181–188.
41. Lee ARYB, Wong SY, Chai LYA, et al. Efficacy of covid-19 vaccines in immunocompromised patients: systematic review and meta-analysis. *BMJ.* 2022;376, e068632.
42. Belongia EA, Simpson MD, King JP, et al. Variable influenza vaccine effectiveness by subtype: a systematic review and meta-analysis of test-negative design studies. *Lancet Infect Dis.* 2016;16(8):942–951.
43. Okoli GN, Racovitan F, Abdulwahid T, Righolt CH, Mahmud SM. Variable seasonal influenza vaccine effectiveness across geographical regions, age groups and levels of vaccine antigenic similarity with circulating virus strains: a systematic review and meta-analysis of the evidence from test-negative design studies after the 2009/10 influenza pandemic. *Vaccine.* 2021;39(8):1225–1240.
44. Clutterbuck EA, Lazarus R, Yu LM, et al. Pneumococcal conjugate, and plain polysaccharide vaccines have divergent effects on antigen-specific B cells. *J Infect Dis.* 2012;205(9):1408–1416.
45. Fiolet T, Kherabi Y, MacDonald CJ, Ghosn J, Peiffer-Smadja N. Comparing COVID-19 vaccines for their characteristics, efficacy and effectiveness against SARS-CoV-2 and variants of concern: a narrative review. *Clin Microbiol Infect.* 2022;28(2):202–221.

46. Minor PD. Live attenuated vaccines: historical successes and current challenges. *Virology.* 2015;479–480:379–392.
47. Del Giudice G, Rappuoli R. Inactivated and adjuvanted influenza vaccines. *Curr Top Microbiol Immunol.* 2015;386:151–180.
48. Delrue I, Verzele D, Madder A, Nauwynck HJ. Inactivated virus vaccines from chemistry to prophylaxis: merits, risks, and challenges. *Expert Rev Vaccines.* 2012;11(6):695–719.
49. Caldera F, Mercer M, Samson SI, Pitt JM, Hayney MS. Influenza vaccination in immunocompromised populations: strategies to improve immunogenicity. *Vaccine.* 2021;39(Suppl. 1):A15–A23.
50. Agrati C, Bartolini B, Bordoni V, et al. Emerging viral infections in immunocompromised patients: a great challenge to better define the role of immune response. *Front Immunol.* 2023;14:1147871.
51. Siegrist CA. Mechanisms by which maternal antibodies influence infant vaccine responses: review of hypotheses and definition of main determinants. *Vaccine.* 2003;21(24):3406–3412.
52. Barug D, Pronk I, van Houten MA, et al. Maternal pertussis vaccination and its effects on the immune response of infants aged up to 12 months in the Netherlands: an open-label, parallel, randomised controlled trial. *Lancet Infect Dis.* 2019;19(4):392–401.
53. Timens W, Boes A, Rozeboom-Uiterwijk T, Poppema S. Immaturity of the human splenic marginal zone in infancy. Possible contribution to the deficient infant immune response. *J Immunol.* 1989;143(10):3200–3206.
54. Siegrist CA. Neonatal and early life vaccinology. *Vaccine.* 2001;19(25–26):3331–3346.
55. Allen JC, Toapanta FR, Chen W, Tennant SM. Understanding immunosenescence and its impact on vaccination of older adults. *Vaccine.* 2020;38(52):8264–8272.
56. DiazGranados CA, Dunning AJ, Kimmel M, et al. Efficacy of high-dose versus standard-dose influenza vaccine in older adults. *N Engl J Med.* 2014;371(7):635–645.
57. Riedel S. Edward Jenner and the history of smallpox and vaccination. *Proc (Baylor Univ Med Cent).* 2005;18(1):21–25.
58. Maertens K, Orije MRP, Van Damme P, Leuridan E. Vaccination during pregnancy: current and possible future recommendations. *Eur J Pediatr.* 2020;179(2):235–242.
59. Skibinski DA, Baudner BC, Singh M, O'Hagan DT. Combination vaccines. *J Global Infect Dis.* 2011;3(1):63–72.
60. Nakashima K, Aoshima M, Ohfuji S, et al. Immunogenicity of simultaneous versus sequential administration of a 23-valent pneumococcal polysaccharide vaccine and a quadrivalent influenza vaccine in older individuals: a randomized, open-label, non-inferiority trial. *Hum Vaccin Immunother.* 2018;14(8):1923–1930.
61. Severance R, Schwartz H, Dagan R, et al. Safety, tolerability, and immunogenicity of V114, a 15-valent pneumococcal conjugate vaccine, administered concomitantly with influenza vaccine in healthy adults aged ≥50 years: a randomized phase 3 trial (PNEU-FLU). *Hum Vaccin Immunother.* 2022;18(1):1–14.
62. Janssen C, Mosnier A, Gavazzi G, et al. Coadministration of seasonal influenza and COVID-19 vaccines: a systematic review of clinical studies. *Hum Vaccin Immunother.* 2022;18(6), 2131166.
63. Quach C, Deeks S. COVID-19 vaccination: why extend the interval between doses? *J Assoc Med Microbiol Infect Dis Can.* 2021;6(2):73–78.
64. CDC. Guidance on the Prioritization of Initial Doses of COVID-19 Vaccine(s). Ottawa: National Advisory Committee on Immunization; 2020. Available from: https://www.canada.ca/en/public-health/services/immunization/national-advisory-committee-on-immunization-naci/guidance-prioritization-initial-doses-covid-19-vaccines.html. Accessed 12 July 2023.
65. CDC. Clinical Guidance for COVID-19 Vaccination. CDC; 2023. Available from: https://www.cdc.gov/vaccines/covid-19/clinical-considerations/interim-considerations-us.html. Accessed 12 July 2023.
66. Rubin LG, Levin MJ, Ljungman P, et al. 2013 IDSA clinical practice guideline for vaccination of the immunocompromised host. *Clin Infect Dis.* 2014;58(3):309–318.
67. Pardi N, Hogan MJ, Porter FW, Weissman D. mRNA vaccines—a new era in vaccinology. *Nat Rev Drug Discov.* 2018;17(4):261–279.
68. Donnelly JJ, Ulmer JB, Shiver JW, Liu MA. DNA vaccines. *Annu Rev Immunol.* 1997;15(1):617–648.
69. Rappuoli R, De Gregorio E, Del Giudice G, et al. Vaccinology in the post-COVID-19 era. *Proc Natl Acad Sci USA.* 2021;118(3):e2020368118.
70. Lauring AS, Tenforde MW, Chappell JD, et al. Clinical severity of, and effectiveness of mRNA vaccines against, covid-19 from omicron, delta, and alpha SARS-CoV-2 variants in the United States: prospective observational study. *BMJ.* 2022;376:e069761.
71. Link-Gelles R, Ciesla AA, Fleming-Dutra KE, et al. Effectiveness of bivalent mRNA vaccines in preventing symptomatic SARS-CoV-2 infection—increasing community access to testing program, United States, September–November 2022. *MMWR Morb Mortal Wkly Rep.* 2022;71(48):1526–1530.
72. Maruggi G, Chiarot E, Giovani C, et al. Immunogenicity and protective efficacy induced by self-amplifying mRNA vaccines encoding bacterial antigens. *Vaccine.* 2017;35(2):361–368.
73. Khan YH, Saifullah A, Mallhi TH. Bacterial vaccines. In: Rezaei N, ed. *Encyclopedia of Infection and Immunity.* Oxford: Elsevier; 2022:530–544. [Internet]. [cited 2023 Jul 13]. Available from: https://www.sciencedirect.com/science/article/pii/B9780128187319001701.
74. Orenstein WA, Bernier RH, Donders TJ, et al. Field evaluation of vaccine efficacy. *Bull World Health Organ.* 1985;63(6):1055–1068.
75. Yang ZR, Jiang YW, Li FX, et al. Efficacy of SARS-CoV-2 vaccines and the dose–response relationship with three major antibodies: a systematic review and

meta-analysis of randomised controlled trials. *Lancet Microbe.* 2023;4(4):e236–e246.
76. Bonten MJM, Huijts SM, Bolkenbaas M, et al. Polysaccharide conjugate vaccine against pneumococcal pneumonia in adults. *N Engl J Med.* 2015;372(12):1114–1125.
77. Smith PG, Rodrigues LC, Fine PE. Assessment of the protective efficacy of vaccines against common diseases using case-control and cohort studies. *Int J Epidemiol.* 1984;13(1):87–93.
78. Greenland S, Frerichs RR. On measures and models for the effectiveness of vaccines and vaccination programmes. *Int J Epidemiol.* 1988;17(2):456–463.
79. Carazo S, Talbot D, Boulianne N, et al. Single-dose messenger RNA vaccine effectiveness against severe acute respiratory syndrome coronavirus 2 in healthcare workers extending 16 weeks postvaccination: a test-negative design from Québec, Canada. *Clin Infect Dis.* 2022;75(1):e805–e813.
80. Ionescu IG, Skowronski DM, Sauvageau C, et al. BNT162b2 effectiveness against Delta and omicron variants of severe acute respiratory syndrome coronavirus 2 in adolescents aged 12-17 years, by dosing interval and duration. *J Infect Dis.* 2023;227(9):1073–1083.
81. Skowronski DM, Setayeshgar S, Zou M, et al. Single-dose mRNA vaccine effectiveness against severe acute respiratory syndrome coronavirus 2 (SARS-CoV-2), including alpha and gamma variants: a test-negative Design in Adults 70 years and older in British Columbia, Canada. *Clin Infect Dis.* 2022;74(7):1158–1165.
82. Orenstein EW, De Serres G, Haber MJ, et al. Methodologic issues regarding the use of three observational study designs to assess influenza vaccine effectiveness. *Int J Epidemiol.* 2007;36(3):623–631.
83. Fukushima W, Hirota Y. Basic principles of test-negative design in evaluating influenza vaccine effectiveness. *Vaccine.* 2017;35(36):4796–4800.
84. De Serres G, Skowronski DM, Wu XW, Ambrose CS. The test-negative design: validity, accuracy and precision of vaccine efficacy estimates compared to the gold standard of randomised placebo-controlled clinical trials. *Euro Surveill.* 2013;18(37):20585.
85. Zhang L, Wei M, Jin P, Li J, Zhu F. An evaluation of a test-negative design for EV-71 vaccine from a randomized controlled trial. *Hum Vaccin Immunother.* 2021;17(7):2101–2106.
86. Schwartz LM, Halloran ME, Rowhani-Rahbar A, Neuzil KM, Victor JC. Rotavirus vaccine effectiveness in low-income settings: an evaluation of the test-negative design. *Vaccine.* 2017;35(1):184–190.
87. Ainslie KEC, Shi M, Haber M, Orenstein WA. On the bias of estimates of influenza vaccine effectiveness from test-negative studies. *Vaccine.* 2017;35(52):7297–7301.
88. Strassburg MA. The global eradication of smallpox. *Am J Infect Control.* 1982;10(2):53–59.
89. Fine PE. Herd immunity: history, theory, practice. *Epidemiol Rev.* 1993;15(2):265–302.
90. Lloyd-Smith JO, Schreiber SJ, Kopp PE, Getz WM. Superspreading and the effect of individual variation on disease emergence. *Nature.* 2005;438(7066):355–359.
91. Zipprich J, Winter K, Hacker J, Xia D, Watt J, Harriman K. Measles outbreak—California, December 2014–February 2015. *MMWR Morb Mortal Wkly Rep.* 2015;64(6):153–154.
92. Sherrard L, Hiebert J, Cunliffe J, Mendoza L, Cutler J. Measles surveillance in Canada: 2015. *Can Commun Dis Rep.* 2016;42(7):139–145.
93. Larson HJ, Gakidou E, Murray CJL. The vaccine-hesitant moment. *N Engl J Med.* 2022;387(1):58–65.
94. Dubé E, Laberge C, Guay M, Bramadat P, Roy R, Bettinger JA. Vaccine hesitancy. *Hum Vaccin Immunother.* 2013;9(8):1763–1773.
95. Cascini F, Pantovic A, Al-Ajlouni Y, Failla G, Ricciardi W. Attitudes, acceptance, and hesitancy among the general population worldwide to receive the COVID-19 vaccines and their contributing factors: a systematic review. *EClinicalMedicine.* 2021;40:101113.
96. Sturgis P, Brunton-Smith I, Jackson J. Trust in science, social consensus, and vaccine confidence. *Nat Hum Behav.* 2021;5(11):1528–1534.
97. Xia S, Nan X. Motivating COVID-19 vaccination through persuasive communication: a systematic review of randomized controlled trials. *Health Commun.* 2023;31:1–24.
98. Institute of Medicine (US) Committee to Study Priorities for Vaccine Development. In: Stratton KR, Durch JS, Lawrence RS, eds. *Vaccines for the 21st Century: A Tool for Decision Making.* Washington, DC, US: National Academies Press; 2000. [Internet]. [cited 2023 Jul 13]. (The National Academies Collection: Reports funded by National Institutes of Health). Available from: http://www.ncbi.nlm.nih.gov/books/NBK233313/.
99. Erickson LJ, De Wals P, Farand L. An analytical framework for immunization programs in Canada. *Vaccine.* 2005;23(19):2470–2476.
100. Piso B, Wild C. Decision support in vaccination policies. *Vaccine.* 2009;27(43):5923–5928.
101. Ismail SJ, Hardy K, Tunis MC, Young K, Sicard N, Quach C. A framework for the systematic consideration of ethics, equity, feasibility, and acceptability in vaccine program recommendations. *Vaccine.* 2020;38(36):5861–5876.
102. Ismail SJ, Zhao L, Tunis MC, Deeks SL, Quach C. National Advisory Committee on immunization. Key populations for early COVID-19 immunization: preliminary guidance for policy. *CMAJ.* 2020;192(48):E1620–E1632.
103. Zhao L, Ismail SJ, Tunis MC. Ranking the relative importance of COVID-19 vaccination strategies in Canada: a priority-setting exercise. *CMAJ Open.* 2021;9(3):E848–E854.
104. Ng S, Wu P, Nishiura H, Ip DK, Lee ES, Cowling BJ. An analysis of national target groups for monovalent 2009 pandemic influenza vaccine and trivalent seasonal influenza vaccines in 2009-10 and 2010-11. *BMC Infect Dis.* 2011;11(1):230.

105. Broadbent AJ, Subbarao K. Influenza virus vaccines: lessons from the 2009 H1N1 pandemic. *Curr Opin Virol.* 2011;1(4):254–262.
106. Dzau VJ, Balatbat CA, Offodile AC. Closing the global vaccine equity gap: equitably distributed manufacturing. *Lancet.* 2022;399(10339):1924–1926.
107. Roozen GVT, Roukens AHE, Roestenberg M. COVID-19 vaccine dose sparing: strategies to improve vaccine equity and pandemic preparedness. *Lancet Glob Health.* 2022;10(4):e570–e573.
108. Skowronski DM, De Serres G. Safety and efficacy of the BNT162b2 mRNA Covid-19 vaccine. *N Engl J Med.* 2021;384(16):1576–1577.
109. Romero-Brufau S, Chopra A, Ryu AJ, et al. Public health impact of delaying second dose of BNT162b2 or mRNA-1273 covid-19 vaccine: simulation agent based modeling study. *BMJ.* 2021;373:n1087.

CHAPTER 24

Vaccines

C. MARY HEALY
Infectious Diseases Section, Baylor College of Medicine, Houston, TX, United States

INTRODUCTION

Historical Context

Infectious diseases have led to catastrophic outbreaks of infections and international pandemics throughout the course of history, with devastating effects on families, communities, and the global population. From historical accounts of the widespread devastation wrought by the bubonic plague, caused by *Yersinia pestis*, that killed 30%–60% of the European population in the middle ages, through local outbreaks of bacterial and viral infections like typhoid fever (*Salmonella typhi*) and influenza, respectively, to name just a few, populations respected and feared disease outbreaks even as the cause was poorly understood.[1] Further tools to control such outbreaks were limited, leading to ostracization of those infected who often suffered and died alone and unaided due to ignorance toward the importance of implemented mitigation and prevention strategies. As recently as the previous century, the 1918 influenza pandemic (known as the "Spanish Flu") occurred at the end of World War I and rampaged worldwide at a time where therapeutic interventions were limited and control measures were primarily nonpharmacologic (use of masks, closure of large events). Although vaccination against diseases such as smallpox was available since 1796, few options were available to prevent infection in the early 20th century, allowing "the great influenza" to infect an estimated third of the world's population and kill an estimated 50 million people.[2,3] The following decades between 1940 and the start of the 21st century were ground-breaking with the advent of safe and effective vaccines, reducing deaths attributable to vaccine-preventable diseases (VPD) by >90% and preventing close to 400 million deaths per year (Table 1).[4] Diseases such as smallpox, polio, and measles, which cast fear into parents' hearts, became less of a threat as safe and effective vaccines were developed. In fact, smallpox has been eradicated, and polio is close to being eradicated.[2,4,5] Excellent uptake of available vaccinations in the primary childhood immunization schedule (e.g., diphtheria, pertussis, and tetanus, *Haemophilus influenzae*, pneumococcal vaccine, measles, mumps, and rubella, and polio vaccines) led to hope that in high and upper middle-income nations, outbreaks and cases of VPDs would be rare. Although VPD outbreaks occurred, the goal was that these be localized in populations who were unvaccinated or undervaccinated and that rapid mobilization of vaccination resources with "shots in arms" would lead to rapid containment. While vaccines impact health, security, and economics (Table 1), inequitable resources and other issues led to persisting and serious rates of childhood morbidity and mortality from VPD, especially in low- and middle-income countries (LMIC), which the World Health Organization (WHO) has made strenuous efforts to address.

In the last decade, the international community has been acutely aware of the need to rapidly mobilize vaccination efforts to contain outbreaks of previously controlled and newly emerging infectious diseases.[5] Yellow fever remains endemic in many countries, and since 2016, numerous outbreaks have occurred in Africa and South America, leading to concerns about vaccine supply.[1,6] Ebola virus disease (EVD, previously known as Ebola hemorrhagic fever) was first identified in 1976, led to a major outbreak in 2014–16 in West Africa, with some rare imported cases into other continents.[7] EVD generated considerable publicity and fear in well-resourced countries due to its high case fatality rate (CFR) of 25%–90% and limited available therapeutic interventions despite vaccines that had been developed to protect against Ebola and to help control outbreaks.[1,7] The discovery of severe acute respiratory coronavirus 2 (SARS-CoV-2) in 2019, the etiological agent of the COVID-19 pandemic, brought these issues to the forefront. The 2019 emergence of SARS-CoV-2 in Wuhan, China, resulted in rapid international spread,

Viral Outbreaks, Biosecurity, and Preparing for Mass Casualty Infectious Diseases Events
https://doi.org/10.1016/B978-0-323-54841-0.00006-8

TABLE 1
Benefits of Vaccines When Routinely Recommended or Recommended in the Settings of Outbreaks, Pandemics, or Bioterrorism Events

	Impact	Examples of Routinely Recommended Vaccines	Examples of Vaccines Used in Bioterrorism and Pandemics
Health	Reduce morbidity and mortality from infectious diseases	Influenza Measles Polio SARS-CoV-2	Anthrax Ebola vaccine Influenza SARS-CoV-2 Smallpox
	Eradicate infectious diseases	Polio Smallpox	Smallpox
	Induce herd immunity	*N. meningitidis* Measles	Ebola vaccine Smallpox
	Reduce complications of vaccine-preventable diseases	Influenza Measles Pertussis Rubella SARS-CoV-2	Influenza SARS-CoV-2 Smallpox
	Prevent cancer	Hepatitis B Human papilloma virus (HPV)	N/A
	Prevent antimicrobial resistance	*S. pneumoniae*	Anthrax
Societal	Equity in care	Diphtheria, tetanus, pertussis (DTP) Hepatitis B HPV SARS-CoV-2	SARS-CoV-2 Influenza
	Strengthen health and social care infrastructure	DTP Polio	SARS-CoV-2 Ebola vaccine
	Enhance life expectancy and its quality	All	Influenza SARS-CoV-2 Smallpox
	Improve safety	Rabies vaccination of animals	MERS-CoV in camels
	Decrease fear	*N. meningitidis* Polio SARS-CoV-2 Tetanus Meningococcal vaccine	Ebola vaccine Smallpox
Economic	Cost-effective preparedness for outbreaks	Measles *N. meningitidis* (in sub-Saharan Africa)	Influenza SARS-CoV-2
	Cost savings	Hepatitis B HPV	Influenza SARS-CoV-2
	Establish vaccine programs	Measles, mumps, rubella DTP	Ebola vaccine SARS-CoV-2 Influenza
	Minimize impact of illness on family/women	Influenza Rotavirus SARS-CoV-2 Tetanus Varicella vaccine	Influenza SARS-CoV-2 Ebola vaccine Smallpox

which was enabled by the ease of international travel. As could be predicted with a novel agent that was highly transmissible, some confusion about the mode of transmission, the severity of infectious complications, and disease burden ensued.[1,8,9] However, as with other agents, it became clear that while mitigation efforts such as strict lockdowns, physical distancing, and universal masking were effective in slowing the spread of this infection, they were not viable as long-term control strategies. Hence, prevention of severe disease and interrupting transmission through effective vaccines was an ultimate tool needed to control the pandemic.[1,10]

VACCINE RESEARCH REGULATION AND MANUFACTURING

Traditional research and development (R&D) of vaccine candidates is a relatively prolonged process, taking a minimum of 5–10 years or longer before entering efficacy trials and subsequently obtaining licensure. While the principles of drug development are similar, vaccine clinical trials commonly require large population cohorts to demonstrate efficacy and complicate the process. After a period of preclinical trial research, vaccine candidates are identified in a process that takes a minimum of 3 months.

Once vaccine candidates are identified, there are three stages of research (called Phases) that must be completed prior to review by regulatory bodies such as the Food and Drug Administration (FDA) (Table 2).[11] Phase I clinical trials generally require 5–6 months and evaluate the vaccine in a small group of healthy volunteers for vaccine safety, potential side effects, and adverse outcomes. Over the next 21–24 months, the research then moves into the Phase II clinical trials, in which the vaccine is tested in hundreds of volunteers to test its effectiveness and to further evaluate the vaccine's safety. Commonly, the efficacy of several different vaccine dosing schedules and vaccine doses is assessed in this phase, usually by measuring immunity, such as neutralizing antibody response levels and their duration. These trials determine the dosage, the adjuvant if needed, and the dosing schedule. Importantly, dose and schedule may vary by age. Next, the most complicated studies begin: the Phase III clinical trials, where the vaccine is tested in thousands of volunteers. These trials assess the vaccine efficacy against infection, monitor for expected and unexpected side effects, and may compare a vaccine to a similar treatment. The data collected from each trial phase is analyzed and evaluated by an independent group of experts, a data safety monitoring board, to assure that efficacy is adequate and safety is not compromised. Data are sent to the regulatory agency for independent analysis to determine if the vaccine can be approved for use in the general population. Once approved, manufacturing

TABLE 2
Description of Clinical Trial Phases to Access Vaccine Efficacy and Safety[a]

Phase	Number of Subjects	Study Cohort	Endpoints Studied
I	20–80	Healthy volunteers	Safety, reactogenicity, side effects. Evaluates if a vaccine induces an immune response
II	100–300	Healthy volunteers	Safety and efficacy. Evaluates the immune response in greater detail. Often evaluates different doses and dosing schedules
III	1000–3000 (often more)	Volunteers who represent the population for whom the vaccine is intended	Safety, effectiveness, monitoring side effects, and often comparing it to no or standard existing vaccines Gathers sufficient data for application for FDA license
IV	Millions	General population	Following FDA approval, Phase IV studies demonstrate ongoing monitoring and surveillance after a vaccine is introduced. These evaluations assess the effectiveness of vaccines in a general population, evaluate the optimal vaccine use, and allow for the detection of rare side effects

FDA, Food and Drug Administration (United States).
[a]Throughout each clinical trial phase, interim and final data are evaluated by an independent data and safety monitoring board or committee to ensure the safety of the volunteers and the integrity of the trial results and their interpretation.
Adapted from National Institutes of Health. *NIH Clinical Research Trials and You*. Available from: https://www.nih.gov/health-information/nih-clinical-research-trials-you/basics. Accessed 25 April 2023.

and distribution require an additional 21–24 months. At each step, the regulatory agency may assess the protocol and make recommendations that may extend the research timeline. Following vaccine licensure, Phase IV clinical studies assess the safety and effectiveness of vaccines as they are used in "real-world" situations and across large populations of individuals for whom it is intended.

While the clinical trial process allows for vaccine assessment beyond effectiveness, including safety and long-term immunogenicity, it is ill-suited for a rapid response when novel or newly adapted infectious agents emerge. Even when vaccine constructs and platforms already exist, the ability to mount a rapid vaccination-based response to a pandemic threat using traditional research and regulatory pathways is limited. For example, it was nevertheless challenging to rapidly deploy effective vaccinations during the 2009 H1N1 influenza pandemic because current influenza vaccine constructs take time to complete the process. New influenza vaccine constructs targeting avian and seasonal influenza utilizing the messenger RNA (mRNA) construct that proved so successful during the COVID-19 pandemic are in preclinical and clinical development, and if successful, these are expected to accelerate this process.[12–14]

There are also inherent inequities in vaccine research, development, and distribution. The COVID-19 pandemic prompted a global response, but effective vaccines were rolled out more rapidly and efficiently in high-income nations, not least because the implementation infrastructure is lacking in LMICs. In addition, VPDs that are rare in high-income nations may not be a priority for study until such time as they spread to these nations, e.g., mpox (formerly known as monkeypox) and EVD. Overall, LMICs lag behind high-income nations in vaccine R&D and implementation of vaccination programs, despite being overrepresented in VPD burden.[1]

VACCINE PREPAREDNESS FOR EMERGING PATHOGENS

In 2002, the original SARS-CoV-1 virus, a novel coronavirus, emerged and generated fears that it would lead to a worldwide pandemic. Despite its high transmissibility and mortality [case fatality rate (CFR) of 10%], the virus was quickly contained with aggressive public health measures and geographically limited, resulting in 813 deaths worldwide and fortunately not re-emerging.[1] Although Phase I vaccine trials were initiated for two candidate vaccines (inactivated and DNA formulations), rapid containment translated into aborting vaccine development.[15,16] This situation where vaccines are not well studied until there is an outbreak or a concern for an infectious agent being used for bioterrorism, and that further R&D is halted once the original crisis has passed, means there are sparse data to guide public health and no developed pipeline to supply preventive vaccines in an emergency.

The 2009 H1N1 influenza pandemic demonstrated a different public health response whereby vaccines were developed, tested, and administered relatively rapidly using vaccine constructs available at that time. However, the rapid response to influenza virus outbreaks and pandemics differs as vaccine manufacturers work with relatively rapid developmental (6–9 month) cycles for influenza vaccines in response to circulating influenza virus in the opposite hemisphere. This compares to typical vaccine R&D timelines, which require years. In addition, the vaccine technology and constructs for influenza vaccines are established, although other constructs that may be deployed more rapidly are in development.[12–14] Regardless, despite these relative advantages, the 2009 H1N1 influenza pandemic caused almost 300,000 deaths, with CFR ranging from 2.9% to 9%, which was up to five-times higher in vulnerable populations.[1,17]

The 2013–16 outbreak of EVD in West Africa between 2014 and 2016, followed by more localized outbreaks in the Democratic Republic of Congo (DRC) in 2017, and more localized outbreaks in subsequent years with smaller numbers of cases (predominantly in travelers from affected areas) resulted in a more concerted effort that had been years in the making. The West African 2014 outbreak resulted in more than 11,000 deaths, yet due to its more prolonged nature, it resulted in the testing of several vaccine candidates, one of which had demonstrated efficacy in clinical trials.[18,19]

The EVD outbreak and response exemplified this phenomenon where vaccine clinical trials were slow to be initiated and, when finally available, vaccines were not distributed rapidly. Although progress was made, the path to regulatory approval and licensure for the Ebola vaccine ended in October 2019, 70 months after the outbreak began, and 56 months after the Phase III trial started in March 2015.[1] Unfortunately, this occurred in June 2016, 15 months after the outbreak was declared over.[1] Following this inadequate response, the WHO urged a more rapid response, with support from Gavi (formally the Global Alliance for Vaccines and Immunization), the vaccine alliance.[19] Such a timeline would obviously be inadequate to deal with a rapidly emerging, highly transmissible pathogen with pandemic potential, such as SARS-CoV-2.

The Coalition for Epidemic Preparedness (CEPI) is a not-for-profit organization dedicated to rapid vaccine development in response to public health emergencies.[20,21] Established to respond to deficiencies in the response to developing and implementing new vaccines, initially CEPI focused on infections that the WHO identified as being of concern, such as Middle Eastern Respiratory Syndrome (MERS-first identified in 2012 with a CFR in excess of 30% but confined to Middle Eastern countries), Lassa fever, Rift Valley fever, Chikungunya, and Zika virus. In advance of worldwide pandemics and outbreaks, CEPI's aim was to advance a variety of vaccine candidates through Phase I clinical trials, establish vaccine and supply vaccine stockpiles in preparation for large outbreaks, or pandemics, and advance rapid response technologies into vaccine development platforms. To minimize the economic risk to vaccine developers and manufacturers, CEPI advanced funding to them to produce vaccines during the COVID-19 pandemic. This funding, in conjunction with the United States-funded Operation Warp Speed (OWS), allowed accelerated R&D of candidate COVID-19 vaccines to be brought quickly into clinical trials.[1,22]

One particular feature of the COVID-19 vaccine response that must be maintained for future outbreaks and pandemics is the ability to rapidly adapt to changing circumstances. During the COVID-19 study, investigators were required to rapidly adapt study designs of clinical trials to dynamic real-world situations. For example, the COVID-19 pandemic response under OWS supported several vaccine clinical trials, including two with competing mRNA constructs. The OWS process allowed for a rapid review of existing data for one clinical trial that had completed enrollment in December 2020. As a result of the promising data, an Emergency Use Authorization (EUA) was issued for this mRNA vaccine candidate and also for its independently developed competitor.[23,24] The CDC recommended a hierarchical distribution of available vaccines initially to those most at risk for infection or severe complications of COVID-19, such as the elderly, nursing home residents, healthcare personnel (HCP), and other frontline workers. However, this process generated ethical concerns for the other ongoing clinical vaccine trials that had enrolled subjects deemed at high risk of getting infection or suffering complications or who had yet to complete enrollment. Hence, other clinical vaccine trials (including the other mRNA study) that were ongoing at the time the first EUA was issued had to adapt, either by unblinding participants to their study assignment or by adjusting enrollment goals to include those at lesser risk of acquiring infection or suffering severe complications, even if this affected the ability of the study to meet predefined study endpoints. One study (PREVENT 19) of an adjuvanted SARS-CoV-2 recombinant spike protein vaccine candidate adopted a crossover design to reduce the chances of behavior change due to unblinding, yet still allowed retention of study subjects.[25,26] For all clinical trials, the emergence of new SARS-CoV-2 variants of special interest and repeat infections meant that vaccine booster doses were considerations as evidence of waning immunity arose. This changing landscape required additional doses of vaccine, longer follow-up periods, and other methodologic considerations for the investigators to incorporate into the study design.[26] This adaptability carries lessons for the future.

COVID-19 VACCINE TRIALS

Vaccine Candidates

WHO, CEPI, and OWS's response to the COVID-19 pandemic focused on mobilizing vaccine R&D and bringing candidate vaccines into clinical trials safely and rapidly. To achieve this goal, a variety of vaccine candidates and technologies were advanced to testing. In contrast to traditional methods, COVID-19 vaccine platforms were those that allowed for rapid development. The first two candidates used mRNA technology, allowing candidate vaccines to be brought to clinical trial within 90 days of the genome sequence of SARS-CoV-2 becoming available. This vaccine technology proved successful, showing safety, short-term efficacy that far exceeded prestudy defined endpoints (in excess of 94% against symptomatic disease),[27,28] and continued protection against severe illness even from variants that were more transmissible than the original Wuhan strain, despite waning immunity and an ongoing need for adaptation to emerging variants and likely booster doses.[29–31] This technology demonstrates undeniable promise for rapid R&D against other viral pathogens,[12–14] however, it is as yet unproven against bacterial and other pathogens, although no theoretical reasons exist to suggest it would not be effective. While an exciting advance in vaccine formulation, the requirements of extremely cold temperature storage limited the ability of these lifesaving vaccines to be distributed and made this vaccine technology a challenge for global distribution, especially in LMICs.

Another vaccine candidate technology was an adjuvanted SARS-CoV-2 recombinant spike protein vaccine where full-length, stabilized, prefusion recombinant spike protein trimers are assembled into nanoparticles co-formulated with a saponin-based adjuvant (matrix M). In Phase III clinical trials, this candidate had impressive efficacy in the range of approximately 85%–90% against symptomatic infection.[25,32] This candidate had the advantage of being stable at 2–8 °C, making it a more viable technology for global distribution.

Other vaccine candidates used nonreplicating viral vectors. One vaccine that received EUA in the United States consisted of a replication-incompetent recombinant adenovirus type 26 vector and expressed the SARS-CoV-2 spike protein in a stabilized conformation.[33] This vaccine had lower reported efficacy than the mRNA constructs but had the advantage of being administered in a single dose. Although protective against severe disease, once introduced to the general population under EUA, this vaccine was associated with rare thrombotic complications (thrombosis and thrombocytopenia syndrome, or TTS), which occurred predominantly in women aged 18–49 years, and some cases of Guillain-Barre syndrome.[34] As of May 7, 2023, this vaccine is no longer available in the United States.[35] Another adenovirus vector candidate was based on chimpanzee adenovirus encoding the SARS-CoV-2 spike glycoprotein (ChAdOx1-S).[33] This 2-dose vaccine had similar efficacy reported as the other candidate but never applied for EUA in the United States. It was also associated with TTS.

Pathway to Licensure

One of the likely enduring consequences of the COVID-19 pandemic is an enhanced pathway to licensure of medical therapeutics, including vaccines. The global pandemic ensured that a worldwide rapid public health response ensued and that therapeutic clinical trials occurred quickly and efficiently using innovative trial design methodologies. In the United States, OWS modeled a private-public partnership with governmental agencies, academic institutions, and private companies, entities working together to ensure vaccine candidates entered well-designed clinical efficacy and safety trials rapidly and minimizing waste. The National Institute of Allergy and Infectious Diseases (NIAID) established the COVID-19 Prevention Network (CoVPN) to coordinate the implementation of Phase III candidate vaccine trials without compromising safety or scientific integrity and drawing on the experience of other agencies and networks involved in HIV and Infectious Diseases Research.[26,36–38] Pharmaceutical companies and vaccine manufacturers partnered with these government agencies and operated as sponsors of clinical trials. Unlike traditional R&D, these clinical trials operated at accelerated speed and in an overlapping fashion in an adaptive model that will be used for future outbreaks and perhaps to accelerate bringing other orphan agents to the marketplace. Phase I trials, which evaluate safety and immunogenicity in healthy volunteers, generally in less than 100 individuals, were initiated first. Once sufficient safety data had been obtained, Phase II trials (performed in hundreds of individuals at risk of disease) started while the Phase I trial continued in parallel. Once sufficient safety and immunogenicity data were obtained from Phase II studies, Phase III trials in thousands of individuals were initiated while earlier phases continued in parallel. This accelerated timeline decreased the time from identifying candidate vaccines to distribution to 11 months, a remarkable achievement. This allowed rapid enrollment of a population that was representative of the general population. In addition, manufacturing of the candidate vaccine occurred concomitantly with the Phase II/III clinical trials, which shortened the time to getting "shots in arms" further.

Harmonization of study endpoints in these situations is critical, especially for a global pandemic, requiring communication among vaccinologists, public health experts, and researchers.[1,26,39] For COVID-19, future viral pandemics and outbreaks, and emerging pathogens, meaningful clinical endpoints (i.e., for Phase III clinical trials) are protection against severe infection or complications of infection, including death and symptomatic infection.[37] While an important endpoint is protection against asymptomatic infection, this may be less important for some outbreaks, for example, viral pathogens, where eradication of infection/colonization may not be possible. Determination of immunogenicity endpoints, and most importantly, a correlate of immunity, which may be serological and cellular, is crucial. These endpoints are critical to determine to assess efficacy in Phase I/II clinical trials, especially when comparing several candidate vaccines. The latter challenge is that the ideal endpoints may only become apparent over time, especially with novel and emerging pathogens. However, for vaccine candidates against known pathogens with immunological correlates of protection, the ability to define the success of vaccination campaigns is more straight forward.

Equity in Vaccine Clinical Trials

One of the most important factors in determining the success of candidate vaccines against new or emerging pathogens is ensuring that the enrolled clinical trial population represents the population at risk of acquiring the infectious agent. This fulfills the ethical principle of justice in clinical trials and increases the likelihood that clinical trial efficacy translates into real-life effectiveness once a vaccine is rolled out for administration in the general population.[1,38] This factor is at the forefront, especially when clinical trials enter Phase 3 (large-scale trials in thousands representing the target population), and how successfully it has been applied is tested when Phase 4 (real-life effectiveness studies done postlicensure) are done.[11] In general terms, justice and equity in clinical trials translates into ensuring the study cohort represents the general population in terms of gender, race, ethnicity, and known risk factors for infection, such as underlying conditions or lifestyle factors that place an individual at risk of acquiring or developing serious infection.[1,38] For example, during the COVID-19 pandemic this meant frequent assessments of study participant demographics, as well as behavior deemed to place individuals at higher risk of acquiring infection, since during lockdown those working remotely and not leaving their household were unlikely to be at risk for infection compared to frontline workers whose roles necessitated contact with numerous persons. It also involved including populations judged to be at high risk of acquiring infection and of developing severe complications of infection, including groups who do not traditionally participate in clinical trials. This type of outreach involves forging partnerships with community leaders and interagency groups and fostering an intercommunity dialog.

The COVID-19 trials were particularly successful in achieving equity, with data demonstrating that 40%–50% of participants across OWS trials were from traditionally underrepresented racial and ethnic minorities.[26] These trials also prioritized enrolling those at high risk of infection through underlying illness, older age groups, and occupational exposure, although other populations such as immunocompromised, pregnant women, and children lagged behind. Overall, however, the efforts at inclusivity and diversity in study populations were useful. Ensuring similarly diverse populations are included in clinical trials is a necessity in future responses, not only to ensure data validity to support licensure and public health interventions, but to facilitate acceptance of vaccine interventions in diverse communities.

POPULATIONS AT SPECIAL RISK

Outbreaks

Any outbreak, mass casualty event (especially those involving displacement), or emerging infection carries inherent risks for those at higher risk of infection or infectious complications. It is known from VPDs, that regular outbreaks are reported in undervaccinated communities. Outbreaks of measles, mumps, and even polio have been reported in high-income countries among communities where vaccine hesitancy is high.[40–42] A measles outbreak in 2014–15 originating from an unvaccinated infected child who visited Disneyland (Anaheim, California) quickly spread across multiple states, leading to public health departments mobilizing vaccination efforts.[43] Similar outbreaks have occurred in Ohio and New York since then, and an international outbreak occurred in Israel in 2018.[42,44,45]

Vaccine hesitancy and undervaccination are not the only reasons behind VPD outbreaks and epidemics; however, in some instances, other factors come into play. Displacement such as occurs in natural disasters may result in evacuation to shelters and cramped living conditions with suboptimal hygiene leading to VPD outbreaks. This is further exacerbated by delays in routinely administered vaccines and the lack of availability of immunization records. In some instances, individuals may not have access to medical care or vaccination due to being under or uninsured. Similarly, natural epidemiological trends that are not always fully understood but are likely related to contact with asymptomatic carriers may lead to outbreaks of infections in communal living settings, including college campuses, with meningococcal disease clusters over the past 20 years.[46] In those instances, interventions such as prophylactic antibiotics and rapid initiation of vaccination campaigns may be needed to stop transmission.[47] A number of pertussis outbreaks were reported in both the United States and the United Kingdom in the last 20 years, resulting in deaths in predominantly infants.[48,49] While vaccine hesitancy played a role in some of those cases, it appears more likely that a major impetus was waning immunity from vaccination, particularly in those who had received only acellular pertussis vaccines.[50] Since immunity from pertussis vaccines or natural infection is not lifelong, individuals become susceptible throughout their lifespan and unrecognized hosts. Ongoing education and robust surveillance to detect outbreaks early and intervene with booster vaccination are needed to prevent and control these events.

Novel and Emerging Pathogens

Children

Specific issues arise with novel and emerging pathogens, with certain groups at risk who have not traditionally been priority groups for vaccine-related clinical trials. The licensure of vaccines for children for established and emerging pathogens persistently lags that in adults, even in adults who are at special risk because of their age or underlying medical conditions. While this is somewhat understandable, as safety and efficacy need to be established in healthy adult populations first, children pose unique issues and challenges in establishing vaccine safety and efficacy. First, pharmacokinetics differ between adults and children, with younger age groups generally, but not always, demonstrating a more robust immune response to vaccine antigens. Second, the safety parameters may not be similar, as evidenced by disproportionately increased rates of myocarditis (although rare and milder than that associated with natural infection) in adolescent male recipients of COVID-19 vaccines compared to other age groups. Third, there is a misperception that because children have lower rates of severe illness and death from novel infections such as COVID-19, vaccine protection is not a priority for this age group. This is misleading because children should not be expected to have similar mortality and morbidity as adults who suffer from numerous co-morbidities and likely have additional risk factors for infection and poor outcomes. Epidemiological data show that as many as 3% of children who develop COVID-19 are hospitalized, and children with COVID-19 have similar hospitalization and risk of intensive care interventions as those with influenza (for which children are recognized as a special risk group).[51–53] Further children are at risk of rare but potentially devastating complications of multisystem inflammatory syndrome (MIS-C) even after mild and symptomatic infection, and vaccination is protective against the latter.[54,55] Finally, while children may not experience severe infection, they may be vectors of transmission, and their vaccination may be critical to establishing effective herd immunity. The lessons learned from the COVID-19 and H1N1 influenza experience should require regulatory agencies to explore rapid responses to evaluate prevention, specifically vaccination, strategies for children in future outbreaks and in evaluation of agents potentially used in bioterrorism.

Pregnant women

Pregnant women are another important yet challenging population when discussing VPD outbreaks and novel pathogens. Pregnant women are uniquely susceptible to respiratory and other infections, not only because of physiological and physical changes that occur during pregnancy, such as reduced respiratory capacity and changes in vascular flow and coagulability, but also because there are immunological adaptations that occur to allow pregnancy to proceed.[56] During the 1918 Spanish Influenza pandemic, pregnant women were recognized as being at particularly high risk for influenza-related complications, with mortality rates as high as 50% reported. In 1964, the CDC recommended that the influenza vaccine be given during pregnancy for protection of the mother.[57] During the 2009 H1N1 pandemic, and notwithstanding the advances in intensive care, pregnant women who were infected with H1N1 had five times higher mortality than their nonpregnant counterparts.[58] Despite these data establishing pregnant women as a group at particular risk of severe influenza, it was many decades before influenza vaccine studies were prioritized in pregnancy, and even when performed, vaccine uptake remains very poor, at slightly above 50%.[56]

During the COVID-19 pandemic, surveillance studies quickly identified pregnant women as a special risk group with higher rates of infection-related complications. Early in the pandemic, the INTERCOVID multinational cohort study evaluated the patient outcomes from 43 institutions in 18 countries and determined that SARS-COV-2-infected pregnant women had up to three times the risk of severe infection, a five-times higher risk of ICU admission, and up to a 22 times higher risk of mortality.[59] More recently, a living systematic review and metaanalysis assessing COVID-19 during pregnancy as a risk factor for adverse maternal and perinatal outcomes determined that despite improved therapeutics and availability of vaccines, infected women had a fivefold and sixfold higher risk of ICU admission and mortality, respectively, with an increased risk of poor perinatal outcome.[60] Despite early recognition of increased risk of severe infection and its complications, pregnant women were not prioritized in early COVID-19 vaccine studies. Although the mRNA vaccines were recommended for pregnant women at the time EUA was granted and this was endorsed by national organizations, the approval and endorsements were based on the lack of theoretical risk. Only 18 pregnant women had received the mRNA vaccine, and in all cases it was prior to the pregnancy being diagnosed.[23,24] Inadequate data likely contributed to early lack of confidence in the vaccine and subsequent poor uptake. Prioritizing pregnant women as a group to include in rapid assessment clinical trials once defined safety endpoints are met in other populations is now firmly established as a priority for the future. This tenet is especially important as this single intervention, vaccination during pregnancy, has the potential to protect both pregnant women and their newborn infants.[61]

Immunocompromized persons

Individuals with compromised immune systems, congenitally acquired, as a result of co-existing illness (e.g., rheumatologic and autoimmune conditions) or functionally immune due to required treatments for underlying illness (e.g., individuals with malignancy, bone marrow and solid-organ transplant recipients, individuals on immune modulating therapies for other illnesses) are another vulnerable group, either for existing pathogens where they have a higher risk of infection or when a novel pathogen emerges.[62,63] They are also a population traditionally excluded from vaccine trials until sufficient safety and immunogenicity data have been gathered in the general population, a process that may take months to years. Although understandable, this model is suboptimal when a novel pathogen, or indeed a bioterrorism event, occurs, as was evidenced during COVID-19. Much like pregnant women, individuals who were functionally moderately to severely immunocompromised were excluded from initial COVID-19 vaccine trials, although those with well-controlled diabetes mellitus or human immunodeficiency virus infection were included.[28,29,32] Surveillance following a mass vaccination program, prioritizing those at highest risk of severe outcome, showed that those with immunocompromising conditions required additional doses of vaccine to achieve acceptable levels of immunity and protection.[64] Similar to pregnant women and children, it is important to develop a system to rapidly perform clinical trials in at-risk populations once adequate safety and immunogenicity data has been obtained in the general population. The model used to rapidly enroll and perform Phase I, II, and III COVID-19 vaccine trials in a parallel, overlapping fashion serves as a model that can be utilized to pivot to populations at risk but in whom studies lag behind, such as immunocompromised children and pregnant women.[26,36–38]

Residents in congregate settings

Residents in congregate settings such as nursing homes and rehabilitation units face a particular challenge during outbreak events and pandemics. This phenomenon was well-described prior to the COVID-19 pandemic, when clusters of infections and outbreaks of VPD occurred. The reasons residents are particularly vulnerable are many. First in many situations, residents in long-term care facilities have underlying co-morbidities that render them unable to live independently and may make them at risk of both acquiring infection and developing severe illness. Second, although residents may be vaccinated, their age and co-morbidities may result in sup-optimal immune responses with a corresponding risk of acquiring infection. Third, living conditions and the multiple social interactions and contacts with different individuals mean that the opportunity for infection is greater. Fourth, when dealing with a novel emerging pathogen, many residents already have co-morbidities that may preclude or delay their participation in clinical trials, and a delay in obtaining data that may be of benefit. During COVID 19, residents in nursing homes were very overrepresented in COVID-related morbidity and mortality.[65,66] Tackling infection outbreaks in this situation is complex and requires a co-ordinated public health response with the ability to rapidly mobilize, operationalize interventions such as enhanced infection prevention measures, provision of prophylactic medications as appropriate, and initiate vaccination campaigns when vaccines are available.[67] This requires investment in the facilities themselves to ensure standards for infection control, including adequate ventilation, are met.[68] Finally, it requires preparedness planning and investment in public health infrastructure to coordinate interventions in an efficient manner.

IMMUNIZATION INFORMATION SYSTEMS

One of the necessary components for a robust public health response to any pathogen of high consequence, VPD, or infectious disease outbreak, whatever the cause, is the presence of a bidirectional immunization information system (IIS) that is accurate, timely, and available to both public health authorities and medical providers. Several model systems exist primarily in European countries where vaccination data are collected using electronic health records (EHR) and are available in real-time.[69] These systems have been shown to decrease data latency and provide more immediate situational awareness. In Europe, the Innovative Medicines Initiative funded the Accelerated Development of VAccine beNefit-risk Collaboration in Europe (ADVANCE) project, a public-private partnership aiming to assess the risk-benefit of vaccines and near real-time assessment of vaccines within weeks of introduction. ADVANCE was succeeded by VAC4EU, a multistakeholder international collaboration from multiple European countries allowing timely study of vaccines with generation of data.[70]

In the United States, there exists an independent network of 61 IIS in 49 states, the District of Columbia, three cities, and eight territories.[71] These IIS capture immunization data for more than 95% of children, 82% of adolescents, and 60% of adults. Unfortunately, there are wide variations in adult vaccination data rates by state that depend upon whether the IIS has an age cut-off or records vaccines across the entire lifespan. In addition, IIS vary by whether they are governed by an "opt-in" process where parents/individuals need to request vaccination data are entered, versus an "opt-out" where individuals are automatically enrolled and need to request their data not be collected. Widely used by pediatricians who advocate for, administer, and record vaccines administered to children in IIS, the National Vaccine Advisory Committee recommends that adult vaccination status also be assessed at all visits and that recommended doses be administered and administration recorded in IIS.[72] This is of particular use when vaccine doses may be administered at different locations, for example, healthcare providers offices, pharmacies, or even health fairs and community events, and less often in the medical homes.

IIS is a comprehensive, confidential repository of vaccinations within a jurisdiction. If used appropriately, it is bidirectional (capable of receiving and imparting information), user-friendly, and interfaces with EHRs used by healthcare organizations and pharmacies. Such systems can create and complete vaccination records, assist with clinical decision-making, forecast when vaccine doses are due and generate reminders, assist with managing vaccine inventory, create reports, and assist with disease surveillance and outbreak response.[71,73] IIS was effective during natural disasters such as Hurricane Katrina in 2005, where large numbers of children were displaced from Louisiana to Texas. Prompt linkage of the Louisiana Immunization Network to the Houston-Harris County Vaccine Registry led to retrieval of records, with cost savings for both vaccines and administration fees.[74]

During the COVID-19 pandemic, particularly earlier in the course, efforts to utilize IIS were undertaken since accurate, bidirectional information is particularly important when vaccine quantities are limited. Lessons can be learned from Europe and other parts of the world, as the United States does not have a single IIS, and as mentioned, there are disparities between existing IIS, particularly for adults. These include linkages into hospital and healthcare EHR systems. Shen and colleagues performed an analysis from peer-reviewed literature and online surveys of existing US IIS in November to December 2021, with a view to enhancing IIS to be ready for the next disease outbreak or pandemic.[73] They made three key recommendations:

1. Financial investment is needed for the long-term needs of users. This includes assistance in financial outlay costs for physicians and healthcare providers to connect to IIS and allow automated data exchange, long-term investments in state and public health authorities supporting staffing and immunization technology infrastructure, and the creation of a secure digital record for parents to access and review records.
2. Expand provider electronic data exchange through incentive programs that promote connections to IIS by a variety of systems (physicians, pharmacies, and long-term care systems).
3. Conduct a systematic review of the IIS reporting mechanism to enhance, quality, type, and efficiency.

SURVEILLANCE AND MONITORING AFTER VACCINATION

The importance of surveillance, both for disease tracking and for ongoing vaccine safety and to assess the efficacy of an intervention, is critical in outbreaks, mass casualties, or pandemics. Such surveillance and analysis both assess whether the effects measured are those expected and help anticipate if any additional adaptations may become necessary. In an outbreak scenario, such as those that have occurred with measles in undervaccinated populations or meningococcal type B clusters experienced on college campuses, surveillance focuses on case finding to determine the efficacy of the vaccine intervention and monitors for vaccine side effects. The intensity of monitoring for either safety or effectiveness of vaccination may vary by pathogen. When outbreaks of infections where vaccines are licensed, recommended in the public health vaccination schedules (e.g., measles, mumps, pertussis) and have established safety and effectiveness, there is no reason to anticipate untoward effects. This contrasts with the second scenario, exemplified by the initial meningococcal group B college outbreaks prior to meningococcal group B vaccines being recommended in the United States. Despite considerable safety and efficacy data from other countries where these vaccines were included in the routine vaccination schedule, in this situation, surveillance needed to focus closely on vaccine safety as well as effectiveness since the collected data obtained from outbreaks would be pivotal in obtaining licensure from federal regulators and influence recommendations for use (through shared decision-making) in situations where an individual's exposure risk was high.[46,47] A third scenario occurred during the 2009 H1N1 influenza pandemic, where although established vaccine platforms/technologies existed, rapid adaptation of the vaccine formulation was needed to target the new variant. Existing surveillance networks were employed to gather timely data.[75] Finally, yet another scenario came into play during the COVID-19 pandemic, where novel vaccine constructs and technologies were used to develop effective vaccines that were widely administered in a rapid fashion. In both cases, monitoring for adverse events or the safety and effectiveness of the vaccine when given to large numbers of individuals was then assessed. Through surveillance, an increased incidence of thromboses with the adenovector-based vaccines led to changes in recommended target groups. In several cases, surveillance data was used to dispel misinformation about vaccines. These data were also used to calculate the vaccine effectiveness in populations while accounting for vaccine-established immunity.

Traditionally, postlicensure surveillance has been achieved through both passive and active surveillance carried out both by both governmental agencies (e.g., the CDC, European Centers for Disease Control [ECDC]) and by vaccine manufacturers. In the United States, an example of passive surveillance is the Vaccine Adverse Event Reporting System (VAERS), co-managed by the CDC and FDA, which accepts and analyzes reports of possible problems after vaccination.[76] VAERS accepts reports from anyone in the public, and healthcare providers and vaccine manufacturers are required to report certain events. The ECDC, the United Kingdom's National Health Service, and countries including Canada have similar surveillance systems. These systems provide a potent early alert or warning system, since when there is a pattern of unusual health reports, this sends a signal that a potential association may exist that requires further study. These systems cannot determine causality, but the signals detected may be investigated further and either result in proven associations, such as occurred with the first rotavirus vaccine, or disproven, such as the reputed link between thrombotic events and the human papillomavirus vaccine. Other surveillance systems, such as Vaccine Safety Datalink (VSD), can react to and investigate signals detected through VAERS and other surveillance databases to determine causality.[77] VSD is a collaborative project between the CDC, integrated health care organizations, and networks across the United States. Through this network, EHR data from participating sites can be used to determine the association between vaccines and medical conditions to confirm or refute signals.

The COVID-19 pandemic and the rapid rollout of vaccines that ensued required robust active surveillance with more timely recognition of potential signals compared to traditional methods. The CDC developed and implemented "v-safe," an after-vaccination electronic checker that allowed individuals to report postvaccination symptoms and health conditions almost in real time through text messages sent to personal devices.[78] Messages were sent daily, weekly, and then monthly, depending on proximity to vaccine doses, and linked to standard short health questionnaires. These types of transactional systems facilitated real-time reporting of reactogenicity, encouraged reporting to more established systems such as VAERS, and also facilitated rapid enrollment into a large pregnancy database. The latter database was urgently needed, and its data was used to reassure pregnant women, who are at higher risk of severe infection and poor outcome but who were excluded from initial Phase III clinical trials. The main limitation of "v-safe" was the likely self-selection of participants who were motivated, younger, and more comfortable with technology, thus potentially leading to underrepresentation of certain segments of the population and communities in the data. There were also issues with compliance with completing data and incomplete questionnaires and structural barriers like blocking messages to participants by spam filters, etc.[78] Despite these limitations, this and other similar technologies were exciting and have considerable promise for rapid, "real-time" surveillance during dynamic situations such as outbreaks or pandemics.

The CDC also implemented disease surveillance systems, such as the Overcoming COVID-19 Network, to track hospitalization data and quickly establish the impact of vaccination. This network was able to rapidly establish the benefits of maternal vaccination in preventing young infant hospitalization and monitor the impact of emerging variants on the intervention's success.[61]

COMMUNICATION (SEE CHAPTER 22 FOR ADDITIONAL DETAILS)

While equally applicable to all aspects of response to outbreaks and casualty events, not only vaccines, one of the most important lessons gained from the recent pandemic is the importance of communication in the face of uncertainty. While this sounds simple, in reality, it is one of the most challenging response components to implement. Yet, it is an essential component of response. A multicomponent risk-communication strategy where public health, academics, and members of the community collaborate is most successful. This facilitates responses, whether an outbreak, mass casualty event, a single case of infection with an agent of high consequence, or pandemic, where events are evolving, and communications need to acknowledge the current uncertainty. The experience of the COVID-19 pandemic shows that further research into effective communication styles and messaging is needed, drawing on expertise in behavioral science theory. Communications need to be simple, at an appropriate level for the target audience, and may need to be tailored to the needs of a specific community. Partnering with trusted messengers in the community is very important in establishing credibility and ensuring the message is heard. The "messengers" who represent public health and the medical community need to be credible and empathetic yet promote factual information, and correct misinformation. Including messengers who are bilingual or represent important cultural aspects of a community is a powerful communication weapon. If possible, establishing a process for bidirectional communication is helpful so that misunderstandings and community-specific concerns can be addressed early. Finally, embracing a myriad of communication mechanisms is important in that some members of the public watch television, others use social media, some research the internet, and others read newspapers—they all need to be targeted. Hence, using all available communication modalities enhances clear singular messaging.

REFERENCES

1. Excler J, Saville M, Berkley S, Kim JH. Vaccine development for emerging infectious diseases. *Nat Med.* 2012;27:591–600.
2 World Health Organization. History of the Small Pox Vaccine; 2024. Available from: History of smallpox vaccination (who.int). Accessed 27 November 2024.
3 Centers for Disease Control and Prevention. 1918 Pandemic (H1N1 Virus); 2023. Available from: https://archive.cdc.gov/#/details?url=https://www.cdc.gov/flu/pandemic-resources/1918-pandemic-h1n1.html. Accessed 27 November 2024.
4. Roush SW, Murphy TV, Vaccine-Preventable Disease Table Working Group. Historical comparisons of morbidity and mortality for vaccine-preventable diseases in the United States. *JAMA.* 2007;298(18):2155–2163.
5. Morens DM, Fauci AS. Emerging infectious diseases: threats to human health and global stability. *PLoS Pathog.* 2013;9(7):e1003467.
6. Sacchetto L, Drumond BP, Han BA, Nogueira ML, Vasilakis N. Re-emergence of yellow fever in the neotropics-quoo vadis? *Emerg Top Life Sci.* 2020;4(4):399–410.
7 World Health Organization. Ebola Virus Disease; 2024. Available from: Ebola virus disease (who.int). Accessed 27 November 2024.
8. Zhu N, Zhang D, Wang W, et al. A novel coronavirus from patients with pneumonia in China. *N Engl J Med.* 2020;382(8):727–733.
9. Huang C, Wang Y, Li X, et al. Clinical features of patients infected with 2019 novel coronavirus in Wuhan, China. *Lancet.* 2020;395(10223):497–506.
10. Friedler A. Sociocultural, behavioural and political factors shaping the COVID-19 pandemic: the need for a biocultural approach to understanding pandemics and (re) emerging pathogens. *Glob Public Health.* 2021;16:17–35.
11. National Institutes of Health. NIH Clinical Research Trials and You. Available from: https://www.nih.gov/health-information/nih-clinical-research-trials-you/basics. Accessed 25 April 2023.
12. Bahl K, Senn JJ, Yuzhakov O, et al. Preclinical and clinical demonstration of immunogenicity by mRNA vaccines against H10N8 and H7N9 influenza viruses. *Mol Ther.* 2017;25(6):1316–1327.
13. Feldman RA, Fuhr R, Smolenov I, et al. mRNA vaccines against H10N8 and H7N9 influenza viruses of pandemic potential are immunogenic and well tolerated in healthy adults in phase 1 randomized clinical trials. *Vaccine.* 2019;37(25):3326–3334.
14. Arevalo CP, Bolton MJ, Le Sage V, et al. A multivalent nucleoside-modified mRNA vaccine against all known influenza virus subtypes. *Science.* 2022;378(6622):899–904.
15. Lin JT, Zhang J, Su N, et al. Safety and immunogenicity from a phase I trial of inactivated severe acute respiratory syndrome coronavirus vaccine. *Antivir Ther.* 2007;12(7):1107–1113.
16. Martin JE, Louder MK, Holman LA, et al. A SARS DNA vaccine induces neutralizing antibody and cellular immune responses in healthy adults in a phase I clinical trial. *Vaccine.* 2008;26(50):6338–6343.
17. Centers for Disease Control and Prevention. Maternal and infant outcomes among severely ill pregnant and postpartum women with 2009 pandemic influenza A (H1N1)—United States, April 2009–August 2010. *MMWR Morb Mortal Wkly Rep.* 2011;60:1193.
18. Jacob ST, Crozier I, Fischer 2nd WA, et al. Ebola virus disease. *Nat Rev Dis Primers.* 2020;6(1):13.
19. Wolf J, Bruno S, Eichberg M, et al. Applying lessons from the Ebola vaccine experience for SARS-CoV-2 and other epidemic pathogens. *npj Vaccines.* 2020;5(1):51.
20. Gouglas D, Christodoulou M, Plotkin SA, Hatchett R. CEPI: driving progress toward epidemic preparedness and response. *Epidemiol Rev.* 2019;41(1):28–33.
21. Røttingen JA, Gouglas D, Feinberg M, et al. New vaccines against epidemic infectious diseases. *N Engl J Med.* 2017;376(7):610–613.
22. Sandbrink JB, Shattock RJ. RNA vaccines: a suitable platform for tackling emerging pandemics? *Front Immunol.* 2020;11:608460.
23. Oliver SE, Gargano JW, Marin M, et al. The Advisory Committee on Immunization Practices' interim recommendation for use of Moderna COVID-19 vaccine—United States, December 2020. *MMWR Morb Mortal Wkly Rep.* 2021;69(5152):1653–1656.
24. Oliver SE, Gargano JW, Marin M, et al. The Advisory Committee on Immunization Practices' interim recom-

mendation for use of Pfizer-BioNTech COVID-19 vaccine—United States, December 2020. *MMWR Morb Mortal Wkly Rep*. 2020;69(50):1922–1924.
25. Dunkle LM, Kotloff KL, Gay CL, et al. Efficacy and safety of NVX-CoV2373 in adults in the United States and Mexico. *N Engl J Med*. 2022;386(6):531–543.
26. Mena Lora AJ, Long JE, Huang Y, et al. Rapid development of an integrated network infrastructure to conduct phase 3 COVID-19 vaccine trials. *JAMA Netw Open*. 2023;6(1):e2251974.
27. Baden LR, El Sahly HM, Essink B, at al. Efficacy and safety of the mRNA-1273 SARS-CoV-2 vaccine. *N Engl J Med*. 2021;384(5):403–416.
28. Polack FP, Thomas SJ, Kitchin N, et al. Safety and efficacy of the BNT162b2 mRNA Covid-19 vaccine. *N Engl J Med*. 2020;383(27):2603–2615.
29. El Sahly HM, Baden LR, Essink B, et al. Efficacy of the mRNA-1273 SARS-CoV-2 vaccine at completion of blinded phase. *N Engl J Med*. 2021;385(19):1774–1785.
30. Thomas SJ, Moreira Jr ED, Kitchin N, et al. Safety and efficacy of the BNT162b2 mRNA Covid-19 vaccine through 6 months. *N Engl J Med*. 2021;385(19):1761–1773.
31. Rosenblum HG, Wallace M, Godfrey M, et al. Interim recommendations from the Advisory Committee on Immunization Practices for the use of bivalent booster doses of COVID-19 vaccines—United States, October 2022. *MMWR Morb Mortal Wkly Rep*. 2022;71(45):1436–1441.
32. Twentyman E, Wallace M, Roper LE, et al. Interim recommendation of the advisory committee on immunization practices for use of the Novavax COVID-19 vaccine in persons aged ≥18 years—United States, July 2022. *MMWR Morb Mortal Wkly Rep*. 2022;71(31):988–992.
33. Fiolet T, Kherabi Y, MacDonald CJ, Ghosn J, Peiffer-Smadja N. Comparing COVID-19 vaccines for their characteristics, efficacy and effectiveness against SARS-CoV-2 and variants of concern: a narrative review. *Clin Microbiol Infect*. 2022;28(2):202–221.
34. Oliver SE, Wallace M, See I, et al. Use of the Janssen (Johnson & Johnson) COVID-19 vaccine: updated interim recommendations from the Advisory Committee on Immunization Practices—United States, December 2021. *MMWR Morb Mortal Wkly Rep*. 2022;71(3):90–95.
35. Centers for Diseases Control and Prevention. Janssen (Johnson & Johnson) COVID-19 Vaccine. Available from: https://www.cdc.gov/vaccines/covid-19/info-by-product/janssen/index.html. Accessed 18 May 2023.
36. Collins FS, Stoffels P. Accelerating COVID-19 therapeutic interventions and vaccines (ACTIV): an unprecedented partnership for unprecedented times. *JAMA*. 2020;323(24):2455–2457.
37. Corey L, Mascola JR, Fauci AS, Collins FS. A strategic approach to COVID-19 vaccine R&D. *Science*. 2020;368(6494):948–950.
38. Collins F, Adam S, Colvis C, et al. The NIH-led research response to COVID-19. *Science*. 2023;379(6631):441–444.
39. Krause P, Fleming TR, Longini I, Henao-Restrepo AM, Peto R, World Health Organization Solidarity Vaccines Trial Expert Group. COVID-19 vaccine trials should seek worthwhile efficacy. *Lancet*. 2020;396(10253):741–743.
40. Phadke VK, Bednarczyk RA, Salmon DA, Omer SB. Association between vaccine refusal and vaccine-preventable diseases in the United States: a review of measles and pertussis. *JAMA*. 2016;315(11):1149–1158.
41. Kauffmann F, Heffernan C, Meurice F, Ota MOC, Vetter V, Casabona G. Measles, mumps, rubella prevention: how can we do better? *Expert Rev Vaccines*. 2021;20(7):811–826.
42. Zucker JR, Rosen JB, Iwamoto M, et al. Consequences of undervaccination—measles outbreak, New York City, 2018–2019. *N Engl J Med*. 2020;382(11):1009–1017.
43. Zipprich J, Winter K, Hacker J, et al. Measles outbreak—California, December 2014–February 2015. *MMWR Morb Mortal Wkly Rep*. 2015;64(6):153–154.
44. Uwishema O, Anis H, El Kassem S, Hamitoglu AE, Essayli D, Nazir A. Recent measles outbreak in unvaccinated children in Ohio: cause and causality—a correspondence. *Int J Surg*. 2023;109(2):196–197.
45. Stein-Zamir C, Abramson N, Shoob H. Notes from the field: large measles outbreak in orthodox Jewish Communities—Jerusalem District, Israel, 2018–2019. *MMWR Morb Mortal Wkly Rep*. 2020;69:562–563.
46. Soeters HM, McNamara LA, Blain AE, et al. University-based outbreaks of meningococcal disease caused by Serogroup B, United States, 2013–2018. *Emerg Infect Dis*. 2019;25(3):434–440.
47. Mbaeyi SA, Bozio CH, Duffy J, et al. Meningococcal vaccination: recommendations of the Advisory Committee on Immunization Practices, United States, 2020. *MMWR Morb Mortal Wkly Rep*. 2020;69(9):1–41.
48. Winter K, Harriman K, Zipprich J, et al. California pertussis epidemic, 2010. *J Pediatr*. 2012;161(6):1091–1096.
49. Amirthalingam G, Andrews N, Campbell H, et al. Effectiveness of maternal pertussis vaccination in England: an observational study. *Lancet*. 2014;384(9953):1521–1528.
50. Misegades LK, Winter K, Harriman K, et al. Association of childhood pertussis with receipt of 5 doses of pertussis vaccine by time since last vaccine dose, California, 2010. *JAMA*. 2012;308(20):2126–2132.
51. Sumner MW, Kanngiesser A, Lotfali-Khani K, et al. Severe outcomes associated with SARS-CoV-2 infection in children: a systematic review and meta-analysis. *Front Pediatr*. 2022;10:916655. https://doi.org/10.3389/fped.2022.916655 [eCollection 2022].
52. Delahoy MJ, Ujamaa D, Taylor CA, et al. Comparison of influenza and COVID-19-associated hospitalizations among children < 18 years old in the United States-FluSurv-NET (October-April 2017-2021) and COVID-NET (October 2020–September 2021). *Clin Infect Dis*. 2023;76(3):e450–e459.
53. Halasa NB, Spieker AJ, Young CC, et al. Life-threatening complications of influenza versus COVID-19 in U.S. children. *Clin Infect Dis*. 2023;76(3):e280–e290.
54. Healy CM. Immune response to SARS-CoV-2 infection in children. *JAMA Pediatr*. 2022;76(11):1075–1076.

55. Nygaard U, Holm M, Hartling UB, et al. Incidence and clinical phenotype of multisystem inflammatory syndrome in children after infection with the SARS-CoV-2 delta variant by vaccination status: a Danish nationwide prospective cohort study. *Lancet Child Adolesc Health.* 2022;6(7):459–465.
56. Healy CM. Vaccines in pregnant women and research initiatives. *Clin Obstet Gynecol.* 2012;55(2):474–486.
57. Burney L. Influenza immunization: statement. *Public Health Rep.* 1960;75(10):944.
58. Centers for Disease Control and Prevention. Maternal and infant outcomes among severely ill pregnant and postpartum women with 2009 pandemic influenza A (H1N1)—United States, April 2009–August 2010. *MMWR Morb Mortal Wkly Rep.* 2011;60(35):1193–1196.
59. Villar J, Ariff S, Gunier RB, et al. COVID-19 in pregnancy is associated with substantially higher maternal morbidity, mortality, preterm birth and severe neonatal complications: the INTERCOVID multinational study. *JAMA Pediatr.* 2021;175(8):817–826.
60. Clinical Manifestations, Risk Factors, and Maternal and Perinatal Outcomes of Coronavirus Disease 2019 in Pregnancy: Living Systematic Review and Meta-Analysis. Available from: www.bmj.com/content/370/bmj.m3320. Accessed 10 March 2023.
61. Halasa NB, Olson SM, Staat MA, et al. Maternal vaccination and risk of hospitalization for Covid-19 among infants. *N Engl J Med.* 2022;387(2):109–119.
62. Centers for Disease Control and Prevention. Altered Immunocompetence. General Best Practice Guidelines for Immunization. https://www.cdc.gov/vaccines/hcp/acip-recs/general-recs/immunocompetence.html. Accessed 21 May 2023.
63. Rubin L, Levin M, Ljungman P, et al. 2013 IDSA clinical practice guideline for vaccination of the immunocompromised host. *Clin Infect Dis.* 2014;58(3):e44–100.
64. Centers for Disease Control and Prevention. COVID-19 Vaccines for People Who Are Moderately or Severely Immunocompromised. Available from: https://www.cdc.gov/coronavirus/2019-ncov/vaccines/recommendations/immuno.html. Accessed 21 May 2023.
65. Bagchi S, Mak J, Li Q, et al. Rates of COVID-19 among residents and staff members in nursing homes—United States, May 25–November 22, 2020. *MMWR Morb Mortal Wkly Rep.* 2021;70(2):52–55.
66. Ma H, Yiu KCY, Baral SD, et al. COVID-19 cases among congregate care facility staff by neighborhood of residence and social and structural determinants: observational study. *JMIR Public Health Surveill.* 2022;8(10):e34927.
67. Nanduri S, Pilishvili T, Derado G, et al. Effectiveness of Pfizer-BioNTech and moderna vaccines in preventing SARS-CoV-2 infection among nursing home residents before and during widespread circulation of the SARS-CoV-2 B.1.617.2 (Delta) variant—National Healthcare Safety Network, March 1–August 1, 2021. *MMWR Morb Mortal Wkly Rep.* 2021;70(34):1163–1166.
68. Zhu X, Lee H, Sang H, et al. Nursing home design and COVID-19: implications for guidelines and regulation. *J Am Med Dir Assoc.* 2022;23(2):272–279.
69. Bollaerts K, de Smedt T, McGee C, et al. ADVANCE: towards near real-time monitoring of vaccination coverage, benefits and risks using European electronic health record databases. *Vaccine.* 2020;38(Suppl. 2):B76–B83.
70. Vaccine Monitoring Collaboration for Europe. Available from: https://vac4eu.org. Accessed 21 May 2023.
71. Trotter AB, Abbott EK, Coyle R, Shen AK. Preparing for COVID-19 vaccination: a call to action for clinicians on immunization information systems. *Ann Intern Med.* 2021;174(5):695–697.
72. National Vaccine Advisory Committee. Recommendations from the National Vaccine Advisory committee: standards for adult immunization practices. *Public Health Rep.* 2014;129:115–123.
73. Shen AK, Sobczyk EA, Coyle R, Tirmal A, Hannan C. How ready was the US vaccination infrastructure and network of immunization information systems for COVID-19 vaccination campaigns: recommendations to strengthen the routine vaccination program and prepare for the next pandemic. *Hum Vaccin Immunother.* 2022;18(5):2088010.
74. Boom JA, Dragsbaek AC, Nelson CS. The success of an immunization information system in the wake of Hurricane Katrina. *Pediatrics.* 2007;119(6):1213–1217.
75. McNeil MM, Gee J, Weintraub ES, et al. The vaccine safety datalink: successes and challenges monitoring vaccine safety. *Vaccine.* 2014;32(42):5390–5398.
76. Centers for Disease Control and Prevention. Vaccine Adverse Event Reporting System (VAERS); 2023. Available from: https://www.cdc.gov/vaccinesafety/ensuringsafety/monitoring/vaers/index.html. Accessed 10 March 2023.
77. Centers for Disease Control and Prevention. Vaccine Safety Datalink (VSD); 2023. Available from: https://www.cdc.gov/vaccinesafety/ensuringsafety/monitoring/vsd/index.html. Accessed 10 March 2023.
78. Myers TR, Marquez PL, Gee JM, et al. The v-safe after vaccination health checker: active vaccine safety monitoring during CDC's COVID-19 pandemic response. *Vaccine.* 2023;41(7):1310–1318.

CHAPTER 25

Therapeutics Overview for Agents of Bioterrorism and Viral Outbreaks

ESTHER Y. GOLNABI[a] • JAMES M. SANDERS[a,b] • CRYSTAL K. HODGE[a,c] • JAMES B. CUTRELL[b]

[a]Department of Pharmacy, University of Texas Southwestern Medical Center, Dallas, TX, United States • [b]Department of Medicine, Division of Infectious Diseases and Geographic Medicine, University of Texas Southwestern Medical Center, Dallas, TX, United States • [c]University of North Texas Health Science Center System College of Pharmacy, Fort Worth, TX, United States

INTRODUCTION

Several notable pathogens represent threats for mass casualties either through dispersal as biological weapons or emerging and re-emerging epidemics. While each of these agents is reviewed in more detail in their respective book chapters, this overview will summarize the therapeutic management for category A bioterrorism agents and key pandemic respiratory viruses. The text will highlight salient principles of treatment in adults, with a special focus on considerations for a pandemic outbreak or bioterror attack. Additional details concerning pediatric and pregnant populations and specific pharmacologic considerations can be found in the accompanying tables. In addition, more detailed information about the pathogens, their epidemiology, microbiology, and prevention can be found in the organism-specific chapters.

CATEGORY A BIOTERRORISM AGENTS

Anthrax (See Chapter 2 for Additional Information)

Treatment of anthrax poses several unique challenges that affect its management: toxin production in vivo, risk of central nervous system (CNS) infection, drug resistance development, and the presence of latent spores requiring a longer duration of therapy. Combined antimicrobial therapy—composed of at least one bactericidal agent and at least one protein synthesis inhibitor—is recommended for treatment of anthrax because combination therapy yields better clinical outcomes than monotherapy (Table 1).[1,22] Theoretically, the bactericidal agent rapidly eradicates the organism while the protein synthesis inhibitor blocks in vivo toxin production. Anthrax-associated meningitis is present in up to one-third of all cases and is associated with high mortality.[23] Therefore, until meningitis is excluded, the default regimen should contain antimicrobials that reach adequate concentration in the central nervous system (CNS). *Bacillus anthracis* isolates are generally susceptible to fluoroquinolones, carbapenems, doxycycline, rifampin, and vancomycin. Due to unpredictable β-lactam resistance in naturally occurring *B. anthracis* and the concern for emergent (or engineered) resistance, empiric β-lactam use is not recommended.[24]

Systemic disease (including meningitis, bacteremia, pleuritis, and sepsis)

In hospitalized patients with systemic anthrax where meningitis cannot be ruled out, at least three antimicrobial drugs, including both bactericidal and protein synthesis inhibitor agents, should be used (Table 1).[1] Among bactericidal agents, fluoroquinolones (ciprofloxacin, levofloxacin, and moxifloxacin) are preferred because they adequately penetrate the CNS and have a lower risk of antimicrobial resistance in naturally occurring *B. anthracis*.[1] Carbapenems (except ertapenem and doripenem due to poor CNS penetration) are usually the second bactericidal option given their high resistance to β-lactamases and excellent CNS penetration. Intravenous vancomycin or a penicillin (if susceptibility is confirmed) are acceptable bactericidal options as well. Options for protein synthesis inhibitors include

Viral Outbreaks, Biosecurity, and Preparing for Mass Casualty Infectious Diseases Events
https://doi.org/10.1016/B978-0-323-54841-0.00018-4

TABLE 1
Treatment and Postexposure Prophylaxis for Category A and Select Category B Bioterrorism Agents and Agents With Pandemic Potential

Agent	Treatment	Postexposure Prophylaxis
CATEGORY A BIOTERRORISM AGENTS		
Anthrax[1,2]	**Systemic Disease** • Antibiotic therapy: initial intravenous (IV) therapy for a minimum of 2 weeks or until clinical stability, followed by oral (PO) follow-up therapy • Use three agents (two bactericidal [usually a fluoroquinolone plus β-lactam] plus one protein synthesis inhibitor) if suspected or confirmed CNS infection, or two agents (one bactericidal plus one protein synthesis inhibitor) if CNS involvement is ruled out • Bactericidal agents o **Adults** ▪ Ciprofloxacin 400 mg IV q8h OR levofloxacin 750 mg IV q24h OR moxifloxacin 400 mg IV q24h OR ▪ Meropenem 2 g IV q8h OR imipenem-cilastatin 1 g IV q6h OR ▪ Vancomycin (dose adjusted per serum drug concentration) ▪ Not recommended if suspected/confirmed meningitis • Doxycycline 100 mg IV or PO q12h OR doripenem 500 mg IV q8h ▪ If confirmed penicillin susceptibility • Penicillin G 4 million units IV q4h OR ampicillin 3 g IV q6h o **Children (1 Month of Age and Older)** ▪ Ciprofloxacin 30 mg/kg/day IV divided into q8h (max 400 mg/dose) OR levofloxacin <50 kg: 16 mg/kg/day IV divided into q12h (max 250 mg/dose); ≥50 kg: 500 mg IV q24h OR moxifloxacin 3 months to <2 years: 12 mg/kg/day IV divided into q12h (max 200 mg/dose); 2–5 year: 10 mg/kg/day IV divided into q12h (max 200 mg/dose); 6–11 year: 8 mg/kg/day IV divided into q12h (max 200 mg/dose); 12–17 year, ≥45 kg: 400 mg IV q24h; 12–17 year, <45 kg: 8 mg/kg/day IV divided into q12h (max 200 mg/dose) OR ▪ Meropenem 120 mg/kg/day IV divided into q8h (max 2 g/dose) OR imipenem-cilastatin 100 mg/kg/day IV divided into q6h (max 1 g/dose) OR ▪ Vancomycin 60 mg/kg/day IV divided into q8h (dose adjusted per serum drug concentration) ▪ If confirmed penicillin susceptibility • Penicillin G 400,000 units/kg/day IV divided into q4h (max 4 million units/dose) OR ampicillin 400 mg/kg/day IV divided into q6h (max 3 g/dose)	**Prophylactic Vaccination** ***Adults and Children*** Start a 3-dose series Anthrax Vaccine Adsorbed (AVA; BioThrax) • Vaccines are administered at diagnosis and 2 and 4 weeks later • Children younger than 6 weeks of age are not candidates for AVA. Antimicrobial prophylaxis should begin immediately, but AVA series should wait until the child reaches 6 weeks of age **Antibiotic Prophylaxis** ***Adults*** • Ciprofloxacin 500 mg PO q12h OR • Doxycycline 100 mg PO q12h OR • Levofloxacin 750 mg PO q24h OR • Moxifloxacin 400 mg PO q24h OR • Clindamycin 600 mg PO q8h OR • If confirmed penicillin susceptibility o Amoxicillin 1 g PO q8h OR o Penicillin VK 500 mg PO q6h • Duration o 42 days OR o 60 days for immunocompromised patients, patients who cannot finish vaccination series, patients >65 years old, pregnant, or breastfeeding ***Children (1 Month of Age and Older)*** • Ciprofloxacin 30 mg/kg/day PO divided into q12h (max 500 mg/dose) OR • Doxycycline <45 kg: 4.4 mg/kg/day PO divided into q12h (max 100 mg/dose); >45 kg: 100 mg PO q12h OR • Clindamycin 30 mg/kg/day PO divided into q8h (max 900 mg/dose) OR • Levofloxacin <50 kg: 16 mg/kg/day PO divided into q12h (max dose 250 mg/dose) >50 kg: 500 mg PO q24h OR • If confirmed penicillin susceptibility o Amoxicillin 75 mg/kg/day PO divided into q8h (max 1 g/dose) o Penicillin VK 50–75 mg/kg/day PO divided into q6h to q8h • Duration: 60 days after exposure

Agent	Treatment	Postexposure Prophylaxis
	• Protein synthesis inhibitor o **Adults** ■ Linezolid 600 mg IV q12h OR ■ Clindamycin 900 mg IV q8h OR ■ Chloramphenicol 1 g IV q6-8h OR ■ Rifampin 600 mg IV q8-12h o Children (1 month of age and older) ■ Linezolid: <12 y old: 30 mg/kg/day IV divided into q8h; ≥12 y old: 30 mg/kg/day IV divided into q12h (max 600 mg/dose) OR ■ Clindamycin 40 mg/kg/day divided into q8h (max 900 mg/dose) OR ■ Rifampin 20 mg/kg/day IV divided into q12h (max 300 mg/dose) OR ■ Chloramphenicol 100 mg/kg/day IV divided into q6h ■ Not recommended if suspected/confirmed meningitis • Doxycycline <45 kg: 4.4 mg/kg/day IV loading dose (max 200 mg/dose); ≥45 kg: 200 mg IV loading dose; then <45 kg: 4.4 mg/kg/day IV divided into q12h (max 100 mg/dose); ≥45 kg: 100 mg IV q12h OR • Consider adding adjunctive antitoxin monoclonal antibody therapy o Human-derived anthrax immune globulin (AIG) OR o Recombinant monoclonal antibodies: obiltoxaximab or raxibacumab • Follow-up oral therapy after initial intravenous therapy o **Adults** ■ Ciprofloxacin 500 mg PO q12h OR levofloxacin 750 mg PO q24h OR moxifloxacin 400 mg PO q24h OR ■ Doxycycline 100 mg PO q12h OR ■ Clindamycin 600 mg PO q8h OR ■ If penicillin susceptibility is confirmed • Amoxicillin 1 g PO q8h OR penicillin VK 500 mg PO q6h o **Children (1 Month of Age or Older)** ■ Use combination therapy for severe anthrax (one bactericidal plus one protein synthesis inhibitor) ■ Bactericidal • Ciprofloxacin 30 mg/kg/day PO divided into q12h (max 500 mg/dose) OR levofloxacin <50 kg: 16 mg/kg/day PO divided into q12h (max 250 mg/dose); ≥50 kg: 500 mg PO q24h OR • If penicillin susceptibility is confirmed o Amoxicillin 75 mg/kg/day PO divided into q8h (max 1 g/dose) OR penicillin VK 50–75 mg/kg/day PO divided into q6h or q8h	

(Continued)

TABLE 1
Treatment and Postexposure Prophylaxis for Category A and Select Category B Bioterrorism Agents and Agents With Pandemic Potential—cont'd

Agent	Treatment	Postexposure Prophylaxis
	▪ Protein synthesis inhibitor • Clindamycin 30 mg/kg/day PO divided into q8h (max 600 mg/dose) OR • Doxycycline <45 kg: 4.4 mg/kg/day PO divided into q12h (max 100 mg/dose); ≥45 kg: 100 mg PO q12h OR • Linezolid (non-CNS dose): <12 years old: 30 mg/kg/day PO divided into q8h; ≥12 years old: 30 mg/kg/day PO divided into q12h (max 600 mg/dose) • Duration: intravenous antibiotics for at least 2 weeks or until clinical stability, then transition to oral therapy to complete 60 days from the onset of illness **Cutaneous Infection Without Systemic Involvement** ***Adults*** • Preferred o Ciprofloxacin 500 mg PO q12h OR doxycycline 100 mg PO q12h OR moxifloxacin 400 mg PO q24h OR levofloxacin 750 mg PO q24h • Others o Clindamycin 600 mg PO q8h OR linezolid 600 mg PO q12h o If penicillin susceptibility is confirmed ▪ Amoxicillin 1 g PO q8h OR penicillin VK 500 mg PO q6h • Duration o If naturally acquired: 7–10 days o Acquired via bioterrorism or aerosol-exposure: 60 days regardless of vaccination history ***Children (1 Month of Age and Older)*** • Any one of the bactericidal or protein synthesis inhibitors recommended for oral follow-up therapy in children (see above) • Duration o 7–10 days for naturally acquired infection o Require additional prophylaxis for inhaled spores to complete an antimicrobial prophylaxis for up to 60 days from the onset of illness	

Agent	Treatment	Postexposure Prophylaxis

Botulism[3]	**Systemic Botulism**
	• Respiratory support + antitoxin × 1 dose
	  o Antitoxin does not reverse ongoing paralysis
	• Available antitoxins in the United States
	  o Heptavalent botulism antitoxin (HBAT): approved for noninfant botulism
	    ■ Available through the local state health department (United States)
	    ■ Total volume depends on the manufacturer lot; refer to the package insert[4]
	  o Human-derived botulism immune globulin (BabyBIG): approved for infant botulism
	    ■ Available through the California Department of Public Health (United States)
	    ■ Dose is specific to the manufactured lot; refer to the package insert[5]
	Wound Botulism
	• Exploration and wound debridement are strongly recommended. Appropriate anaerobic cultures should be obtained
	• In infants, do not administer antibiotics unless for indications other than botulism
	• Antibiotics: Administer after antitoxin administration
	  o *Adults*: Penicillin G 3 million units IV q4h OR metronidazole 500 mg q8h (if allergic to penicillin)
	  o *Children*: Penicillin G IV 250,000 to 400,000 units/kg/day OR metronidazole (if allergic to penicillin)
	  o Duration: 10–14 days
		None

Plague[6,7]	**Adults**
	Preferred
	• Streptomycin 1 g IM q12h
	• Gentamicin 5 mg/kg IM or IV q24h OR 2 mg/kg loading dose followed by 1.7 mg/kg q8h
	Alternatives
	• Levofloxacin 500 mg IV or PO q24h
	• Ciprofloxacin 400 mg IV q8-12h OR 500–750 mg PO q12h
	• Doxycycline 100 mg IV or PO q12h OR 200 mg IV or PO q24h
	• Moxifloxacin 400 mg IV or PO q24h
	• Chloramphenicol 25 mg/kg IV q6h
	Pregnant Women
	Preferred
	• Gentamicin 5 mg/kg IM or IV q24h OR 2 mg/kg loading dose followed by 1.7 mg/kg q8h
	Alternatives
	• Ciprofloxacin 400 mg IV q8-12h OR 500–750 mg PO q12h
	• Doxycycline 100 mg IV or PO q12h OR 200 mg IV or PO q24h
		Adults
		Preferred
		• Doxycycline 100 mg PO q12h
		Alternative
		• Ciprofloxacin 500 mg PO q12h
		Pregnant Women
		• **Same as adults**
		Children
		Preferred
		• Doxycycline (for children ≥8 years)
		  o Weight < 45 kg: 2.2 mg/kg PO q12h (maximum daily dose, 200 mg)
		  o Weight ≥ 45 kg: same as adult dose
		Alternative
		• Ciprofloxacin 20 mg/kg PO q12h (maximum daily dose, 1 g)
		Duration: 7 days

(Continued)

TABLE 1
Treatment and Postexposure Prophylaxis for Category A and Select Category B Bioterrorism Agents and Agents With Pandemic Potential—cont'd

Agent	Treatment	Postexposure Prophylaxis

	Children[a]
	Preferred
	• Streptomycin 15 mg/kg IM q12h (maximum 2 g/day)
	• Gentamicin 2.5 mg/kg/dose IM or IV q8h
	Alternatives
	• Levofloxacin 8 mg/kg/dose IV or PO q12h (max 250 mg per dose)
	• Ciprofloxacin 15 mg/kg/dose IV q12h (maximum 400 mg/dose) OR 20 mg/kg/dose PO q12h (maximum 500 mg/dose)
	• Doxycycline
	  o Weight < 45 kg: 2.2 mg/kg IV or PO q12h (maximum daily dose, 200 mg)
	  o Weight ≥ 45 kg: same as adult dose
	• Chloramphenicol (for children >2 years) 25 mg/kg IV q6h (maximum daily dose, 4 g)
	Duration: 10 to 14 days, or until 2 days after fever subsides	

Smallpox, Nonvariola orthopoxvirus (e.g., monkeypox [MPox])[8,9]	**Adults**
	• Variola virus (smallpox)
	  o FDA-approved
	    ▪ Tecovirimat: 600 mg PO q12h × 14 days
	    ▪ Brincidofovir
	      • <10 kg: 6 mg/kg PO once weekly × 2 doses
	      • 10–47 kg: 4 mg/kg PO once weekly × 2 doses
	      • 48 kg+: 200 mg PO once weekly × 2 doses
	  o Investigational
	    ▪ Cidofovir/probenecid via FDA for emergency use
	• Vaccinia virus (vaccine)
	  o 1st line: Vaccinia immune globulin intravenous (VGIV) 6000 units/kg IV × 1
	  o 2nd line: Tecovirimat OR Cidofovir OR Brincidofovoir
		Adults
		• Postexposure prophylactic vaccinations should be administered as soon as possible after a known exposure to maximize efficacy
		• JYNNEOS vaccine given subcutaneously (0.5 mL/dose), or intradermally (0.1 mL/dose) × 2 doses given 4 weeks apart; booster dose may be given every 2 years for persons at continued risk of exposure
		• ACAM2000 vaccine given by scarification

Agent	Treatment	Postexposure Prophylaxis
	• Nonvariola orthopoxvirus (e.g., monkeypox) (off-label) o Tecovirimat ■ IV • 35 to <120 kg: 200 mg IV q12h • ≥120 kg: 300 mg IV q12h ■ PO • 40 to <120 kg: 600 mg PO q12h • ≥120 kg: 600 mg PO q8h ■ Duration is usually 14 days but adjusted based on clinical response and drug tolerance o Brincidofovir: 200 mg PO once weekly for up to three doses (limited data) o Alternatives: vaccinia immune globulin intravenous (VIGIV), cidofovir **Children** • Variola virus (smallpox) o Tecovirimat ■ 13–25 kg: 200 mg q12h × 14 days ■ 25–40 kg: 400 mg q12h × 14 days ■ 40 kg +: 600 mg q12h × 14 days o Brincidofovir ■ <10 kg: 6 mg/kg PO once weekly × 2 doses ■ 10–47 kg: 4 mg/kg PO once weekly × 2 doses ■ 48 kg +: 200 mg PO once weekly × 2 doses • Vaccinia virus (vaccines) o Not established	
Tularemia[10]	**Adults** Preferred[b] • Streptomycin 1 g IM q12h • Gentamicin 5 mg/kg IM or IV q24h (with desired levels of at least 5 μg/mL) Alternatives • Ciprofloxacin 400 mg IV OR 500 mg PO q12h[c] • Doxycycline 100 mg IV or PO q12h **Pregnant Women** • **Same as adults** **Children** Preferred[b] • Streptomycin 15 mg/kg IM q12h (maximum 2 g/day) • Gentamicin 2.5 mg/kg/dose IM or IV q8h[d] Alternatives • Ciprofloxacin 15 mg/kg/dose IV or PO q12h (maximum 800 mg/d IV and 1 g/d PO PO) Duration: minimum of 10 days for streptomycin and gentamicin; 10–14 days for ciprofloxacin; and 14 days for doxycycline	**Adults** Preferred • Doxycycline 100 mg PO q12h Alternative • Ciprofloxacin 500 mg PO q12h **Pregnant Women** • **Same as adults** **Children** Preferred • Doxycycline (for children ≥8 years) o Weight < 45 kg: 2.2 mg/kg PO q12h (maximum daily dose, 200 mg) o Weight ≥ 45 kg: same as adult dose Alternative • Ciprofloxacin 15 mg/kg PO q12h (maximum daily dose, 1 g) Duration: 14 days

(Continued)

TABLE 1
Treatment and Postexposure Prophylaxis for Category A and Select Category B Bioterrorism Agents and Agents With Pandemic Potential—cont'd

Agent	Treatment	Postexposure Prophylaxis
Viral hemorrhagic fevers[11]	**Adults** Lassa fever/Crimean Congo HF/Possibly Rift Valley Fever • Ribavirin o Loading dose: 30 mg/kg (max of 2 g) IV o Regimen: 16 mg/kg (max of 1 g per dose) IV q6h × 4 days, then 8 mg/kg (max 500 mg per dose) IV q8h × 6 days o Duration: 10 days Argentinian HF/Bolivian HF • Convalescent plasma Ebola • Atoltivimab/maftivimab/odesivimab-ebgn IV 50 mg/50 mg/50 mg per kg × 1 dose OR • Ansuvimab-zykl 50 mg/kg × 1 • Duration: 1 dose **Children** Argentinian HF/Bolivian HF • Convalescent plasma Ebola • Atoltivimab/maftivimab/odesivimab-ebgn IV 50 mg/50 mg/50 mg per kg × 1 dose OR • Ansuvimab-zykl 50 mg/kg × 1 • Duration: 1 dose Duration: Lassa fever/Crimean Congo HF/Rift Valley Fever treated with ribavirin for 10 days; Ebola monoclonal antibodies: 1 dose	**Adults** Lassa fever/Crimean Congo HF/Possibly Rift Valley Fever • Ribavirin 500 mg PO q6h × 7 days OR • Ribavirin loading dose 2 g PO × 1 then 600 mg (if weight ≤ 75 kg then 400 mg in am and 600 mg in pm) PO q12h x 10 days Duration: 7–10 days depending on dosing strategy
CATEGORY B BIOTERRORISM AGENTS		
Brucellosis[12]	**Adults** • Doxycycline 100 mg PO or IV q12h PLUS rifampin 600–900 mg PO or IV daily OR • Doxycycline 100 mg PO or IV q12h PLUS gentamicin 5 mg/kg IV q24h for the first 14 days OR • Ciprofloxacin 400 mg IV q12h PLUS rifampin 600–900 mg PO or IV daily OR • Ceftriaxone 1–2 g q12h PLUS rifampin 600–900 mg PO or IV daily (for CNS disease) • Duration: 4 to 6 weeks **Children** • Doxycycline 2–4 mg/kg/day (max dose 200 mg/day, in two divided doses) PLUS rifampin 15–20 mg/kg/day (up to 600–900 mg/day) OR • TMP-SMX 10 mg/kg (TMP component) PO q12h (up to 480 mg TMP/day) • Duration: 4 to 6 weeks	**Adults** Doxycycline 100 mg IV or PO q12h AND rifampin 600–900 mg/day IV or PO **Children** Doxycycline 2–4 mg/kg PO q12h (up to 200 mg/day) PLUS rifampin 15–20 mg/kg/day (up to 600 mg/day) **Pregnant Women** • TMP-SMX (TMP 6–8 mg/kg/day divided into q8h to q12h) PLUS rifampin 600–900 mg/day IV or PO Duration: 3 weeks from exposure

Agent	Treatment	Postexposure Prophylaxis
	Pregnant Women • Avoid doxycycline • TMP-SMX (TMP 6–8 mg/kg/day divided into q8h to q12h) PLUS streptomycin 1 g IM daily for the first 14 days OR gentamicin 5 mg/kg/day for the first 14 days Duration: 4 to 6 weeks (may be extended for 4 to 6 months for life-threatening complications, such as meningitis or endocarditis)	
Cholera[13,14]	**Adults** Doxycycline 300 mg PO once OR azithromycin 1 g PO once OR ciprofloxacin 1 g PO once **Children (<12 years)** Doxycycline 2–4 mg/kg PO once OR azithromycin 20 mg/kg (max 1 g) PO once OR ciprofloxacin 20 mg/kg (max 1 g) PO once	None
Q fever[15–17]	**Pneumonia** **Adults** • Doxycycline 100 mg q12h (preferred) OR • Azithromycin OR clarithromycin PLUS rifampin OR fluoroquinolones • Duration: 14 days **Pregnant Women** • TMP-SMX 1 DS tablet PO q12h through entire pregnancy **Children** • Regardless of age, doxycycline 2.2 mg/kg (max 100 mg/dose) PO q12h for 14 days • If still febrile after 5 days of therapy, convert to TMP-SMX 4–20 mg/kg q12h for 14 days **Hepatitis**: doxycycline 100 mg PO q12h for 14 days **Endocarditis**: Doxycycline 100 mg PO or IV q12h PLUS hydroxychloroquine 200 mg q8h for at least 18 months (indefinitely or until phase I IgG <1:200) **Pregnant women**: Long-term TMP-SMX 1 DS tablet PO q12h through the entire pregnancy and may need to remain on therapy (convert to doxycycline PLUS hydroxychloroquine postpartum) if titers remain elevated >12 months after delivery (immunoglobulin G phase I titer ≥1:1024)	None
Viral encephalitis[18]	Supportive therapy, such as IV therapy and anticonvulsants	None
Respiratory Viruses With Pandemic Potential		
Coronaviruses		
SARS-CoV-1	No currently recommended specific therapies; refer to text for details on potential agents	None
MERS-CoV	No currently recommended specific therapies; one RCT supports the use of IFN beta-1b eight million IU SQ every other day plus lopinavir/ritonavir 400/100 mg PO q12 hours for 14 days or until discharge	None

(Continued)

TABLE 1
Treatment and Postexposure Prophylaxis for Category A and Select Category B Bioterrorism Agents and Agents With Pandemic Potential—cont'd

Agent	Treatment	Postexposure Prophylaxis
SARS-CoV-2 (113)	**Hospitalized** Adults *Mild to moderate disease (no supplemental oxygen requirement)* • Supportive care and symptomatic treatment • Corticosteroids NOT recommended • Remdesivir not routinely recommended but may be considered in those at high risk for progression *Severe disease requiring supplemental oxygen* • Remdesivir 200 mg IV × 1, then 100 mg IV daily for a total of 5 days PLUS • Dexamethasone 6 mg PO/IV daily for up to 10 days or until discharge *Severe disease requiring high-flow oxygen or noninvasive ventilation* • Remdesivir 200 mg IV × 1, then 100 mg IV daily for a total of 5 days PLUS • Dexamethasone 6 mg PO/IV[18] daily for up to 10 days or until discharge PLUS • Baricitinib 4 mg PO daily for up to 14 days (dose reduce for eGFR ≤60) OR tocilizumab 8 mg/kg IV (maximum dose 800 mg) × 1 *if recently hospitalized and evidence of rapid progression and systemic inflammation* *Critical disease (mechanical ventilation or ECMO)* • Dexamethasone 6 mg PO/IV daily for up to 10 days or until discharge PLUS • Tocilizumab 8 mg/kg IV (maximum dose 800 mg) × 1 *if within 24 h of ICU admission* • Remdesivir NOT recommended in critical disease but may complete the course if already on therapy Pregnant women: Should be generally managed the same as nonpregnant adults, with shared decision-making to discuss the risks and benefits of specific therapies Children: In general, management in children is extrapolated from adult clinical trial data. Dexamethasone should be used in all children with severe disease requiring higher levels of supplemental oxygen, noninvasive ventilation, or mechanical ventilation. Remdesivir should be used in children >12 requiring supplemental oxygen with risk factors for progression; children <12 may be considered on a case-by-case basis. There is insufficient evidence for or against the use of baricitinib or tocilizumab in children	Although several SARS-CoV-2 monoclonal antibodies were previously authorized for use in PEP, there are none currently authorized for use due to the prevalence of circulating SARS-CoV-2 variants with in vitro high-level resistance to previously available agents Ongoing trials are evaluating currently authorized direct oral antivirals and novel agents for use in PEP in high-risk patient populations

Agent	Treatment	Postexposure Prophylaxis
	Multisystem inflammatory syndrome in children (MIS-C) is a rare, delayed complication of COVID-19 seen in a minority of children and young adults. Although the optimal treatment regimen is not established, intravenous immunoglobulins and corticosteroids are first-line therapies. Consultation with a multidisciplinary team is recommended **Outpatient** Adults *Mild to moderate disease (no supplemental oxygen requirement) in patients without risk factors for progression* • Supportive care with symptomatic treatments and close outpatient follow-up recommended • Corticosteroids or remdesivir NOT recommended • Oral antiviral therapies not currently authorized for patients without risk factors for progression *Mild to moderate disease (no supplemental oxygen requirement) in patients at high risk for progression to severe disease (treatments listed in order of preference and based on timing from symptom onset)* • *Within 5 days of symptom onset:* Nirmatrelvir 300 mg plus ritonavir 100 mg oral twice daily for 5 days (**Must closely review drug-drug interactions prior to use**; renal dose adjustment required for eGFR 30–60 mL/min; not currently recommended in eGFR <30 mL/min) OR • *Within 7 days of symptom onset:* Remdesivir 200 mg IV × 1 then 100 mg IV daily for total of 3 days OR • *Within 5 days of symptom onset:* Molnupiravir 800 mg oral twice daily for 5 days (only if no alternative outpatient treatments available) • High-titer convalescent plasma may be considered on a case-by-case basis in immunocompromised patients not expected to have an adequate antibody response • Corticosteroids NOT recommended Pregnant women*:* Management should be generally managed the same as nonpregnant adults, with shared decision-making to discuss the risks and benefits of specific therapies. Molnupiravir is contraindicated in pregnancy Children*:* There are no randomized trials of outpatient SARS-CoV-2 treatments in children, so data is largely extrapolated from adults. Nirmatrelvir plus ritonavir is authorized for use in children 12 years of age and older who are at high risk for progression. Children under 12 may be considered for remdesivir on a case-by-case basis. Molnupiravir is contraindicated in children under the age of 18	

(Continued)

TABLE 1
Treatment and Postexposure Prophylaxis for Category A and Select Category B Bioterrorism Agents and Agents With Pandemic Potential—cont'd

Agent	Treatment	Postexposure Prophylaxis
Influenza Viruses		

Influenza[19,20]	**Adults**
	Hospitalized
	• Oseltamivir 75mg PO q12h
	Outpatient
	• Oseltamivir 75mg PO q12h OR Zanamivir 10mg (2×5mg) inhaled q12h OR Peramivir 600mg IV×1 dose OR Baloxavir 40mg (<80kg) or 80mg (≥80kg) PO×1 dose
	Pregnant Women
	• Oseltamivir 75mg PO q12h
	Children
	Hospitalized
	• Oseltamivir
	  o If younger than 1 year old use postmenstrual age (PMA)
	    ▪ PMA < 38 weeks: 1 mg/kg/dose PO q12h
	    ▪ PMA 38–40 weeks: 1.5 mg/kg/dose PO q12h
	    ▪ PMA >40 weeks: 3 mg/kg/dose PO q12h
	  o If 1 year or older, the dose varies by child's weight
	    ▪ 15kg or less: 30mg PO q12h
	    ▪ >15 to 23kg: 45mg PO q12h
	    ▪ >23 to 40kg: 60mg PO q12h
	    ▪ >40kg: 75mg PO q12h
	Outpatient
	• Oseltamivir (see hospitalized) OR
	• Zanamivir (children 7 years or older) 10mg (2×5mg) inhaled q12h OR
	• Peramivir OR
	  o 2 to 12 years of age:
	    ▪ 12mg/kg dose IV×1 dose (maximum 600mg)
	  o ≥13 years of age
	    ▪ 600mg IV×1 dose
	• Baloxavir (children 12 years or older): 40mg (<80kg) or 80mg (≥80kg) PO×1 dose
	Duration: 5 days (1 day for peramivir and baloxavir)
		Adults
		• Oseltamivir 75mg PO q24h OR Zanamivir 10mg (2×5mg) inhaled q24h OR Baloxavir 40mg (<80kg) or 80mg (≥80kg) PO×1 dose
		Pregnant Women
		• Oseltamivir 75mg PO q24h
		Children
		• Oseltamivir OR
		  o If younger than 1 year old use age:
		    ▪ <3 months not recommended
		    ▪ Term 3–8 months: 3mg/kg/dose PO q24h
		    ▪ 9–11 months: 3.5mg/kg/dose PO q24h
		  o If 1 year or older, dose varies by weight
		    ▪ 15kg or less: 30mg PO q24h
		    ▪ >15 to 23kg: 45mg PO q24h
		    ▪ >23 to 40kg: 60mg PO q24h
		    ▪ >40kg: 75mg PO q24h
		• Zanamivir (children 7 years or older) 10mg (2×5mg) inhaled q24h OR
		• Baloxavir (children 12 years or older) 40mg (<80kg) or 80mg (≥80kg) PO×1 dose
		Duration: 7 days after last exposure (1 day for baloxavir)

Agent	Treatment	Postexposure Prophylaxis
Avian Influenza[21]	**Adults** Hospitalized • Oseltamivir 75 mg PO q12h Outpatient *Severe, progressive, or complicated* • Oseltamivir 75 mg PO q12h *Uncomplicated* • Oseltamivir 75 mg PO q12h OR Zanamivir 10 mg (2 × 5 mg) inhaled q12h OR Peramivir 600 mg IV q24 **Pregnant Women** • Oseltamivir 75 mg PO q12h **Children** Hospitalized • Oseltamivir o If younger than 1 year old use PMA ■ PMA < 38 weeks: 1 mg/kg/dose PO q12h ■ PMA 38–40 weeks: 1.5 mg/kg/dose PO q12h ■ PMA >40 weeks: 3 mg/kg/dose PO q12h o If 1 year or older, dose varies by child's weight ■ 15 kg or less: 30 mg PO q12h ■ >15 to 23 kg: 45 mg PO q12h ■ >23 to 40 kg: 60 mg PO q12h ■ >40 kg: 75 mg PO q12h Outpatient *Severe, progressive, or complicated* • Oseltamivir (see hospitalized) *Uncomplicated* • Oseltamivir (see hospitalized) OR • Zanamivir (children 7 years or older) 10 mg (2 × 5 mg) inhaled q12h OR • Peramivir o 2 to 12 years of age: 12 mg/kg dose IV q24h (maximum 600 mg) o ≥ 13 years of age: 600 mg IV q24 Duration: minimum of 10 days for inpatient; 5 days for outpatient	**Adults** • Oseltamivir 75 mg PO q12h OR Zanamivir 10 mg (2 × 5 mg) inhaled q12h **Pregnant Women** • Oseltamivir 75 mg PO q12h **Children** • Oseltamivir OR o If younger than 1 year old use age ■ <3 months not recommended ■ Term 3–8 months: 3 mg/kg/dose PO q24h ■ 9–11 months: 3.5 mg/kg/dose PO q24h o If 1 year or older, dose varies by weight ■ 15 kg or less: 30 mg PO q12h ■ >15 to 23 kg: 45 mg PO q12h ■ >23 to 40 kg: 60 mg PO q12h ■ >40 kg: 75 mg PO q12h • Zanamivir (children 7 years or older) 10 mg (2 × 5 mg) inhaled q12h Duration: 5–10 days

yo, years old; *yrs*, years; *PO*, oral; *IV*, intravenous; *PMA*, postmenstrual age.
[a]All recommended antimicrobials have relative contraindications for use in children; however, use is justified in life-threatening situations.
[b]Chloramphenicol may be added to treat meningitis.
[c]Preferred in mass causality situation.
[d]Once-daily dosing could be considered in consultation with a pediatric infectious disease specialist and a pharmacist.

linezolid (preferred) or clindamycin. Clindamycin does not reliably reach adequate CNS concentration and should be avoided if there is suspicion for meningitis. Rifampin is an alternative to linezolid and has historically been used for treatment of anthrax based on potential synergy when combined with other antibiotics. Doxycycline is not recommended due to its poor CNS penetration.[1] Despite the lack of randomized controlled trials specific to human anthrax, intravenous dexamethasone with initial antibiotic therapy is recommended in the setting of suspected or confirmed anthrax meningitis.[1]

In systemic anthrax without concern for meningitis, CNS penetration is no longer a factor in therapeutic choice. In this setting, combined antimicrobial therapy of ≥2 agents with a bactericidal agent and a protein synthesis inhibitor are recommended.[1] Due to potential delayed infection from latent spores, the treatment duration is prolonged, for up to 60 days. Initially, intravenous therapy should be administered for at least 2 weeks or until clinical stability, whichever is longer. Then, patients can be transitioned to a single oral agent to finish the course.[1]

Limited cutaneous anthrax

Patients with cutaneous anthrax without systemic involvement, can be appropriately treated with oral antimicrobial agents initially. A single oral antimicrobial regimen has historically been used successfully for cutaneous anthrax (Table 1). Either oral fluoroquinolones or doxycycline are first-line agents. If both first-line agents are contraindicated, other acceptable oral agents include clindamycin, linezolid, or, if susceptible, amoxicillin or penicillin VK. A shorter duration of therapy of 7–10 days is appropriate if the cutaneous anthrax is naturally acquired. If acquired via bioterrorism or aerosol-exposure, then the recommended duration is 60 days regardless of vaccination history. If requiring the longer duration, long-term side effects of certain antibiotics (e.g., linezolid) should be considered by the prescribing provider.

Anthrax prophylaxis

The US Food and Drug Administration (FDA) approved Anthrax Vaccine Adsorbed (AVA) (BioThrax) for preexposure prophylaxis (PrEP) for adults aged 18–65 years who are at high risk for exposure to *B. anthracis* and for postexposure prophylaxis (PEP) for adults with suspected or known exposure to aerosolized *B. anthracis* spores.

For PEP in patients who are exposed to anthrax but are asymptomatic, a prophylactic antibiotic regimen should be started as soon as possible, as delays are associated with poorer outcomes. Current recommendations are for a 42-day antimicrobial monotherapy regimen (60 days, if immunocompromised) and a three-dose adsorbed anthrax vaccine (AVA; BioThrax) series.[25] If the AVA series cannot be completed, antimicrobial therapy should be continued for 60 days. The Advisory Committee on Immunization Practices (ACIP) to the Centers for Disease Control and Prevention (CDC), suggests that in situations where subcutaneous vaccine administration is not feasible, intramuscular administration can be utilized as there was no significant difference in serologic or clinical outcomes between the two routes.[26]

The ACIP, recommends vaccine boosters at 12-month intervals for PEP (Table 1). For PrEP, they recommend a booster dose to be given at 12 and 18 months and annually, thereafter, in individuals who are at high risk for exposure. For those who are not at high risk for exposure and have previously finished the three-dose primary and two-dose AVA booster series, additional booster doses are recommended every 3 years (specific dose schedules: Table 1).[2,26]

Anthrax antitoxins

Three anthrax antitoxins are licensed and available from the United States Strategic National Stockpile (SNS): (1) anthrax immune globulin intravenous (AIGIV), (2) obiltoxaximab (Anthim), and (3) raxibacumab (ABthrax). The antitoxins bind to the protective antigen, which is necessary to transport toxins into cells. All three antitoxins are indicated to treat inhalational anthrax in adults and children in combination with antimicrobial agents. Obiltoxaximab and raxibacumab are also indicated for PEP when no other alternative therapies are available. AIGIV does not have an indication for PEP and should not be co-administered with AVA due to possible reduced immunogenicity of the vaccine. Raxibacumab was not shown to adversely impact immunogenicity when co-administered with AVA.[27]

Botulism

Botulism is a neuroparalytic syndrome caused by neurotoxin produced by *Clostridium botulinum* or rarely by *C. butyricum* or *C. baratii*.[28] The most common types include infant botulism (77%), foodborne botulism (10%), wound botulism (10%), and botulism of unknown origin.[29] According to the CDC's National Botulism Surveillance Summary, there were 182 laboratory-confirmed botulism cases reported in 2017.[29] Due to its potential to cause widespread fatal disease, botulinum toxin could be used in a biological attack, but has not been reported in bioterrorism-associated events to date.[29]

Symptomatic persons with suspected botulism should be hospitalized for appropriate management, which includes respiratory support, source control such as wound debridement, and therapeutic interventions (antitoxins, antimicrobials).[3] Two antitoxins are currently available and bind botulism toxin in the blood and prevent the toxin from binding to the postsynaptic cholinergic receptors. Because the antitoxins only bind to free toxins present in the blood, they are unable to reverse active paralysis. Equine heptavalent botulinum antitoxin (HBAT) is approved by the FDA for noninfant botulism and contains antibodies specific to the seven serotypes of botulism exotoxins (A to G). Human-derived botulism immune globulin (BabyBIG) is an orphan drug also approved by the FDA for the treatment of infant botulism types A and B.[30] Based on multiple systematic reviews, HBAT is safe and effective in both adult and pediatric patients with botulism.[31–33] Administration of HBAT within 2 days of symptom onset significantly shortens hospital and intensive care unit length of stay.[33] Although severe anaphylactic reactions to HBAT are rare, the CDC recommends conducting a skin test prior to its administration. The package insert also advises slowing the rate of administration to less than 0.01 mL/minute for individuals at high risk for a hypersensitivity reaction (Table 1).[34]

For wound botulism, anaerobic tissue cultures and wound debridement are recommended. Although lacking clinical trial data, adjunctive antimicrobials have historically been used and should be administered after antitoxin administration (Table 1). Appropriate options include penicillin G or metronidazole in both adults and children.[35] In infants with botulism, antibiotics are generally not administered due to the risk of botulism neurotoxin release during cell lysis unless indicated for other reasons (e.g., pneumonia).[28]

Plague (See Chapter 4 for Additional Information)

Plague caused by the bacterium *Yersinia pestis* infects humans via a flea bite. Bubonic plague represents the most common clinical form of the infection, followed rarely by primary septicemic and pneumonic forms. In contrast, the most likely method for its use in bioterrorism would be via aerosol dissemination, with the potential for high rates of pneumonic plague.[6]

Rapid treatment of patients with plague ensures optimal outcomes. Aminoglycosides and tetracyclines are the two most common antimicrobial classes used in its treatment.[6,36] A recent review of antimicrobial treatment patterns reports the increased use of fluoroquinolones over time despite limited clinical evidence.[36] Currently, the CDC recommends one of several aminoglycosides (streptomycin, gentamicin), fluoroquinolones (levofloxacin, ciprofloxacin, moxifloxacin), doxycycline, and chloramphenicol as treatment options (Table 1). The choice of agent must take into consideration patient co-morbidities, allergies, and clinical presentation. Gentamicin is the treatment of choice for severe pneumonic or septic presentations due to demonstrated clinical efficacy and the limited availability of streptomycin.[37,38] In contrast for bubonic plague, an alternative or combination therapy is recommended due to poor penetration of gentamicin into abscesses. In patients with suspected meningitis, antimicrobials that penetrate into the CNS should be selected, and this is an indication for chloramphenicol.[6] Sulfonamides, rifampin, and beta-lactams are alternatives and should be used with caution due to variable activity and efficacy.[39] The recommended treatment duration is 10 to 14 days or until clinical defervescence.[6]

Existing efficacy data primarily evaluates aminoglycosides and tetracyclines for the treatment of plague. A small randomized clinical trial (RTC, $n=65$) demonstrated that both doxycycline and gentamicin effectively treated patients with plague.[38] Two agents are typically recommended for patients with an underlying abscess, although a small series of 50 cases demonstrated similar outcomes among patients who received gentamicin monotherapy versus those who received gentamicin plus doxycycline.[37] More recently, two systematic reviews that included treatment publications from 1937 to 2019 found the lowest case fatality rates among patients treated with aminoglycosides, tetracyclines, and chloramphenicol.[7,40] An assessment of 533 plague cases in the United States, found that the use of either aminoglycosides or tetracyclines significantly improved survival.[36] Case fatality rates were comparable when treatment included fluoroquinolones; however, studies primarily included fluoroquinolones in combination with another agent, limiting the recommendation for fluoroquinolone monotherapy.[40] Alternative antimicrobials, such as sulfonamides or those that are penicillin-based, led to poorer outcomes; hence, their use is limited to those unable to take the preferred regimens.[7,40]

Mass causality situations arising may limit access to parenteral antimicrobials, making enteral agents (e.g., fluoroquinolones and doxycycline) attractive options for stockpiling and mass distribution. Consensus recommendations for contained and mass casualty situations mirror the treatment of naturally occurring infections, with the caveat that logistics may necessitate enteral therapy (Table 1).[39] Postexposure prophylaxis (PEP) is recommended for asymptomatic individuals in close contact (≤2 m) with individuals with untreated pneumonic plague. Doxycycline is preferred for prophylaxis for a total of 7 days, with fluoroquinolones as the alternative agent. Symptomatic individuals who were within two meters of an untreated pneumonic plague case should be evaluated for infection and treated as above.

Among pregnant populations, the risks and benefits of prophylaxis and treatment for plague should be weighed.[41] The preferred treatments all have relative contraindications in pregnancy; thus, risks of teratogenicity must be considered; the risk of plague-related complications and outbreak containment may outweigh relative theoretical risks in these patients (Tables 1 and 2).[6]

Orthopoxviruses [Smallpox, Monkeypox (Now Called Mpox); See Chapter 6 for Additional Information]

Smallpox is caused by the variola virus from the *Orthopoxvirus* genera of the Poxviridae family. It is an enveloped, double-stranded DNA virus that replicates and matures within infected cells.[46] There are several related smallpox viruses that infect humans, including the vaccinia virus used in the smallpox vaccine and monkeypox, now called Mpox.[46]

Tecovirimat

Tecovirimat (TPOXX) is one of two FDA-approved medications for the treatment of human smallpox and is included in the SNS.[8,44,46,47] Tecovirimat inhibits the VP37 protein, which is key to maturation of the virion's envelope.[46,48] Without the envelope, the immature virus will not be released from the infected cell, limiting the spread of the virus to other healthy cells.[8,46,47,49] Tecovirimat received FDA approval via the Animal Efficacy Rule, which allows for approval based on animal efficacy models and human safety data without additional human efficacy data. Thus, because of the global eradication of smallpox, there is currently no human efficacy data available.[8,47] However, with the evolution of the global public health emergency of Mpox, increasing reports of its use and efficacy in humans are emerging. To obtain tecovirimat from the SNS, providers are referred to their local health department to begin the Expanded Access Investigational New Drug (EA-IND) protocol paperwork for the CDC.[50]

Tecovirimat is approved for both adults and children weighing at least 13 kg (Table 1). Doses should be taken within 30 min of a full moderate-to-high-fat meal. The capsules can be opened, and the contents mixed with 30 mL of liquid or soft food.[47,48] An intravenous formulation is also available if patients cannot absorb or take oral medications. While animal model data suggested that 5 days of therapy was sufficient, a 14-day regimen was chosen to prevent recrudescence.[48] The current CDC protocol for use of tecovirimat for the treatment of Mpox also uses a duration of 14 days.[51] In some immunocompromised hosts, the duration of treatment has been extended. Other considerations include animal data suggesting that efficacy may be decreased in patients with immunocompromising conditions. For drug-drug interactions, tecovirimat is a weak inducer of cytochrome P450 enzyme (CYP) 3A and a weak inhibitor of CYP 2C8 and 2C19. If co-administered with the live smallpox vaccine, animal data suggests the efficacy of the vaccine may be limited as tecovirimat will inhibit the vaccinia virus in the vaccine, leading to less immunogenicity.[47,52]

Human safety data were based on an expanded randomized controlled trial with four participants receiving tecovirimat for every one participant receiving placebo for adults aged 18–79.[48] Among the healthy 361 tecovirimat and 91 placebo recipients, 10% of patients were older than 65 years of age. This population may not be representative of the response to tecovirimat in patients with either smallpox or Mpox (Table 1).[47,48] To illustrate the differences in patient populations, an international case series of 528 persons diagnosed with monkeypox had a median age of 38 years old, were >99% male, and largely came from Europe (90%).[48] Additionally, 96% of the reported cases identified as homosexual, 41% were HIV positive, and 29% had a confirmed concomitant sexually transmitted infection. Only 5% received monkeypox-specific therapy.

Brincidofovir/cidofovir

Brincidofovir is a prodrug of cidofovir, a nucleotide analog, designed to provide a more favorable pharmacokinetic and side effect profiles. The FDA approved this drug to treat smallpox in June of 2021 using the Animal Efficacy Rule previously mentioned.[9,44] The lipid conjugate of oral brincidofovir allows for greater passive diffusion across host cell membranes of the intestines and greater intracellular concentrations than intravenous cidofovir. This nucleotide analog competes with cytosine for incorporation into replicating DNA strands, ultimately causing DNA synthesis inhibition.[44,45,53] Based on this mechanism, these agents are considered to have a wide spectrum of antiviral activity, including against the variola virus. Other potential mechanisms of action of cidofovir include impaired genome encapsulation and virion assembly.

TABLE 2
Key Characteristics of Select Pharmacologic Agents Used for Discussed Infectious Agents[42,43]

Drug (Routes of Administration)	Renal and Hepatic Dose Adjustment	Considerations in Pregnant and/or Breastfeeding Mothers and Pediatrics	Key Adverse Drug Reactions	Safety Laboratory Monitoring Parameters	Key Drug-Drug or -Food Interactions
ANTIBIOTICS					
Aminoglycosides					
Gentamicin (IV/IM) Streptomycin (IV/IM)	• Serum drug concentration monitoring is recommended in persons with renal impairment	• Use caution • Reports of total irreversible bilateral congenital deafness in children whose mothers received streptomycin during pregnancy. Gentamicin seems to be a safer choice than streptomycin in pregnant women; however, it may still carry a risk for fetal harm • Present in breast milk	Risks are higher in persons with concomitant renal impairment • Nephrotoxicity • Neurotoxicity (e.g., ototoxicity [vestibular or auditory]) could be irreversible	• Serum drug concentrations • Renal function test and changes in urine output • Hearing and vestibular function	• Avoid concurrent systemic use of other potentially neurotoxic and/or nephrotoxic drugs
Beta-lactams					
Ampicillin (IV)	• Requires renal dose adjustment	• Safe for use during pregnancy • Present in breast milk	Beta-lactam class effects • Hypersensitivity reactions (immediate and delayed) • Pancytopenia with prolonged use and higher doses • Gastrointestinal side effects (diarrhea, vomiting, nausea) • *Clostridioides difficile* infections Antibiotic-specific effects • Ceftriaxone—Kernicterus in neonates, resulting from hyperbilirubinemia • Imipenem-cilastatin and meropenem: risk of seizures • Penicillin G: phlebitis, Jarisch-Herxheimer reactions, seizures (with higher doses and renal impairment)	• Renal, hepatic, and hematologic function tests (CMP, CBC with diff)	• Allopurinol: may enhance hypersensitivity reaction or rash to ampicillin
Ceftriaxone (IV/IM)	• Does not require renal dose adjustment • May require dose adjustment in persons with concurrent severe hepatic and renal impairment			• Renal, hepatic, and hematologic function tests (CMP, CBC with diff)	
Imipenem-cilastatin (IV)	• Requires renal dose adjustment			• Renal, hepatic, and hematologic function tests (CMP, CBC with diff)	• Valproic acid: carbapenems decrease Valproic acid serum concentrations significantly
Meropenem (IV)	• Requires renal dose adjustment				

(Continued)

TABLE 2
Key Characteristics of Select Pharmacologic Agents Used for Discussed Infectious Agents—cont'd

Drug (Routes of Administration)	Renal and Hepatic Dose Adjustment	Considerations in Pregnant and/or Breastfeeding Mothers and Pediatrics	Key Adverse Drug Reactions	Safety Laboratory Monitoring Parameters	Key Drug-Drug or -Food Interactions
Penicillin G aqueous (IV)	• Requires renal dose adjustment			• Renal, hepatic, and hematologic function tests (CMP, CBC with diff)	
Penicillin V potassium (PO)	• Does not require renal dose adjustment			• Renal and hematologic function tests (BMP, CBC with diff)	
Chloramphenicol (IV)	• Serum drug concentration monitoring is recommended in persons with renal or hepatic impairment	• Safe for use during pregnancy but avoid near term due to the potential of "gray baby syndrome" • Present in breast milk	• Bone marrow suppression (associated with higher serum concentrations) • Rare: fatal aplastic anemia (not dose-related), "gray baby syndrome," optic neuritis, peripheral neuropathy	• Renal, hepatic, and hematologic function tests (CMP, CBC with diff) • Serum drug concentrations	• HIV protease inhibitors, phenobarbital, and rifampin: may decrease chloramphenicol serum concentrations
Fluoroquinolones					
Ciprofloxacin Levofloxacin Moxifloxacin	• Requires renal dose adjustment • Requires renal dose adjustment • Does not require renal dose adjustment	• Use caution—animal studies suggested teratogenicity (joint malformation); the effect appears to be the greatest in the 1st trimester • Safety data of levofloxacin in pediatric patients are limited to 14-day courses[2]	• Tendinitis and tendon rupture, arthralgia and myalgia, peripheral neuropathy, QTc prolongation, CNS toxicity, *Clostridioides difficile* infections, hepatotoxicity, aortic aneurysm and rupture of aortic aneurysm, hypoglycemia	• Renal (not with moxifloxacin), hepatic, and hematologic function tests (CMP, CBC with diff)	• Avoid concurrent administration with food or medications that contain multivalent cations (e.g., antacids, sucralfate, rube feeds, multivitamins) • Ciprofloxacin is an inhibitor of CYP1A2 and may increase serum concentrations of agents that are metabolized by CYP1A2 (e.g., propranolol, duloxetine) • QTc-prolonging effect may be enhanced with concurrent use with other QTc-prolonging agents

Drug (Routes of Administration)	Renal and Hepatic Dose Adjustment	Considerations in Pregnant and/or Breastfeeding Mothers and Pediatrics	Key Adverse Drug Reactions	Safety Laboratory Monitoring Parameters	Key Drug-Drug or -Food Interactions
Tetracyclines					
Doxycycline (IV/PO)	• Does not require renal or hepatic dose adjustment	• Avoid during pregnancy and lactation • A course of doxycycline for up to 14 days in pediatrics is likely not related to tooth staining[2]	• Rash, nausea, esophageal irritation, photosensitivity • Stains and deforms teeth in children <8 years old (including fetuses when given to pregnant women)	• Renal, hepatic, and hematologic function tests (CMP, CBC with diff)	• Avoid concurrent administration with food or medications that contain multivalent cations (e.g., antacids, sucralfate, rube feeds, multivitamins)
Tetracycline (PO)	• Avoid in severe renal impairment • Does not require hepatic dose adjustment				
Other Antibacterials					
Clindamycin	• Does not require renal or hepatic dose adjustment	• Safe for pregnancy	• Gastrointestinal side effects (diarrhea, vomiting, nausea) • *Clostridium difficile* infections	• Renal, hepatic, and hematologic function tests (CMP, CBC with diff)	
Clarithromycin	• Requires renal dose adjustment	• Depends on trimester—No evidence of teratogenicity was found during human pregnancy, but embryocidal effects were found following exposure during the 1st trimester	• Metallic taste • QTc prolongation	• Renal, hepatic, and hematologic function tests (CMP, CBC with diff)	• Clarithromycin is a CYP3A4 inhibitor and can increase serum concentrations of agents that are metabolized by CYP3A4
Linezolid (IV/PO)	• Does not require renal or hepatic dose adjustment	• Insufficient data	• Bone marrow suppression (associated with long-term therapy [> 3 weeks]) • Optic neuritis, irreversible sensory motor polyneuropathy (associated with long-term therapy [>3 weeks]) • Lactic acidosis	• Hematologic test (CBC with diff)	• Serotonergic agents due to concern for serotonin syndrome (risk is higher when multiple interacting serotonergic agents are administered together)

(Continued)

TABLE 2
Key Characteristics of Select Pharmacologic Agents Used for Discussed Infectious Agents—cont'd

Drug (Routes of Administration)	Renal and Hepatic Dose Adjustment	Considerations in Pregnant and/or Breastfeeding Mothers and Pediatrics	Key Adverse Drug Reactions	Safety Laboratory Monitoring Parameters	Key Drug-Drug or -Food Interactions
Rifampin (IV/PO)	• Does not require renal or hepatic dose adjustment • Use caution in patients with hepatic impairment	• Safe during pregnancy	• Red-orange discoloration of bodily fluids • Gastrointestinal side effects • Hypersensitivity reactions • Hepatotoxicity (LFT elevation) • Hematologic abnormalities (thrombocytopenia, hemolytic anemia)	• Hematologic and hepatic function test (CMP, CBC with diff)	• Rifampin is an inducer of CYP3A4 (strong), CYP2B6, 2C8, 2C19, and 2D6. Medications that are metabolized by the enzymes require dose adjustment
Trimethoprim/ sulfamethoxazole (TMP/SMX) (IV/PO)	• Require renal dose adjustment • Does not require hepatic dose adjustment	• Depends on trimester—Teratogenic and embryocidal effects were found in animal studies when used during the 1st trimester	• Hypersensitivity reaction (rash, toxic epidermal necrolysis [TEN]), Stevens Johnson Syndrome [SJS], Sweet's syndrome • Gastrointestinal side effects • Clinically nonsignificant elevation in serum creatinine • Hyperkalemia with higher doses • Photosensitivity • Myelosuppression with higher doses • Aseptic meningitis	• Renal, hepatic, and hematologic function tests (CMP, CBC with diff)	• Warfarin, phenytoin, sulfonylureas, procainamide, methotrexate, angiotensin converting enzyme inhibitors, angiotensin receptor blockers, potassium-containing agents
Vancomycin (IV)	• Require renal dose adjustment (serum drug concentration should be monitored) • Does not require hepatic dose adjustment	• Safe during pregnancy • Present in breast milk	• Nephrotoxicity, ototoxicity, vancomycin infusion reaction • Thrombocytopenia (rare)	• Renal and hematologic function tests (CMP, CBC with diff) • Serum drug concentration	• Avoid concurrent systemic use of other potentially nephrotoxic medications
ANTIVIRALS					
Baloxavir marboxil (PO)	• Does not require renal or hepatic dose adjustment	• Due to insufficient data, baloxavir is not recommended to be used during pregnancy • Unknown presence in breast milk	• Gastrointestinal side effects		• No known drug interactions

Drug (Routes of Administration)	Renal and Hepatic Dose Adjustment	Considerations in Pregnant and/or Breastfeeding Mothers and Pediatrics	Key Adverse Drug Reactions	Safety Laboratory Monitoring Parameters	Key Drug-Drug or -Food Interactions
Brincidofovir[44]	• Does not require renal or hepatic dose adjustment	• In animal studies: carcinogenic, teratogenic, and potential irreversible infertility • Unknown presence in breast milk • Weight based pediatric dose	• Gastrointestinal side effects • Increased risk for mortality with prolonged durations	• LFTs including bilirubin at baseline and during treatment • Pregnancy testing	• Take on an empty stomach (tab and suspension) or with a low-fat meal (tab only) • Increased concentrations when administered with OATP1B1 and 1B3 inhibitors
Cidofovir (IV)[45]	• Avoid use in patients with renal impairment (contraindicated for SCr > 1.5 mg/dL, CrCl ≤55 mL/min, urine protein ≥100 mg/dL) • Does not require hepatic dose adjustment	• In animal studies: carcinogenic, teratogenic, hypospermia • Unknown presence in breast milk	• Nephrotoxicity (dose dependent) • Neutropenia • Metabolic acidosis • Uveitis/Iritis (rare) and decreased intraocular pressure	• Renal and hematologic function tests (CMP, CBC with diff) with serum magnesium and phosphorus and urine protein	• Avoid concurrent systemic use of other potentially nephrotoxic medications • Substrate of OAT1 • Administered with probenecid, which has significant drug-drug interactions
Lopinavir/ritonavir	• Does not require renal or hepatic dose adjustment	• Insufficient data	• Increase in serum alanine aminotransferase • Gastrointestinal side effects (diarrhea) • Increased triglycerides and cholesterol • QTc prolongation	• CBC with diff, CMP	• Ritonavir is a strong inhibitor of CYP3A4. Medications that are metabolized by the enzymes require dose adjustment
Molnupiravir (PO)	• Does not require renal or hepatic dose adjustment	• Animal studies suggest possible fetal harm with in-utero exposure	• Hypersensitivity and dermatologic reactions (e.g., rash)		
Nirmatrelvir/ritonavir (PO)	• Require renal dose adjustment • Avoid use in severe renal and/or hepatic impairment	• Possible embryo-fetal developmental toxicities	• Dysgeusia, diarrhea, myalgia		• Ritonavir is a strong inhibitor of CYP3A4. Medications that are metabolized by the enzymes require dose adjustment

(Continued)

TABLE 2
Key Characteristics of Select Pharmacologic Agents Used for Discussed Infectious Agents—cont'd

Drug (Routes of Administration)	Renal and Hepatic Dose Adjustment	Considerations in Pregnant and/or Breastfeeding Mothers and Pediatrics	Key Adverse Drug Reactions	Safety Laboratory Monitoring Parameters	Key Drug-Drug or -Food Interactions
Oseltamivir (PO)	• Require renal dose adjustment • Does not require hepatic dose adjustment	• Safe during pregnancy (preferred neuraminidase inhibitor for the treatment and prophylaxis of influenza during pregnancy) • Present in breast milk	• Gastrointestinal side effects, headache • Neuropsychiatric events (e.g., confusion, delirium, hallucination): rare		• Dichlorphenamide and probenecid (can increase serum concentration of oseltamivir)
Peramivir (IV)	• Require renal dose adjustment • Does not require hepatic dose adjustment	• Insufficient data in use during pregnancy • Unknown presence in breast milk	• Hypertension, GI side effects, increased serum glucose, increased creatine phosphokinase in blood specimen	• Renal function test	• No known drug interactions
Remdesivir (IV)	• Avoid use in patients with severe renal impairment (estimated GFR < 30 mL/min/m^2) unless benefit outweighs the risk • Avoid use in patients with ALT ≥ five times the upper limit of normal at baseline	• Insufficient data	• Gastrointestinal side effects • Infusion-related reactions • Hypokalemia, hypoglycemia • Anemia, thrombocytopenia • Rash • Elevated transaminases and bilirubin • Prothrombin time elevation without a change in INR	• Renal, hepatic, and hematologic function tests (CMP, CBC with diff)	• Remdesivir is a substrate of CYP2C8, CYP2D6, CYP3A4, OAPT1B1, and P-glycoprotein transporter. It is also an inhibitor of CYP3A4, OATP1B1, BSEP, MRP4, and NTCP
Ribavirin	• Requires renal dose adjustment; contraindicated for CrCl <50 mL/min • Use is contraindicated in patients with hepatic decompensation (Child-Pugh classes B and C) with hepatitis C infected patients or autoimmune hepatitis	• Teratogenic; testicular toxicity • Avoid pregnancy during therapy and for 6 months after completion of treatment in both female and female partners of male patients who are taking ribavirin therapy	• Hemolytic anemia (dose-related) • Pancreatitis, pulmonary disorders, ophthalmologic disorders, psychiatric disorders • Dyspepsia, insomnia, headache, fatigue, nausea, gout, alopecia • Flu-like symptoms	• Renal and hematologic function tests (CMP, CBC with diff) • Hepatic function tests, including bilirubin • TSH, HCV, dental exam, EKG • Pregnancy testing	• Capsules should be taken with food • Abacavir, didanosine, zidovudine, azathioprine, dapsone, ganciclovir, amphotericin B, pyrimethamine, warfarin

Drug (Routes of Administration)	Renal and Hepatic Dose Adjustment	Considerations in Pregnant and/or Breastfeeding Mothers and Pediatrics	Key Adverse Drug Reactions	Safety Laboratory Monitoring Parameters	Key Drug-Drug or -Food Interactions
Tecovirimat	• Does not require renal or hepatic dose adjustment	• Insufficient data	• Gastrointestinal side effects, headache		• Take within 30 min of a full meal of moderate-to-high fat • Tecovirimat is a weak inhibitor of CYP2C8 and CYP2C19, and a weak inducer of CYP3A4 • Hypoglycemia with repaglinide • Decreases efficacy of midazolam • Capsules contain gelatin, lactose, and cellulose • Presumed drug interaction with smallpox vaccine
Zanamivir (INH)	• Does not require renal or hepatic dose adjustment	• Zanamivir use during pregnancy has not been shown to increase the risk of adverse outcomes • Unknown presence in breast milk	• Sore throat, cough, tonsil disease, sinusitis		• No known drug interactions
ANTITOXINS					
Heptavalent botulinum antitoxin (HBAT)	• Does not require renal or hepatic dose adjustment	• Insufficient data	Pruritus, urticarial, headache, nausea, fever, skin rash		• No known drug interactions
MONOCLONAL ANTIBODIES (MABS)					
Atoltivimab/ maftivimab/ odesivimab (IV)	• Does not require renal or hepatic dose adjustment	• Insufficient data but expected to cross the placenta	• Hypersensitivity and infusion-related reactions • Pyrexia, chills, tachycardia, tachypnea, vomiting	• Renal and hepatic function tests	• Presumed drug interaction with Ebola vaccine

(Continued)

TABLE 2
Key Characteristics of Select Pharmacologic Agents Used for Discussed Infectious Agents—cont'd

Drug (Routes of Administration)	Renal and Hepatic Dose Adjustment	Considerations in Pregnant and/or Breastfeeding Mothers and Pediatrics	Key Adverse Drug Reactions	Safety Laboratory Monitoring Parameters	Key Drug-Drug or -Food Interactions
Ansuvimab (IV)	• Does not require renal or hepatic dose adjustment	• Insufficient data but expected to cross the placenta	• Hypersensitivity and infusion-related reactions • Pyrexia, tachycardia, gastrointestinal, hypotension, tachypnea, chills	• Renal and hepatic function tests	• Presumed drug interaction with Ebola vaccine
Raxibacumab (IV)	• Does not require renal or hepatic dose adjustment	• Insufficient data	• Infusion site reaction, rash		• No known drug interactions
Obiltoxaximab (IV)	• Does not require renal or hepatic dose adjustment	• Insufficient data	• Headache, pruritus, upper respiratory tract infection, hypersensitivity reaction		• No known drug interactions
OTHERS					
Anthrax vaccine adsorbed (AVA [BioThrax]) (IM [preferred]/SubQ)	• Does not require renal or hepatic dose adjustment	• Insufficient data	• Injection site reactions, fatigue, headache		• No known drug interactions
Baricitinib (PO)	• Requires renal dose adjustment; not recommended in patients with estimated GFR below 15 mL/min/1.73 m^2	• Insufficient data	• Potentially increases infection risk and thrombosis; concomitant Janus kinase inhibitor (JAK) inhibitors or disease-modifying antirheumatic drugs (DMARDs)	• Renal and hepatic function tests; CBC with diff	• Dose reductions required with strong OAT inhibitors (e.g., probenecid)
Dexamethasone (IV/PO)		• Not recommended for use during pregnancy and lactation	• Potentially increases infection risk; hyperglycemia; GI side effects		• Dexamethasone is a major CYP3A4 substrate and a minor P-glycoprotein substrate

Drug (Routes of Administration)	Renal and Hepatic Dose Adjustment	Considerations in Pregnant and/or Breastfeeding Mothers and Pediatrics	Key Adverse Drug Reactions	Safety Laboratory Monitoring Parameters	Key Drug-Drug or -Food Interactions
Hydroxychloroquine (PO)	• Does not require renal or hepatic dose adjustment	• Safe during pregnancy and lactation	• Gastrointestinal side effects (dose-related), headache, dizziness, tinnitus, rash, pruritus, hypoglycemia, prolongation of QTc, QRS, and PR, retinal toxicity (dose-related)	• Hematologic and hepatic function tests • G6PD	• Antacids, antidiabetic drugs, antiepileptic drugs, digoxin, cyclosporine, QTc-prolonging agents
Tocilizumab (IV)	• Does not require renal or hepatic dose adjustment	• Safe during pregnancy and lactation	• Contraindicated in patients with known hypersensitivity to tocilizumab • Do not administer tocilizumab during any other concurrent active infections • Use caution in diverticulitis, GI perforation, immunosuppressed (particularly on biologic immunomodulating drugs), neutropenic and thrombocytopenic patients, LFTs >5–10× ULN	• Any development of new infection • Hepatic function tests and CBC with diff	• Inhibition of IL-6 may lead to increased metabolism of drugs that are CYP450 substrates
Vaccinia immune globulin intravenous (VIGIV) (IV)	• Caution in patients with renal insufficiency or at risk of renal insufficiency	• Insufficient data	• Headache, nausea, rigors, dizziness • Thrombotic events, aseptic meningitis, hemolysis, and transfusion-related reactions • Contraindicated for isolated vaccinia keratitis, history of severe reactions to immunoglobulin products, immunoglobulin A deficiency	• Renal function and urine output • Consider thrombotic evaluation prior to starting therapy, including fasting triglycerides • Some adverse reactions may be associated with the infusion rate	• Maltose in VIGIV can cause falsely high glucose with some glucose testing • Can interfere with serologic testing • Interacts with live vaccines

Abbreviations: *ALT*, alanine transaminase; *BMP*, basic metabolic panel; *BUN*, blood urea nitrogen; *CBC with diff*, complete blood count with differentials; *CMP*, comprehensive metabolic panel; *CrCl*, creatinine clearance; *CNS*, central nervous system; *EKG*, electrocardiogram; *G6PD*, glucose-6-phosphate dehydrogenase; *GFR*, glomerular filtration rate; *GI*, gastrointestinal; *HCV*, hepatitis C virus; *IM*, intramuscular use; *INH*, oral inhalation; *IV*, intravenous; *OAT*, organic anion transporter; *PO*, oral use; *SCr*, serum creatinine; *SubQ*, subcutaneous use; *TSH*, thyroid stimulating hormone; *ULN*, upper limit of normal.

Brincidofovir is available as a once weekly oral tablet and suspension that allows for targeted delivery of the drug to the virus within the infected cells instead of concentrating in the organic anion transporters in the kidney tubules like cidofovir (Table 1).[44,54] In addition, brincidofovir has demonstrated up to 100-fold higher potency compared to cidofovir.[54–56] In a retrospective case series from the United Kingdom, three patients received brincidofovir at 200 mg once or two doses separated by a week. No patient tolerated the recommended three weekly doses from the manufacturer.[57] With a lack of renal accumulation, brincidofovir is less likely to cause dose-limiting nephrotoxicity and does not require co-administration with probenecid. While not as toxic as cidofovir to the patient, it is considered a potential carcinogen and should be handled with care. It should not be administered concomitantly with intravenous cidofovir or the smallpox vaccine.[44]

Cidofovir is rarely used in clinical practice due to limitations in available formulations, significant toxicities, and drug-drug interactions. Cidofovir was originally approved for the treatment of cytomegalovirus retinitis in persons living with acquired immunodeficiency syndrome (AIDS) when co-administered with probenecid.[45] The addition of probenecid to cidofovir creates a drug-drug interaction that increases and prolongs the levels of cidofovir. Cidofovir carries several black box warnings from the FDA, including nephrotoxicity, neutropenia, and carcinogenicity/teratogenicity. The risk of nephrotoxicity remains substantial despite mitigation strategies such as prehydration and co-administration of probenecid. Dosing of cidofovir to treat smallpox is not established, but the medication could be made available through the CDC's expanded access protocol from the SNS.[9,50] To treat smallpox vaccine adverse reactions, cidofovir is a potential second-line therapy. The early Mpox case series included 12 persons (2%) that were treated with cidofovir.[58]

Vaccinia immune globulin intravenous

CNJ-016 (also known as VIGIV) are immunoglobulins collected from the sera of individuals that have been vaccinated against smallpox.[59] Since the smallpox vaccine contains the vaccinia virus instead of the wild-type variola virus, the immunoglobulins provide passive immunity to the vaccinia virus. This product is licensed for the treatment of acute complications from the vaccine, including eczema vaccinatum, progressive vaccinia, severe generalized vaccinia, or for patients with vaccinia infections and select skin conditions. Vaccinia immune globulin intravenous (VIGIV) is not effective for postvaccinia encephalitis (Table 1).[59] While there is no guidance on repeat doses, there are phase one data supporting safety for up to 24,000 units/kg. This medication should be administered as soon as symptoms appear with an infusion rate of 2 mL/min.[59] The CDC has an active EA-IND to use VIGIV for treatment of orthopoxviruses, including both smallpox and Mpox.[9]

Tularemia (See Chapter 3 for Additional Information)

The diverse clinical presentations of tularemia all manifest following exposure to the bacterium *Francisella tularensis*.[10] The route of exposure ultimately determines the clinical presentation of the disease. Naturally occurring tularemia occurs by direct inoculation from a bite (e.g., tick bite) or contact with an infected animal host (i.e., skin and eye contact, ingestion, and inhalation). The most relevant bioterrorism exposure would be via aerosol-exposure leading to inhalational tularemia with progression to the pneumonic form of the infection.[60]

Tularemia is treated primarily with three antimicrobial classes: aminoglycosides, fluoroquinolones, and tetracyclines. The CDC recommends streptomycin, gentamicin, ciprofloxacin, and doxycycline as preferred treatment options for adults (Table 1). Of note, neither gentamicin nor ciprofloxacin is approved by the FDA for the treatment of tularemia. Antimicrobial selection depends on patient characteristics, including age, underlying medical conditions (e.g., kidney disease) or pregnancy, availability of agents, and clinical presentation. Limited availability of streptomycin often requires using alternative agents such as gentamicin or other antimicrobial classes. Therefore, gentamicin has been used preferentially for naturally occurring infections and is recommended in casualty situations. However, during times of mass causality, limitations on parenteral therapy access and the ability to provide therapeutic monitoring favor the use of enteral agents over the aminoglycosides. In this case, ciprofloxacin and doxycycline are preferred for both adults and children. Due to reported higher rates of treatment failure with tetracyclines, some experts recommend ciprofloxacin preferentially in this circumstance. Specific considerations for use of certain antimicrobial agents include utilizing an aminoglycoside for severe presentations of tularemia and the addition of chloramphenicol for treatment of meningitis. Therapy for a minimum of 10 days is recommended for most agents, except doxycycline, which should be administered for at least 14 days. In the event of a known attack, PEP may be initiated with doxycycline or ciprofloxacin for exposed people who are within the incubation period. No PEP is necessary for close contacts.[10,60]

In pregnancy, the treatment of tularemia requires weighing the potential teratogenicity of the preferred agents (see Tables 1 and 2) with the risk of developing infection in the exposed individual. During a mass casualty event, the risk of exposure to and from the infection outweighs the risk of toxicity, leading to recommendations for ciprofloxacin and doxycycline in this patient population. Limited case series have shown the safety and efficacy of ciprofloxacin for the treatment of tularemia in pregnancy.[61]

Viral Hemorrhagic Fevers (Additional Information in Chapter 5)

Numerous "old world" and "new world" viral families, including *Arenaviridae, Bunyaviridae, Filoviridae, Flaviviridae,* and *Paramyxoviridae*, cause viral hemorrhagic fevers (VHF).[62] Despite a long list of viruses that can cause VHF, supportive care remains the mainstay of therapy, and there are limited antiviral options available, with only two that are FDA-approved specifically for Ebola virus infection (Table 1).[11,63–65] For viruses within its spectrum of activity, such as arenaviruses (excluding *Filoviridae* and *Flaviviridae* viruses), intravenous ribavirin is the recommended treatment. The quantity and quality of evidence for treatment vary significantly for the various different VHF virus's.[11] Other potential therapeutics include convalescent plasma and numerous investigational agents that are beyond the scope of this chapter.

Ebolavirus monoclonal antibodies

There are two FDA-approved monoclonal antibody formulations for the treatment of one Ebolavirus species, *Zaire ebolavirus* (Ebola): Inmazeb (REGN-EB3) and Ebanga (MAb114).[64–66] Inmazeb, the first to be FDA-approved, contains a cocktail of three monoclonal IgG1 antibodies, atoltivimab, maftivimab, and odesivimab, that specifically target the *Zaire ebolavirus* glycoprotein. The glycoprotein targeted is important for viral attachment and incorporation into the host cell and is also expressed on the surface of Ebola-infected host cells. The three monoclonal antibodies can bind simultaneously and noncompetitively. The pharmacokinetics of these agents in patients with Ebola are presumed to be altered, yet the available pharmacokinetic data for this monoclonal antibody combination product is derived from healthy individuals.[64]

An open label controlled clinical trial of four different potential therapies (ZMapp [the control group], the antiviral agent remdesivir, the single human-derived monoclonal antibody MAb114 [Ebanga], or the triple monoclonal antibody REGN-EB3 [Inmazeb]), 681 adults and children with confirmed Ebolavirus infections were randomized to one of the study arms.[67] There was a 17.8% decrease in mortality among the 155 patients who received Inmazeb compared to 169 who received an investigational control monoclonal antibody, ZMapp[68] (95% confidence interval [CI] −28.9 to −2.9, $P = .002$). In addition, among those receiving Inmazeb, the median time to a negative Ebola PCR (from blood) was 15 days compared to 20–30 for the other treatment arm. When comparing Inmazeb to ZMapp, the odds ratio of death 28 days after infusion was 79% lower (OR = 0.21; 95% CI 0.08 to 0.53).

Ebanga (or ansuvimab-zykl; MAb114) is a single monoclonal antibody targeting the glycan cap subunit of the *Zaire ebolavirus* glycoprotein and thus inhibits viral entry into host cells.[65] In a separate study arm of this same randomized controlled trial, patients receiving ansuvimab-zykl had a 28-day mortality of 35.1% (mortality difference −14.6; 95% CI −25.2 to −1.7, $P = .007$) compared to 49.7% (95% CI 0.1–0.61) in the group that received the control, ZMapp.[68] The mortality rates were similar to those reported in the Inmazeb group, as was the time to negative blood PCR at 16 days. Importantly, receipt of the Ebola vaccine or other baseline disease severity and comorbid conditions impacted all study arms and may modulate mortality based on the multivariable models.

Ribavirin

Although ribavirin is commercially available as an oral and inhaled formulation, the intravenous formulation must be obtained through a compassionate use program from the FDA.[67,69,70] It is a guanine analog that has been in use for various antiviral indications since the 1970s. Despite decades of use, its mechanism of action remains poorly understood.[71] Of the viruses that can present as a VHF, ribavirin has either in vitro or in vivo data to support activity against *Lassa* virus, *Junin* virus (known as Argentine HF), *Machupo* virus (known as Bolivian HF), *Lujo* virus, Crimean Congo HF virus, Rift Valley Fever, and *Hantavirus*. If one of the former viruses is suspected and the patient presents with severe signs and symptoms, intravenous ribavirin can be considered for treatment. Ribavirin should not be used for the major VHF pathogens in the *Filoviruses* and *Flaviviruses* families.[62,63,72]

Ribavirin dosing recommendations are primarily derived from a 1986 pragmatic, adaptive design study comparing intravenous ribavirin, oral ribavirin, or convalescent plasma to no therapy for Lassa fever.[73] Because the case fatality rate in the arms where patients received intravenous ribavirin alone or intravenous ribavirin plus convalescent plasma were similar, the results were combined. Among the 108 participants, the case fatality rate was 76% for those with untreated Lassa fever, 57% when treated with convalescent plasma,

32% when treated with intravenous ribavirin (with or without convalescent plasma), and 30% when treated with oral ribavirin. The decrease in case fatality was most profound when treatment was initiated within the first 6 days of symptoms.[73] In addition to this clinical prospective study examining ribavirin treatment for *Lassa* virus, a 2019 systematic review and metaanalysis identified five additional retrospective cohorts and estimated the odds of death as 0.13 (95% CI 0.04 to 0.4) when ribavirin was administered in addition to supportive care vs. supportive care alone.[74] Based on these data, ribavirin is recommended for treatment and PEP in both guidance from the CDC and the World Health Organization (WHO) for any VHF not caused by Ebola or Marburg viruses (Table 1).[11,75–77]

Convalescent plasma

Persons who have recovered from a VHF can donate plasma to convalescent plasma banks. When infused into a patient with an active infection, the convalescent plasma with immunoglobulins specific to the infection should, theoretically, provide passive immunity. For the treatment of VHF, convalescent plasma has conflicting efficacy results depending on the specific viral etiology.[62,78,79] A double-blind placebo-controlled trial demonstrated the efficacy of 500 mL of convalescent plasma in treating *Junin* virus, the cause of Argentine HF.[80] If convalescent plasma was administered within 8 days of symptom onset, the case fatality rate decreased from 16.5% to 1.1% when compared to those receiving control plasma.[80]

Other investigational agents

Due to the persistent global threat of VHF, there have been numerous attempts to find safe therapeutic treatment options for the varied viral organisms and species. Despite these efforts, supportive intensive care largely remains the mainstay of treatment for VHF. Other potential agents that have limited data and are under investigation include favipiravir, interferon alpha, ivermectin, chloroquine, pentoxifylline, convalescent plasma for other VHF, monoclonal antibodies, and intravenous immunoglobulins (IVIG).[62,63,71,72,81]

VIRAL RESPIRATORY DISEASES WITH PANDEMIC POTENTIAL

Influenza and Avian Influenza

Influenza (see Chapters 7 and 8 for additional information)

Influenza represents a common cause of seasonal and occasionally pandemic respiratory illness throughout the world (e.g., H1N1, H2N3). The spectrum of the disease varies, and more severe forms of the disease are seen in high-risk groups and with certain usually emerging strains. High-risk groups that warrant priority for antiviral treatment include hospitalized patients, patients with severe, complicated, or progressive illness, and individuals at higher risk for influenza complications (e.g., underlying immunosuppression or respiratory disease, pregnancy, etc.). Those at high risk require expedited treatment for suspected or confirmed influenza. Generally, antiviral treatment initiation should occur within 48 h of illness to optimize antiviral efficacy, and treatment following longer onset periods may be considered for more severely ill and immunocompromised patients.[19,20]

The treatment of influenza consists of supportive care, administration of antivirals, and in some instances, secondary bacterial infections. Routine use of corticosteroids should be avoided due to associated prolonged viral shedding and increased mortality unless corticosteroids are indicated for another underlying medical condition.[20] The two recommended pharmacologic treatment categories for influenza are neuraminidase inhibitors (oseltamivir, zanamivir, and peramivir) and cap-dependent endonuclease inhibitors (baloxavir). Underlying medical conditions (e.g., respiratory disease for inhaled zanamivir, renal dysfunction for peramivir and oseltamivir, etc.) should be considered when choosing and dosing antiinfluenza agents. Adamantanes (amantadine and rimantadine) are not currently recommended due to high levels of circulating resistance in influenza A viruses and lack of activity against influenza B viruses.

Hospitalized patients should receive the appropriate neuraminidase inhibitor based on the preponderance of efficacy data in this subset of influenza patients and continued low levels of circulating resistance.[19,20] Retrospective studies demonstrate that hospitalized patients treated with baloxavir have similar clinical outcomes as with neuraminidase inhibitors.[82] For patients unable to swallow, an alternative enteral formulation of oseltamivir (i.e., oral suspension) is available for administration via nasogastric tube. If enteral administration is not feasible, intravenous peramivir may be utilized, although there is limited evidence defining its efficacy in hospitalized patients.[83,84] The unique mechanism of action of baloxavir and synergy with neuraminidase inhibitors makes combination therapy an attractive option in severe influenza cases; however, the benefits of dual therapy remain unknown pending larger studies.[85] On the other hand, zanamivir, when combined with oseltamivir or peramivir, is antagonistic.[19,86]

For outpatients with uncomplicated influenza infection, oseltamivir, inhaled zanamivir, intravenous peramivir, or baloxavir may be considered. Available formulations vary among these antivirals, and administration is optimized based on treatment setting and patient characteristics. Potential advantages of baloxavir are reduced viral shedding duration, suggesting a potential public health benefit by preventing the spread of influenza, and the single dose lessens potential medication compliance issues.[87] Oseltamivir and inhaled zanamivir are administered for 5 days, while baloxavir and peramivir require 1 day of treatment; extended durations may be considered for severe infection or in certain patient populations (e.g., immunosuppressed).[19,20]

Antiviral selection may differ from recommendations above in select populations (see Table 1) and during a pandemic. Oseltamivir remains the preferred medication in pregnancy based on multiple studies demonstrating safety and efficacy.[19] Higher doses of oseltamivir have been used for the treatment of influenza, especially for pandemic H1N1 strains. Increased doses are not recommended for seasonal influenza due to clinical trials demonstrating no benefit.[20,88,89] During a pandemic, novel influenza strains may predominate and display unique antiviral resistance profiles, leading to different recommendations of agents, dosing, and the need for combination therapy.[90]

Routine chemoprophylaxis for preexposure (PrEP) and PEP prophylaxis is not recommended to avoid the potential to select for resistance. For example, oseltamivir use leads to the development of resistance, particularly in H1N1 and subtherapeutic doses (e.g., chemoprophylaxis), and underlying immunosuppression with prolonged viral replication increases the risk for developing resistance.[20,91] Notably, in outbreak settings (e.g., long-term care facilities), more liberal administration of antivirals such as PrEP and PEP is recommended.[92] In addition, PrEP or PEP may be recommended including for adults or children with a high risk of developing complications or individuals in close contact with another individual at high risk for developing complications when vaccination is contraindicated, unavailable, delayed, or expected to have low efficacy for the at-risk individual.[20] Agents for chemoprophylaxis include inhaled zanamivir, oseltamivir, and baloxavir.[19] The recommended duration for PrEP is for the duration of community influenza activity until 7 days after the last known exposure, whereas the recommended duration for PEP is 7 days after the most recent exposure for zanamivir and oseltamivir (or 1 day if baloxavir is used).[19,20]

Avian influenza (see Chapter 8 for additional information)

Novel influenza A viruses arise in both wild and domesticated avian species. The two most prominent strains identified are the highly pathogenic avian influenza (HPAI) A (H5N1) virus and low-pathogenic avian influenza (LPAI) A (H7N9) virus. Due to their potential threat for triggering global pandemics, these, along with other avian influenza viruses (e.g., other H5 variants), require careful epidemiological monitoring and further studies to identify optimal treatment.[21]

For hospitalized patients with an avian influenza strain, initiate treatment in all confirmed, probable, and cases under investigation. Therapy initiation should occur as soon as possible and should be initiated regardless of time from illness onset to patient presentation.[21] Avian influenza viruses demonstrate prolonged viral shedding resulting from higher viral loads and sustained viral replication necessitating a prolonged treatment initiation window.[93] This commonly requires input from local, regional, or national public health experts. For patients in the outpatient setting, treatment may be withheld from cases under investigation or those limited to only travel exposure without exposure to a human case or infected bird.

Avian influenza treatment is treated similarly to seasonal influenza. Most of the data exists for oseltamivir, which is the preferred therapy, especially for severe, progressive, or complicated illnesses, while intravenous peramivir or inhaled zanamivir are alternatives. A global registry of H5N1 influenza A infections demonstrated that providing at least one dose of oseltamivir increased the crude survival from 24% to 60%.[94] Double-dose oseltamivir is not routinely recommended based on insufficient evidence. A randomized controlled trial, that included 5.2% influenza A H5N1 cases assessed viral clearance or clinical outcomes for the treatment of severe influenza and found no benefit of increased doses of oseltamivir.[89] The efficacy of intravenous peramivir and zanamivir in treating novel influenza viruses is reported in cases series.[95] Baloxavir has in vitro activity against a wide array of influenza strains, including avian influenza viruses; however, no clinical efficacy is currently available.[96] The necessity or effectiveness of combination therapy has not been well studied and is not recommended. The optimal duration of therapy remains unknown. A minimum of 10 days is recommended for severely ill hospitalized patients.[21] Higher doses of oseltamivir are not routinely recommended based on insufficient evidence. A randomized controlled trial that included 5.2% influenza A H5N1 cases assessed viral clearance or clinical outcomes for the treatment of severe influenza and found no benefit of increased doses of oseltamivir.[89] Adamantanes (amantadine and rimantadine) should be avoided due to circulating resistance among novel influenza viruses. Corticosteroids should not be given due to insufficient evidence to support use. Limited data suggests corticosteroids prolong viral shedding, increase antiviral resistance, and increase mortality.[95,97]

PEP can be considered for all exposed individuals, especially among those at high risk for complications (e.g., immunosuppressed, chronic respiratory disease, etc.) and those within the highest-risk exposure category (i.e., household, or close family member contacts of a confirmed or probable case). Chemoprophylaxis should be initiated preferably within 48 h of exposure using either oral oseltamivir or inhaled zanamivir twice daily for 5–10 days. The shorter duration is recommended for time-limited exposures and patients without ongoing exposures, whereas 10 days is recommended for ongoing (e.g., household) exposure.[21]

Severe Acute Respiratory Syndrome (See Chapter 9 for Additional Information)

The original novel severe acute respiratory syndrome (SARS) coronavirus (SARS-CoV-1), an enveloped, positive-sense ribonucleic acid (RNA) beta-coronavirus, was implicated in a worldwide outbreak between November 2002 and August 2003, where 8096 probable cases were recorded with 774 deaths from 29 countries, centered primarily in Southeast Asia.[98] This novel virus is thought to have originated as an endemic bat coronavirus before making the jump to an intermediate animal host, likely palm civets, and ultimately into humans. The resultant disease, SARS, is characterized by a febrile respiratory syndrome and atypical pneumonia, which can progress to acute respiratory distress syndrome (ARDS) in approximately 15% of patients. Overall mortality was reported around 10% but reached as high as 50% in those over age 60.

Despite the rapid and dramatic spread of SARS, an aggressive global public health response controlled the epidemic such that no additional cases have been reported since 2004. Therefore, large randomized controlled interventional trials were not performed, and no consensus on therapeutic management was reached.[98] The mainstay of therapy remains supportive care, including intensive care and mechanical ventilation for those who progress to respiratory failure. No specific therapy has proven effective, although clinical experiences during the epidemic and therapies with efficacy against subsequent epidemic coronaviruses may provide clues as to potential effective therapies should SARS re-emerge.

Ribavirin was one of the most commonly used therapies, alone or in combination, during the SARS pandemic. Case series and retrospective observational studies suggested possible benefits from ribavirin, but results were confounded by a lack of controls and concomitant use of other therapies. The sole RTC in Guangdong, China, evaluated multiple treatment arms and failed to show benefit with low-dose ribavirin (400–600 mg/day) compared to steroids and interferon alfa.[99] Moreover, in vitro testing subsequently demonstrated an inability to achieve inhibition of SARS-CoV-1 replication at therapeutically achievable levels of ribavirin.[98] These findings, along with the drug's substantial toxicities at higher doses, limit its potential utility for SARS.

The HIV protease inhibitor combination lopinavir/ritonavir was also utilized during the pandemic, with a signal of decreased progression to ARDS or death seen in retrospective evaluation compared to historical matched controls.[100] Another study compared outcomes with lopinavir/ritonavir as initial therapy or salvage rescue therapy with matched controls as part of a protocol including steroids and ribavirin for all patients.[101] This study found that initial treatment with lopinavir/ritonavir resulted in a statistically significant reduction in mortality and progression to mechanical ventilation. Delayed use as salvage therapy failed to demonstrate the same benefit. Other protease inhibitors and antiviral compounds, including fusion inhibitors, small-molecule inhibitors of ACE2 receptor binding, niclosamide, glycyrrhizin, and small interfering RNAs, have been evaluated in vitro or with experimental animal models, but human clinical data are lacking.[98]

Immunomodulatory therapy with steroids and type 1 interferon (IFN) was commonly deployed in treatment. High-dose corticosteroids were added to target ARDS and immune hyperactivity, which are often seen in those patients with SARS who demonstrated clinical deterioration with anecdotal success.[98] However, the retrospective nature, lack of control groups, and frequent combination with other therapies such as ribavirin prevented any definitive conclusions about the role of steroids in SARS. Counterbalancing the uncertain efficacy, concerns regarding prolonged viral shedding and toxicities such as avascular necrosis and secondary bacterial and mold infections were associated with steroid use. Additional immunotherapy in the form of IVIG and SARS convalescent plasma was utilized, with inconclusive results observed.

A seminal 2006 systematic review of the major proposed SARS treatments commissioned by the WHO evaluated 54 SARS treatment studies, 15 in vitro studies, and three ARDS management studies.[102] The in vitro studies demonstrated that ribavirin, lopinavir/ritonavir, and type 1 IFN could inhibit SARS-CoV in tissue culture. However, no therapy conclusively demonstrated benefit in human clinical trials (ribavirin: 26 studies inconclusive, four possible harms; corticosteroids: 25 studies inconclusive, four possible harms; type 1 IFN: three studies inconclusive; lopinavir/ritonavir: two studies inconclusive; convalescent plasma or IVIG: seven studies inconclusive). Since this review was published, therapeutics such as the antivirals remdesivir and nirmatrelvir/ritonavir, monoclonal antibodies targeting the spike protein, and corticosteroids in the treatment of the related virus SARS-CoV-2 that have been developed and tested could alter treatment recommendations and clinical trial design priorities should SARS re-emerge.

In terms of prevention, extensive efforts to develop effective vaccines against SARS-CoV-1 have been undertaken using a variety of platforms, including viral vectors, recombinant DNA, and inactivated vaccines.[98] Most vaccines targeted the spike glycoprotein on the surface of the virus, with extensive animal model data demonstrating neutralizing antibody responses. However, the observation of vaccine-associated enhanced respiratory disease in animals raised concerns about possible paradoxical severe disease from a natural infection following vaccination. More encouragingly, the recent development of highly effective vaccines against SARS-CoV-2 across various vaccine platforms provides strong proof of concept for active immunization, and recent work has focused on developing a potential mRNA vaccine with broad protection against all beta-coronaviruses.[103]

Middle East Respiratory Syndrome (See Chapter 10 for Additional Information)

Middle East respiratory syndrome (MERS) coronavirus (MERS-CoV) was the second novel epidemic betacoronavirus of the 21st century and was first identified in 2012 in a patient with severe respiratory illness in Jeddah, the Kingdom of Saudi Arabia (KSA). Since 2012, over 2400 cases of MERS have been reported to the WHO, primarily in the Arabian Peninsula or linked to infected travelers returning from the region. Unlike SARS-CoV-1, MERS-CoV continues to cause sporadic cases and endemic disease primarily in the Arabian Peninsula due to its ongoing animal reservoir, the dromedary camels. Unlike SARS, MERS can present with asymptomatic infection and, like SARS, can produce severe respiratory and multiorgan failure and has a higher associated case fatality rate of approximately 40%.[104] The updated 2019 WHO treatment guidelines prioritize early recognition and diagnosis, rigorous infection prevention and control measures, and meticulous supportive care, including intensive care ventilatory management and organ support.[105] No specific antiviral therapies are recommended outside of the context of clinical interventional trials.

The most promising treatment data comes from a randomized, adaptive, double-blind, placebo-controlled trial of IFN beta-1b plus lopinavir/ritonavir for 14 days versus placebo in hospitalized MERS patients.[106] Conducted at nine sites in the KSA, in 95 patients the trial demonstrated a reduction in 90-day mortality associated with combination therapy (28% vs 44%; one-sided P value = .024). A prespecified subgroup analysis demonstrated that benefit was primarily in those receiving treatment within 7 days of symptom onset, although early trial cessation may have led to an overestimation of the treatment effect size. Other antiviral combinations, such as IFN alpha-2a plus ribavirin, have demonstrated significant mortality reduction by day 14 but not day 28 in a retrospective cohort of critically ill MERS patients.[104] Other experimental antivirals or repurposed drugs have been proposed based on in vitro data, such as MERS-CoV fusion inhibitors, cyclosporine, chloroquine, nitazoxanide, and mycophenolate.[104]

Steroid therapy is frequently used for severe or critically ill patients with MERS, but clinical trials have not documented its efficacy. Retrospective, observational data in 309 adults treated with steroids demonstrated no mortality benefit and suggested longer duration of viral spreading, prompting recommendations to avoid their use in MERS.[107] Other immunomodulatory therapies such as monoclonal antibodies, convalescent plasma, and polyclonal human immunoglobulins are under investigation. Again, the development and demonstrated success of SARS-CoV-2 therapeutics, including the antivirals remdesivir and nirmatrelvir/ritonavir, monoclonal antibodies, and steroids, may alter treatment decisions and clinical trial priorities if a large MERS outbreak starts.

Regarding prevention, ongoing efforts to develop effective vaccines against MERS-CoV have tested recombinant modified vaccine Ankara (MVA), vesicular stomatitis viral vector vaccines, DNA vaccines, and other vaccine platforms in nonhuman primate studies. Another prevention strategy that has been investigated involves immunizing camels to break the cycle of transmission. Given the success of the SARS-CoV-2 vaccines, renewed efforts in MERS-CoV and pan-beta-coronavirus vaccine development have recently garnered scientific attention.[103,108]

Coronavirus Disease 2019 (COVID-19) (See Chapter 11 for Additional Information)

SARS-CoV-2 is the causative agent of COVID-19 and the third novel beta-coronavirus emerging in the 21st century. First identified in Wuhan, China, in late 2019, this pathogen caused a global pandemic with over 640 million reported cases and 6.6 million deaths as of December 2022. Given the duration and magnitude of the pandemic, an array of observational and randomized interventional trials was conducted to evaluate both novel and repurposed drug treatments for COVID-19. Prior work on SARS-CoV-1 and MERS-CoV and rapidly expanding scientific understanding of this novel agent have identified key therapeutic targets from the virus lifecycle as well as the host immune and inflammatory response.[109] The following section briefly summarizes recommended treatment options as of December 2022 through the rapidly evolving treatment paradigms that require reference to continuously updated guidelines from groups such as the WHO (https://www.who.int/publications/i/item/WHO-2019-nCoV-therapeutics-2022.4), the US National Institutes of Health (NIH; https://www.covid19treatmentguidelines.nih.gov/), or the Infectious Diseases Society of America (https://www.idsociety.org/practice-guideline/covid-19-guideline-treatment-and-management/) for the latest recommendations.

A guiding principle of clinical approaches to COVID-19 management is categorizing patients by disease severity and stage of illness to optimize the efficacy and timing of therapeutic interventions.[110] Disease severity is generally stratified as asymptomatic infection, mild disease (no signs or symptoms of lower respiratory disease), moderate disease (evidence of lower respiratory disease and oxygen saturation ≥ 94% on room air [RA]), severe disease (lower respiratory tract disease plus RA oxygen saturation < 94%), and critical illness (respiratory failure, shock, or multiorgan dysfunction). However, an individual patient's clinical severity can change with the unpredictable and highly variable tempo of disease. Disease stages are typically divided into the preexposure, incubation, and early viral phases when most symptoms are driven by viral replication, followed in some patients with a hyperinflammatory phase when host immune and inflammatory responses drive disease pathogenesis. Finally, a substantial fraction of patients' experiences, prolonged symptoms of postacute sequelae of COVID-19 (PASC) that are still poorly understood. Understanding the severity, phase, and tempo of an individual patient's disease can assist clinicians in timing specific therapeutic interventions within the context of the care delivery setting and available resources.[110]

Inpatient COVID-19 management

The best studied interventions for COVID-19 are in the management of hospitalized COVID-19 patients, often derived from large national or multinational, adaptive platform clinical trials. These therapeutics can largely be divided into three categories: antivirals, passive immunity, and immunomodulatory therapy.

The first and only FDA-approved antiviral for the treatment of hospitalized COVID-19 patients is remdesivir, a nucleoside triphosphate prodrug that inhibits viral RNA polymerase. Based on prior in vitro studies in other coronaviruses, this agent was quickly moved into clinical trials to evaluate its efficacy against COVID-19. The NIH-sponsored ACTT-1 trial was a randomized, double-blind, placebo-controlled trial in 1062 patients, which demonstrated that 10 days of remdesivir significantly reduced time to recovery by 5 days and increased the odds of clinical improvement (odds ratio 1.5; 95% CI 1.2–1.9) by day 15 compared to placebo.[111] Subgroup analyses suggested that those presenting within 10 days of symptom onset and receiving lower levels of oxygen derived the most benefit from remdesivir. Importantly, this trial was not adequately powered to demonstrate a mortality benefit with remdesivir. Subsequent clinical trials have shown equivalent outcomes comparing a 5 versus 10-day treatment course.[112] Although other early clinical trials individually failed to show a mortality benefit when remdesivir was compared to standard of care,[111,112] the final report of the WHO-sponsored SOLIDARITY trial in over 14,000 patients demonstrated a 13% reduction (RR 0.87 [0.76–0.99], $P = .03$) in in-hospital mortality in hospitalized patients on oxygen but not mechanically ventilated.[113] No clinical benefit was seen in patients already on mechanical ventilation. A combined metaanalysis of all randomized trials of remdesivir in hospitalized patients showed similar results.[113] Although differences in trial design, outcome measures, and evolving standards of care make head-to-head comparisons difficult, the current data suggests remdesivir offers a clinical benefit in hospitalized patients who are not yet mechanically ventilated.[114] Remdesivir does generally appear to be well tolerated but requires monitoring of hepatic transaminases and renal function for toxicity.[110]

Passive immunity is provided by both monoclonal antibodies (mAbs) targeting the SARS-CoV-2 spike protein and convalescent plasma from recovered COVID-19 patients. Although mAbs have played a major role in outpatient management (discussed below), their efficacy in hospitalized patients has been limited. The largest trial to date, the RECOVERY trial, randomized 9785 hospitalized patients to receive standard of care with or without a single 8000 mg dose of the mAb cocktail casirivimab/imdevimab and demonstrated no difference in 28-day all-cause mortality, time to hospital discharge, or disease progression.[115] Unfortunately, with the continued evolution of the SARS-CoV-2 virus leading to new variants (such as the Omicron subvariants BQ.1, BQ.1.1, and XBB) that escape the available mAbs, in December 2022, there are no authorized mAbs available for treatment. Similarly, convalescent plasma (CP) has been studied and not demonstrated significant benefit in hospitalized patients despite initial enthusiasm, including a US-based CP registry that treated over 100,000 patients early in the pandemic. Multiple RCTs evaluating CP and a systematic review and metaanalysis show no difference in all-cause mortality or other clinical benefits in hospitalized patients.[116,117]

The most effective class of interventions thus far for hospitalized COVID-19 patients have been immunomodulatory therapies, targeting the hyperinflammatory host response often present in patients with clinical disease progression. The paradigm-shifting RECOVERY trial demonstrated a significant mortality reduction (22.9% vs 25.7%, age-adjusted risk ratio 0.83; $P < .001$) when the corticosteroid dexamethasone 6 mg daily for up to 10 days was administered compared to standard of care in hospitalized patients.[118] The strongest benefit was seen in patients on mechanical ventilation or supplemental oxygen, while no benefit and possible harm was seen in those not requiring oxygen. Other clinical trials, many stopped early after the publication of the RECOVERY trial, confirmed this benefit so that corticosteroid use has become the standard of care for all hospitalized patients requiring oxygen or ventilatory support.[119] Further research studies to clarify the optimal corticosteroid agent, dose, and duration for specific patient populations are still ongoing.

Two other classes of immunomodulatory therapies—interleukin-6 receptor antagonists (IL-6-RA) and the Janus kinase inhibitor, baricitinib—also improve outcomes in those with severe COVID-19 disease. Following initial discordant results from earlier clinical trials, two large, adaptive platform trials, REMAP-CAP and RECOVERY, demonstrated that the addition of IL-6-RA tocilizumab to corticosteroids reduced 28-day all-cause or in-hospital mortality.[120,121] Of note, the inclusion criteria for both studies specifically targeted patients with signs of hyperinflammation and clinical progression to higher levels of oxygen or ventilatory support despite receipt of corticosteroids. In the ACTT-2 trial, the JAK1/2 inhibitor, baricitinib, when added to remdesivir compared to remdesivir alone decreased the time to clinical recovery, particularly in the group requiring high-flow oxygen or noninvasive ventilation.[122] More importantly, the COV-Barrier trial found that hospitalized patients receiving baricitinib compared to those receiving placebo added to standard of care (about 80% of patients in both groups received a systemic corticosteroid) had a significantly reduced mortality.[123] Current NIH and IDSA treatment guidelines recommend the addition of either tocilizumab or baricitinib to corticosteroids in patients requiring higher levels of oxygen or ventilatory support and showing signs of clinical progression. Supportive but less robust data demonstrated similar benefits with the IL-6-RA sarilumab and the JAK inhibitor tofacitinib, suggesting a broader class effect.[124] More clinical data derived from head-to-head comparisons of different immunomodulator combinations and longer-term studies of their risks, including secondary infections, are still needed.

Outpatient COVID-19 management

Despite less attention in initial clinical trials, effective outpatient treatments for early stage COVID-19 to prevent clinical disease progression requiring hospitalization are essential for individual patients and to preserve the healthcare system. In the early stages of the pandemic, the most effective outpatient therapeutics were the monoclonal antibodies (mAbs) targeting the SARS-CoV-2 spike protein. In the United States, a total of four mAbs received emergency use authorization (EUA) for use in outpatients with risk factors for disease progression and with mild-to-moderate COVID-19: the combination products casirivimab/imdevimab and bamlanivimab/etesevimab, and the single agents sotrovimab and bebtelovimab. The first three products were studied in "Phase 3" RCTs among outpatients that have mild to moderate COVID-19 with risk factors for disease progression and significantly reduced the risk of hospitalization or death from COVID-19.[125–127] However, all three products were subsequently removed from clinical use due to emergent viral resistance. Bebtelovimab was authorized based on more limited clinical trial data and in vitro studies demonstrating activity against the Omicron variant (B1.1.529) of SARS-CoV-2. However, with the arrival of newer Omicron subvariants (BQ.1, BQ.1.1, and XBB), which demonstrate high-level resistance to bebtelovimab in vitro, its EUA was revoked, leaving no available mAbs for treatment as of December 2022.[128] On the other hand, high-titer polyclonal antibody therapy in the form of CP could still play a role in early outpatient treatment, although significant logistical challenges of screening plasma and CP administration remain. A recent RCT demonstrated a 3.4% absolute risk reduction (1.0%–5.8%; $P=.005$) and a 54% relative risk reduction in 28-day hospitalization in patients receiving CP within 9 days of symptom onset, although most were unvaccinated.[129]

Given the logistical challenges of passive immune therapies, affordable and effective oral antiviral treatments are a significant unmet need, particularly for low and middle-income countries.[130] Early studies with oral repurposed agents such as hydroxychloroquine, chloroquine, azithromycin, lopinavir/ritonavir, nitazoxanide, and ivermectin showed no benefit when studied in larger, rigorous trials.[110,124] Several novel direct antivirals are efficacious in early outpatient treatment of COVID-19. Ritonavir-boosted nirmatrelvir, a novel oral antiviral combination that targets the viral protease inhibitor, is authorized under EUA and the preferred therapy for outpatients over 12 years of age who are at high risk for progression to severe COVID-19 and within 5 days of symptom onset. The EPIC-HR trial, a phase 2/3 study in 2246 unvaccinated high-risk participants, demonstrated a 5.81% absolute risk reduction (95% CI [−7.78% to −3.84%], $P<.001$; 88.9% relative risk reduction) in 28-day COVID-19-related hospitalization or death.[131] However, the parallel study conducted in much lower-risk patients (EPIC-SR) failed to demonstrate a significant benefit with early treatment. Moreover, all randomized trials studied unvaccinated patients and predated the current Omicron variants, leaving unanswered the question of benefit in contemporary patients. Nevertheless, recent observational data from the Omicron era supports that higher-risk patients, particularly those 65 years of age or older, have lower hospitalization or death rates with ritonavir-boosted nirmatrelvir treatment, regardless of vaccination status or prior SARS-CoV-2 immunity.[132] The medication is dosed as 300 mg nirmatrelvir, plus 100 mg ritonavir twice daily for 5 days in those with normal renal function; a dose adjustment to 150 mg nirmatrelvir is required for an estimated glomerular filtration rate (GFR) between 30 and 60 mL/min.[133] It is not currently recommended in patients with severe liver dysfunction (CTP class C) or an estimated GFR < 30 mL/min. The other major consideration for its use is the extensive potential drug-drug interactions due to the pharmacokinetic boosting effects of ritonavir. This may limit its use in some populations, and prescribers should consult with available drug interaction resources such as the University of Liverpool COVID-19 Drug Interaction Tool (https://www.covid19-druginteractions.org/).

While intravenous remdesivir is primarily used for inpatient COVID-19 treatment, its utility in high-risk outpatients was shown in a Phase 3 RTC (PINETREE) comparing 3 days of remdesivir (200 mg IV load followed by 100 mg infusions on 2 following days) to placebo within 7 days of symptom onset. This study found an 87% relative reduction (HR 0.13; 95% CI 0.03–0.59; $P=.008$) in the risk of COVID-19 related hospitalization or death at day 28.[134] The major barriers to its widespread deployment are the medication cost and logistics of three consecutive daily IV infusions given on an outpatient basis.

Molnupiravir, an oral prodrug of a ribonucleoside analog that interferes with viral replication, is currently authorized under EUA for outpatients with mild-to-moderate COVID-19 at high risk for progression within 5 days of symptom onset. This approval was based on the phase three MOVe-OUT study, which randomized 1433 patients to receive either molnupiravir 800 mg twice daily for 5 days or a placebo. The results showed an absolute risk reduction of 3% (95% CI −5.9% to −0.1%; relative risk reduction 30%) in hospitalization or death by day 29 with molnupiravir treatment.[135] Based on this lower demonstrated efficacy, molnupiravir is only recommended when other outpatient COVID-19 treatments are not available. Importantly, due to concerns about the teratogenicity and mutagenic potential of molnupiravir, the drug is not recommended for use in those who are pregnant, and effective contraception should be used during and following treatment.

Prevention

The cornerstone of COVID-19 prevention is active vaccination with one of several approved SARS-CoV-2 vaccines (see Chapter 20 for additional information). While a comprehensive review of the data supporting active vaccination is beyond the scope of this chapter, several SARS-CoV-2 vaccines across different platforms, including mRNA, adenoviral vector, and protein subunit vaccines, have demonstrated remarkable efficacy at reducing symptomatic disease, hospitalization, or death due to COVID-19.[136] Additionally, vaccination has been shown to reduce asymptomatic infection and transmission, although to lesser degrees and with more rapid waning efficacy against milder disease. The efficacy of the vaccines has varied with the variants. The efficacy of the vaccines has decreased somewhat with the emergence of the Omicron variant and subvariants. Much work remains to define the optimal number of vaccine doses and intervals for long-term immune protection and to understand the impact of emerging SARS-CoV-2 variants on the need for updated vaccine boosters to optimize protection. Additionally, addressing the challenges of global vaccine distribution and equity and overcoming vaccine hesitancy remain paramount concerns.

Research on the use of drug therapies for PrEP and PEP in COVID-19 has demonstrated mixed results. Most early studies of chemoprophylaxis focused on hydroxychloroquine, which was not shown to have any efficacy in this setting.[137] Other trials of chemoprophylaxis agents such as ritonavir-boosted nirmatrelvir or molnupiravir are either still underway or have been negative. There is hope that novel oral antivirals under development against coronaviruses could also have utility when used for PrEP or PEP. The mAbs against SARS-CoV-2 have previously demonstrated efficacy in the PrEP and PEP settings, preventing symptomatic COVID-19 among persons with close contact with COVID-19-infected individuals. For example, a trial of mAbs for PEP showed a reduction in rates of symptomatic infection following a household exposure with casirivimab/imdevimab compared to placebo (29% for the mAb arm and 42% for the placebo arm; $P=.038$).[138] Similarly, Cohen and colleagues demonstrated a reduction in symptomatic disease for residents or staff in skilled nursing or assisted living facilities with the use of bamlanivimab monotherapy as PrEP compared to placebo (8.5% for the mAb arm and 15.2% for the placebo arm; $P<.001$) in the prevaccine period.[139] Unfortunately, as of December 2022, the emergent viral resistance with the new Omicron subvariants discussed above has rendered the previously available mAbs ineffective for PEP.

While active vaccination has obviated the need for PrEP in most immunocompetent patients, moderately to severely immunocompromised patients remain at higher risk for infection despite vaccination. In this special population, the development of mAbs with an extended half-life, such as the combination tixagevimab/cilgavimab, has served as an important tool for the prevention of COVID-19. This product received EUA for PrEP in those 12 years of age and older who are moderate or severely immunocompromised and not expected to mount an adequate immune response to vaccination or who are not able to receive the vaccine due to prior adverse reactions. The phase 3 PROVENT randomized clinical trial demonstrated that use of intramuscular tixagevimab/cilgavimab (at a lower dose of 150/150 mg) had a 77% relative risk reduction (95% CI, 46%–90%) of developing symptomatic COVID-19.[140] With the arrival of the original Omicron variant of concern (BA.1), the FDA recommended an increased dose of 300/300 mg due to the mAbs reduced in vitro activity. Based on the original pharmacokinetic studies, the FDA currently recommends repeat dosing every 6 months with tixagevimab/cilgavimab. Finally, many of the newest emerging Omicron subvariants (including BA.4.6, BQ.1, BQ.1.1, among others) demonstrate resistance to tixagevimab/cilgavimab in vitro, suggesting that this product's utility for PrEP is waning quickly and vulnerable patients should still practice recommended nonpharmacologic precautions even after receiving it.

REFERENCES

1. Hendricks KA, Wright ME, Shadomy SV, et al. Centers for disease control and prevention expert panel meetings on prevention and treatment of anthrax in adults. *Emerg Infect Dis.* 2014;20(2), e130687. https://doi.org/10.3201/eid2002.130687.
2. Bradley JS, Peacock G, Krug SE, et al. Pediatric anthrax clinical management: executive summary. *Pediatrics.* 2014;133(5):940–942.
3. Sobel J, Rao AK. Making the best of the evidence: toward national clinical guidelines for botulism. *Clin Infect Dis.* 2017;66(suppl_1):S1–S3.
4. BAT (Botulism Antitoxin Heptavalent [A, B, C, D, E, F, G]—[Equine] Solution for Injection) [Product Monograph]. Winnipeg, Manitoba, Canada: Emergent BioSolutions Canada; September 2019.
5. BabyBIG (BIG-IV) (Botulism Immune Globulin) [Prescribing Information]. Temecula, CA: FFF Enterprises; 2015. September.
6. Centers for Disease Control and Prevention. Plague. Clinical Care of Plague (Updated May 15, 2024). https://www.cdc.gov/plague/hcp/clinical-care/index.html [Accessed 6 November 2024].
7. Nelson CA, Meaney-Delman D, Fleck-Derderian S, Cooley KM, Yu PA, Mead PS. Antimicrobial treatment and prophylaxis of plague: recommendations for naturally acquired infections and bioterrorism response. *MMWR Recomm Rep.* 2021;70(RR-3):1–27. https://doi.org/10.15585/mmwr.rr7003a1.
8. CDC. Smallpox For Clinicians Treatment; 2020. https://www.cdc.gov/smallpox/clinicians/treatment.html. Updated July 2, 2020. Accessed 9 May 2021.
9. Prevention CfDCa. Treatment Information for Healthcare Professionals; 2022. Updated July 28, 2022. Available from: https://www.cdc.gov/poxvirus/monkeypox/clinicians/treatment.html.
10. Centers for Disease Control and Prevention. Tularemia. Clinical Care of Tularemia (Updated May 15, 2024). https://www.cdc.gov/tularemia/hcp/clinical-care/?CDC_AAref_Val=https://www.cdc.gov/tularemia/clinicians/index.html [Accessed 6 November 2024].

11. CDC. Management of patients with suspected viral hemorrhagic fever. *MMWR*. 1988;37(S-3):1–16.
12. Al-Tawfiq JA. Therapeutic options for human brucellosis. *Expert Rev Anti-Infect Ther*. 2008;6(1):109–120.
13. Shane AL, Mody RK, Crump JA, et al. 2017 Infectious Diseases Society of America clinical practice guidelines for the diagnosis and management of infectious diarrhea. *Clin Infect Dis*. 2017;65(12):1963–1973.
14. Wong KK, Burdette E, Mahon BE, Mintz ED, Ryan ET, Reingold AL. Recommendations of the Advisory Committee on Immunization Practices for use of cholera vaccine. *MMWR Morb Mortal Wkly Rep*. 2017;66(18):482–485.
15. Anderson A, Bijlmer H, Fournier PE, et al. Diagnosis and management of Q fever—United States, 2013: recommendations from CDC and the Q FeverWorking Group. *MMWR Recomm Rep*. 2013;62(RR-03):1–30.
16. Mandell LA, Wunderink RG, Anzueto A, et al. Infectious Diseases Society of America/American Thoracic Society consensus guidelines on the management of community-acquired pneumonia in adults. *Clin Infect Dis*. 2007;44(Suppl. 2):S27–S72.
17. Fenollar F, Fournier PE, Carrieri MP, et al. Risks factors and prevention of Q fever endocarditis. *Clin Infect Dis*. 2001;33(3):312–316.
18. Tunkel AR, Glaser CA, Bloch KC, et al. The management of encephalitis: clinical practice guidelines by the Infectious Diseases Society of America. *Clin Infect Dis*. 2008;47(3):303–327.
19. Centers for Disease Control and Prevention. Seasonal Influenza (Flu): Treatment; 2024. https://www.cdc.gov/flu/treatment/index.html. Accessed 30 November 2021.
20. Uyeki TM, Bernstein HH, Bradley JS, et al. Clinical practice guidelines by the Infectious Diseases Society of America: 2018 update on diagnosis, treatment, chemoprophylaxis, and institutional outbreak Management of Seasonal Influenza A. *Clin Infect Dis*. 2019;68(6):e1–e47.
21. Centers for Disease Control and Prevention. Avian Flu: Health Care & Laboratorian Guidance. https://www.cdc.gov/flu/avianflu/treatment-prophylaxis.htm. Accessed 30 November 2021.
22. Holty J-EC, Bravata DM, Liu H, Olshen RA, McDonald KM, Owens DK. Systematic review: a century of inhalational anthrax cases from 1900 to 2005. *Ann Intern Med*. 2006;144(4):270–280.
23. Katharios-Lanwermeyer S, Holty J-E, Person M, et al. Identifying meningitis during an anthrax mass casualty incident: systematic review of systemic anthrax since 1880. *Clin Infect Dis*. 2016;62(12):1537–1545.
24. Turnbull PCB, Sirianni NM, LeBron CI, et al. MICs of selected antibiotics for *Bacillus anthracis*, *Bacillus cereus*, *Bacillus thuringiensis*, and *Bacillus mycoides* from a range of clinical and environmental sources as determined by the Etest. *J Clin Microbiol*. 2004;42(8):3626–3634.
25. Bower WA, Schiffer J, Atmar RL, et al. Use of anthrax vaccine in the United States: recommendations of the Advisory Committee on Immunization Practices. *MMWR Recomm Rep*. 2019;68(RR-4):1–14. https://doi.org/10.15585/mmwr.rr6804a1.
26. Wright JG, Plikaytis BD, Rose CE, et al. Effect of reduced dose schedules and intramuscular injection of anthrax vaccine adsorbed on immunological response and safety profile: a randomized trial. *Vaccine*. 2014;32:1019–1028.
27. Malkevich NV, Basu S, Rudge Jr TL, et al. Effect of anthrax immune globulin on response to BioThrax (anthrax vaccine adsorbed) in New Zealand white rabbits. *Antimicrob Agents Chemother*. 2013;57:5693–5696.
28. Jeffery LA, Karim S. Botulism. In: *StatPearls*. Treasure Island, FL: StatPearls Publishing; 2021. January [Internet]. [Updated 2020 Jul 19]. Available from: https://www.ncbi.nlm.nih.gov/books/NBK459273/.
29. Centers for Disease Control and Prevention (CDC). Botulism Annual Summary, 2017. Atlanta, Georgia: US Department of Health and Human Services, CDC; 2019.
30. Arnon SS, Schechter R, Maslanka SE, Jewell NP, Hatheway CL. Human botulism immune globulin for the treatment of infant botulism. *N Engl J Med*. 2006;354(5):462–471.
31. Griese SE, Kisselburgh HM, Bartenfeld MT, et al. Pediatric botulism and use of equine botulinum antitoxin in children: a systematic review. *Clin Infect Dis*. 2017;66:S17–S29.
32. O'Horo JC, Harper EP, El Rafei A, et al. Efficacy of antitoxin therapy in treating patients with foodborne botulism: a systematic review and meta-analysis of cases, 1923–2016. *Clin Infect Dis*. 2017;66:S43–S56.
33. Yu PA, Lin NH, Mahon BE, et al. Safety and improved clinical outcomes in patients treated with new equine-derived heptavalent botulinum antitoxin. *Clin Infect Dis*. 2018;66(suppl_1):S57–S64.
34. Ni SA, Brady MF. Botulism antitoxin. In: *StatPearls*. Treasure Island, FL: StatPearls Publishing; 2021. January. [Internet]. [Updated 2020 Sep 27]. Available from: https://www.ncbi.nlm.nih.gov/books/NBK534807/.
35. Carrillo-Marquez MA. Botulism. *Pediatr Rev*. 2016;37(5):183–192.
36. Kugeler KJ, Mead PS, Campbell SB, Nelson CA. Antimicrobial treatment patterns and illness outcome among United States patients with plague, 1942-2018. *Clin Infect Dis*. 2020;70(70 Suppl. 1):S20–S26.
37. Boulanger LL, Ettestad P, Fogarty JD, Dennis DT, Romig D, Mertz G. Gentamicin and tetracyclines for the treatment of human plague: review of 75 cases in new Mexico, 1985-1999. *Clin Infect Dis*. 2004;38(5):663–669.
38. Mwengee W, Butler T, Mgema S, et al. Treatment of plague with gentamicin or doxycycline in a randomized clinical trial in Tanzania. *Clin Infect Dis*. 2006;42(5):614–621.
39. Inglesby TV, Dennis DT, Henderson DA, et al. Plague as a biological weapon: medical and public health management. Working Group on Civilian Biodefense. *JAMA*. 2000;283(17):2281–2290.
40. Godfred-Cato S, Cooley KM, Fleck-Derderian S, et al. Treatment of human plague: a systematic review of published aggregate data on antimicrobial efficacy, 1939-2019. *Clin Infect Dis*. 2020;70(70 Suppl. 1):S11–S19.
41. Meaney-Delman D, Oussayef NL, Honein MA, Nelson CA. Plague and pregnancy: why special consider-

ations are needed. *Clin Infect Dis.* 2020;70(70 Suppl. 1):S27–S29.
42. Lexi-Drugs Online. Waltham, MA: UpToDate, Inc; December 1, 2021. https://online.lexi.com. Accessed 1 December 2021.
43. Micromedex Solutions. Greenwood Village, CO: Truven Health Analytics; 2021. http://micromedex.com/. Updated December 1, 2021. Accessed 1 December 2021.
44. Tembexa (Brincidofovir) [Package Insert]. Whippany, NJ: Chimerix; 2021. Revised 06/2021.
45. Vistide (Cidofovir Injection) [Package Insert]. Foster City, CA: Gilead Sciences; 2000. Updated 09/2000.
46. Petersen BW, Damon IK. Orthopoxviruses vaccinia (smallpox vaccine), variola (smallpox), monkeypox, and cowpox. In: *Mandell, Douglas, and Bennett's Principles and Practice of Infectious Diseases.* 9th ed. Philadelphia, PA: Elsevier; 2020:1809–1817.e3. [chapter 132].
47. TPOXX (Tecovirimat) [Package Insert]. Winchester, KY: Catalent Pharma Solutions; 2018. Revised 07/2018.
48. Grosenbach DW, Honeychurch K, Rose EA, et al. Oral tecovirimat for the treatment of smallpox. *N Engl J Med.* 2018;379(1):44–53.
49. SIGA Technologies Inc. TPOXX-tecovirimat monohydrate injection, solution, concentrate. In: *DailyMed [Internet].* Bethesda (MD): National Library of Medicine (US); 2018 [rev. 2024 Apr; cited 2024 Nov]. Available from: https://dailymed.nlm.nih.gov/dailymed/fda/fdaDrugXsl.cfm?setid=fce826ab-4d6a-4139-a2ee-a304a913a253&type=display.
50. (CDC) CfDCaP. Information for Healthcare Providers on Obtaining and Using TPOXX (Tecovirimat) for Treatment of Monkeypox; 2022. Updated August 18, 2022. Available from: https://www.cdc.gov/poxvirus/monkeypox/clinicians/obtaining-tecovirimat.html.
51. (CDC) CfDCaP. Expanded Access IND Protocol: Use of Tecovirimat (TPOXX®) for Treatment of Human Non-Variola Orthopoxvirus Infections in Adults and Children. IND No. 116,039. CDC IRB No. 6402. Available from: https://www.cdc.gov/poxvirus/monkeypox/pdf/Tecovirimat-IND-Protocol-CDC-IRB.pdf.
52. Russo AT, Berhanu A, Bigger CB, et al. Co-administration of tecovirimat and ACAM2000 in non-human primates: effect of tecovirimat treatment on ACAM2000 immunogenicity and efficacy versus lethal monkeypox virus challenge. *Vaccine.* 2020;38(3):644–654.
53. Drugs.com. Chimerix Announces FDA Acceptance of New Drug Application for Brincidofovir as a Medical Countermeasure for Smallpox; 2020. https://www.drugs.com/nda/brincidofovir_201207.html. December 7, 2020. Accessed 9 May 2021.
54. Painter W, Robertson A, Trost LC, Godkin S, Lampert B, Painter G. First pharmacokinetic and safety study in humans of the novel lipid antiviral conjugate CMX001, a broad-spectrum oral drug active against double-stranded DNA viruses. *Antimicrob Agents Chemother.* 2012;56(5):2726–2734.
55. Delaune D, Iseni F. Drug development against smallpox: present and future. *Antimicrob Agents Chemother.* 2020;64(4), e01683-19.
56. Olson VA, Smith SK, Foster S, et al. In vitro efficacy of brincidofovir against variola virus. *Antimicrob Agents Chemother.* 2014;58(9):5570–5571.
57. Adler H, Gould S, Hine P, et al. Clinical features and management of human monkeypox: a retrospective observational study in the UK. *Lancet Infect Dis.* 2022;22(8):1153–1162.
58. Thornhill JP, Barkati S, Walmsley S, et al. Monkeypox virus infection in humans across 16 countries—April-June 2022. *N Engl J Med.* 2022;387(8):679–691.
59. CNJ-016, Vaccinia Immune Globulin Intravenous (Human), Sterile Solution [Package Insert]. Cangene Corporation; 2010. Revised 01/2010.
60. Dennis DT, Inglesby TV, Henderson DA, et al. Tularemia as a biological weapon: medical and public health management. *JAMA.* 2001;285(21):2763–2773.
61. Yesilyurt M, Kilic S, Celebsmall i UB, Gul S. Tularemia during pregnancy: report of four cases. *Scand J Infect Dis.* 2013;45(4):324–328.
62. Ippolito G, Feldmann H, Lanini S, et al. Viral hemorrhagic fevers: advancing the level of treatment. *BMC Med.* 2012;10:31.
63. Kilgore PE, Grabenstein JD, Salim AM, Rybak M. Treatment of Ebola virus disease. *Pharmacotherapy.* 2015;35(1):43–53.
64. Inmazeb (Atoltivimab, Maftivimab, and Odesivimab-Ebgn) [Package Insert]. Tarrytown, NT: Regeneron; 2020. Revised 10/2020. Accessed 11 May 2021.
65. Ebanga (asuvimab-zykl) [Package Insert]. Miami, Fl: Ridgeback Biotherapeutics, LP; 2020. Revised 12/2020. Accessed 11 May 2021.
66. CDC. Ebola (Ebola Virus Disease) Treatment; 2021. https://www.cdc.gov/vhf/ebola/treatment/index.html. Revised February 26, 2021. Accessed 11 May 2021.
67. Shoemaker T, Choi M. Travel-related infectious diseases viral hemorrhagic fevers. In: *CDC Yellow Book 2020: Health Information for International Travel.* New York: Oxford University Press; 2019 [chapter 4].
68. Mulangu S, Dodd LE, Davey Jr RT, et al. A randomized, controlled trial of Ebola virus disease therapeutics. *N Engl J Med.* 2019;381(24):2293–2303.
69. Rebetol® (ribavirin) [Package Insert]. Whitehouse Station, NJ: Merck & CO; 2013. Revised 11/2013. Accessed 10 May 2021.
70. Virazole® (Ribavirin for Inhalation Solution) [Package Insert]. Bridgewater, NJ: Hospira; 2019. Revised 05/2019. Accessed 10 May 2021.
71. De Clercq E. New nucleoside analogues for the treatment of hemorrhagic fever virus infections. *Chem Asian J.* 2019;14(22):3962–3968.
72. Iannetta M, Di Caro A, Nicastri E, et al. Viral hemorrhagic fevers other than Ebola and Lassa. *Infect Dis Clin N Am.* 2019;33(4):977–1002.
73. McCormick JB, King IJ, Webb PA, et al. Lassa fever effective therapy with ribavirin. *N Engl J Med.* 1986;314:20–26.
74. Eberhardt KA, Mischlinger J, Jordan S, Groger M, Gunther S, Ramharter M. Ribavirin for the treatment of Lassa fever: a systematic review and meta-analysis. *Int J Infect Dis.* 2019;87:15–20.

75. World Health Organization. Clinical Management of Patients With Viral Haemorrhagic Fever: A Pocket Guide for Front-Line Health Workers Interim Emergency Guidance for Country Adaptation; 2016. https://apps.who.int/iris/bitstream/handle/10665/205570/9789241549608_eng.pdf. Published February 2016. Accessed 10 May 2021.
76. Borio L, Inglesby T, Peters CJ, et al. Hemorrhagic fever viruses as biological weapons medical and public health management. *JAMA.* 2002;287:2391–2405.
77. Hadi CM, Goba A, Khan SH, et al. Ribavirin for Lassa fever postexposure prophylaxis. *Emerg Infect Dis.* 2010;16(12):2009–2011.
78. Centers for Disease Control and Prevention. Viral Hemorrhagic Fevers (VHFs) (Updated April 15, 2024). https://www.cdc.gov/viral-hemorrhagic-fevers/about/index.html [Accessed 10 May 2021].
79. Braden JB, Duchin JS. Instructor's Manual Preparing for and Responding to Bioterrorism: Information for Primary Care Clinicians Tularemia and Viral Hemorrhagic Fevers; 2002. Revised July 2002. Accessed 10 May 2021.
80. Enria DA, Briggiler AM, Sanchez Z. Treatment of argentine hemorrhagic fever. *Antivir Res.* 2008;78:132–139.
81. Thomas SJ, Endy TP, Rothman AL, Barrett AD. Flaviviruses (dengue, yellow fever, Japanese encephalitis, West Nile Encephaliis, Usutu encephalitis, St. Lois encephalitis, tick-borne encephalitis, Kyasanur Forest disease, Alkhurma hemorrhagic fever, Zika). In: *Mandell, Douglas, and Bennett's Principles and Practice of Infectious Diseases.* 9th ed. Philadelphia, PA: Elsevier; 2020:2013–2039.e7.
82. Shah S, McManus D, Bejou N, et al. Clinical outcomes of baloxavir versus oseltamivir in patients hospitalized with influenza a. *J Antimicrob Chemother.* 2020;75(10):3015–3022.
83. de Jong MD, Ison MG, Monto AS, et al. Evaluation of intravenous peramivir for treatment of influenza in hospitalized patients. *Clin Infect Dis.* 2014;59(12):e172–e185.
84. Lee JS, Lee MS, Park Y, Lee J, Joo EJ, Eom JS. Clinical effectiveness of intravenous peramivir versus oseltamivir for the treatment of influenza in hospitalized patients. *Infect Drug Resist.* 2020;13:1479–1484.
85. Fukao K, Noshi T, Yamamoto A, et al. Combination treatment with the cap-dependent endonuclease inhibitor baloxavir marboxil and a neuraminidase inhibitor in a mouse model of influenza A virus infection. *J Antimicrob Chemother.* 2019;74(3):654–662.
86. Duval X, van der Werf S, Blanchon T, et al. Efficacy of oseltamivir-zanamivir combination compared to each monotherapy for seasonal influenza: a randomized placebo-controlled trial. *PLoS Med.* 2010;7(11):e1000362.
87. Hayden FG, Sugaya N, Hirotsu N, et al. Baloxavir marboxil for uncomplicated influenza in adults and adolescents. *N Engl J Med.* 2018;379(10):913–923.
88. Lee N, Hui DS, Zuo Z, et al. A prospective intervention study on higher-dose oseltamivir treatment in adults hospitalized with influenza a and B infections. *Clin Infect Dis.* 2013;57(11):1511–1519.
89. South East Asia Infectious Disease Clinical Research Network. Effect of double dose oseltamivir on clinical and virological outcomes in children and adults admitted to hospital with severe influenza: double blind randomised controlled trial. *BMJ.* 2013;346:f3039.
90. CDC. Pandemic Influenza Plan: 2017. Update https://www.cdc.gov/flu/pandemic-resources/pdf/pan-flu-report-2017v2.pdf.
91. Graitcer SB, Gubareva L, Kamimoto L, et al. Characteristics of patients with oseltamivir-resistant pandemic (H1N1) 2009, United States. *Emerg Infect Dis.* 2011;17(2):255–257.
92. (CDC) CfDCaP. Guidance: Outbreak Management in Long-Term Care Facilities; 2022. [updated November 21, 2022. Available from: https://www.cdc.gov/flu/professionals/infectioncontrol/ltc-facility-guidance.htm.
93. Yu L, et al. Clinical, virological, and histopathological manifestations of fatal human infections by avian influenza A(H7N9) virus. *Clin Infect Dis.* 2013;57(10):1449–1457.
94. Adisasmito W, et al. Effectiveness of antiviral treatment in human influenza A(H5N1) infections: analysis of a Global Patient Registry. *J Infect Dis.* 2010;202(8):1154–1160.
95. Hu Y, et al. Association between adverse clinical outcome in human disease caused by novel influenza A H7N9 virus and sustained viral shedding and emergence of antiviral resistance. *Lancet.* 2013;381(9885):2273–2279.
96. Noshi T, Kitano M, Taniguchi K, et al. In vitro characterization of baloxavir acid, a first-in-class cap-dependent endonuclease inhibitor of the influenza virus polymerase PA subunit. *Antivir Res.* 2018;160:109–117.
97. Sivanandy P, et al. A review on current trends in the treatment of human infection with H7N9-avian influenza A. *J Infect Public Health.* 2019;12(2):153–158.
98. Groneberg DA, Poutanen SM, Low DE, Lode H, Welte T, Zabel P. Treatment and vaccines for severe acute respiratory syndrome. *Lancet Infect Dis.* 2005;5(3):147–155.
99. Zhao Z, Zhang F, Xu M, et al. Description and clinical treatment of an early outbreak of severe acute respiratory syndrome (SARS) in Guangzhou, PR China. *J Med Microbiol.* 2003;52(Pt 8):715–720.
100. Chu CM, Cheng VC, Hung IF, et al. Role of lopinavir/ritonavir in the treatment of SARS: initial virological and clinical findings. *Thorax.* 2004;59(3):252–256.
101. Chan KS, Lai ST, Chu CM, et al. Treatment of severe acute respiratory syndrome with lopinavir/ritonavir: a multicentre retrospective matched cohort study. *Hong Kong Med J.* 2003;9(6):399–406.
102. Stockman LJ, Bellamy R, Garner P. SARS: systematic review of treatment effects. *PLoS Med.* 2006;3(9):e343.
103. Saunders KO, Lee E, Parks R, et al. Neutralizing antibody vaccine for pandemic and pre-emergent coronaviruses. *Nature.* 2021;594(7864):553–559.
104. Zumla A, Hui DS, Perlman S. Middle East respiratory syndrome. *Lancet.* 2015;386(9997):995–1007.
105. World Health Organization. Middle East Respiratory Syndrome Coronavirus (MERS-CoV). https://www.who.int/health-topics/middle-east-respiratory-syndrome-coronavirus-mers#tab=tab_1. Accessed 26 November 2021.

106. Arabi YM, Asiri AY, Assiri AM, et al. Interferon beta-1b and lopinavir-ritonavir for Middle East respiratory syndrome. *N Engl J Med.* 2020;383(17):1645–1656.
107. Arabi YM, Mandourah Y, Al-Hameed F, et al. Corticosteroid therapy for critically ill patients with Middle East respiratory syndrome. *Am J Respir Crit Care Med.* 2018;197(6):757–767.
108. Modjarrad K, Roberts CC, Mills KT, et al. Safety and immunogenicity of an anti-Middle East respiratory syndrome coronavirus DNA vaccine: a phase 1, open-label, single-arm, dose-escalation trial. *Lancet Infect Dis.* 2019;19(9):1013–1022.
109. Sanders JM, Monogue ML, Jodlowski TZ, Cutrell JB. Pharmacologic treatments for coronavirus disease 2019 (COVID-19): a review. *JAMA.* 2020;323(18):1824–1836.
110. Bae E, Sanders JM, Johns M, et al. Therapeutic options for coronavirus disease 2019 (COVID-19): where are we now? *Curr Infect Dis Rep.* 2021;23(12):28. https://doi.org/10.1007/s11908-021-00769-8. [Epub 2021 Dec 11].
111. Beigel JH, Tomashek KM, Dodd LE, et al. Remdesivir for the treatment of Covid-19—final report. *N Engl J Med.* 2020;383(19):1813–1826.
112. Goldman JD, Lye DCB, Hui DS, et al. Remdesivir for 5 or 10 days in patients with severe Covid-19. *N Engl J Med.* 2020;383(19):1827–1837.
113. Department of error. *Lancet.* 2022;400(10362):1512.
114. Ansems K, Grundeis F, Dahms K, et al. Remdesivir for the treatment of COVID-19. *Cochrane Database Syst Rev.* 2021;8:CD014962.
115. Horby PW, Mafham M, Peto L, et al. Casirivimab and imdevimab in patients admitted to hospital with COVID-19 (RECOVERY): a randomised, controlled, open-label, platform trial. *medRxiv.* 2021. https://doi.org/10.1101/2021.06.15.21258542. 2021.06.15.21258542.
116. Group RC. Convalescent plasma in patients admitted to hospital with COVID-19 (RECOVERY): a randomised controlled, open-label, platform trial. *Lancet.* 2021;397(10289):2049–2059.
117. Axfors C, Janiaud P, Schmitt AM, et al. Association between convalescent plasma treatment and mortality in COVID-19: a collaborative systematic review and meta-analysis of randomized clinical trials. *BMC Infect Dis.* 2021;21(1):1170.
118. Group RC, Horby P, Lim WS, et al. Dexamethasone in hospitalized patients with Covid-19. *N Engl J Med.* 2021;384(8):693–704.
119. Group WHOREAfC-TW, Sterne JAC, Murthy S, et al. Association between Administration of Systemic Corticosteroids and Mortality among critically ill patients with COVID-19: a meta-analysis. *JAMA.* 2020;324(13):1330–1341.
120. Abani O, Abbas A, Abbas F, et al. Tocilizumab in patients admitted to hospital with COVID-19 (recovery): a randomised, controlled, open-label, platform trial. *Lancet.* 2021;397(10285):1637–1645.
121. The REMAP-CAP Investigators. Interleukin-6 receptor antagonists in critically ill patients with covid-19. *N Engl J Med.* 2021;384(16):1491–1502. https://doi.org/10.1056/NEJMoa2100433.
122. Kalil AC, Patterson TF, Mehta AK, et al. Baricitinib plus remdesivir for hospitalized adults with covid-19. *N Engl J Med.* 2021;384(9):795–807.
123. Marconi VC, Ramanan AV, de Bono S, et al. Efficacy and safety of baricitinib for the treatment of hospitalised adults with COVID-19 (COV-BARRIER): a randomised, double-blind, parallel-group, placebo-controlled phase 3 trial. *Lancet Respir Med.* 2021;9(12):1407–1418. https://doi.org/10.1016/S2213-2600(21)00331-3. [Epub 2021 Sep 1].
124. COVID-19 Treatment Guidelines Panel. Coronavirus Disease 2019 (COVID-19) Treatment Guidelines. National Institutes of Health; 2021. https://www.covid19treatmentguidelines.nih.gov/. Accessed 20 November 2021.
125. Gupta A, Gonzalez-Rojas Y, Juarez E, et al. Early covid-19 treatment with SARS-CoV-2 neutral izing antibody sotrovimab. *medRxiv.* 2021. https://doi.org/10.1101/2021.05.27.21257096. 2021.05.27.21257096.
126. Gottlieb RL, Nirula A, Chen P, et al. Efect of bamlanivimab as monotherapy or in combination with etesevimab on viral load in patients with mild to moderate COVID-19: a randomized clinical trial. *JAMA.* 2021;325(7):632–644. https://doi.org/10.1001/jama.2021.0202.
127. Weinreich DM, Sivapalasingam S, Norton T, et al. REGN-COV2, a neutralizing antibody cocktail, in outpatients with Covid-19. *N Engl J Med.* 2021;384(3):238–251. https://doi.org/10.1056/NEJMoa2035002.
128. Imai M, Ito M, Kiso M, et al. Efficacy of antiviral agents against omicron subvariants BQ.1.1 and XBB. *N Engl J Med.* 2023;388(1):89–91. https://doi.org/10.1056/NEJMc2214302. [Epub 2022 Dec 7].
129. Sullivan DJ, Gebo KA, Shoham S, et al. Early outpatient treatment for covid-19 with convalescent plasma. *N Engl J Med.* 2022;386(18):1700–1711.
130. Maxwell D, Sanders KC, Sabot O, et al. COVID-19 therapeutics for low- and middle-income countries: a review of candidate agents with potential for near-term use and impact. *Am J Trop Med Hyg.* 2021;105(3):584–595.
131. Hammond J, Leister-Tebbe H, Gardner A, et al. Oral nirmatrelvir for high-risk, nonhospitalized adults with covid-19. *N Engl J Med.* 2022;386(15):1397–1408.
132. Arbel R, Wolff Sagy Y, Hoshen M, et al. Nirmatrelvir use and severe covid-19 outcomes during the omicron surge. *N Engl J Med.* 2022;387(9):790–798.
133. Fact Sheet for Healthcare Providers: Emergency Use Authorization for Paxlovid [Internet]; 2022. [cited December 11, 2022]. Available from: https://www.fda.gov/media/155050/download.
134. Gottlieb RL, Vaca CE, Paredes R, et al. Early remdesivir to prevent progression to severe covid-19 in outpatients. *N Engl J Med.* 2022;386(4):305–315.
135. Jayk Bernal A, Gomes da Silva MM, Musungaie DB, et al. Molnupiravir for oral treatment of covid-19 in nonhospitalized patients. *N Engl J Med.* 2022;386(6):509–520.
136. Sharif N, Alzahrani KJ, Ahmed SN, Dey SK. Efficacy, immunogenicity and safety of COVID-19 vaccines: a systematic review and meta-analysis. *Front Immunol.* 2021;12, 714170.

137. Bartoszko JJ, Siemieniuk RAC, Kum E, et al. Prophylaxis against covid-19: living systematic review and network meta-analysis. *BMJ.* 2021;373, n949.
138. O'Brien MP, Forleo-Neto E, Musser BJ, et al. Subcutaneous REGEN-COV antibody combination to prevent covid-19. *N Engl J Med.* 2021;385(13):1184–1195.
139. Cohen MS, Nirula A, Mulligan MJ, et al. Effect of bamlanivimab vs placebo on incidence of COVID-19 among residents and staff of skilled nursing and assisted living facilities: a randomized clinical trial. *JAMA.* 2021;326(1):46–55.
140. Levin MJ, Ustianowski A, De Wit S, et al. Intramuscular AZD7442 (Tixagevimab-Cilgavimab) for prevention of covid-19. *N Engl J Med.* 2022;386(23):2188–2200.

CHAPTER 26

Ethical Issues in Preparing for and Responding to Infectious Outbreaks and Bioterror Attacks

MATTHEW WYNIA[a,b] • JEAN ABBOTT[a] • CHARLES M. LITTLE[b,c]
[a]Center for Bioethics and Humanities, University of Colorado, Anschutz Medical Campus, Aurora, CO, United States • [b]University of Colorado School of Medicine and Colorado School of Public Health, Aurora, CO, United States • [c]University of Colorado Hospital, Aurora, CO, United States

[Dr. Rieux] knew that the tale he had to tell...could be only the record of what had to be done, and what assuredly would have to be done again in the never-ending fight against terror and its relentless onslaughts, despite their personal afflictions, by all who, while unable to be saints but refusing to bow down to pestilences, strive their utmost to be healers.

—ALBERT CAMUS, *THE PLAGUE* (1991, P. 308).

INTRODUCTION

In the last 20 years, health professionals around the world have faced a variety of naturally occurring viral outbreaks and bioterrorist threats, including the 2001 US anthrax attacks that killed two postal workers; the 2003 SARS epidemic that sickened and killed more than 800 people; the MERS CoV epidemic that started in 2012 and is ongoing, having killed over 400 people to date; the Chikungunya and Zika virus outbreaks across the Americas; the 2014 Ebola outbreak in West Africa that killed more than 11,000 people; and, of course, the ongoing COVID-19 pandemic, which has brought to the forefront ethical dilemmas not confronted since the influenza pandemic of 1918. In our never-ending attempt to peacefully coexist with our human and microbiological neighbors, there is no doubt that new threats will continue to emerge and old threats will come back to afflict humans in epidemic fashion.

Across these widely varying events, a few core ethical challenges are faced by those charged with being prepared for and responding to viral outbreaks and bioterror attacks. The framing of this chapter is around three general types of ethical challenges that have repeatedly been seen as important across various outbreaks and attacks. Namely, there are ethical issues related to: (1) using the so-called "police powers" of public health to restrict individual or organizational liberties in efforts to protect the larger community; (2) ensuring that health professionals and other critical personnel show up for work in the face of greater than usual levels of risk, sometimes called "duty to treat" challenges; and (3) resource allocation during outbreaks or attacks in which the need for services or resources dramatically overwhelms available capacity, forcing painful triage decisions. These three categories of ethical challenges have been called the three Rs of ethics in epidemic response:

Restrictions, Responsibilities, and Rationing

To facilitate our discussion, two cases will introduce each section of the chapter. These cases are fictional, combining several problems that have been experienced by those planning for and responding to outbreaks and attacks, but they are intended to present realistic instances that illustrate how considerations of ethics can and should affect preparedness and response activities. The cases use two recently epidemic diseases: Ebola and a novel influenza virus with pandemic potential. We have avoided using the ongoing COVID-19

Viral Outbreaks, Biosecurity, and Preparing for Mass Casualty Infectious Diseases Events
https://doi.org/10.1016/B978-0-323-54841-0.00014-7

pandemic as a primary example for several reasons: we continue to learn lessons from the COVID-19 response, it remains politically charged, and the ethical principles underlying public health responses are easier to tease apart in the context of a more limited outbreak.

Our discussion will make use of some key ethical principles in preparing for and responding to epidemics and bioterror attacks. In recent decades, it has become common in biomedical ethics to think in terms of just four principles (autonomy, justice, beneficence, and nonmaleficence), but additional principles often come into play in catastrophic disasters, and some of the traditional four principles tend to get reduced in emphasis. Table 1 presents a set of principles that are often raised in analyzing ethical issues during disasters.

TABLE 1
Ethical Principles to Guide Epidemic and Bioterror Preparedness and Response

Substantive principles: Ethical norms to guide decisions	
Fairness	• Seek fair allocation of resources and fair distribution of benefits and burdens • Give special attention to vulnerable communities more likely to suffer excess harm in disasters • Ensure fairness of decision-making processes (below), tracking and mitigating unequal outcomes where possible
Duty	• Accept the professional duty to treat, even at some risk to oneself • Promote respect for the dying, treat them as you would wish to be treated • Deliver the best care possible given available resources
Leadership	• Recognize the role of leader involves stewardship of shared resources, which may be very limited • Make decisions with input from others; do not make difficult ethical decisions alone • Respect and support first responders and other professionals working under extreme stress
Proportionality	• Ensure good situational awareness before making triage or other rationing decisions • Use the least restrictive means to achieve legitimate public health aims • Use best-available data to assess benefits and harms
Protection	• Strive to maintain social order during the disaster; be a role model of civility and mutual respect • Seek to ensure continuation of a good society after the disaster; recovery starts with preparation and response • Minimize the economic impact of the disaster; use best-available data about short- and long-term costs
Procedural principles: Ethical processes to follow when making decisions	
Inclusion	• Engage affected stakeholders in both planning and response to the extent possible given the circumstances • Update and share knowledge with relevant stakeholders as the situation evolves
Transparency	• Develop and share principles for guiding difficult decisions with all stakeholders, both before and during disaster • Openly acknowledge that autonomy, ownership of resources, and fidelity in the patient-professional relationship are often less dominant (but still not ignored) values during catastrophic disasters
Consistency	• Use the same decision process over time when possible; the information used in decision-making will evolve • Like circumstances should be treated alike, while differences are respected and integrated in decisions when relevant
Accountability	• Optimize due process, use formal notice of decisions, and provide opportunities to voice objections to a neutral arbiter • Be clear about who is responsible for making specific decisions • Balance personal accountability with compassion for those forced to make heart-wrenching decisions

While it is common in biomedical ethics to think in terms of just four principles (autonomy, justice, beneficence, and nonmaleficence), a number of more detailed and often overlapping principles often come into play in catastrophic disasters, and some of the traditional four principles may be reduced in emphasis. This table presents principles that can be helpful in analyzing issues and making ethically justifiable decisions during disasters. These are derived from several sources, including Moskop/Iserson: Triage in medicine, Part II: Underlying values and principles.; CSC (2009); and Refs. 1–3.

Finally, three caveats before we dive in. First, this chapter (like the larger book) focuses on issues related to preparedness and initial response and does not directly examine ethical issues related to long-term recovery from outbreaks or attacks. For example, the ongoing COVID-19 pandemic has highlighted some ethical challenges related to an extremely prolonged disaster with an uncertain recovery trajectory, such as evolving areas of resource scarcity as well as social trust and political considerations, which are outside the scope of this chapter. We note, however, that better preparation can be an important component of building community resilience, including the capacity for a speedy and full recovery. In fact, in a best-case scenario, communities that prepare and respond effectively to disasters can come out of the experience stronger, more cohesive, and better prepared for the next emergency. In this regard, a general ethical rule of thumb is to always engage the community in conversations about ethical challenges during disasters—in advance if it is possible to do so. Not only can working with the community on these thorny ethical issues help with preparedness, but it might also help during and after the response, through its creation of better lines of communication, greater social trust, and stronger community coherence.[4,5]

Second, this chapter focuses on epidemics or bioterror attacks with agents that pose a contagious threat. These disasters pose some unique ethical challenges, but much of the ethical guidance we provide can also be applied in disasters such as earthquakes, floods, nuclear events, or storms, even though these do not carry the same element of possible contagion.

Third, we focus in this chapter on ethical issues arising while preparing for and responding to epidemics and bioterrorism attacks, recognizing that larger ethical issues can also be at play in the development of such emergencies to begin with. There are important ethical and social policy challenges related to the origins of terrorism, for example, that are not in scope for this chapter.[6] Similarly, there are structural issues of social justice and inequities that consistently set some communities up to experience epidemics and to have worse outcomes when epidemics arise.[7–9] These broader ethical issues relate to educational, housing, transportation, environmental exposure, and other disparities that comprise social determinants of infectious disease outbreaks. These issues certainly deserve attention in any conversation about public health preparedness, since addressing them could prevent outbreaks before they start. Yet, to adequately explore responses to the social determinants of epidemics would require an entire additional chapter, or even a book. Consequently, we focus this chapter on ethical challenges in responding to an outbreak once it has begun, though we will include some discussion of the ethical responsibility during an epidemic response to address the needs of more vulnerable individuals and communities.

PART 1. RESTRICTIONS ON LIBERTY: THE ETHICS OF ISOLATION, QUARANTINE, AND SOCIAL DISTANCING

There is no force on earth strong enough to force Americans to do something they do not believe is in their own best interests or that of their families.

—FMR SEN. SAM NUNN, WHO PLAYED THE PRESIDENT FOR THE DARK WINTER BIOTERRORISM EXERCISE, IN WHICH AN ATTEMPTED MASS QUARANTINE FAILED, AS QUOTED IN REF. [10], P. 19.

Ebola case: Karen Marks is a nurse and the mother of two school-aged children. She was deployed to Sierra Leone as an aid worker by her church when the Ebola outbreak emerged. She stayed for a month, taking appropriate precautions against infection. On her return, she is met at the airport by her husband and children, as well as some members of the local media. She is feeling well, and a blood test for Ebola is taken and sent to the Centers for Disease Control and Prevention. The initial blood test comes back negative the next day, but the governor of her state proposes to hold both her and her family in home-based quarantine under armed guard for the next month, or "until we know what's going on."

Pandemic influenza case: A novel form of influenza has broken out, with initial cases in several countries across Central and South America. Currently, available vaccines are ineffective. A traveler to an affected area has returned to a mid-sized town in the United States and was just admitted to the local hospital for what appears to be influenza pneumonia. He has been home for just over a week and had been ill for several days prior to presenting to the emergency department, during which time he attended a baseball game and ate out at two different restaurants. Several additional probable cases have been reported in the last 24 h, and the local public health department has told the restaurants to close while all employees are tested. The baseball team is instructed to cancel an upcoming home game.

The outbreak of a contagious illness often leads to consideration of whether and how to implement restrictive measures to prevent spread. Restrictive strategies can generally be categorized as three types: isolation, quarantine, and social distancing measures, and each of these can be ethically appropriate or problematic.

Isolation is the restriction of individuals who are known to have an illness, often in a particular room in a hospital that may be equipped with specialized air filtration systems and negative pressure. It is undoubtedly the most used strategy that restricts individual liberty to protect the larger community from infection, since isolation of individuals with contagious illnesses is very common in hospitals worldwide. It also tends to cause fewer ethical problems. Typically, people who are placed in isolation are exhibiting symptoms of illness, so they tend to be willing to be in isolation as a condition of receiving treatment. They also pose an obvious risk to others, which makes it less likely that they will choose to put others in harm's way. But that is not always the case; during the SARS outbreak, some ill individuals refused to stay in isolation,[11] and similar flouting of isolation protocols has arisen during the COVID-19 pandemic.[12] As a result, bioterror training scenarios have worked under the assumption that some patients will refuse isolation.[13,14]

There are legitimate concerns from individuals placed in isolation that should be considered in planning. For instance, patients in isolation may report lower satisfaction scores and receive fewer nurse visits compared to patients with similar conditions who are not isolated.[15] Many patients in isolation for COVID-19 suffered and sometimes died without family present, in nursing homes and in hospitals, creating enormous moral distress for families and professional caregivers alike.[16] These negative consequences of isolation do not mean it is always unwarranted, but that it must be well justified. In addition, there is an obligation to specifically track and mitigate these potential harms to the extent possible.[17]

In some cases, concerns about isolation protocols might relate to a more fundamental unwillingness to sacrifice individual liberty—whether due to misunderstanding or ideology—even when health professionals are quite certain that such a sacrifice is necessary to protect the larger community. Perhaps the most infamous example of this, historically, is the case of Mary Mallon, who refused to stop working as a cook despite repeated attempts by public health authorities to convince her to do so; eventually, these officials concluded that "only isolation for the remainder of her life would effectively control the risk of typhoid transmission."[18] While most people will not act like "Typhoid Mary," there is a strain of libertarian push-back against mandatory public health interventions that remains strong both in the US and elsewhere and which has been on vivid display throughout the COVID-19 pandemic.

In fact, medical and public health professionals hold several constitutional "police powers," including the right to hold patients against their will. These powers should be exercised with caution, but they can and should be used when necessary to prevent contagious patients from spreading a dangerous disease. In general, the legal and ethical standard is that public health police powers may be invoked to restrict an individual's liberty if there is a compelling state interest, if the restriction is well-targeted, using the least restrictive means necessary, and if there is an opportunity for an appeals process. So, just as psychiatrists are empowered to hold dangerously psychotic patients against their will, it is possible for health professionals to enforce isolation when necessary to protect the public and if there are mechanisms to ensure timely judicial review of these decisions.[11]

Even if they are legally solid, decisions to impose restrictions on liberties pose ethical challenges for many health professionals, who are accustomed to putting the preferences and values of individual patients at the forefront of their ethical thinking. Over the last 50 years, the undeniable emphasis in American medical ethics has been on respect for patient autonomy. This emphasis and the complementary push against any form of "paternalism" in health care have multiple and powerful roots, and it should not be rejected lightly. But the deeper origins of professionalism in health care lie in a recognition that health professionals serve individual patients in the context of also serving important social roles, including the task of protecting the community from contagious illness.[11,19] In this respect, contemplating and planning for a serious outbreak presents an important opportunity for health professionals to examine their professional ethics, the larger meaning of their work, and the possible protective role they can play in society.[20]

Quarantine is distinct from isolation in that the people being asked to sacrifice their liberty through being placed under quarantine *are not ill*. Quarantine is the separation of healthy people who might have been exposed to a contagious illness, but who are not yet sick. If they become sick, they would presumably be placed in isolation. In fact, the great majority of people placed in quarantine typically turn out not to have been infected. For instance, Taiwan quarantined over 130,000 people during the SARS outbreak, of whom only two were eventually confirmed as having severe acute respiratory syndrome (SARS) (another 132 were "probable" or "suspected" cases).[18] None of the many returning health care workers or others quarantined in the US after "possible" exposure to Ebola turned out to have the disease, though one returning doctor who was undergoing self-monitoring (but not quarantine) did.[21] During the COVID-19 pandemic, some entire cities, regions, or nations have experienced "lockdowns," which are effectively attempts at imposing a universal quarantine in attempts to limit the spread of the virus.

Also, quarantine can carry a significantly higher cost than isolation because it often encompasses many more people, and those people are otherwise well and productive citizens. Asking people who feel healthy to stay in a quarantine facility or even to quarantine at home can be costly. In addition to obvious economic costs, various other costs should be considered, including that people placed in quarantine are sometimes stigmatized and even traumatized by the experience. Almost one-third of the people placed under quarantine for possible SARS exposure in Toronto reported symptoms of posttraumatic stress disorder after the event.[18] Also, in our Ebola example above, public health authorities worried that if health professionals were forced to stay in quarantine after returning home, it could dissuade them from volunteering to help address the outbreak at its source, delaying eventual control of the epidemic.[21] And as the COVID-19 pandemic has shown, people (including children) placed in quarantine also may face challenges related to continuing their schooling, experiencing social isolation, and other downstream effects. On the other hand, the fact that "essential workers" were sometimes exempt from quarantine requirements (i.e., compelled to work despite the risk) has sometimes proven devastating to their health and has exacerbated social disparities.[22]

The challenges of quarantine raise a very basic ethical dilemma in deciding to implement a quarantine: while isolation of people who are ill and contagious has obvious clinical and public health utility, quarantine might not. That is, quarantine might not be a "proportionate" response, with benefits that outweigh its harms, and it might not be the "least restrictive means necessary" to achieve a benefit, as called for under both law and ethics.[23]

The "harm principle" of the libertarian philosopher, J.S. Mill, states that "...the only purpose for which (state) power can be rightfully exercised over any member of a civilized community, against his will, is to prevent harm to others."[24] In this light, the first task in making an ethical analysis of whether or not to implement a quarantine is to determine with some certainty that it will be effective at halting or slowing the spread of the outbreak.

Unfortunately, determining the utility of a proposed quarantine can be a challenge, since disease spread is affected by a wide variety of factors. Some factors are biological, and they might be known at the outset, or they can be determined over time, such as the transmissibility of the agent, mode of transmission, the duration of transmissibility, recovery rates, and correlations, between symptoms and infectiousness (see Chapter 18 for additional details). For example, smallpox is extremely contagious while anthrax is virtually not transmissible from person to person. And it turned out that SARS was not readily transmissible until after the patient was febrile, as is also true of Ebola; but this is not true for influenza or for COVID-19, which can be transmitted a day or more prior to first symptoms and may be completely asymptomatic in some carriers. For those making decisions about quarantine, these biological factors are critical to understand. Restrictions should be proportionate, using the best knowledge available at the time, and should be adjusted as understanding of biologic characteristics evolves. In our pandemic influenza scenario, as with the current COVID-19 pandemic, public health recommendations at the onset may well be found overly restrictive with hindsight; prompt modification and transparent communication are required for ongoing epidemics as understanding of transmissibility improves.

Meanwhile, there are also several nonbiological, social factors that can make quarantine more or less effective, and these are even more challenging to calculate. These social factors include the levels of community cohesion, social trust, and public understanding of the situation. These factors can easily make attempts at quarantine not merely ineffective and costly but dangerous. To be very blunt, a quarantine done poorly can lead individuals—some of whom might be contagious—to ignore public health advisories or even flee the area, dispersing into the population and spreading the contagion more rapidly and more widely than it might otherwise have spread. In addition, as in the Ebola vignette above, an unwarranted, prolonged quarantine of health professionals returning home from caring for Ebola patients could prevent health professionals from joining the fight where it most needs to be fought.[21]

There are many real-world examples of inadvertent harms associated with quarantine efforts. For instance, early in the SARS epidemic, when the police arrived to place the Amoy Gardens apartment complex in Hong Kong under quarantine, they found half of the apartments to be empty, and in one after-action summary, Taiwan officials said they believed their "aggressive use of quarantine contributed to public panic."[18] When the city of Wuhan was locked down in late January 2020, at the outset of the COVID-19 pandemic, for a variety of reasons almost half of the population was no longer in the city.[25] The COVID-19 pandemic has also been marked by increases in some types of "deaths of despair," such as overdose deaths, presumably exacerbated by the isolating conditions of lockdowns.[26]

On the other hand, there are instances where quarantine can work, even if initial considerations might argue against it. For instance, unlike SARS, both COVID-19 and flu spread easily and before symptoms arise, so citywide or regional quarantines probably cannot completely halt spread; by the time it is apparent these viral infections are in one area, with modern travel patterns they will have already spread to other areas. Yet, mathematical modeling still suggests that a quarantine for influenza in which only half of the people complied could still cut transmission rates notably.[27,28] Moreover, in one (pre-COVID-19) survey, 94% of Americans said they would accept a voluntary 7- to 10-day quarantine if they thought they might have been exposed to a pandemic flu,[29] suggesting that voluntary quarantine actions might sometimes be as or more effective than legally enforced quarantine might be. The COVID-19 pandemic has also shown that even modest reductions in transmission rates can "smooth the curve" and ease the response burden—that is, even if the same number of people get infected in the end, at least they do not all need hospital care at the same time. Experiences with "voluntary" implementation of different types of lockdowns during COVID-19 have been variable, but broadly suggest that quarantines and other social distancing measures can reduce local transmission rates.[30]

The survey data mentioned above also illustrate that, at least historically, public cooperation and social cohesion rise during disasters, despite the attention given to outlier behavior in entertainment and the news. As Edelson[31] summarizes the research from the field, "It is a canard sometimes used to justify authoritarian actions that the public responds to emergencies by losing control and panicking; indeed, it is the consensus of social scientists that people in emergency situations tend to be more cooperative and more generous toward others than they may normally be." In this light, it is a special ethical responsibility of public health professionals to follow the best-available evidence, which might mean guarding against political pressures leading toward the inappropriate and counterproductive uses of police powers in some situations,[2] while in other situations it might require urging reluctant politicians to implement restrictive measures that are likely to be effective in mitigating the effects of an outbreak, even though these measures might be politically unpopular.[32]

Finally, there are a variety of additional ways in which public health authorities can seek to prevent social interactions that might lead to disease transmission, which are collectively known as "social distancing measures." Common examples include forcing the cancellation of public events, such as sporting, theatrical, or musical events; school or daycare closures; implementing holiday schedules or closing mass transit; and encouraging telecommuting. Of these, school closures are probably the best studied, and there is some evidence they can be effective at mitigating disease transmission rates.[30,33–36] But in all these cases, there are economic and social costs to distancing measures, and as such, the same ethical considerations should be applied that have been mentioned above. For instance, there should be evidence suggesting that the social distancing intervention will be effective and not counterproductive, there should be adequate supports provided to those being asked to give up their freedom to protect the larger community, and there should be meaningful mechanisms to ensure due process around these decisions. Regarding due process, this does not necessarily entail access to a judge and a jury of one's peers; during an acute epidemic or bioterror attack, this level of due process might not be feasible. But that does not mean due process is simply jettisoned. Rather, it will often be possible to provide some of the important aspects of due process, such as adequate notice of the action with a written order, an opportunity to have one's objections heard by a neutral decision-maker in a timely manner, and some level of access to legal counsel to help formulate one's objections.[1,37] And in an extended disaster like the COVID-19 pandemic, repeated assessments based on the best data available at the time will be necessary.

PART 2. RESPONSIBILITY: PROFESSIONAL AND INSTITUTIONAL PERSPECTIVES ON THE "DUTY TO TREAT"

It is our vocation to save life. It involves risk, but when we serve with love, that is when the risk does not matter so much. When we believe our mission is to save lives, we have got to do our work.

—DR. MATTHEW LUKWIYA, SUPERINTENDENT OF A UGANDAN MISSIONARY HOSPITAL; DIED OF EBOLA HEMORRHAGIC FEVER, IN DECEMBER 2000.[38]

Ebola case: Ms. Marks agreed to stay in quarantine at home, and a guard was initially placed outside her front door, but she felt healthy and did not want her children to stay with her in case she was to become ill. After discussion between the governor and the head of the state department of public health, her children were allowed to stay with their father, and the guard was removed. Ms. Marks was asked to limit social interactions, monitor her temperature three times a day, and call the department of public health if she developed a fever. Sadly, 3 days later she did develop fever and abdominal pain, and she was brought to the local hospital emergency department by ambulance. The ambulance crew called ahead, and the Emergency Department (ED) staff were notified that a patient might be arriving with an Ebola infection. On hearing this, three ED nurses told their supervisor they were feeling ill and wanted to go home.

Pandemic influenza case: In the past week, the local hospital has been swamped with ill citizens and ill staff. A tent has been sent up for additional triage outside the ED, and a "surge emergency" has been called. The hospital administration has extended shift hours and asked for all staff to cancel vacations and days off. The dietary and environmental staff is pushing back due to fear for themselves and their families; they are threatening to call in sick, even if they themselves are not sick....yet.

The challenge of getting health workers and others to continue providing care when there is a sudden escalation of personal risk has been described in both theoretical studies and in evidence from epidemics. For example, Qureshi and colleagues conducted a survey of health workers in the New York City area and found that hypothetical willingness to respond varied according to the type of hypothesized disaster, with 48% of workers being willing to respond during a SARS outbreak but higher willingness for other disasters, citing barriers of fear, family concerns, and concerns for self.[39] In a pre-SARS survey, Wynia and Alexander found that most physicians (85%) reported being willing to take on some risk in caring for patients with "an unknown but potential deadly illness," but this dropped as the risk increased, and most physicians felt unprepared for playing a role in managing a contagious outbreak.[40] These challenges are longstanding and persistent[20,41,42]: in 1988, 25% of house staff in one survey said they would refuse to care for patients with AIDS if given the option,[43] and a similar percent of health professionals in 2016 said it would be ethical to refuse to care for patients with Ebola virus disease.[44] Furthermore, in real scenarios of contagious threats, including the recent SARS and Ebola outbreaks, there have been highly publicized cases of health workers refusing to show up for work. In Taiwan, more than 160 health workers either quit or refused to work on SARS wards, despite the government threatening to revoke their professional licenses; in China, at least six doctors were banned from practice for life when they refused to care for patients with SARS; and in Canada, some nurses refused to work in SARS wards despite a doubling of their wages.[45] By contrast, the experience early in the COVID-19 pandemic was often of increased camaraderie and volunteerism among health professionals, despite the risk and often despite inadequate supplies of personal protective equipment (PPE). However, at the time of this writing, while camaraderie remains, volunteerism has often given way to burnout, frustration, and clinicians leaving their professions as the pandemic has worn on.[46,47]

Refusals to work in the face of extreme risk can be well-founded. While uncertainty about dangers to health professionals can be particularly high in the initial days of a crisis—when the "fog" of early, mixed, and uncoordinated messages can make understanding the threats to personnel and the efficacy of protective procedures unclear—the risk can also remain substantial as the crisis evolves. In Taiwan, over 90% of those infected with SARS were health workers,[48] and in Toronto, where 44 people died of SARS, 45% of probable or suspect cases were among health professionals.[49] The WHO reports that health workers in the African nations affected by the 2014 Ebola virus outbreak were "between 21 and 32 times more likely to be infected with Ebola than people in the general adult population," and two-thirds of the health workers who were infected died.[50] Early in the COVID-19 pandemic, especially when PPE was in short supply, health care workers faced considerably higher risk of infection, serious illness, and death compared to others not in front-line jobs,[51] and these early risks have presumably evolved to include risks of long-term COVID, psychological sequelae, and burnout.[52,53]

Despite the apparent, if intermittent, dangers in being a health professional, and the challenge of getting some health professionals to show up for work during times of higher levels of personal risk, the health workers' "duty to treat," or professional responsibility to provide care despite some risk to oneself, is based on longstanding ethical principles and traditions. And regarding disaster response, this duty applies not just to health workers, but to police, prehospital personnel, and other public servants vital to a public health response. Moreover, the COVID-19 pandemic has necessitated the articulation of ethical arguments to support some level of duty among the public to take actions to protect oneself and others, demonstrating the interconnection between issues of "responsibility" in this section and those discussed above under "restrictions."

For physicians, the call to treat the sick despite personal risk was perhaps first codified in the original AMA Code of Medical Ethics from 1847: "...when pestilence prevails, it is (the physicians') duty to face the danger, and to continue their labors for the alleviation of the suffering, even at the jeopardy of their own lives," and the phrase, "and without regard to remuneration" was added in 1912.[20] Over history, professional adherence to the duty to treat seems to have waxed and waned, but the frequency of health professionals declining to show up for work during recent epidemics, including SARS and Ebola, has demonstrated a particular need to reaffirm the "moral center" of the medical profession today.[54]

The basic principle of a fiduciary responsibility, i.e., the commitment to care for the ill and injured and to put the welfare of patients above one's own, is a bedrock of professionalism and central to public trust in health professionals,[20] but it is not unlimited. Table 2 lists several key ethical considerations that can either support or limit a health professional's duty to provide care in the face of personal risk. For example, considerations supporting the duty to treat include the many privileges afforded health care professionals by society, which are granted in exchange for professionals upholding several implicit and explicit social promises. Health professionals' privileges include not just a relatively elevated economic and social status but also the ability to self-regulate and to hold the monopoly that society grants them regarding treatment decisions, authorization to prescribe medications, and general authority over medical matters in both nondisaster and disaster situations. These privileges are balanced in the existing "social contract" by professionals' responsibilities to treat patients fairly, put patient needs first, practice to the best of their abilities, and provide care even when doing so poses some danger. In a related vein, maintaining and enhancing public trust in the healing professions is an important element of the social commitment of health professionals. The COVID pandemic has been especially notable for its illustration of how important trust in medicine and public health can be in disaster situations, where difficult decisions have been required that involve medical and public health professionals acting to establish and enforce isolation, quarantine, and social distancing restrictions for the good of the larger community, as discussed in Section "Part 1. Restrictions on Liberty: The Ethics of Isolation, Quarantine, and Social Distancing." In some instances, mistrust (and misinformation) has sparked overt anger toward and even abuse of health professionals, doubtlessly contributing to professional burnout.[55]

TABLE 2
Considerations Supporting and Limiting a Health Professional's Duty to Treat in the Face of Personal Risk

Considerations supporting a health professional's duty to treat

- Social contract
- Specialized training and expertise
- Fairness or nondiscrimination
- Maintaining public trust
- Obligations to community

Considerations that may limit a health professional's duty to treat

- Level of risk (no obligation to become a martyr)
- Ability to provide benefit to victims
- Professional obligations to other patients
- Relevance of professional expertise
- Obligations to family
- Availability of others to respond

In some circumstances, the duty to treat is an established legal obligation based on an actual contract. So, for example, trained fire personnel are expected to respond to fires and explosions, as are prehospital emergency responders, even though such events clearly pose some risk to the responder. But Table 2 also suggests that the responsibility to respond in a crisis can sometimes be thought of as existing on a spectrum. For example, the level of obligation might vary according to the specialized training and expertise that a particular HCP possesses. Hence, an individual who specializes in emergency medicine is expected to respond to medical emergencies, and the infectious disease specialist is expected to apply his/her expertise to an infection-related crisis, while those with different types of medical training might hold a lesser obligation to respond. This increased obligation according to one's specific role derives in part from the fact that specialized training and expertise can make responding somewhat less dangerous for these professionals than it would be for untrained individuals and somewhat more effective.[56]

Role-related responsibilities can also vary depending on the individual's proximity to the event, the severity of the emergency, the opportunity to benefit survivors, and the number of other providers available to respond.[56] For example, in the Ebola vignette above, emergency medical services (EMS) professionals are clearly expected to transport Mrs. Marks, and ED personnel are expected to receive her, assess her, and provide interventions appropriate to her illness. Their response should be done with as much personal and institutional preparation in understanding Ebola and providing necessary protection of responders as is possible at the time.[57]

On the other hand, the issue of whether nurses and physicians should, for example, attempt resuscitation if Mrs. Marks were to suffer a cardiopulmonary arrest exemplifies the potential pitfalls of an overly simplistic understanding of the duty to treat. If the cardiac arrest were to occur where sufficient protections were not available to staff (making cardiopulmonary resuscitation (CPR) more dangerous) and if it were most likely the result of terminal Ebola (making CPR much less likely to succeed), then attempting CPR would not be ethically obligatory and might simply be foolhardy. At the other extreme, once Mrs. Marks is admitted and the designated staff is already wearing adequate personal protective equipment (PPE) and in a controlled isolation unit, and if the arrest were to arise from a critically low potassium level, which can be reversed, CPR would be indicated as possible and an ethical responsibility for the health professionals providing her care.[58] These two extreme cases demonstrate how an unconditional procedure-based rule (whether "always provide CPR" or "never provide CPR" to patients with Ebola) can be problematic.[59]

Our point in discussing CPR policies is not to say that developing uniform policies about whether, when, and how to provide CPR to patients with Ebola virus disease (or COVID-19) is unwise, but to emphasize that such policies should be clinically and ethically nuanced, and they must be flexible and change as circumstances evolve. The latter point is particularly important during disaster response. During a specific crisis, the understanding of potential risks to personnel and the benefits of interventions to patients are very likely to change and evolve over time (e.g., early wariness about using noninvasive ventilation for patients with COVID-19, based partly on the risk of exposure for medical personnel, soon evolved to a preference for using such ventilation techniques for these patients, based on increasing evidence of patient benefit).[60] Rules and policies regarding the duty to treat should be modified according to this evolving understanding of risk to personnel and benefits to patients.

This discussion also implies that the risks that must be assumed by medical personnel in response to epidemics are not limitless. That is, the duty to treat is not absolute, and responders are not required to be foolhardy or to become martyrs when responding entails exposure to life-threatening hazards for themselves, especially if doing so is unlikely to provide benefit to the patient. This is consistent with the guidance provided to other first responders—so, for example, the prehospital professionals who respond to a car accident with a downed electrical wire are expected to secure their own safety before rescuing a victim.[61]

In this light, Table 2 lists not only a set of common justifications for the "duty to treat" among health professionals, but also a list of some competing obligations that healthcare personnel (HCP) must confront as they respond, particularly to situations in which a sharp escalation of professional risk is involved. For instance, Mrs. Marks in the Ebola vignette above appears now to have an active infection (putting her in much greater danger and making her care much riskier), and providers who care for her after she is admitted to a special isolation unit will be unable to fulfill care obligations to other assigned patients (meaning they must balance her needs with those of other patients). Further, if the assessment of Mrs. Marks' condition were to be that she is very unlikely to survive, then these health professionals would also have limited ability to benefit her. There might also be a surfeit of health professionals who would volunteer to care for her. Factors like these would mitigate against a strict duty to treat being applied to any particular health professional. And if the scenario were to evolve in this way, the hospital would be ethically justified in making her care a volunteer activity rather than a mandatory one for health professionals at the hospital.

Family obligations are often the most pressing concerns of those declining to report to work during epidemics and deserve specific attention. These concerns might include childcare, elder care, pet care, or other obligations, and it is common for both adults in a family to work (both might even be "essential workers"). Virtually all medical personnel will have important responsibilities outside of their professional roles, so decisions about whom to allow to opt out of risky work can be contentious, and there is no simple algorithm to determine the ethically "correct" answer. The best course is to establish a process for making these decisions that does not leave the entire decision to a single person, that will allow the decision to be revisited when circumstances change, and that engages the relevant stakeholders in the discussion. Ideally, such conversations should also have started in advance of the disaster, through such mechanisms as disaster drills, tabletop exercises, and role play scenarios.

In the pandemic influenza vignette, the challenge to the institution is increased, with a need to fulfill core responsibilities to the community in the face of the threat of a loss of health workers to illness, fear, and increased and stressful workloads. While resource allocation challenges are discussed in Section "Part 3. Rationing: What to Do When Not Everyone Can Get What They Need" below (e.g., what to do if there are not enough staff to care for all the patients who need it), this case raises the fact that there are clear ethical policy choices for institutions and public health, which can encourage an affirmative response by personnel to the call to duty. How can institutions and society provide the safest work environment possible in the face of a disaster? How can attrition be prevented or minimized? What are the responsibilities of institutions and the community to the families of those workers who heed the call and perish? When should institutions, including employers, professional societies, and licensing boards, sanction those who don't respond? These questions do not have easy answers, but the response to HCPs who seek to opt out of providing care under circumstances of greater than usual risk should be informed by consideration of the ethical principles in Table 1, including that the policy response should be proportional, transparent, and backed by the best evidence available.[62,63] And, as the COVID-19 pandemic has taught, institutions might need to provide additional layers of support and reconsider approaches to retention of front-line workers as a disaster plays out over time.

Two general components of institutional response are ethically required (Table 3). The first is in the arena of advance planning in this era when threats are likely to become more common; the so-called duty to plan.[64] Planning starts with the education of trainees and employees in understanding the ethical underpinnings of their profession and the inherent and sometimes extraordinary risks that come with their chosen career. Tabletop exercises supplemented by education on ethical frameworks are used by FEMA and others to help responders work through choices they might be required to make in a disaster.[65] The general public also should be informed about difficult choices that may be required in the event of a crisis. In Maryland, prior to COVID-19, a set of deliberative conversations on triage choices around pandemic influenza encouraged citizens to grapple with the difficult choices faced by medical personnel in hypothetical scenarios.[66] In Canada, a series of townhall meetings was held to engage the public in a post-SARS deliberation around the duty to care and found that participants were able to grasp legitimate limits but also expectations of health care practitioners during disasters.[67] Getting "buy in" from the public and from HCPs involves convening key stakeholders, both in the abstract and as the threat of pandemics or other crises loom, to maximize solidarity as difficult choices need to be made.[68]

TABLE 3
Institutional Ethical Responsibilities Related to High-Risk Work

- Frequent and accurate updates about known and unknown aspects of disease, risks, and protections
- Provide training about disease, risks, and protections, modified as knowledge evolves
- Adequate/optimal supplies for personal protection and environmental risk mitigation
- Special response teams designated and trained
- Danger pay for those taking on excess risk
- Survivor benefits for families of those ill or killed in the response
- Preferential access to supportive or therapeutic services for those who become infected
- Family support (day care, release of a second parent, pet care)
- Transparent and participatory policy development

The second core administrative responsibility is the ethical obligation to mitigate increased risk and directly address the fears of health care personnel. Organizations can do this by providing the safest work environment possible, including by providing adequate PPE (assuming it is available) and creating a culture of safety in the workplace. When adequate PPE supplies are not available, organizations will be required to adopt ethically reasonable rationing strategies (see the "Rationing" section below), as has occurred during the COVID-19 pandemic. Some specific interventions to be considered to protect HCPs and mitigate risk during epidemics or bioterror attacks are listed in Table 3.

Finally, the extent and limits of the "duty to treat" in our society, which emphasizes individualism, need to be discussed openly. Expectations to respond in crises should be part of training and of ongoing discussions among professionals as we anticipate new or recurring crises in the future. Enforcement of the professional duty to treat largely relies on moral suasion rather than the law, since the prospect of carrying out threatened penalties is hard to imagine for most policy planners.[69] Inculcating ethical expectations as a part of caring professions, socialization of community obligations, and self-monitoring are the primary means of "soft" enforcement. Meanwhile, institutional and community recognition of individuals who are assuming risks (such as the nightly noisemaking to express gratitude toward health care workers that took place early in the COVID-19 pandemic) can also encourage participation, at least in the short term. Meanwhile, it bears noting that societal demonstration of solidarity with health professionals and workers, including by honoring public health advisories and mandates, can also be construed as an ethical responsibility, albeit one that has become frayed in the extended COVID-19 pandemic.

PART 3. RATIONING: WHAT TO DO WHEN NOT EVERYONE CAN GET WHAT THEY NEED

I didn't know if I was doing the right thing. But I did not have time. I had to make snap decisions, under the most appalling circumstances, and I did what I thought was right.

—"UNNAMED FEMALE DOCTOR" IN AN INTERVIEW WITH THE MAIL ON SUNDAY ABOUT THE FLOODING OF MEMORIAL HOSPITAL FOLLOWING HURRICANE KATRINA, AS QUOTED IN SHERI FINK'S PULITZER PRIZE-WINNING BOOK, *FIVE DAYS AT MEMORIAL* (FINK,[70] P. 277.)

Ebola case: Karen Marks has been back from Sierra Leone for 12 days. For the last 2 days she has had high fevers, nausea, and vomiting. Her repeat Ebola PCR test was positive, and she has been transferred to a hospital designated as a regional Ebola Treatment Center. As she is currently the only infected person receiving care at that site, there will not be a shortage of typical supportive care for her, but she and her family would like for her to receive an experimental therapy if it can be obtained. There are several such treatments being advanced, though none has been proven in scientific studies. The one she is most likely to get is a new experimental agent, but only 200 doses exist, and the manufacturer is convening a group to consider the ethics of making these doses available to patients in the US (where the treatment was developed and funded) compared to people in the outbreak zone in Sierra Leone (where stemming the outbreak is an urgent priority). They are also considering requiring that all doses be administered in the context of a randomized clinical trial with a placebo arm.

In the meantime, this morning Mrs. Marks suffered a cardiopulmonary arrest in the context of profuse diarrhea and a low serum potassium level. She received emergent CPR, but during the code several of her ribs were heard to crack. She survived the code, but over the last hour she has become increasingly short of breath. An urgent supine portable chest film showed only several rib fractures, but the team is worried that she might have a hemothorax. A small amount of fluid is seen on portable ultrasound, but before inserting a chest tube, which carries risks to the patient and the team, the physician caring for her has ordered an emergent CT scan of the chest. If this were to be done, it would require moving her across the hospital to the CT scan area, which would essentially close that area to other patients for the day. The company that services the CT scanner also says they will no longer maintain it if it has been used by someone infected with Ebola, perhaps removing it from service completely and causing a high expense to replace it. The head of radiology calls the Chief Medical Officer to ask her to intervene and cancel the scan.

Pandemic influenza case: Since the outbreak was first reported over a month ago, the local hospital and all other hospitals, clinics, and physician offices across the region and nationwide have been inundated with requests for a prescription for oseltamivir. While physician offices and pharmacies were essentially wiped out of their stocks in the first few weeks, some hospitals have been rationing access to this medication using various, locally developed allocation protocols and have some remaining drug in stock. The state department of public health was just granted access to a limited amount of the drug from the strategic national stockpile, but the amount to be released will be far less than the demand.

In the meantime, the novel variant of influenza is now recognized as a new pandemic strain with mortality higher than typical seasonal influenza. The vaccine is being rushed into production, but there is a serious shortage compared to demand. Hospitals have a 25% absentee rate due to illness and fear of infection in staff. They are advocating that their staff should receive priority in receiving vaccines so that they can continue to provide care. The State Office of Emergency Management is very concerned about absenteeism in other vital infrastructure sectors, such as power and water treatment facilities, and they wish to prioritize these critical workers. And with higher-than-normal fatalities in children, advocates are calling for a vaccine prioritization protocol that will "save the children."

To make matters even worse, hospitals nationwide are rapidly filling with patients, some of whom require invasive mechanical ventilation. In some parts of the country, more than 95% of intensive care unit beds are full, even after hospitals have halted all elective procedures. Most are also already implementing plans to discharge as many people from the hospitals as possible, but even with these steps, the best-available models of pandemic growth suggest that within 3 weeks there will be more people needing mechanical ventilation than there are ventilators and the highly-trained staff needed to operate them.

Major outbreaks virtually always create resource shortages of one form or another for some period of time across some geographic area. The resources needed to respond to disasters, including outbreaks, comprise three broad categories, which are referred to in colloquial shorthand among disaster response professionals: staff, stuff, and space. *Staff* resources include care providers (such as nurses and doctors) and also critical personnel in housekeeping, engineering, and so on. Severe shortages of staff often result in difficult decisions about whether or not to require staff to perform tasks that are outside their usual scope of practice or to take on greater than usual patient care burdens, which comprises less safe medical care and also creates physical, psychological, and moral distress for the staff involved. *Space* concerns often focus on treatment spaces, such as rooms and beds (especially critical care beds), and severe shortages of space may require decisions about whether to use nontraditional spaces, including hallways and exterior spaces, to house patients. And *stuff* includes items such as ventilators, personal protective equipment (PPE), medications, resuscitation fluids, and even oxygen or oxygen tubing (as has been seen during severe COVID-19 surges in some areas). Severe shortages of supplies like these can force heart-wrenching triage decisions, with those denied access to needed supplies suffering and even dying from conditions that might not usually result in death if adequate resources were available. In addition, shortages may ripple to degrade symptom management for palliative and hospice patients at the end of life.[71]

While it is common to think of resources as being either present or absent, adequate or inadequate, it is helpful to recognize that during disasters (and, in fact, during normal operations too), there is a wide continuum of resource needs in relation to resource availability, ranging from having plenty of a resource (whether staff, stuff, or space) to meet all current and foreseeable future needs on the one extreme to having none of that resource at the other extreme (Fig. 1). As an outbreak or attack unfolds and resource demands surge, there are likely to be progressively increasing shortages of various resources in relation to demand, which will force increasingly difficult decisions about the allocation of these resources by some decision-maker or group of decision-makers.[72,73] With regard to staff shortages, one can often "flex" existing staff to work more hours and cover more patients, at least for a period of time. But the COVID-19 pandemic has also taught that staff cannot be stretched beyond their limits; spreading staff too thinly increases safety risks and can exhaust the pool of available staff as individuals fall ill or become overworked, burned out, and leave the field. Consequently, when planning for a prolonged event, staffing must be considered as potentially comprising a "hard ceiling" that might require triage decisions of withholding services that require heavy staff resources (Colorado Healthcare Staffing: https://drive.google.com/file/d/1sDLT42s1nTJGSrDZkKakuvsY8HSK6geQ/view).

The figure shows in pictorial form the gradual degradation of quality of care that can be delivered as resource needs gradually (or suddenly) outstrip resource availability, including some of the operational strategies that are commonly used to "stretch" existing resources and maintain adequate quality of care despite shortages. The concepts and strategies of contingency and crisis standards of care are beyond the scope of this chapter and book and are not addressed in detail. Our point with this figure is to note that (a) care quality degrades along a spectrum and ethical responses should be attuned to this while recognizing the importance of setting discrete lines, or triggers, for making certain important decisions.[73] And (b) it is important to recognize, as the health care system degrades from normal to crisis care, that the ethical framework for health professionals making resource allocation decisions also must gradually shift from focusing on providing all resources necessary for every individual to a distribution of resources that primarily aims to provide maximal benefit to a population.

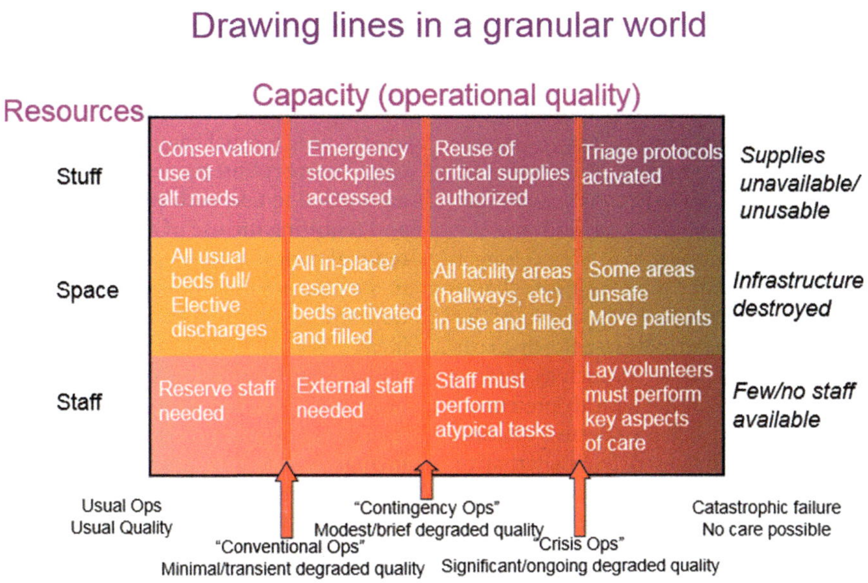

FIG. 1 The gradual degradation of quality as resource scarcity worsens. This figure illustrates the granular nature of care quality as it gradually degrades from usual to conventional, contingency, and then crisis operations, with examples of strategies used by organizations to maintain optimal quality of care at each stage despite increasingly severe shortages of staff, space, and supplies.

When operating at "conventional capacity," there is typically enough staff, space, and stuff to operate at usual levels of quality, if appropriate adjustments are made. Operating in "conventional capacity" (as opposed to normal operations) in the setting of a resource shortage (or looming shortage) should be proactively managed by the emergency management structure of the organizations affected. This early level of emergency operations often provides new and additional resources for use (e.g., by accessing stockpiles), which can help to maintain care at usual levels of quality despite an increased demand. Still, some changes that may be thought of as within conventional capacity operations can have effects on patients. For example, if bed shortages are expected, conventional operations might require that "elective" surgical cases be deferred. However, while some elective surgeries, such as primary resection of colon cancer, are not emergencies, per se, delaying such operations more than briefly might well worsen the patient's outcome. As such, strategies like delaying elective services can easily morph into "contingency" or even "crisis" standard of care strategies, depending on the expected impacts on patient outcomes.[74,75]

When operating at conventional capacity, the use of spaces, staff, and supplies remains generally consistent with daily practices within the institution. That said, even during normal operations, it is common to have one or more resources that are in shortage relative to demand. Multiple examples of medications and other resource shortages arose prior to the COVID-19 pandemic, including normal saline bags, ketamine, bumetanide, fluorescein strips, and many others, and the Food and Drug Administration and similar agencies in other countries keep up-to-date lists of current drug shortages on their websites.[76] These shortage situations are sometimes unavoidable and often tragic; but for hospitals and health systems they also present an invaluable opportunity to develop and test protocols for establishing how to make ethical allocation decisions under resource scarcity, and they should be used for this purpose.[77–79] In a similar way, the annual influenza vaccination campaign provides an opportunity to practice how to get a new vaccine to large numbers of people, with certain populations being targeted for early access.[3] It is incumbent on organizations and systems to use the existence of situations one might call "routine shortages" to develop, test, and practice their capacity to respond to future crisis situations in which other resource shortages are expected to arise. Similarly, during the COVID-19 pandemic, resource shortages on multiple fronts have forced many hospitals and health systems to develop and implement contingency and even crisis care strategies; there is an ethical obligation to learn from these experiences to inform future response strategies.

When dealing with a routine drug shortage (i.e., not during an acute and overwhelming crisis), organizations are often forced to move from "conventional" operations to "contingency" operations as regards that specific resource. Under contingency operations, the spaces, staff, and/or supplies being used are no longer of usual quality, but institutions can provide care that is functionally near-equivalent to usual. Alterations of the use of space, for example, may involve overflowing critical care patients into procedure areas, such as cardiac catheterization labs. Similarly, if the typical "preferred" antibiotic is in short supply, but an effective alternative is available, it will be substituted. Such alternative spaces, supplies, or practices may be used temporarily during a major mass casualty incident or on a more sustained basis during an ongoing pandemic, as has occurred with the COVID-19 pandemic. As institutions move into contingency care, some staff might need to carry out tasks that are on the margins or even just outside their usual scope of practice; typically, all "elective" procedures and surgeries will be canceled, and reuse of critical supplies might be authorized. These alterations should be acknowledged as likely to result in some discrete reductions in the quality of care, but the aim remains to keep these reductions to a minimum.[74,80]

As resource shortages worsen and an organization is forced to move from "contingency operations" into "crisis operations" mode, the quality of care that is provided to some patients—and sometimes to all patients—will be significantly decreased. During crisis operations, spaces, staff, and/or supplies will not be consistent with usual quality standards, and the focus will move toward providing sufficient care to as many people as possible given the context of a catastrophic disaster (i.e., provide the best possible care to patients given the circumstances and resources available). Importantly, however, as Gostin and Hanfling note, "ethical norms do not change during disasters—professionals remain obligated to providing the best care reasonable in these circumstances."[81] But because operating in crisis capacity constitutes a major adjustment to the quality of care that can be provided and is expected to result in significantly worse outcomes than under normal care, at least for some patients, this mode of operation should be officially endorsed through the declaration of a state of emergency or disaster by officials who are authorized to make such a declaration.[72,73,81,82]

As the system degrades from normal operations through conventional, then contingency, and finally crisis operations, a proactive plan to address resource allocation dilemmas is needed. In the setting of conventional care, the emergency management team should be monitoring resource use and adjusting as possible to stay near normal care. In the setting of contingency care, a more robust process is needed, which should be authorized to take such actions as deferring procedures and requiring the use of alternative medications or the reuse of critical supplies. These decisions must be made in a coordinated fashion to maintain a similar level of care and equity for patients across an institution or, ideally, across a region. The monitoring of patients in nonstandard care areas, such as procedure units, must be closely watched to avoid adverse outcomes. And sometimes simple processes such as minimizing documentation requirements can be used to free health care workers to provide more direct patient care. Monitoring of bedside decisions after the fact may also be needed to assure that the important principles in Table 1 are maintained and that fair allocation occurs, even when (perhaps especially when) formal invocation of Crisis Standards has not occurred.[75,80]

As the system degrades into crisis operations, some resource allocation decisions might result in the near-term death or poor outcomes of patients who are denied access to limited resources. These decisions should not be left on the shoulders of a single person, and they should not be made in an ad hoc fashion. Rather, the institution should implement a proactive plan to form resource triage allocation teams and follow some type of objective process in evaluating patients for therapies. This plan should be cognizant of key ethical principles in Table 1. During a disaster such as that which occurs when an institution runs out of ventilators to treat patients with acute respiratory failure (as in the vignette above), such allocation teams can help assure fairness and use of the best medical information available to distribute the ventilators according to a transparent, equitable plan.[83]

The US National Academy of Medicine (formerly, the Institute of Medicine, or IOM) has developed a formal definition of "Crisis Standards of Care," which reads as follows:

> *"Crisis standards of care" is defined as a substantial change in usual health care operations and the level of care it is possible to deliver, which is made necessary by a pervasive (e.g., pandemic influenza) or catastrophic (e.g., earthquake, hurricane) disaster. This change in the level of care delivered is justified by specific circumstances and is formally declared by a state government, in recognition that crisis operations will be in effect for a sustained period. The formal declaration that crisis standards of care are in operation*

enables specific legal/regulatory powers and protections for healthcare personnel in the necessary tasks of allocating and using scarce medical resources and implementing alternate care facility operations.

IOM[82]

Once operating within a crisis standards framework, there are several substantive principles, or rules, that have been proposed to guide the rationing of limited resources, but we find all of these to be overly simplistic for use in practice. Proposed substantive allocation rules include: saving the most lives by treating those most likely to survive; saving the most life years (e.g., giving preference to younger people); saving the most quality or disability-adjusted life years; saving women and children first; allocating resources based on the principle of "first come, first served"; giving preference to those who can help others (medical, EMS, and other public servants); or some kind of market-based scheme based on ability to buy care. In reality, we see these proposed rule-based resource allocation ideas as attempts to simplify what are inherently complex and heart-wrenching rationing decisions, which require attention to multiple principles. As such, while each proposed substantive decision rule reflects an important value, none of them should always trump the others. Therefore, it is very important to also consider ways to make the decision-making *process* more ethical. In this regard, the principles of procedural justice in the second half of Table 1, such as transparency, involvement of all stakeholders, and providing mechanisms to ensure accountability, are worthy of considerable attention when developing and implementing mechanisms for making difficult allocation decisions.[3] In other words, being ready for the ethical implementation of a triage system may be more important than coming to agreement in advance on specific allocation rules, such as whether children should receive priority for accessing vaccines.

While this chapter is not focused on legal issues, there are some important legal implications of implementing a triage system that deserve specific consideration in advance. First, health professionals might be worried about malpractice or of running afoul of their respective professional licensure boards if they provide less than their usual quality of care, even during a crisis. But in the United States, the concept of a local standard of care generally applies when determining if medical decisions are appropriate. This comes down to a general agreement that the standard of care is always what a similar "reasonable" physician would do *under similar circumstances*. Ethically, it is interesting to note that the "reasonable professional" standard is an extension of the "ought-implies-can" argument long made by ethicists and philosophers; namely, that it cannot be an ethical requirement to do something that it is impossible to do (or, conversely, it cannot be unethical to do something that one is forced to do, such as rationing limited resources). These notions of not being legally or ethically required to do what is impossible, or even anything other than what any other well-trained person caught in the same circumstance would do, are central to the ethics of triage during crises.

As such, if one is forced to make triage decisions, the first ethical obligation is to ensure that triage decision-making really is required, and the second should be to ensure that the triage decision-making process has been formally authorized. In this regard, as in the circumstances described in Sections "Restriction on Liberty" and "Responsibility" above, legal and ethical problems related to resource allocation decisions are most likely to arise if there has been a lack of advance planning or if there is no formal declaration of a crisis.

Several steps should be taken to assure an appropriate legal and ethical climate for medical personnel who may be forced to make triage decisions during crises. The first step should be the declaration of a "disaster" or "public health emergency" by the healthcare entity, as well as by the county or state. Unfortunately, the COVID-19 pandemic has shown that there can be considerable reluctance among leaders to acknowledge when rationing is becoming necessary or even already happening (Mehta, Persoff). Failing to declare a disaster does not make it any less calamitous, of course, and it does not prevent rationing from taking place: implementing rationing strategies is not a choice; it is a tragic circumstance one is thrust into. Hence, in the absence of a formal declaration promoting use of ethical rationing strategies, unethical strategies (such as misleading patients about the "futility" of treatments that are in short supply) become more appealing. This is partly because formal guidance is more likely to be well-considered than ad hoc decisions, but also because formal declarations allowing adoption of crisis standards of care can bring a group of legal protections to bear, which will depend on a variety of state laws and regulations. Detailed guidance has been provided by the National Academy of Medicine to help states in developing "Crisis Standards of Care" plans.[72,73,82] Implementation of a preestablished formal crisis standard of care plan by the state is particularly important for ensuring equitable application of the process across the state. These plans often include draft executive orders for the Governor to sign with the onset of specific types of crises, which can provide specific direction as

TABLE 4
Actions That Can Facilitate the Implementation of More Ethical Resource Triage and Rationing

- Declaration of disaster by healthcare entities and local and state governments
- Implementation of emergency operations plans by relevant entities
- Implementation of an incident management system
- Legal authorization of explicit triage strategies by government
- Prior and ongoing implementation of lower-risk contingency strategies for scarce resources, including minimization of use, reuse, and use of alternate items
- Activation of resource triage teams to make allocation decisions
- Use of preplanned resource allocation tools
- Implementation of alternative/palliative care strategies for those denied resources

well as legal and regulatory protections for health care workers. These protections may be an important factor in convincing personnel to stay at work (as noted in Section "Responsibility"), which can help to mitigate the crisis and prevent shortages of personnel. Other actions that can or should be taken during crises that might facilitate better decision-making regarding resource allocation (Table 4), and each of these should be addressed in advance when developing crisis standards of care plans at the local and state level.

The advance development of triage teams that can be rapidly assembled during crises is especially important for several reasons (see Chapters 14, 19, and 27 for more detail). First, individual nurses and physicians are ethically obligated to advocate for their patients. This causes inherent conflict with other care providers over whose patient should receive scarce resources, which an independent triage team can mediate. Second, the evaluation of complex medical cases will benefit from a triage team including multiple viewpoints, including medical, nursing, ethics, and others. Third, shared team decision-making prevents any one individual from being forced to make decisions that will potentially lead directly to a patient dying, thus mitigating (but not eliminating) the moral distress of practicing triage.

The allocation of critical care beds and critical items such as ventilators can be particularly difficult, even for teams of decision-makers. While one would never remove a ventilator from a patient during usual care except by the consent of the patient or their proxy, during a crisis it can be ethically appropriate to remove a ventilator from one patient to provide it to another patient with significantly better odds of near-term survival. Similarly, it might be ethically appropriate to deny use of a CT scanner to one patient if doing so will preserve use of that scanner for many other patients who need it, as in the Ebola case above.

When such complex decisions arise, the use of objective criteria to guide decision-making is appealing, though users should recognize the inherent imprecision and potential biases of seemingly objective scoring systems.[84] For example, the use of the Sequential Organ Failure Assessment (SOFA) score forms part of a common framework for ICU bed and ventilator allocation[85] (White/Lo). But the SOFA score was found to have limited predictive value for COVID-19,[84,86] and it is biased against racial minorities due to both higher rates of comorbid conditions in these communities and common race-adjustments to lab values included in the score.[87] On the other hand, even if imperfect, scoring systems might still be better than some other available triage options, such as a first-come, first-served strategy or leaving decisions to individual clinicians and their personal biases. Moreover, scoring systems can help create the necessary ethical and practical framework to allow withdrawal of a resource from one patient when it is not likely to benefit that patient and has a better chance of benefiting another. Such decisions are undeniably difficult, but when faced with a forced choice and only bad options, it is ethically appropriate to choose the least bad option.

Finally, it has long been recognized that disasters tend to hit marginalized communities hardest, and this was seen in the COVID-19 pandemic.[88] To mitigate the exacerbation of racial, ethnic, geographic, and other health disparities during outbreaks, explicit attention to equity and the social determinants of health should be incorporated into resource allocation strategies. This often means sending additional resources to harder-hit neighborhoods. In the COVID-19 pandemic, it also sometimes meant giving priority in rationing strategies to "essential workers," who were often placed at greater risk of infection by virtue of their work and who tended to be from disadvantaged minority communities.

CONCLUSIONS

This chapter has reviewed several types of ethical challenges faced by those charged with being prepared for and responding to viral outbreaks and bioterror attacks. Such challenges are seen repeatedly in a wide variety of such situations and have been called the three Rs of ethics in epidemic response: restrictions, responsibilities, and rationing. While the ways in which these challenges arise will differ across different scenarios, ethical lessons that have been learned from recent outbreaks, including the COVID-19 pandemic, can highlight ethical complexities and provide practical guidance for future challenges.

REFERENCES

1. Wynia MK. Ethics and public health emergencies: encouraging responsibility. *Am J Bioethics.* 2007;7(4):1–4.
2. Wynia MK. Ethics and public health emergencies: restrictions on liberties. *Am J Bioethics.* 2007;7(2):1–5.
3. Wynia MK. Ethics and public health emergencies: rationing vaccines. *Am J Bioethics.* 2006;6(6):4–7.
4. FEMA. A Whole Community Approach to Emergency Management: Principles, Themes and Pathways to Action; 2011. FDOC 104-008-1. Available from https://www.fema.gov/media-library-data/20130726-1813-25045-0649/whole_community_dec2011__2_.pdf. Accessed 18 February 2018.
5. Wells KB, Springgate BF, Lizaola E, et al. Community engagement in disaster preparedness and recovery: a tale of two cities - Los Angeles and New Orleans. *Psychiatr Clinic North Amer.* 2013;36(3):451–466.
6. Burgoon B. On welfare and terror: social welfare policies and political-economic roots of terrorism. *J Conflict Resol.* 2006;50(2):176–203.
7. Braveman P. Accumulating knowledge on the social determinants of health and infectious diseases. *Public Health Rep.* 2011;126(suppl 3):28–30.
8. Semenva JC, Suk JE, Tsolova S. Social determinants of infectious diseases: a public health priority. *Euro Surveill.* 2010;15(27):2–4.
9. White DB, Lo B. A framework for rationing ventilators and critical care beds during the COVID-19 Pandemic. *JAMA.* 2020;323(18):1773–1774. https://doi.org/10.1001/jama.2020.5046.
10. Annas GJ. The statue of security: Human rights and post-9/11 epidemics. In: Balint J, Philpott S, Baker R, Strosberg M, eds. *Ethics and Epidemics.* Amsterdam, Neth: Elsevier Press; 2006:3–28.
11. Wynia MK, Gostin LO. Ethical challenges in preparing for bioterrorism: barriers within the health care system. *Am J Public Health.* 2004;94(7):1096–1102.
12. Tseng CW, Roh Y, DeJong C, et al. Patients' compliance with quarantine requirements for exposure or potential symptoms of COVID-19. *Hawaii J Health Soc Welf.* 2021;80(11):276–282.
13. Inglesby T, Grossman R, O'Toole T. A plague on your city: observations from TOPOFF. *Clin Infect Dis.* 2001;32(3):436–445.
14. Johns Hopkins Center for Civilian Biodefense, Center for Strategic and International Studies, ANSER, Memorial Institute for the Prevention of Terrorism. Final Script: Dark Winter: Bioterrorism Exercise, Andrews Air Force Base. June 22-23, Baltimore: Johns Hopkins Center for Civilian Biodefense; 2001. Available at: http://www.centerforhealthsecurity.org/our-work/events/2001_dark-winter/about.html. Accessed 18 February 2018.
15. Stelfox HT, Bates DW, Redelmeier DA. Safety of patients isolated for infection control. *JAMA.* 2003;290(14):1899–1905.
16. Anderson-Shaw LK, Zar FA. COVID-19, Moral conflict, distress, and dying alone. *J Bioeth Inq.* 2020;17(4):777–782. https://doi.org/10.1007/s11673-020-10040-9.
17. Bowling JE, Taylor BS. Isolation precautions for hospitalized patients: the challenges of identifying unintended individual consequences and measuring the prevention of community harm. *J Gen Intern Med.* 2017;32:238–240. doi. https://doi.org/10.1007/s11606-016-3926-5.
18. Rothstein MA, Alcalde MG, Elster NR, et al. Quarantine and isolation: lessons learned from SARS. A report to the Centers for Disease Control and Prevention. Louisville KY: Institute for Bioethics, Health Policy and Law, University of Louisville School of Medicine; 2003. Available at: https://biotech.law.lsu.edu/blaw/cdc/SARS_REPORT.pdf. Accessed 17 February 2018.
19. Wynia MK, Kurlander JE, Green SK. Chapter 6. Physician professionalism and preparing for epidemics: Challenges and opportunities. In: Balint J, Philpott S, Baker R, Martin Strosberg M, eds. *Ethics and Epidemics (Advances in Bioethics, Volume 9).* Somerville, Mass: Emerald Group Publishing Limited; 2006:135–161.
20. Huber SJ, Wynia MK. When pestilence prevails... physician responsibilities in epidemics. *Am J Bioeth.* 2004;4(1):W5–11. https://doi.org/10.1162/152651604773067497.
21. Drazen JM, Kanapathipillai R, Campion EW, et al. Ebola and quarantine. *N Engl J Med.* 2014;371(21):2029–2030.
22. Dineen KK, Lowe A, Kass NE, et al. Treating workers as essential too: an ethical framework for public health interventions to prevent and control COVID-19 infections among meat-processing facility workers and their communities in the United States. *J Bioeth Inq.* 2022;19(2):301–314. https://doi.org/10.1007/s11673-022-10170-2.
23. Siracusa Principles. Siracusa Principles on the Limitation and Derogation Provisions in the International Covenant on Civil and Political Rights. International Commission of Jurists; 1984. Available at: https://www.icj.org/siracusa-principles-on-the-limitation-and-derogation-provisions-in-the-international-covenant-on-civil-and-political-rights/. Accessed 17 February 2018.
24. Mill JS. On Liberty; 1859.
25. Gibbs H, Liu Y, Pearson CAB, et al. Changing travel patterns in China during the early stages of the COVID-19 pandemic. *Nat Commun.* 2020;11:5012. https://doi.org/10.1038/s41467-020-18783-0.
26. Arena PJ, Malta M, Rimoin AW, et al. Race, COVID-19 and deaths of despair. *EClinicalMedicine.* 2020;25:100485. https://doi.org/10.1016/j.eclinm.2020.100485.
27. Sattenspiel L, Herring DA. Simulating the effect of quarantine on the spread of the 1918-19 flu in Central Canada. *Bull Math Biol.* 2003;65(1):1–26.

28. Markel H, Lipman HB, Navarro JA. Nonpharmacological interventions implemented by US cities during the 1918-1919 influenza pandemic. *JAMA.* 2007;298(6):644–654.
29. Blendon RJ, Koonin LM, Benson JM, et al. Public response to community mitigation measures for pandemic influenza. *Emerg Infect Dis.* 2008;14(5):778–786.
30. Talic S, Shah S, Wild H, et al. Effectiveness of public health measures in reducing the incidence of covid-19, SARS-CoV-2 transmission, and covid-19 mortality: systematic review and meta-analysis. *BMJ.* 2021;375, e068302. https://doi.org/10.1136/bmj-2021-068302 [Erratum in: BMJ. 2021 Dec 3;375:n2997. https://doi. org/10.1136/bmj.n2997. PMID: 34789505; PMCID: PMC9423125].
31. Edelson PJ. Quarantine and civil liberties. In: Balint J, Philpott S, Baker R, Strosberg M, eds. *Ethics and Epidemics (Advances in Bioethics, Volume 9).* Somerville MA: Emerald Group Publishing Limited; 2006:29–42.
32. Hick JL, Hanfling D, Wynia M, et al. Crisis Standards of Care and COVID-19: What Did We Learn? How Do We Ensure Equity? What Should We Do? NAM Perspectives (Discussion). Washington, DC: National Academy of Medicine; 2021. https://doi.org/10.31478/202108e.
33. Cauchemez S, Valleron AJ, Boelle PY, et al. Estimating the impact of school closure on influenza transmission from sentinel data. *Nature.* 2008;452(7188):750–754.
34. Heymann A, Chodick G, Reichman B, et al. Influence of school closure on the incidence of viral respiratory diseases among children and on health care utilization. *Pediatr Infect Dis J.* 2004;23(7):675–677.
35. Kahn LH. Pandemic influenza school closure policies. *Emerg Infect Dis.* 2007;13(2):344–345.
36. Sasaki A, Hoen AG, Ozonoff AI, et al. Evidence-based tool for triggering school closures during influenza outbreaks, Japan. *Emerg Infect Dis.* 2009;15(11):1841–1843.
37. Cetron MS. Quarantine, isolation and community mitigation: battling 21st century pandemics with a 14th century toolbox. In: *Presented at Legal and Ethical Aspects of Pandemic Preparedness.* Washington DC: Institute of Medicine; 2006. Available at: http://www.nationalacademies.org/hmd/~/media/Files/Activity%20Files/PublicHealth/MicrobialThreats/cetron_Qethicsseminar_IOM2.pdf. Accessed 17 February 2018.
38. Harden BD. Matthew's Passion. NY Times Magazine; 2001. Feb 18. Available electronically at: http://www.nytimes.com/2001/02/18/magazine/dr-matthew-s-passion.html.
39. Qureshi K, Gershon RR, Sherman MF, et al. Health care workers' ability and willingness to report to duty during catastrophic disasters. *J Urban Health.* 2005;82(3):378–388.
40. Alexander GC, Wynia MK. Ready and willing? Physician readiness and willingness to treat potential victims of bioterror. *Health Aff.* 2003;22(5):189–197.
41. Ruderman C, Tracy CS, Bensimon CM, et al. On pandemics and the duty to care: whose duty? Who cares? *BMC Med Ethics.* 2006;7:E5.
42. Minkoff H, Ecker J. Physicians' obligations to patients infected with Ebola: echoes of acquired immune deficiency syndrome. *Am J Obstet Gynecol.* 2015;212(4). https://doi.org/10.1016/j.ajog.2014.12.026. 456.e1-4.
43. Link RN, Feingold AR, Charap MH, et al. Concerns of medical and pediatric house staff about contracting AIDS from their patients. *Am J Public Health.* 1988;78(4):455–459. https://doi.org/10.2105/ajph.78.4.455.
44. Narasimhulu DM, Edwards V, Chazotte C, et al. Health care workers' attitudes toward patients with Ebola virus disease in the United States. *Open Forum Infect Dis.* 2016;3(1). ofv192.
45. Knobler S, Mahmoud A, Lemon S, et al, eds. Learning from SARS: Preparing for the next disease outbreak. In: *Workshop Summary.* Washington, DC: Institute of Medicine, National Academy of Sciences; 2004. Institute of Medicine (US) Forum on Microbial Threats; Washington (DC): National Academies Press (US); 2004.
46. Christianson J, Johnson N, Nelson A, et al. Work-related burnout, compassion fatigue, and nurse intention to leave the profession during COVID-19. *Nurse Lead.* 2023;21(2):244–251. https://doi.org/10.1016/j.mnl.2022.06.007.
47. Magnavita N, Chirico F, Garbarino S, et al. SARS/MERS/SARS-CoV-2 outbreaks and burnout syndrome among healthcare workers. An umbrella systematic review. *Int J Environ Res Public Health.* 2021;18(8):4361. https://doi.org/10.3390/ijerph18084361.
48. Sande MA, Ronald AR. Update in infectious diseases. *Ann Intern Med.* 2004;140(4):290–295.
49. McDonald LC, Simor AE, Su IJ, et al. SARS in healthcare facilities, Toronto and Taiwan. *Emerg Infect Dis.* 2004;10(5):777–781.
50. World Health Organization (WHO). Health worker Ebola infections in Guinea, Liberia and Sierra Leone; 2015. Preliminary Report. WHO/EVD/SDS/REPORT/2015.1. Available at http://www.who.int/csr/resources/publications/ebola/health-worker-infections/en/. Accessed 18 February 2018.
51. Nguyen LH, Drew DA, Graham MS, et al. Risk of COVID-19 among front-line health-care workers and the general community: a prospective cohort study. *Lancet Public Health.* 2020;5(9):e475–e483. https://doi.org/10.1016/S2468-2667(20)30164-X.
52. Norman SB, Feingold JH, Kaye-Kauderer H, et al. Moral distress in frontline healthcare workers in the initial epicenter of the COVID-19 pandemic in the United States: relationship to PTSD symptoms, burnout, and psychosocial functioning. *Depress Anxiety.* 2021;38(10):1007–1017. https://doi.org/10.1002/da.23205.
53. Burrowes SAB, Casey SM, Pierre-Joseph N, et al. COVID-19 pandemic impacts on mental health, burnout, and longevity in the workplace among healthcare workers: a mixed methods study. *J Res Interprof Pract Educ.* 2023;32:100661. https://doi.org/10.1016/j.xjep.2023.100661.
54. Emanuel EJ. The lessons of SARS. *Ann Intern Med.* 2003;139(7):589–591.
55. García-Zamora S, Pulido L, Miranda-Arboleda AF, et al. Aggression, micro-aggression, and abuse against health

care providers during the COVID-19 pandemic. A Latin American survey. *Curr Probl Cardiol.* 2022;47(10):101296. https://doi.org/10.1016/j.cpcardiol.2022.101296.
56. Macpherson CC, Wynia MK. Should health professionals speak up to reduce the health risks of climate change? *AMA J Ethics.* 2017;19:1202–1210.
57. Yakubu A, Folayan MO, Sani-Gwarzo N, et al. The Ebola outbreak in Western Africa: ethical obligations for care. *J Med Ethics.* 2016;42(4):209–210. https://doi.org/10.1136/medethics-2014-102434.
58. Halpern SD, Emanuel EJ. Ethical guidance on the use of life-sustaining therapies for patients with Ebola in developed countries. *Ann Intern Med.* 2015;162(4):304–305.
59. Torabi-Parzini P, Davey RT, Suffredini AF, et al. Ethical and practical considerations in providing critical care to patients with ebola virus disease. *Chest.* 2015;147(6):1460–1466.
60. Cappuccio FP. Confusion over CPR in patients with covid-19. *BMJ.* 2020;369, m1805. https://doi.org/10.1136/bmj.m1805.
61. Iserson KV, Heine CE, Larkin GL, et al. Fight or flight: the ethics of emergency physician disaster response. *Ann Emerg Med.* 2008;51(4):345–353.
62. Lor A, Thomas JC, Barrett DH, et al. Key ethical issues discussed at CDC-sponsored international, regional meetings to explore cultural perspectives and contexts on pandemic influenza preparedness and response. *Int J Health Policy Manag.* 2016;5(11):653–662.
63. National Academies of Sciences, Engineering, and Medicine. Evidence-Based Practice for Public Health Emergency Preparedness and Response. Washington, DC: The National Academies Press; 2020. https://doi.org/10.17226/25650.
64. Hick JL, Hanfling D, Wynia MK. Duty to plan: health care, crisis standards of care, and novel coronavirus SARS-CoV-2. *NAM Perspect.* 2020;2020. https://doi.org/10.31478/202003b.
65. FEMA. Emergency Planning Exercises. (Last Updated 4.13.17); 2017. Available from https://www.fema.gov/emergency-planning-exercises. Accessed 2 October 2018.
66. Fink S. Whose Lives Should be Saved? Researchers Ask Public. New York Times; 2016. August 22 https://www.nytimes.com/2016/08/22/us/whose-lives-should-be-saved-to-help-shape-policy-researchers-in-maryland-ask-the-public.html. Accessed 2 October 2018.
67. Bensimon C, Smith MJ, Pisartchik D, et al. The duty to care in an influenza pandemic: a qualitative study of Canadian public perspectives. *Soc Sci Med.* 2012;75(12):2425–2430.
68. Thompson AK, Faith K, Gibson JL, Upshur REG. Pandemic influenza preparedness: an ethical framework to guide decision-making. *BMC Med Ethics.* 2006;7:E12.
69. Coleman CH, Reis A. Potential penalties for healthcare professionals who refuse to work during a pandemic. *JAMA.* 2008;299(12):1471–1473.
70. Fink S. Five Days at Memorial. Life and Death in a Storm Ravaged Hospital. New York NY: Crown Publishers; 2013.
71. Abbott J, Johnson D, Wynia M. Ensuring adequate palliative and hospice care during COVID-19 surges. *JAMA.* 2020;324(14):1393–1394. https://doi.org/10.1001/jama.2020.16843.
72. IOM (Institute of Medicine). Volume 1 - Introduction and CSC framework. In: *Crisis Standards of Care: A Systems Framework for Catastrophic Disaster Response.* Washington (DC): National Academies Press (US); 2012. https://doi.org/10.17226/13351. Mar 21. Available from: https://www.ncbi.nlm.nih.gov/books/NBK201063/.
73. IOM (Institute of Medicine). Crisis Standards of Care: A Toolkit for Indicators and Triggers. Washington, DC: The National Academies Press; 2013.
74. Persoff J, Wynia MK. Ethically navigating the murky waters of "Contingency Standards of Care". *Am J Bioeth.* 2021;21(8):20–21. https://doi.org/10.1080/15265161.2021.1939810.
75. Mehta AB, Wynia MK. Crisis standards of care-more than just a thought experiment? *Hastings Cent Rep.* 2021;51(5):53–55. https://doi.org/10.1002/hast.1288.
76. United States Food and Drug Administration. Drug Shortages; 2024. Available at: https://www.fda.gov/drugs/drug-safety-and-availability/drug-shortages. Accessed 3 November 2024.
77. Lipworth W, Kerridge I. Why drug shortages are an ethical issue. *Australas Med J.* 2013;6(11):556–559.
78. Singleton R, Chubbs K, Flynn J, et al. From framework to the frontline: designing a structure and process for drug supply shortage planning. *Healthc Manage Forum.* 2013;26(1):41–45.
79. DeJong C, Chen AH, Lo B. An ethical framework for allocating scarce inpatient medications for COVID-19 in the US. *JAMA.* 2020;323(23):2367–2368. https://doi.org/10.1001/jama.2020.8914.
80. Alfandre D, Sharpe VA, Geppert C, et al. Between usual and crisis phases of a public health emergency: the mediating role of contingency measures. *Am J Bioeth.* 2021;21(8):4–16. https://doi.org/10.1080/15265161.2021.1925778.
81. Gostin LO, Hanfling D. National preparedness for a catastrophic emergency: crisis standards of care. *JAMA.* 2009;302(21):2365–2366.
82. IOM (Institute of Medicine). Guidance for Establishing Crisis Standards of Care for use in Disaster Situations: A Letter Report. Washington (DC): National Academies Press (US); 2009. Available from: https://doi.org/10.17226/12749.
83. Vawter DE, Garrett JE, Gervais KG, et al. Attending to social vulnerability when rationing pandemic resources. *J Clin Ethics.* 2011;22(1):42–53.
84. Wynia MK. Crisis triage-attention to values in addition to efficiency. *JAMA Netw Open.* 2020;3(12), e2029326. https://doi.org/10.1001/jamanetworkopen.2020.29326 [Erratum in: JAMA Netw Open. 2021 Feb 1;4(2):e212183. https://doi.org/10.1001/jamanetworkopen.2021.2183. PMID: 33315107].
85. Christian MD, Sprung CL, King MA, et al. Triage: care of the critically ill and injured during pandemics and disasters: CHEST consensus statement. *Chest.* 2014;146(4 Suppl):e61S–74S.

86. Wunsch H, Hill AD, Bosch N, et al. Comparison of 2 triage scoring guidelines for allocation of mechanical ventilators. *JAMA Netw Open.* 2020;3(12), e2029250. https://doi.org/10.1001/jamanetworkopen.2020.29250 [Erratum in: JAMA Netw Open. 2021 Feb 1;4(2):e212183. https://doi.org/10.1001/jamanetworkopen.2021.2183. PMID: 33315112; PMCID: PMC7737087].
87. Sarkar R, Martin C, Mattie H, et al. Performance of intensive care unit severity scoring systems across different ethnicities in the USA: a retrospective observational study. *Lancet Digit Health.* 2021;3(4):e241–e249. https://doi.org/10.1016/S2589-7500(21)00022-4.
88. Acosta AM, Garg S, Pham H, et al. Racial and ethnic disparities in rates of COVID-19-associated hospitalization, intensive care unit admission, and in-hospital death in the United States from March 2020 to February 2021. *JAMA Netw Open.* 2021;4(10), e2130479. https://doi.org/10.1001/jamanetworkopen.2021.30479.

CHAPTER 27

Strategies for Successful Communications During Health Emergencies: Insights From Journalists Turned Public Relations Experts

JENNIFER DOREN[a] • HEATHER SVOKOS[b]
[a]Communications, Marketing, and Public Affairs, UT Southwestern Medical Center, Dallas, TX, United States • [b]Employee Communications and Engagement, UT Southwestern Medical Center, Dallas, TX, United States

THE CHALLENGE

During a public health emergency, health risk communication is vital.[1] Lessons from previous influenza pandemics, events with high-consequence pathogens, and outbreaks highlight the importance of communication in garnering cooperation with proposed public health mitigation strategies.[1] The quality of the response is influenced by the ability to coordinate messaging, engage different populations, and effectively impart and exchange information. However, universal challenges in communication can arise and can be summarized as the following:

1. Evolving information may require a shifting of public health mitigation messages and strategies;
2. Information and data are misconstrued, misunderstood, or falsely reported, leading to an epidemic of misinformation that needs to be corrected;
3. There is uncertainty around the severity, trajectory, and duration of the epidemic, as well as the clinical outcomes of those infected;
4. Information is conflicting;
5. Public expectations are unrealistic about how much is known, what can be predicted and with what certainty, and what measures will need to be implemented to curb transmission.

These challenges are likely to surface not only for your organization and the community you serve but within your workplace too. "As leaders do everything in their power to beat COVID-19 and ensure their hospitals survive the crisis, they must urgently safeguard employees' needs," wrote Vibhas Ratanjee and Dan Foy of Gallup.[2] "Leaders must facilitate healthcare workers' success."[2] Ratanjee and Foy were interpreting results from an online, probability-based Gallup Panel survey conducted March 13-April 14, 2020, which revealed that:

- Only 36% of healthcare personnel strongly agree that they are confident they will be safe if they follow their organization's health policies.
- 47% of healthcare workers strongly agree that their employer has communicated a clear plan of action for COVID-19.
- 78% of healthcare workers feel that COVID-19 will have a somewhat negative or very negative effect on their workplace.

As with previous infectious disease events, whether Ebola or H1N1, what that data underscores is that in the early days of the COVID-19 pandemic, there were widespread communications problems that impacted individual institutions, cities, states, and the larger national public perception. How authorities and leaders adapted their response awakened a deeper appreciation for the importance of knowledgeable, engaged, and supported employees, patients, and community members. We learned the value of having our healthcare personnel become our most vocal ambassadors for helping to dispel myths and fear and disseminate accurate information about public health or medical emergencies on a broader scale (for additional details on communication from the public health perspective, see Chapter 13).

Viral Outbreaks, Biosecurity, and Preparing for Mass Casualty Infectious Diseases Events
https://doi.org/10.1016/B978-0-323-54841-0.00027-5

THE RESPONSE

The Health and Safety of Our Community, Including Our Workforce, Remain Our Top Priority

One of the most essential, if not most important, messages you can impart during a viral outbreak, biosecurity, or mass casualty infectious disease event is what you read just above. The health and safety of our community, including our workforce, remains the organizational top priority. That line should form the underpinning of all internal and external communications and continuously be reinforced. Think of it as your mantra and stick to it.

When structuring your communications approach, focus on three "Ps:" process, people, and partners.[1] The process requires multiple strategies utilizing print, broadcast, electronic, and social media. The effectiveness of each of these communication outlets may depend on the population targeted, specifically their access to news, educational level, and beliefs. When promoting messaging, look for people who are respected in your community, as well as those who are trusted and dependable sources of reliable scientific information. Credible community leaders, including those in ministries and part of professional groups, can help build bridges to those of different cultures, cultural expectations, languages, and beliefs. They may also help address any barriers to access to care. Engaging these experts facilitates a sustainable response that can more organically reach the masses and is the focus of our experience. Finally, there is a need for partners who can be ambassadors of these messages. This is especially necessary for the setting of a pandemic, where communication requires a prolonged effort to reach myriad communities. These individuals or organizations are known and recognized entities and have reach and influence within their communities.

When incorporating the three "P's" of process, people, and partners, a five-point plan can be used as a guide for your organization to achieve effective messaging:

1. Communicate early, often, and across multiple channels.
2. Provide two-way communication.
3. Promote clarity over complexity.
4. Establish trust through transparency.
5. Demonstrate empathy and compassion.

Cutting across all the five-point plan components listed above are four audience factors that should be considered when any communication strategy is being developed and implemented.[1] First, it is important to be mindful of environmental circumstances such as people's access to healthcare and underlying medical conditions. Second, there are social and cultural considerations, including religious beliefs, education, and healthcare literacy. Third, we must adapt communications to meet language preferences. Fourth and final, there are pre-existing knowledge, beliefs, and attitudes about the recommended public health or medical interventions within a community. Keeping these four factors in mind, we will now walk through the five-point plan outlined above and then summarize and synthesize this information with a case study.

COMMUNICATE EARLY, OFTEN, AND ACROSS MULTIPLE CHANNELS

Frequent communication matters. Distributing factual, timely information—oftentimes daily—helps to reduce the risk of transmission during infectious disease emergencies.[3] To instill trust in public health messaging, it is valuable to reference epidemiological models that provide data from a central source, if available. Information should be shared broadly as early as possible without sacrificing accuracy or wading into the dangerous waters of inference and conjecture (see rule #3 from "Promote Clarity over Complexity" below). Communications and behavioral scientists have long demonstrated that the most effective way to engage and educate the public is through face-to-face interaction.[4] Naturally, you may find yourself asking how to do that when a pandemic creates physical separation. COVID-19 forced all of us to find creative ways to remain informed and connected in a controlled way that minimized risk while steering us to safe practices.

One such tactic was leaning more heavily on video, which captures attention quickly and typically holds it for longer than written communications. When we watch something on TV or on our portable digital devices, the content is oftentimes palatable and engaging. Video helps to humanize leaders, grow trust, and move people from awareness to action. Video content accounts for an overwhelming majority of all global internet traffic—about 82% in 2022. Such knowledge can be used to inform approaches to communications.

Remember Your Audience

The way we communicate translates through words and images and can either reflect a commitment to equity and inclusion or make others feel insignificant or peripheral. Think critically about whom you are trying to reach the most with your messaging—who is at the highest risk and who has the least access to help or information—and make smart choices about the individuals you put forward to reach them.

Multiple factors influence how messages are received and accepted and should guide internal and external communication strategies. For example, environmental, social, and cultural characteristics frame populations that benefit from messaging.[1] In the case of COVID-19, research revealed early on that minority communities—specifically Black and Latinx—were disproportionately affected and suffered more severe consequences from the disease. A randomized controlled clinical trial was designed based on that information to evaluate the effectiveness of video messages about the pandemic. The videos varied by physician race or ethnicity and the degree to which the physician acknowledged the difficulties faced by communities of color in accessing health services.[5] A large number ($n = 14,267$) of self-identified Black or Latinx adults were randomly assigned to either watch three video messages about COVID-19 and then answer questions, or answer questions first and then watch the videos. Information seeking—in other words, clicking links that provided additional information on COVID-19—was higher among Black participants who viewed messages from Black physicians. However, this trend was not observed among the Latinx participants.

A prominent researcher, whose work focuses on healthcare disparities, stated, "I think it's incumbent on all of us to realize that the health of all of us depends on the health of each of us".[6,7] No two people are the same. Each of us comes from varying backgrounds and households that speak different languages. Dr. Alicia Fernandez's quote reminds us that language preferences and translation can be important in communicating factual and evidence-based scientific information and minimizing misinformation.[1] For example, multilingual public service announcements presented by a diverse pool of experts provide information and promote cultural sensitivity. Organizations must be nimble and creative in their messaging, given that there are large portions of the global community with multiple language preferences other than English.

PROVIDE TWO-WAY COMMUNICATION

Whether addressing your employees, patients, or community members, the objectives are the same. To effectively inform, you must also remind your reader or viewer that communication goes both ways. Organizations should develop a way for employees to conveniently pose questions that are on their minds and then be reassured that they'll be addressed and answered. Creating dialogue builds trust and signals that an organization is committed to transparency and is sensitive to the needs of its community. In the first few weeks of any event, as data and institutional processes are rapidly evolving, producing clear and concise communications and responding to questions that naturally arise are necessary.

Examples of effective two-way communication include open forums or "town hall"-style meetings. It is also beneficial to set up dedicated email inboxes for questions from internal (employee) and external (public) audiences and to expeditiously address questions and comments. Frequent updates and dialogue echo that key statement previously mentioned: *The health and safety of our community, including our workforce, remain our top priority.* That messaging should be amplified on social media channels, which leads us to another important point when developing effective communications: understand news consumption and adapt to it.

Power of Social Media

How we receive and share news is changing at a whirlwind pace. When you couple the rapid rise of citizen journalism with the widespread use of social media, it can be tough to discern fact from fiction. That makes the work of health officials even more challenging and critical. In 2021, more than 80% of adult Americans consumed news through digital devices.[8] About half of U.S. adults (53%) relied heavily on social platforms like Facebook (36%), YouTube (23%), and X (15%) as regular news sources. Unfortunately, however, the speed of sharing new information comes at a cost. Social platforms allow messages to be amplified quickly, and sometimes the wrong information gets out. On X (formerly Twitter), falsehoods are 70% more likely to be retweeted than truths. That misinformation also reaches the first 1500 people six times faster.[9] In addition, a cross-sectional online survey of a convenience sample of adults found that COVID-19 knowledge correlated with whether the participants obtained information from a reliable source such as the Centers for Disease Control and Prevention or a local public health department website. Hence, what participants viewed as the "most trusted" news source influenced whether they could correctly answer factual questions about COVID-19.[10] Those who relied on television news for health information during the early days of COVID-19 were the most misinformed. The second least knowledgeable were those who obtained their information from Facebook ($P = 0.05$).

As former journalists, we find the results of that survey both troubling and incredibly telling of the work we as healthcare workers and academic professionals are charged with doing. No matter which country was surveyed, people who were more susceptible to misinformation during the pandemic were less likely to comply with public health recommendations and less likely to get vaccinated.[11,12] As each unit on a Likert scale increased by one, the authors showed that the individual's susceptibility to misinformation increased by 23% and was 28% less likely to get vaccinated or recommend vaccination. Furthermore, if individuals trusted scientists, the odds of getting vaccinated and recommending the vaccine to others increased. It is imperative that we counter misinformation and what's been dubbed the COVID-19 "infodemic".[12,13] What that phrase refers to is "a mix of evolving and conflicting findings, factual errors, rumors, and conspiracy theories, spread lightning-fast through all forms of media, often to promote political agendas rather than public health".[13]

Care providers and clinical researchers have a moral obligation to inform the public and advise policymakers. Part of that responsibility means ensuring the media are accurately reporting. We can also control the dialogue by directly answering questions, debunking myths, and sharing reliable and timely health information. For example, develop a medical blog such as was done to debunk some of the questions about masks (https://utswmed.org/medblog/covid19-mask-myths-realities/). While it is critical to communicate early and often, being first is not always best. That is true always and especially during viral outbreaks. As many reporters have learned the hard way throughout their careers, racing to push information out the fastest does not always win you awards or earn you additional points with the public. You will likely lose points quicker than you gain them if that information hasn't been effectively vetted and confirmed accurate. In the case of viral outbreaks and high-consequence pathogens, science and data should trump assumptions. If you're waiting to learn more, be honest and say just that.

Social media, while a potential breeding ground for misinformation, can also be crucial for promoting truth and nurturing two-way communication. Post updates and fact-based information, often on your organization's pages, and make sure private messages are closely monitored. Examples of this can be seen in the case study (Fig. 1). Create an autoreply so those who take the time to reach out know you value their doing so and are aware you will circle back with an additional response, if necessary. During COVID-19, we anticipated frequently asked questions and provided links to pertinent information as part of our organization's autoreply.

PROMOTE CLARITY OVER COMPLEXITY

To build trust, communicate clearly, or you risk causing unnecessary confusion. Think back to when you were in elementary school and first learned the importance of the "5W's"—who, what, when, where, and why. Knowing the answers to those simple questions helps readers and listeners understand the full scope of the topic at hand. Get back to the basics.

In the case of TV reporters, they want 10-s soundbites. If an interview isn't live, they will frequently stitch together portions of what you say to hook the viewer. Print reporters also favor straightforward information. For any interaction with media, live or recorded, remember this 10-point checklist:

1. Keep it short (10-s soundbites).
2. Explain what you're talking about as you would to your neighbor. Remove medical, technical, and scientific jargon from your messaging.
3. Focus on the facts. Stick with what you know is accurate today.
4. Don't imply and avoid projections.
5. Reinforce your internal messaging and the content you have on your websites.
6. If you misspeak during an interview, back up and correct yourself.
7. There is no "off the record." If you don't want to read it or hear it in the media, don't say it.
8. Practice.
9. Practice.
10. Practice again, in front of a mirror. Focus on your facial expressions and how you sound.

Some people, including specific patient populations that are at heightened risk, may want more granular details. You can be mindful of that, but don't make them run to a dictionary to make sense of the details. Frequently asked questions (FAQs) are an effective way of sharing key facts and figures. Presenting that information on a dedicated webpage, where you can easily make updates, is essential (Figs. 1–3). That website should become a central resource for all material and include references to additional resources for those who may be seeking more. These materials can and should also be shared in places of worship, schools, businesses, and other spots that members of the community frequent and trust. Printing materials also makes it possible to reach those who may not have internet access.

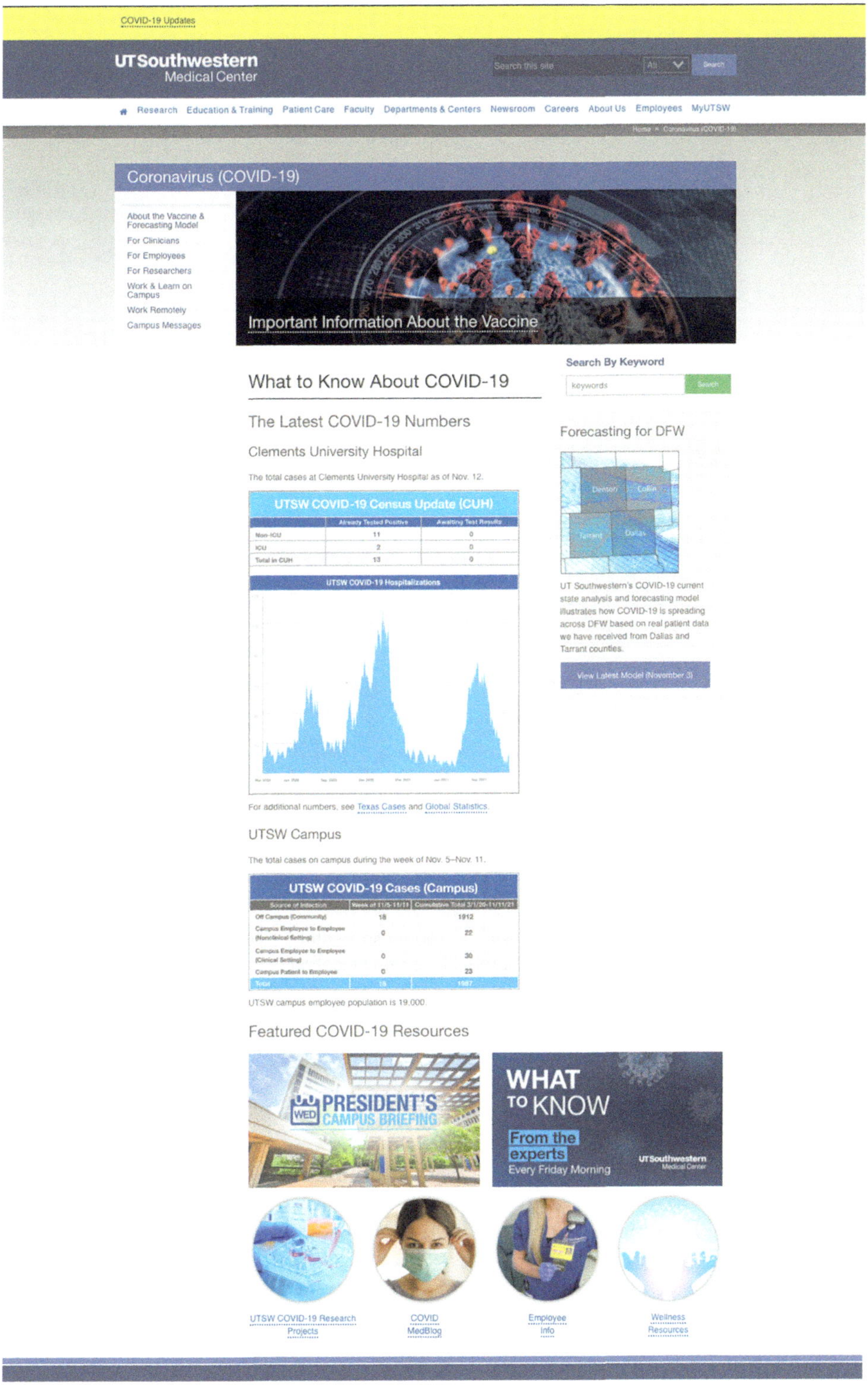

FIG. 1 Example of a website linking to multiple communications used during COVID-19. Website visualizes links to data, lectures, town halls. Note *yellow* banner to help with navigation.

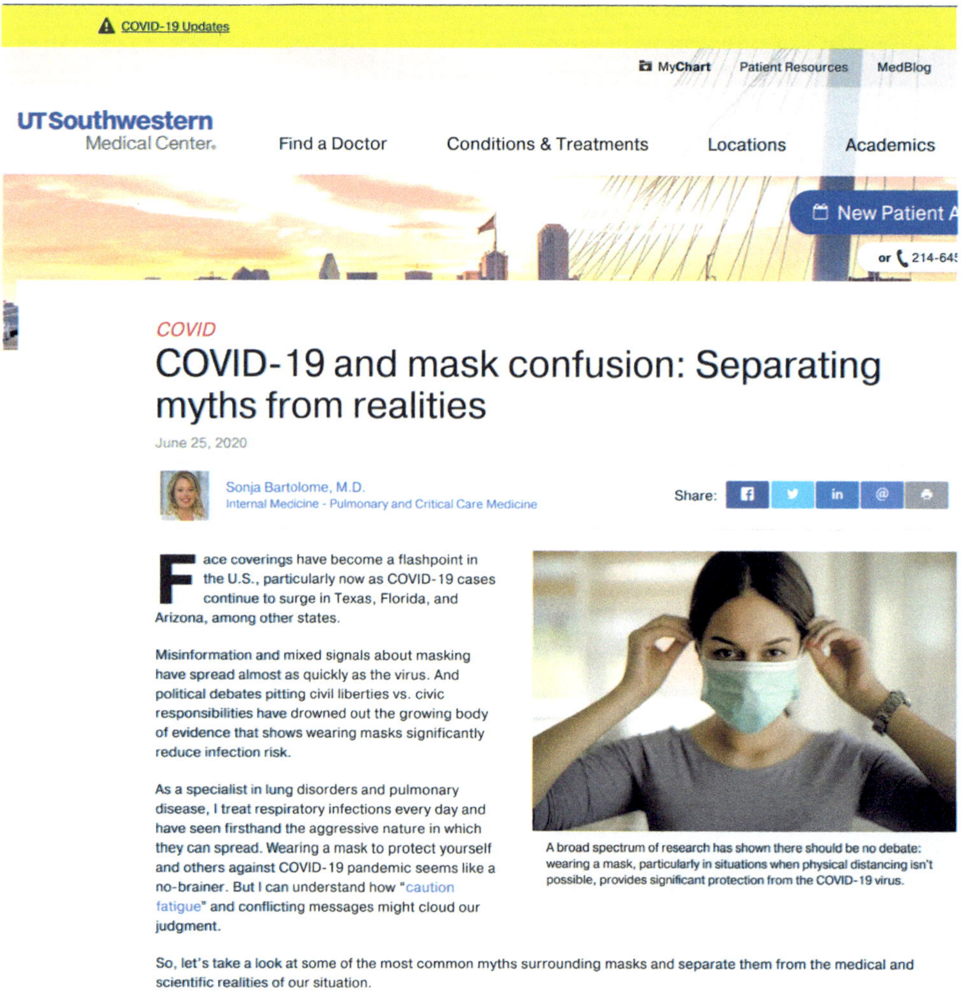

COVID-19 Updates

MyChart | Patient Resources | MedBlog

UTSouthwestern Medical Center.

Find a Doctor | Conditions & Treatments | Locations | Academics

New Patient A

or 214-64

COVID

COVID-19 and mask confusion: Separating myths from realities

June 25, 2020

Sonja Bartolome, M.D.
Internal Medicine - Pulmonary and Critical Care Medicine

Share:

Face coverings have become a flashpoint in the U.S., particularly now as COVID-19 cases continue to surge in Texas, Florida, and Arizona, among other states.

Misinformation and mixed signals about masking have spread almost as quickly as the virus. And political debates pitting civil liberties vs. civic responsibilities have drowned out the growing body of evidence that shows wearing masks significantly reduce infection risk.

As a specialist in lung disorders and pulmonary disease, I treat respiratory infections every day and have seen firsthand the aggressive nature in which they can spread. Wearing a mask to protect yourself and others against COVID-19 pandemic seems like a no-brainer. But I can understand how "caution fatigue" and conflicting messages might cloud our judgment.

A broad spectrum of research has shown there should be no debate: wearing a mask, particularly in situations when physical distancing isn't possible, provides significant protection from the COVID-19 virus.

So, let's take a look at some of the most common myths surrounding masks and separate them from the medical and scientific realities of our situation.

FIG. 2 Strategy to counter misinformation using a blog on an institutional website. https://utswmed.org/medblog/covid19-mask-myths-realities/. Example of a communication that is countering misinformation on the web.

UTSW Campus COVID-19 Cases

Source of Infection	Week of 10/30-11/5	Cumulative Total 3/1-11/5
Off Campus (Community)	28	381
Campus Employee to Employee (Nonclinical Setting)	0	10
Campus Employee to Employee (Clinical Setting)	0	15
Campus Patient to Employee	0	14
Total	28	420

FIG. 3 Example of communicating information to Healthcare personnel during the COVID-19 pandemic.

ESTABLISH TRUST THROUGH TRANSPARENCY

Revealing a peek behind the curtain can go a long way in improving trust and understanding. To become a leader in the community, transparency goes a long way in relationship-building.

How Bad Is It Now?

Show me the numbers. Whether it's your employees, your community, or the media, everyone feeds on facts. Public health authorities publish data, but to further enhance communication, organizational leaders can publicize additional data and amplify existing figures that illuminate the scope of the current problem. For example, during the COVID-19 pandemic, when healthcare resources were severely stretched, our academic medical center published daily—both internally and on a public-facing website (Fig. 1)—data about the following:

- Hospital census
- Number of COVID-19-positive patients admitted to our hospital in the intensive care units and on the hospital wards
- Number of patients awaiting test results
- Numbers of employees affected by COVID-19 (both in isolation and quarantine) and where and how they acquired their infection (i.e., community exposure vs. on campus in a clinical or non-clinical setting)

While city and county COVID-19 case counts informed the public, employee transmission data provided a sense of how well the campus and its workforce followed and enforced safety protocols. Furthermore, this information was reassuring to employees, in particular healthcare personnel, and proved throughout the pandemic that they were largely protected in clinical settings. The greatest struggle and risk to the institution was through exposure outside the institution, which informed the focus of other communications.

How Bad Is It Going To Get?

Uncertainty in the evolution and trajectory of infectious disease outbreaks is one of the communication challenges. Providing factual data and information and putting it into context is important. Partnering with researchers who can offer data and interpretation, as well as work on predictive modeling and genomic sequencing, adds valuable insight into the direction of the outbreak. For example, to determine the regional COVID-19 epidemiology, scientists at several universities made regional data publicly available and on institutional websites. The goal was to inform the public and keep the region, especially policymakers, ahead of the virus.

DEMONSTRATE EMPATHY AND COMPASSION

Much of your messaging will necessarily be filled with prescriptive, need-to-know information and tips for staying safe. But don't forget the human connection. During the COVID-19 pandemic, there were scores of day-to-day human struggles: stress, exhaustion, anxiety, grief, and staff attrition from sickness, childcare demands, and at-home learning.

If you consider the meaning of the word compassion, Merriam-Webster defines it as "sympathetic consciousness of other's distress together with a desire to alleviate it." The combination of being aware of the concerns of others with a goal to ease them is what helps to separate good leaders from great ones. Here is how you can accomplish that and cultivate compassion through written, verbal, and multimedia communications:

- Acknowledge people's concerns and anxieties about the health and safety of themselves, their families, and their co-workers.
- Express pride and gratitude for a job well done under extreme conditions.
- Remind your colleagues that they play an integral role in continuing the company's mission and in supporting the well-being of each other.
- Let them know you're there to help and encourage them to seek support if needed.
- In addition to promoting your two-way communications channels, be sure to assemble a collection of the various support and wellness resources available and guide your audience there.

Infusing humanity into your messaging will help your workforce feel heard, valued, and united in carrying out the mission of your organization and promoting public health messaging.

A CASE STUDY: UT SOUTHWESTERN AND THE COVID-19 PANDEMIC

To synthesize the five-point plan and four factors affecting messaging acceptance discussed above, a case study from Dallas, Texas, can be instructive. The city of 1.3 million is diverse and multilingual, with 42% of the residents being Hispanic or Latino, and just 42% of its people speak a language other than English at home. The city is home to UT Southwestern Medical Center, one of two academic medical centers in the North Texas region and well-regarded for its research, education, and clinical care. Throughout the COVID-19 pandemic, UT Southwestern leaders, infectious diseases experts, and faculty used a multifaceted communication approach to address issues around the COVID-19 pandemic and mitigation strategies. Keeping in mind our four factors outlined above, we gathered several concrete strategy examples that can be reviewed in Table 1. These can be of great reference when developing a strategy that ensures all components of the communication plan are successfully addressed.

(1) Communicate early, often, and across multiple channels

Within the early weeks of the pandemic, UT Southwestern launched a weekly—later turned bi-weekly—video series called "What To Know," hosted by the Executive Vice President for Health System Affairs/Chief Executive Officer of the Health System. As host, the senior leader sent a powerful message to the community that the pandemic required a collaborative, all-hands-on-deck response. He felt a responsibility and duty to be available and responsive to community concerns and needs, which again underscores the value of two-way communication. The pre-recorded series provided several dozen credible content experts with a platform for addressing timely topics and an opportunity to quickly reach people not only locally, but globally. Guests countered fear with facts, answered recurring questions, and explored the latest scientific research and advances in clinical care. Topics were varied and strategically chosen. They ranged, in part, from why COVID-19 hits men harder than women and how to manage the rise in anxiety and depression to understanding pregnancy and cancer care during a pandemic and developing new therapies for the SARS-CoV-2 virus. The producers from the communications and marketing team made certain that each of the discussions featured a diverse panel of scientists, physicians, and institutional and community leaders who could confidently present late-breaking information and, when necessary, field questions in English and Spanish.

Similarly, shortly after the first cases of COVID-19 appeared in Dallas-Fort Worth, the communications team launched a standing daily meeting and, among several deliverables, collaborated to record and edit more than a dozen multilingual public service announcements. These were short, roughly 30-s videos that drove home the importance of masking, physical distancing, and hand hygiene in reducing the spread of the virus. Each video featured a different expert speaking in languages including, Amharic, Arabic, English, French, Gujarati, Hindi, Igbo, Korean, Mandarin, Somali, Spanish, Telugu, Vietnamese, and Yoruba, among many others. The goal was to reinforce comprehensive messaging and make sure all populations felt valued, engaged, and heard.

(2) Provide two-way communication

In response to COVID-19, a dedicated institutional resource email box was created, which allowed employees to ask COVID-19-related questions. The questions were answered by experts or, in some cases, by a medical center senior leader during a weekly audio briefing that included 15 min of curated Q&A. All employees, students, and trainees had to do was write "Question for the President" in the subject line of an email. All questions to that box were addressed by a team of content experts in infectious diseases, occupational health, quality and safety, pediatrics, and more. This activity continued several years into the pandemic, demonstrating an appreciation for ongoing communication.

If we look back on the early weeks of the pandemic, twice-daily emails were also sent to the entire campus as a means of sharing evolving information and details on our campus response. In addition to those campus-wide messages, hyper-targeted and specific communications were developed and distributed to care teams, so they could track changes in safety protocols, take required training, be informed on supply chain issues, and hear about other operational updates. We created a library of tip sheets housed on our employee health system portal for easy access by staff and faculty. We frequently directed them to our web pages, where new videos and tip sheets were also being added. We wanted everyone to know that we were aware of their questions and that we were doing our best to address them quickly and accurately, so no one was left guessing what to do next. Again, all this echoes that key statement: *The health and safety of our community, including our workforce, remain our top priority.* That messaging was amplified on our social media channels, along with occasional myth-busting content (Fig. 2).

(3) Promote clarity over complexity

As previously mentioned, when developing communications, there's great value in getting back to the basics of the "5W's" —who, what, when, where, and why. When messaging patients, we kept our messages concise and frequently directed them to the latest FAQs on our website, where facts

TABLE 1

Factors that Affect Acceptance of Public Health and Medical Messaging and Examples of a Multifaceted Approach to a Communication Strategy

Factor	Description	Communication Strategies	Example(s)
Environmental circumstances	Populations at risk because of environmental factors such as gender, immune status, underlying medical conditions, and access to healthcare	• Websites, dashboards • Targeted tip sheets, FAQs (in written and video format), and protocol guidance for healthcare personnel, patients, and the public. • Patient-centric messages with pertinent updates sent via a secure, online health management portal. • Targeted informational emails.	• See Figs. 1, 3 • https://www.cdc.gov/coronavirus/2019-ncov/communication/print-resources.html • https://www.utsouthwestern.edu/covid-19/ • https://covid-harriscounty.hub.arcgis.com/ • https://www.dallascounty.org/covid-19/need-to-know-cdc.php • https://www.utsouthwestern.edu/covid-19/about-virus-and-testing/faqs-espanol.html • https://es.parklandhealthplan.com/viviendo-bien/blog/articulos/preguntas-frecuentes-sobre-la-vacuna-covid-19/?_gl=1*edjldh*_ga*MTg4NzYzNjk1OC4xNjgwMTI3NTUw*_ga_Z5GFN7R08T*MTY4MDEyNzU0OS4xLjEuMTY4MDEyNzU3Mi4wLjAuMA. • https://www.utsouthwestern.edu/covid-19/employees/ • https://www.utsouthwestern.edu/covid-19/messages/archive/2020june22.html • https://www.dallascounty.org/covid-19/ • https://www.dallascounty.org/departments/dchhs/2019-novel-coronavirus.php • https://covid19.who.int • https://coronavirus.jhu.edu/map.html
Social and cultural	Group differences such as generational differences, religious beliefs, health literacy, education	• Virtual employee town hall meetings with live Q&A session. • Press conferences with multilingual experts. • Weekly and bi-weekly leadership briefings via podcast, Zoom, and/or meeting platforms. • Two-way communication strategies.	• https://www.utsouthwestern.edu/covid-19/messages/ • What to Know Bi-weekly video • email box: COVID-19Questions@utsouthwestern.edu • Link to press conference • https://www.mavs.com/mavericks-utsw-vaccine-initiative/ • https://www.dallascounty.org/departments/dchhs/2019-novel-coronavirus/schools-universities.php • https://www.youtube.com/watch?v=T98laYk2Dzw • https://www.who.int/campaigns/vaccine-equity
Language preferences	Appropriate language and translation of information are important; culturally and educationally sensitive	• Targeted and subject specific webpages updated frequently in multiple languages (e.g., English and Spanish)	• https://www.youtube.com/watch?v=KSf2OzfFaLc • https://www.utsouthwestern.edu/covid-19/about-virus-and-testing/faqs-espanol.html • https://www.michigan.gov/coronavirus/-/media/Project/Websites/coronavirus/Vaccine-Page/Vaccine-Hesitancy-Toolkit.pdf?rev=d1c9bdb3f5fa47068a604a973afbfdf7
Knowledge, attitudes, and beliefs about recommended public health or medical interventions	Increase the understanding of recommended mitigation strategies, including vaccination and medical therapies	• Visuals to make finding information easy: A yellow emergency banner across the top of all web pages, which took you to pertinent updates in a single click. • Expert-driven video interview series and blog posts.	• Link to information on vaccine hesitancy • https://www.cdc.gov/vaccines/covid-19/vaccinate-with-confidence.html • https://www.youtube.com/watch?v=JftNMuKodLQ • https://emergency.cdc.gov/han/index.asp • https://emergency.cdc.gov/coca/

Adapted from Vaughan E, Tinker T. Effective health risk communication about pandemic influenza for vulnerable populations. *Am J Public Health*. 2009 Oct;99 (Suppl 2):S324–32. https://doi.org/10.2105/AJPH.2009.162537. PMID: 19797744; PMCID: PMC4504362.

and figures were clearly presented and regularly reviewed and updated by our research and clinical faculty. Video messages were also linked that explored certain subjects in greater detail, like the safety of schools and holiday travel during COVID-19. We remained focused on developing such communications in multiple languages. Additionally, bilingual pamphlets and brochures on the value of vaccination were produced and distributed throughout the community.

(4) Establish trust through transparency
Our organization was extremely transparent about important pieces of information, including the daily COVID-19 hospital census and the impact of the community spread of the virus on our workforce. Figs. 1 and 3 provide examples of sharing detailed internal information to help establish trust through transparency. We also summarized regional data and developed a weekly slide deck that provided information about the impact on the community, including the number of cases, hospitalizations, and ICU admissions in North Texas, and the trajectory of the pandemic.

(5) Demonstrate empathy and compassion
It is very easy for messaging to fall on deaf ears. While leadership is essential for building trust during a crisis, people appreciate sincerity, humility, and gratitude, too. Community members want assurance that you have their best interests. Employees want to feel recognized and appreciated for their extra work. In general, the theme is "we're in this together." Here is just one example of effective communication during a surge of COVID-19 in 2020 from the top executive of an academic medical center. This is a portion of an audio briefing (https://www.utsouthwestern.edu/about-us/office-of-the-president/messages/assets/podolsky-briefing-23dec2020-transcript.pdf): "I've come to realize in the 12-plus years I've been President that year after year, there's exceptional work and commitment that goes out on the campus. And so, in that sense, there's nothing exceptional about being exceptional this year, except this was extraordinary. And extraordinary how you all have learned to adapt, to find the resilience, to carry on the work of the university—whether that's caring for our patients, continuing to see their students and other learners get the training and the foundations they need to be the caregivers of tomorrow—and, of course ... impactful research, much of it this year focused on the problem at hand, COVID-19. But in parallel with that, really important discoveries across the many areas of unmet medical need. And I'm enormously proud of that, and I'm incredibly grateful."[14]

CONCLUSION: *BE A SOURCE OF GUIDING LIGHT*

Within journalism circles, there's a certain, tongue-in-cheek way to refer to someone who leaves the field for a communications or public relations job. That person is gently mocked for "going over to the dark side." But what we've both learned is that when it comes to communicating with an audience, there's more similarity than difference between the two fields. In a time of crisis, all communication should be useful, timely, relevant, factual, and sometimes inspirational. That holds whether it's a news story, a video, a press release, a social media post, or an email from the Chief Executive Officer.

When that moment presents itself, remember that your community craves reliable information, reassurance, and connection. You are experts in medicine, science, health, and healing. When you join forces with your communications colleagues, you have the aptitude to promote what you're doing to keep your community safe. Consider it a privilege and seize it.

REFERENCES

1. Vaughan E, Tinker T. Effective health risk communication about pandemic influenza for vulnerable populations. *Am J Public Health.* 2009;99(Suppl 2):S324–S332. https://doi.org/10.2105/AJPH.2009.162537.
2. Ratanjee V, Foy D. What Healthcare Workers Need from Leaders in COVID-19 Crisis. Gallup at Work: Gallup; 2020.
3. Bernardin A, Martinez AJ, Perez-Acle T. On the effectiveness of communication strategies as non-pharmaceutical interventions to tackle epidemics. *PloS One.* 2021;16(10), e0257995. https://doi.org/10.1371/journal.pone.0257995.
4. Ransom A, LaGrant B, Spiteri A, Kushnir T, Anderson AK, De Rosa E. Face-to-face learning enhances the social transmission of information. *PloS One.* 2022;17(2), e0264250. https://doi.org/10.1371/journal.pone.0264250.
5. Alsan M, Stanford FC, Banerjee A, et al. Comparison of knowledge and information-seeking behavior after general COVID-19 public health messages and messages tailored for black and Latinx communities : a randomized controlled trial. *Ann Intern Med.* 2021;174(4):484–492. https://doi.org/10.7326/M20-6141.

6. Fernandez A. In: Chang A, Brown A, Burnett E, eds. *Drastic Drop in Life Expectancy Is Far Steeper for Black and Latino Populations.* National Public Radio; 2021. NPR.
7. Riley AR, Chen YH, Matthay EC, et al. Excess mortality among Latino people in California during the COVID-19 pandemic. *SSM Popul Health.* 2021;15, 100860. https://doi.org/10.1016/j.ssmph.2021.100860.
8. Shearer. More than Eight-in Ten Americans Get News from Digital Devices. Pew Research Center; 2021.
9. Vosoughi S, Roy D, Aral S. The spread of true and false news online. *Science.* 2018;359(6380):1146–1151. https://doi.org/10.1126/science.aap9559.
10. Sakya SM, Scoy LJV, Garman JC, et al. The impact of COVID-19-related changes in media consumption on public knowledge: results of a cross-sectional survey of Pennsylvania adults. *Curr Med Res Opin.* 2021;37(6):911–915. https://doi.org/10.1080/03007995.2021.1901679.
11. Roozenbeek J, Schneider CR, Dryhurst S, et al. Susceptibility to misinformation about COVID-19 around the world. *R Soc Open Sci.* 2020;7(10), 201199. https://doi.org/10.1098/rsos.201199.
12. van der Linden S, Roozenbeek J, Compton J. Inoculating against fake news about COVID-19. *Front Psychol.* 2020;11, 566790. https://doi.org/10.3389/fpsyg.2020.566790.
13. Bansal P. Covid-19 - the Infodemic. *J Family Med Prim Care.* 2020;9(10):5388. https://doi.org/10.4103/jfmpc.jfmpc_1797_20.
14. https://www.utsouthwestern.edu/about-us/office-of-the-president/messages/assets/podolsky-briefing-23dec2020-transcript.pdf.

CHAPTER 28

Recovery From Biological Disasters: Bioterrorism, Outbreaks of Emerging Infectious Diseases, and Pandemics

TERRI REBMANN[a] • RACHEL CHARNEY[b]
[a]Institute for Biosecurity, College for Public Health and Social Justice, Saint Louis University • [b]School of Medicine, Saint Louis University, ST. Louis, MO, United States

Disaster recovery is a long-term process that begins soon after the onset of an event and may continue for many years, even as the agency or organization returns to day-to-day functioning. Traditional activities that occur during disaster recovery include restoration, rebuilding, and reconstruction. The length and extent of the recovery period will vary, depending upon the size and scope of the disaster and the effectiveness of the response. Better-prepared facilities and communities will be more resilient and are more likely to have a shorter recovery period.[1] According to the Federal Emergency Management Agency (FEMA), disaster recovery is led by local efforts, and all external resources obtained for recovery should be considered supplemental.[2] Therefore, recovery planning is an essential component of making an agency or organization more resilient.

Planning for recovery prior to and after an event allows an agency or organization to partner with collaborators and identify a common vision and recovery priorities, including ethical distribution of resources, sustainability, and projects that will help the community reach the shared vision, and improve resilience for future events.[1,2] Recovery planning is very different from disaster planning, and the plans have different content and formats. A study of state recovery plans found that most recovery plans consist of a description of funding sources, administrative avenues for seeking funding after an event, protocols for declaring a disaster, and procedures to set up joint field offices.[1] Most state recovery plans outlined stakeholders that need to be involved in recovery activities but did not identify how the agencies' and organizations' actions should be coordinated.[1] No studies were found that have examined agency or organization recovery plans, and little information is available on what should be included in such a plan except to indicate that agency and organization recovery planning is vital to success.[1] However, even with predisaster planning, recovery is often the longest of the four phases of any disaster: mitigation, preparedness, response, and recovery.[2] Researchers have estimated that recovery lasts 10 times longer than response to the event,[3] and that does not even factor in the long-term recovery process associated with the disaster's psychological effects.[4] Local public health departments will play a critical role in disaster recovery, and their responsibilities will include providing healthcare services to the underserved, conducting surveillance, and communicating with the public through health advisories and other mechanisms.[5]

Biological disasters, such as outbreaks of emerging infectious diseases, pandemics, and bioterrorism, pose unique challenges to the recovery process. Prior biological disasters, such as the 2014 to 2016 Ebola Virus Disease outbreak and the 2009 H1N1 pandemic, illustrated how an influx of contagious patients has a profound impact on healthcare and public health systems, even when the event involves only a single individual or a low mortality rate. Healthcare personnel (HCP) often become victims of the event, stockpiled supplies quickly become depleted, and the psychological impacts from the event can be long-lasting. Many biological disasters are not even classified as a *disaster* per se.

Viral Outbreaks, Biosecurity, and Preparing for Mass Casualty Infectious Diseases Events
https://doi.org/10.1016/B978-0-323-54841-0.00029-9

For example, FEMA's report on Lessons in Community Recovery summarized events between 2004 and 2011, but did not include even a single biological event, despite the fact that the 2009 H1N1 pandemic occurred in this time period and was declared an official public health emergency.[2] Perhaps most challenging of all: very little research—and no consensus—exists on exactly how healthcare facilities and public health organizations should recover from large-scale biological disasters.[6a]

Of note, the strategies used to respond to a biological disaster may shape behavior longer term. For example, during the COVID-19 pandemic, a significant number of U.S. citizens reported the intention of adopting long-term public face covering use. A national survey conducted in early 2021 found that 72% of Americans planned to continue wearing masks in public, 80% intended to avoid crowds, and 90% planned to continue increased hand hygiene usage after the pandemic ends.[6b] Other sociological and behavioral changes may also remain long-term. There may be a shift toward a larger segment of the population working remotely and/or students who choose remote learning or home-schooling, strategies that began as pandemic responses but may shift into a new norm.[6c] For healthcare facilities and systems, extended use and long-term use of PPE may also continue long past recovery, especially in areas where personal protective equipment (PPE) access is limited.

The U.S.'s *National Disaster Recovery Framework* identifies eight principles that guide recovery support activities and six recovery support functions.[7] However, this framework focuses heavily on repairing infrastructure and restoring healthcare and public health systems. A major gap continues to be the lack of focus and coordination of efforts to address the long-term physical and mental health consequences of disasters.[4] In addition, it is challenging to differentiate the response from the recovery period. There are often no clear indicators when one phase ends and the other begins. Furthermore, recovery efforts are often slowed by the overlapping recovery needs for multiple events at once and/or the development of new disasters.[4] For example, the long-term effects of the 2001 anthrax bioterrorism attack were still being addressed when the severe acute respiratory syndrome coronavirus (SARS-CoV) first emerged in 2003. Another example was the winter storms that occurred throughout the United States in February of 2021, resulting in significant snowfalls and large-scale electrical grid failure in Texas.[6d] These storms significantly interrupted COVID-19 vaccine delivery and distribution. Healthcare and public health will be facing new outbreaks and challenges even as they continue to manage the long-term medical issues associated with Ebola and Zika virus infections long after those outbreaks have ended.

Just as during the response period, healthcare facilities and public health agencies will need to continue to provide day-to-day services as much as possible throughout the recovery period, and this requires prior planning.[8] The recovery period should also include mitigation of future events in terms of returning physical structures and systems back to baseline, such as restocking medical supplies and pharmaceutical products used during the event, as well as building staff and supply surge capacity for future events. The recovery period itself may also include a secondary surge due to the exacerbation of chronic medical conditions as a result of medical infrastructure breakdown during disaster response.[9a] This was seen in the COVID-19 pandemic, when out-of-hospital cardiac arrest rates rose, presumably due to healthcare avoidance.[9b] These secondary surges strain medical and public health systems that are struggling to recover from the disaster and may prolong the time needed to return to routine services.[9a] It will also be more challenging to return to routine functioning during recovery from biological disasters than from natural disasters due to the unique strain to healthcare and public health posed by the event. Biological disasters disproportionately affect healthcare and public health systems, and this will make it very challenging to return to baseline functioning. For example, the development and shipment of seasonal influenza vaccines were severely delayed during the 2009 H1N1 pandemic due to the need to use vaccine production infrastructure to create a pandemic vaccine. Hospitals and healthcare facilities in West Africa struggled to respond to routine communicable diseases and provide basic healthcare services while recovering from the Ebola outbreak.[10]

It is also important to note that our understanding of how individuals, agencies, and communities recover from disaster and exactly what constitutes a *full recovery* continues to evolve.[2,11] Though researchers have postulated a definition of *life recovery* for individuals after a disaster that is based on a socioecological model (housing stability, stable economic resources, good mental and physical health, and positive social role adaptation),[11] no such definition of recovery exists for agencies or organizations. Furthermore, researchers have postulated two different approaches to measuring recovery: (1) to return to a predisaster baseline, or (2) to attain a state that would have existed if the disaster had never occurred.[2,12] This chapter will use a socioecological

TABLE 1
Checklist of Activities Hospitals Need to Perform During the Recovery Period

- Return physical plant to previous/normal configuration
- Perform thorough environmental decontamination
- Conduct environmental sampling as needed to ensure contamination has been eliminated before reopening areas or using equipment
- Manage any remaining medical waste, following applicable laws and regulations
- Determine if the hospital will invest in improving buildings' HVAC systems before the next event
- Evaluate the hospital disaster and recovery plans using lessons learned, and revise as needed
- Evaluate existing MOAs to determine if new MOAs are needed
- Evaluate existing crisis standards of care for utility and determine if new standards are needed
- Examine impact of the event on the healthcare workforce and consider investment strategies to return to baseline or improve surge capacity before the next event
- Document financial costs associated with the event and file paperwork for reimbursement
- Replace depleted stockpile supplies that were used during the event
- Evaluate stockpile purchasing priorities before future event
- Implement a PR campaign to regain or improve hospital reputation, when applicable
- Rapidly restore medical homes or deploy mobile medical clinics, as needed
- Prepare for a secondary surge that is expected during disaster recovery
- Conduct surveillance for physical and mental health negative outcomes associated with the event
- Implement interventions to decrease stigma among healthcare personnel and the community
- Address the specific needs of vulnerable populations
- Implement Crisis and Emergency Risk Communication (CERC) practices to share information with the public and employees
- Develop interventions using positive psychology for use among hospital patients and staff
- Provide preevent training to staff to prepare for future events

MOA = memorandum of agreement.
HVAC = heating, ventilation, and air conditioning.
PR = public relations.

model that is based on the construct of *life recovery* as the foundation to describe agency recovery from biological disasters to return to baseline functioning. Physical structure stability, disaster plan evaluation and revision, stable economic resources, good mental and physical health, and posttraumatic growth and/or positive social role adaptation will all be described from the perspective of healthcare and public health systems affected by a biological disaster. Agencies and organizations will have a large number of goals in place to achieve recovery. It will be important for stakeholders to prioritize which goals most define recovery and align staff and efforts to achieving these goals foremost.[13] A list of activities hospitals need to perform during recovery from biological events is outlined in Table 1.

PHYSICAL STRUCTURE RECOVERY

The first step in disaster recovery is to assess the damages that occurred during the event so that restoration can begin. Recovery from natural disasters primarily deals with infrastructure recovery, such as the need to rebuild the Joplin Mercy Hospital after it was hit by an EF5 tornado in 2011.[14] Recovery from a biological disaster is inherently different due to the nature of the event. Biological disasters generally do not harm the physical structure of a hospital or healthcare facility. During the recovery period, healthcare facilities should be able to return the physical plant to its previous/normal configuration if it had been altered to respond to the event. For example, during disaster response, some facilities will need to convert large open areas to temporary negative pressure rooms to accommodate an influx of patients infected with an airborne spread disease, such as during a smallpox bioterrorism attack or an outbreak of Middle East Respiratory Syndrome Coronavirus (MERS CoV).[15] Creating these temporary negative pressure rooms or areas may involve the erection of makeshift walls or barriers that will need to be disassembled and the area disinfected during the recovery period when returning the space to its predisaster state.[16]

An important intervention during disaster recovery to restore physical infrastructure is to replace any depleted stockpile supplies that were used during the event. Research indicates that many hospitals, healthcare systems, and regions are developing stockpiles of supplies, equipment, and medication.[17–19] The intent of these stockpiles is to meet surge capacity needs during a disaster to enable a maximized localized response. It is critical that used/removed supplies be replaced as soon as feasible after disaster response to ensure that the stockpile is ready to be deployed for the next event.[20] The supplies most likely to be used during a biological disaster include personal protective equipment (PPE), isolation-related supplies, vaccines, and antiinfective therapy, such as antivirals or antibiotics.[17,20] In addition to replacing used supplies and medication or vaccines, it is important for healthcare facilities and regional disaster planning agencies to reevaluate their stockpile purchasing and maintenance processes during disaster recovery.[21] It is useful during disaster recovery to examine the amount and types of supplies and medication that were used during the event as well as the effectiveness of the deployment. This can help inform the agency about more cost-effective purchasing and stockpile management practices that will improve the cache before the next event.[21] For example, disaster planners should evaluate the cost-effectiveness and feasibility of using alternative approaches to stockpiling materials and medications, such as implementing a vendor-managed inventory (VMI) system.[22] VMI systems involve having the vendor store, rotate, and replace supplies and medication, which eliminates hospitals' costs associated with storing and managing the stockpile.[22] An outline of procedures for evaluating a hospital stockpile for biological disasters is provided in Table 2.

REMEDIATION ISSUES DURING DISASTER RECOVERY

A major component of recovery from natural disasters involves debris removal and management.[23] Debris removal or management is generally not an issue for biological disasters, except as it pertains to handling biological waste. Medical waste management is anticipated to be a major challenge during recovery from biological disasters, and appropriate procedures are critical for hospitals because improperly managed infectious waste can lead to occupational exposure and illness.[24] The risk posed by medical and infectious waste is particularly high for events involving bioterrorism or an outbreak of an emerging infectious disease, because these events are likely to involve an agent that produces category A infectious waste, such as plague or Ebola, and few facilities are willing to accept such waste due to its risk of life-threatening illness or death after exposure.[24–26] Though most medical and infectious waste is expected to be generated during disaster response, managing the waste is likely to extend into the recovery period due to time needed to transport the waste to another facility. For example, the Ebola patient seen in a Dallas, Texas hospital during the 2014 Ebola crisis died almost 2 weeks before the medical waste generated from his care was transported to another facility for management.[27] Waste management will likely extend into the recovery period even if the healthcare facility chooses to purchase an autoclave sufficient to manage category A substances due to the time needed to install and validate/test the new equipment.[28] Having sufficient waste management plans in place prior to

TABLE 2
Evaluating a Hospital's Stockpiling Practices and Purchases for Biological Disasters During Disaster Recovery

- Determine the amount of deployable materials, medications, and vaccines remaining in the stockpile
- Evaluate whether investment is needed in stockpile management infrastructure
- Calculate how much and which types of materials and medications or vaccines were removed from the stockpile or obtained from vendors and MOAs
- Determine purchasing priorities to replenish the stockpile
- Evaluate stockpile deployment performance that occurred during the event and determine if improvement is needed
- Determine if the stockpile location is working or if it needs to be relocated
- Calculate the cost-effectiveness and feasibility of using alternative approaches to stockpiling materials and medications
- Determine if a VMI system may be a more cost-effective approach to stockpiling

MOA = memorandum of agreement.
VMI = vendor-managed inventory.

an event, such as developing a memorandum of agreement with a facility willing to accept this type of waste, can greatly reduce costs during the recovery period.[23]

Remediation in the form of environmental sampling, cleaning, and decontamination may be a substantial component of disaster recovery, depending on the size and scope of the event and the infectious agent involved.[5,8,29] Bioterrorism attacks are the biological disaster most likely to result in the need for extensive environmental remediation, though the type and amount of remediation needed will vary. The 2001 Amerithrax bioterrorism attack, which involved the mailing of letters containing anthrax to various political and media outlets, resulted in extensive contamination of postal facilities that processed the letters. Decontaminating these facilities and its associated equipment and conducting environmental sampling to ensure safety lasted long into the recovery phase of the attack and resulted in costs estimated at $320 million.[29] Remediation following other bioterrorism attacks could involve very different procedures, depending on how the agent was released, the agent involved, and the size of the event. Mathematical modeling examining various approaches to an indoor release of anthrax spores estimates that the use of HEPA air cleaners and vacuums could reduce remediation time and avoid the need to permanently close down the affected space, though this process would still require 6–12 months of the recovery period and is not recommended for hospitals, long-term care facilities, or buildings housing other high-risk or critical individuals.[30] Substantially more aggressive remediation would be required for hospitals, daycares, and long-term care facilities due to the preponderance of vulnerable patients in these settings.[30]

Remediation of outdoor spaces following a bioterrorism attack poses the largest potential challenge during disaster recovery.[31] If anthrax or another biological agent is released in aerosol form and results in the contamination of the outside of buildings or the environment, it would be very expensive and time-consuming to effectively remediate the event. The biggest challenge is the lack of evidence-based approaches to addressing this type of scenario. Historically, a large-scale release of anthrax has only happened twice: on Gruinard Island when anthrax spores were released as part of offensive weapons testing, and in Sverdlovsk in the former Soviet Union when anthrax was accidentally released from a military facility. Decontamination of Gruinard Island involved removing the top layer of soil and then spraying sporicidal chemical solutions over the island.[32] Information on the remediation following the release of anthrax in Sverdlovsk is limited but included environmental sampling and decontaminating of victims' homes, washing/spraying of trees, and paving roads as a minimum.[33]

If the biological disaster involves a bioterrorism attack consisting of an aerosolized release of an infectious agent, it will be critical to have effective heating, ventilation, and air conditioning (HVAC) systems to remove the agent from the air and reduce the risk of aerosol inhalation.[34] Improving buildings' HVAC systems not only mitigates the risk from bioterrorism attacks but also reduces respiratory diseases and improves worker performance during routine times.[34] In addition to removing pathogens from the air following a bioterrorism attack involving an aerosol release in order to reduce the risk of inhalation, extensive environmental decontamination of surfaces will be required to remove the risk of infection due to direct contact with the agent. This is because infectious particles settle on the physical environment, such as furniture, floors, and other work surfaces, after falling out of suspension.[34] Removal of the agent from the air will most likely occur during disaster response, but the longer-term remediation needed for decontaminating the indoor environment due to the aerosol release will extend long into the recovery period.

Deciding on the exact remediation procedures needed for any particular biological disaster is complex due to the lack of knowledge and research surrounding this area.[31] If a hospital becomes the site of a bioterrorism attack, hospital administrators should partner with public health officials and federal investigators to determine the best approach to decontaminating their facility. It is essential that any potential threat from environmental contamination be mitigated or eliminated before reopening that portion of the facility for business. Likewise, if public areas become contaminated during a bioterrorism attack, public health officials should partner with federal investigators to determine the best approach to decontaminating the area and ensure that the environmental threat is minimized or eliminated before allowing the general public into that space. Environmental testing, consisting of surface swabs and air sampling, will likely be needed throughout the recovery period until there is strong evidence that environmental decontamination has been effective and the risk of infection is eliminated.[35] The time and resources needed to remediate an area, building, or space are expected to extend into the recovery period during biological events and could pose one of the most challenging aspects of recovery.[31] Additionally, it is recommended that these remediation steps be very visible to the public to provide reassurance that care is being taken to ensure public safety.[36]

DISASTER AND RECOVERY PLAN EVALUATION AND REVISION

It is critical that healthcare facilities and public health agencies assess the effectiveness of their disaster and recovery plans before, during, and after an event. Postevent plan evaluation occurs during the recovery period. It is at this time that facilities and agencies need to examine which components of their disaster plan worked well during the event and which need improvement before another disaster occurs. In addition, it is critical that agencies and organizations examine their disaster recovery plans after an event and revise the plan as needed.[1]

Mutual aid agreements, such as memoranda of agreement (MOA), that were in place prior to the event need to be evaluated during recovery for utility and feasibility for future disasters. In doing so, it is important to evaluate the utility of both MOAs that were deployed and those that were not honored. Some MOAs may need to be revised to adequately reflect facility surge capacity needs. Particular attention needs to be paid to MOAs that were not honored during the event. If the MOA was not honored due to a lack of available resources, it may be reasonable to keep that MOA. However, MOAs that were not honored due to an unwillingness of partners to uphold the MOA may need to be revoked.[17] The unwillingness of partners to uphold MOAs was a common occurrence during the 2009 H1N1 pandemic, leading to a lack of personal protective equipment (PPE), antiviral medication, and other critical supplies when facilities and vendors refused to share resources as outlined in the MOA.[17] Having unusable MOAs in place may provide the hospital with a false sense of preparedness and could contribute to disease spread during a biological disaster.

In addition to examining the utility of MOAs, hospital disaster planners should review their facility's crisis standards of care (CSC) during the recovery period. CSCs are developed for use during disaster response when supplies and medications are limited or depleted and ethical decisions need to be made about how to allocate available resources.[37] During biological disasters, hand hygiene products, negative pressure rooms/areas, PPE, ventilators, vaccines, and antimicrobial therapy are all resources that are likely to be limited or unavailable due to an influx of contagious patients.[38–42] Many of these patients may require long-term ventilator care, and this could extend into the recovery period, meaning that supply shortages may not end after the response period is over; in addition, a secondary surge is expected during disaster recovery, and this may involve continued use of CSCs.[9a] Although many institutions are developing CSCs, the utility and effective implementation of these protocols need to be evaluated during disaster recovery. CSCs may need to be revised to better reflect the ethical framework on which they were written or to be more in line with the community's priorities before the next biological disaster occurs.[38]

Hospitals and healthcare facilities may find it very challenging to recover from a biological disaster if their workforce is negatively affected by the event. HCPs are often disproportionately at risk during a bioterrorism attack, pandemic, or outbreak of an emerging infectious pathogen if the disease is contagious. This puts a tremendous strain on healthcare systems during disaster response, when HCP may not be able to work due to illness. Limited HCP availability may extend into the recovery period if the biological disaster resulted in a high mortality rate. For example, healthcare systems in West Africa were even more understaffed than normal following the Ebola crisis of 2014 to 2016 due to the very high number of HCP deaths that occurred during the outbreak; more than 800 HCP died in West Africa during the outbreak.[10,43a] HCP were also disproportionately affected during the SARS-CoV outbreak in Canada and East Asia.[44a] Due to the close contact between HCP and patients during care delivery, it is expected that HCP will always be one of the highest risk groups during any future biological disaster that involves a contagious disease. This adds strain on healthcare and public health systems while recovering from these events. It also means that it could take years for a community to rebuild its HCP infrastructure after a biological disaster if a large number of personnel died during the event.[43a] Beyond death, a prolonged disaster may also drive HCP to other careers. In one survey conducted in January 2021, 26% of United States based HCPs were considering leaving their job, with 14% stating that they might leave the profession entirely.[44b,c]

ECONOMIC RECOVERY

Economic recovery of hospitals, healthcare systems, and public health are essential to the recovery of the community. Therefore, it is critical that communities resume usual healthcare and public health processes as soon as possible. Economic recovery from a biologic disaster varies from a physical disaster, as there are typically fewer structural concerns after an infectious disease event. While some structural modifications may have been made to the building to accommodate an influx of contagious patients, the main structure of the building most likely will remain intact. An exception to this might be in the case of significant societal distress, where the public may have caused physical damage. Alternatively, structures may need long-term modification to prepare for the next biological disaster, such as HVAC alterations made to decrease COVID-19 spread.[44d] Beyond the physical building and systems, however, biologic disasters open a hospital up to significant economic recovery needs. Reimbursement is often a time-consuming and difficult process, with the potential for prolonged waits as insurance and governmental entities struggle with limited staffing to process claims.[45] Preplanning that includes appropriate documentation and tracking to ensure that claims will be paid is essential to hospital recovery. Additionally, reimbursements may be hindered if local jobs are lost as a result of the disaster, causing a subsequent loss of health insurance.[45]

During a biologic event, staffing is likely to be of concern in both the immediate and long-term recovery. Staffing is likely to be diminished after the event as HCP recovers from the same or higher levels of morbidity and mortality as the public. Patients are likely to continue to present in increased volumes during the recovery period if outpatient practices have been disrupted by the illness, and hospitals are essential to regaining the baseline health of the population. The duration, mortality rate, and scope of the biologic event all impact the ability to retain and regain HCP during disaster recovery. Long term, there may be a diminished availability of HCP due to disruption of schools, resulting in lower levels of graduating HCP. Creative staffing solutions may be needed to bridge that gap.

During the recovery period, hospitals will need to restock supplies, a costly and time-consuming process that may be prolonged if other hospitals are seeking the same supplies or if the supplying companies were negatively affected by the biologic outbreak.[21] Obtaining supplies from a variety of sources with differing geographic locations can be useful in this instance. It is also important to check if multiple local healthcare organizations are planning to use the same suppliers, as it is not infrequent for a supplying corporation to make MOUs with all of them without the ability to meet all of the needs should they come up at once.[17]

Some biological disasters can bring publicity to the responding hospital, and this can have major negative financial implications. If the hospital is the care site for one or more of the victims of the biological event, the hospital may suffer stigma from the contagion and lose significant desirability to the public. For example, Texas Health Presbyterian Hospital in Dallas, Texas became known as the "Ebola Hospital" while treating Thomas Duncan, an Ebola-infected patient.[46] The hospital was then shunned by local citizens, costing the hospital over $20 million in just the 2 months following admission of Mr. Duncan, though the hospital recovered financially within a few months.[46]

Funding for disaster recovery is covered under the Stafford Act, consisting of the Public Assistance Program (PA) and the Individual Assistance Program (IA).[8] The IA program only covers individuals. The PA program can provide funding for hospital disaster recovery, assuming the event is declared a disaster at the federal level.[47] FEMA recommends that hospitals and healthcare systems have a written plan in place for seeking reimbursement, as such a plan may result in more comprehensive reimbursement for the facility/agency.[47] The PA program funds physical labor as well as some staffing costs, these are defined as reasonable costs tied to the performance of eligible work. FEMA outlines the full formal process for obtaining reimbursement through the PA program.[48] Yale New Haven Health developed an abbreviated checklist describing the PA program and processes for obtaining reimbursement during disaster recovery[47]; disaster managers might consider following this guide to ease the reimbursement process. In addition to the PA program, there is specific pandemic coverage covered under the Stafford Act, which can include reimbursement for medical care, temporary healthcare facilities, supplies, and public health risk reduction.[49] It is important to note that only public and nonprofit hospitals qualify for FEMA disaster recovery funding. For-profit hospitals may seek low-interest loans via the U.S. Small Business Administration to help cover disaster costs.[50] Additionally, FEMA funding is only to be used after insurance and other funding options have been utilized to their fullest extent.

Documentation is critical during the recovery process.[8,43a] Poor documentation during response to the event can also have a negative impact on recovery from the disaster. This documentation pertains to patient care, supplies used during the event, structural costs associated with the disaster, and staffing costs.[51] A lack of documentation can affect reimbursement and follow-up for survivors.[43a] Legal counsel should be involved in the planning of disaster recovery funding, as the reimbursement systems may vary by state and over time, and be administered by a variety of agencies; details of this are beyond the scope of this chapter.[52]

RESTORATION OR MAXIMIZATION OF PHYSICAL AND MENTAL HEALTH

Disaster planners, HCPs, and public health professionals have invested a great deal of time and money in developing plans to restore the physical infrastructure of communities and respond to the immediate health impacts after a disaster. For example, many HCPs and public health professionals willingly volunteer to assist in disaster response. However, historically significantly less planning and resources have been focused on aiding individuals and communities during disaster recovery, such as addressing the long-term physical and mental health challenges that arise following disasters.[4,5] This is even truer when examining the impact of biological disasters, because experts are continuously learning more about the long-term effects of these events. Despite this, physical restoration of a community is usually completed months or years before the physical and mental health impacts from the event have ended.[4] Much more investment needs to be made in addressing the psychological impact from biological disasters as well as the long-term physical consequences of these events. This shift appears to be underway as the *National Disaster Recovery Framework* now lists psychological and emotional restoration as a core element of disaster recovery.[7]

Researchers have asserted that one solution to returning postdisaster communities to their baseline is to rapidly restore medical homes.[6a] The medical home model is a multidisciplinary patient-centered approach to healthcare that increases access to care, ensures continuity of care, and manages communication between the patient and HCP. The primary aim is to better coordinate care while increasing quality and decreasing costs. Though there is conflicting research on the cost-savings associated with the use of medical homes, there is strong evidence that this model is effective for underserved children.[6a] Coordinated care is important during routine times, but even more critical during disasters when healthcare and public health services may be disrupted. For example, outpatient clinics may be over capacity or closed down during recovery from a biological disaster due to a secondary surge or loss of HCP who are ill or died from the event. Mobile clinics using a medical home model were found to be effective in past disasters, though they have only been implemented during natural disasters.[6a] The utility of medical homes during a biological disaster has thus far been untested, though theoretically it could help coordinate care as communities are transitioning from alternate care sites used during disaster response back to traditional healthcare systems during recovery.

Some diseases that could be involved in a bioterrorism attack or outbreak of an emerging infectious pathogen can have long-term medical effects. For example, the Ebola virus has been detected in the semen of previously infected men up to 18 months after recovery from infection.[53] In addition, survivors of Ebola may experience arthralgia, myalgia, vision problems, hearing loss, psychological issues, and confusion for up to a year after recovering from the disease.[43a,54,55] In addition, Ebola survivors who experience long-term chronic pain due to arthralgia and myalgia are more likely to report depression.[54] Other diseases that could be associated with a biological disaster can also result in long-term medical sequelae, such as the very extensive scarring that is common after smallpox infection.[56]

Surveillance will be an essential function of healthcare facilities and local public health departments during recovery from a biological disaster.[5] Disease surveillance includes the collection and analysis of health-related data to identify individual cases of illness, clusters of infection, or potential outbreaks.[57] One of the most critical types of surveillance needed will be to continue to monitor for a return of the disease involved in the biological disaster, as it is possible for there to be a break in cases that makes it appear that the outbreak is over when it is really only a serial interval between cases or clusters instead. It will also be critical for local public health to conduct surveillance for routine communicable conditions during the recovery period when community members are at increased risk from these diseases. This increased risk of illness is due to the shifting of priorities that occurs during disaster response. When resources are focused on responding to the disaster, routine practices are often delayed or eliminated.[10] For example, mobilizing healthcare and public health to distribute mass medical countermeasures during a bioterrorism attack may mean that routine immunization or communicable disease surveillance is not performed or is greatly delayed. This can leave the community at risk from routine vaccine preventable diseases, tuberculosis, or other communicable disease risks long after the disaster response ends while the healthcare and public health systems are recovering from the event. For example, during the 2014 Ebola crisis, uptake of the measles vaccine dropped from 71% to 55% due to a lack of workers available to provide immunization; this resulted in increased numbers of measles cases throughout Liberia, Sierra Leone, and Guinea while these countries were recovering from the Ebola outbreak.[10] In addition to surveillance for the disease involved in the disaster and the monitoring of routine communicable diseases, it is essential that public health departments conduct surveillance to rapidly identify a potential new outbreak during the recovery period. This surveillance is most likely to consist of syndromic surveillance, the collection and analysis of prediagnostic health criteria to identify a bioterrorism attack or outbreak of an emerging infectious disease.[58]

In addition to physical impacts, disasters are likely to result in long-term negative psychological effects. Researchers have found that the most common mental health problems associated with disasters include posttraumatic stress disorder (PTSD), depression, and anxiety,[59–61] and that those with low income, those who have health disparities, and/or disaster recovery workers are significantly more likely to suffer from negative psychological effects.[60,61] Psychological issues associated with biological disasters have been found to be similar. As mentioned previously, depression is common among Ebola survivors, especially those who experience long-term chronic pain.[54] Depression, anxiety, and PTSD were expected to occur even among those who were never infected with Ebola but who had provided care to an Ebola-infected friend or family member.[62] HCPs who provided care to Ebola-infected patients did not report higher levels of anxiety, depression, or fatigue compared to HCPs who did not treat infected patients, but those who had direct contact with Ebola patients reported significantly more social isolation and the need to work shorter shifts.[63] Negative psychological effects are expected for biological disasters involving other diseases, too. For example, increased psychological distress was identified 8 months after the 2001 anthrax bioterrorism attack among those who were not involved in the attack in any way (i.e., not exposed to or infected with anthrax).[64] In another example, the extensive scarring among smallpox survivors was often associated with extreme stigma and psychological distress; if a smallpox bioterrorism attack were to occur, the psychological impact due to the terrorism event and the subsequent medical sequela could be profound.[56]

A common negative psychological effect from biological disasters is stigma. Stigma is caused by fear surrounding severe outbreaks and can be related to the necessary public health control measures implemented during the event to prevent disease spread, such as isolation, quarantine, or participating in environmental decontamination after an event.[46,65] Stigma most often affects those who are infected, but can even occur among the exposed or those perceived as being exposed during a biological disaster. For example, HCPs who provided care to SARS-CoV patients in Canada reported feeling stigmatized by their neighbors.[66] Even HCPs who had not actually provided care to SARS-infected patients but were known by their neighbors as being HCPs reported feeling stigmatized and rejected.[66] Many HCP also feared becoming infected, and 15% of those in one study reported not going home after work as a way of preventing exposure to their family members.[66] Members of the sanitation crew who cleaned up the apartment of the first U.S. Ebola case in 2014 reported being stigmatized by friends and neighbors.[46] The sanitation crew also indicated that their children were stigmatized simply by being related to someone who had been involved in cleaning the apartment of the Ebola patient; they mentioned that their children faced stigma at school and in their extracurricular teams.[46]

During past biological disasters, individuals placed on quarantine have reported feeling stigmatized, even long after the quarantine has ended. This stigma can last into the recovery period and could have negative impacts on interpersonal relationships.[67] Stigma not only harms interpersonal relationships, but may also lead to increased disease spread, most notably when fear of being stigmatized leads infected individuals to avoid medical treatment.[65]

Though almost everyone can be at risk during a disaster, certain groups of individuals are considered vulnerable populations (i.e., at higher risk than others). Vulnerable groups are more likely to be affected by disasters and to have long-term physical and mental health consequences due to the event.[4,9a] Vulnerable groups are not only at higher risk of morbidity and mortality during disaster response, but remain at higher risk throughout the recovery period when medical and public health systems struggle to address secondary surge capacity needs while attempting to return to routine functioning.[9a] This is especially true for biological disasters. Although the epidemiology—and thus high-risk groups—varies by the disease involved in the outbreak, some groups of individuals are almost always vulnerable populations during biological disasters. Very young children (especially newborns and those born prematurely), the elderly, those who are immunocompromised or have comorbidities, and pregnant women are examples of common vulnerable populations during biological disasters.[68] In addition, socioeconomic factors, such as income, access to healthcare or insurance, homelessness, and illiteracy, can affect the risk of becoming infected or the severity of illness/length of recovery during biological disasters.[9a]

Pregnant women and newborns, both high-risk groups during routine times, are disproportionately negatively affected during many disasters, especially if the woman is a minority or has low income.[60] Pregnant women and newborns are affected even more negatively when the disaster involves an infectious disease. For example, pregnant women are at significantly higher risk of illness and death during an influenza pandemic or SARS-CoV outbreak compared to nonpregnant women.[69,70] During the 1918 influenza epidemic, pregnant women had a mortality rate between 30% and 50%, while the mortality rate for nonpregnant individuals was closer to 5%.[69] Pregnant women also had higher rates of hospitalization and longer hospital stays compared to nonpregnant individuals during past influenza pandemics[69] and during outbreaks of avian influenza.[71]

Newborns are also at high risk of complications from infection and death during biological disasters, and these issues can extend into the recovery period. For example, newborns infected with seasonal and pandemic influenza are more likely to require ventilator support and for longer periods of time compared to older children and adults.[72] Some negative outcomes associated with infection during biological disasters have profound long-term effects on the child's life, such as developing microcephaly after exposure to the Zika virus before birth.[70] Babies born to mothers infected with influenza during the 1918 Spanish Flu pandemic were found to have significant negative health impacts many years later; as adults, these individuals were more likely to have hypertension, heart or renal disease, and cancer.[73] Exposure to Ebola is even more severe; only one infant born from an Ebola-infected mother has survived longer than 3 weeks.[70,74]

Elderly individuals are also disproportionately affected during biological disasters and may have extended recovery periods and higher mortality rates compared to younger individuals. For example, the mortality rate for SARS was about 10% overall but was close to 50% among the elderly.[75] During influenza pandemics, those over the age of 60 are likely to be at higher risk for needing ventilator support and for longer periods of time compared to younger individuals.[72] Even the use of a vaccine can increase the risk of long-term negative outcomes among the elderly, depending on the event. For example, use of the smallpox vaccine has been found to be associated with myocarditis and pericarditis among those who have underlying cardiac issues, most of whom are elderly, and treating such infections would extend into disaster recovery.[76]

As mentioned previously, HCP are expected to be one of the highest risk groups during any biological disaster that involves a contagious disease. This impacts not only the healthcare system and healthcare surge capacity, but also the physical and psychological health of the HCP themselves. Research indicates that disaster recovery workers, including HCP, are at increased risk for PTSD, depression, and anxiety after some disasters.[59] In addition, HCP are at risk of developing empathy exhaustion, burnout, and acute stress disorder, especially if the HCP are placed on quarantine.[66,77] Negative psychological outcomes among HCP are expected to be higher when the biological disaster is man-made (i.e., a bioterrorism event), though there is limited research in this area.[77]

During any type of disaster, individuals with low income or other health disparities are disproportionately at risk from morbidity and mortality due to a lack of access to insurance and/or health care services.[9a] Individuals with health disparities often have chronic medical conditions that can put them at higher risk of complications from infectious diseases, and this can be exacerbated during recovery from biological disasters.[9a] For example, diabetic individuals are more likely to experience severe complications of influenza during pandemics[78,79] and those with a low income are more likely to be diabetic or have uncontrolled diabetes. In addition, those with health disparities may be unable to obtain routine care during disaster recovery due to the secondary healthcare surge that occurs, and this may exacerbate their condition.[9a]

To address the unique needs of vulnerable populations during disaster recovery, it is critical to factor them into preevent disaster and recovery planning.[9a,60] It is also critical that healthcare and public health assist in developing programs that build resilience during disaster recovery, especially among the most vulnerable groups.[60] Building resilience and preventing illness is more effective than trying to mitigate the long-term negative outcomes associated with infection among these high-risk groups. Important interventions include prioritizing these groups for immunization, vaccinating those around the vulnerable individual in an attempt to limit exposure, prioritizing them for prophylaxis and treatment, rapidly identifying and treating illness when it occurs, providing psychological first aid soon after the event occurs, and using population-based interventions.[70,77] It is also critical for healthcare and public health systems to plan for the anticipated secondary surge that occurs during disaster recovery; planning for this secondary surge may enhance the community's resilience and improve healthcare delivery.[9a] A more comprehensive plan is needed to address psychological resilience among HCPs and the general public.[4] Public health, healthcare, and disaster planners need to work together to develop effective strategies and communications that limit fear and stigmatization during biological disasters.

COMMUNICATION NEEDS DURING RECOVERY

As mentioned earlier, some biological disasters can bring publicity to the responding hospital, and this can negatively affect the hospital's reputation if the facility becomes known as the "Ebola hospital" or "smallpox hospital." In these situations, robust risk communication can make the difference between success and failure in terms of maintaining a positive reputation. Despite the challenges of being the responding hospital during a biological disaster, facilities and healthcare systems can leverage these events to their advantage if handled correctly. If the hospital communicates the message that they have the expertise to manage complex cases—such as Ebola—successfully, it can increase patient revenue in the long run.[46] An active public relations (PR) program will be necessary to recover from this type of reputational loss, especially in a geographic location where there are multiple hospital options for the public. For example, due to an aggressive PR campaign, Texas Health effectively recovered their reputation and rebounded from their revenue loss due to managing the Ebola patient within just a few months.[46]

Analysis of this process points out the importance of communication and transparency with the community following a biologic event, even if mistakes are made.[36] Hospitals may find themselves in a position of reputation recovery due to chance, as in the prior case, or in a wider disaster where they are assigned to be a cohorting hospital. Communication with the community during recovery is essential to hospital resilience. One PR professional has asserted that communication coming directly from clinical staff—physicians or nurses—may be perceived as more trustworthy than messages from hospital administrators, and it could provide additional reassurance to the public.[80] The CDC recommends that Crisis and Emergency Risk Communication (CERC) practices be used during response and recovery from a biological disaster and that hospital administrators and public health officials ensure that their messages are accurate, empathetic, action-oriented, and respectful.[81]

Beyond reputational repair, recovery information will need to be shared with the public. Determination of what type of information should be shared (resumed services, cleaning operations, etc.) and the vehicle through which that information is shared will need to be determined. Communication through news agencies, social media, and the internet is all likely, and the type of news and method may vary depending on the audience. Examples of stakeholders to receive recovery information include the general public, partnering agencies, and patients. Each stakeholder group will be in search of information as it relates to them, so targeted and tailored messages will be vital to communicating information regarding risk related to the event, impact on jobs, safety, and other considerations.[82]

Ongoing communication with staff will also be integral to the recovery process. Staff will have concerns about safety, compensation, and the security of their ongoing employment. Addressing these questions rapidly and transparently will ensure staff morale and better ensure staff retention. This communication should be bidirectional, sending information down to staff as well as collecting information on staff concerns, needs, and questions.[83] One primary objective of communication with staff should be to identify key operational goals of the hospital, especially when resources are limited and staff diminished, so that all employees are focused on the top priorities of the hospital.[83] Further information on this topic can be found in Chapter 22, "Communication Strategies and the Media."

POSTTRAUMATIC GROWTH (POSITIVE SOCIAL ROLE ADAPTATION)

Though biological disasters pose great challenges and threats to healthcare and public health systems, recovery from such events grants facilities and agencies the opportunity to improve their preparedness for the next incident.[84] It is critical that facilities and agencies utilize lessons learned from past events to prepare for the inevitable future disaster. While all methods of future mitigation may be beyond the scope of initial recovery, some rebuilding, such as improving hospital airflow systems and stockpiling locations, may be worked into existing plans. Two large components of disaster recovery involve responding to the secondary healthcare surge and preparing for the next event.[9a] Specific to outbreaks of emerging infectious diseases, pandemics, and bioterrorism, it is critical that facilities and agencies have plans in place to increase availability of primary care providers,[9a] rapidly recognize potential threats, identify contagious patients, and implement control measures to reduce infection spread.

An important factor that affects how well an individual, agency, or community recovers from any type of disaster is resilience.[59,84] *Resilience* refers to the adaptive strengths and skills that aid in recovering from adversity. Healthcare, public health, and disaster planners are recognizing the importance of cultivating resilience preevent to maximize response to a disaster. Resilient individuals and agencies may even experience posttraumatic growth after a disaster.[84] Posttraumatic growth among the general public after terrorist attacks and disasters has most often been associated with a greater sense of purpose in life by encouraging healthy behaviors and increasing social interactions.[85] Researchers have found that the use of positive psychology after disasters has been very effective at reducing negative psychological outcomes and increasing posttraumatic growth among children and adolescents.[86] Specific to the disaster recovery phase, this includes addressing minors' age-related needs and concerns, repairing or rebuilding a sense of safety, teaching or encouraging techniques for calming or self-soothing, and promoting self-efficacy.[86] It has also been suggested that interventions to reduce the negative psychological impact of disasters on children or adolescents be targeted at parents, as evidence shows that poor or dysfunctional parenting styles have been associated with increased vulnerability among children after a disaster.[87] Healthcare and public health agencies should partner with crisis counselors and disaster mental health professionals to develop a comprehensive screening and response plan to address psychological issues that may arise during disaster recovery.[87]

Researchers have found that an increased sense of control and perceived self-efficacy are protective against adverse outcomes, including the negative psychological impacts of disasters.[88] This has been found to be especially true among disaster workers, whose resilience is highly impacted by the individual's perceived self-efficacy (i.e., their belief that certain behaviors will have a positive effect on their health).[5] As stated earlier, disaster workers are at high risk of anxiety, depression, and PTSD due to prolonged and repeated exposure to stressors during disaster response, especially if they overextend themselves.[84] Increased self-efficacy in the form of believing that one has gained improved coping skills gained by surviving past traumatic events has been found to be protective against negative outcomes from stressors experienced during future disasters.[89]

In relation to disaster recovery, *self-efficacy* also refers to *response efficacy*, which is the belief that certain actions performed during a disaster will have a positive effect on the individual's health or the health of others.[90] The higher an emergency responder's response efficacy, the more willing they are to report to work during disasters and perceive their role as important during an event.[90,91] It may also have a protective effect against PTSD, depression, and anxiety, though there is still a lack of evidence in this area.

An important way to increase HCP and public health professionals' response efficacy is to train them preevent.[91] Recommendations on important training topics for HCP[92–94] and public health professionals[93,95–97] in relation to bioterrorism, pandemics, and outbreaks of emerging pathogens are outlined in Tables 3 and 4, respectively. Preevent training is preferred to just-in-time (JIT) training provided during an event, though JIT training can play a vital role in responding to any disaster. It is particularly important to provide JIT training related to the disease involved in the event during a biological disaster. Even if HCP and public

TABLE 3
Training Topics for Healthcare Professionals That Are Specific to Bioterrorism Attacks, Pandemics, and Outbreaks of Emerging Infectious Diseases

- Patient decontamination procedures
- Isolation
- Selection and appropriate use of personal protective equipment
- Environmental decontamination
- Vulnerable populations
- Identification of bioterrorism attack and pandemic
- Reporting procedures
- Role during an event
- Biological agents of greatest threat
- Chain of custody procedures
- Mental health impact of event
- Psychosocial needs during disasters
- Dispersion methods of bioterrorism
- Phases of emergency management
- Quarantine
- Disease control measures
- Pharmacological interventions
- Nonpharmacological interventions
- Patient and staff cohorting
- Safe specimen handling and management
- Epidemiology of pathogens that may be used in acts of bioterrorism
- Personal preparedness
- Clinical presentation of potential pathogens
- Role and contents of Strategic National Stockpile (SNS)
- Back-up equipment needed for a surge of contagious patients
- Surveillance and screening procedures to identify potentially contagious individuals
- Altered standards of care
- Self-screening for illness
- Social distancing
- Handling potentially contaminated items or equipment
- Occupational exposure reporting, evaluation, and treatment
- Infectious waste management procedures

TABLE 4
Training Topics for Public Health Professionals That Are Specific to Bioterrorism Attacks, Pandemics, and Outbreaks of Emerging Infectious Diseases

- Role during an event
- Chain of command during an event
- Chain of custody procedures
- Training to work in a point of dispensing (POD)
  - o Collecting personal identification
  - o Assessing POD clients for medication contraindications
  - o Screening for identifying symptomatic individuals
  - o Interpreting antibiotic dosing per protocol
  - o Vaccine administration procedures
  - o Medication administration procedures
  - o Cold chain techniques for handling vaccines
  - o Adverse events reporting procedures
  - o Labeling of medication
  - o Repackaging of medication
- Infection prevention in the POD
- Epidemiology of pathogens that may be used in acts of bioterrorism
- Use of communication equipment used during events
- Development of risk communication messages
- Identification of bioterrorism attack, pandemic or emerging infectious disease
- Public health laws applicable during disasters
- Public health triage principles
- Selection and appropriate use of personal protective equipment
- Indicators of mass exposure
- Outbreak investigation procedures
- Surveillance activities specific to biological disasters
- Psychosocial needs during disasters
- Population-based infection prevention
- Health education related to infectious diseases
- Role and contents of Strategic National Stockpile (SNS)
- Patient decontamination procedures
- Home isolation
- Quarantine
- Altered standards of care
- Self-screening for illness
- Social distancing
- Handling potentially contaminated items or equipment
- Occupational exposure reporting, evaluation, and treatment
- Environmental cleaning/disinfection
- Infectious waste management procedures
- Safe food handling

health staff are trained on infectious diseases preevent, situation-specific information will need to be communicated to staff during an outbreak. For example, the epidemiology of a disease may be different than what was anticipated based on past outbreaks, and it is critical that this information be communicated to HCPs and public health professionals so that informed decision-making can be made mid-event. An example of this was the unusual epidemiology of H1N1 during the 2009 pandemic. Pediatric patients and pregnant women were disproportionately affected during the H1N1 pandemic, and this led to these groups being prioritized for the pandemic vaccine when it first became available[98,99] Another example was the need to communicate the CDC's guideline change related to personal protective equipment usage when providing clinical care to patients with Ebola; mid-outbreak, the CDC recommended the use of expanded PPE along with an observer as HCP donned and doffed the PPE.[100]

CONCLUSION

Though the recovery period is the longest of any phase of a disaster, research and planning are lacking to address the unique needs of individuals, facilities, and communities during recovery from disasters. In particular, the long-term physical and mental health challenges posed by biological disasters need to be addressed by healthcare and public health systems. Learning from past disasters and using those lessons to plan and train for future events enhances physical and emotional preparedness. Positive social role adaptation and training are key to strategies to mitigate the impact of disasters by facilitating recovery and preservation and impactful utilization of supplies, equipment, and personnel.

REFERENCES

1. Sandler D, Smith G. Assessing the quality of state disaster recovery plans: implications for policy and practice. *J Emerg Manage.* 2013;11(4):281–291.
2. Federal Emergency Management Agency. Lessons in Community Recovery: Seven Years of Emergency Support Function # 14 Long-Term Community Recovery From 2004–2011; 2011. https://www.fema.gov/pdf/rebuild/ltrc/2011_report.pdf. Accessed 6 November 2024.
3. Kates RW, Pijawka D. Chapter 1: From Rubble to Monument: The Pace of Reconstruction. *Reconstruction Following Disaster*. Cambridge, MA: MIT Press; 1977:1–23.
4. Chandra A, Acosta JD. Disaster recovery also involves human recovery. *JAMA.* 2010;304(14):1608–1609.

5. Walsh L, Garrity S, Rutkow L, et al. Applying a behavioral model framework for disaster recovery research in local public health agencies: a conceptual approach. *Disaster Med Public Health Prep.* 2015;9(4):403–408.
6. (a) Kanter R.K., Abramson D.M., Redlener I., Gracy D. The medical home and care coordination in disaster recovery: Hypothesis for interventions and research. Disaster Med Public Health Prep 2015;9(4):337–343; (b) http://osuwmc.multimedia-newsroom.com/index.php/2021/02/08/survey-most-americans-will-continue-health-precautions-after-covid-19/. (c) https://www.edweek.org/policy-politics/home-schooling-is-way-up-with-covid-19-will-it-last/2020/11. (d) https://www.nbcnews.com/news/us-news/power-outage-forces-texas-officials-scramble-administer-covid-19-vaccine-n1257999. Accessed March 28, 2021.
7. U.S. Department of Homeland Security. National Disaster Recovery Framework. U.S. Department of Homeland Security; 2016. https://www.fema.gov/media-library/assets/documents/117794 Accessed January 8, 2018.
8. Federal Emergency Management Agency. IS-558: Public Works and Disaster Recovery. Federal Emergency Management Agency; 2013. https://training.fema.gov/is/courseoverview.aspx?code=IS-558 Accessed January 6, 2018.
9. (a) Runkle JD, Brock-Martin A, Karmaus W, Svendsen ER. Secondary surge capacity: a framework for understanding long-term access to primary care for medically vulnerable populations in disaster recovery. *Am J Public Health.* 2012;102(12):e24–e32. (b) Rashid Hons M, Gale Hons CP, Curzen Hons N, et al. Impact of Coronavirus Disease 2019 Pandemic on the Incidence and Management of Out-of-Hospital Cardiac Arrest in Patients Presenting With Acute Myocardial Infarction in England. *J Am Heart Assoc.* 2020;9(22), e018379.
10. Edelstein M, Angelides P, Heymann DL. Ebola: the challenging road to recovery. *Lancet.* 2015;385(9984):2234–2235.
11. Abramson DM, Stehling-Ariza T, Park YS, Walsh L, Culp D. Measuring individual disaster recovery: a socio-ecological framework. *Disaster Med Public Health Prep.* 2010;4(Suppl 1):S46–S54.
12. Cheng S, Ganapati E, Ganapati S. Measuring disaster recovery: bouncing back or reaching the counterfactual state? *Disasters.* 2015;39(3):427–446.
13. Harvard School of Public Health Emergency Preparedness and Response Exercise Program Essential functions and considerations for hospital recovery; 2014. https://massgeneral.org/assets/mgh/pdf/emergency-medicine/hsph-emergency-preparedness-response-exercise-program_hospital-recovery.pdf. Accessed 8 January 2018.
14. Corbit N. Mercy Hospital Joplin Built to Stand Against Nature; 2015. https://www.mercy.net/newsroom/2015-02-28/mercy-hospital-joplin-built-to-stand-against-nature/. Accessed January 10, 2018.
15. Rebmann T. Management of patients infected with airborne-spread diseases: an algorithm for infection control professionals. *Am J Infect Control.* 2005;33(10):571–579.
16. Rebmann T, Wilson R, Alexander S, Cloughessy M, Moroz D, Citarella B. et al. Infection Prevention and Control for Shelters During Disasters; 2009. http://www.apic.org2008. Accessed August 14, 2009.
17. Rebmann T, Wagner W. Infection preventionists' experience during the first months of the 2009 novel H1N1 influenza a pandemic. *Am J Infect Control.* 2009;37(10):e5–e16.
18. Rebmann T, Carrico R, English JF. Hospital infectious disease emergency preparedness: a survey of infection control professionals. *Am J Infect Control.* 2007;35(1):25–32.
19. Adini B, Goldberg A, Laor D, Cohen R, Zadok R, Bar-Dayan Y. Assessing levels of hospital emergency preparedness. *Prehosp Disaster Med.* 2006;21(6):451–457.
20. Rebmann T, McPhee K, Haas GA, et al. Findings from an assessment and inventory of a regional, decentralized stockpile. *Health Secur.* 2018;16(2):1–8.
21. Rebmann T, McPhee K, Osborne L, Gillen DP, Haas GA. Best practices for healthcare facility and regional stockpile maintenance and sustainment: a literature review. *Health Secur.* 2017;15(4):409–417.
22. Nicholson A, Wollek S, Kahn B, Hermann J. The nation's medical countermeasurec stockpile: Opportunities to improve the efficiency, effectiveness, and sustainability of the CDC Strategic National Stockpile: Workshop summary; 2016. http://www.nap.edu/235322016. Accessed 8 January 2018.
23. Crowley J. A measurement of the effectiveness and efficiency of pre-disaster debris management plans. *Waste Manag.* 2017;62:262–273.
24. Le AB, Hoboy S, Germain A, et al. A pilot survey of the U.S. medical waste industry to determine training needs for safely handling highly infectious waste. *Am J Infect Control.* 2018;46(2):133–138.
25. Lemieux P, Wood J, Drake J, et al. Analysis of waste management issues arising from a field study evaluating decontamination of a biological agent from a building. *J Air Waste Manag Assoc.* 2016;66(1):17–27.
26. Garibaldi BT, Reimers M, Ernst N, et al. Validation of autoclave protocols for successful decontamination of category a medical waste generated from care of patients with serious communicable diseases. *J Clin Micro.* 2017;55(2):545–551.
27. Archer P. Ebola Waste From Dallas Hospital Arrives at UTMB-Galveston; 2014. https://www.click2houston.com/news/ebola-waste-from-dallas-hospital-arrives-at-utmb-galveston_20151124022056869. Accessed February 10, 2018.
28. Centers for Disease Control & Prevention. Ebola-Associated Waste Management; 2015. https://www.cdc.gov/vhf/ebola/healthcare-us/cleaning/waste-management.html. Accessed February 10, 2018.
29. Schmitt K, Zacchia NA. Total decontamination cost of the anthrax letter attacks. *Biosecur Bioterror.* 2012;10(1):98–107.
30. Wein LM, Liu Y, Leighton TJ. HEPA/vaccine plan for indoor anthrax remediation. *Emerg Infect Dis.* 2005;11(1):69–76.

31. Campbell CG, Kirvel RD, Love AH, et al. Decontamination after a release of B. anthracis spores. *Biosecur Bioterror.* 2012;10(1):108–122.
32. Manchee RJ, Broster MG, Anderson IS, Henstridge RM, Melling J. Decontamination of bacillus anthracis on Gruinard Island? *Nature.* 1983;303(5914):239–240.
33. Meselson M, Guillemin J, Hugh-Jones M, et al. The Sverdlovsk anthrax outbreak of 1979. *Science.* 1994;266(5188):1202–1208.
34. Hitchcock PJ, Mair M, Inglesby TV, et al. Improving performance of HVAC systems to reduce exposure to aerosolized infectious agents in buildings; recommendations to reduce risks posed by biological attacks. *Biosecur Bioterror.* 2006;4(1):41–54.
35. Trafny EA, Lewandowski R, Stepinska M, Kaliszewski M. Biological threat detection in the air and on the surface: how to define the risk. *Arch Immunol Ther Exp (Warsz).* 2014;62(4):253–261.
36. Lewton KL. 'Reputation Recovery': The Ebola Patient Crisis in Dallas. http://apps.prsa.org/Intelligence/TheStrategist/Articles/view/10923/1104/Reputation_Recovery_The_Ebola_Patient_Crisis_in_Da - .WoIV2YJG0UE2014. Accessed January 28, 2018.
37. Leider JP, DeBruin D, Reynolds N, Koch A, Seaberg J. Ethical guidance for disaster response, specifically around crisis standards of care: a systematic review. *Am J Public Health.* 2017;107(9):e1–e9.
38. Zaza S, Koonin LM, Ajao A, et al. A conceptual framework for allocation of federally stockpiled ventilators during large-scale public health emergencies. *Health Secur.* 2016;14(1):1–6.
39. Ajao A, Nystrom SV, Koonin LM, et al. Assessing the capacity of the US health care system to use additional mechanical ventilators during a large-scale public health emergency. *Disaster Med Public Health Prep.* 2015;9(6):634–641.
40. Gall C, Wetzel R, Kolker A, Kanter RK, Toltzis P. Pediatric triage in a severe pandemic: maximizing survival by establishing triage thresholds. *Crit Care Med.* 2016;44(9):1762–1768.
41. Abramovich MN, Hershey JC, Callies B, Adalja AA, Tosh PK, Toner ES. Hospital influenza pandemic stockpiling needs: a computer simulation. *Am J Infect Control.* 2017;45(3):272–277.
42. Radonovich LJ, Magalian PD, Hollingsworth MK, Baracco G. Stockpiling supplies for the next influenza pandemic. *Emerg Infect Dis.* 2009;15(6), e1.
43. (a) Green A. West African countries focus on post-Ebola recovery plans. Lancet 2016;388(10059):2463-2465;. (b) Kennedy, M.S. (2021). Where do we go from here? Am J Nurs, 121(3): 7. https://doi.org/10.1097/01.NAJ.0000737220.28816.3e;. (c) https://assets.morningconsult.com/wp-uploads/2021/01/24220044/210101_crosstabs_MC_HEALTH_HEALTH_CARE_WORKERS_Health_Care_Workers_v1.pdf.
44. (a) McDonald LC, Simor AE, Su IJ, et al. SARS in healthcare facilities, Toronto and Taiwan. *Emerg Infect Dis.* 2004;10(5):777–781. (b) Kennedy MS. Where do we go from here? *Am J Nurs.* 2021;121(3):7. https://doi.org/10.1097/01.NAJ.0000737220.28816.3e. (c) https://assets.morningconsult.com/wp-uploads/2021/01/24220044/210101_crosstabs_MC_HEALTH_HEALTH_CARE_WORKERS_Health_Care_Workers_v1.pdf;. (d) Sun C, Zhai Z. The efficacy of social distance and ventilation effectiveness in preventing COVID-19 transmission. *Sustain Cities Soc.* 2020;62:102390.
45. Weeks E. After the catastrophe: disaster relief for hospitals. *NC L Rev.* 2006;85:223–300.
46. Silverman L. After Ebola, Some Businesses Suffered, While Others Profited; 2014. http://stories.kera.org/surviving-ebola/2015/09/07/north-texas-businesses-suffered-and-profited-from-ebola/?_ga=2.12253623.247538084.1517935930-539216897.1517935929 Accessed February 11, 2018.
47. Yale New Haven Health System Center for Emergency Preparedness and Disaster Response. A Quick Guide: FEMA Reimbursement for Acute Care Hospitals; 2012. http://www.calhospitalprepare.org/sites/main/files/file-attachments/fema-ach_reimbursementguide.pdf2012. Accessed January 14, 2018.
48. Federal Emergency Management Agency. Public Assistance Program and Policy Guide. FP 104-009-2; 2020. https://www.fema.gov/media-library/assets/documents/111781 2017.
49. Federal Emergency Management Agency. Emergency Assistance for Human Influenza Pandemic Disaster Assistance Policy. DAP9523.17; 2009. http://www.nasemso.org/Resources/documents/H1N1Policy9523.17112509.pdf2009. Accessed January 24, 2018.
50. U.S. Small Business Association. Disaster Assistance; 2017. https://www.sba.gov/disaster-assistance. Accessed February 2, 2018.
51. Texas Hospital Association. Filing Claims With FEMA; 2018. https://www.tha.org/Harvey/Filing-Claims-With-FEMA. Accessed January 16, 2018.
52. Association of State and Territorial Health Officials (ASTHO). Disaster Recovery for Public Health; 2007. http://www.astho.org/Programs/Preparedness/Disaster-Recovery-for-Public-Health/2007. Accessed January 30, 2018.
53. Deen GF, Broutet N, Xu W, et al. Ebola RNA persistence in semen of Ebola virus disease survivors—final report. *N Engl J Med.* 2017;377(15):1428–1437.
54. Pers YM, Sow MS, Taverne B, et al. Characteristics of the musculoskeletal symptoms observed among survivors of Ebola virus disease in the Postebogui cohort in Guinea. *Rheumatology (Oxford).* 2017;56(12):2068–2072.
55. Clark DV, Kibuuka H, Millard M, et al. Long-term sequelae after Ebola virus disease in Bundibugyo, Uganda: a retrospective cohort study. *Lancet Infect Dis.* 2015;15(8):905–912.
56. Burgdorf WH, Hoenig LJ. Pockmarked. *JAMA Derm.* 2016;152(1):114.
57. World health Organization. Health Topics: Public Health Surveillance; 2015. http://www.who.int/topics/public_health_surveillance/en/. Accessed 02/12/2015. Accessed May 6, 2016.

58. Rebmann T, Kunerth AK, Zelicoff A, Elliott MB, Wieldt HF. Missouri K-12 school collection and reporting of school-based syndromic surveillance data: a cross sectional study. *BMC Public Health.* 2016;16:103.
59. Hansel TC, Osofsky HJ, Langhinrichsen-Rohling J, et al. Gulf Coast resilience coalition: an evolved collaborative built on shared disaster experiences, response, and future preparedness. *Disaster Med Public Health Prep.* 2015;9(6):657–665.
60. Giarratano G, Harville EW, Barcelona de Mendoza V, Savage J, Parent CM. Healthy start: description of a safety net for perinatal support during disaster recovery. *Mater Child Hlth J.* 2015;19(4):819–827.
61. Lowe SR, Kwok RK, Payne J, Engel LS, Galea S, Sandler DP. Why does disaster recovery work influence mental health?: Pathways through physical health and household income. *Am J Community Psychol.* 2016;58(3–4):354–364.
62. Shultz JM, Baingana F, Neria Y. The 2014 Ebola outbreak and mental health: current status and recommended response. *JAMA.* 2015;313(6):567–568.
63. Lehmann M, Bruenahl CA, Lowe B, et al. Ebola and psychological stress of health care professionals. *Emerg Infect Dis.* 2015;21(5):913–914.
64. Dougall AL, Hayward MC, Baum A. Media exposure to bioterrorism: stress and the anthrax attacks. *Psychiatry.* 2005;68(1):28–42.
65. Person B, Sy F, Holton K, Govert B, Liang A. National Center for Infectious diseases SCOT. Fear and stigma: the epidemic within the SARS outbreak. *Emerg Infect Dis.* 2004;10(2):358–363.
66. Bai Y, Lin CC, Lin CY, Chen JY, Chue CM, Chou P. Survey of stress reactions among health care workers involved with the SARS outbreak. *Psychiatr Serv.* 2004;55(9):1055–1057.
67. Wynia MK. Ethics and public health emergencies: encouraging responsibility. *Am J Bioethics.* 2007;7(4):1–4.
68. Rebmann T. Infectious disease disasters: Bioterrorism, emerging infections, and pandemics. In: Grota P, ed. *APIC Text of Infection Control and Epidemiology.* 4th ed. Washington, DC: Association of Professionals in Infection Control and Epidemiology; 2014.
69. Ramsey PS, Ramin KD. Pneumonia in pregnancy. *Obstet Gynecol Clin North Am.* 2001;28(3):553–569.
70. Beigi RH. Emerging infectious diseases in pregnancy. *Ob Gyn.* 2017;129(5):896–906.
71. Liu S, Sha J, Yu Z, et al. Avian influenza virus in pregnancy. *Rev Med Vir.* 2016;26(4):268–284.
72. von der Beck D, Seeger W, Herold S, Gunther A, Loh B. Characteristics and outcomes of a cohort hospitalized for pandemic and seasonal influenza in Germany based on nationwide inpatient data. *PloS One.* 2017;12(7), e0180920.
73. Almond D, Mazumder B. The 1918 influenza pandemic and subsequent health outcomes: an analysis of SIPP data. *Am Econ Rev.* 2005;95(2):258–262.
74. Last Ebola patient, a baby girl named Nubia, recovers [press release]. https://www.nbcnews.com/storyline/ebola-virus-outbreak/last-ebola-patient-baby-girl-named-nubia-recovers-n4654812016. Accessed January 30, 2018.
75. World Health Organization. Consensus Document on the Epidemiology of Severe Acute Respiratory Syndrome (SARS). WHO; 2003. http://www.who.int/csr/sars/en/WHOconsensus.pdf2003. Accessed July 6, 2005.
76. Ortega-Sanchez IR, Sniadack MM, Mootrey GT. Economics of cardiac adverse events after smallpox vaccination: lessons from the 2003 US Vaccination Program. *Clin Infect Dis.* 2008;46(Suppl 3):S168–S178.
77. Benedek DM, Fullerton C, Ursano RJ. First responders: mental health consequences of natural and human-made disasters for public health and public safety workers. *Annu Rev Public Health.* 2007;28:55–68.
78. Mertz D, Kim TH, Johnstone J, et al. Populations at risk for severe or complicated influenza illness: systematic review and meta-analysis. *BMJ.* 2013;347, f5061.
79. Jimenez-Garcia R, Hernandez-Barrera V, Rodriguez-Rieiro C, et al. Hospitalizations from pandemic influenza [A(H1N1)pdm09] infections among type 1 and 2 diabetes patients in Spain. *Influenza Resp Viruses.* 2013;7(3):439–447.
80. Yasmin S, Railey K. Texas Health Presbyterian Begins Public Relations Effort to Restore; 2014. https://www.dallasnews.com/news/news/2014/10/17/texas-health-presbyterian-begins-public-relations-effort-to-restore-trust. Accessed February 1, 2018.
81. Sell TK. When the next disease strikes: how to communicate (and how not to). *Hlth Sec.* 2017;15(1):28–30.
82. U.S. Department of Homeland Security. Ready.Gov. Crisis Communications Plan; 2018. https://www.ready.gov/business/implementation/crisis. Accessed February 8, 2018.
83. Tibbo B. Leadership in the Eye of the Storm: Putting your People First in a Crisis. Toronto, Canada: Rotman-Utp Publishing; 2016.
84. Southwick SM, Satodiya R, Pietrzak RH. Disaster mental health and positive psychology: an afterward to the special issue. *J Clin Psychol.* 2016;72(12):1364–1368.
85. Schulenberg SE, Smith CV, Drescher CF, Buchanan EM. Assessment of meaning in adolescents receiving clinical services in Mississippi following the deepwater horizon oil spill: an application of the purpose in life test-short form (PIL-SF). *J Clin Psychol.* 2016;72(12):1279–1286.
86. Vernberg EM, Hambrick EP, Cho B, Hendrickson ML. Positive psychology and disaster mental health: strategies for working with children and adolescents. *J Clin Psychol.* 2016;72(12):1333–1347.
87. Cobham VE, McDermott B, Haslam D, Sanders MR. The role of parents, parenting and the family environment in children's post-disaster mental health. *Curr Psych Rep.* 2016;18(6):53.
88. Maier SF. Behavioral control blunts reactions to contemporaneous and future adverse events: medial prefrontal cortex plasticity and a corticostriatal network. *Neurobiol Stress.* 2015;1:12–22.

89. Tsai J, Mota NP, Southwick SM, Pietrzak RH. What doesn't kill you makes you stronger: a national study of U.S. military veterans. *J Affect Disord.* 2016;189:269–271.
90. Barnett DJ, Balicer RD, Thompson CB, et al. Assessment of local public health workers' willingness to respond to pandemic influenza through application of the extended parallel process model. *PloS One.* 2009;4(7), e6365.
91. Barnett DJ, Thompson CB, Errett NA, et al. Determinants of emergency response willingness in the local public health workforce by jurisdictional and scenario patterns: a cross-sectional survey. *BMC Public Health.* 2012;12:164.
92. Rebmann T, Mohr LB. Bioterrorism knowledge and educational participation of nurses in Missouri. *J Contin Educ Nurs.* 2010;41(2):67–76.
93. Polivka BJ, Stanley SA, Gordon D, Taulbee K, Kieffer G, McCorkle SM. Public health nursing competencies for public health surge events. *Public Health Nurs.* 2008;25(2):159–165.
94. Jorgensen AM, Mendoza GJ, Henderson JL. Emergency preparedness and disaster response core competency set for perinatal and neonatal nurses. *J Obstet Gynecol Neonatal Nurs.* 2010;39(4):450–465. quiz 465–457.
95. Rebmann T, Loux TM, Swick Z, et al. A national study examining closed points of dispensing (PODs): existence, preparedness, exercise participation, and training provided. *Biosecur Bioterror.* 2014;12(4):208–216.
96. Centers for Disease Control & Prevention. Bioterrorism & Emergency Readiness: Competencies for all Public Health Workers; 2002. https://training.fema.gov/emiweb/downloads/bioterrorism and emergency readiness.pdf2002. Accessed November 3, 2004.
97. Rebmann T, Coll B. Emergency preparedness committee. Infection prevention in points of dispensing. *Am J Infect Control.* 2009;37(9):695–702.
98. Haaheim LR, Madhun AS, Cox R. Pandemic influenza vaccines—the challenges. *Viruses.* 2009;1(3):1089–1109.
99. Rebmann T, Zelicoff A. Vaccination against influenza: role and limitations in pandemic intervention plans. *Exp Rev Vacc.* 2012;11(8):1009–1019.
100. Centers for Disease Control & Prevention. Frequently Asked Questions for Guidance on Personal Protective Equipment to be Used by Healthcare Workers During Management of Patients With Confirmed Ebola or Persons Under Investigation (PUI) for Ebola Who Are Clinically Unstable or Have Bleeding, Vomiting or Diarrhea in U.S. Hospitals, Including Procedures for Donning and Doffing; 2015. https://www.cdc.gov/vhf/ebola/healthcare-us/ppe/faq.html. Accessed April 3, 2016.

Index

Note: Page numbers followed by *f* indicate figures, *t* indicate tables, and *b* indicate boxes.

H

I

J

L

M

9780323548410